Essentials of
Medical Physiology

Essentials of
Medical Physiology

Sixth Edition

K Sembulingam PhD
and
Prema Sembulingam PhD
Madha Medical College & Research Institute
Kundrathur Main Road, Kovur, Thandalam (Near Porur)
Chennai, Tamil Nadu, India

Formerly
MR Medical College
Gulbarga, Karnataka, India

Sri Ramachandra Medical College and Research Institute
Chennai, Tamil Nadu, India

School of Health Sciences, Universiti Sains Malaysia
Kelantan, Malaysia

Sri Lakshmi Narayana Institute of Medical Sciences
Puducherry, India

Sri Manakula Vinayagar Medical College and Hospital
Puducherry, India
and
Shri Sathya Sai Medical College and Research Institute
Kanchipuram, Tamil Nadu, India

JAYPEE BROTHERS MEDICAL PUBLISHERS (P) LTD

New Delhi • Panama City • London • Dhaka • Kathmandu

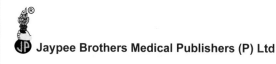 Jaypee Brothers Medical Publishers (P) Ltd

Headquarters
Jaypee Brothers Medical Publishers (P) Ltd
4838/24, Ansari Road, Daryaganj
New Delhi 110 002, India
Phone: +91-11-43574357
Fax: +91-11-43574314
Email: jaypee@jaypeebrothers.com

Overseas Offices

J.P. Medical Ltd
83 Victoria Street, London
SW1H 0HW (UK)
Phone: +44-2031708910
Fax: +02-03-0086180
Email: info@jpmedpub.com

Jaypee Brothers Medical Publishers (P) Ltd
17/1-B Babar Road, Block-B, Shaymali
Mohammadpur, Dhaka-1207
Bangladesh
Mobile: +08801912003485
Email: jaypeedhaka@gmail.com

Jaypee-Highlights Medical Publishers Inc.
City of Knowledge, Bld. 237, Clayton
Panama City, Panama
Phone: + 507-301-0496
Fax: + 507-301-0499
Email: cservice@jphmedical.com

Jaypee Brothers Medical Publishers (P) Ltd
Shorakhute, Kathmandu
Nepal
Phone: +00977-9841528578
Email: jaypee.nepal@gmail.com

Website: www.jaypeebrothers.com
Website: www.jaypeedigital.com

© 2013, Jaypee Brothers Medical Publishers

Essentials of Medical Physiology

First Edition: 1999
Second Edition: 2000
Third Edition: 2004
Fourth Edition: 2006
Fifth Edition: 2010
Sixth Edition: **2013**

ISBN 978-93-5025-936-8

Printed at: Ajanta Offset & Packagings Ltd., New Delhi

Dedicated to

Our beloved students

Foreword to the Sixth Edition

MADHA MEDICAL COLLEGE & RESEARCH INSTITUTE

Approved by Medical Council of India, New Delhi,
Affiliated to Tamil Nadu Dr. M.G.R. Medical University, Chennai, Proc. No. Affln. III (3)/4206/2010

Thandalam, Kovur (Near Porur), Chennai-600 122. Phone : 044 - 2478 0333, 2478 0055
E-mail: madhahospital@gmail.com

Dr S MADAN KUMAR MD, Dip. A & E
Director

It is my privilege and pleasure to give this foreword to sixth edition of the textbook *Essentials of Medical Physiology* written by two of our dedicated and renowned teachers Dr K Sembulingam and Dr Prema Sembulingam. Since the publication of first edition in the year 1999, this book has been accepted by the faculty of many universities in and out of country. It has become popular among medical, dental and paramedical students because of its elegant presentation, simple language and clear illustrations with diagrams, flow charts and tables.

The authors have taken concerted efforts to improve the contents and update the information in every subsequent edition of this book. This sixth edition with newly formatted and updated tables, flow charts and self-explanatory diagrams will help the students in better understanding and performance in various types of examinations. Clinical physiology with updated information in this edition will help the students for their clinical knowledge to a great extent.

I congratulate Dr K Sembulingam and Dr Prema Sembulingam on their great effort in bringing sixth edition of this book.

Dr S Madan Kumar MD, Dip. A & E
Director
Madha Medical College & Research Institute
Thandalam, Kovur (Near Porur)
Chennai, Tamil Nadu, India

Foreword to the First Edition

SRI RAMACHANDRA MEDICAL COLLEGE AND RESEARCH INSTITUTE (DEEMED UNIVERSITY)

1, RAMACHANDRA NAGAR, PORUR, CHENNAI-600 116

Dr TK PARTHA SARATHY FRCS (C) FACS

Diplomate of the American Board of Surgery

VICE-CHANCELLOR

Off : 4828027-29, 31-33

Fax : 091-44-48277008

Telex : 41-25050 PCO IN

It is indeed with a great sense of pleasure and privilege that I give this foreword to the book *Essentials of Medical Physiology* written by two of our dedicated teachers Dr K Sembulingam and Dr Prema Sembulingam. The students have always appreciated the efforts of these two teachers and their ability to make physiology easily comprehended and interesting. Why one more book in physiology, is what I asked myself first before I reviewed the book. The book has been largely directed to the broad and specific needs of the undergraduate students, and simplicity and clarity have been emphasized. The students can easily assimilate the logical sequence in which the subjects have been presented not only for them to understand the same but also perform well in the various types of objective and routine examinations.

Several readily understandable diagrams and tables have been included to make subject comprehension and revision easy. Applied physiology, clinical importance and altered situations in pediatrics, geriatrics and pregnancy have been well brought out. The approach utilized in dealing with the subject of physiology would be appreciated by other teachers as well. I have no doubts that this will be a valuable addition to the armamentarium of a student of physiology who is preparing for examination and is seeking a strong foundation to build further on.

Here at Sri Ramachandra Medical College and Research Institute (Deemed University), Chennai, Tamil Nadu, India, the faculty involved in writing and editing books of this nature are greatly appreciated, and I as its Vice-Chancellor wish to congratulate the Sembulingams on their great effort.

TK Partha Sarathy FRCS (C) FACS
Diplomate of the American Board of Surgery
Vice-Chancellor
Sri Ramachandra Medical College and Research
Institute (Deemed University)
Porur, Chennai, Tamil Nadu, India

Preface to the Sixth Edition

With this Sixth edition, Sembulingam's *Essentials of Medical Physiology* enters into its second decade and the core subject matter with updated physiological information remain as green as ever. We live in an era where the thirst for knowledge and urge for learning is so much increased that even a layman knows the fundamentals of common disorders like diabetes mellitus, hypertension, jaundice, etc. So, it becomes doubly important to fulfill the expectations of the educated mass, especially in medical field.

We are humbly thankful and heavenly happy for the popularity of this book among the undergraduate and postgraduate students of medical, dental and paramedical courses, doctors and other health professionals in and out of our country.

Like many other successful textbooks, this book also has sailed through the years smoothly, fruitfully and successfully. May be because, it meets the needs of every group of the readers. Students are happy because it is student-friendly while reading, and exam-friendly while revising. Knowledge seekers are happy because they get the updated and recent developments in the field of physiology. Doctors are happy because applied aspects are covered adequately.

Our thirst for improving this textbook is growing every year by seeing outright acceptance of this book by the students, and the appreciation and overwhelming support given by our fellow teachers. The most comments and the suggestions, we receive from our readers, are responsible for better shaping of this book in every edition.

This edition is enriched with addition of many more flow charts, tables and descriptive diagrams to make the subject matter easier and approachable for all class of students. Many chapters are upgraded as per the suggestions from our colleagues and fellow teachers from various institutes and universities in and out of India.

Our thirst for improving this book is still alive. The improvement is possible only by the comments and suggestions expressed by the readers. So, we welcome the opinions, comments and valuable suggestions from one and all who happen to come across this book.

K Sembulingam
ksembu@yahoo.com

Prema Sembulingam
prema_sembu@yahoo.com

Preface to the First Edition

The need for having a simple book with basic principles of Medical Physiology has been felt since long. A sincere and maiden attempt has been made with the idea of fulfilling the requirements of present-day curriculum. The script of the book is formatted in such a way that it will be suitable not only for medical students, but also for dental students and the students of allied health subjects like Physiotherapy, Occupational Therapy, Pharmacy, Nursing, Speech, Hearing and Language, etc.

Written in a textbook form, this book encompasses the knowledge of basic principles of physiology in each system. An attempt is also made to describe the applied physiology in each system.

To give an idea of the matters to be studied, the topics are listed at the beginning of each chapter. Most of the figures are given in schematic form to enable students to understand and reproduce the facts. The probable questions given for each section will help the students preparing for examinations. However, it will be ideal for the students to read each section thoroughly before referring to the questions.

We will be very happy to receive opinions, comments and valuable suggestions from all our senior colleagues, fellow teachers and students so that, every aspect of the book can be reviewed in succeeding editions.

K Sembulingam
Prema Sembulingam

Acknowledgments

We express our profound gratitude to Late Mr NPV Ramasamy Udayar, Founder Chancellor, Sri Ramachandra Medical College and Research Institute (Deemed University), Chennai, Tamil Nadu, India for his keen interest in all the academic activities of the faculty members.

We would like to express our sincere gratitude to Sri VR Venkatachalam, the Chancellor of Sri Ramachandra Medical College and Research Institute (Deemed University) for accepting to grace the occasion of 'Book Releasing Ceremony' of *Essentials of Medical Physiology*—first edition and for releasing the book. We are very much thankful to the former Vice-Chancellor of this University Dr TK Partha Sarathy, who honored us by attending the function and received the first copy of the book. We are also overwhelmed by his magnanimity for his encouragement and for going through the entire script before giving the foreword.

We sincerely thank Mrs Radha Venkatachalam, Registrar and Administrative Director, Sri Ramachandra Medical College and Research Institute (Deemed University), who always encouraged the faculty of the university for publications.

We thank Dr Sylvia Walter, Professor Emeritus, Department of Physiology, Sri Ramachandra Medical College and Research Institute (Deemed University), who is the inspiration for us to bring out this book. We are also indebted to her for giving many valuable clues to modify the script in many chapters. Our special thanks to Dr V Srinivasan, Former Professor and Head, Department of Physiology, Sri Ramachandra Medical College and Research Institute (Deemed University) for his strong belief in this project, constant encouragement and valuable suggestions. We are very much grateful to Dr V Srinivasan for his keen interest and valuable suggestions for upgrading the script in each edition.

We thank all our fellow teachers and senior professors from various institutes and universities in and out of India for their comments and suggestions, which enabled us to bring out each edition of the book successfully.

We are deeply indebted to our students of Sri Ramachandra Medical College and Research Institute (Deemed University), Chennai, Tamil Nadu, India and MR Medical College, Gulbarga, Karnataka, India who were the spirit behind the idea of bringing out this book.

Our special thanks to Dr M Chandrasekar, Vice-Principal and Head, Department of Physiology, Meenakshi Medical College, Kanchipuram, Tamil Nadu, India for writing a review article on this book in the Journal 'Biomedicine' (Vol 20, No. 1). Many valuable suggestions from him enabled us to upgrade the book in each edition.

We are grateful to Professor Mafauzy Mohamad, Director, Health Campus, Universiti Sains Malaysia, Kelantan, Malaysia for providing the photos of endocrine disorder patients. We are thankful to Dr Nivaldo Medeiros, Former Director of Hematology and Cytology Services, Central Laboratory, University of São Paulo, School of Medicine, USA for giving us the hematology pictures.

Our profound thanks are due to Dr S Peter, Founder and Chairman, Madha Group of Academic Institutions for the recognition, appreciation and encouragement given to us in bringing out this edition. We are thankful to Dr S Madan Kumar, Director, Madha Medical College & Research Institute for his keen interest in publishing this edition. We also thank him for accepting and rendering foreword for this edition. We thank Dr K Gajendran, Principal, Madha Medical College & Research Institute for his constant encouragement in bringing out this edition.

We are thankful to Shri Jitendar P Vij (CEO), Mr Tarun Duneja (Director-Publishing) and Mr KK Raman (Production Manager) of M/s Jaypee Brothers Medical Publishers (P) Ltd, New Delhi, India for publishing the book in the same format as we wanted. We thank Ms Chetna Malhotra Vohra (Senior Business Executive Manager) for coordinating the processing of this edition. We thank Ms Sajini SV (Project Leader), Ms Hemalata Malini B and Mr Samiulla (DTP Operators); Ms Nandini N, Ms Ramya VR, Ms Bhavya M, and Ms Nikita G (Proofreaders) of Bengaluru Production Unit, M/s Jaypee Brothers Medical Publishers (P) Ltd, Bengaluru Branch, for their wholehearted contribution while formatting the book. We also thank Ms Shilpa K Bhat (Graphic Designer), of Bengaluru Production Unit for making the figures attractive.

Special Acknowledgments

We sincerely acknowledge the following fellow teachers for their valuable suggestions. All the points suggested by them were acknowledged and incorporated in this edition.

1. **Dr M Chandrasekar**
   Vice Principal and Head
   Department of Physiology
   Meenakshi Medical College
   Kanchipuram, Tamil Nadu, India

2. **Dr P Sai Kumar**
   Vice Principal and Professor
   Department of Physiology
   Sri Balaji Medical College and Hospital
   Chennai, Tamil Nadu, India

3. **Dr B Vishwanatha Rao**
   Professor
   Department of Physiology
   Madras Medical College
   Chennai, Tamil Nadu, India

4. **Dr K Sarayu**
   Professor and Head
   Department of Physiology
   KAT Viswanathan Government Medical College
   Trichy, Tamil Nadu, India

5. **Dr D Venkatesh**
   Professor
   Department of Physiology
   MS Ramaiah Medical College
   Bengaluru, Karnataka, India

6. **Dr S Manikandan**
   Associate Professor
   Department of Physiology
   Tagore Medical College
   Chennai, Tamil Nadu, India

7. **Dr NV Mishra**
   Associate Professor
   Department of Physiology
   Medical College
   Nagpur (MS), Maharashtra, India

8. **Dr KS Udayashankar**
   Professor and Head
   Department of Physiology
   Sri Rajarajeshwari Medical College and Hospital
   Bengaluru, Karnataka, India

9. **Dr MG Hymavthi**
   Professor
   Department of Physiology
   Sri Rajarajeshwari Medical College and Hospital
   Bengaluru, Karnataka, India

Contents

SECTION 3
MUSCLE PHYSIOLOGY

SECTION 4
DIGESTIVE SYSTEM

SECTION 5
RENAL PHYSIOLOGY AND SKIN

SECTION 6

ENDOCRINOLOGY

SECTION 7

REPRODUCTIVE SYSTEM

SECTION 8
CARDIOVASCULAR SYSTEM

SECTION 9
RESPIRATORY SYSTEM AND ENVIRONMENTAL PHYSIOLOGY

SECTION 10
NERVOUS SYSTEM

SECTION 11
SPECIAL SENSES

Introduction

Physiology is the most fascinating and ancient branch of science. It is fascinating because, it unfolds the mystery of complicated functional aspects of individual organs in the body. It is ancient because, it exists ever since the origin of life. Even before knowing the language, culture and society, man knew about the hunger, thirst, pain and fear which are the basics of physiology.

Physiology is defined as the study of functions of various systems and different organs of the body. Physiology is of different types namely, Human Physiology, Animal Physiology and Plant Physiology. Human Physiology and Animal Physiology are very much inter-related. Knowledge of Human Physiology is essential to understand the other allied subjects like Biochemistry, Pharmacology, Pathology, Medicine, etc. However, it is worthwhile to have a brief knowledge of anatomy of different systems and various organs to understand the principles of Human Physiology.

The basic physiological functions include, provision of oxygen and nutrients, removal of metabolites and other waste products, maintenance of blood pressure and body temperature, hunger and thirst, locomotor functions, special sensory functions, reproduction and the higher intellectual functions like learning and memory.

In the unicellular organisms, all the physiological functions are carried out by simple diffusion through the cell membrane. Because of the evolutionary and ecological changes over the years, individual system is developed for each function such as digestive system, cardiovascular system, respiratory system, excretory system, etc. Every system in the body is independent structurally and functionally yet, all the systems are interdependent.

Human Physiology is usually studied under the following headings:

1. General Physiology
2. Blood and Body Fluids
3. Muscle Physiology
4. Digestive System
5. Renal Physiology and Excretion
6. Endocrinology
7. Reproductive System
8. Cardiovascular System
9. Respiratory System and Environmental Physiology
10. Nervous System
11. Special Senses

Section

1

General Physiology

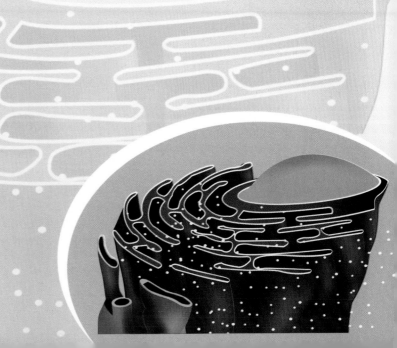

Cell

Chapter 1

- ■ INTRODUCTION
- ■ STRUCTURE OF THE CELL
- ■ CELL MEMBRANE
- ■ CYTOPLASM
- ■ ORGANELLES IN CYTOPLASM
- ■ ORGANELLES WITH LIMITING MEMBRANE
- ■ ORGANELLES WITHOUT LIMITING MEMBRANE
- ■ NUCLEUS
- ■ DEOXYRIBONUCLEIC ACID
- ■ GENE
- ■ RIBONUCLEIC ACID
- ■ GENE EXPRESSION
- ■ GROWTH FACTORS
- ■ CELL DEATH
- ■ CELL ADAPTATION
- ■ CELL DEGENERATION
- ■ CELL AGING
- ■ STEM CELLS

■ INTRODUCTION

■ CELL

All the living things are composed of cells. A single cell is the smallest unit that has all the characteristics of life. Cell is defined as the structural and functional unit of the living body.

General Characteristics of Cell

Each cell in the body:
1. Needs nutrition and oxygen
2. Produces its own energy necessary for its growth, repair and other activities
3. Eliminates carbon dioxide and other metabolic wastes
4. Maintains the medium, i.e. the environment for its survival

5. Shows immediate response to the entry of invaders like bacteria or toxic substances into the body
6. Reproduces by division. There are some exceptions like neuron, which do not reproduce.

■ TISSUE

Tissue is defined as the group of cells having similar function. There are many types of tissues in the body. All the tissues are classified into four major types which are called the **primary tissues**. The primary tissues include:
1. Muscle tissue (skeletal muscle, smooth muscle and cardiac muscle)
2. Nervous tissue (neurons and supporting cells)
3. Epithelial tissue (squamous, columnar and cuboidal epithelial cells)
4. Connective tissue (connective tissue proper, cartilage, bone and blood).

■ ORGAN

An organ is defined as the structure that is formed by two or more primary types of tissues, which execute the functions of the organ. Some organs are composed of all the four types of primary tissues. The organs are of two types, namely tubular or **hollow organs** and compact or **parenchymal organs.** Some of the organs in the body are brain, heart, lungs, stomach, intestine, liver, gallbladder, pancreas, kidneys, endocrine glands, etc.

■ SYSTEM

The organ system is defined as group of organs that work together to carry out specific functions of the body.

Each system performs a specific function. Digestive system is concerned with digestion of food particles. Excretory system eliminates unwanted substances. Cardiovascular system is responsible for transport of substances between the organs. Respiratory system is concerned with the supply of oxygen and removal of carbon dioxide. Reproductive system is involved in the reproduction of species. Endocrine system is concerned with growth of the body and regulation and maintenance of normal life. Musculoskeletal system is responsible for stability and movements of the body. Nervous system controls the locomotion and other activities including the intellectual functions.

■ STRUCTURE OF THE CELL

Each cell is formed by a **cell body** and a membrane covering the cell body called the cell membrane. Cell body has two parts, namely nucleus and cytoplasm surrounding the nucleus (Fig. 1.1). Thus, the structure of the cell is studied under three headings:
1. Cell membrane
2. Cytoplasm
3. Nucleus.

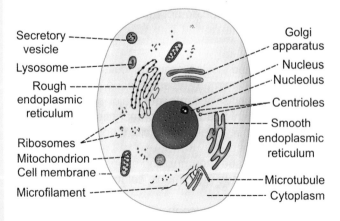

FIGURE 1.1: Structure of the cell

■ CELL MEMBRANE

Cell membrane is a protective sheath, enveloping the cell body. It is also known as **plasma membrane** or **plasmalemma**. This membrane separates the fluid outside the cell called extracellular fluid (ECF) and the fluid inside the cell called intracellular fluid (ICF). The cell membrane is a semipermeable membrane. So, there is free exchange of certain substances between ECF and ICF. Thickness of the cell membrane varies from 75 to 111Å (Fig. 1.2).

■ COMPOSITION OF CELL MEMBRANE

Cell membrane is composed of three types of substances:
1. Proteins (55%)
2. Lipids (40%)
3. Carbohydrates (5%).

■ STRUCTURE OF CELL MEMBRANE

On the basis of structure, cell membrane is called a **unit membrane** or a three-layered membrane. The electron microscopic study reveals three layers of cell membrane, namely, one central **electron-lucent layer** and two **electron-dense layers.** The two electron-dense layers are placed one on either side of the central layer. The central layer is a lipid layer formed by lipid substances. The other two layers are protein layers formed by proteins. Cell membrane contains some carbohydrate molecules also.

Structural Model of the Cell Membrane

1. *Danielli-Davson model*

'Danielli-Davson model' was the first proposed basic model of membrane structure. It was proposed by James F Danielli and Hugh Davson in 1935. And it was accepted by scientists for many years. This model was basically a **'sandwich of lipids'** covered by proteins on both sides.

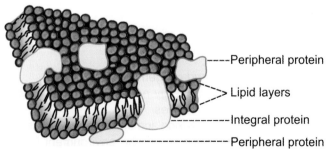

FIGURE 1.2: Diagram of the cell membrane

2. Unit membrane model

In 1957, JD Robertson replaced 'Danielli-Davson model' by 'Unit membrane model' on the basis of electron microscopic studies.

3. Fluid mosaic model

Later in 1972, SJ Singer and GL Nicholson proposed 'The fluid mosaic model'. According to them, the membrane is a fluid with mosaic of proteins (mosaic means pattern formed by arrangement of different colored pieces of stone, tile, glass or other such materials). This model is accepted by the scientists till now. In this model, the proteins are found to float in the lipid layer instead of forming the layers of the sandwich-type model.

Lipid Layers of the Cell Membrane

The central lipid layer is a bilayered structure. This is formed by a thin film of lipids. The characteristic feature of lipid layer is that, it is fluid in nature and not a solid structure. So, the portions of the membrane move from one point to another point along the surface of the cell. The materials dissolved in lipid layer also move to all areas of the cell membrane.

Major lipids are:
1. Phospholipids
2. Cholesterol.

1. Phospholipids

Phospholipids are the lipid substances containing phosphorus and fatty acids. **Aminophospholipids, sphingomyelins, phosphatidylcholine, phosphatidyletholamine, phosphatidylglycerol, phosphatidylserine** and **phosphatidylinositol** are the phospholipids present in lipid layer of cell membrane.

Phospholipid molecules are arranged in two layers (Fig. 1.3). Each phospholipid molecule resembles the headed pin in shape. The outer part of the phospholipid molecule is called the **head portion** and the inner portion is called the **tail portion.**

Head portion is the polar end and it is soluble in water and has strong affinity for water **(hydrophilic).** Tail portion is the non-polar end. It is insoluble in water and repelled by water **(hydrophobic).**

Two layers of phospholipids are arranged in such a way that the hydrophobic tail portions meet in the center of the membrane. Hydrophilic head portions of outer layer face the ECF and those of the inner layer face ICF (cytoplasm).

2. Cholesterol

Cholesterol molecules are arranged in between the phospholipid molecules. Phospholipids are soft and oily structures and cholesterol helps to 'pack' the phospholipids in the membrane. So, cholesterol is responsible for the structural integrity of lipid layer of the cell membrane.

Functions of Lipid Layer in Cell Membrane

Lipid layer of the cell membrane is a semipermeable membrane and allows only the fat-soluble substances to pass through it. Thus, the fat-soluble substances like oxygen, carbon dioxide and alcohol can pass through this lipid layer. The water-soluble substances such as glucose, urea and electrolytes cannot pass through this layer.

Protein Layers of the Cell Membrane

Protein layers of the cell membrane are electron-dense layers. These layers cover the two surfaces of the central lipid layer. Protein layers give protection to the central lipid layer. The protein substances present in these layers are mostly glycoproteins.

Protein molecules are classified into two categories:
1. Integral proteins or transmembrane proteins.
2. Peripheral proteins or peripheral membrane proteins.

1. Integral proteins

Integral or transmembrane proteins are the proteins that pass through entire thickness of cell membrane from one side to the other side. These proteins are tightly bound with the cell membrane.

Examples of integral protein:
   i. Cell adhesion proteins
   ii. Cell junction proteins
   iii. Some carrier (transport) proteins
   iv. Channel proteins
   v. Some hormone receptors
   vi. Antigens
   vii. Some enzymes.

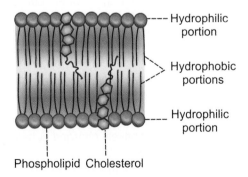

FIGURE 1.3: Lipids of the cell membrane

2. *Peripheral proteins*

Peripheral proteins or peripheral membrane proteins are the proteins which are partially embedded in the outer and inner surfaces of the cell membrane and do not penetrate the cell membrane. Peripheral proteins are loosely bound with integral proteins or lipid layer of cell membrane. So, these protein molecules dissociate readily from the cell membrane.

Examples of peripheral proteins:
  i. Proteins of cytoskeleton
  ii. Some carrier (transport) proteins
  iii. Some enzymes.

Functions of Proteins in Cell Membrane

1. Integral proteins provide the structural integrity of the cell membrane
2. Channel proteins help in the diffusion of water-soluble substances like glucose and electrolytes
3. Carrier or transport proteins help in the transport of substances across the cell membrane by means of active or passive transport
4. Pump: Some carrier proteins act as pumps, by which ions are transported actively across the cell membrane
5. Receptor proteins serve as the receptor sites for hormones and neurotransmitters
6. Enzymes: Some of the protein molecules form the enzymes and control chemical (metabolic) reactions within the cell membrane
7. Antigens: Some proteins act as antigens and induce the process of antibody formation
8. Cell adhesion molecules or the integral proteins are responsible for attachment of cells to their neighbors or to basal lamina.

Carbohydrates of the Cell Membrane

Some of the carbohydrate molecules present in cell membrane are attached to proteins and form **glycoproteins (proteoglycans).** Some carbohydrate molecules are attached to lipids and form glycolipids.

Carbohydrate molecules form a thin and loose covering over the entire surface of the cell membrane called **glycocalyx.**

Functions of Carbohydrates in Cell Membrane

1. Carbohydrate molecules are negatively charged and do not permit the negatively charged substances to move in and out of the cell
2. Glycocalyx from the neighboring cells helps in the tight fixation of cells with one another

3. Some carbohydrate molecules function as the receptors for some hormones.

■ FUNCTIONS OF CELL MEMBRANE

1. *Protective function*: Cell membrane protects the cytoplasm and the organelles present in the cytoplasm
2. *Selective permeability:* Cell membrane acts as a semipermeable membrane, which allows only some substances to pass through it and acts as a barrier for other substances
3. *Absorptive function:* Nutrients are absorbed into the cell through the cell membrane
4. *Excretory function:* Metabolites and other waste products from the cell are excreted out through the cell membrane
5. *Exchange of gases:* Oxygen enters the cell from the blood and carbon dioxide leaves the cell and enters the blood through the cell membrane
6. *Maintenance of shape and size of the cell:* Cell membrane is responsible for the maintenance of shape and size of the cell.

■ CYTOPLASM

Cytoplasm of the cell is the jelly-like material formed by 80% of water. It contains a clear liquid portion called **cytosol** and various particles of different shape and size. These particles are proteins, carbohydrates, lipids or electrolytes in nature. Cytoplasm also contains many organelles with distinct structure and function.

Cytoplasm is made up of two zones:
1. Ectoplasm: Peripheral part of cytoplasm, situated just beneath the cell membrane
2. Endoplasm: Inner part of cytoplasm, interposed between the ectoplasm and the nucleus.

■ ORGANELLES IN CYTOPLASM

Cytoplasmic organelles are the cellular structures embedded in the cytoplasm. Organelles are considered as small organs of the cell. Some organelles are bound by limiting membrane and others do not have limiting membrane (Box 1.1). Each organelle is having a definite structure and specific functions (Table 1.1).

■ ORGANELLES WITH LIMITING MEMBRANE

■ ENDOPLASMIC RETICULUM

Endoplasmic reticulum is a network of tubular and microsomal vesicular structures which are interconnected with one another. It is covered by a limiting membrane which is formed by proteins and bilayered lipids. The lumen

BOX 1.1: Cytoplasmic organelles

Organelles with limiting membrane
1. Endoplasmic reticulum
2. Golgi apparatus
3. Lysosome
4. Peroxisome
5. Centrosome and centrioles
6. Secretory vesicles
7. Mitochondria
8. Nucleus
Organelles without limiting membrane
1. Ribosomes
2. Cytoskeleton

of endoplasmic reticulum contains a fluid medium called **endoplasmic matrix.** The diameter of the lumen is about 400 to 700Å. The endoplasmic reticulum forms the link between nucleus and cell membrane by connecting the cell membrane with the nuclear membrane.

Types of Endoplasmic Reticulum

Endoplasmic reticulum is of two types, namely rough endoplasmic reticulum and smooth endoplasmic reticulum. Both the types are interconnected and continuous with one another. Depending upon the activities of the cells, the rough endoplasmic reticulum changes to smooth endoplasmic reticulum and vice versa.

Rough Endoplasmic Reticulum

It is the endoplasmic reticulum with rough, bumpy or bead-like appearance. Rough appearance is due to the attachment of granular ribosomes to its outer surface. Hence, it is also called the **granular endoplasmic**

TABLE 1.1: Functions of cytoplasmic organelles

Organelles	Functions
Rough endoplasmic reticulum	1. Synthesis of proteins 2. Degradation of worn-out organelles
Smooth endoplasmic reticulum	1. Synthesis of lipids and steroids 2. Role in cellular metabolism 3. Storage and metabolism of calcium 4. Catabolism and detoxification of toxic substances
Golgi apparatus	1. Processing, packaging, labeling and delivery of proteins and lipids
Lysosomes	1. Degradation of macromolecules 2. Degradation of worn-out organelles 3. Removal of excess of secretory products 4. Secretion of perforin, granzymes, melanin and serotonin
Peroxisomes	1. Breakdown of excess fatty acids 2. Detoxification of hydrogen peroxide and other metabolic products 3. Oxygen utilization 4. Acceleration of gluconeogenesis 5. Degradation of purine to uric acid 6. Role in the formation of myelin 7. Role in the formation of bile acids
Centrosome	1. Movement of chromosomes during cell division
Mitochondria	1. Production of energy 2. Synthesis of ATP 3. Initiation of apoptosis
Ribosomes	1. Synthesis of proteins
Cytoskeleton	1. Determination of shape of the cell 2. Stability of cell shape 3. Cellular movements
Nucleus	1. Control of all activities of the cell 2. Synthesis of RNA 3. Sending genetic instruction to cytoplasm for protein synthesis 4. Formation of subunits of ribosomes 5. Control of cell division 6. Storage of hereditary information in genes (DNA)

reticulum (Fig. 1.4). Rough endoplasmic reticulum is vesicular or tubular in structure.

Functions of Rough Endoplasmic Reticulum

1. *Synthesis of proteins*

Rough endoplasmic reticulum is concerned with the synthesis of proteins in the cell. It is involved with the synthesis of mainly those proteins which are secreted from the cells such as insulin from β-cells of islets of Langerhans in pancreas and antibodies from B lymphocytes.

Ribosomes arrange the amino acids into small units of proteins and transport them into the rough endoplasmic reticulum. Here, the carbohydrates are added to the protein units forming the **glycosylated proteins** or **glycoproteins,** which are arranged in the form of reticular vesicles. These vesicles are transported mainly to Golgi apparatus for further modification and processing. Few vesicles are transported to other cyto-plasmic organelles.

2. *Degradation of worn-out organelles*

Rough endoplasmic reticulum also plays an important role in the degradation of worn-out cytoplasmic orga-nelles like mitochondria. It wraps itself around the worn-out organelles and forms a vacuole which is often called the **autophagosome.** Autophagosome is digested by lysosomal enzymes (see below for details).

Smooth Endoplasmic Reticulum

It is the endoplasmic reticulum with smooth appearance. It is also called **agranular reticulum.** It is formed by many interconnected tubules. So, it is also called **tubular endoplasmic reticulum.**

Functions of Smooth Endoplasmic Reticulum

1. *Synthesis of non-protein substance*

Smooth endoplasmic reticulum is responsible for syn-thesis of non-protein substances such as cholesterol and steroid. This type of endoplasmic reticulum is abundant in cells that are involved in the synthesis of lipids, phospholipids, lipoprotein substances, steroid hormones, sebum, etc. In most of the other cells, smooth endoplasmic reticulum is less extensive than the rough endoplasmic reticulum.

2. *Role in cellular metabolism*

Outer surface of smooth endoplasmic reticulum contains many enzymes which are involved in various metabolic processes of the cell.

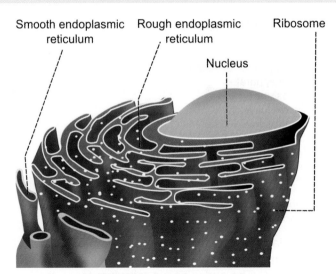

FIGURE 1.4: Endoplasmic reticulum

3. *Storage and metabolism of calcium*

Smooth endoplasmic reticulum is the major site of storage and metabolism of calcium. In skeletal muscle fibers, it releases calcium which is necessary to trigger the muscle contraction.

4. *Catabolism and detoxification*

Smooth endoplasmic reticulum is also concerned with catabolism and detoxification of toxic substances like some drugs and **carcinogens** (cancer-producing substances) in the liver.

■ GOLGI APPARATUS

Golgi apparatus or Golgi body or Golgi complex is a membrane-bound organelle, involved in the processing of proteins. It is present in all the cells except red blood cells. It is named after the discoverer Camillo Golgi. Usually, each cell has one Golgi apparatus. Some of the cells may have more than one Golgi apparatus. Each Golgi apparatus consists of 5 to 8 flattened membranous sacs called the **cisternae.**

Golgi apparatus is situated near the nucleus. It has two ends or faces, namely **cis face** and **trans face.** The cis face is positioned near the endoplasmic reticulum. Reticular vesicles from endoplasmic reticulum enter the Golgi apparatus through cis face. The trans face is situated near the cell membrane. The processed substances make their exit from Golgi apparatus through trans face (Fig. 1.5).

Functions of Golgi Apparatus

Major functions of Golgi apparatus are processing, packing, labeling and delivery of proteins and other molecules like lipids to different parts of the cell.

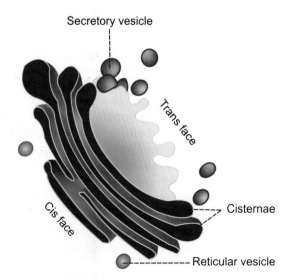

FIGURE 1.5: Golgi apparatus

1. Processing of materials

Vesicles containing glycoproteins and lipids are transported into Golgi apparatus. Here, the glycoproteins and lipids are modified and processed.

2. Packaging of materials

All the processed materials are packed in the form of secretory granules, secretory vesicles and lysosomes, which are transported either out of the cell or to another part of the cell. Because of this, Golgi apparatus is called the **'post office of the cell'**.

3. Labeling and delivery of materials

Finally, the Golgi apparatus sorts out the processed and packed materials and labels them (such as phosphate group), depending upon the chemical content for delivery (distribution) to their proper destinations. Hence, the Golgi apparatus is called **'shipping department of the cell'**.

■ LYSOSOMES

Lysosomes are the membrane-bound vesicular organelles found throughout the cytoplasm. The lysosomes are formed by Golgi apparatus. The enzymes synthesized in rough endoplasmic reticulum are processed and packed in the form of small vesicles in the Golgi apparatus. Then, these vesicles are pinched off from Golgi apparatus and become the lysosomes.

Among the organelles of the cytoplasm, the lysosomes have the thickest covering membrane. The membrane is formed by a bilayered lipid material. It has many small granules which contain hydrolytic enzymes.

Types of Lysosomes

Lysosomes are of two types:
1. Primary lysosome, which is pinched off from Golgi apparatus. It is inactive in spite of having hydrolytic enzymes
2. Secondary lysosome, which is the active lysosome. It is formed by the fusion of a primary lysosome with phagosome or endosome (see below).

Functions of Lysosomes

Lysosomes are often called **'garbage system'** of the cell because of their degradation activity. About 50 different hydrolytic enzymes, known as acid **hydroxylases** are present in the lysosomes, through which lysosomes execute their functions.

Important lysosomal enzymes

1. Proteases, which hydrolyze the proteins into amino acids
2. Lipases, which hydrolyze the lipids into fatty acids and glycerides
3. Amylases, which hydrolyze the polysaccharides into glucose
4. Nucleases, which hydrolyze the nucleic acids into mononucleotides.

Mechanism of lysosomal function

Lysosomal functions involve two mechanisms:
1. Heterophagy: Digestion of extracellular materials engulfed by the cell via endocytosis
2. Autophagy: Digestion of intracellular materials such as worn-out cytoplasmic organelles.

Specific functions of lysosomes

1. Degradation of macromolecules

Macromolecules are engulfed by the cell by means of endocytosis (phagocytosis, pinocytosis or receptor-mediated endocytosis: Chapter 3). The macromolecules such as bacteria, engulfed by the cell via phagocytosis are called **phagosomes** or **vacuoles**. The other macromolecules taken inside via pinocytosis or receptor-mediated endocytosis are called **endosomes**. The **primary lysosome** fuses with the phagosome or endosome to form the **secondary lysosome**. The pH in the secondary lysosome becomes acidic and the lysosomal enzymes are activated. The bacteria and the other macromolecules are digested and degraded by these enzymes. The secondary lysosome containing these degraded waste products moves through cytoplasm and fuses with cell membrane. Now the waste products are eliminated by exocytosis.

2. *Degradation of worn-out organelles*

The rough endoplasmic reticulum wraps itself around the worn-out organelles like mitochondria and form the vacuoles called **autophagosomes.** One primary lysosome fuses with one autophagosome to form the secondary lysosome. The enzymes in the secondary lysosome are activated. Now, these enzymes digest the contents of autophagosome.

3. *Removal of excess secretory products in the cells*

Lysosomes in the cells of the secretory glands remove the excess secretory products by degrading the secretory granules.

4. *Secretory function – secretory lysosomes*

Recently, lysosomes having secretory function called secretory lysosomes are found in some of the cells, particularly in the cells of immune system. The conventional lysosomes are modified into secretory lysosomes by combining with secretory granules (which contain the particular secretory product of the cell).

Examples of secretory lysosomes:
  i. Lysosomes in the cytotoxic T lymphocytes and natural killer (NK) cells secrete perforin and **granzymes,** which destroy both viral-infected cells and tumor cells. Perforin is a pore-forming protein that initiates cell death. Granzymes belong to the family of serine proteases (enzymes that dislodge the peptide bonds of the proteins) and cause the cell death by **apoptosis**
  ii. Secretory lysosomes of melanocytes secrete melanin
  iii. Secretory lysosomes of mast cells secrete serotonin, which is a vasoconstrictor substance and inflammatory mediator.

■ PEROXISOMES

Peroxisomes or microbodies are the membrane limited vesicles like the lysosomes. Unlike lysosomes, peroxisomes are pinched off from endoplasmic reticulum and not from the Golgi apparatus. Peroxisomes contain some oxidative enzymes such as catalase, urate oxidase and D-amino acid oxidase.

Functions of Peroxisomes

Peroxisomes:
  i. Breakdown the fatty acids by means of a process called beta-oxidation: This is the major function of peroxisomes
  ii. Degrade the toxic substances such as hydrogen peroxide and other metabolic products by means of **detoxification.** A large number of peroxisomes are present in the cells of liver, which is the major organ for detoxification. Hydrogen peroxide is formed from poisons or alcohol, which enter the cell. Whenever hydrogen peroxide is produced in the cell, the peroxisomes are ruptured and the oxidative enzymes are released. These oxidases destroy hydrogen peroxide and the enzymes which are necessary for the production of hydrogen peroxide
  iii. Form the major site of oxygen utilization in the cells
  iv. Accelerate gluconeogenesis from fats
  v. Degrade purine to uric acid
  vi. Participate in the formation of myelin
  viii. Play a role in the formation of bile acids.

■ CENTROSOME AND CENTRIOLES

Centrosome is the membrane-bound cellular organelle situated almost in the center of cell, close to nucleus. It consists of two cylindrical structures called centrioles which are made up of proteins. Centrioles are responsible for the movement of chromosomes during cell division.

■ SECRETORY VESICLES

Secretory vesicles are the organelles with limiting membrane and contain the secretory substances. These vesicles are formed in the endoplasmic reticulum and are processed and packed in Golgi apparatus. Secretory vesicles are present throughout the cytoplasm. When necessary, these vesicles are ruptured and secretory substances are released into the cytoplasm.

■ MITOCHONDRION

Mitochondrion (plural = mitochondria) is a membrane-bound cytoplasmic organelle concerned with production of energy. It is a rod-shaped or oval-shaped structure with a diameter of 0.5 to 1 μ. It is covered by a bilayered membrane (Fig. 1.6). The outer membrane is smooth and encloses the contents of mitochondrion. This membrane contains various enzymes such as acetyl-CoA synthetase and glycerolphosphate acetyltransferase.

The inner membrane is folded in the form of shelf-like inward projections called **cristae** and it covers the inner matrix space. Cristae contain many enzymes and other protein molecules which are involved in respiration and synthesis of adenosine triphosphate (ATP). Because of these functions, the enzymes and other protein molecules

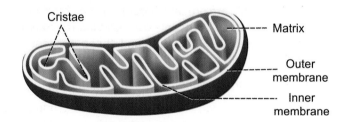

FIGURE 1.6: Structure of mitochondrion

in cristae are collectively known as respiratory chain or electron transport system.

Enzymes and other proteins of respiratory chain

  i. Succinic dehydrogenase
  ii. Dihydronicotinamide adenine dinucleotide (NADH) dehydrogenase
  iii. Cytochrome oxidase
  iv. Cytochrome C
  v. ATP synthase.

Inner cavity of mitochondrion is filled with matrix which contains many enzymes. Mitochondrion moves freely in the cytoplasm of the cell. It is capable of reproducing itself. Mitochondrion contains its own deoxyribonucleic acid (DNA), which is responsible for many enzymatic actions. In fact, mitochondrion is the only organelle other than nucleus, which has its own DNA.

Functions of Mitochondrion

1. Production of energy

Mitochondrion is called the **'power house'** or **'power plant'** of the cell because it produces the energy required for cellular functions. The energy is produced during the oxidation of digested food particles like proteins, carbohydrates and lipids by the oxidative enzymes in cristae. During the oxidative process, water and carbon dioxide are produced with release of energy. The released energy is stored in mitochondria and used later for synthesis of ATP.

2. Synthesis of ATP

The components of respiratory chain in mitochondrion are responsible for the synthesis of ATP by utilizing the energy by oxidative phosphorylation. ATP molecules diffuse throughout the cell from mitochondrion. Whenever energy is needed for cellular activity, the ATP molecules are broken down.

3. Apoptosis

Cytochrome C and second mitochondria-derived activator of caspases (SMAC)/diablo secreted in mitochondria are involved in apoptosis (see below).

4. Other functions

Other functions of mitochondria include storage of calcium and detoxification of ammonia in liver.

■ ORGANELLES WITHOUT LIMITING MEMBRANE

■ RIBOSOMES

Ribosomes are the organelles without limiting membrane. These organelles are granular and small dot-like structures with a diameter of 15 nm. Ribosomes are made up of 35% of proteins and 65% of ribonucleic acid (RNA). RNA present in ribosomes is called ribosomal RNA (rRNA). Ribosomes are concerned with protein synthesis in the cell.

Types of Ribosomes

Ribosomes are of two types:
  i. Ribosomes that are attached to rough endoplasmic reticulum
  ii. Free ribosomes that are distributed in the cytoplasm.

Functions of Ribosomes

Ribosomes are called **'protein factories'** because of their role in the synthesis of proteins. Messenger RNA (mRNA) carries the **genetic code** for protein synthesis from nucleus to the ribosomes. The ribosomes, in turn arrange the amino acids into small units of proteins.

Ribosomes attached to rough endoplasmic reticulum are involved in the synthesis of proteins such as the enzymatic proteins, hormonal proteins, lysosomal proteins and the proteins of the cell membrane.

Free ribosomes are responsible for the synthesis of proteins in hemoglobin, peroxisome and mitochondria.

■ CYTOSKELETON

Cytoskeleton is the cellular organelle present throughout the cytoplasm. It determines the shape of the cell and gives support to the cell. It is a complex network of structures with varying sizes. In addition to determining the shape of the cell, it is also essential for the cellular movements and the response of the cell to external stimuli.

Cytoskeleton consists of three major protein components:
1. Microtubule
2. Intermediate filaments
3. Microfilaments.

1. Microtubules

Microtubules are the straight, hollow and tubular structures of the cytoskeleton. These organelles without the limiting membrane are arranged in different bundles. Each tubule has a diameter of 20 to 30 nm. Length of microtubule varies and it may be 1000 times more than the thickness.

Structurally, the microtubules are formed by bundles of globular protein called **tubulin** (Fig. 1.7). Tubulin has two subunits, namely α-subunit and β-subunit.

Functions of microtubules

Microtubules may function alone or join with other proteins to form more complex structures like cilia, flagella or centrioles and perform various functions. Microtubules:
- i. Determine the shape of the cell
- ii. Give structural strength to the cell
- iii. Act like conveyer belts which allow the movement of granules, vesicles, protein molecules and some organelles like mitochondria to different parts of the cell
- iv. Form the spindle fibers which separate the chromosomes during mitosis
- v. Are responsible for the movement of centrioles and the complex cellular structures like cilia.

2. Intermediate Filaments

Intermediate filaments are the structures that form a network around the nucleus and extend to the periphery of the cell. Diameter of each filament is about 10 nm. The intermediate filaments are formed by rope-like polymers, which are made up of **fibrous proteins** (Fig. 1.8).

Subclasses of intermediate filaments

Intermediate filaments are divided into five subclasses:
- i. Keratins (in epithelial cells)
- ii. Glial filaments (in astrocytes)
- iii. Neurofilaments (in nerve cells)
- iv. Vimentin (in many types of cells)
- v. Desmin (in muscle fibers).

Functions of intermediate filaments

Intermediate filaments help to maintain the shape of the cell. These filaments also connect the adjacent cells through desmosomes.

3. Microfilaments

Microfilaments are long and fine thread-like structures with a diameter of about 3 to 6 nm. These filaments are made up of non-tubular contractile proteins called actin and myosin. Actin is more abundant than myosin.

Microfilaments are present throughout the cytoplasm. The microfilaments present in ectoplasm contain only actin molecules (Fig. 1.9) and those present in endoplasm contain both actin and myosin molecules.

Functions of microfilaments

Microfilaments:
- i. Give structural strength to the cell
- ii. Provide resistance to the cell against the pulling forces
- iii. Are responsible for cellular movements like contraction, gliding and cytokinesis (partition of cytoplasm during cell division).

■ NUCLEUS

Nucleus is the most prominent and the largest cellular organelle. It has a diameter of 10 μ to 22 μ and occupies about 10% of total volume of the cell.

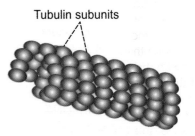

FIGURE 1.7: Microtubule

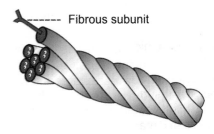

FIGURE 1.8: Intermediate filament

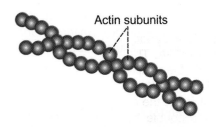

FIGURE 1.9: Microfilament of ectoplasm

Nucleus is present in all the cells in the body except the red blood cells. The cells with nucleus are called **eukaryotes** and those without nucleus are known as **prokaryotes**. Presence of nucleus is necessary for cell division.

Most of the cells have only one nucleus (**uninucleated cells**). Few types of cells like skeletal muscle cells have many nuclei (**multinucleated cells**). Generally, the nucleus is located in the center of the cell. It is mostly spherical in shape. However, the shape and situation of nucleus vary in some cells.

■ STRUCTURE OF NUCLEUS

Nucleus is covered by a membrane called **nuclear membrane** and contains many components. Major components of nucleus are **nucleoplasm, chromatin** and nucleolus.

Nuclear Membrane

Nuclear membrane is double layered and porous in nature. This allows the nucleoplasm to communicate with the cytoplasm. The outer layer of nuclear membrane is continuous with the membrane of endoplasmic reticulum. The space between the two layers of nuclear membrane is continuous with the lumen of endoplasmic reticulum.

Pores of the nuclear membrane are guarded (lined) by protein molecules. Diameter of the pores is about 80 to 100 nm. However, it is decreased to about 7 to 9 nm because of the attachment of protein molecules with the periphery of the pores. Exchange of materials between nucleoplasm and cytoplasm occurs through these pores.

Nucleoplasm

Nucleoplasm is a highly viscous fluid that forms the ground substance of the nucleus. It is similar to cytoplasm present outside the nucleus.

Nucleoplasm surrounds chromatin and nucleolus. It contains dense fibrillar network of proteins called the nuclear matrix and many substances such as nucleotides and enzymes. The nuclear matrix forms the structural framework for organizing chromatin. The soluble liquid part of nucleoplasm is known as nuclear hyaloplasm.

Chromatin

Chromatin is a thread-like material made up of large molecules of DNA. The DNA molecules are compactly packed with the help of a specialized basic protein called histone. So, chromatin is referred as **DNA-histone complex.** It forms the major bulk of nuclear material.

DNA is a double helix which wraps around central core of eight histone molecules to form the fundamental packing unit of chromatin called **nucleosome.** Nucleosomes are packed together tightly with the help of a histone molecule to form a chromatin fiber.

Just before cell division, the chromatin condenses to form chromosome.

Chromosomes

Chromosome is the rod-shaped nuclear structure that carries a complete blueprint of all the hereditary characteristics of that species. A chromosome is formed from a single DNA molecule coiled around histone molecules. Each DNA contains many genes.

Normally, the chromosomes are not visible in the nucleus under microscope. Only during cell division, the chromosomes are visible under microscope. This is because DNA becomes more tightly packed just before cell division, which makes the chromosome visible during cell division.

All the dividing cells of the body except reproductive cells contain 23 pairs of chromosomes. Each pair consists of one chromosome inherited from mother and one from father. The cells with 23 pairs of chromosomes are called **diploid cells.** The reproductive cells called gametes or sex cells contain only 23 single chromosomes. These cells are called **haploid cells.**

Nucleolus

Nucleolus is a small, round granular structure of the nucleus. Each nucleus contains one or more nucleoli. The nucleolus contains RNA and some proteins, which are similar to those found in ribosomes. The RNA is synthesized by five different pairs of chromosomes and stored in the nucleolus. Later, it is condensed to form the subunits of ribosomes. All the subunits formed in the nucleolus are transported to cytoplasm through the pores of nuclear membrane. In the cytoplasm, these subunits fuse to form ribosomes, which play an essential role in the formation of proteins.

■ FUNCTIONS OF NUCLEUS

Major functions of nucleus are the control of cellular activities and storage of hereditary material. Several processes are involved in the nuclear functions.

Functions of nucleus:

1. Control of all the cell activities that include metabolism, protein synthesis, growth and reproduction (cell division)
2. Synthesis of RNA
3. Formation of subunits of ribosomes
4. Sending genetic instruction to the cytoplasm for protein synthesis through messenger RNA (mRNA)

5. Control of the cell division through genes
6. Storage of hereditary information (in genes) and transformation of this information from one generation of the species to the next.

■ DEOXYRIBONUCLEIC ACID

Deoxyribonucleic acid (DNA) is a nucleic acid that carries the genetic information to the offspring of an organism. DNA forms the chemical basis of hereditary characters. It contains the instruction for the synthesis of proteins in the ribosomes. Gene is a part of a DNA molecule.

DNA is present in the nucleus (chromosome) and mitochondria of the cell. The DNA present in the nucleus is responsible for the formation of RNA. RNA regulates the synthesis of proteins by ribosomes. DNA in mitochondria is called **non-chromosomal DNA.**

■ STRUCTURE OF DNA

DNA is a double-stranded complex nucleic acid. It is formed by deoxyribose, phosphoric acid and four types of bases. Each DNA molecule consists of two polynucleotide chains, which are twisted around one another in the form of a double helix. The two chains are formed by the sugar deoxyribose and phosphate. These two substances form the backbone of DNA molecule. Both chains of DNA are connected with each other by some organic bases (Fig. 1.10).

Each chain of DNA molecule consists of many nucleotides. Each nucleotide is formed by:
1. Deoxyribose – sugar
2. Phosphate
3. One of the following organic (nitrogenous) bases:

Purines	– Adenine (A)
	– Guanine (G)
Pyrimidines	– Thymine (T)
	– Cytosine (C)

The strands of DNA are arranged in such a way that both are bound by specific pairs of bases. The adenine of one strand binds specifically with thymine of opposite strand. Similarly, the cytosine of one strand binds with guanine of the other strand.

DNA forms the component of chromosomes, which carries the hereditary information. The hereditary information that is encoded in DNA is called **genome.** Each DNA molecule is divided into discrete units called genes.

■ GENE

Gene is a portion of DNA molecule that contains the message or code for the synthesis of a specific protein from amino acids. It is like a book that contains the information necessary for protein synthesis. Gene is considered as the basic hereditary unit of the cell.

In the nucleotide of DNA, three of the successive base pairs are together called a triplet or a **codon.** Each codon codes or forms code word (information) for one amino acid. There are 20 amino acids and there is separate code for each amino acid. For example, the triplet CCA is the code for glycine and GGC is the code for proline.

Thus, each gene forms the code word for a particular protein to be synthesized in ribosome (outside the nucleus) from amino acids.

■ GENETIC DISORDERS

A genetic disorder is a disorder that occurs because of the abnormalities in an individual's genetic material (genome). Genetic disorders are either hereditary disorders or due to defect in genes.

Causes of Gene Disorders

Genetic disorders occur due to two causes:
1. *Genetic variation:* Presence of a different form of gene
2. *Genetic mutation:* Generally, mutation means an alteration or a change in nature, form, or quality. Genetic mutation refers to change of the DNA sequence within a gene or chromosome of an organism, which results in the creation of a new character.

Classification of Genetic Disorders

Genetic disorders are classified into four types:
1. Single gene disorders
2. Multifactorial genetic disorders
3. Chromosomal disorders
4. Mitochondrial DNA disorders.

1. Single Gene Disorders

Single gene disorders or Mendelian or monogenic disorders occur because of variation or mutation in one single gene. Examples include sickle cell anemia and Huntington's disease.

2. Multifactorial Genetic Disorders

Multifactorial genetic disorders or polygenic disorders are caused by combination of environmental factors and mutations in multiple genes. Examples are coronary heart disease, Alzheimer's disease, arthritis and diabetes.

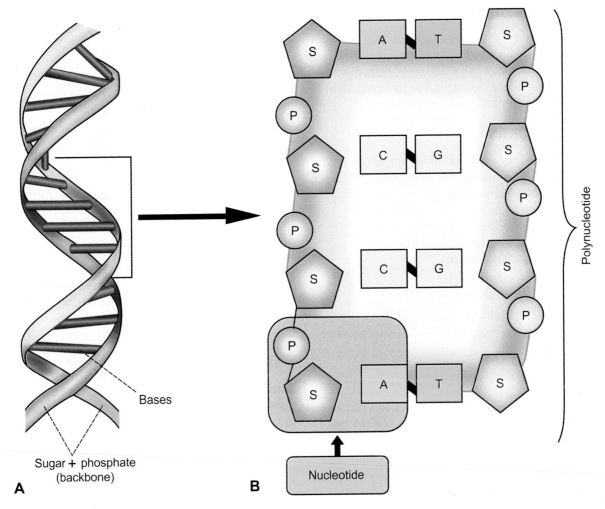

FIGURE 1.10: Structure of DNA. **A.** Double helical structure of DNA; **B.** Magnified view of the components of DNA.
A = Adenine, C = Cytocine, G= Guanine, P = Phosphate, S = Sugar, T = Thymine.

3. Chromosomal Disorders

Chromosomal disorder is a genetic disorder caused by abnormalities in chromosome. It is also called chromosomal abnormality, anomaly or aberration. It often results in genetic disorders which involve physical or mental abnormalities. Chromosomal disorder is caused by numerical abnormality or structural abnormality.

Chromosomal disorder is classified into two types:

i. Structural abnormality (alteration) of chromosomes which leads to disorders like chromosome instability syndromes (group of inherited diseases which cause malignancies)

ii. Numerical abnormality of chromosomes which is of two types:

a. **Monosomy** due to absence of one chromosome from normal diploid number. Example is Turner's syndrome, which is characterized by physical disabilities

b. **Trisomy** due to the presence of one extra chromosome along with normal pair of chromosomes in the cells. Example is **Down syndrome,** which is characterized by physical disabilities and mental retardation.

4. Mitochondrial DNA Disorders

Mitochondrial DNA disorders are the genetic disorders caused by the mutations in the DNA of mitochondria (non-chromosomal DNA). Examples are **Kearns-Sayre syndrome** (neuromuscular disorder characterized by myopathy, cardiomyopathy and paralysis of ocular muscles) and **Leber's hereditary optic neuropathy** (disease characterized by degeneration of retina and loss of vision).

■ RIBONUCLEIC ACID

Ribonucleic acid (RNA) is a nucleic acid that contains a long chain of nucleotide units. It is similar to DNA but contains ribose instead of deoxyribose. Various functions coded in the genes are carried out in the cytoplasm of the cell by RNA. RNA is formed from DNA.

■ STRUCTURE OF RNA

Each RNA molecule consists of a single strand of polynucleotide unlike the double-stranded DNA. Each nucleotide in RNA is formed by:

1. Ribose – sugar.
2. Phosphate.
3. One of the following organic bases:
   Purines   – Adenine (A)
                  – Guanine (G)
   Pyrimidines – Uracil (U)
                  – Cytosine (C).

Uracil replaces the thymine of DNA and it has similar structure of thymine.

■ TYPES OF RNA

RNA is of three types. Each type of RNA plays a specific role in protein synthesis. The three types of RNA are:

1. Messenger RNA (mRNA)

Messenger RNA carries the genetic code of the amino acid sequence for synthesis of protein from the DNA to the cytoplasm.

2. Transfer RNA (tRNA)

Transfer RNA is responsible for decoding the genetic message present in mRNA.

3. Ribosomal RNA (rRNA)

Ribosomal RNA is present within the ribosome and forms a part of the structure of ribosome. It is responsible for the assembly of protein from amino acids in the ribosome.

■ GENE EXPRESSION

Gene expression is the process by which the information (code word) encoded in the gene is converted into functional gene product or document of instruction (RNA) that is used for protein synthesis.

Gene expression involves two steps:
1. Transcription.
2. Translation.

■ TRANSCRIPTION OF GENETIC CODE

The word transcription means copying. It indicates the copying of genetic code from DNA to RNA. The proteins are synthesized in the ribosomes which are present in the cytoplasm. However, the synthesis of different proteins depends upon the information (sequence of codon) encoded in the genes of the DNA which is present in the nucleus. Since DNA is a macromolecule, it cannot pass through the pores of the nuclear membrane and enter the cytoplasm. But, the information from DNA must be sent to ribosome. So, the gene has to be transcribed (copied) into mRNA which is developed from DNA.

Thus, the first stage in the protein synthesis is transcription of genetic code, which occurs within the nucleus. It involves the formation of mRNA and simultaneous copying or transfer of information from DNA to mRNA. The mRNA enters the cytoplasm from the nucleus and activates the ribosome resulting in protein synthesis. The formation of mRNA from DNA is facilitated by the enzyme RNA polymerase.

■ TRANSLATION OF GENETIC CODE

Translation is the process by which protein synthesis occurs in the ribosome of the cell under the direction of genetic instruction carried by mRNA from DNA. Or, it is the process by which the mRNA is read by ribosome to produce a protein. This involves the role of other two types of RNA, namely tRNA and rRNA.

The mRNA moves out of nucleus into the cytoplasm. Now, a group of ribosomes called **polysome** gets attached to mRNA. The sequence of **codons** in mRNA are exposed and recognized by the complementary sequence of base in tRNA. The complementary sequence of base is called **anticodon.** According to the sequence of bases in anticodon, different amino acids are transported from the cytoplasm into the ribosome by tRNA that acts as a carrier. With the help of rRNA, the protein molecules are assembled from amino acids. The protein synthesis occurs in the ribosomes which are attached to rough endoplasmic reticulum.

■ GROWTH FACTORS

Growth factors are proteins which act as cell signaling molecules like cytokines (Chapter 17) and hormones (Chapter 65). These factors bind with specific surface receptors of the target cell and activate proliferation, differentiation and/or maturation of these cells.

Often, the term growth factor is interchangeably used with the term **cytokine.** But growth factors are distinct from cytokines. Growth factors act on the cells of the growing tissues. But cytokines are concerned with the cells of immune system and hemopoietic cells.

Many growth factors are identified. The known growth factors are:

1. Platelet-derived growth factor – PDGF (Chapter 18)
2. Colony stimulating factors – CSF (Chapter 16)
3. Nerve growth factors – NGF (Chapter 134)
4. Neurotropins (Chapter 134)
5. Erythropoietin (Chapter 10)
6. Thrombopoietin (Chapter 18)
7. Insulin-like growth factors – IGF (Chapter 66)
8. Epidermal growth factor – present in keratinocytes and fibroblasts. It inhibits growth of hair follicles and cancer cells
9. Basic fibroblast growth factor – present in blood vessels. It is concerned with the formation of new blood vessels
10. Myostatin – present in skeletal muscle fibers. It controls skeletal muscle growth
11. Transforming growth factors (TGF) – present in transforming cells (cells undergoing differentiation) and in large quantities in tumors and cancerous tissue. TGF is of two types:
    i. TGF-α secreted in brain, keratinocytes and macrophages. It is concerned with growth of epithelial cells and wound healing
    ii. TGF-β secreted by hepatic cells, T lymphocytes, B lymphocytes, macrophages and mast cells. When the liver attains the maximum size in adults, it controls liver growth by inhibiting pro-liferation of hepatic cells. TGF-β also causes immunosuppression.

■ CELL DEATH

Cell death occurs by two distinct processes:
1. Apoptosis
2. Necrosis.

■ APOPTOSIS

Apoptosis is defined as the natural or **programed death** of the cell under genetic control. Originally, apoptosis refers to the process by which the leaves fall from trees in autumn (In Greek, apoptosis means 'falling leaves'). It is also called **'cell suicide'** since the genes of the cell play a major role in the death.

This type of programmed cell death is a normal phenomenon and it is essential for normal development of the body. In contrast to necrosis, apoptosis usually does not produce inflammatory reactions in the neighboring tissues.

Functional Significance of Apoptosis

The purpose of apoptosis is to remove unwanted cells without causing any stress or damage to the neighboring cells. The functional significance of apoptosis:

1. Plays a vital role in cellular homeostasis. About 10 million cells are produced everyday in human body by mitosis. An equal number of cells die by apoptosis. This helps in cellular homeostasis.
2. Useful for removal of a cell that is damaged beyond repair by a virus or a toxin
3. An essential event during the development and in adult stage.

Examples:

i. A large number of neurons are produced during the development of central nervous system. But up to 50% of the neurons are removed by apoptosis during the formation of synapses between neurons
ii. Apoptosis is responsible for the removal of tissues of webs between fingers and toes during developmental stage in fetus
iii. It is necessary for regression and disappearance of duct systems during sex differentiation in fetus (Chapter 74)
iv. The cell that looses the contact with neighboring cells or basal lamina in the epithelial tissue dies by apoptosis. This is essential for the death of old enterocytes that shed into the lumen of intestinal glands (Chapter 41)
v. It plays an important role in the cyclic sloughing of the inner layer of endometrium, resulting in menstruation (Chapter 80)
vi. Apoptosis removes the autoaggressive T cells and prevents autoimmune diseases.

Activation of Apoptosis

Apoptosis is activated by either withdrawal of positive signals (survival factors) or arrival of negative signals.

Withdrawal of positive signals

Positive signals are the signals which are necessary for the long-time survival of most of the cells. The positive signals are continuously produced by other cells or some chemical stimulants. Best examples of chemical stimulants are:

i. Nerve growth factors (for neurons)
ii. Interleukin-2 (for cells like lymphocytes).

The absence or withdrawal of the positive signals activates apoptosis.

Arrival of negative signals

Negative signals are the external or internal stimuli which initiate apoptosis. The negative signals are produced during various events like:
1. Normal developmental procedures
2. Cellular stress
3. Increase in the concentration of intracellular oxidants
4. Viral infection
5. Damage of DNA
6. Exposure to agents like chemotherapeutic drugs, X-rays, ultraviolet rays and the death-receptor ligands.

Death-receptor ligands and death receptors

Death-receptor ligands are the substances which bind with specific cell membrane receptors and initiate the process of apoptosis. The common death-receptor ligands are tumor necrosis factors (TNF- α, TNF- β) and Fas ligand (which binds to the receptor called Fas).

Death-receptors are the cell membrane receptors which receive the death-receptor ligands. Well-charact-erized death receptors are TNF receptor-1 (TNFR1) and TNF-related apoptosis inducing ligand (TRAIL) receptors called DR4 and DR5.

Role of mitochondria in apoptosis

External or internal stimuli initiate apoptosis by activating the proteases called **caspases** (cysteinyl-dependent aspartate-specific proteases). Normally, caspases are suppressed by the inhibitor protein called **apoptosis inhibiting factor (AIF).**

When the cells receive the apoptotic stimulus, mitochondria releases two protein materials. First one is **Cytochrome C** and the second protein is called second mitochondria-derived activator of caspases (SMAC) or its homologudiablo.

SMAC/diablo inactivates AIF so that the inhibitor is inhibited. During this process, SMAC/diablo and AIF aggregate to form **apoptosome** which activates caspases. Cytochrome C also facilitates caspase activation.

Apoptotic Process

Cell shows sequence of characteristic morphological changes during apoptosis, viz.:
1. Activated caspases digest the proteins of cyto-skeleton and the cell shrinks and becomes round
2. Because of shrinkage, the cell losses the contact with neighboring cells or surrounding matrix
3. Chromatin in the nucleus undergoes degradation and condensation

4. Nuclear membrane becomes discontinuous and the DNA inside nucleus is cleaved into small fragments
5. Following the degradation of DNA, the nucleus breaks into many discrete nucleosomal units, which are also called chromatin bodies
6. Cell membrane breaks and shows bubbled appearance
7. Finally, the cell breaks into several fragments containing intracellular materials including chromatin bodies and organelles of the cell. Such cellular fragments are called vesicles or apoptotic bodies
8. Apoptotic bodies are engulfed by phagocytes and dendritic cells.

Abnormal Apoptosis

Apoptosis within normal limits is beneficial for the body. However, too much or too little apoptosis leads to abnormal conditions.

Common abnormalities due to too much apoptosis:

1. Ischemic-related injuries
2. Autoimmune diseases like:
   i. Hemolytic anemia
   ii. Thrombocytopenia
   iii. Acquired immunodeficiency syndrome (AIDS)
3. Neurodegenerative diseases like Alzheimer's disease.

Common abnormalities due to too little apoptosis:

1. Cancer
2. Autoimmune lymphoproliferative syndrome (ALPS).

■ NECROSIS

Necrosis (means 'dead' in Greek) is the uncontrolled and **unprogramed death** of cells due to unexpected and accidental damage. It is also called **'cell murder'** because the cell is killed by extracellular or external events. After necrosis, the harmful chemical substances released from the dead cells cause damage and inflammation of neighboring tissues.

Causes for Necrosis

Common causes of necrosis are injury, infection, inflammation, infarction and cancer. Necrosis is induced by both physical and chemical events such as heat, radiation, trauma, hypoxia due to lack of blood flow and exposure to toxins.

Necrotic Process

Necrosis results in lethal disruption of cell structure and activity. The cell undergoes a series of characteristic changes during necrotic process, viz.

1. Cell swells causing damage of the cell membrane and appearance of many holes in the membrane
2. Intracellular contents leak out into the surrounding environment
3. Intracellular environment is altered
4. Simultaneously, large amount of calcium ions are released by the damaged mitochondria and other organelles
5. Presence of calcium ions drastically affects the organization and activities of proteins in the intracellular components
6. Calcium ions also induce release of toxic materials that activate the lysosomal enzymes
7. Lysosomal enzymes cause degradation of cellular components and the cell is totally disassembled resulting in death
8. Products broken down from the disassembled cell are ingested by neighboring cells.

Reaction of Neighboring Tissues after Necrosis

Tissues surrounding the necrotic cells react to the breakdown products of the dead cells, particularly the derivatives of membrane phospholipids like the arachidonic acid. Along with other materials, arachidonic acid causes the following inflammatory reactions in the surrounding tissues:

1. Dilatation of capillaries in the region and thereby increasing local blood flow
2. Increase in the temperature leading to reddening of the tissues
3. Release of histamine from these tissues which induces pain in the affected area
4. Migration of leukocytes and macrophages from blood to the affected area because of increased capillary permeability
5. Movement of water from blood into the tissues causing local edema
6. Engulfing and digestion of cellular debris and foreign materials like bacteria by the leukocytes and macrophages
7. Activation of immune system resulting in the removal of foreign materials
8. Formation of pus by the dead leukocytes during this process
9. Finally, tissue growth in the area and wound healing.

■ CELL ADAPTATION

Cell adaptation refers to the changes taking place in a cell in response to environmental changes.

Normal functioning of the cell is always threatened by various factors such as stress, chemical agents, diseases and environmental hazards. Yet, the cell survives and continues the function by means of adaptation. Only during extreme conditions, the cell fails to withstand the hazardous factors which results in destruction and death of the cell.

Cellular adaptation occurs by any of the following mechanisms.

1. Atrophy
2. Hypertrophy
3. Hyperplasia
4. Dysplasia
5. Metaplasia.

■ ATROPHY

Atrophy means decrease in size of a cell. Atrophy of more number of cells results in decreased size or wasting of the concerned tissue, organ or part of the body.

Causes of Atrophy

Atrophy is due to one or more number of causes such as:

  i. Poor nourishment
 ii. Decreased blood supply
iii. Lack of workload or exercise
 iv. Loss of control by nerves or hormones
  v. Intrinsic disease of the tissue or organ.

Types of Atrophy

Atrophy is of two types, physiological atrophy and pathological atrophy. Examples of physiological atrophy are the atrophy of thymus in childhood and tonsils in adolescence. The pathological atrophy is common in skeletal muscle, cardiac muscle, sex organs and brain.

■ HYPERTROPHY

Hypertrophy is the increase in the size of a cell. Hypertrophy of many cells results in enlargement or overgrowth of an organ or a part of the body. Hypertrophy is of three types.

1. Physiological Hypertrophy

Physiological hypertrophy is the increase in size due to increased workload or exercise. The common physiological hypertrophy includes:

i. *Muscular hypertrophy:* Increase in bulk of skeletal muscles that occurs in response to strength training exercise

ii. *Ventricular hypertrophy:* Increase in size of ventricular muscles of the heart which is advantageous only if it occurs in response to exercise.

2. Pathological Hypertrophy

Increase in cell size in response to pathological changes is called pathological hypertrophy. Example is the ventricular hypertrophy that occurs due to pathological conditions such as high blood pressure, where the workload of ventricles increases.

3. Compensatory Hypertrophy

Compensatory hypertrophy is the increase in size of the cells of an organ that occurs in order to compensate the loss or dysfunction of another organ of same type. Examples are the hypertrophy of one kidney when the other kidney stops functioning; and the increase in muscular strength of an arm when the other arm is dysfunctional or lost.

■ HYPERPLASIA

Hyperplasia is the increase in number of cells due to increased cell division (mitosis). It is also defined as abnormal or unusual proliferation (multiplication) of cells due to constant cell division. Hyperplasia results in gross enlargement of the organ. Hyperplasia involves constant cell division of the normal cells only. Hyperplasia is of three types.

1. Physiological Hyperplasia

Physiological hyperplasia is the momentary adaptive response to routine physiological changes in the body. For example, during the proliferative phase of each menstrual cycle, the endometrial cells in uterus increase in number.

2. Compensatory Hyperplasia

Compensatory hyperplasia is the increase in number of cells in order to replace the damaged cells of an organ or the cells removed from the organ.

Compensatory hyperplasia helps the tissues and organs in regeneration. It is common in liver. After the surgical removal of the damaged part of liver, there is increase in the number of liver cells resulting in regeneration. Compensatory hyperplasia is also common in epithelial cells of intestine and epidermis.

3. Pathological Hyperplasia

Pathological hyperplasia is the increase in number of cells due to abnormal increase in hormone secretion. It is also called hormonal hyperplasia. For example, in gigantism, hypersecretion of growth hormone induces hyperplasia that results in overgrowth of the body.

■ DYSPLASIA

Dysplasia is the condition characterized by the abnormal change in size, shape and organization of the cell. Dysplasia is not considered as true adaptation and it is suggested as related to hyperplasia. It is common in epithelial cells of cervix and respiratory tract.

■ METAPLASIA

Metaplasia is the condition that involves replacement of one type of cell with another type of cell. It is of two types.

1. Physiological Metaplasia

Replacement of cells in normal conditions is called physiological metaplasia. Examples are transformation of cartilage into bone and transformation of monocytes into macrophages.

2. Pathological Metaplasia

Pathological metaplasia is the irreversible replacement of cells due to constant exposure to harmful stimuli. For example, chronic smoking results in transformation of normal mucus secreting ciliated columnar epithelial cells into non-ciliated squamous epithelial cells, which are incapable of secreting mucus. These transformed cells may become cancerous cells if the stimulus (smoking) is prolonged.

■ CELL DEGENERATION

Cell degeneration is a process characterized by damage of the cells at cytoplasmic level, without affecting the nucleus. Degeneration may result in functional impairment or deterioration of a tissue or an organ. It is common in metabolically active organ like liver, heart and kidney. Degenerative changes are reversible in most of the cells.

Causes for Cell Degeneration

Common causes for cell degeneration:
1. Atrophy, hypertrophy, hyperplasia and/or dysplasia of cell

2. Fluid accumulation in the cell
3. Fat infiltration into the cell
4. Calcification of cellular organelles.

■ CELL AGING

Cell aging is the gradual structural and functional changes in the cells that occur over the passage of time. It is now suggested that cell aging is due to damage of cellular substances like DNA, RNA, proteins and lipids, etc. when the cell becomes old. When more cellular substances are damaged, the cellular function decreases. This causes deterioration of tissues, organs or parts of the body. Finally, the health of the body starts declining and this leads to death. So, the cell aging determines the health and life span of the body.

■ STEM CELLS

Stem cells are the primary cells capable of reforming themselves through mitotic division and differentiating into specialized cells. These cells serve as repair system of the body and are present in all multicellular organisms.

■ TYPES OF STEM CELLS

Stem cells are of two types:
1. Embryonic stem cells derived from embryo
2. Adult stem cells derived from adults.

1. Embryonic Stem Cells

Embryonic stem cells are derived from the inner cell mass of a blastocyst which is an early stage of embryo. It takes about 4 to 5 days after fertilization to reach the blastocyst stage and it has about 30 to 50 cells. Embryonic stem cells have two important qualities:
   i. Self-renewal capacity
   ii. Pluripotent nature, i.e. these cells are capable of differentiating into all types of cells in ectodermal, endodermal and mesodermal layers.

Because of these two qualities, the embryonic stem cells can be used therapeutically for regeneration or replacement of diseased or destroyed tissues. In fact, embryonic pluripotent stem cells are now cultured and lot of research is going on to explore the possibility of using these cells in curing the disorders like diabetes mellitus by cell replacement technique. But, ethical issues arise because the embryo has to be destroyed to collect the stem cells.

Stem cells from umbilical cord blood

Stem cells in umbilical cord blood are collected from the placenta or umbilical cord. Use of these stem cells for research and therapeutic purposes does not create any ethical issue because it does not endanger the life of the fetus or newborn. Because of vitality and easy availability, the umbilical cord blood stem cells are becoming a potent resource for transplant therapies. Nowadays, these stem cells are used to treat about 70 diseases and are used in many transplants worldwide.

2. Adult Stem Cells

Embryonic stem cells do not disappear after birth. But remain in the body as adult stem cells and play a role in repair of damaged tissues. However, their number becomes less. Adult stem cells are the undifferentiated multipotent progenitor cells found in growing children and adults. These are also known as **somatic stem cells** and are found everywhere in the body. These cells are capable of dividing and reforming the dying cells and regenerating the damaged tissues. So, these stem cells can also be used for research and therapeutic purposes.

Adult stem cells are collected from bone marrow. Two types of stem cells are present in bone marrow:
   i. **Hemopoietic stem cells,** which give rise to blood cells (Chapter 10)
   ii. **Bone marrow stromal cells,** which can differentiate into cardiac and skeletal muscle cells.

■ ADVANTAGES OF STEM CELLS

Adult stem cells from bone marrow are used in bone marrow transplant to treat leukemia and other blood disorders since 30 years. Recently, it is known that these stem cells can develop into nerve cells, liver cells, skeletal muscle cells and cardiac muscle cells.

Recent discoveries also reveal that the stem cells are present in several tissues which include blood, blood vessels, skeletal muscle, liver, skin and brain. It is also found that these cells are capable of differentiating into multiple cell types. So, the cell-based therapy using stem cells may be possible to treat many diseases such as heart diseases, diabetes, Parkinson's disease, Alzheimer's disease, spinal cord injury, stroke and rheumatoid arthritis.

Cell Junctions

■ DEFINITION AND CLASSIFICATION

Cell junction is the connection between the neighboring cells or the contact between the cell and extracellular matrix. It is also called **membrane junction.**

Cell junctions are classified into three types:
1. Occluding junctions
2. Communicating junctions
3. Anchoring junctions.

■ OCCLUDING JUNCTIONS

Cell junctions which prevent intercellular exchange of substances are called occluding junctions, i.e. these junctions prevent the movement of ions and molecules from one cell to another cell. Tight junctions belong to this category.

■ TIGHT JUNCTION

Tight junction is the intercellular occluding junction that prevents the passage of large molecules. It is also called **zonula occludens.** It is the region where the cell membranes of the adjacent cells fuse together firmly. This type of junction is present in the **apical margins** of epithelial and endothelial cells in intestinal mucosa, wall of renal tubule, capillary wall and choroid plexus.

Structure of Tight Junction

Tight junction is made up of a **ridge** which has two halves. One half of the ridge is from one cell and another half is from the other cell. Both halves of the ridge fuse with each other very tightly and occupy the space between the two cells (Fig. 2.1). Each half of the ridge consists of **tight junction strands.**

Proteins of tight junction

Proteins involved in the formation of tight junctions are classified into two types:
1. Tight junction **membrane proteins** or integral membrane proteins, such as occludin, claudin and **junctional adhesion molecules (JAMs)**

2. **Scaffold** (framework or platform) proteins or peripheral membrane proteins or cytoplasmic **plaque proteins** such as cingulin, symplekin and ZO-1, 2, 3.

Tight junction membrane protein molecules are anchored in the strands of the ridge and attach with their counterparts of neighboring cell, so that both the cells are held together. The scaffold (platform) proteins are attached with the tight junction membrane proteins and strengthen the anchoring in the ridges.

Functions of Tight Junction

1. *Strength and stability:* The tight junction holds the neighboring cells of the tissues firmly and thus provides strength and stability to the tissues.
2. *Selective permeability* **(gate function):** The tight junction forms a selective barrier for small molecules and a total barrier for large molecules.

   In the epithelial and endothelial cells, tight junction is the most apical intercellular junction, which functions as selective (semipermeable) diffusion barriers between the neighboring cells. This function is called barrier or gate function. **Barrier function** of tight junction regulates the interchange of ions, water and varieties of macromolecules between the cells. The magnitude of this function varies in different tissues. In some epithelial cells, few substances pass through the tight junction (by diffusion or active transport). In other cells, no substance passes through the tight junction.
3. *Fencing function:* Tight junction prevents the lateral movement of proteins (integral membrane proteins) and lipids in cell membrane and thus acts as a fence. The fencing function maintains the different composition of proteins and lipids between the apical and basolateral plasma membrane domains. Because of this function, the tight junction is sometimes referred as impermeable junction.
4. *Maintenance of cell polarity:* Fencing function of the tight junction maintains the cell polarity by keeping the proteins in the apical region of the cell membrane.
5. *Blood-brain barrier:* Tight junction in the brain capillaries forms the blood-brain barrier, which prevents the entrance of many substances from capillary blood into brain tissues. Only lipid-soluble substances like drugs and steroid hormones can pass through the blood-brain barrier.

■ APPLIED PHYSIOLOGY

Diseases caused by mutation of genes encoding proteins of tight junction:

1. Hereditary deafness
2. Ichthyosis (scaly skin)
3. Sclerosing cholangitis (inflammation of bile duct causing obstruction)
4. Hereditary hypomagnesemia (low level of magnesium in the blood)
5. Synovial sarcoma (soft tissue cancer)

Functions of tight junction are affected by some bacteria and viruses also.

■ COMMUNICATING JUNCTIONS

Cell junctions which permit the intercellular exchange of substances are called communicating junctions, i.e. these junctions permit the movement of ions and molecules from one cell to another cell. Gap junction and chemical synapse are the communicating junctions.

■ GAP JUNCTION

Gap junction is the intercellular junction that allows passage of ions and smaller molecules between the cells. It is also called **nexus**. It is present in heart, basal part of epithelial cells of intestinal mucosa, etc.

Structure of Gap Junction

Membranes of the two adjacent cells lie very close to each other and the intercellular space is reduced from the usual size of 2.5 to 3 nm. Cytoplasm of the two cells is connected by the channels formed by the membranes of both cells. So, the molecules move from one cell to another cell directly through these channels, without having contact with extracellular fluid (ECF).

Each channel consists of two halves. Each half belongs to one of the two adjacent cells. Each half of the

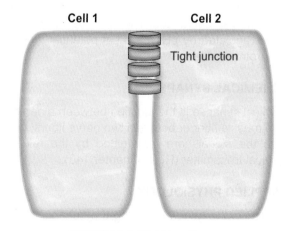

FIGURE 2.1: Tight junction

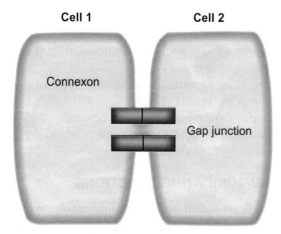

FIGURE 2.2: Gap junction

channel is surrounded by 6 subunits of proteins which are called **connexins** or **connexons** (Fig. 2.2).

Functions of Gap Junction

1. Diameter of the channel in the gap junction is about 1.5 to 3 nm. So, the channel permits the passage of glucose, amino acids, ions and other substances, which have a molecular weight less than 1,000
2. It helps in the exchange of chemical messengers between the cells
3. It helps in rapid propagation of action potential from one cell to another cell.

Regulation of the Diameter of Channels in Gap Junction

In the gap junctions, the diameter of each channel is regulated by the intracellular calcium ions. When the concentration of intracellular calcium ion increases, the protein subunits of connexin surrounding the channel come close to each other by sliding. Thus, the diameter of the channel decreases. The diameter of the channel is also regulated by pH, electrical potential, hormones or neurotransmitter.

■ CHEMICAL SYNAPSE

Chemical synapse is the junction between a nerve fiber and a muscle fiber or between two nerve fibers, through which the signals are transmitted by the release of chemical transmitter (Refer Chapter 140).

■ APPLIED PHYSIOLOGY

Mutation in the genes encoding the connexins causes diseases such as:

1. Deafness
2. Keratoderma (thickening of skin on palms and soles)
3. Cataract (opacity of lens in eye)
4. Peripheral neuropathy (damage to the nerves of peripheral nervous system)
5. Charcot-Marie-Tooth disease (a form of neuropathy)
6. Heterotaxia (abnormal arrangement of organs or parts of the body in relation to left-right symmetry).

■ ANCHORING JUNCTIONS

Anchoring junctions are the junctions, which provide strength to the cells by acting like mechanical attachments, i.e. these junctions provide firm structural attachment between two cells or between a cell and the extracellular matrix (Fig. 2.3). Anchoring junctions are responsible for the **structural integrity** of the tissues and are present in the tissues like heart muscle and epidermis of skin, which are subjected to severe mechanical stress.

The firm attachment between two cells or between a cell and the **extracellular matrix** is provided by either actin filaments or the intermediate filaments. Depending upon this, anchoring junctions are classified into four types:

1. Actin filament attachment
   i. Adherens junction (cell to cell)
   ii. Focal adhesion (cell to matrix)
2. Intermediate filament attachment
   i. Desmosome (cell to cell)
   ii. Hemidesmosome (cell to matrix)

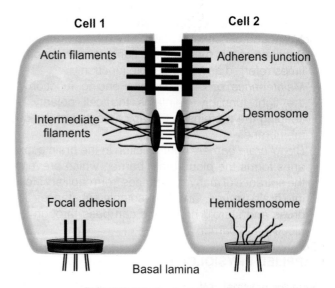

FIGURE 2.3: Anchoring junctions

■ ADHERENS JUNCTION

Adherens junction is the cell to cell junction, which connects the actin filaments of one cell to those of another cell. In some places like epithelial linings, this junction forms a continuous adhesion **(zonula adherens)** just below the tight junctions. In adherens junction, the membranes of the adjacent cells are held together by some transmembrane proteins called cadherins.

Adherens junction provides strong mechanical attachments of the adjacent cells. Adherens junction is present in the **intercalated disks** between the branches of cardiac muscles (Chapter 89). During the contractions and relaxation of heart, the cardiac muscle fibers are held together tightly by means of this junction. The adherens junction present in epidermis helps the skin to withstand the mechanical stress.

■ FOCAL ADHESION

Focal adhesion is the cell to matrix junctions, which connects the actin filaments of the cell to the extracellular matrix. In epithelia of various organs, this junction connects the cells with their basal lamina. The transmembrane proteins, which hold the cell membrane and the matrix are called **integrins.**

■ DESMOSOME

Desmosome is a cell to cell junction, where the intermediate filaments connect two adjacent cells. Desmosome is also called **macula adherens.** The membranes of two adjacent cells, which oppose each other, are thickened and become spot-like patches. Intermediate filaments are attached with the thickened patches. Some of these filaments are parallel to the membrane and others are arranged in radiating fashion. Desmosomes function like tight junctions. The transmembrane proteins involved in desmosome are mainly cadherins.

■ HEMIDESMOSOME

Hemidesmosome is a cell to matrix junction, which connects the intermediate filaments of the cell to the extracellular matrix. This type of cell junction is like half desmosome and the thickening of membrane of only one cell occurs. So, this is known as hemidesmosome or half desmosome. Mostly, the hemidesmosome connects the cells with their **basal lamina.** The proteins involved in this are integrins (Table 2.1).

■ APPLIED PHYSIOLOGY

1. Dysfunction of adherens junction and focal junction in colon due to mutation of proteins results in **colon cancer.** It also leads to **tumor metastasis** (spread of cancer cells from a primary tumor to other parts of the body)
2. Dysfunction of desmosome causes **bullous pemphigoid** (autoimmune disease with tense blistering

TABLE 2.1: Cell junctions

Junction type	Proteins involved	Function	Example
Tight junction	Occludin Claudin JAMs Cingulin Symplekin ZO-1, 2, 3	Strength and stability to tissues Selective permeability Fencing function Maintenance of cell polarity Formation of blood-brain barrier	Epithelial lining of intestinal mucosa and renal tubule Endothelium in capillary wall and choroid plexus
Gap junction	Connexins	Allows passage of small molecules, ions and chemical messengers Propagation of action potential	Epithelial lining Heart Intestine
Adherens junction	Cadherins	Cell to cell attachment	Epithelial lining Heart Epidermis
Focal adhesions	Integrins	Cell attachment to Basal lamina Extracellular matrix	Epithelial lining
Desmosome	Cadherins	Cell to cell attachment	Epithelial lining Skin
Hemidesmosome	Integrins	Cell attachment to Basal lamina Extracellular matrix	Epithelial lining

eruptions of the skin). The patients with this disease develop antibodies against cadherins
3. Dysfunction of hemidesmosome also causes bullous pemphigoid. The patients develop antibodies against integrins.

■ CELL ADHESION MOLECULES

Cell adhesion molecules (CAMs) or cell adhesion proteins are the protein molecules, which are responsible for the attachment of cells to their neighbors or to basal lamina (or basal membrane). CAMs form the important structures of intercellular connections and are responsible for structural organization of tissues.

■ TYPES OF CELL ADHESION MOLECULES

Cell adhesion molecules are classified into four types:
1. **Cadherins,** which form the molecular limbs between neighboring cells. These CAMs form adherens junction and desomosome
2. **Integrins,** which form the focal adhesion and hemidesmosome
3. **IgG super family,** which form the cell adhesion molecules in nervous system
4. **Selectins,** which act as receptors for carbohydrates (ligand or mucin) and are found in platelets and endothelial cells.

Transport through Cell Membrane

- ■ INTRODUCTION
- ■ BASIC MECHANISM OF TRANSPORT
- ■ PASSIVE TRANSPORT
- ■ SPECIAL TYPES OF PASSIVE TRANSPORT
- ■ ACTIVE TRANSPORT
- ■ SPECIAL TYPES OF ACTIVE TRANSPORT
- ■ MOLECULAR MOTORS
- ■ APPLIED PHYSIOLOGY

■ INTRODUCTION

All the cells in the body must be supplied with essential substances like nutrients, water, electrolytes, etc. Cells also must get rid of many unwanted substances like waste materials, carbon dioxide, etc. The cells achieve these by means of transport mechanisms across the cell membrane.

Structure of the cell membrane is well suited for the transport of substances in and out of the cell. Lipids and proteins of cell membrane play an important role in the transport of various substances between extracellular fluid (ECF) and intracellular fluid (ICF). Refer Chapter 1 for details of lipids and proteins of the cell membrane.

■ BASIC MECHANISM OF TRANSPORT

Two types of basic mechanisms are involved in the transport of substances across the cell membrane:
1. Passive transport mechanism
2. Active transport mechanism.

■ PASSIVE TRANSPORT

Passive transport is the transport of substances along the **concentration gradient** or **electrical gradient** or both **(electrochemical gradient)**. It is also known as **diffusion** or **downhill movement.** It does not need energy. Passive transport is like swimming in the direction of water flow in a river. Here, the substances

move from region of higher concentration to the region of lower concentration. Diffusion is of two types, namely simple diffusion and facilitated diffusion.

Simple diffusion of substances occurs either through lipid layer or protein layer of the cell membrane. Facilitated diffusion occurs with the help of the carrier proteins of the cell membrane. Thus, the diffusion can be discussed under three headings:
1. Simple diffusion through lipid layer
2. Simple diffusion through protein layer
3. Facilitated or carrier-mediated diffusion.

■ SIMPLE DIFFUSION THROUGH LIPID LAYER

Lipid layer of the cell membrane is permeable only to lipid-soluble substances like oxygen, carbon dioxide and alcohol. The diffusion through the lipid layer is directly proportional to the solubility of the substances in lipids (Fig. 3.1A).

■ SIMPLE DIFFUSION THROUGH PROTEIN LAYER

Protein layer of the cell membrane is permeable to water-soluble substances. Mainly, electrolytes diffuse through the protein layer.

Protein Channels or Ion Channels

Throughout the central lipid layer of the cell membrane, there are some **pores.** Integral protein molecules of protein layer invaginate into these pores from either surface of the cell membrane. Thus, the pores present in the central lipid layer are entirely lined up by the integral protein molecules. These pores are the hypothetical pores and form the channels for the diffusion of water, electrolytes and other substances, which cannot pass through the lipid layer. As the channels are lined by protein molecules, these are called **protein channels** for water-soluble substances.

Types of Protein Channels or Ion Channels

Characteristic feature of the protein channels is the selective permeability. That is, each channel can permit only one type of ion to pass through it. Accordingly, the channels are named after the ions which diffuse through these channels such as sodium channels, potassium channels, etc.

Regulation of the Channels

Some of the protein channels are continuously opened and most of the channels are always closed. Continuously opened channels are called **ungated channels** (Fig. 3.1B). Closed channels are called **gated channels.** These channels are opened only when required (Fig. 3.1C).

Gated Channels

Gated channels are divided into three categories:
  i. Voltage-gated channels
  ii. Ligand-gated channels
  iii. Mechanically gated channels.

i. Voltage-gated channels

Voltage-gated channels are the channels which open whenever there is a change in the electrical potential. For example, in the neuromuscular junction, when action potential reaches axon terminal, the calcium channels are opened and calcium ions diffuse into the interior of the axon terminal from ECF (Chapter 32).

Similarly, in the muscle during the **excitation-contraction coupling,** the action potential spreads through the transverse tubules of the sarcotubular system. When the action potential reaches the cisternae, large number of calcium ions diffuse from cisternae into sarcoplasm.

ii. Ligand-gated channels

Ligand-gated channels are the type of channels which open in the presence of some hormonal substances. The hormonal substances are called ligands and the channels are called ligand-gated channels. During the transmission of impulse through the neuromuscular junction, acetylcholine is released from the vesicles. The acetylcholine moves through the presynaptic membrane (membrane of the axon terminal) and reaches the synaptic cleft. Then, the acetylcholine molecules cause opening of sodium channels in the postsynaptic membrane and sodium ions diffuse into the neuromuscular junction from ECF.

iii. Mechanically gated channels

Mechanically gated channels are the channels which are opened by some mechanical factors. Examples are, channels present in the pressure receptors (Pacinian corpuscles) and the receptor cells (hair cells) of organ

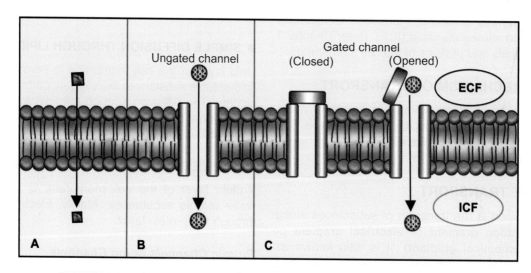

FIGURE 3.1: Hypothetical diagram of simple diffusion through the cell membrane.
A. Diffusion through lipid layer; **B.** Diffusion through ungated channel; **C.** Diffusion through gated channel.

of Corti and vestibular apparatus. When a Pacinian corpuscle is subjected to pressure, it is compressed resulting in deformation of its core fiber. This deformation causes opening of sodium channel and development of receptor potential (Chapter 139).

Sound waves cause the movement of cilia of hair cells in organ of Corti (cochlea), which is the receptor organ in the ear. Movements of the cilia cause opening of potassium channels leading to the development of receptor potential (Chapter 174). Similar mechanism prevails in hair cells of vestibular apparatus also (Chapter 158).

Ion Channel Diseases

Refer applied physiology of this chapter.

■ FACILITATED OR CARRIER-MEDIATED DIFFUSION

Facilitated or carrier-mediated diffusion is the type of diffusion by which the water-soluble substances having larger molecules are transported through the cell membrane with the help of a carrier protein. By this process, the substances are transported across the cell membrane faster than the transport by simple diffusion.

Glucose and amino acids are transported by facilitated diffusion. Glucose or amino acid molecules cannot diffuse through the channels because the diameter of these molecules is larger than the diameter of the channels. Molecule of these substances binds with carrier protein. Now, some conformational change occurs in the carrier protein. Due to this change, the molecule reaches the other side of the cell membrane (Fig. 3.2).

■ FACTORS AFFECTING RATE OF DIFFUSION

Rate of diffusion of substances through the cell membrane is affected by the following factors:

1. Permeability of the Cell Membrane

Rate of diffusion is directly proportional to the permeability of cell membrane. Since the cell membrane is selectively permeable, only limited number of substances can diffuse through the membrane.

2. Temperature

Rate of diffusion is directly proportional to the body temperature. Increase in temperature increases the rate of diffusion. This is because of the thermal motion of molecules during increased temperature.

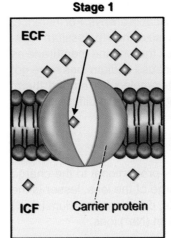
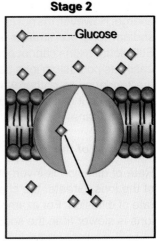

FIGURE 3.2: Hypothetical diagram of facilitated diffusion from higher concentration (ECF) to lower concentration (ICF). Stage 1. Glucose binds with carrier protein. Stage 2. Conformational change occurs in the carrier protein and glucose is released into ICF.

3. Concentration Gradient or Electrical Gradient of the Substance across the Cell Membrane

Rate of diffusion is directly proportional to the concentration gradient or electrical gradient of the diffusing substances across the cell membrane. However, facilitated diffusion has some limitation beyond certain level of concentration gradient.

4. Solubility of the Substance

Diffusion rate is directly proportional to the solubility of substances, particularly the lipid-soluble substances. Since oxygen is highly soluble in lipids, it diffuses very rapidly through the lipid layer.

5. Thickness of the Cell Membrane

Rate of diffusion is inversely proportional to the thickness of the cell membrane. If the cell membrane is thick, diffusion of the substances is very slow.

6. Size of the Molecules

Rate of diffusion is inversely proportional to the size of the molecules. Thus, the substances with smaller molecules diffuse rapidly than the substances with larger molecules.

7. Size of the Ions

Generally, rate of diffusion is inversely proportional to the size of the ions. Smaller ions can pass through the membrane more easily than larger ions with the same charge. However, it is not applicable always. For instance, sodium ions are smaller in size than potassium ions. Still, sodium ions cannot pass through the membrane as easily as potassium ions because sodium ions have got the tendency to gather water molecules around them. This makes it difficult for sodium ions to diffuse through the membrane.

8. Charge of the Ions

Rate of diffusion is inversely proportional to the charge of the ions. Greater the charge of the ions, lesser is the rate of diffusion. For example, diffusion of calcium (Ca^{++}) ions is slower than the sodium (Na^+) ions.

■ SPECIAL TYPES OF PASSIVE TRANSPORT

In addition to diffusion, there are some special types of passive transport, viz.
1. Bulk flow
2. Filtration
3. Osmosis.

■ BULK FLOW

Bulk flow is the diffusion of large quantity of substances from a region of high pressure to the region of low pressure. It is due to the pressure gradient of the substance across the cell membrane.

Best example for bulk flow is the exchange of gases across the respiratory membrane in lungs. Partial pressure of oxygen is greater in the alveolar air than in the alveolar capillary blood. So, oxygen moves from alveolar air into the blood through the respiratory membrane. Partial pressure of carbon dioxide is more in blood than in the alveoli. So, it moves from the blood into the alveoli through the respiratory membrane (Chapter 124).

■ FILTRATION

Movement of water and solutes from an area of high hydrostatic pressure to an area of low hydrostatic pressure is called filtration. Hydrostatic pressure is developed by the weight of the fluid. Filtration process is seen at arterial end of the capillaries, where movement of fluid occurs along with dissolved substances from blood into the interstitial fluid (Chapter 27). It also occurs in glomeruli of kidneys (Chapter 52).

■ OSMOSIS

Osmosis is the special type of diffusion. It is defined as the movement of water or any other solvent from an area of lower concentration to an area of higher concentration of a solute, through a semipermeable membrane (Fig. 3.3). The semipermeable membrane permits the passage of only water or other solvents but not the solutes.

Osmosis can occur whenever there is a difference in the solute concentration on either side of the membrane. Osmosis depends upon osmotic pressure.

Osmotic Pressure

Osmotic pressure is the pressure created by the solutes in a fluid. During osmosis, when water or any other solvent moves from the area of lower concentration to the area of higher concentration, the solutes in the area of higher concentration get dissolved in the solvent. This creates a pressure which is known as osmotic pressure. Normally, the osmotic pressure prevents further movement of water or other solvent during osmosis.

Reverse Osmotic Pressure

Reverse osmosis is a process in which water or other solvent flows in reverse direction (from the area of higher concentration to the area of lower concentration of the solute), if an external pressure is applied on the area of higher concentration.

Colloidal Osmotic Pressure and Oncotic Pressure

The osmotic pressure exerted by the colloidal substances in the body is called the colloidal osmotic pressure. And, the osmotic pressure exerted by the colloidal substances

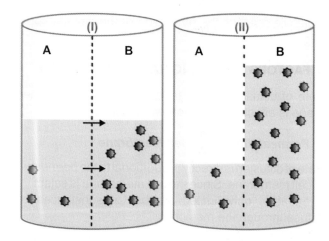

FIGURE 3.3: Osmosis. Red objects = solute, Yellow shade = water, Green dotted line = semipermeable membrane. In (I), concentration of solute is high in compartment B and low in compartment A. So, water moves from A to B through semipermeable membrane. In (II), entrance of water into B exerts osmotic pressure.

(proteins) of the plasma is known as oncotic pressure and it is about 25 mm Hg.

Types of Osmosis

Osmosis across the cell membrane is of two types:
1. Endosmosis: Movement of water into the cell
2. Exosmosis: Movement of water out of the cell.

■ ACTIVE TRANSPORT

Active transport is the movement of substances against the chemical or electrical or electrochemical gradient. It is like swimming against the water tide in a river. It is also called **uphill transport.** Active transport requires energy, which is obtained mainly by breakdown of high energy compounds like **adenosine triphosphate (ATP).**

Active Transport vs Facilitated Diffusion

Active transport mechanism is different from facilitated diffusion by two ways:
1. Carrier protein of active transport needs energy, whereas the carrier protein of facilitated diffusion does not need energy
2. In active transport, the substances are transported against the concentration or electrical or electrochemical gradient. In facilitated diffusion, the substances are transported along the concentration or electrical or electrochemical gradient.

■ CARRIER PROTEINS OF ACTIVE TRANSPORT

Carrier proteins involved in active transport are of two types:
1. Uniport
2. Symport or antiport.

1. Uniport

Carrier protein that carries only one substance in a single direction is called uniport. It is also known as **uniport pump.**

2. Symport or Antiport

Symport or antiport is the carrier protein that transports two substances at a time.

Carrier protein that transports two different substances in the same direction is called symport or **symport pump.** Carrier protein that transports two different substances in opposite directions is called antiport or **antiport pump.**

■ MECHANISM OF ACTIVE TRANSPORT

When a substance to be transported across the cell membrane comes near the cell, it combines with the carrier protein of the cell membrane and forms substance-protein complex. This complex moves towards the inner surface of the cell membrane. Now, the substance is released from the carrier proteins. The same carrier protein moves back to the outer surface of the cell membrane to transport another molecule of the substance.

■ SUBSTANCES TRANSPORTED BY ACTIVE TRANSPORT

Substances, which are transported actively, are in ionic form and non-ionic form. Substances in ionic form are sodium, potassium, calcium, hydrogen, chloride and iodide. Substances in non-ionic form are glucose, amino acids and urea.

■ TYPES OF ACTIVE TRANSPORT

Active transport is of two types:
1. Primary active transport
2. Secondary active transport.

■ PRIMARY ACTIVE TRANSPORT

Primary active transport is the type of transport mechanism in which the energy is liberated directly from the breakdown of ATP. By this method, the substances like sodium, potassium, calcium, hydrogen and chloride are transported across the cell membrane.

Primary Active Transport of Sodium and Potassium: Sodium-Potassium Pump

Sodium and potassium ions are transported across the cell membrane by means of a common carrier protein called sodium-potassium (Na^+-K^+) pump. It is also called **Na^+-K^+ ATPase pump** or **Na^+-K^+ ATPase.** This pump transports sodium from inside to outside the cell and potassium from outside to inside the cell. This pump is present in all the cells of the body.

Na^+-K^+ pump is responsible for the distribution of sodium and potassium ions across the cell membrane and the development of resting membrane potential.

Structure of Na^+-K^+ pump

Carrier protein that constitutes Na^+-K^+ pump is made up of two protein subunit molecules, an α-subunit with a molecular weight of 100,000 and a β-subunit with a molecular weight of 55,000. Transport of Na^+ and K^+

occurs only by α-subunit. The β-subunit is a glycoprotein the function of which is not clear.

α-subunit of the Na⁺-K⁺ pump has got six sites:

i. Three receptor sites for sodium ions on the inner (towards cytoplasm) surface of the protein molecule

ii. Two receptor sites for potassium ions on the outer (towards ECF) surface of the protein molecule

iii. One site for enzyme adenosine triphosphatase (ATPase), which is near the sites for sodium.

Mechanism of action of Na⁺-K⁺ pump

Three sodium ions from the cell get attached to the receptor sites of sodium ions on the inner surface of the carrier protein. Two potassium ions outside the cell bind to the receptor sites of potassium ions located on the outer surface of the carrier protein (Fig. 3.4, Stage 1).

Binding of sodium and potassium ions to carrier protein activates the enzyme ATPase. ATPase causes breakdown of ATP into adenosine diphosphate (ADP) with the release of one high energy phosphate. Now, the energy liberated causes some sort of conformational change in the molecule of the carrier protein. Because of this, the outer surface of the molecule (with potassium ions) now faces the inner side of the cell. And, the inner surface of the protein molecule (with sodium ions) faces the outer side of the cell (Fig. 3.4, Stage 2). Now, dissociation and release of the ions take place so that the sodium ions are released outside the cell (ECF) and the potassium ions are released inside the cell (ICF). Exact mechanisms involved in the dissociation and release of ions are not yet known.

Electrogenic activity of Na⁺-K⁺ pump

Na⁺-K⁺ pump moves three sodium ions outside the cell and two potassium ions inside cell. Thus, when the pump works once, there is a net loss of one positively charged ion from the cell. Continuous activity of the sodium-potassium pumps causes reduction in the number of positively charged ions inside the cell leading to increase in the negativity inside the cell. This is called the electrogenic activity of Na⁺-K⁺ pump.

Abnormalities of Na⁺-K⁺ Pump

Refer applied physiology of this Chapter.

Transport of Calcium Ions

Calcium is actively transported from inside to outside the cell by calcium pump. Calcium pump is operated by a separate carrier protein. Energy is obtained from ATP

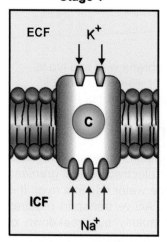
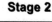
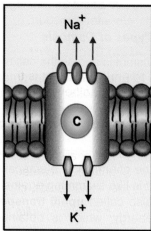

FIGURE 3.4: Hypothetical diagram of sodium-potassium pump. C = carrier protein. Stage 1: Three Na⁺ from ICF and two K⁺ from ECF bind with 'C'. Stage 2: Conformational change occurs in 'C' followed by release of Na⁺ into ECF and K⁺ into ICF

by the catalytic activity of ATPase. Calcium pumps are also present in some organelles of the cell such as sarcoplasmic reticulum in the muscle and the mitochondria of all the cells. These pumps move calcium into the organelles.

Transport of Hydrogen Ions

Hydrogen ion is actively transported across the cell membrane by the carrier protein called hydrogen pump. It also obtains energy from ATP by the activity of ATPase. The hydrogen pumps that are present in two important organs have some functional significance.

1. *Stomach:* Hydrogen pumps in parietal cells of the gastric glands are involved in the formation of hydrochloric acid (Chapter 38)

2. *Kidney:* Hydrogen pumps in epithelial cells of distal convoluted tubules and collecting ducts are involved in the secretion of hydrogen ions from blood into urine (Chapter 54).

■ SECONDARY ACTIVE TRANSPORT

Secondary active transport is the transport of a substance with sodium ion, by means of a common carrier protein. When sodium is transported by a carrier protein, another substance is also transported by the same protein simultaneously, either in the same direction (of sodium movement) or in the opposite direction. Thus, the transport of sodium is coupled with transport of another substance.

Secondary active transport is of two types:
1. Cotransport
2. Counter transport.

Sodium Cotransport

Sodium cotransport is the process in which, along with sodium, another substance is transported by a carrier protein called symport. Energy for movement of sodium is obtained by breakdown of ATP. And the energy released by the movement of sodium is utilized for movement of another substance.

Substances carried by sodium cotransport are glucose, amino acids, chloride, iodine, iron and urate.

Carrier protein for sodium cotransport

Carrier protein for the sodium cotransport has two receptor sites on the outer surface.

Among the two sites, one is for binding of sodium and another site is for binding of other substance.

Sodium cotransport of glucose

One sodium ion and one glucose molecule from the ECF bind with the respective receptor sites of carrier protein of the cell membrane. Now, the carrier protein is activated. It causes conformational changes in the carrier protein, so that sodium and glucose are released into the cell (Fig. 3.5).

Sodium cotransport of glucose occurs during absorption of glucose from the intestine and reabsorption of glucose from the renal tubule.

Sodium cotransport of amino acids

Carrier proteins for the transport of amino acids are different from the carrier proteins for the transport of glucose. For the transport of amino acids, there are five sets of carrier proteins in the cell membrane. Each one carries different amino acids depending upon the molecular weight of the amino acids.

Sodium cotransport of amino acids also occurs during the absorption of amino acids from the intestine and reabsorption from renal tubule.

Sodium Counter Transport

Sodium counter transport is the process by which the substances are transported across the cell membrane in exchange for sodium ions by carrier protein called antiport.

Various counter transport systems are:
   i. Sodium-calcium counter transport: In this, sodium and calcium ions move in opposite directions with the help of a carrier protein. This type of transport of sodium and calcium ions is present in all the cells

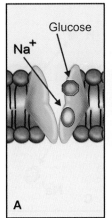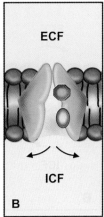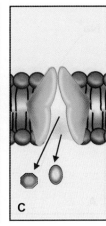

FIGURE 3.5: Sodium cotransport. **A.** Na⁺ and glucose from ECF bind with carrier protein; **B.** Conformational change occurs in the carrier protein; **C.** Na⁺ and glucose are released into ICF.

   ii. Sodium-hydrogen counter transport: In this system, the hydrogen ions are exchanged for sodium ions and this occurs in the renal tubular cells. The sodium ions move from tubular lumen into the tubular cells and the hydrogen ions move from tubular cell into the lumen (Figs 3.6 and 3.7)
   iii. Other counter transport systems: Other counter transport systems are sodium-magnesium counter transport, sodium-potassium counter transport, calcium-magnesium counter transport, calcium-potassium counter transport, chloride-bicarbonate counter transport and chloride-sulfate counter transport.

■ SPECIAL TYPES OF ACTIVE TRANSPORT

In addition to primary and secondary active transport systems, there are some special categories of active transport which are generally called the vesicular transport.

Special categories of active transport:
1. Endocytosis
2. Exocytosis
3. Transcytosis.

■ ENDOCYTOSIS

Endocytosis is defined as a transport mechanism by which the **macromolecules** enter the cell. Macromolecules (substances with larger molecules) cannot pass through the cell membrane either by active or by passive transport mechanism. Such substances are transported into the cell by endocytosis.

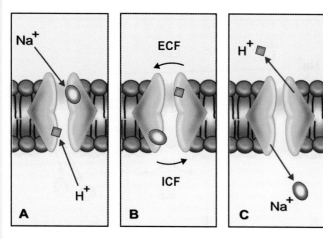

FIGURE 3.6: Sodium counter transport. **A.** Na⁺ from ECF and H⁺ from ICF bind with carrier protein; **B.** Conformational change occurs in the carrier protein; **C.** Na⁺ enters ICF and H⁺ enters ECF.

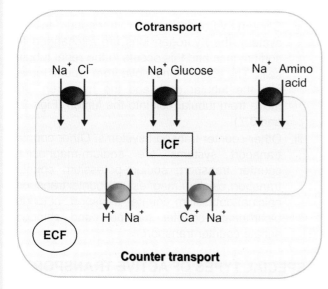

FIGURE 3.7: Sodium cotransport and counter transport by carrier proteins

Endocytosis is of three types:
1. Pinocytosis
2. Phagocytosis
3. Receptor-mediated endocytosis.

1. *Pinocytosis*

Pinocytosis is a process by which macromolecules like bacteria and antigens are taken into the cells. It is otherwise called the **cell drinking.**

Mechanism of pinocytosis

Pinocytosis involves following events:

   i. Macromolecules (in the form of droplets of fluid) bind to the outer surface of the cell membrane
   ii. Now, the cell membrane evaginates around the droplets
   iii. Droplets are engulfed by the membrane
   iv. Engulfed droplets are converted into vesicles and vacuoles, which are called endosomes (Fig. 3.8)
   v. Endosome travels into the interior of the cell
   vi. Primary lysosome in the cytoplasm fuses with endosome and forms secondary lysosome
   vii. Now, hydrolytic enzymes present in the secondary lysosome are activated resulting in digestion and degradation of the endosomal contents.

2. *Phagocytosis*

Phagocytosis is the process by which particles larger than the macromolecules are engulfed into the cells. It is also called **cell eating.** Larger bacteria, larger antigens and other larger foreign bodies are taken inside the cell by means of phagocytosis. Only few cells in the body like neutrophils, monocytes and the tissue macrophages show phagocytosis. Among these cells, the macrophages are the largest phagocytic cells.

Mechanism of phagocytosis

   i. When bacteria or foreign body enters the body, first the phagocytic cell sends cytoplasmic extension **(pseudopodium)** around bacteria or foreign body
   ii. Then, these particles are engulfed and are converted into endosome like vacuole. Vacuole is very large and it is usually called the phagosome
   iii. Phagosome travels into the interior of cell
   iv. Primary lysosome fuses with this phagosome and forms secondary lysosome
   v. Hydrolytic enzymes present in the secondary lysosome are activated resulting in digestion and degradation of the phagosomal contents (Fig. 3.9).

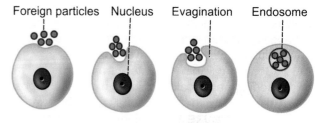

FIGURE 3.8: Process of pinocytosis

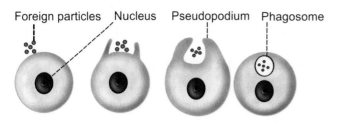

FIGURE 3.9: Process of phagocytosis

3. *Receptor-mediated Endocytosis*

Receptor-mediated endocytosis is the transport of macromolecules with the help of a receptor protein. Surface of cell membrane has some pits which contain a receptor protein called **clathrin.** Together with a receptor protein (clathrin), each pit is called **receptor-coated pit.** These receptor-coated pits are involved in the receptor-mediated endocytosis (Fig. 3.10).

Mechanism of receptor-mediated endocytosis

i. Receptor-mediated endocytosis is induced by substances like ligands (Fig. 3.10-i)

ii. Ligand molecules approach the cell and bind to receptors in the coated pits and form ligand-receptor complex (Fig. 3.10-ii)

iii. Ligand-receptor complex gets aggregated in the coated pits. Then, the pit is detached from cell membrane and becomes the coated vesicle. This coated vesicle forms the endosome (Fig. 3.10-iii)

iv. Endosome travels into the interior of the cell. Primary lysosome in the cytoplasm fuses with endosome and forms secondary lysosome (Fig. 3.10-iv)

v. Now, the hydrolytic enzymes present in secondary lysosome are activated resulting in release of ligands into the cytoplasm (Fig. 3.10-v)

vi. Receptor may move to a new pit of the cell membrane (Fig. 3.10-vi).

Receptor-mediated endocytosis play an important role in the transport of several types of macromolecules into the cells, viz.

i. Hormones: Growth hormone, thyroid stimulating hormone, luteinizing hormone, prolactin, insulin, glucagon, calcitonin and catecholamines

ii. Lipids: Cholesterol and low-density lipoproteins (LDL)

iii. Growth factors (GF): Nerve GF, epidermal GF, platelet-derived GF, interferon

iv. Toxins and bacteria: Cholera toxin, diphtheria toxin, pseudomonas toxin, recin and concanavalin A

v. Viruses: Rous sarcoma virus, semliki forest virus, vesicular stomatitis virus and adenovirus

vi. Transport proteins: Transferrin and transcobalamine

vii. Antibodies: IgE, polymeric IgG and maternal IgG.

Some of the receptor-coated pits in cell membrane are coated with another protein called **caveolin** instead of clathrin. Caveolin-coated pits are concerned with the transport of vitamins into the cell.

■ EXOCYTOSIS

Exocytosis is the process by which the substances are expelled from the cell. In this process, the substances are extruded from cell without passing through the cell membrane. This is the reverse of endocytosis.

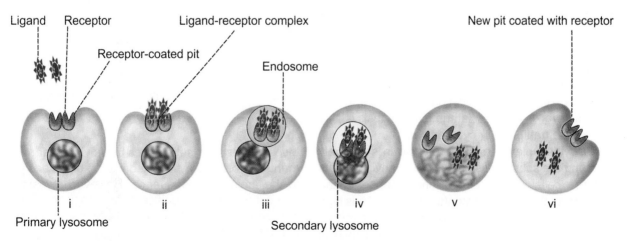

FIGURE 3.10: Mechanism of receptor-mediated endocytosis. The numbering of each figure corresponds with the numbers used in the text.

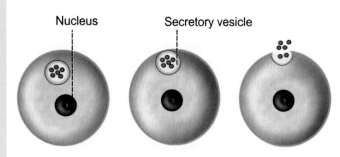

FIGURE 3.11: Process of exocytosis

Mechanism of Exocytosis

Exocytosis is involved in the release of secretory substances from cells. Secretory substances of the cell are stored in the form of secretory vesicles in the cytoplasm. When required, the vesicles approach the cell membrane and get fused with the cell membrane. Later, the contents of the vesicles are released out of the cell (Fig. 3.11).

Role of Calcium in Exocytosis

Calcium ions play an important role during the release of some secretory substances such as neurotransmitters. The calcium ions enter the cell and cause exocytosis. However, the exact mechanism of exocytosis is not clear.

■ TRANSCYTOSIS

Transcytosis is a transport mechanism in which an extracellular macromolecule enters through one side of a cell, migrates across cytoplasm of the cell and exits through the other side.

Mechanism of Transcytosis

Cell encloses the extracellular substance by invagination of the cell membrane to form a vesicle. Vesicle then moves across the cell and thrown out through opposite cell membrane by means of exocytosis. Transcytosis involves the receptor-coated pits as in receptor-mediated endocytosis. Receptor protein coating the pits in this process is caveolin and not clathrin. Transcytosis is also called, vesicle trafficking or cytopempsis.

Transcytosis plays an important role in selectively transporting the substances between two environments across the cells without any distinct change in the composition of these environments. Example of this type of transport is the movement of proteins from capillary blood into interstitial fluid across the endothelial cells of the capillary. Many pathogens like human immunodeficiency virus (HIV) are also transported by this mechanism.

■ MOLECULAR MOTORS

Molecular motors are the protein-based molecular machines that perform intracellular movements in response to specific stimuli.

■ FUNCTIONS OF MOLECULAR MOTORS

1. Transport of synaptic vesicles containing neurotransmitters from the nerve cell body to synaptic terminal
2. Role in cell division (mitosis and meiosis) by pulling the chromosomes
3. Transport of viruses and toxins to the interior of the cell for its own detriment.

■ TYPES OF MOLECULAR MOTORS

Molecular motors are classified into three super families:
1. Kinesin
2. Dynein
3. Myosin.

1. Kinesin

Kinesin transports substances by moving over the microtubules. Each kinesin molecule has two heads and a tail portion. One of the heads hydrolyses ATP to obtain energy. By utilizing this energy, the other head swings continuously causing movement of the whole kinesin molecule (Fig. 3.12). End portion of the tail carries the cargo (substances to be transported). Kinesin is responsible for **anterograde transport** (transport of substances towards the positive end of microtubule).

2. Dynein

Dynein is almost similar to kinesin and transports substances by moving over the microtubules. But it is responsible for **retrograde transport** (transport of substances towards the negative end of microtubule).

3. Myosin

Myosin transports substances by moving over microfilaments. Myosins are classified into 18 types according to the amino acid sequence. However, myosin II and V are functionally significant. Myosin II is involved in muscle contraction (Chapter 31). Myosin V is involved in transport of vesicles.

■ APPLIED PHYSIOLOGY

■ ABNORMALITIES OF SODIUM-POTASSIUM PUMP

Abnormalities in the number or function of Na^+-K^+ pump are associated with several pathological conditions. Important examples are:

1. Reduction in either the number or concentration of Na^+-K^+ pump in myocardium is associated with cardiac failure
2. Excess reabsorption of sodium in renal tubules is associated with hypertension.

■ CHANNELOPATHIES OR ION CHANNEL DISEASES

Channelopathies or ion channel diseases are caused by mutations in genes that encode the ion channels.

1. *Sodium Channel Diseases*

Dysfunction of sodium channels leads to muscle spasm and **Liddle's syndrome** (dysfunction of sodium channels in kidney resulting in increased osmotic pressure in the blood and hypertension).

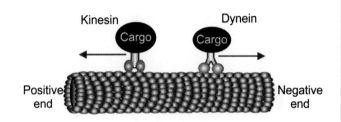

FIGURE 3.12: Kinesin and dynein motor molecules

2. *Potassium Channel Diseases*

Potassium channel dysfunction causes disorders of heart, inherited deafness and epileptic seizures in newborn.

3. *Chloride Channel Diseases*

Dysfunction of chloride channels results in formation of renal stones and **cystic fibrosis.** Cystic fibrosis is a generalized disorder affecting the functions of many organs such as lungs (due to excessive mucus), exocrine glands like pancreas, biliary system and immune system.

Homeostasis

- ■ **INTRODUCTION**
- ■ **ROLE OF VARIOUS SYSTEMS OF THE BODY IN HOMEOSTASIS**
- ■ **COMPONENTS OF HOMEOSTATIC SYSTEM**
- ■ **MECHANISM OF ACTION OF HOMEOSTATIC SYSTEM**
  - ■ **NEGATIVE FEEDBACK**
  - ■ **POSITIVE FEEDBACK**

■ INTRODUCTION

'Homeostasis' refers to the maintenance of constant internal environment of the body (homeo = same; stasis = standing). Importance of internal environment was notified by the great biologist of 19th century Claude Bernard. He enlightened the fact that multicellular organisms including man live in a perfectly organized and controlled internal environment, which he called **'milieu interieur'.** The word 'homeostasis' was introduced by Harvard Professor, Walter B Cannon in 1930.

Internal environment in the body is the **extracellular fluid (ECF)** in which the cells live. It is the fluid outside the cell and it constantly moves throughout the body. It includes blood, which circulates in the vascular system and fluid present in between the cells called **interstitial fluid.** ECF contains nutrients, ions and all other substances necessary for the survival of the cells.

Normal healthy living of large organisms including human beings depends upon the constant maintenance of internal environment within the physiological limits. If the internal environment deviates beyond the **set limits,** body suffers from malfunction or dysfunction. Therefore, the ultimate goal of an organism is to have a normal healthy living, which is achieved by the maintenance of internal environment within set limits.

The concept of homeostasis forms basis of physiology because it explains why various physiological functions are to be maintained within a normal range and in case if any function deviates from this range how it is

brought back to normal. Understanding the concept of homeostasis also forms the basis for clinical diagnostic procedures. For example, increased body temperature beyond normal range as in the case of fever, indicates that something is wrong in the heat production-heat loss mechanism in the body. It induces the physician to go through the diagnostic proceedings and decide about the treatment.

For the functioning of homeostatic mechanism, the body must recognize the deviation of any physiological activity from the normal limits. Fortunately, body is provided with appropriate **detectors** or **sensors,** which recognize the deviation. These detectors sense the deviation and alert the **integrating center.** The integrating center immediately sends information to the concerned **effectors** to either accelerate or inhibit the activity so that the normalcy is restored.

■ ROLE OF VARIOUS SYSTEMS OF THE BODY IN HOMEOSTASIS

One or more systems are involved in homeostatic mechanism of each function. Some of the functions in which the homeostatic mechanism is well established are given below:

1. The pH of the ECF has to be maintained at the critical value of 7.4. The tissues cannot survive if it is altered. Thus, the decrease in pH (acidosis) or increase in pH (alkalosis) affects the tissues markedly. The respiratory system, blood and kidney help in the regulation of pH.

2. Body temperature must be maintained at 37.5°C. Increase or decrease in temperature alters the metabolic activities of the cells. The skin, respiratory system, digestive system, excretory system, skeletal muscles and nervous system are involved in maintaining the temperature within normal limits.

3. Adequate amount of nutrients must be supplied to the cells. Nutrients are essential for various activities of the cell and growth of the tissues. These substances also form the source of energy required for various activities of the cells. Nutrients must be digested, absorbed into the blood and supplied to the cells. Digestive system and circulatory system play major roles in the supply of nutrients.

4. Adequate amount of oxygen should be made available to the cells for the metabolism of the nutrients. Simultaneously, the carbon dioxide and other metabolic end products must be removed. Respiratory system is concerned with the supply of oxygen and removal of carbon dioxide. Kidneys and other excretory organs are involved in the excretion of waste products.

5. Many hormones are essential for the metabolism of nutrients and other substances necessary for the cells. Hormones are to be synthesized and released from the endocrine glands in appropriate quantities and these hormones must act on the body cells appropriately. Otherwise, it leads to abnormal signs and symptoms.

6. Water and electrolyte balance should be maintained optimally. Otherwise it leads to dehydration or water toxicity and alteration in the osmolality of the body fluids. Kidneys, skin, salivary glands and gastrointestinal tract take care of this.

7. For all these functions, the blood, which forms the major part of internal environment, must be normal. It should contain required number of normal red blood cells and adequate amount of plasma with normal composition. Only then, it can transport the nutritive substances, respiratory gases, metabolic and other waste products.

8. Skeletal muscles are also involved in homeostasis. This system helps the organism to move around in search of food. It also helps to protect the organism from adverse surroundings, thus preventing damage or destruction.

9. Central nervous system, which includes brain and spinal cord also, plays an important role in homeostasis. Sensory system detects the state of the body or surroundings. Brain integrates and interprets the pros and cons of these information and commands the body to act accordingly through

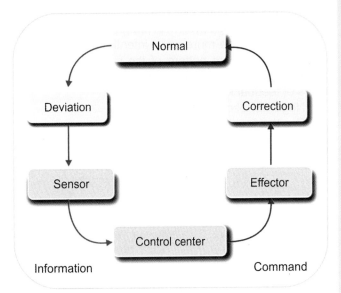

FIGURE 4.1: Components of homeostatic system

motor system so that, the body can avoid the damage.

10. Autonomic nervous system regulates all the vegetative functions of the body essential for homeostasis.

■ COMPONENTS OF HOMEOSTATIC SYSTEM

Homeostatic system in the body acts through self-regulating devices, which operate in a cyclic manner (Fig. 4.1). This cycle includes four components:
1. **Sensors** or **detectors,** which recognize the deviation
2. Transmission of this message to a **control center**
3. Transmission of information from the control center to the effectors for correcting the deviation

 Transmission of the message or information may be an electrical process in the form of impulses through nerves or a chemical process mainly in the form of hormones through blood and body fluids
4. **Effectors,** which correct the deviation.

■ MECHANISM OF ACTION OF HOMEOSTATIC SYSTEM

Homeostatic mechanism in the body is responsible for maintaining the normalcy of various body systems. Whenever there is any change in behavioral pattern of any system, the effectors bring back the normalcy either by inhibiting and reversing the change or by supporting and accelerating the change depending upon requirement of the situation. This is achieved by means of **feedback signals.**

Feedback is a process in which some proportion of the output signal of a system is fed (passed) back to the input. This is done more often intentionally in order to control the behavior pattern of the system. Whenever any change occurs, system receives and reacts to two types of feedback:

1. Negative feedback
2. Positive feedback.

■ NEGATIVE FEEDBACK

Negative feedback is the one to which the system reacts in such a way as to arrest the change or reverse the direction of change. After receiving a message, effectors send negative feedback signals back to the system. Now, the system stabilizes its own function and makes an attempt to maintain homeostasis.

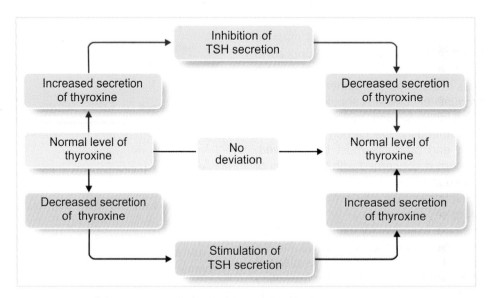

FIGURE 4.2: Negative feedback mechanism – secretion of thyroxine.
TSH = Thyroid-stimulating hormone.

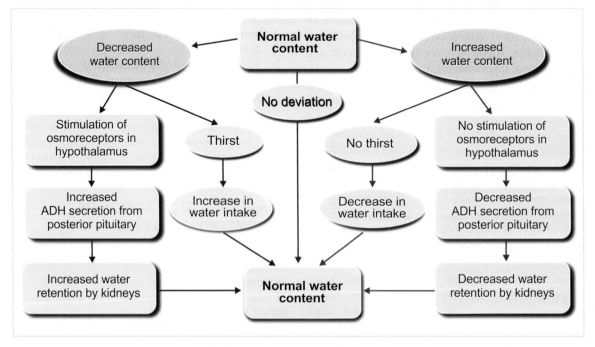

FIGURE 4.3: Negative feedback mechanism – maintenance of water balance.
ADH = Antidiuretic hormone.

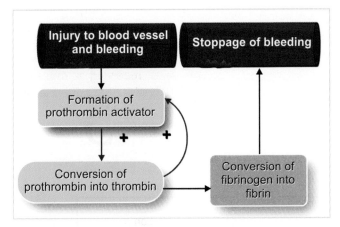

FIGURE 4.4: Positive feedback mechanism – coagulation of blood. Once formed, thrombin induces the formation of more prothrombin activator.

Many homeostatic mechanisms in the body function through negative feedback. For example, thyroid-stimulating hormone (TSH) released from pituitary gland stimulates thyroid gland to secrete thyroxine. When thyroxine level increases in blood, it inhibits the secretion of TSH from pituitary so that, the secretion of thyroxin from thyroid gland decreases (Fig. 4.2). On the other hand, if thyroxine secretion is less, its low blood level induces pituitary gland to release TSH. Now, TSH stimulates thyroid gland to secrete thyroxine (Refer Chapter 67 for details). Another example for negative feedback mechanism is maintenance of water balance in the body (Fig. 4.3).

■ POSITIVE FEEDBACK

Positive feedback is the one to which the system reacts in such a way as to increase the intensity of the change in the same direction. Positive feedback is less common than the negative feedback. However, it has its own significance particularly during emergency conditions.

One of the positive feedbacks occurs during the blood clotting. Blood clotting is necessary to arrest bleeding during injury and it occurs in three stages.

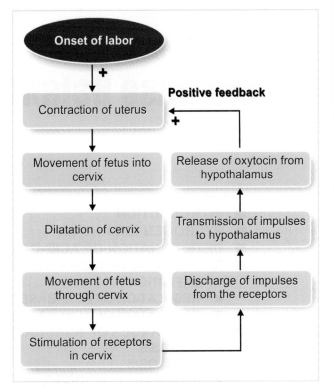

FIGURE 4.5: Positive feedback mechanism – parturition

The three stages are:
  i. Formation of prothrombin activator
 ii. Conversion of prothrombin into thrombin
iii. Conversion of fibrinogen into fibrin.

Thrombin formed in the second stage stimulates the formation of more prothrombin activator in addition to converting fibrinogen into fibrin (Fig. 4.4). It causes formation of more and more amount of prothrombin activator so that the blood clotting process is accelerated and blood loss is prevented quickly (Chapter 20). Other processes where positive feedback occurs are milk ejection reflex (Chapter 66) and parturition (Fig. 4.5) (Chapter 84) and both the processes involve oxytocin secretion.

Acid-base Balance

Chapter 5

- ■ **INTRODUCTION**
- ■ **HYDROGEN ION AND pH**
- ■ **DETERMINATION OF ACID-BASE STATUS**
- ■ **REGULATION OF ACID-BASE BALANCE**
  - ■ **DEFINITION**
  - ■ **REGULATION OF ACID-BASE BALANCE BY RESPIRATORY MECHANISM**
  - ■ **REGULATION OF ACID-BASE BALANCE BY RENAL MECHANISM**
- ■ **DISTURBANCES OF ACID-BASE STATUS**
  - ■ **ACIDOSIS**
  - ■ **ALKALOSIS**
  - ■ **RESPIRATORY ACIDOSIS**
  - ■ **RESPIRATORY ALKALOSIS**
  - ■ **METABOLIC ACIDOSIS**
  - ■ **METABOLIC ALKALOSIS**
- ■ **CLINICAL EVALUATION – ANION GAP**

■ INTRODUCTION

Acid-base balance is very important for the homeostasis of the body and almost all the physiological activities depend upon the acid-base status of the body. Acids are constantly produced in the body. However, the acid production is balanced by the production of bases so that the acid-base status of the body is maintained.

An acid is the **proton donor** (the substance that liberates hydrogen ion). A base is the **proton acceptor** (the substance that accepts hydrogen ion).

In spite of continuous production of acids in the body, the concentration of free hydrogen ion is kept almost constant at a pH of 7.4 with slight variations.

■ HYDROGEN ION AND pH

Hydrogen ion (H^+) contains only a single proton (positively charged particle), which is not orbited by any electron. Therefore, it is the smallest ionic particle. However, it is highly reactive. Because of this, the H^+ shows severe effects on the physiological activities of the body even at low concentrations. The normal H^+ concentration in the extracellular fluid (ECF) is 38 to 42 nM/L.

The pH is another term for H^+ concentration that is generally used nowadays instead of 'hydrogen ion concentration'. The pH scale was introduced in order to simplify the mathematical handling of large numbers.

Negative logarithm of H^+ concentration is taken for calculating the pH as given below.

$$pH = \log \frac{1}{H^+}$$

An increase in H^+ ion concentration decreases the pH (acidosis) and a reduction in H^+ concentration increases the pH (alkalosis). An increase in pH by one-fold requires a tenfold decrease in H^+ concentration (Table 5.1).

In a healthy person, the pH of the ECF is 7.40 and it varies between 7.38 and 7.42. The maintenance of acid-base status is very important for homeostasis, because even a slight change in pH below 7.38 or above 7.42 will cause serious threats to many physiological functions.

TABLE 5.1: Hydrogen ion concentration and pH

H+ (nM/L)	pH
10,000	5.0
1,000	6.0
100	7.0
10	8.0
1	9.0

■ DETERMINATION OF ACID-BASE STATUS

It is difficult to determine the acid-base status in the ECF by direct methods. So, an indirect method is followed by using **Henderson-Hasselbalch equation.** In this, to determine the pH of a fluid, the concentration of bicarbonate ions (HCO_3^-) and the CO_2 dissolved in the fluid are measured. The pH is calculated as follows:

$$pH = pK + \log\frac{HCO_3^-}{CO_2}$$

Where, pK is constant with pH of 6.1
Thus,

$$pH = 6.1 + \log\frac{HCO_3^-}{CO_2}$$

In addition to this, the pH of plasma is also determined by using an instrument called pH meter.

Normal acid-base ratio is 1:20, i.e. the ratio of 1 part of CO_2 (derived from H_2CO_3) and 20 parts of HCO_3^-. If this ratio is altered, the pH also is altered leading to either acidosis or alkalosis.

Thus, the pH of arterial blood is an indirect measurement of H+ concentration and it reflects the balance of CO_2 and HCO_3^-.

■ REGULATION OF ACID-BASE BALANCE

Body is under constant threat of acidosis because of the production of large amount of acids. Generally, two types of acids are produced in the body:
1. Volatile acids
2. Non-volatile acids.

1. *Volatile Acids*

Volatile acids are derived from CO_2. Large quantity of CO_2 is produced during the metabolism of carbohydrates and lipids. This CO_2 is not a threat because it is almost totally removed through expired air by lungs.

2. *Non-volatile Acids*

Non-volatile acids are produced during the metabolism of other nutritive substances such as proteins. These acids are real threat to the acid-base status of the body. For example, sulfuric acid is produced during the metabolism of sulfur containing amino acids such as **cysteine** and **metheonine;** hydrochloric acid is produced during the metabolism of lysine, arginine and histidine. Fortunately, body is provided with the best regulatory mechanisms to prevent the hazards of acid production.

Compensatory Mechanism

Whenever there is a change in pH beyond the normal range, some compensatory changes occur in the body to bring the pH back to normal level. The body has three different mechanisms to regulate acid-base status:
1. Acid-base buffer system, which binds free H+
2. Respiratory mechanism, which eliminates CO_2
3. Renal mechanism, which excretes H+ and conserves the bases (HCO_3^-).

Among the three mechanisms, the acid-base buffer system is the fastest one and it readjusts the pH within seconds. The respiratory mechanism does it in minutes. Whereas, the renal mechanism is slower and it takes few hours to few days to bring the pH back to normal. However, the renal mechanism is the most powerful mechanism than the other two in maintaining the acid-base balance of the body fluids.

■ REGULATION OF ACID-BASE BALANCE BY ACID-BASE BUFFER SYSTEM

■ DEFINITION

An acid-base buffer system is the combination of a weak acid **(protonated substance)** and a base – the salt **(unprotonated substance).** Buffer system is the one, which acts immediately to prevent the changes in pH. Buffer system maintains pH by binding with free H+.

Types of Buffer Systems

Body fluids have three types of buffer systems, which act under different conditions:
1. Bicarbonate buffer system
2. Phosphate buffer system
3. Protein buffer system.

1. *Bicarbonate Buffer System*

Bicarbonate buffer system is present in ECF (plasma). It consists of the protonated substance, carbonic acid (H_2CO_3) which is a weak acid and the unprotonated substance, HCO_3^- which is a weak base. HCO_3^- is in the form of salt, i.e. sodium bicarbonate ($NaHCO_3$).

Mechanism of action of bicarbonate buffer system

Bicarbonate buffer system prevents the fall of pH in a fluid to which a strong acid like hydrochloric acid (HCl) is added.

Normally, when HCl is mixed with a fluid, pH of that fluid decreases quickly because the strong HCl dissociates into H^+ and Cl^-.

But, if bicarbonate buffer system ($NaHCO_3$) is added to the fluid with HCl, the pH is not altered much. This is because the H^+ dissociated from HCl combines with HCO_3^- of $NaHCO_3$ and forms a weak H_2CO_3. This H_2CO_3 in turn dissociates into CO_2 and H_2O.

$$HCl + NaHCO_3 \rightarrow H_2CO_3 + NaCl$$
$$\downarrow$$
$$CO_2 + H_2O$$

Bicarbonate buffer system also prevents the increase in pH in a fluid to which a strong base like sodium hydroxide (NaOH) is added.

Normally, when a base (NaOH) is added to a fluid, pH increases. It is prevented by adding H_2CO_3, which dissociates into H^+ and HCO_3^-. The hydroxyl group (OH) of NaOH combines with H^+ and forms H_2O. And Na^+ combines with HCO_3^- and forms $NaHCO_3$. $NaHCO_3$ is a weak base and it prevents the increase in pH by the strong NaOH.

As sodium bicarbonate is a very weak base, its association with H^+ is poor. So the rise in pH of the fluid is very mild.

Importance of bicarbonate buffer system

Bicarbonate buffer system is not powerful like the other buffer systems because of the large difference between the pH of ECF (7.4) and the pK of bicarbonate buffer system (6.1). But this buffer system plays an important role in maintaining the pH of body fluids than the other buffer systems. It is because the concentration of two components (HCO_3^- and CO_2) of this buffer system is regulated separately by two different mechanisms.

Concentration of HCO_3^- is regulated by kidney and the concentration of CO_2 is regulated by the respiratory system. These two regulatory mechanisms operate constantly and simultaneously, making this system more effective.

2. Phosphate Buffer System

This system consists of a weak acid, the dihydrogen phosphate (H_2PO_4 – protonated substance) in the form of sodium dihydrogen phosphate (NaH_2PO_4) and the base, hydrogen phosphate (HPO_4 – unprotonated substance) in the form of disodium hydrogen phosphate (Na_2HPO_4).

Phosphate buffer system is useful in the intracellular fluid (ICF), in red blood cells or other cells, as the concentration of phosphate is more in ICF than in ECF.

Mechanism of phosphate buffer system

When a strong acid like hydrochloric acid is mixed with a fluid containing phosphate buffer, sodium dihydrogen phosphate (NaH_2PO_4 – weak acid) is formed. This permits only a mild change in the pH of the fluid.

$$\underset{\text{(strong acid)}}{HCl} + Na_2HPO_4 \rightarrow \underset{\text{(weak acid)}}{NaH_2PO_4} + NaCl$$

If a strong base such as sodium hydroxide (NaOH) is added to the fluid containing phosphate buffer, a weak base called disodium hydrogen phosphate (Na_2HPO_4) is formed. This prevents the changes in pH.

$$\underset{\text{(strong base)}}{NaOH} + NaH_2PO_4 \rightarrow \underset{\text{(weak base)}}{NaHPO_4} + H_2O$$

Importance of phosphate buffer system

Phosphate buffer system is more powerful than bicarbonate buffer system as it has a pK of 6.8, which is close to the pH of the body fluids, i.e. 7.4. In addition to ICF, phosphate buffer is useful in tubular fluids of kidneys also. It is because more phosphate ions are found in tubular fluid.

In the red blood cells, the potassium ion concentration is higher than the sodium ion concentration. So, the elements of phosphate buffer inside the red blood cells are in the form of potassium dihydrogen phosphate (KH_2PO_4) and dipotassium hydrogen phosphate (K_2HPO_4).

3. Protein Buffer System

Protein buffer systems are present in the blood; both in the plasma and erythrocytes.

Protein buffer systems in plasma

Elements of proteins, which form the weak acids in the plasma are:
  i. C-terminal carboxyl group, N-terminal amino group and side-chain carboxyl group of glutamic acid
  ii. Side-chain amino group of lysine
  iii. Imidazole group of histidine.

Protein buffer systems in plasma are more powerful because of their high concentration in plasma and because of their pK being very close to 7.4.

Protein buffer system in erythrocytes (Hemoglobin)

Hemoglobin is the most effective protein buffer and the major buffer in blood. Due to its high concentration than the plasma proteins, hemoglobin has about six times more buffering capacity than the plasma proteins. The deoxygenated hemoglobin is a more powerful buffer than oxygenated hemoglobin because of the higher pK. When a hemoglobin molecule becomes deoxygenated in the capillaries, it easily binds with H^+, which are released when CO_2 enters the capillaries. Thus, hemoglobin prevents fall in pH when more and more CO_2 enters the capillaries.

■ REGULATION OF ACID-BASE BALANCE BY RESPIRATORY MECHANISM

Lungs play an important role in the maintenance of acid-base balance by removing CO_2 which is produced during various metabolic activities in the body. This CO_2 combines with water to form carbonic acid.

Since carbonic acid is unstable, it splits into H^+ and HCO_3^-.

$$CO_2 + H_2O \rightarrow H_2CO_3 \rightarrow H^+ + HCO_3^-$$

Entire reaction is reversed in lungs when CO_2 diffuses from blood into the alveoli of lungs.

$$H^+ + HCO_3^- \rightarrow H_2CO_3 \rightarrow CO_2 + H_2O$$

And CO_2 is blown off by ventilation (Chapter 125).

When metabolic activities increase, more amount of CO_2 is produced in the tissues and the concentration of H^+ increases as seen above. Increased H^+ concentration increases the pulmonary ventilation (hyperventilation) by acting through the chemoreceptors (Chapter 126). Due to hyperventilation, the excess of CO_2 is removed from the body.

■ REGULATION OF ACID-BASE BALANCE BY RENAL MECHANISM

Kidney maintains the acid-base balance of the body by the secretion of H^+ and by the retention of HCO_3^- (Fig. 5.1). Details are given in Chapter 54.

■ APPLIED PHYSIOLOGY – DISTURBANCES OF ACID-BASE STATUS

■ ACIDOSIS

Acidosis is the reduction in pH (increase in H^+ concentration) below normal range.

Acidosis is produced by:
1. Increase in partial pressure of CO_2 in the body fluids particularly in arterial blood
2. Decrease in HCO_3^- concentration.

■ ALKALOSIS

Alkalosis is the increase in pH (decrease in H^+ concentration) above the normal range (Table 5.2).

Alkalosis is produced by:
1. Decrease in partial pressure of CO_2 in the arterial blood
2. Increase in HCO_3^- concentration.

Since the partial pressure of CO_2 (pCO_2) in arterial blood is controlled by lungs, the acid-base disturbances produced by the change in arterial pCO_2 are called the respiratory disturbances.

On the other hand, the disturbances in acid-base status produced by the change in HCO_3^- concentration are generally called the metabolic disturbances.

Thus the acid-base disturbances are:
1. Respiratory acidosis
2. Respiratory alkalosis
3. Metabolic acidosis
4. Metabolic alkalosis.

■ RESPIRATORY ACIDOSIS

Respiratory acidosis is the acidosis that is caused by alveolar hypoventilation. During hypoventilation the lungs fail to expel CO_2, which is produced in the tissues. CO_2 is the major end product of oxidation of carbohydrates, proteins and fats.

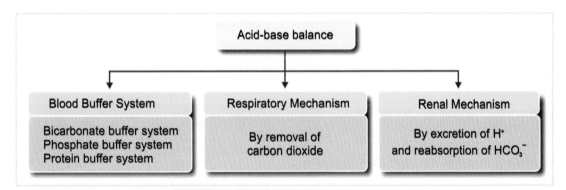

FIGURE 5.1: Regulation of acid-base balance

CO_2 accumulates in blood where it reacts with water to form carbonic acid, which is called **respiratory acid.** Carbonic acid dissociates into H^+ and HCO_3^-. The increased H^+ concentration in blood leads to decrease in pH and acidosis.

Normal partial pressure of CO_2 in arterial blood is about 40 mm Hg. When it increases above 60 mm Hg acidosis occurs.

Causes of Excess CO_2 in the Body

Hypoventilation (decreased ventilation) is the primary cause for excess CO_2 in the body. Some of the conditions when increase in pCO_2 and respiratory acidosis occur due to hypoventilation are listed in Table 5.3.

■ RESPIRATORY ALKALOSIS

Respiratory alkalosis is the alkalosis that is caused by alveolar hyperventilation. Hyperventilation causes excess loss of CO_2 from the body. Loss of CO_2 leads to decreased formation of carbonic acid and decreased release of H^+. Decreased H^+ concentration increases the pH leading to respiratory alkalosis.

When the partial pressure of CO_2 in arterial blood decreases below 20 mm Hg, alkalosis occurs.

Causes of Decrease in CO_2 in the Body

Hyperventilation is primary cause for loss of excess CO_2 from the body because during hyperventilation, lot of CO_2 is expired through respiratory tract leading to decreased pCO_2. Some of the conditions when decreased pCO_2 and respiratory alkalosis occur due to hyperventilation are given in Table 5.4.

■ METABOLIC ACIDOSIS

Metabolic acidosis is the acid-base imbalance characterized by excess accumulation of **organic acids** in the body, which is caused by abnormal metabolic processes. Organic acids such as lactic acid, ketoacids and uric acid are formed by normal metabolism. The quantity of these acids increases due to abnormality in the metabolism.

Causes of Metabolic Acidosis

Lactic acid

The amount of lactic acid increases during anaerobic glycolysis in some abnormal conditions such as circulatory shock.

TABLE 5.2: Biochemical changes in arterial blood during acid-base disturbance

Parameter	Acidosis		Alkalosis	
	Respiratory	Metabolic	Respiratory	Metabolic
H^+	Increases	Increases	Decreases	Decreases
pH	Decreases	Decreases	Increases	Increases
pCO_2	Increases	Decreases	Decreases	Increases
HCO_3^-	Increases slightly	Decreases very much	Decreases slightly	Increases very much

TABLE 5.3: Causes of acidosis

Respiratory acidosis	Metabolic acidosis
1. Airway obstruction due to bronchitis, bronchospasm, emphysema, etc.	1. Lactic acidosis as in circulatory shock
2. Lung diseases like fibrosis, pneumonia, etc.	2. Ketoacidosis as in diabetes mellitus
3. Respiratory center depression by anesthetics, sedatives, cerebral trauma, tumors, etc.	3. Uric acidosis as in renal failure
4. Extrapulmonary thoracic diseases like flail chest, kyphosis and scoliosis	4. Acid poisoning
5. Neural diseases like polymyelitis, paralysis of respiratory muscles	5. Renal tubular acidosis due to decreased H^+ excretion
	6. Loss of excess HCO_3^- due to diarrhea and pancreatic, intestinal, or biliary fistula

TABLE 5.4: Causes of alkalosis

Respiratory alkalosis	Metabolic alkalosis
1. Hypoxia as in high altitude, severe anemia and pulmonary diseases like edema and embolism	1. Vomiting and congenital diarrhea
2. Increased respiratory drive due to cerebral disturbances, voluntary hyperventilation and psychological and emotional trauma	2. Endocrine disorders such as Cushing's syndrome and Conn's syndrome
	3. Diuretic therapy

TABLE 5.5: Variations in anion gap

Increase in anion gap	Decrease in anion gap
1. Metabolic disorder (inability to metabolize lactic acid)	1. Hyperchloremic acidosis (increased chloride level in blood)
2. Dehydration	2. Hypoalbuminemia (low albumin level in blood)
3. Diabetes, starvation, alcoholism (due to increased production of ketoacid)	3. Multiple myeloma (due to accumulation of anionic proteins)
4. Renal disease (failure to excrete acids – phosphate and sulfate)	4. Hyponatremia (low blood sodium level)
5. Respiratory disease (production of excess lactic acid due to inadequate oxygen supply to tissues)	5. Renal disease (loss of excess sodium or potassium through urine)
6. Genetic disorder (involving enzymes of carbohydrate metabolism)	6. Hyperthyroidism
7. Nutritional deficiencies	7. Toxicity due to lithium or bromide

Ketoacids

The amount of ketoacids increases because of insulin deficiency as in the case of diabetes mellitus. In diabetes mellitus, glucose is not utilized due to lack of insulin. So, lipids are utilized for liberation of energy resulting in production of excess acetoacetic acid and beta hydroxybutyric acid.

Uric acid

The amount of uric acid increases in the body due to the failure of excretion. Normally uric acid is excreted by kidneys. But in renal diseases, the kidneys fail to excrete the uric acid.

Some of the conditions when the metabolic acids increase in the body resulting in metabolic acidosis are listed in Table 5.3.

■ METABOLIC ALKALOSIS

Metabolic alkalosis is the acid-base imbalance caused by loss of excess H^+ resulting in increased HCO_3^- concentration. Some of the endocrine disorders, renal tubular disorders, etc. cause metabolic disorders leading to loss of H^+. It increases HCO_3^- and pH in the body leading to metabolic alkalosis.

Some of the conditions when excess H^+ is lost and HCO_3^- content increases leading to metabolic alkalosis are given in Table 5.4.

■ CLINICAL EVALUATION OF DISTURBANCES IN ACID-BASE STATUS – ANION GAP

Anion gap is an important measure in the clinical evaluation of disturbances in acid-base status. Only few cations and anions are measured during routine clinical investigations. Commonly **measured cation** is sodium and the **unmeasured cations** are potassium, calcium and magnesium. Usually measured anions are chloride and bicarbonate. The unmeasured anions are phosphate, sulfate, proteins in anionic form such as albumin and other organic anions like lactate.

Difference between concentrations of unmeasured anions and unmeasured cations is called anion gap.

It is calculated as:

$$\text{Anion gap} = [Na^+] - [HCO_3^-] - [Cl^-]$$
$$= 144 - 24 - 108 \text{ mEq/L}$$
$$= 12 \text{ mEq/L}$$

Normal value of anion gap is 9 to 15 mEq/L. It increases when concentration of unmeasured anion increases and decreases when concentration of unmeasured cations decreases.

Anion gap is a useful measure in the differential diagnosis (diagnosis of the different causes) of acid-base disorders particularly the metabolic acidosis. Variations of anion gap are given in Table 5.5.

QUESTIONS IN GENERAL PHYSIOLOGY

■ LONG QUESTIONS

1. Describe the mechanism of active transport of substances through cell membrane.
2. Describe the mechanism of passive transport of substances through cell membrane.
3. Explain the regulation of acid-base balance. Add a note on disturbances of acid-base balance.
4. Explain the homeostasis in the body with suitable examples.

■ SHORT QUESTIONS

1. Cell membrane.
2. Proteins of cell membrane.
3. Organelles present in the cytoplasm of the cell.
4. Endoplasmic reticulum.
5. Ribosomes.
6. Mitochondria.
7. Golgi apparatus.
8. RNA.
9. DNA.
10. Cellular organelles taking part in protective function.
11. Apoptosis.
12. Cellular necrosis.
13. Tight junctions.
14. Gap junctions.
15. Passive transport.
16. Active transport.
17. Primary active transport.
18. Secondary active transport.
19. Sodium-potassium pump.
20. Simple diffusion through cell membrane.
21. Facilitated diffusion or carrier-mediated diffusion.
22. Ion channels.
23. Factors affecting diffusion.
24. Pinocytosis.
25. Phagocytosis.
26. Transcytosis.
27. Receptor-mediated endocytosis.
28. Homeostasis.
29. Components of homeostasis.
30. Negative feedback.
31. Positive feedback.
32. Acid-base buffer system.
33. Role of blood in the maintenance of acid-base balance or acid-base buffer system.
34. Role of lungs in the maintenance of acid-base balance.
35. Role of kidneys in the maintenance of acid-base balance.
36. Acidosis.
37. Alkalosis.
38. Anion gap.

Section

2

Blood and Body Fluids

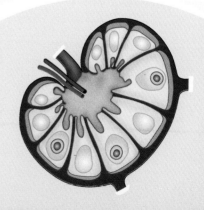

Body Fluids

- ■ INTRODUCTION
- ■ SIGNIFICANCE
- ■ COMPARTMENTS
- ■ COMPOSITION
- ■ MEASUREMENT
- ■ CONCENTRATION
- ■ MAINTENANCE OF WATER BALANCE
- ■ APPLIED PHYSIOLOGY

■ INTRODUCTION

Body is formed by solids and fluids. Fluid part is more than two third of the whole body. Water forms most of the fluid part of the body.

In human beings, the total body water varies from 45% to 75% of body weight. In a normal young adult male, body contains 60% to 65% of water and 35% to 40% of solids. In a normal young adult female, the water is 50% to 55% and solids are 45% to 50%. In females, water is less because of more amount of subcutaneous adipose tissue. In thin persons, water content is more than that in obese persons. In old age, water content is decreased due to increase in adipose tissue. Total quantity of body water in an average human being weighing about 70 kg is about 40 L.

■ SIGNIFICANCE OF BODY FLUIDS

■ IN HOMEOSTASIS

Body cells survive in the fluid medium called **internal environment** or **'milieu interieur'**. Internal environment contains substances such as glucose, amino acids, lipids, vitamins, ions, oxygen, etc. which are essential for growth and functioning of the cell. Water not only forms the major constituent of internal environment but also plays an important role in homeostasis.

■ IN TRANSPORT MECHANISM

Body water forms the transport medium by which nutrients and other essential substances enter the cells; and unwanted substances come out of the cells. Water forms an important medium by which various enzymes, hormones, vitamins, electrolytes and other substances are carried from one part to another part of the body.

■ IN METABOLIC REACTIONS

Water inside the cells forms the medium for various metabolic reactions, which are necessary for growth and functional activities of the cells.

■ IN TEXTURE OF TISSUES

Water inside the cells is necessary for characteristic form and texture of various tissues.

■ IN TEMPERATURE REGULATION

Water plays a vital role in the maintenance of normal body temperature.

■ COMPARTMENTS OF BODY FLUIDS – DISTRIBUTION OF BODY FLUIDS

Total water in the body is about 40 L. It is distributed into two major compartments:

1. *Intracellular fluid (ICF):* Its volume is 22 L and it forms 55% of the total body water
2. *Extracellular fluid (ECF):* Its volume is 18 L and it forms 45% of the total body water.
   ECF is divided into 5 subunits:
   i. Interstitial fluid and lymph (20%)
   ii. Plasma (7.5%)
   iii. Fluid in bones (7.5%)
   iv. Fluid in dense connective tissues like cartilage (7.5%)
   v. Transcellular fluid (2.5%) that includes:
      a. Cerebrospinal fluid
      b. Intraocular fluid
      c. Digestive juices
      d. Serous fluid – intrapleural fluid, pericardial fluid and peritoneal fluid
      e. Synovial fluid in joints
      f. Fluid in urinary tract.

Volume of interstitial fluid is about 12 L. Volume of plasma is about 2.75 L. Volume of other subunits of ECF is about 3.25 L. Water moves between different compartments (Fig. 6.1).

■ COMPOSITION OF BODY FLUIDS

Body fluids contain water and solids. Solids are organic and inorganic substances.

■ ORGANIC SUBSTANCES

Organic substances are glucose, amino acids and other proteins, fatty acids and other lipids, hormones and enzymes.

■ INORGANIC SUBSTANCES

Inorganic substances present in body fluids are sodium, potassium, calcium, magnesium, chloride, bicarbonate, phosphate and sulfate.

ECF contains large quantity of sodium, chloride, bicarbonate, glucose, fatty acids and oxygen. ICF contains large quantities of potassium, magnesium, phosphates, sulfates and proteins. The pH of ECF is 7.4. The pH of ICF is 7.0. Differences between ECF and ICF are given in Table 6.1.

■ MEASUREMENT OF BODY FLUID VOLUME

Total body water and the volume of different compartments of the body fluid are measured by indicator dilution method or dye dilution method.

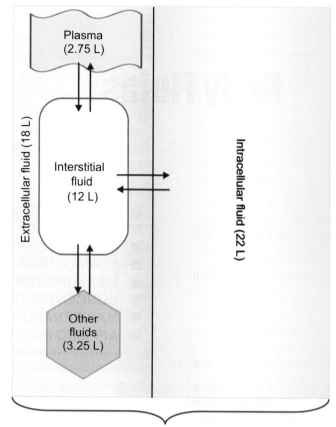

Total body water = 40 L

FIGURE 6.1: Body fluid compartments and movement of fluid between different compartments. Other fluids = Transcellular fluid, fluid in bones and fluid in connective tissue.

■ INDICATOR DILUTION METHOD

Principle

A known quantity of a substance such as a dye is administered into a specific body fluid compartment. These substances are called the marker substances or indicators. After administration into the fluid compartment, the substance is allowed to mix thoroughly with the fluid. Then, a sample of fluid is drawn and the concentration of the marker substance is determined. Radioactive substances or other substances whose concentration can be determined by using colorimeter are generally used as marker substances (Table 6.2).

Formula to Measure the Volume of Fluid by Indicator Dilution Method

Quantity of fluid in the compartment is measured using the formula:

$$V = \frac{M}{C}$$

V = Volume of fluid in the compartment.

M = Mass or total quantity of marker substance injected.

C = Concentration of the marker substance in the sample fluid

Correction factor

Some amount of marker substance is lost through urine during distribution. So, the formula is corrected as follows:

$$\text{Volume} = \frac{M - \text{Amount of substance excreted}}{C}$$

Uses of Indicator Dilution Method

Indicator dilution or dye dilution method is used to measure ECF volume, plasma volume and the volume of total body water.

Characteristics of Marker Substances

Dye or any substance used as a marker substance should have the following qualities:

1. Must be nontoxic

2. Must mix with the fluid compartment thoroughly within reasonable time
3. Should not be excreted rapidly
4. Should be excreted from the body completely within reasonable time
5. Should not change the color of the body fluid
6. Should not alter the volume of the body fluid.

Marker Substances Used to Measure Fluid Compartments

Marker substances used to measure different fluid compartment are listed in Table 6.2.

■ MEASUREMENT OF TOTAL BODY WATER

Volume of total body water (fluid) is measured by using a marker substance which is distributed through all the compartments of body fluid. Such substances are listed in Table 6.2.

Deuterium oxide and **tritium oxide** mix with fluids of all the compartments within few hours after injection. Since plasma is part of total body fluid, the concentration of marker substances can be obtained from sample of plasma. The formula for indicator dilution method is applied to calculate total body water.

Antipyrine is also used to measure total body water. But as it takes longer time to penetrate various fluid compartments, the value obtained is slightly low.

■ MEASUREMENT OF EXTRACELLULAR FLUID VOLUME

Substances which pass through the capillary membrane but do not enter the cells, are used to measure ECF volume. Such marker substances are listed in Table 6.2.

These substances remain only in ECF and do not enter the cell (ICF). When any of these substances is injected into blood, it mixes with the fluid of all subcompartments of ECF within 30 minutes to 1 hour. Indicator dilution method is applied to calculate ECF volume. Since ECF includes plasma, the concentration of marker substance can be obtained in the sample of plasma.

Some of the marker substances like sodium, chloride, inulin and sucrose diffuse more evenly throughout all subcompartments of ECF. So, the measured volume of ECF by using these substances is referred as **sodium space, chloride space, inulin space** and **sucrose space.**

Example for Measurement of ECF Volume

Quantity of sucrose injected (Mass)	: 150 mg
Urinary excretion of sucrose	: 10 mg
Concentration of sucrose in plasma	: 0.01 mg/mL

TABLE 6.1: Differences between extracellular fluid (ECF) and intracellular fluid (ICF)

Substance	ECF	ICF
Sodium	142 mEq/L	10 mEq/L
Calcium	5 mEq/L	1 mEq/L
Potassium	4 mEq/L	140 mEq/L
Magnesium	3 mEq/L	28 mEq/L
Chloride	103 mEq/L	4 mEq/L
Bicarbonate	28 mEq/L	10 mEq/L
Phosphate	4 mEq/L	75 mEq/L
Sulfate	1 mEq/L	2 mEq/L
Proteins	2 g/dL	16 g/dL
Amino acids	30 mg/dL	200 mg/dL
Glucose	90 mg/dL	0-20 mg/dL
Lipids	0.5 g/dL	2-95 g/dL
Partial pressure of oxygen	35 mm Hg	20 mm Hg
Partial pressure of carbon dioxide	46 mm Hg	50 mm Hg
Water	15 to 20 L (18)	20 to 25 L (22)
pH	7.4	7.0

$$V = \frac{M}{C}$$

$$\text{Sucrose space} = \frac{\text{Mass} - \text{Amount lost in urine}}{\text{Concentration of sucrose in plasma}}$$

$$= \frac{150 - 10 \text{ mg}}{0.01 \text{ mg/mL}}$$

$$= 14,000 \text{ mL}$$

Therefore, the ECF volume = 14 L.

■ MEASUREMENT OF PLASMA VOLUME

The substance which binds with plasma proteins strongly and diffuses into interstitium only in small quantities or does not diffuse is used to measure plasma volume. Such substances are listed in Table 6.2.

(Measurement of plasma volume and blood volume is explained in chapter 23).

■ MEASUREMENT OF INTERSTITIAL FLUID VOLUME

Volume of interstitial fluid cannot be measured directly. It is calculated from the values of ECF volume and plasma volume.

Interstitial fluid volume =
ECF volume – Plasma volume

■ MEASUREMENT OF INTRACELLULAR FLUID VOLUME

Volume of ICF cannot be measured directly. It is calculated from the values of total body water and ECF.

ICF volume = Total fluid volume – ECF volume.

■ CONCENTRATION OF BODY FLUIDS

Concentration of body fluids is expressed in three ways:
1. Osmolality
2. Osmolarity
3. Tonicity.

■ OSMOLALITY

Measure of a fluid's capability to create osmotic pressure is called osmolality or osmotic (osmolar) concentration of a solution. In simple words, it is the concentration of osmotically active substance in the solution. Osmolality is expressed as the number of particles (osmoles) per kilogram of solution (osmoles/kg H_2O).

TABLE 6.2: Marker substances used to measure body fluid compartments

Fluid compartment	Marker substances
Total body water	1. Deuterium oxide (D_2O) 2. Tritium oxide (T_2O) 3. Antipyrine
Extracellular fluid	1. Radioactive sodium, chloride, bromide, sulfate and thiosulfate. 2. Non-metabolizable saccharides like inulin, mannitol, raffinose and sucrose
Plasma	1. Radioactive iodine (^{131}I) 2. Evans blue (T-1824)

■ OSMOLARITY

Osmolarity is another term to express the osmotic concentration. It is the number of particles (osmoles) per liter of solution (osmoles/L).

Osmotic pressure in solutions depends upon osmolality. However, in practice, the osmolarity and not osmolality is considered to determine the osmotic pressure because of the following reasons:
  i. Measurement of weight (kilogram) of water in solution is a difficult process
  ii. Difference between osmolality and osmolarity is very much negligible and it is less than 1%.

Often, these two terms are used interchangeably. Change in osmolality of ECF affects the volume of both ECF and ICF. When osmolality of ECF increases, water moves from ICF to ECF. When the osmolality decreases in ECF, water moves from ECF to ICF. Water movement continues until the osmolality of these two fluid compartments becomes equal.

Mole and Osmole

A mole (mol) is the molecular weight of a substance in gram. Millimole (mMol) is 1/1000 of a mole. One osmole (Osm) is the expression of amount of osmotically active particles. It is the molecular weight of a substance in grams divided by number of freely moving particles liberated in solution of each molecule. One milliosmole (mOsm) is 1/1000 of an osmole.

■ TONICITY

Usually, movement of water between the fluid compartments is not influenced by small molecules like urea and alcohol, which cross the cell membrane very rapidly. These small molecules are called ineffective osmoles. On the contrary, the larger molecules like sodium and glucose, which cross the cell membrane slowly, can influence the movement of water. Therefore, such molecules are called effective osmoles. Osmolality that causes the movement of water from one compartment to another is called effective osmolality and the effective osmoles are responsible for this.

Tonicity is the measure of effective osmolality. In terms of tonicity, the solutions are classified into three categories:

    i. Isotonic fluid
   ii. Hypertonic fluid
  iii. Hypotonic fluid.

i. *Isotonic Fluid*

Fluid which has the same effective osmolality (tonicity) as body fluids is called isotonic fluid. Examples are 0.9% sodium chloride solution (normal saline) and 5% glucose solution.

Red blood cells or other cells placed in isotonic fluid (normal saline) neither gain nor lose water by osmosis (Fig. 6.2). This is because of the **osmotic equilibrium** between inside and outside the cell across the cell membrane.

ii. *Hypertonic Fluid*

Fluid which has greater effective osmolality than the body fluids is called hypertonic fluid. Example is 2% sodium chloride solution.

When red blood cells or other cells are placed in hypertonic fluid, water moves out of the cells (exosmosis) resulting in shrinkage of the cells (crenation). Refer Figure 6.2

iii. *Hypotonic Fluid*

Fluid which has less effective osmolality than the body fluids is called hypotonic fluid. Example is 0.3% sodium chloride solution.

When red blood cells or other cells are placed in hypotonic fluid, water moves into the cells (endosmosis) and causes swelling of the cells (Fig. 6.2). Now the red blood cells become globular (sphereocytic) and get ruptured (hemolysis).

■ MAINTENANCE OF WATER BALANCE

Body has several mechanisms which work together to maintain the water balance. The important mechanisms involve hypothalamus (Chapters 4, 149) and kidneys (Chapter 53).

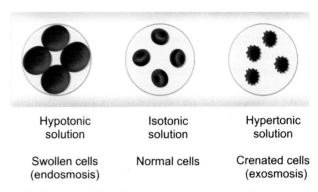

Hypotonic solution	Isotonic solution	Hypertonic solution
Swollen cells (endosmosis)	Normal cells	Crenated cells (exosmosis)

FIGURE 6.2: Effect of isotonic, hypertonic and hypotonic solutions on red blood cells

■ APPLIED PHYSIOLOGY

■ DEHYDRATION

Definition

Dehydration is defined as excessive loss of water from the body. Body requires certain amount of fluid intake daily for normal functions. Minimum daily requirement of water intake is about 1 L. This varies with the age and activity of the individual. The most active individuals need 2 to 3 L of water intake daily. Dehydration occurs when fluid loss is more than what is consumed.

Classification

Basically, dehydration is of three types:

1. *Mild dehydration:* It occurs when fluid loss is about 5% of total body fluids. Dehydration is not very serious and can be treated easily by rehydration.
2. *Moderate dehydration:* It occurs when fluid loss is about 10%. Dehydration becomes little serious and immediate treatment should be given by rehydration.
3. *Severe dehydration:* It occurs when fluid loss is about 15%. Dehydration becomes severe and requires hospitalization and emergency treatment. When fluid loss is more than 15%, dehydration becomes very severe and life threatening.

On the basis of ratio between water loss and sodium loss, dehydration is classified into three types:

1. *Isotonic dehydration:* Balanced loss of water and sodium as in the case of diarrhea or vomiting.
2. *Hypertonic dehydration:* Loss of more water than sodium as in the case of fever.
3. *Hypotonic dehydration:* Loss of more sodium than water as in the case of excess use of diuretics.

Causes

1. Severe diarrhea and vomiting due to gastrointestinal disorders
2. Excess urinary output due to renal disorders
3. Excess loss of water through urine due to endocrine disorders such as diabetes mellitus, diabetes insipidus and adrenal insufficiency
4. Insufficient intake of water
5. Prolonged physical activity without consuming adequate amount of water in hot environment
6. Excess sweating leading to heat frustration (extreme loss of water, heat and energy). Severe sweating and dehydration occur while spending longer periods on regular basis in the saunas
7. Use of laxatives or diuretics in order to lose weight quickly. This is common in athletes.

Signs and Symptoms

Mild and moderate dehydration

1. Dryness of the mouth
2. Excess thirst
3. Decrease in sweating
4. Decrease in urine formation
5. Headache
6. Dizziness
7. Weakness
8. Cramps in legs and arms.

Severe dehydration

1. Decrease in blood volume
2. Decrease in cardiac output
3. Low blood pressure
4. Hypovolemic cardiac shock
5. Fainting.

Very severe dehydration

1. Damage of organs like brain, liver and kidneys
2. Mental depression and confusion
3. Renal failure
4. Convulsions
5. Coma.

Dehydration in Infants

Infants suffering from severe diarrhea and vomiting caused by bacterial or viral infection, develop dehydration. It becomes life threatening if the lost body fluids are not replaced. This happens when parents are unable to recognize the signs.

Aging Effects on Dehydration

Elders are at higher risk for dehydration even if they are healthy. It is because of increased fluid loss and decreased fluid intake. In some cases, severe dehydration in old age may be fatal.

Treatment

Treatment depends upon the severity of dehydration. In mild dehydration, the best treatment is drinking of water and stopping fluid loss. However, in severe dehydration drinking water alone is ineffective because it cannot compensate the salt loss. So the effective treatment for severe dehydration is oral rehydration therapy.

Oral rehydration therapy

Oral rehydration therapy (ORT) is the treatment for dehydration in which a **oral rehydration solution (ORS)** is administered orally. ORS was formulated by World Health Organization (WHO). This solution contains anhydrous glucose, sodium chloride, potassium chloride and trisodium citrate.

In case of very severe dehydration, proper treatment is the intravenous administration of necessary water and electrolytes.

■ WATER INTOXICATION OR OVERHYDRATION

Definition

Water intoxication is the condition characterized by great increase in the water content of the body. It is also called overhydration, hyperhydration, water excess or water poisoning.

Causes

Water intoxication occurs when more fluid is taken than that can be excreted. Water intoxication due to drinking excess water is rare when the body's systems are functioning normally. But there are some conditions that can produce water intoxication.

1. Heart failure in which heart cannot pump blood properly
2. Renal disorders in which kidney fails to excrete enough water in urine
3. Hypersecretion of antidiuretic hormone as in the case of syndrome of inappropriate hypersecretion of antidiuretic hormone (SIADH)
4. Intravenous administration of unduly large amount of medications and fluids than the person's body can excrete

5. Infants have greater risk of developing water intoxication in the first month of life, when the filtration mechanism of the kidney is underdeveloped and cannot excrete the fluid rapidly
6. Water intoxication is also common in children having swimming practice, since they are more prone to drink too much of water while swimming
7. An adult (whose heart and kidneys are functioning normally) can develop water intoxication, if the person consumes about 8 L of water everyday regularly.

Signs and Symptoms

1. Since the brain is more vulnerable to the effects of water intoxication, behavioral changes appear first
2. Person becomes drowsy and inattentive
3. Nausea and vomiting occur
4. There is sudden loss of weight, followed by weakness and blurred vision
5. Anemia, acidosis, cyanosis, hemorrhage and shock are also common

6. Muscular symptoms such as weakness, cramps, twitching, poor coordination and paralysis develop
7. Severe conditions of water intoxication result in:
   i. Delirium (extreme mental condition characterized by confused state and illusion)
   ii. Seizures (sudden uncontrolled involuntary muscular contractions)
   iii. Coma (profound state of unconsciousness, in which the person fails to respond to external stimuli and cannot perform voluntary actions).

Treatment

Mild water intoxication requires only fluid restriction. In very severe cases, the treatment includes:
1. Diuretics to increase water loss through urine
2. Antidiuretic hormone (ADH) receptor antagonists to prevent ADH-induced reabsorption of water from renal tubules
3. Intravenous administration of saline to restore sodium.

Blood

Chapter 7

- ■ **INTRODUCTION**
- ■ **PROPERTIES**
- ■ **COMPOSITION**
    - ■ **BLOOD CELLS**
    - ■ **PLASMA**
    - ■ **SERUM**
- ■ **FUNCTIONS**
    - ■ **NUTRITIVE FUNCTION**
    - ■ **RESPIRATORY FUNCTION**
    - ■ **EXCRETORY FUNCTION**
    - ■ **TRANSPORT OF HORMONES AND ENZYMES**
    - ■ **REGULATION OF WATER BALANCE**
    - ■ **REGULATION OF ACID-BASE BALANCE**
    - ■ **REGULATION OF BODY TEMPERATURE**
    - ■ **STORAGE FUNCTION**
    - ■ **DEFENSIVE FUNCTION**

■ INTRODUCTION

Blood is a connective tissue in fluid form. It is considered as the **'fluid of life'** because it carries oxygen from lungs to all parts of the body and carbon dioxide from all parts of the body to the lungs. It is known as **'fluid of growth'** because it carries nutritive substances from the digestive system and hormones from endocrine gland to all the tissues. The blood is also called the **'fluid of health'** because it protects the body against the diseases and gets rid of the waste products and unwanted substances by transporting them to the excretory organs like kidneys.

■ PROPERTIES OF BLOOD

1. *Color:* Blood is red in color. Arterial blood is scarlet red because it contains more oxygen and venous blood is purple red because of more carbon dioxide.

2. *Volume:* Average volume of blood in a normal adult is 5 L. In a newborn baby, the volume is 450 ml. It increases during growth and reaches 5 L at the time of puberty. In females, it is slightly less and is about 4.5 L. It is about 8% of the body weight in a normal young healthy adult, weighing about 70 kg.

3. *Reaction and pH:* Blood is slightly alkaline and its pH in normal conditions is 7.4.

4. *Specific gravity:*
   Specific gravity of total blood : 1.052 to 1.061
   Specific gravity blood cells   : 1.092 to 1.101
   Specific gravity of plasma   : 1.022 to 1.026

5. *Viscosity:* Blood is five times more viscous than water. It is mainly due to red blood cells and plasma proteins.

■ COMPOSITION OF BLOOD

Blood contains the blood cells which are called formed elements and the liquid portion known as plasma.

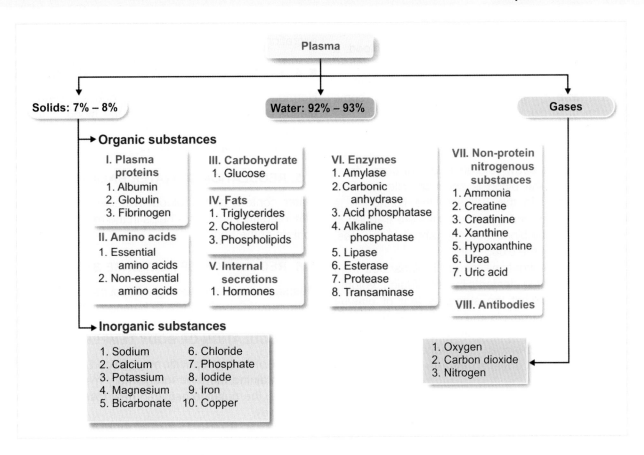

FIGURE 7.1: Composition of plasma

■ BLOOD CELLS

Three types of cells are present in the blood:
1. Red blood cells or erythrocytes
2. White blood cells or leukocytes
3. Platelets or thrombocytes.

Hematocrit Value

If blood is collected in a hematocrit tube along with a suitable anticoagulant and centrifuged for 30 minutes at a speed of 3000 revolutions per minute (rpm), the red blood cells settle down at the bottom having a clear plasma at the top. Plasma forms 55% and red blood cells form 45% of the total blood. Volume of red blood cells expressed in percentage is called the hematocrit value or packed cell volume (PCV). In between the plasma and the red blood cells, there is a thin layer of **white buffy coat.** This white buffy coat is formed by the aggregation of white blood cells and platelets (see Fig. 12.1).

TABLE 7.1: Normal values of some important substances in blood

Substance	Normal value
Glucose	100 to 120 mg/dL
Creatinine	0.5 to 1.5 mg/dL
Cholesterol	Up to 200 mg/dL
Plasma proteins	6.4 to 8.3 g/dL
Bilirubin	0.5 to 1.5 mg/dL
Iron	50 to 150 µg/dL
Copper	100 to 200 mg/dL
Calcium	9 to 11 mg/dL 4.5 to 5.5 mEq/L
Sodium	135 to 145 mEq/L
Potassium	3.5 to 5.0 mEq/L
Magnesium	1.5 to 2.0 mEq/L
Chloride	100 to 110 mEq/L
Bicarbonate	22 to 26 mEq/L

■ PLASMA

Plasma is a straw-colored clear liquid part of blood. It contains 91% to 92% of water and 8% to 9% of solids. The solids are the organic and the inorganic substances (Fig. 7.1). Table 7.1 gives the normal values of some important substances in blood.

■ SERUM

Serum is the clear straw-colored fluid that oozes from blood clot. When the blood is shed or collected in a container, it clots. In this process, the fibrinogen is converted into fibrin and the blood cells are trapped in this fibrin forming the blood clot. After about 45 minutes, serum oozes out of the blood clot.

For clinical investigations, serum is separated from blood cells and clotting elements by centrifuging. Volume of the serum is almost the same as that of plasma (55%). It is different from plasma only by the absence of fibrinogen, i.e. serum contains all the other constituents of plasma except fibrinogen. Fibrinogen is absent in serum because it is converted into fibrin during blood clotting. Thus,

Serum = Plasma – Fibrinogen

■ FUNCTIONS OF BLOOD

■ 1. NUTRITIVE FUNCTION

Nutritive substances like glucose, amino acids, lipids and vitamins derived from digested food are absorbed from gastrointestinal tract and carried by blood to different parts of the body for growth and production of energy.

■ 2. RESPIRATORY FUNCTION

Transport of respiratory gases is done by the blood. It carries oxygen from alveoli of lungs to different tissues and carbon dioxide from tissues to alveoli.

■ 3. EXCRETORY FUNCTION

Waste products formed in the tissues during various metabolic activities are removed by blood and carried to the excretory organs like kidney, skin, liver, etc. for excretion.

■ 4. TRANSPORT OF HORMONES AND ENZYMES

Hormones which are secreted by ductless (endocrine) glands are released directly into the blood. The blood transports these hormones to their target organs/tissues. Blood also transports enzymes.

■ 5. REGULATION OF WATER BALANCE

Water content of the blood is freely interchangeable with interstitial fluid. This helps in the regulation of water content of the body.

■ 6. REGULATION OF ACID-BASE BALANCE

Plasma proteins and hemoglobin act as buffers and help in the regulation of acid-base balance (Chapter 5).

■ 7. REGULATION OF BODY TEMPERATURE

Because of the high specific heat of blood, it is responsible for maintaining the thermoregulatory mechanism in the body, i.e. the balance between heat loss and heat gain in the body.

■ 8. STORAGE FUNCTION

Water and some important substances like proteins, glucose, sodium and potassium are constantly required by the tissues. Blood serves as a readymade source for these substances. And, these substances are taken from blood during the conditions like starvation, fluid loss, electrolyte loss, etc.

■ 9. DEFENSIVE FUNCTION

Blood plays an important role in the defense of the body. The white blood cells are responsible for this function. Neutrophils and monocytes engulf the bacteria by phagocytosis. Lymphocytes are involved in development of immunity. Eosinophils are responsible for detoxification, disintegration and removal of foreign proteins (Chapters 16 and 17).

Plasma Proteins

- ■ INTRODUCTION
- ■ NORMAL VALUES
- ■ SEPARATION
- ■ PROPERTIES
- ■ ORIGIN
- ■ FUNCTIONS
- ■ PLASMAPHERESIS
- ■ VARIATIONS IN PLASMA PROTEIN LEVEL

■ INTRODUCTION

Plasma proteins are:
1. Serum albumin
2. Serum globulin
3. Fibrinogen.

Serum (Chapter 7) contains only albumin and globulin. Fibrinogen is absent in serum because, it is converted into fibrin during blood clotting. Because of this, the albumin and globulin are usually called serum albumin and serum globulin.

■ NORMAL VALUES

Normal values of the plasma proteins are:

Total proteins : 7.3 g/dL (6.4 to 8.3 g/dL)
Serum albumin : 4.7 g/dL
Serum globulin : 2.3 g/dL
Fibrinogen : 0.3 g/dL

■ ALBUMIN/GLOBULIN RATIO

Ratio between plasma level of albumin and globulin is called albumin/globulin (A/G) ratio.

It is an important indicator of some diseases involving liver or kidney.

Normal A/G ratio is 2 : 1.

■ SEPARATION OF PLASMA PROTEINS

Plasma proteins are separated by the following methods.

■ 1. PRECIPITATION METHOD

Proteins in the serum are separated into albumin and globulin. This is done by precipitating globulin with 22% sodium sulfate solution. Albumin remains in solution.

■ 2. SALTING-OUT METHOD

Serum globulin is separated into two fractions called **euglobulin** and **pseudoglobulin** by salting out with different solutions. Euglobulin is salted out by full saturation with sodium chloride solution; half saturation with magnesium sulfate solution and one-third saturation with ammonium sulfate solution. It is insoluble in water. Pseudoglobulin is salted out by full saturation with magnesium sulfate and, half saturation with ammonium sulfate. It is soluble in water but it cannot be salted out by sodium chloride solution.

■ 3. ELECTROPHORETIC METHOD

In this, the plasma proteins are separated depending on their differences in electrical charge and the rate of migration. It is done in a **Tiselius apparatus** by using paper or cellulose or starch block. By this method, the proteins are separated into albumin (55%), alpha globulin (13%), beta globulin (14%), gamma globulin (11%) and fibrinogen (7%).

■ 4. COHN'S FRACTIONAL PRECIPITATION METHOD

By this method, plasma proteins are separated into albumin and different fractions of globulin, depending upon their solubility.

■ 5. ULTRACENTRIFUGATION METHOD

In this method, albumin, globulin and fibrinogen are separated depending upon their density. This method is also useful in determining the molecular weight of these proteins.

■ 6. GEL FILTRATION CHROMATOGRAPHY

Gel filtration chromatography is a column chromatographic method by which the proteins are separated on the basis of size. Protein molecules are separated by passing through a bed of porous beads. The diffusion of different proteins into the beads depends upon their size.

■ 7. IMMUNOELECTROPHORETIC METHOD

By this method, the proteins are separated on the basis of electrophoretic patterns formed by precipitation at the site of antigen-antibody reactions. This technique provides valuable quantitative measurement of different proteins.

■ PROPERTIES OF PLASMA PROTEINS

■ MOLECULAR WEIGHT

Albumin   :   69,000
Globulin   : 1,56,000
Fibrinogen : 4,00,000

Thus, the molecular weight of fibrinogen is greater than that of other two proteins.

■ ONCOTIC PRESSURE

Plasma proteins are responsible for the oncotic or osmotic pressure in the blood. Osmotic pressure exerted by proteins in the plasma is called **colloidal osmotic (oncotic) pressure** (Chapter 3). Normally, it is about 25 mm Hg. Albumin plays a major role in exerting oncotic pressure.

■ SPECIFIC GRAVITY

Specific gravity of the plasma proteins is 1.026.

■ BUFFER ACTION

Acceptance of hydrogen ions is called buffer action. The plasma proteins have 1/6 of total buffering action of the blood.

■ ORIGIN OF PLASMA PROTEINS

■ IN EMBRYO

In embryonic stage, the plasma proteins are synthesized by the **mesenchyme cells.** The albumin is synthesized first and other proteins are synthesized later.

■ IN ADULTS

In adults, the plasma proteins are synthesized mainly from **reticuloendothelial cells** of liver. The plasma proteins are synthesized also from spleen, bone marrow, disintegrating blood cells and general tissue cells. Gamma globulin is synthesized from B lymphocytes.

■ FUNCTIONS OF PLASMA PROTEINS

Plasma proteins are very essential for the body. Following are the functions of plasma proteins:

■ 1. ROLE IN COAGULATION OF BLOOD

Fibrinogen is essential for the coagulation of blood (Chapter 20).

■ 2. ROLE IN DEFENSE MECHANISM OF BODY

Gamma globulins play an important role in the defense mechanism of the body by acting as antibodies (immune substances). These proteins are also called immuno-globulins (Chapter 17). Antibodies react with antigens of various microorganisms, which cause diseases like diphtheria, typhoid, streptococcal infections, mumps, influenza, measles, hepatitis, rubella, poliomyelitis, etc.

■ 3. ROLE IN TRANSPORT MECHANISM

Plasma proteins are essential for the transport of various substances in the blood. Albumin, alpha globulin and beta globulin are responsible for the transport of the hormones, enzymes, etc. The alpha and beta globulins play an important role in the transport of metals in the blood.

■ 4. ROLE IN MAINTENANCE OF OSMOTIC PRESSURE IN BLOOD

At the capillary level, most of the substances are exchanged between the blood and the tissues. However, because of their large size, the plasma proteins cannot pass through the capillary membrane easily and remain in the blood. In the blood, these proteins exert the colloidal osmotic (oncotic) pressure. Osmotic pressure exerted by the plasma proteins is about 25 mm Hg.

Since the concentration of albumin is more than the other plasma proteins, it exerts maximum pressure. Globulin is the next and fibrinogen exerts least pressure.

Importance of Osmotic Pressure – Starling's Hypothesis

Osmotic pressure exerted by the plasma proteins plays an important role in the exchange of various substances between blood and the cells through capillary membrane. According to Starling's hypothesis, the net filtration through capillary membrane is proportional to the hydrostatic pressure difference across the membrane minus the oncotic pressure difference (Chapter 27).

■ 5. ROLE IN REGULATION OF ACID-BASE BALANCE

Plasma proteins, particularly the albumin, play an important role in regulating the acid-base balance in the blood. This is because of the virtue of their buffering action (Chapter 5). Plasma proteins are responsible for 15% of the buffering capacity of blood.

■ 6. ROLE IN VISCOSITY OF BLOOD

Plasma proteins provide viscosity to the blood, which is important to maintain the blood pressure. Albumin provides maximum viscosity than the other plasma proteins.

■ 7. ROLE IN ERYTHROCYTE SEDIMENTATION RATE

Globulin and fibrinogen accelerate the tendency of rouleaux formation by the red blood cells. **Rouleaux formation** is responsible for ESR, which is an important diagnostic and prognostic tool (Chapter 12).

■ 8. ROLE IN SUSPENSION STABILITY OF RED BLOOD CELLS

During circulation, the red blood cells remain suspended uniformly in the blood. This property of the red blood cells is called the suspension stability. Globulin and fibrinogen help in the suspension stability of the red blood cells.

■ 9. ROLE IN PRODUCTION OF TREPHONE SUBSTANCES

Trephone substances are necessary for nourishment of tissue cells in culture. These substances are produced by leukocytes from the plasma proteins.

■ 10. ROLE AS RESERVE PROTEINS

During fasting, inadequate food intake or inadequate protein intake, the plasma proteins are utilized by the body tissues as the last source of energy. Plasma proteins are split into amino acids by the tissue macrophages. Amino acids are taken back by blood and distributed throughout the body to form cellular protein molecules. Because of this, the plasma proteins are called the reserve proteins.

■ PLASMAPHERESIS

■ DEFINITION

Plasmapheresis is an experimental procedure done in animals to demonstrate the importance of plasma proteins. Earlier, this was called **Whipple's experiment** because it was established by George Hoyt Whipple.

■ PROCEDURE

Plasmapheresis is demonstrated in dogs. Blood is removed completely from the body of the dog. Red blood cells are separated from plasma and are washed in saline and reinfused into the body of the same dog along with a physiological solution called Locke's solution.

Due to sudden lack of proteins, the animal undergoes a state of shock. If the animal is fed with diet containing sufficiently high quantity of proteins, the normal level of plasma proteins is restored within seven days and the animal survives. The new plasma proteins are synthesized by the liver of the dog.

If the experiment is done in animals after removal of liver, even if the diet contains adequate quantity of proteins, the plasma proteins are not produced. The shock persists in the animal and leads to death.

Thus, the experiment 'plasmapheresis' is used to demonstrate:
1. Importance of plasma proteins for survival
2. Synthesis of plasma proteins by the liver.

■ CLINICAL SIGNIFICANCE OF PLASMAPHERESIS – THERAPEUTIC PLASMA EXCHANGE

Plasmapheresis is used as a blood purification procedure for an effective temporary treatment of many auto-

TABLE 8.1: Variations in plasma protein level

Plasma Protein	Conditions when increases	Conditions when decreases
Total proteins	Hyperproteinemia: 1. Dehydration 2. Hemolysis 3. Acute infections like acute hepatitis and acute nephritis 4. Respiratory distress syndrome 5. Excess of glucocorticoids 6. Leukemia 7. Rheumatoid arthritis 8. Alcoholism	Hypoproteinemia: 1. Diarrhea 2. Hemorrhage 3. Burns 4. Pregnancy 5. Malnutrition 6. Prolonged starvation 7. Cirrhosis of liver 8. Chronic infections like chronic hepatitis or chronic nephritis
Albumin	1. Dehydration 2. Excess of glucocorticoids 3. Congestive cardiac failure	1. Malnutrition 2. Cirrhosis of liver 3. Burns 4. Hypothyroidism 5. Nephrosis 6. Excessive intake of water
Globulin	1. Cirrhosis of liver 2. Chronic infections 3. Nephrosis 4. Rheumatoid arthritis	1. Emphysema 2. Acute hemolytic anemia 3. Glomerulonephritis 4. Hypogammaglobulinemia
Fibrinogen	1. Acute infections 2. Rheumatoid arthritis 3. Glomerulonephritis 4. Myocardial infarction 5. Stroke 6. Trauma	1. Liver dysfunction 2. Use of anabolic steroids 3. Use of phenobarbital
A/G ratio	1. Hypothyroidism 2. Excess of glucocorticoids 3. Hypogammaglobulinemia 4. Intake of high carbohydrate or protein diet	1. Liver dysfunction 2. Nephrosis

immune diseases. It is also called therapeutic plasma exchange.

In an autoimmune disease, the immune system attacks the body's own tissues through antibodies (Chapter 17). The antibodies that are proteins in nature circulate in the bloodstream before attacking the target tissues. Plasmapheresis is used to remove these antibodies from the blood.

Procedure

Venous blood is removed from the patient and blood cells are separated from plasma by the equipment called cell separator. This equipment works on the principle of a centrifuge. An anticoagulant is used to prevent the clotting of blood when it is removed from the body. After the separation of blood cells, the plasma is discarded. The blood cells are returned to the bloodstream of the

patient by mixing with a substitute fluid (saline) and sterilized human albumin protein.

Uses of Plasmapheresis

Though plasmapheresis is used to remove antibodies from the blood, it cannot prevent the production of antibodies by the immune system of the body. So, it can provide only a temporary benefit of protecting the tissues from the antibodies. The patients must go for repeated sessions of this treatment.

Plasmapheresis is an effective temporary treatment for the following diseases:

1. Myasthenia gravis – autoimmune disease causing muscle weakness (Chapter 17)
2. Thrombocytopenic purpura – bleeding disorder (Chapter 20)

3. Paraproteinemic peripheral neuropathy – dysfunction of peripheral nervous system due to an abnormal immunoglobulin called paraprotein.

4. Chronic demyelinating polyneuropathy – neurological disorder characterized by progressive weakness and impaired sensory function in the legs and arms due to the damage of myelin sheath in peripheral nerves.

5. Guillain-Barré syndrome – autoimmune disease causing weakness, abnormal sensations (like tingling) in the limbs and paralysis.

6. Lambert-Eaton myasthenic syndrome – autoimmune disorder of the neuromuscular junction.

■ VARIATIONS IN PLASMA PROTEIN LEVEL

Level of plasma proteins vary independently of one another. However, in several conditions, the quantity of albumin and globulin change in opposite direction. Elevation of all fractions of plasma proteins is called **hyperproteinemia** and decrease in all fractions of plasma proteins is called **hypoproteinemia.** Variations in the level of plasma proteins are given in Table 8.1.

Red Blood Cells

Chapter 9

- ■ INTRODUCTION
- ■ NORMAL VALUE
- ■ MORPHOLOGY
- ■ PROPERTIES
- ■ LIFESPAN
- ■ FATE
- ■ FUNCTIONS
- ■ VARIATIONS IN NUMBER
- ■ VARIATIONS IN SIZE
- ■ VARIATIONS IN SHAPE
- ■ VARIATIONS IN STRUCTURE

■ INTRODUCTION

Red blood cells (RBCs) are the **non-nucleated** formed elements in the blood. Red blood cells are also known as erythrocytes (erythros = red). Red color of the red blood cell is due to the presence of the coloring pigment called hemoglobin. RBCs play a vital role in transport of respiratory gases. RBCs are larger in number compared to the other two blood cells, namely white blood cells and platelets.

■ NORMAL VALUE

RBC count ranges between 4 and 5.5 million/cu mm of blood. In adult males, it is 5 million/cu mm and in adult females, it is 4.5 million/cu mm.

■ MORPHOLOGY OF RED BLOOD CELLS

■ NORMAL SHAPE

Normally, the RBCs are disk shaped and biconcave (dumbbell shaped). Central portion is thinner and periphery is thicker. The biconcave contour of RBCs has some mechanical and functional advantages.

Advantages of Biconcave Shape of RBCs

1. Biconcave shape helps in equal and rapid diffusion of oxygen and other substances into the interior of the cell.
2. Large surface area is provided for absorption or removal of different substances.
3. Minimal tension is offered on the membrane when the volume of cell alters.
4. Because of biconcave shape, while passing through minute capillaries, RBCs squeeze through the capillaries very easily without getting damaged.

■ NORMAL SIZE

Diameter   : 7.2 μ (6.9 to 7.4 μ).
Thickness   : At the periphery it is thicker with 2.2 μ and at the center it is thinner with 1 μ (Fig. 9.1). This difference in thickness is because of the biconcave shape.
Surface area : 120 sq μ.
Volume   : 85 to 90 cu μ.

■ NORMAL STRUCTURE

Red blood cells are non-nucleated. Only mammal, which has nucleated RBC is camel. Because of the

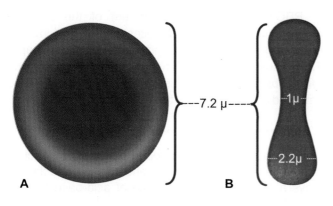

FIGURE 9.1: Dimensions of RBC.
A. Surface view, B. Sectioned view.

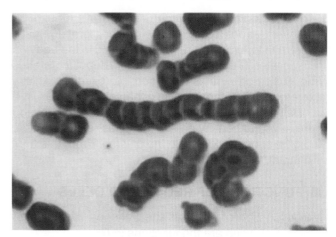

FIGURE 9.2: Rouleau formation
(*Courtesy:* Dr Nivaldo Medeiros)

absence of nucleus in human RBC, the DNA is also absent. Other organelles such as mitochondria and Golgi apparatus also are absent in RBC. Because of absence of mitochondria, the energy is produced from glycolytic process. Red cell does not have insulin receptor and so the glucose uptake by this cell is not controlled by insulin.

RBC has a special type of **cytoskeleton,** which is made up of **actin** and **spectrin.** Both the proteins are anchored to transmembrane proteins by means of another protein called **ankyrin.** Absence of spectrin results in hereditary spherocytosis. In this condition, the cell is deformed, losses its biconcave shape and becomes globular (spherocytic). The spherocyte is very fragile and easily ruptured (hemolyzed) in hypotonic solutions.

■ PROPERTIES OF RED BLOOD CELLS

■ ROULEAUX FORMATION

When blood is taken out of the blood vessel, the RBCs pile up one above another like the pile of coins. This property of the RBCs is called rouleaux (pleural = rouleau) formation (Fig. 9.2). It is accelerated by plasma proteins globulin and fibrinogen.

■ SPECIFIC GRAVITY

Specific gravity of RBC is 1.092 to 1.101.

■ PACKED CELL VOLUME

Packed cell volume (PCV) is the proportion of blood occupied by RBCs expressed in percentage. It is also called hematocrit value. It is 45% of the blood and the plasma volume is 55% (Chapters 7 and 13).

■ SUSPENSION STABILITY

During circulation, the RBCs remain suspended uniformly in the blood. This property of the RBCs is called the suspension stability.

■ LIFESPAN OF RED BLOOD CELLS

Average lifespan of RBC is about 120 days. After the lifetime the senile (old) RBCs are destroyed in reticuloendothelial system.

Determination of Lifespan of Red Blood Cells

Lifespan of the RBC is determined by radioisotope method. RBCs are tagged with radioactive substances like radioactive iron or radioactive chromium. Life of RBC is determined by studying the rate of loss of radio-active cells from circulation.

■ FATE OF RED BLOOD CELLS

When the cells become older (120 days), the cell membrane becomes more fragile. Diameter of the capillaries is less or equal to that of RBC. Younger RBCs can pass through the capillaries easily. However, because of the fragile nature, the older cells are destroyed while trying to squeeze through the capillaries. The destruction occurs mainly in the capillaries of red pulp of spleen because the diameter of splenic capillaries is very small. So, the spleen is called **'graveyard of RBCs'.**

Destroyed RBCs are fragmented and hemoglobin is released from the fragmented parts. Hemoglobin is immediately phagocytized by macrophages of the body, particularly the macrophages present in liver **(Kupffer cells),** spleen and bone marrow.

Hemoglobin is degraded into iron, globin and porphyrin. Iron combines with the protein called apoferritin to form ferritin, which is stored in the body and reused later. Globin enters the protein depot for later use (Fig. 9.3). Porphyrin is degraded into bilirubin, which is excreted by liver through bile (Chapter 40).

Daily 10% RBCs, which are senile, are destroyed in normal young healthy adults. It causes release of about 0.6 g/dL of hemoglobin into the plasma. From this 0.9 to 1.5 mg/dL bilirubin is formed.

■ FUNCTIONS OF RED BLOOD CELLS

Major function of RBCs is the transport of respiratory gases. Following are the functions of RBCs:

1. *Transport of Oxygen from the Lungs to the Tissues*

Hemoglobin in RBC combines with oxygen to form **oxyhemoglobin.** About 97% of oxygen is transported in blood in the form of oxyhemoglobin (Chapter 125).

2. *Transport of Carbon Dioxide from the Tissues to the Lungs*

Hemoglobin combines with carbon dioxide and form **carbhemoglobin.** About 30% of carbon dioxide is transported in this form.

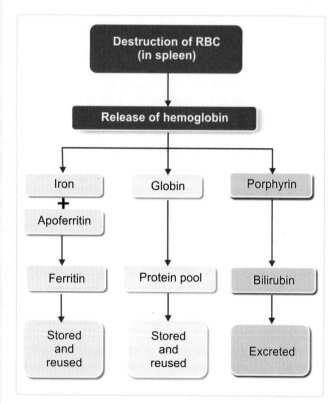

FIGURE 9.3: Fate of RBC

RBCs contain a large amount of the **carbonic anhydrase.** This enzyme is necessary for the formation of bicarbonate from water and carbon dioxide (Chapter 125). Thus, it helps to transport carbon dioxide in the form of bicarbonate from tissues to lungs. About 63% of carbon dioxide is transported in this form.

3. *Buffering Action in Blood*

Hemoglobin functions as a good buffer. By this action, it regulates the hydrogen ion concentration and thereby plays a role in the maintenance of acid-base balance (Chapter 5).

4. *In Blood Group Determination*

RBCs carry the **blood group antigens** like A antigen, B antigen and Rh factor. This helps in determination of blood group and enables to prevent reactions due to incompatible blood transfusion (Chapter 21).

■ VARIATIONS IN NUMBER OF RED BLOOD CELLS

■ PHYSIOLOGICAL VARIATIONS

A. *Increase in RBC Count*

Increase in the RBC count is known as **polycythemia.** It occurs in both physiological and pathological conditions. When it occurs in physiological conditions it is called physiological polycythemia. The increase in number during this condition is marginal and temporary. It occurs in the following conditions:

1. *Age*

At birth, the RBC count is 8 to 10 million/cu mm of blood. The count decreases within 10 days after birth due to destruction of RBCs causing **physiological jaundice** in some newborn babies. However, in infants and growing children, the cell count is more than the value in adults.

2. *Sex*

Before puberty and after menopause in females the RBC count is similar to that in males. During reproductive period of females, the count is less than that of males (4.5 million/cu mm).

3. *High altitude*

Inhabitants of mountains (above 10,000 feet from mean sea level) have an increased RBC count of more than 7 million/cu mm. It is due to **hypoxia** (decreased oxygen supply to tissues) in high altitude. Hypoxia stimulates kidney to secrete a hormone called **erythropoietin.** The erythropoietin in turn stimulates the bone marrow to produce more RBCs (Fig. 9.4).

4. Muscular exercise

There is a temporary increase in RBC count after exercise. It is because of mild hypoxia and contraction of spleen. Spleen stores RBCs (Chapter 25). Hypoxia increases the sympathetic activity resulting in secretion of adrenaline from adrenal medulla. Adrenaline contracts spleen and RBCs are released into blood (Fig. 9.5).

5. Emotional conditions

RBC count increases during the emotional conditions such as anxiety. It is because of increase in the sympathetic activity as in the case of muscular exercise (Fig. 9.5).

6. Increased environmental temperature

Increase in atmospheric temperature increases RBC count. Generally increased temperature increases all the activities in the body including production of RBCs.

7. After meals

There is a slight increase in the RBC count after taking meals. It is because of need for more oxygen for metabolic activities.

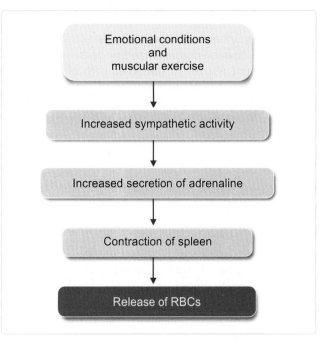

FIGURE 9.5: Physiological polycythemia in emotional conditions and exercise

B. Decrease in RBC Count

Decrease in RBC count occurs in the following physiological conditions:

1. High barometric pressures

At high barometric pressures as in deep sea, when the oxygen tension of blood is higher, the RBC count decreases.

2. During sleep

RBC count decreases slightly during sleep and immediately after getting up from sleep. Generally all the activities of the body are decreased during sleep including production of RBCs.

3. Pregnancy

In pregnancy, the RBC count decreases. It is because of increase in ECF volume. Increase in ECF volume, increases the plasma volume also resulting in hemodilution. So, there is a relative reduction in the RBC count.

■ PATHOLOGICAL VARIATIONS

Pathological Polycythemia

Pathological polycythemia is the abnormal increase in the RBC count. Red cell count increases above 7 million/cu mm of the blood. Polycythemia is of two types, the primary polycythemia and secondary polycythemia.

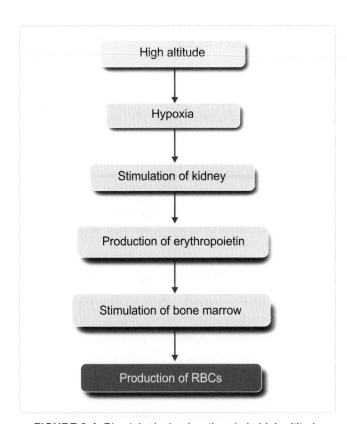

FIGURE 9.4: Physiological polycythemia in high altitude

Primary Polycythemia – Polycythemia Vera

Primary polycythemia is otherwise known as polycythemia vera. It is a disease characterized by persistent increase in RBC count above 14 million/cu mm of blood. This is always associated with increased white blood cell count above 24,000/cu mm of blood. Polycythemia vera occurs in **myeloproliferative disorders** like malignancy of red bone marrow.

Secondary Polycythemia

This is secondary to some of the pathological conditions (diseases) such as:
1. Respiratory disorders like emphysema.
2. Congenital heart disease.
3. Ayerza's disease (condition associated with hypertrophy of right ventricle and obstruction of blood flow to lungs).
4. Chronic carbon monoxide poisoning.
5. Poisoning by chemicals like phosphorus and arsenic.
6. Repeated mild hemorrhages.

All these conditions lead to hypoxia which stimulates the release of erythropoietin. Erythropoietin stimulates the bone marrow resulting in increased RBC count.

Anemia

Abnormal decrease in RBC count is called anemia. This is described in Chapter 14.

■ VARIATIONS IN SIZE OF RED BLOOD CELLS

Under physiological conditions, the size of RBCs in venous blood is slightly larger than those in arterial blood. In pathological conditions, the variations in size of RBCs are:
1. Microcytes (smaller cells)
2. Macrocytes (larger cells)
3. Anisocytes (cells with different sizes).

■ MICROCYTES

Microcytes are present in:
   i. Iron-deficiency anemia
  ii. Prolonged forced breathing
 iii. Increased osmotic pressure in blood.

■ MACROCYTES

Macrocytes are present in:
   i. Megaloblastic anemia
  ii. Decreased osmotic pressure in blood.

■ ANISOCYTES

Anisocytes occurs in pernicious anemia.

■ VARIATIONS IN SHAPE OF RED BLOOD CELLS

Shape of RBCs is altered in many conditions including different types of anemia.
1. *Crenation:* Shrinkage as in hypertonic conditions.
2. *Spherocytosis:* Globular form as in hypotonic conditions.
3. *Elliptocytosis:* Elliptical shape as in certain types of anemia.
4. *Sickle cell:* Crescentic shape as in sickle cell anemia.
5. *Poikilocytosis:* Unusual shapes due to deformed cell membrane. The shape will be of flask, hammer or any other unusual shape.

■ VARIATIONS IN STRUCTURE OF RED BLOOD CELLS

■ PUNCTATE BASOPHILISM

Striated appearance of RBCs by the presence of dots of **basophilic materials** (porphyrin) is called punctate basophilism. It occurs in conditions like **lead poisoning.**

■ RING IN RED BLOOD CELLS

Ring or twisted strands of basophilic material appear in the periphery of the RBCs. This is also called the **Goblet ring.** This appears in the RBCs in certain types of anemia.

■ HOWELL-JOLLY BODIES

In certain types of anemia, some nuclear fragments are present in the ectoplasm of the RBCs. These nuclear fragments are called Howell-Jolly bodies.

Erythropoiesis

- ■ **DEFINITION**
- ■ **SITE OF ERYTHROPOIESIS**
  - ■ **IN FETAL LIFE**
  - ■ **IN NEWBORN BABIES, CHILDREN AND ADULTS**
- ■ **PROCESS OF ERYTHROPOIESIS**
  - ■ **STEM CELLS**
  - ■ **CHANGES DURING ERYTHROPOIESIS**
  - ■ **STAGES OF ERYTHROPOIESIS**
- ■ **FACTORS NECESSARY FOR ERYTHROPOIESIS**
  - ■ **GENERAL FACTORS**
  - ■ **MATURATION FACTORS**
  - ■ **FACTORS NECESSARY FOR HEMOGLOBIN FORMATION**

■ DEFINITION

Erythropoiesis is the process of the origin, development and maturation of erythrocytes. Hemopoiesis or hematopoiesis is the process of origin, development and maturation of all the blood cells.

■ SITE OF ERYTHROPOIESIS

■ IN FETAL LIFE

In fetal life, the erythropoiesis occurs in three stages:

1. *Mesoblastic Stage*

During the first two months of intrauterine life, the RBCs are produced from **mesenchyme** of yolk sac.

2. *Hepatic Stage*

From third month of intrauterine life, **liver** is the main organ that produces RBCs. **Spleen** and **lymphoid organs** are also involved in erythropoiesis.

3. *Myeloid Stage*

During the last three months of intrauterine life, the RBCs are produced from red **bone marrow** and **liver.**

■ IN NEWBORN BABIES, CHILDREN AND ADULTS

In newborn babies, growing children and adults, RBCs are produced only from the red bone marrow.

1. *Up to the age of 20 years:* RBCs are produced from red bone marrow of all bones (**long bones** and all the **flat bones**).
2. *After the age of 20 years:* RBCs are produced from **membranous bones** like vertebra, sternum, ribs, scapula, iliac bones and skull bones and from the ends of long bones. After 20 years of age, the shaft of the long bones becomes yellow bone marrow because of fat deposition and looses the erythropoietic function.

In adults, liver and spleen may produce the blood cells if the bone marrow is destroyed or fibrosed. Collectively bone marrow is almost equal to liver in size and weight. It is also as active as liver. Though bone marrow is the site of production of all blood cells, comparatively 75% of the bone marrow is involved in the production of leukocytes and only 25% is involved in the production of erythrocytes.

But still, the leukocytes are less in number than the erythrocytes, the ratio being 1:500. This is mainly because of the lifespan of these cells. Lifespan of erythrocytes is 120 days whereas the lifespan of leukocytes is very short ranging from one to ten days. So the leukocytes need larger production than erythrocytes to maintain the required number.

■ PROCESS OF ERYTHROPOIESIS

■ STEM CELLS

Stem cells are the primary cells capable of self-renewal and differentiating into specialized cells (Chapter 1). Hemopoietic stem cells are the primitive cells in the bone marrow, which give rise to the blood cells.

Hemopoietic stem cells in the bone marrow are called uncommitted pluripotent hemopoietic stem cells (PHSC). PHSC is defined as a cell that can give rise to all types of blood cells. In early stages, the PHSC are not designed to form a particular type of blood cell. And it is also not possible to determine the blood cell to be developed from these cells: hence, the name uncommitted PHSC (Fig. 10.1). In adults, only a few number of these cells are present. But the best source of these cells is the umbilical cord blood.

When the cells are designed to form a particular type of blood cell, the uncommitted PHSCs are called committed PHSCs. Committed PHSC is defined as a cell, which is restricted to give rise to one group of blood cells.

Committed PHSCs are of two types:
1. Lymphoid stem cells (LSC) which give rise to lymphocytes and natural killer (NK) cells
2. Colony forming blastocytes, which give rise to myeloid cells. Myeloid cells are the blood cells other than lymphocytes. When grown in cultures, these cells form colonies hence the name colony forming blastocytes.

Different units of colony forming cells are:
   i. Colony forming unit-erythrocytes (CFU-E) – Cells of this unit develop into erythrocytes
   ii. Colony forming unit-granulocytes/monocytes (CFU-GM) – These cells give rise to granulocytes (neutrophils, basophils and eosinophils) and monocytes
   iii. Colony forming unit-megakaryocytes (CFU-M) – Platelets are developed from these cells.

■ CHANGES DURING ERYTHROPOIESIS

Cells of CFU-E pass through different stages and finally become the matured RBCs. During these stages four important changes are noticed.
1. Reduction in size of the cell (from the diameter of 25 to 7.2 μ)
2. Disappearance of nucleoli and nucleus

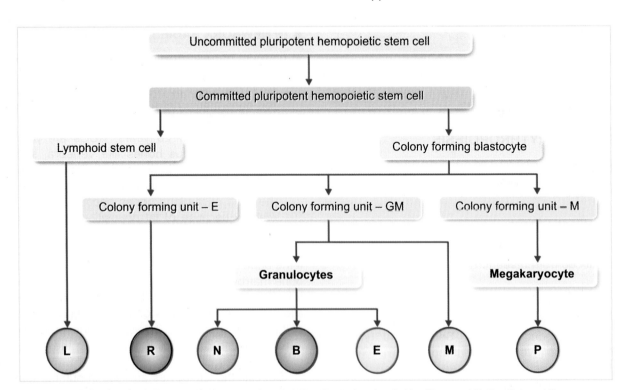

FIGURE 10.1: Stem cells. L = Lymphocyte, R = Red blood cell, N = Neutrophil, B = Basophil, E = Eosinophil, M = Monocyte, P = Platelet.

3. Appearance of hemoglobin
4. Change in the staining properties of the cytoplasm.

■ **STAGES OF ERYTHROPOIESIS**

Various stages between CFU-E cells and matured RBCs are (Fig. 10.2):
1. Proerythroblast
2. Early normoblast
3. Intermediate normoblast.

4. Late normoblast
5. Reticulocyte
6. Matured erythrocyte.

1. *Proerythroblast (Megaloblast)*

Proerythroblast or megaloblast is the first cell derived from CFU-E. It is very large in size with a diameter of about 20 µ. Its nucleus is large and occupies the cell almost completely. The nucleus has two or more nucleoli

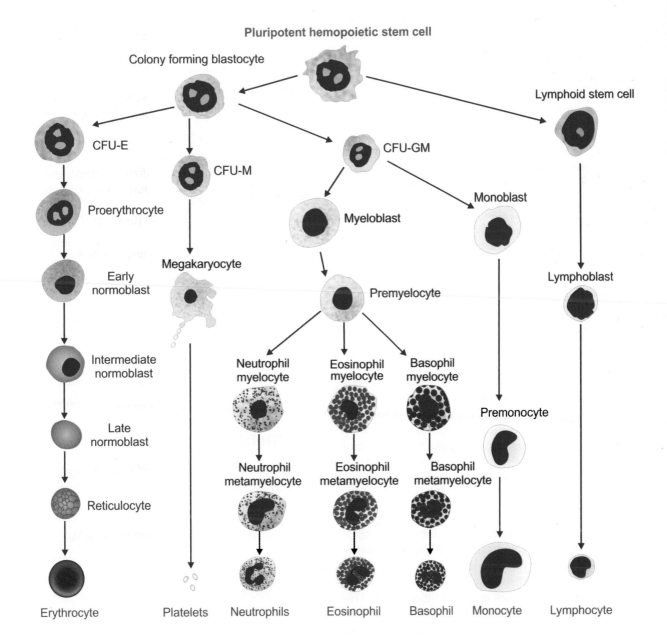

FIGURE 10.2: Stages of erythropoiesis. CFU-E = Colony forming unit-erythrocyte, CFU-M = Colony forming unit-megakaryocyte, CFU-GM = Colony forming unit-granulocyte/monocyte.

and a reticular network. Proerythroblast does not contain hemoglobin. The cytoplasm is basophilic in nature. Proerythroblast multiplies several times and finally forms the cell of next stage called early normoblast. Synthesis of hemoglobin starts in this stage. However, appearance of hemoglobin occurs only in intermediate normoblast.

2. Early Normoblast

The early normoblast is little smaller than proerythroblast with a diameter of about 15 μ. In the nucleus, the nucleoli disappear. Condensation of chromatin network occurs. The condensed network becomes dense. The cytoplasm is basophilic in nature. So, this cell is also called **basophilic erythroblast.** This cell develops into next stage called intermediate normoblast.

3. Intermediate Normoblast

Cell is smaller than the early normoblast with a diameter of 10 to 12 μ. The nucleus is still present. But, the chromatin network shows further condensation. The hemoglobin starts appearing.

Cytoplasm is already basophilic. Now, because of the presence of hemoglobin, it stains with both acidic as well as basic stains. So this cell is called polychromophilic or **polychromatic erythroblast.** This cell develops into next stage called late normoblast.

4. Late Normoblast

Diameter of the cell decreases further to about 8 to 10 μ. Nucleus becomes very small with very much condensed chromatin network and it is known as ink-spot nucleus.

Quantity of hemoglobin increases. And the cytoplasm becomes almost acidophilic. So, the cell is now called orthochromic erythroblast. In the final stage of late normoblast just before it passes to next stage, the nucleus disintegrates and disappears. The process by which nucleus disappears is called **pyknosis.** The final remnant is extruded from the cell. Late normoblast develops into the next stage called reticulocyte.

5. Reticulocyte

Reticulocyte is otherwise known as immature RBC. It is slightly larger than matured RBC. The cytoplasm contains the reticular network or reticulum, which is formed by remnants of disintegrated organelles. Due to the reticular network, the cell is called reticulocyte. The reticulum of reticulocyte stains with supravital stain.

In newborn babies, the reticulocyte count is 2% to 6% of RBCs, i.e. 2 to 6 reticulocytes are present for every 100 RBCs. The number of reticulocytes decreases during the first week after birth. Later, the reticulocyte count remains constant at or below 1% of RBCs. The number increases whenever production and release of RBCs increase.

Reticulocyte is basophilic due to the presence of remnants of disintegrated Golgi apparatus, mitochondria and other organelles of cytoplasm. During this stage, the cells enter the blood capillaries through capillary membrane from site of production by diapedesis. Important events during erythropoiesis is given in Table 10.1

6. Matured Erythrocyte

Reticular network disappears and the cell becomes the matured RBC and attains the biconcave shape. The cell decreases in size to 7.2 μ diameter. The matured RBC is with hemoglobin but without nucleus.

It requires 7 days for the development and maturation of RBC from proerythroblast. It requires 5 days up to the stage of reticulocyte. Reticulocyte takes 2 more days to become the matured RBC.

TABLE 10.1: Important events during erythropoiesis

Stage of erythropoiesis	Important event
Proerythroblast	Synthesis of hemoglobin starts
Early normoblast	Nucleoli disappear
Intermediate normoblast	Hemoglobin starts appearing
Late normoblast	Nucleus disappears
Reticulocyte	Reticulum is formed. Cell enters capillary from site of production
Matured RBC	Reticulum disappears Cell attains biconcavity

■ FACTORS NECESSARY FOR ERYTHROPOIESIS

Development and maturation of erythrocytes require variety of factors, which are classified into three categories:
1. General factors
2. Maturation factors
3. Factors necessary for hemoglobin formation.

■ GENERAL FACTORS

General factors necessary for erythropoiesis are:
    i. Erythropoietin
   ii. Thyroxine
  iii. Hemopoietic growth factors
   iv. Vitamins.

i. *Erythropoietin*

Most important general factor for erythropoiesis is the hormone called erythropoietin. It is also called hemopoietin or erythrocyte stimulating factor.

Chemistry

Erythropoietin is a glycoprotein with 165 amino acids.

Source of secretion

Major quantity of erythropoietin is secreted by peritubular capillaries of kidney. A small quantity is also secreted from liver and brain.

Stimulant for secretion

Hypoxia is the stimulant for the secretion of erythropoietin.

Actions of erythropoietin

Erythropoietin causes formation and release of new RBCs into circulation. After secretion, it takes 4 to 5 days to show the action.

Erythropoietin promotes the following processes:
   a. Production of proerythroblasts from CFU-E of the bone marrow
   b. Development of proerythroblasts into matured RBCs through the several stages – early normoblast, intermediate normoblast, late normoblast and reticulocyte
   c. Release of matured erythrocytes into blood. Even some reticulocytes (immature erythrocytes) are released along with matured RBCs.

Blood level of erythropoietin increases in anemia.

ii. *Thyroxine*

Being a general metabolic hormone, thyroxine accelerates the process of erythropoiesis at many levels. So, hyperthyroidism and polycythemia are common.

iii. *Hemopoietic Growth Factors*

Hemopoietic growth factors or growth inducers are the interleukins and stem cell factor (steel factor). Generally these factors induce the proliferation of PHSCs. Interleukins (IL) are glycoproteins, which belong to the cytokines family.

Interleukins involved in erythropoiesis:
   a. Interleukin-3 (IL-3) secreted by T-cells
   b. Interleukin-6 (IL-6) secreted by T-cells, endothelial cells and macrophages
   c. Interleukin-11 (IL-11) secreted by osteoblast.

iv. *Vitamins*

Some vitamins are also necessary for the process of erythropoiesis. Deficiency of these vitamins cause anemia associated with other disorders.

Vitamins necessary for erythropoiesis:
   a. *Vitamin B:* Its deficiency causes anemia and pellagra (disease characterized by skin lesions, diarrhea, weakness, nervousness and dementia).
   b. *Vitamin C:* Its deficiency causes anemia and scurvy (ancient disease characterized by impaired collagen synthesis resulting in rough skin, bleeding gum, loosening of teeth, poor wound healing, bone pain, lethargy and emotional changes).
   c. *Vitamin D:* Its deficiency causes anemia and rickets (bone disease – Chapter 68).
   d. *Vitamin E:* Its deficiency leads to anemia and malnutrition.

■ MATURATION FACTORS

Vitamin B12, intrinsic factor and folic acid are necessary for the maturation of RBCs.

1. *Vitamin B12 (Cyanocobalamin)*

Vitamin B12 is the maturation factor necessary for erythropoiesis.

Source

Vitamin B12 is called **extrinsic factor** since it is obtained mostly from diet. Its absorption from intestine requires the presence of **intrinsic factor of Castle.** Vitamin B12 is stored mostly in liver and in small quantity in muscle. When necessary, it is transported to the bone marrow to promote maturation of RBCs. It is also produced in the large intestine by the intestinal flora.

Action

Vitamin B12 is essential for synthesis of DNA in RBCs. Its deficiency leads to failure in maturation of the cell and reduction in the cell division. Also, the cells are larger with fragile and weak cell membrane resulting in macrocytic anemia.

Deficiency of vitamin B12 causes **pernicious anemia.** So, vitamin B12 is called antipernicious factor.

2. *Intrinsic Factor of Castle*

Intrinsic factor of castle is produced in gastric mucosa by the parietal cells of the gastric glands. It is essential for the absorption of vitamin B12 from intestine. In the absence of intrinsic factor, vitamin B12 is not absorbed from intestine. This leads to pernicious anemia.

Deficiency of intrinsic factor occurs in:
  i. Severe gastritis
  ii. Ulcer
  iii. Gastrectomy.

Hematinic principle

Hematinic principle is the principle thought to be produced by the action of intrinsic factor on extrinsic factor. It is also called or **antianemia principle.** It is a maturation factor.

3. Folic Acid

Folic acid is also essential for maturation. It is required for the synthesis of DNA. In the absence of folic acid, the synthesis of DNA decreases causing failure of maturation. This leads to anemia in which the cells are larger and appear in megaloblastic (proerythroblastic) stage. And, anemia due to folic acid deficiency is called **megaloblastic anemia.**

■ FACTORS NECESSARY FOR HEMOGLOBIN FORMATION

Various materials are essential for the formation of hemoglobin in the RBCs. Deficiency of these substances decreases the production of hemoglobin leading to anemia.

Such factors are:

1. *First class proteins and amino acids:* Proteins of high biological value are essential for the formation of hemoglobin. Amino acids derived from these proteins are required for the synthesis of protein part of hemoglobin, i.e. the globin.

2. *Iron:* Necessary for the formation of heme part of the hemoglobin.

3. *Copper:* Necessary for the absorption of iron from the gastrointestinal tract.

4. *Cobalt and nickel:* These metals are essential for the utilization of iron during hemoglobin formation.

5. *Vitamins:* Vitamin C, riboflavin, nicotinic acid and pyridoxine are also essential for the formation of hemoglobin.

Hemoglobin and Iron Metabolism

- ■ INTRODUCTION
- ■ NORMAL HEMOGLOBIN CONTENT
- ■ FUNCTIONS
- ■ STRUCTURE
- ■ TYPES OF NORMAL HEMOGLOBIN
- ■ ABNORMAL HEMOGLOBIN
- ■ ABNORMAL HEMOGLOBIN DERIVATIVES
- ■ SYNTHESIS
- ■ DESTRUCTION
- ■ IRON METABOLISM

■ INTRODUCTION

Hemoglobin (Hb) is the iron containing coloring matter of red blood cell (RBC). It is a chromoprotein forming 95% of dry weight of RBC and 30% to 34% of wet weight. Function of hemoglobin is to carry the respiratory gases, oxygen and carbon dioxide. It also acts as a buffer. Molecular weight of hemoglobin is 68,000.

■ NORMAL HEMOGLOBIN CONTENT

Average hemoglobin (Hb) content in blood is 14 to 16 g/dL. However, the value varies depending upon the age and sex of the individual.

Age

At birth	:	25 g/dL
After 3rd month	:	20 g/dL
After 1 year	:	17 g/dL
From puberty onwards	:	14 to 16 g/dL

At the time of birth, hemoglobin content is very high because of increased number of RBCs (Chapter 9).

Sex

In adult males	:	15 g/dL
In adult females	:	14.5 g/dL

■ FUNCTIONS OF HEMOGLOBIN

■ TRANSPORT OF RESPIRATORY GASES

Main function of hemoglobin is the transport of respiratory gases:
1. Oxygen from the lungs to tissues.
2. Carbon dioxide from tissues to lungs.

1. Transport of Oxygen

When oxygen binds with hemoglobin, a physical process called **oxygenation** occurs, resulting in the formation of oxyhemoglobin. The iron remains in ferrous state in this compound. Oxyhemoglobin is an unstable compound and the combination is reversible, i.e. when more oxygen is available, it combines with hemoglobin and whenever oxygen is required, hemoglobin can release oxygen readily (Chapter 125).

When oxygen is released from oxyhemoglobin, it is called reduced hemoglobin or ferrohemoglobin.

2. Transport of Carbon Dioxide

When carbon dioxide binds with hemoglobin, carbhemoglobin is formed. It is also an unstable compound and the combination is reversible, i.e. the carbon dioxide can be released from this compound. The affinity of hemoglobin for carbon dioxide is 20 times more than that for oxygen (Chapter 125).

■ BUFFER ACTION

Hemoglobin acts as a buffer and plays an important role in acid-base balance (Chapter 5).

■ STRUCTURE OF HEMOGLOBIN

Hemoglobin is a conjugated protein. It consists of a protein combined with an iron-containing pigment. The protein part is globin and the iron-containing pigment is **heme.** Heme also forms a part of the structure of **myoglobin** (oxygen-binding pigment in muscles) and **neuroglobin** (oxygen-binding pigment in brain).

■ IRON

Normally, it is present in ferrous (Fe^{2+}) form. It is in unstable or loose form. In some abnormal conditions, the iron is converted into ferric (Fe^{3+}) state, which is a stable form.

■ PORPHYRIN

The pigment part of heme is called porphyrin. It is formed by four pyrrole rings (tetrapyrrole) called, I, II, III and IV. The **pyrrole rings** are attached to one another by methane (CH_4) bridges.

The iron is attached to 'N' of each pyrrole ring and 'N' of globin molecule.

■ GLOBIN

Globin contains four polypeptide chains. Among the four polypeptide chains, two are chains and two are α-chains (Refer Table 11.1 for molecular weight and number of amino acids in the polypeptide chains).

TABLE 11.1: Molecular weight and number of amino acids of polypeptide chains of globin

Polypeptide chain	Molecular weight	Amino acids
α-chain	15,126	141
β-chain	15,866	146

■ TYPES OF NORMAL HEMOGLOBIN

Hemoglobin is of two types:
1. Adult hemoglobin – HbA
2. Fetal hemoglobin – HbF

Replacement of fetal hemoglobin by adult hemoglobin starts immediately after birth. It is completed at about 10th to 12th week after birth. Both the types of hemoglobin differ from each other structurally and functionally.

Structural Difference

In adult hemoglobin, the globin contains two α-chains and two β-chains. In fetal hemoglobin, there are two α chains and two γ-chains instead of β-chains.

Functional Difference

Functionally, fetal hemoglobin has more affinity for oxygen than that of adult hemoglobin. And, the oxygen-hemoglobin dissociation curve of fetal blood is shifted to left (Chapter 125).

■ ABNORMAL HEMOGLOBIN

Abnormal types of hemoglobin or hemoglobin variants are the pathologic mutant forms of hemoglobin. These variants are produced because of structural changes in the polypeptide chains caused by mutation in the genes of the globin chains. Most of the mutations do not produce any serious problem. Occasionally, few mutations result in some disorders.

There are two categories of abnormal hemoglobin:
1. Hemoglobinopathies
2. Hemoglobin in thalassemia and related disorders.

1. *Hemoglobinopathies*

Hemoglobinopathy is a genetic disorder caused by abnormal polypeptide chains of hemoglobin.

Some of the hemoglobinopathies are:
i. *Hemoglobin S:* It is found in sickle cell anemia. In this, the α-chains are normal and β-chains are abnormal.
ii. *Hemoglobin C:* The β-chains are abnormal. It is found in people with hemoglobin C disease, which is characterized by mild hemolytic anemia and splenomegaly.
iii. *Hemoglobin E:* Here also the β-chains are abnormal. It is present in people with hemoglobin E disease which is also characterized by mild hemolytic anemia and splenomegaly.
iv. *Hemoglobin M:* It is the abnormal hemoglobin present in the form of methemoglobin. It occurs due to mutation of genes of both in α and β chains, resulting in abnormal replacement of amino acids. It is present in babies affected by hemoglobin M disease or blue baby syndrome. It is an inherited disease, characterized by methemoglobinemia.

2. Hemoglobin in Thalassemia and Related Disorders

In thalassemia, different types of abnormal hemoglobins are present. The polypeptide chains are decreased, absent or abnormal. In α-thalassemia, the α-chains are decreased, absent or abnormal and in β-thalassemia, the β-chains are decreased, absent or abnormal (Chapter 14). Some of the abnormal hemoglobins found in thalassemia are hemoglobin G, H, I, Bart's, Kenya, Lepore and constant spring.

■ ABNORMAL HEMOGLOBIN DERIVATIVES

'Hemoglobin derivatives' refer to a blood test to detect and measure the percentage of abnormal hemoglobin derivatives.

Hemoglobin is the only carrier for transport of oxygen, without which tissue death occurs within few minutes. When hemoglobin is altered, its oxygen carrying capacity is decreased resulting in lack of oxygen. So, it is important to know about the causes and the effects of abnormal hemoglobin derivatives.

Abnormal hemoglobin derivatives are formed by carbon monoxide (CO) poisoning or due to some drugs like nitrites, nitrates and sulphanamides.

Abnormal hemoglobin derivatives are:

1. Carboxyhemoglobin
2. Methemoglobin
3. Sulfhemoglobin.

Normal percentage of hemoglobin derivatives in total hemoglobin:

Carboxyhemoglobin : 3% to 5 %
Methemoglobin : less than 3%
Sulfhemoglobin : trace (undetectable).

Abnormally high levels of hemoglobin derivates in blood produce serious effects. These derivatives prevent the transport of oxygen resulting in oxygen lack in tissues, which may be fatal.

■ CARBOXYHEMOGLOBIN

Carboxyhemoglobin or carbon monoxyhemoglobin is the abnormal hemoglobin derivative formed by the combination of carbon monoxide with hemoglobin. Carbon monoxide is a colorless and odorless gas. Since hemoglobin has 200 times more affinity for carbon monoxide than oxygen, it hinders the transport of oxygen resulting in tissue hypoxia (Chapter 127).

Normally, 1% to 3% of hemoglobin is in the form of carboxyhemoglobin.

Sources of Carbon Monoxide

1. Charcoal burning
2. Coal mines
3. Deep wells
4. Underground drainage system
5. Exhaust of gasoline engines
6. Gases from guns and other weapons
7. Heating system with poor or improper ventilation
8. Smoke from fire
9. Tobacco smoking.

Signs and Symptoms of Carbon Monoxide Poisoning

1. While breathing air with less than 1% of CO, the Hb saturation is 15% to 20% and mild symptoms like headache and nausea appear
2. While breathing air with more than 1% CO, the Hb saturation is 30% to 40%. It causes severe symptoms like:
   i. Convulsions
   ii. Cardiorespiratory arrest
   iii. Unconsciousness and coma.
3. When Hb saturation increases above 50%, death occurs.

■ METHEMOGLOBIN

Methemoglobin is the abnormal hemoglobin derivative formed when iron molecule of hemoglobin is oxidized from normal ferrous state to ferric state. Methemoglobin is also called **ferrihemoglobin.**

Normal methemoglobin level is 0.6% to 2.5% of total hemoglobin.

Under normal circumstances also, body faces the threat of continuous production of methemoglobin. But it is counteracted by erythrocyte protective system called **nicotinamide adenine dinucleotide (NADH)** system, which operates through two enzymes:

1. Diaphorase I (nicotinamide adenine dinucleotide phosphate [NADPH]-dependent reductase): Responsible for 95% of the action.
2. Diaphorase II (NADPH-dependent methemoglobin reductase): Responsible for 5% of the action.

These two enzymes prevent the oxidation of ferrous iron into ferric iron.

Methemoglobinemia

Methemoglobinemia is the disorder characterized by high level of methemoglobin in blood. It leads to tissue hypoxia, which causes cyanosis and other symptoms.

Causes of methemoglobinemia

Methemoglobinemia is caused by variety of factors:

1. *Common factors of daily life:*

   i. Well water contaminated with nitrates and nitrites
   ii. Fires
   iii. Laundry ink
   iv. Match sticks and explosives
   v. Meat preservatives (which contain nitrates and nitrites)
   vi. Mothballs (naphthalene balls)
   vii. Room deodorizer propellants.

2. *Exposure to industrial chemicals such as:*

   i. Aromatic amines
   ii. Fluorides
   iii. Irritant gases like nitrous oxide and nitrobenzene
   iv. Propylene glycol dinitrate.

3. *Drugs:*

   i. Antibacterial drugs like sulfonamides
   ii. Antimalarial drugs like chloroquine
   iii. Antiseptics
   iv. Inhalant in cyanide antidote kit
   v. Local anesthetics like benzocaine.

4. *Hereditary trait:*

Due to deficiency of NADH-dependant reductase or presence of abnormal hemoglobin M. Hemoglobin M is common in babies affected by blue baby syndrome (a pathological condition in infants, characterized by bluish skin discoloration (cyanosis), caused by congenital heart defect).

■ SULFHEMOGLOBIN

Sulfhemoglobin is the abnormal hemoglobin derivative, formed by the combination of hemoglobin with hydrogen sulfide. It is caused by drugs such as phenacetin or sulfonamides.

Normal sulfhemoglobin level is less than 1% of total hemoglobin.

Sulfhemoglobin cannot be converted back into hemoglobin. Only way to get rid of this from the body is to wait until the affected RBCs with sulfhemoglobin are destroyed after their lifespan.

Blood Level of Sulfhemoglobin

Normally, very negligible amount of sulfhemoglobin is present in blood which is nondetectable. But when its level rises above 10 gm/dL, cyanosis occur. Usually, serious toxic effects are not noticed.

■ SYNTHESIS OF HEMOGLOBIN

Synthesis of hemoglobin actually starts in proerythroblastic stage (Fig. 11.1). However, hemoglobin appears in the intermediate normoblastic stage only. Production of hemoglobin is continued until the stage of reticulocyte.

Heme portion of hemoglobin is synthesized in mitochondria. And the protein part, globin is synthesized in ribosomes.

■ SYNTHESIS OF HEME

Heme is synthesized from succinyl-CoA and the glycine. The sequence of events in synthesis of hemoglobin:

1. First step in heme synthesis takes place in the mitochondrion. Two molecules of succinyl-CoA combine with two molecules of glycine and condense to form δ-aminolevulinic acid (ALA) by ALA synthase.
2. ALA is transported to the cytoplasm. Two molecules of ALA combine to form porphobilinogen in the presence of ALA dehydratase.
3. Porphobilinogen is converted into uroporphobilinogen I by uroporphobilinogen I synthase.
4. Uroporphobilinogen I is converted into uroporphobilinogen III by porphobilinogen III cosynthase.
5. From uroporphobilinogen III, a ring structure called coproporphyrinogen III is formed by uroporphobilinogen decarboxylase.
6. Coproporphyrinogen III is transported back to the mitochondrion, where it is oxidized to form protoporphyrinogen IX by coproporphyrinogen oxidase
7. Protoporphyrinogen IX is converted into protoporphyrin IX by protoporphyrinogen oxidase.
8. Protoporphyrin IX combines with iron to form heme in the presence of ferrochelatase.

■ FORMATION OF GLOBIN

Polypeptide chains of globin are produced in the ribosomes. There are four types of polypeptide chains namely, alpha, beta, gamma and delta chains. Each of these chains differs from others by the amino acid sequence. Each globin molecule is formed by the combination of 2 pairs of chains and each chain is made of 141 to 146 amino acids. Adult hemoglobin contains two alpha chains and two beta chains. Fetal hemoglobin contains two alpha chains and two gamma chains.

■ CONFIGURATION

Each polypeptide chain combines with one heme molecule. Thus, after the complete configuration, each

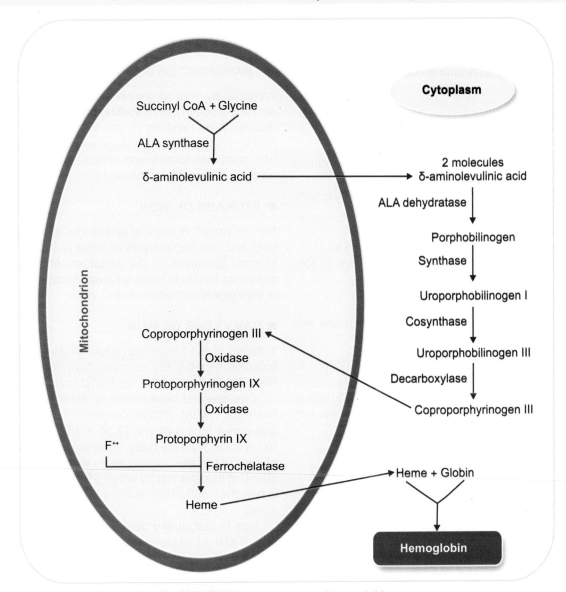

FIGURE 11.1: Synthesis of hemoglobin

hemoglobin molecule contains 4 polypeptide chains and 4 heme molecules.

■ SUBSTANCES NECESSARY FOR HEMOGLOBIN SYNTHESIS

Various materials are essential for the formation of hemoglobin in the RBC (Refer Chapter 10 for details).

■ DESTRUCTION OF HEMOGLOBIN

After the lifespan of 120 days, the RBC is destroyed in the reticuloendothelial system, particularly in spleen and the hemoglobin is released into plasma. Soon, the hemoglobin is degraded in the reticuloendothelial cells and split into globin and heme.

Globin is utilized for the resynthesis of hemoglobin. Heme is degraded into iron and porphyrin. Iron is stored in the body as ferritin and hemosiderin, which are reutilized for the synthesis of new hemoglobin. Porphyrin is converted into a green pigment called biliverdin. In human being, most of the biliverdin is converted into a yellow pigment called bilirubin. Bilirubin and biliverdin are together called the bile pigments (Details of bile pigments are given in Chapter 40).

■ IRON METABOLISM

■ IMPORTANCE OF IRON

Iron is an essential mineral and an important component of proteins, involved in oxygen transport. So, human body needs iron for oxygen transport. Iron is important for the formation of hemoglobin and myoglobin. Iron is also necessary for the formation of other substances like **cytochrome, cytochrome oxidase, peroxidase** and **catalase.**

■ NORMAL VALUE AND DISTRIBUTION OF IRON IN THE BODY

Total quantity of iron in the body is about 4 g. Approximate distribution of iron in the body is as follows:

In the hemoglobin	: 65% to 68%
In the muscle as myoglobin	: 4%
As intracellular oxidative heme compound	: 1%
In the plasma as transferrin	: 0.1%
Stored in the reticuloendothelial system	: 25% to 30%

■ DIETARY IRON

Dietary iron is available in two forms called heme and nonheme.

Heme Iron

Heme iron is present in fish, meat and chicken. Iron in these sources is found in the form of heme. Heme iron is absorbed easily from intestine.

Non-heme Iron

Iron in the form of nonheme is available in vegetables, grains and cereals. Non-heme iron is not absorbed easily as heme iron. Cereals, flours and products of grains which are enriched or fortified (strengthened) with iron become good dietary sources of non-heme iron, particularly for children and women.

■ ABSORPTION OF IRON

Iron is absorbed mainly from the small intestine. It is absorbed through the intestinal cells (enterocytes) by pinocytosis and transported into the blood. Bile is essential for the absorption of iron.

Iron is present mostly in ferric (Fe^{3+}) form. It is converted into ferrous form (Fe^{2+}) which is absorbed into the blood. Hydrochloric acid from gastric juice makes the ferrous iron soluble so that it could be converted into ferric iron by the enzyme ferric reductase from enterocytes. From enterocytes, ferric iron is transported into blood by a protein called ferroportin. In the blood, ferric iron is converted into ferrous iron and transported.

■ TRANSPORT OF IRON

Immediately after absorption into blood, iron combines with a β-globulin called **apotransferrin** (secreted by liver through bile) resulting in the formation of **transferrin.** And iron is transported in blood in the form of transferrin. Iron combines loosely with globin and can be released easily at any region of the body.

■ STORAGE OF IRON

Iron is stored in large quantities in reticuloendothelial cells and liver hepatocytes. In other cells also it is stored in small quantities. In the cytoplasm of the cell, iron is stored as ferritin in large amount. Small quantity of iron is also stored as hemosiderin.

■ DAILY LOSS OF IRON

In males, about 1 mg of iron is excreted everyday through feces. In females, the amount of iron loss is very much high. This is because of the menstruation.

One gram of hemoglobin contains 3.34 mg of iron. Normally, 100 mL of blood contains 15 gm of hemoglobin and about 50 mg of iron (3.34 × 15). So, if 100 mL of blood is lost from the body, there is a loss of about 50 mg of iron. In females, during every menstrual cycle, about 50 mL of blood is lost by which 25 mg of iron is lost. This is why the iron content is always less in females than in males.

Iron is lost during hemorrhage and blood donation also. If 450 mL of blood is donated, about 225 mg of iron is lost.

■ REGULATION OF TOTAL IRON IN THE BODY

Absorption and excretion of iron are maintained almost equally under normal physiological conditions. When the iron storage is saturated in the body, it automatically reduces the further absorption of iron from the gastro-intestinal tract by feedback mechanism.

Factors which reduce the absorption of iron:
1. Stoppage of apotransferrin formation in the liver, so that the iron cannot be absorbed from the intestine.
2. Reduction in the release of iron from the transferrin, so that transferrin is completely saturated with iron and further absorption is prevented.

Erythrocyte Sedimentation Rate

```
■ DEFINITION
■ DETERMINATION
    ■ WESTERGREN'S METHOD
    ■ WINTROBE'S METHOD
■ NORMAL VALUES
■ SIGNIFICANCE OF DETERMINING ESR
■ VARIATIONS OF ESR
    ■ PHYSIOLOGICAL VARIATION
    ■ PATHOLOGICAL VARIATION
■ FACTORS AFFECTING ESR
    ■ FACTORS INCREASEING ESR
    ■ FACTORS DECREASEING ESR
```

■ DEFINITION

Erythrocyte sedimentation rate (ESR) is the rate at which the erythrocytes settle down. Normally, the red blood cells (RBCs) remain suspended uniformly in circulation. This is called suspension stability of RBCs. If blood is mixed with an anticoagulant and allowed to stand on a vertical tube, the red cells settle down due to gravity with a supernatant layer of clear plasma.

ESR is also called sedimentation rate, **sed rate** or **Biernacki reaction.** It was first demonstrated by Edmund Biernacki in 1897.

■ DETERMINATION OF ESR

There are two methods to determine ESR.
1. Westergren method
2. Wintrobe method

■ WESTERGREN METHOD

In this method, Westergren tube is used to determine ESR.

Westergren Tube

The tube is 300 mm long and opened on both ends (Fig. 12.1A). It is marked 0 to 200 mm from above downwards. Westergren tube is used only for determining ESR.

1.6 mL of blood is mixed with 0.4 mL of 3.8% sodium citrate (anticoagulant) and loaded in the Westergren tube. The ratio of blood and anticoagulant is 4:1. The tube is fitted to the stand vertically and left undisturbed. The reading is taken at the end of 1 hour.

■ WINTROBE METHOD

In this method, Wintrobe tube is used to determine ESR.

Wintrobe Tube

Wintrobe tube is a short tube opened on only one end (Fig. 12.1B). It is 110 mm long with 3 mm bore. Wintrobe tube is used for determining ESR and PCV. It is marked on both sides. On one side the marking is from 0 to 100 (for ESR) and on other side from 100 to 0 (for PCV).

About 1 mL of blood is mixed with anticoagulant, ethylenediaminetetraacetic acid (EDTA). The blood is loaded in the tube up to '0' mark and the tube is placed on the Wintrobe stand. And, the reading is taken after 1 hour.

■ NORMAL VALUES OF ESR

By Westergren Method

In males	:	3 to 7	mm in 1 hour
In females	:	5 to 9	mm in 1 hour
Infants	:	0 to 2	mm in 1 hour

By Wintrobe Method

In males	:	0 to 9	mm in 1 hour
In females	:	0 to 15	mm in 1 hour
Infants	:	0 to 5	mm in 1 hour

■ SIGNIFICANCE OF DETERMINING ESR

Erythrocyte sedimentation rate (ESR) is an easy, inexpensive and non-specific test, which helps in diagnosis as well as prognosis. It is non-specific because it cannot indicate the exact location or cause of disease. But, it helps to confirm the diagnosis. Prognosis means monitoring the course of disease and response of the patient to therapy. Determination of ESR is especially helpful in assessing the progress of patients treated for certain chronic inflammatory disorders such as:

1. Pulmonary tuberculosis (Chapter 14)
2. Rheumatoid arthritis (Chapter 14)
3. Polymyalgia rheumatica (inflammatory disease characterized by pain in shoulder and hip)
4. Temporal arteritis (inflammation of arteries of head).

■ VARIATIONS OF ESR

■ PHYSIOLOGICAL VARIATION

1. *Age:* ESR is less in children and infants because of more number of RBCs.
2. *Sex:* It is more in females than in males because of less number of RBCs.
3. *Menstruation:* The ESR increases during menstruation because of loss of blood and RBCs
4. *Pregnancy:* From 3rd month to parturition, ESR increases up to 35 mm in 1 hour because of hemodilution.

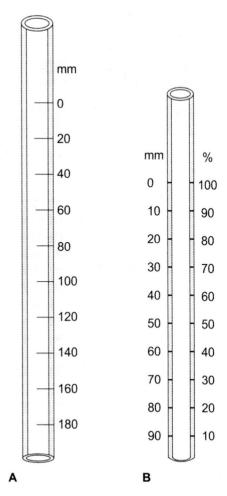

FIGURE 12.1: A. Westergren tube: This is used for determining ESR; **B.** Wintrobe tube: This is used to determine ESR and PCV.

■ PATHOLOGICAL VARIATION

ESR increases in diseases such as the following conditions:

1. Tuberculosis
2. All types of anemia except sickle cell anemia
3. Malignant tumors
4. Rheumatoid arthritis
5. Rheumatic fever
6. Liver diseases.

ESR decreases in the following conditions:

1. Allergic conditions
2. Sickle cell anemia

3. Peptone shock
4. Polycythemia
5. Severe leukocytosis.

■ FACTORS AFFECTING ESR

■ FACTORS INCREASEING ESR

1. *Specific Gravity of RBC*

When the specific gravity of the RBC increases, the cells become heavier and sedimentation is fast. So ESR increases.

2. *Rouleaux Formation*

Rouleaux formation increases the ESR. Globulin and fibrinogen accelerate the rouleaux formation.

3. *Increase in Size of RBC*

When the size of RBC increases (macrocyte), ESR also increases.

■ FACTORS DECREASING ESR

1. *Viscosity of Blood*

Viscosity offers more resistance for settling of RBCs. So when the viscosity of blood increases, the ESR decreases.

2. *RBC count*

When RBC count increases, the viscosity of blood is increased and ESR decreases. And when the RBC count decreases, ESR increases.

Packed Cell Volume and Blood Indices

Chapter **13**

- ■ DEFINITION
- ■ METHOD OF DETERMINATION
- ■ SIGNIFICANCE OF DETERMINING
- ■ NORMAL VALUES
- ■ VARIATIONS
- ■ BLOOD INDICES
- ■ IMPORTANCE OF BLOOD INDICES
- ■ DIFFERENT BLOOD INDICES
- ■ CALCULATION OF BLOOD INDICES

■ DEFINITION

Packed cell volume (PCV) is the proportion of blood occupied by RBCs, expressed in percentage. It is the volume of RBCs packed at the bottom of a hematocrit tube when the blood is centrifuged. It is also called **hematocrit value** or **erythrocyte volume fraction (EVF)**.

■ METHOD OF DETERMINATION

Blood is mixed with the anticoagulant ethylenediamine-tetraacetic acid (EDTA) or heparin and filled in hematocrit or Wintrobe tube (110 mm long and 3 mm bore) up to 100 mark. The tube with the blood is centrifuged at a speed of 3000 revolutions per minute (rpm) for 30 minutes.

RBCs packed at the bottom form the packed cell volume and the plasma remains above this. In between the RBCs and the plasma, there is a **white buffy coat,** which is formed by white blood cells and the platelets (Fig. 13.1).

In the laboratories with modern equipments, hematocrit is not measured directly but calculated indirectly by autoanalyzer. It is determined by multiplying RBC count by mean cell volume. However, some amount of plasma is always trapped between the RBCs. So, accurate value is obtained only by direct measurement of PCV.

■ SIGNIFICANCE OF DETERMINING PCV

Determination of PCV helps in:
1. Diagnosis and treatment of anemia
2. Diagnosis and treatment of polycythemia
3. Determination of extent of dehydration and recovery from dehydration after treatment
4. Decision of blood transfusion.

■ NORMAL VALUES OF PCV

Normal PCV:
In males = 40% to 45%
In females = 38% to 42%

■ VARIATIONS IN PCV

■ INCREASE IN PCV

PCV increases in:
1. Polycythemia
2. Dehydration
3. Dengue shock syndrome: Dengue fever (tropical disease caused by flavivirus transmitted by mosquito *Aedes aegypti*) of grade III or IV severity.

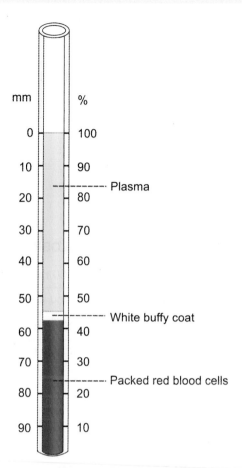

FIGURE 13.1: Packed cell volume

■ DECREASE IN PCV

PCV decreases in:
1. Anemia
2. Cirrhosis of liver (Chapter 40)
3. Pregnancy
4. Hemorrhage due to **ectopic pregnancy** (pregnancy due to implantation of fertilized ovum in tissues other than uterine wall), which is characterized by vaginal bleeding.

■ BLOOD INDICES

Blood indices are the calculations derived from RBC count, hemoglobin content of blood and PCV.

■ IMPORTANCE OF BLOOD INDICES

Blood indices help in diagnosis of the type of anemia.

■ DIFFERENT BLOOD INDICES

Blood indices include:
1. Mean corpuscular volume (MCV).
2. Mean corpuscular hemoglobin (MCH).
3. Mean corpuscular hemoglobin concentration (MCHC).
4. Color Index (CI).

1. Mean Corpuscular Volume (MCV)

MCV is the average volume of a single RBC and it is expressed in cubic microns (cu μ). Normal MCV is 90 cu μ (78 to 90 cu μ).

When MCV is normal, the RBC is called normocyte. When MCV increases, the cell is known as a macrocyte and when it decreases, the cell is called microcyte.

In pernicious anemia and megaloblastic anemia, the RBCs are macrocytic in nature. In iron deficiency anemia the RBCs are microcytic.

2. Mean Corpuscular Hemoglobin (MCH)

MCH is the quantity or amount of hemoglobin present in one RBC. It is expressed in micro-microgram or picogram (pg). Normal value of MCH is 30 pg (27 to 32 pg).

3. Mean Corpuscular Hemoglobin Concentration (MCHC)

MCHC is the concentration of hemoglobin in one RBC. It is the amount of hemoglobin expressed in relation to the volume of one RBC. So, the unit of expression is percentage. This is the most important absolute value in the diagnosis of anemia. Normal value of MCHC is 30% (30% to 38%).

When MCHC is normal, the RBC is normochromic. When the MCHC decreases, the RBC is known hypochromic. In pernicious anemia and megaloblastic anemia, RBCs are macrocytic and normochromic or hypochromic. In iron deficiency anemia, RBCs are microcytic and hypochromic. A single RBC cannot be hyperchromic because, the amount of hemoglobin cannot increase beyond normal.

4. Color Index (CI)

Color index is the ratio between the percentage of hemoglobin and the percentage of RBCs in the blood. Actually, it is the average hemoglobin content in one cell of a patient compared to the average hemoglobin content in one cell of a normal person. Normal color index is 1.0 (0.8 to 1.2). It was widely used in olden days. However, it is useful in determining the type of anemia. It increases in macrocytic (pernicious) anemia and megaloblastic anemia. It is reduced in iron deficiency anemia. And, it is normal in normocytic normochromic anemia.

■ CALCULATION OF BLOOD INDICES

Blood indices are calculated by using different formula. These calculations require the values of RBC count, hemoglobin content and PCV.

For example, in the blood of a male subject:

RBC count	=	4 million/cu mm.
Hemoglobin content	=	8 g/dL
PCV	=	30%

Color index, MCV, MCH and MCHC are calculated as follows:

■ COLOR INDEX

Color index is calculated by dividing the hemoglobin percentage by the RBC count percentage.

$$\text{Thus, color index} = \frac{\text{Hemoglobin \%}}{\text{RBC \%}}$$

Hemoglobin %

$$= \frac{\text{Hemoglobin content in the subject}}{\text{Hemoglobin content in normal persons}} \times 100$$

$$= \frac{8 \text{ g/dL}}{15 \text{ g/dL}} \times 100 = 53.3\%$$

RBC %

$$= \frac{\text{RBC count in the subject}}{\text{RBC count in normal persons}} \times 100$$

$$= \frac{4 \text{ million/cu mm}}{5 \text{ million/cu mm}} \times 100 = 80\%$$

By using these two values, CI is calculated

$$\text{Color Index} = \frac{\text{Hemoglobin\%}}{\text{RBC\%}} = \frac{53.3\%}{80\%} = 0.67$$

Thus, color index = 0.67

■ MEAN CORPUSCULAR VOLUME

$$MCV = \frac{\text{PCV in mL / 1,000 mL of blood}}{\text{RBC count in million/cu mm of blood}}$$

$$= \frac{\text{PCV in 1000 mL or in 100 mL} \times 10}{\text{RBC count in million/cu mm}} \text{ cu } \mu$$

$$MCV = \frac{30 \times 10}{4} = 75 \text{ cu } \mu.$$

Thus, MCV = 75 cu μ

■ MEAN CORPUSCULAR HEMOGLOBIN

$$MCH = \frac{\text{Hemoglobin in gram per 1000 ml of blood}}{\text{RBC count in million/cu mm}}$$

$$MCH = \frac{\text{Hemoglobin in gram per 100 ml of blood} \times 10}{\text{RBC count in million/cu mm}}$$

$$= \frac{80}{4} \text{ pg.}$$

Thus, MCH = 20 pg or micro-micro gram.

■ MEAN CORPUSCULAR HEMOGLOBIN CONCENTRATION

$$MCHC = \frac{\text{Hemoglobin in gram/100 mL of blood}}{\text{PCV in 100 mL of blood}} \times 100$$

$$= \frac{8}{30} \times 100$$

$$= \frac{800}{30} \%$$

Thus, MCHC = 26.67%.

■ RESULTS

CI	=	0.67	(Normal = 0.8 to1.2)
MCV	=	75 cu μ	(Normal = 78 to 90 cu μ)
MCH	=	20 pg	(Normal = 27 to 32 pg)
MCHC	=	26.67%	(Normal = 30% to 38%)

Results of these indices indicate that the person is suffering from microcytic hypochromic anemia, which commonly occurs during iron deficiency.

Anemia

```
■ INTRODUCTION
■ CLASSIFICATION
■ SIGNS AND SYMPTOMS
```

■ INTRODUCTION

Anemia is the blood disorder, characterized by the reduction in:
1. Red blood cell (RBC) count
2. Hemoglobin content
3. Packed cell volume (PVC).

Generally, reduction in RBC count, hemoglobin content and PCV occurs because of:
1. Decreased production of RBC
2. Increased destruction of RBC
3. Excess loss of blood from the body.

All these incidents are caused either by inherited disorders or environmental influences such as nutritional problem, infection and exposure to drugs or toxins.

■ CLASSIFICATION OF ANEMIA

Anemia is classified by two methods:
1. Morphological classification
2. Etiological classification.

■ MORPHOLOGICAL CLASSIFICATION

Morphological classification depends upon the size and color of RBC. Size of RBC is determined by mean corpuscular volume (MCV). Color is determined by mean corpuscular hemoglobin concentration (MCHC). By this method, the anemia is classified into four types (Table 14.1):

1. Normocytic Normochromic Anemia

Size (MCV) and color (MCHC) of RBCs are normal. But the number of RBC is less.

2. Macrocytic Normochromic Anemia

RBCs are larger in size with normal color. RBC count is less.

3. Macrocytic Hypochromic Anemia

RBCs are larger in size. MCHC is less, so the cells are pale (less colored).

4. Microcytic Hypochromic Anemia

RBCs are smaller in size with less color.

■ ETIOLOGICAL CLASSIFICATION

On the basis of etiology (study of cause or origin), anemia is divided into five types (Table 14.2):
1. Hemorrhagic anemia
2. Hemolytic anemia
3. Nutrition deficiency anemia
4. Aplastic anemia
5. Anemia of chronic diseases.

TABLE 14.1: Morphological classification of anemia

Type of anemia	Size of RBC (MCV)	Color of RBC (MCHC)
Normocytic normochromic	Normal	Normal
Normocytic hypochromic	Normal	Less
Macrocytic hypochromic	Large	Less
Microcytic hypochromic	Small	Less

1. *Hemorrhagic Anemia*

Hemorrhage refers to excessive loss of blood (Chapter 115). Anemia due to hemorrhage is known as hemorrhagic anemia. It occurs both in acute and chronic hemorrhagic conditions.

Acute hemorrhage

Acute hemorrhage refers to sudden loss of a large quantity of blood as in the case of accident. Within about 24 hours after the hemorrhage, the plasma portion of blood is replaced. However, the replacement of RBCs does not occur quickly and it takes at least 4 to 6 weeks. So with less number of RBCs, hemodilution occurs. However, morphologically the RBCs are normocytic and normochromic.

Decreased RBC count causes hypoxia, which stimulates the bone marrow to produce more number of RBCs. So, the condition is corrected within 4 to 6 weeks.

Chronic hemorrhage

It refers to loss of blood by internal or external bleeding, over a long period of time. It occurs in conditions like peptic ulcer, purpura, hemophilia and menorrhagia.

Due to continuous loss of blood, lot of iron is lost from the body causing iron deficiency. This affects the synthesis of hemoglobin resulting in less hemoglobin content in the cells. The cells also become small. Hence, the RBCs are microcytic and hypochromic (Table 14.2).

2. *Hemolytic Anemia*

Hemolysis means destruction of RBCs. Anemia due to excessive hemolysis which is not compensated by increased RBC production is called hemolytic anemia. It is classified into two types:
  A. Extrinsic hemolytic anemia.
  B. Intrinsic hemolytic anemia.

A. *Extrinsic hemolytic anemia:* It is the type of anemia caused by destruction of RBCs by external factors. Healthy RBCs are hemolyzed by factors outside the blood cells such as antibodies, chemicals and drugs. Extrinsic hemolytic anemia is also called **autoimmune hemolytic anemia.**

Common causes of external hemolytic anemia:
  i. Liver failure
  ii. Renal disorder

TABLE 14.2: Etiological classification of anemia

Type of anemia	Causes	Morphology of RBC
Hemorrhagic anemia	Acute loss of blood	Normocytic, normochromic
	Chronic loss of blood	Microcytic, hypochromic

Hemolytic anemia	Extrinsic hemolytic anemia:
	  i. Liver failure
	  ii. Renal disorder
	  iii. Hypersplenism
	  iv. Burns
	  v. Infections – hepatitis, malaria and septicemia
	  vi. Drugs – Penicillin, antimalarial drugs and sulfa drugs
	  vii. Poisoning by lead, coal and tar
	  viii. Presence of isoagglutinins like anti Rh
	  xi. Autoimmune diseases – rheumatoid arthritis and ulcerative colitis
		Normocytic normochromic

	Intrinsic hemolytic anemia: Hereditary disorders	Sickle cell anemia: Sickle shape
		Thalassemia: Small and irregular
Nutrition deficiency anemia	Iron deficiency	Microcytic, hypochromic
	Protein deficiency	Macrocytic, hypochromic
	Vitamin B12	Macrocytic, normochromic/hypochromic
	Folic acid	Megaloblastic, hypochromic
Aplastic anemia	Bone marrow disorder	Normocytic, normochromic
Anemia of chronic diseases	i. Non-infectious inflammatory diseases – rheumatoid arthritis ii. Chronic infections – tuberculosis iii. Chronic renal failure iv. Neoplastic disorders – Hodgkin's disease	Normocytic, normochromic

iii. Hypersplenism

iv. Burns

v. Infections like hepatitis, malaria and septicemia

vi. Drugs such as penicillin, antimalarial drugs and sulfa drugs

vii. Poisoning by chemical substances like lead, coal and tar

viii. Presence of isoagglutinins like anti-Rh

ix. Autoimmune diseases such as rheumatoid arthritis and ulcerative colitis.

B. *Intrinsic hemolytic anemia:* It is the type of anemia caused by destruction of RBCs because of the defective RBCs. There is production of unhealthy RBCs, which are short lived and are destroyed soon. Intrinsic hemolytic anemia is often inherited and it includes sickle cell anemia and thalassemia.

Because of the abnormal shape in sickle cell anemia and thalassemia, the RBCs become more fragile and susceptible for hemolysis.

Sickle cell anemia

Sickle cell anemia is an inherited blood disorder, characterized by sickle-shaped red blood cells. It is also called **hemoglobin SS disease** or **sickle cell disease.** It is common in people of African origin.

Sickle cell anemia is due to the abnormal hemoglobin called hemoglobin S (sickle cell hemoglobin). In this, α-chains are normal and β-chains are abnormal. The molecules of hemoglobin S polymerize into long chains and precipitate inside the cells. Because of this, the RBCs attain sickle (crescent) shape and become more fragile leading to hemolysis (Fig. 14.1). Sickle cell anemia occurs when a person inherits two abnormal genes (one from each parent).

In children, hemolyzed sickle cells aggregate and block the blood vessels, leading to infarction (stoppage of blood supply). The infarction is common in small bones. The infarcted small bones in hand and foot results in varying length in the digits. This condition is known as **hand and foot syndrome.** Jaundice also occurs in these children.

Thalassemia

Thalassemia is an inherited disorder, characterized by abnormal hemoglobin. It is also known as **Cooley's anemia** or **Mediterranean anemia.** It is more common in Thailand and to some extent in Mediterranean countries.

Thalassemia is of two types:

i. α-thalassemia

ii. β-thalassemia.

The β-thalassemia is very common among these two.

In normal hemoglobin, number of α and β polypeptide chains is equal. In thalassemia, the production of these chains become imbalanced because of defective synthesis of globin genes. This causes the precipitation of the polypeptide chains in the immature RBCs, leading to disturbance in erythropoiesis. The precipitation also occurs in mature red cells, resulting in hemolysis.

α-Thalassemia

α-thalassemia occurs in fetal life or infancy. In this α-chains are less, absent or abnormal. In adults, β-chains are in excess and in children, γ-chains are in excess. This leads to defective erythropoiesis and hemolysis. The infants may be stillborn or may die immediately after birth.

β-Thalassemia

In β-thalassemia, β-chains are less in number, absent or abnormal with an excess of α-chains. The α-chains precipitate causing defective erythropoiesis and hemolysis.

3. *Nutrition Deficiency Anemia*

Anemia that occurs due to deficiency of a nutritive substance necessary for erythropoiesis is called nutrition deficiency anemia. The substances which are necessary for erythropoiesis are iron, proteins and vitamins like C, B12 and folic acid. The types of nutrition deficiency anemia are:

Iron deficiency anemia

Iron deficiency anemia is the most common type of anemia. It develops due to inadequate availability of iron for hemoglobin synthesis. RBCs are microcytic and hypochromic.

Causes of iron deficiency anemia:

i. Loss of blood

ii. Decreased intake of iron

iii. Poor absorption of iron from intestine

iv. Increased demand for iron in conditions like growth and pregnancy.

Features of iron deficiency anemia: Features of iron deficiency anemia are brittle nails, spoon-shaped nails **(koilonychias),** brittle hair, atrophy of papilla in tongue and **dysphagia** (difficulty in swallowing).

Protein deficiency anemia

Due to deficiency of proteins, the synthesis of hemoglobin is reduced. The RBCs are macrocytic and hypochromic.

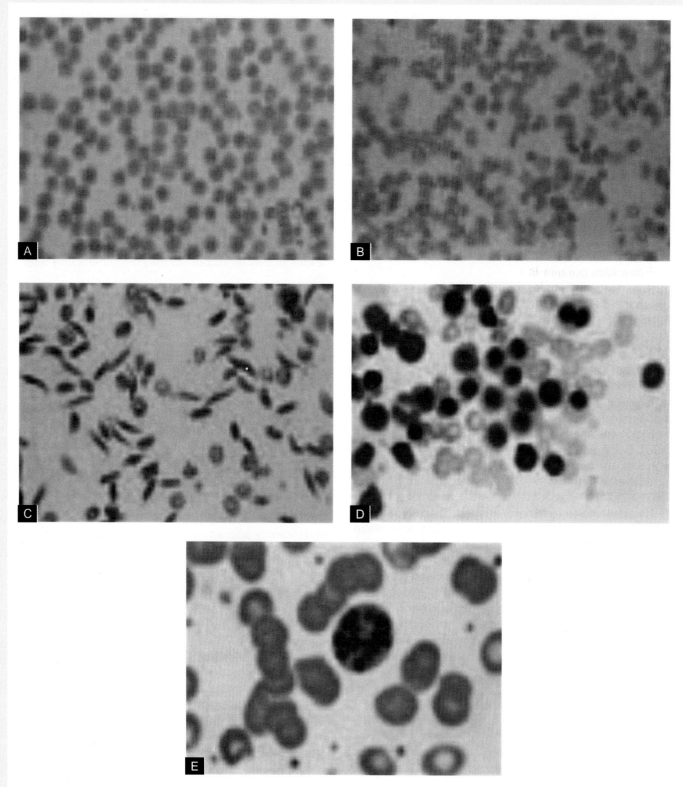

FIGURE 14.1: A. Normal RBC; **B.** Hypochromic anemia; **C.** Sickle cell anemia; **D.** Thalassemia;
E. Megaloblastic anemia (*Courtesy:* Dr Nivaldo Medeiros).

Pernicious anemia or Addison's anemia

Pernicious anemia is the anemia due to deficiency of vitamin B12. It is also called Addison's anemia. It is due to atrophy of the gastric mucosa because of autoimmune destruction of parietal cells. The gastric atrophy results in decreased production of intrinsic factor and poor absorption of vitamin B12, which is the maturation factor for RBC. RBCs are larger and immature with almost normal or slightly low hemoglobin level. Synthesis of hemoglobin is almost normal in this type of anemia. So, cells are macrocytic and normochromic/hypochromic.

Before knowing the cause of this anemia, it was very difficult to treat the patients and the disease was considered to be fatal. So, it was called pernicious anemia.

Pernicious anemia is common in old age and it is more common in females than in males. It is associated with other autoimmune diseases like disorders of thyroid gland, Addison's disease, etc. Characteristic features of this type of anemia are lemon yellow color of skin (due to anemic paleness and mild jaundice) and red sore tongue. Neurological disorders such as **paresthesia** (abnormal sensations like numbness, tingling, burning, etc.), **progressive weakness** and **ataxia** (muscular incoordination) are also observed in extreme conditions.

Megaloblastic anemia

Megaloblastic anemia is due to the deficiency of another maturation factor called folic acid. Here, the RBCs are not matured. The DNA synthesis is also defective, so the nucleus remains immature. The RBCs are megaloblastic and hypochromic.

Features of pernicious anemia appear in megaloblastic anemia also. However, neurological disorders may not develop.

4. *Aplastic Anemia*

Aplastic anemia is due to the disorder of red bone marrow. Red bone marrow is reduced and replaced by fatty tissues. Bone marrow disorder occurs in the following conditions:
   i. Repeated exposure to X-ray or gamma ray radiation.
   ii. Presence of bacterial toxins, quinine, gold salts, benzene, radium, etc.
   iii. Tuberculosis.
   iv. Viral infections like hepatitis and HIV infections.
   In aplastic anemia, the RBCs are normocytic and normochromic.

5. *Anemia of Chronic Diseases*

Anemia of chronic diseases is the second common type of anemia (next to iron deficiency anemia). It is characterized by short lifespan of RBCs, caused by disturbance in iron metabolism or resistance to erythropoietin action. Anemia develops after few months of sustained disease. RBCs are normocytic and normochromic.

   Common causes anemia of chronic diseases:
   i. Non-infectious inflammatory diseases such as **rheumatoid arthritis** (chronic inflammatory autoimmune disorder affecting joints).
   ii. Chronic infections like tuberculosis (infection caused by *Mycobacterium tuberculosis*) and abscess (collection of pus in the infected tissue) in lungs.
   iii. Chronic renal failure, in which the erythropoietin secretion decreases (since erythropoietin is necessary for the stimulation of bone marrow to produce RBCs, its deficiency causes anemia).
   iv. Neoplastic disorders (abnormal and disorganized growth in tissue or organ) such as **Hodgkin's disease** (malignancy involving lymphocytes) and cancer of lung and breast.

   RBCs are generally normocytic and normochromic in this type of anemia. However, in progressive disease associated with iron deficiency the cells become microcytic and hypochromic.

■ SIGNS AND SYMPTOMS OF ANEMIA

■ SKIN AND MUCOUS MEMBRANE

Color of the skin and mucous membrane becomes pale. Paleness is more constant and prominent in buccal and pharyngeal mucous membrane, conjunctivae, lips, ear lobes, palm and nail bed. Skin looses the elasticity and becomes thin and dry. Thinning, loss and early grayness of hair occur. The nails become brittle and easily breakable.

■ CARDIOVASCULAR SYSTEM

There is an increase in heart rate (tachycardia) and cardiac output. Heart is dilated and cardiac murmurs are produced. The velocity of blood flow is increased.

■ RESPIRATION

There is an increase in rate and force of respiration. Sometimes, it leads to breathlessness and dyspnea (difficulty in breathing). Oxygen-hemoglobin dissociation curve is shifted to right.

■ DIGESTION

Anorexia, nausea, vomiting, abdominal discomfort and constipation are common. In pernicious anemia, there is atrophy of papillae in tongue. In aplastic anemia, necrotic lesions appear in mouth and pharynx.

■ METABOLISM

Basal metabolic rate increases in severe anemia.

■ KIDNEY

Renal function is disturbed. Albuminuria is common.

■ REPRODUCTIVE SYSTEM

In females, the menstrual cycle is disturbed. There may be menorrhagia, oligomenorrhea or amenorrhea (Chapter 80).

■ NEUROMUSCULAR SYSTEM

Common neuromuscular symptoms are increased sensitivity to cold, headache, lack of concentration, restlessness, irritability, drowsiness, dizziness or vertigo (especially while standing) and fainting. Muscles become weak and the patient feels lack of energy and fatigued quite often and quite easily.

Hemolysis and Fragility of Red Blood Cells

- ■ **DEFINITION**
- ■ **PROCESS OF HEMOLYSIS**
- ■ **FRAGILITY TEST**
- ■ **CONDITIONS WHEN HEMOLYSIS OCCURS**
- ■ **HEMOLYSINS**
  - ■ **CHEMICAL SUBSTANCES**
  - ■ **SUBSTANCES OF BACTERIAL ORIGIN OR SUBSTANCES FOUND IN BODY**

■ DEFINITION

1. Hemolysis: Hemolysis is the destruction of formed elements. To define more specifically, it is the process, which involves the breakdown of red blood cells (RBCs) and liberation of hemoglobin.
2. Fragility: Susceptibility (to be affected) of RBC to hemolysis or tendency to break easily is called fragility (Fragile = easily broken).

   Fragility is of two types:
   i. **Osmotic fragility,** which occurs due to exposure to hypotonic saline
   ii. **Mechanical fragility,** which occurs due to mechanical trauma (wound or injury).

   Under normal conditions, only old RBCs are destroyed in the reticuloendothelial system. Abnormal hemolysis is the process by which even younger RBCs are destroyed in large number by the presence of hemolytic agents or hemolysins.

■ PROCESS OF HEMOLYSIS

Normally, plasma and RBCs are in osmotic equilibrium. When the osmotic equilibrium is disturbed, the cells are affected. For example, when the RBCs are immersed in hypotonic saline the cells swell and rupture by bursting because of **endosmosis** (Chapter 4). The hemoglobin is released from the ruptured RBCs.

■ FRAGILITY TEST

Fragility test is a test that measures the resistance of erythrocytes in hypotonic saline solution. It is done by using sodium chloride solution at different concentrations from 1.2% to 0.2%. The solutions at different concentrations are taken in series of Cohn's tubes. Then one drop of blood to be tested is added to each tube. The sodium chloride solution and the blood in each tube are mixed well and left undisturbed for some time.

Results can be analyzed by observing the tubes directly or by centrifuging the tubes after 15 minutes.

Direct observations

1. If there is no hemolysis: Fluid in the tube appears turbid
2. If hemolysis is started: Turbidity is reduced
3. If hemolysis is completed: Fluid becomes clear.

Observations after centrifugation

1. If there is no hemolysis: Cells sediment at the bottom with clear colorless fluid above
2. If hemolysis is started: Cell sedimentation is less and the fluid becomes slightly reddish because of the release of small amount of hemoglobin from few hemolyzed RBCs
3. If hemolysis is completed: Fluid becomes more reddish without any sedimentation due to release of

more amount of hemoglobin from all the hemolyzed cells.

Index for Fragility

After 20 minutes:

No hemolysis	=	up to 0.6%
Onset of hemolysis	=	around 0.45%
Completion of hemolysis	=	around 0.35%

At 0.45%, only the older cells are destroyed because, their membrane is fragile. So, these cells cannot withstand this hypotonicity. But, younger cells are not affected. At 0.35%, even the younger cells are destroyed.

■ CONDITIONS WHEN HEMOLYSIS OCCURS

1. Hemolytic jaundice
2. Antigen-antibody reactions
3. Poisoning by chemicals or toxins
4. While using artificial kidney for hemodialysis or heart-lung machine during cardiac surgery (rare occasions).

■ HEMOLYSINS

Hemolysins or hemolytic agents are the substances, which cause destruction of RBCs. The hemolysins are of two types:
A. Chemical substances
B. Substances of bacterial origin or substances found in body.

■ A. CHEMICAL SUBSTANCES

1. Alcohol
2. Benzene
3. Chloroform
4. Ether
5. Acids
6. Alkalis
7. Bile salts
8. Saponin
9. Chemical poisons like:
   i. Arsenial preparations
   ii. Carbolic acid
   iii. Nitrobenzene
   iv. Resin.

■ B. SUBSTANCES OF BACTERIAL ORIGIN OR SUBSTANCES FOUND IN BODY

1. Toxic substances or toxins from bacteria:
   i. *Streptococcus*
   ii. *Staphylococcus*
   iii. Tetanus bacillus, etc.
2. Venom of poisonous snakes like cobra
3. Hemolysins from normal tissues.

White Blood Cells

Chapter 16

- ■ INTRODUCTION
- ■ CLASSIFICATION
- ■ MORPHOLOGY
- ■ NORMAL COUNT
- ■ VARIATIONS
- ■ LIFESPAN
- ■ PROPERTIES
- ■ FUNCTIONS
- ■ LEUKOPOIESIS

■ INTRODUCTION

White blood cells (WBCs) or leukocytes are the colorless and nucleated formed elements of blood (leuko is derived from Greek word leukos = white). Alternate spelling for leukocytes is leucocytes.

Compared to RBCs, the WBCs are larger in size and lesser in number. Yet functionally, these cells are important like RBCs because of their role in defense mechanism of body and protect the body from invading organisms by acting like soldiers.

WBCs Vs RBCs

WBCs differ from RBCs in many aspects. The differences between WBCs and RBCs are given in Table 16.1.
1. Larger in size.
2. Irregular in shape.
3. Nucleated.
4. Many types.
5. Granules are present in some type of WBCs.
6. Lifespan is shorter.

■ CLASSIFICATION

Some of the WBCs have granules in the cytoplasm. Based on the presence or absence of granules in the cytoplasm, the leukocytes are classified into two groups:
1. Granulocytes which have granules.
2. Agranulocytes which do not have granules.

1. Granulocytes

Depending upon the staining property of granules, the granulocytes are classified into three types:
   i. Neutrophils with granules taking both acidic and basic stains.
   ii. Eosinophils with granules taking acidic stain.
   iii. Basophils with granules taking basic stain.

2. Agranulocytes

Agranulocytes have plain cytoplasm without granules. Agranulocytes are of two types:
   i. Monocytes.
   ii. Lymphocytes.

■ MORPHOLOGY OF WHITE BLOOD CELLS

■ NEUTROPHILS

Neutrophils which are also known as polymorphs have fine or small granules in the cytoplasm. The granules take acidic and basic stains. When stained with **Leishman's stain** (which contains acidic eosin and basic methylene blue) the granules appear violet in color.

Nucleus is multilobed (Fig. 16.1). The number of lobes in the nucleus depends upon the age of cell. In younger cells, the nucleus is not lobed. And in older neutrophils, the nucleus has 2 to 5 lobes. The diameter

TABLE 16.1: Differences between WBCs and RBCs

Feature	WBCs	RBCs
Color	Colorless	Red
Number	Less: 4,000 to 11,000/cu mm	More: 4.5 to 5.5 million/cu mm
Size	Larger Maximum diameter = 18 μ	Smaller Maximum diameter = 7.4 μ
Shape	Irregular	Disk-shaped and biconcave
Nucleus	Present	Absent
Granules	Present in some types	Absent
Types	Many types	Only one type
Lifespan	Shorter ½ to 15 days	Longer 120 days

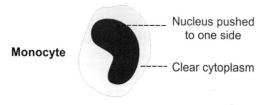

Neutrophil — Fine granules with eosin and methylene blue stain

— Multilobed nucleus

Eosinophil — Coarse granules with eosin stain

— Bilobed nucleus

Basophil — Coarse granules with methylene blue stain

— Bilobed nucleus

Monocyte — Nucleus pushed to one side

— Clear cytoplasm

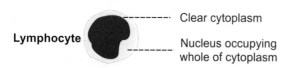

Lymphocyte — Clear cytoplasm

— Nucleus occupying whole of cytoplasm

FIGURE 16.1: Different white blood cells

of cell is 10 to 12 μ (Table 16.2). The neutrophils are ameboid in nature.

■ EOSINOPHILS

Eosinophils have coarse (larger) granules in the cytoplasm, which stain pink or red with eosin. Nucleus is bilobed and spectacle-shaped. Diameter of the cell varies between 10 and 14 μ.

■ BASOPHILS

Basophils also have coarse granules in the cytoplasm. The granules stain purple blue with methylene blue. Nucleus is bilobed. Diameter of the cell is 8 to 10 μ.

■ MONOCYTES

Monocytes are the largest leukocytes with diameter of 14 to 18 μ. The cytoplasm is clear without granules. Nucleus is round, oval and horseshoe shaped, bean shaped or kidney shaped. Nucleus is placed either in the center of the cell or pushed to one side and a large amount of cytoplasm is seen.

■ LYMPHOCYTES

Like monocytes, the lymphocytes also do not have granules in the cytoplasm. Nucleus is oval, bean-shaped or kidney-shaped. Nucleus occupies the whole of the cytoplasm. A rim of cytoplasm may or may not be seen.

Types of Lymphocytes

Depending upon the size, lymphocytes are divided into two groups:
1. *Large lymphocytes:* Younger cells with a diameter of 10 to 12 μ.
2. *Small lymphocytes:* Older cells with a diameter of 7 to 10 μ.

Depending upon the function, lymphocytes are divided into two types:
1. *T lymphocytes:* Cells concerned with cellular immunity.
2. *B lymphocytes:* Cells concerned with humoral immunity.

TABLE 16.2: Diameter and lifespan of WBCs

WBC	Diameter (μ)	Lifespan (days)
Neutrophils	10 to 12	2 to 5
Eosinophils	10 to 14	7 to 12
Basophils	8 to 10	12 to 15
Monocytes	14 to 18	2 to 5
Lymphocytes	7 to 12	½ to 1

■ NORMAL WHITE BLOOD CELL COUNT

1. Total WBC count (TC): 4,000 to 11,000/cu mm of blood.
2. Differential WBC count (DC): Given in Table 16.3.

■ VARIATIONS IN WHITE BLOOD CELL COUNT

Leukocytosis

Leukocytosis is the increase in total WBC count. Leukocytosis occurs in both physiological and pathological conditions.

Leukopenia

Leukopenia is the decrease in total WBC count. The term leukopenia is generally used for pathological conditions only.

Granulocytosis

Granulocytosis is the abnormal increase in the number of granulocytes.

Granulocytopenia

Granulocytopenia is the abnormal reduction in the number of granulocytes.

Agranulocytosis

Agranulocytosis is the acute pathological condition characterized by absolute lack of granulocytes.

■ PHYSIOLOGICAL VARIATIONS

1. *Age:* WBC count is about 20,000 per cu mm in infants and about 10,000 to 15,000 per cu mm of blood in children. In adults, it ranges between 4,000 and 11,000 per cu mm of blood.
2. *Sex:* Slightly more in males than in females.
3. *Diurnal variation:* Minimum in early morning and maximum in the afternoon.

TABLE 16.3: Normal values of different WBCs

WBC	Percentage	Absolute value per cu mm
Neutrophils	50 to 70	3,000 to 6,000
Eosinophils	2 to 4	150 to 450
Basophils	0 to 1	0 to 100
Monocytes	2 to 6	200 to 600
Lymphocytes	20 to 30	1,500 to 2,700

4. *Exercise:* Increases slightly.
5. *Sleep:* Decreases.
6. *Emotional conditions like anxiety:* Increases.
7. *Pregnancy:* Increases.
8. *Menstruation:* Increases.
9. *Parturition:* Increases.

■ PATHOLOGICAL VARIATIONS

All types of leukocytes do not share equally in the increase or decrease of total leukocyte count. In general, the neutrophils and lymphocytes vary in opposite directions.

Leukocytosis

Leukocytosis is the increase in total leukocyte (WBC) count. It occurs in conditions such as:
1. Infections
2. Allergy
3. Common cold
4. Tuberculosis
5. Glandular fever.

Leukemia

Leukemia is the condition which is characterized by abnormal and uncontrolled increase in leukocyte count more than 1,000,000/cu mm. It is also called blood cancer.

Leukopenia

Leukopenia is the decrease in the total WBC count. It occurs in the following pathological conditions:
1. Anaphylactic shock
2. Cirrhosis of liver
3. Disorders of spleen
4. Pernicious anemia
5. Typhoid and paratyphoid
6. Viral infections.

Variation in Differential Leukocyte Count

Differential leukocyte count varies in specific diseases. Details are given in Table 16.4.

Neutrophilia

Neutrophilia or neutrophilic leukocytosis is the increase in neutrophil count. It occurs in the following conditions:
1. Acute infections
2. Metabolic disorders
3. Injection of foreign proteins

4. Injection of vaccines
5. Poisoning by chemicals and drugs like lead, mercury, camphor, benzene derivatives, etc.
6. Poisoning by insect venom
7. After acute hemorrhage.

Eosinophilia

Eosinophilia is the increase in eosinophil count and it occurs in:

1. Asthma and other allergic conditions
2. Blood parasitism (malaria, filariasis)

TABLE 16.4: Pathological variations in different types of WBCs

Disorder	Variation	Conditions
Neutrophilia or neutrophilic leukocytosis	Increase in neutrophil count	1. Acute infections 2. Metabolic disorders 3. Injection of foreign proteins 4. Injection of vaccines 5. Poisoning by chemicals and drugs like lead, mercury, camphor, benzene derivatives, etc. 6. Poisoning by insect venom 7. After acute hemorrhage
Neutropenia	Decrease in neutrophil count	1. Bone marrow disorders 2. Tuberculosis 3. Typhoid 4. Autoimmune diseases
Eosinophilia	Increase in eosinophil count	1. Allergic conditions like asthma 2. Blood parasitism (malaria, filariasis) 3. Intestinal parasitism 4. Scarlet fever
Eosinopenia	Decrease in eosinophil count	1. Cushing's syndrome 2. Bacterial infections 3. Stress 4. Prolonged administration of drugs like steroids, ACTH and epinephrine
Basophilia	Increase in basophil count	1. Smallpox 2. Chickenpox 3. Polycythemia vera
Basopenia	Decrease in basophil count	1. Urticaria (skin disorder) 2. Stress 3. Prolonged exposure to chemotherapy or radiation therapy
Monocytosis	Increase in monocyte count	1. Tuberculosis 2. Syphilis 3. Malaria 4. Kala-azar
Monocytopenia	Decrease in monocyte count	Prolonged use of prednisone (immunosuppressant steroid)
Lymphocytosis	Increase in lymphocyte count	1. Diphtheria 2. Infectious hepatitis 3. Mumps 4. Malnutrition 5. Rickets 6. Syphilis 7. Thyrotoxicosis 8. Tuberculosis
Lymphocytopenia	Decrease in lymphocyte count	1. AIDS 2. Hodgkin's disease (cancer of lymphatic system) 3. Malnutrition 4. Radiation therapy 5. Steroid administration

3. Intestinal parasitism
4. Scarlet fever.

Basophilia

Basophilia is the increase in basophil count and it occurs in:
1. Smallpox
2. Chickenpox
3. Polycythemia vera.

Monocytosis

Monocytosis is the increase in monocyte count and it occurs in:
1. Tuberculosis
2. Syphilis
3. Malaria
4. Kala-azar
5. Glandular fever.

Lymphocytosis

Lymphocytosis is the increase in lymphocyte count and it occurs in:
1. Diphtheria
2. Infectious hepatitis
3. Mumps
4. Malnutrition
5. Rickets
6. Syphilis
7. Thyrotoxicosis
8. Tuberculosis.

Neutropenia

Neutropenia is the decrease in neutrophil count. It occurs in:
1. Bone marrow disorders
2. Tuberculosis
3. Typhoid
4. Vitamin deficiencies
5. Autoimmune diseases.

Eosinopenia

Decrease in eosinophil count is called eosinopenia. It occurs in:
1. Cushing's syndrome
2. Bacterial infections
3. Stress
4. Prolonged administration of drugs such as steroids, ACTH, epinephrine.

Basopenia

Basopenia or basophilic leukopenia is the decrease in basophil count. It occurs in:
1. Urticaria (skin disorder)
2. Stress
3. Prolonged exposure to chemotherapy or radiation therapy.

Monocytopenia

Monocytopenia is the decrease in monocyte count. It occurs in:
1. Prolonged use of prednisone (immunosuppressant steroid)
2. AIDS
3. Chronic lymphoid leukemia.

Lymphocytopenia

Lymphocytopenia is the decrease in lymphocytes. It occurs in:
1. AIDS
2. Hodgkin's disease (cancer of the lymphatic system)
3. Malnutrition
4. Radiation therapy
5. Steroid administration.

■ LIFESPAN OF WHITE BLOOD CELLS

Lifespan of WBCs is not constant. It depends upon the demand in the body and their function. Lifespan of these cells may be as short as half a day or it may be as long as 3 to 6 months. Lifespan of WBCs is given in Table 16.2.

■ PROPERTIES OF WHITE BLOOD CELLS

1. Diapedesis

Diapedesis is the process by which the leukocytes squeeze through the narrow blood vessels.

2. Ameboid Movement

Neutrophils, monocytes and lymphocytes show amebic movement, characterized by protrusion of the cytoplasm and change in the shape.

3. Chemotaxis

Chemotaxis is the attraction of WBCs towards the injured tissues by the chemical substances released at the site of injury.

4. *Phagocytosis*

Neutrophils and monocytes engulf the foreign bodies by means of phagocytosis (Chapter 3).

■ FUNCTIONS OF WHITE BLOOD CELLS

Generally, WBCs play an important role in defense mechanism. These cells protect the body from invading organisms or foreign bodies, either by destroying or inactivating them. However, in defense mechanism, each type of WBCs acts in a different way.

■ NEUTROPHILS

Neutrophils play an important role in the defense mechanism of the body. Along with monocytes, the neutrophils provide the first line of defense against the invading microorganisms. The neutrophils are the free cells in the body and wander freely through the tissue and practically, no part of the body is spared by these leukocytes.

Substances Present in Granules and Cytoplasm of Neutrophils

Granules of neutrophils contain enzymes like proteases, myeloperoxidases, elastases and metalloproteinases (Table 16.5). These enzymes destroy the microorganisms. The granules also contain antibody like peptides called **cathelicidins** and **defensins,** which are antimicrobial peptides and are active against bacteria and fungi.

Membrane of neutrophils contains an enzyme called **NADPH oxidase** (dihydronicotinamide adenine dinucleotide phosphate oxidase). It is activated by the toxic metabolites released from infected tissues. The activated NADPH oxidase is responsible for bactericidal action of neutrophils (see below).

All these substances present in the granules and cell membrane make the neutrophil a powerful and effective killer machine.

Neutrophils also secrete **platelet-activating factor (PAF),** which is a cytokine. It accelerates the aggregation of platelets during injury to the blood vessel, resulting in prevention of excess loss of blood.

Mechanism of Action of Neutrophils

Neutrophils are released in large number at the site of infection from the blood. At the same time, new neutrophils are produced from the progenitor cells. All the neutrophils move by diapedesis towards the site of infection due to chemotaxis.

Chemotaxis occurs due to the attraction by some chemical substances called **chemoattractants,** which are released from the infected area. After reaching the area, the neutrophils surround the area and get adhered to the infected tissues. Chemoattractants increase the adhesive nature of neutrophils so that all the neutrophils become sticky and get attached firmly to the infected area. Each neutrophil can hold about 15 to 20 microorganisms at a time. Now, the neutrophils start destroying the invaders. First, these cells engulf the bacteria and then destroy them by means of phagocytosis (Chapter 3).

Respiratory Burst

Respiratory burst is a rapid increase in oxygen consumption during the process of phagocytosis by neutrophils and other phagocytic cells. Nicotinamide adenine dinucleotide phosphate (NADPH) oxidase is responsible for this phenomenon. During respiratory burst, the free radical O_2^- is formed. $2O_2^-$ combine with $2H^+$ to form H_2O_2 (hydrogen peroxide). Both O_2^- and H_2O_2 are the oxidants having potent bactericidal action.

Pus and Pus Cells

Pus is the whitish yellow fluid formed in the infected tissue by the dead WBCs, bacteria or foreign bodies and cellular debris. It consists of white blood cells, bacteria or other foreign bodies and cellular debris. The dead WBCs are called pus cells.

During the battle against the bacteria, many WBCs are killed by the toxins released from the bacteria. The dead cells are collected in the center of infected area. The dead cells together with plasma leaked from the blood vessel, liquefied tissue cells and RBCs escaped from damaged blood vessel (capillaries) constitute the pus.

■ EOSINOPHILS

Eosinophils play an important role in the defense mechanism of the body against the parasites. During parasitic infections, there is a production of a large number of eosinophils which move towards the tissues affected by parasites. Eosinophil count increases also during allergic diseases like asthma.

Eosinophils are responsible for detoxification, disintegration and removal of foreign proteins.

Mechanism of Action of Eosinophils

Eosinophils are neither markedly motile nor phagocytic like the neutrophils. Some of the parasites are larger in size. Still eosinophils attack them by some special type of cytotoxic substances present in their granules. When

TABLE 16.5: Substances secreted by WBCs

WBC	Substance secreted	Action
Neutrophil	Proteases	Destruction of microorganisms
	Myeloperoxidases	
	Elastases	
	Metalloproteinases	
	Defensins	Antimicrobial action Anti-inflammatory action Wound healing Chemotaxis
	Cathelicidins	Antimicrobial action
	NADPH oxidase	Bactericidal action
	Platelet-activating factor	Aggregation of platelets
Eosinophil	Eosinophil peroxidase	Destruction of worms, bacteria and tumor cells
	Major basic protein	Destruction of worms
	Eosinophil cationic protein	Destruction of worms Neurotoxic action
	Eosinophil-derived neurotoxin	Neurotoxic action
	Interleukin-4 and 5	Acceleration of inflammatory response Destruction of invading organisms
Basophil	Heparin	Prevention of intravascular blood clotting
	Histamine	
	Bradykinin	Production of acute hypersensitivity reactions
	Serotonin	
	Proteases	Destruction of microorganisms
	Myeloperoxidases	
	Interleukin-4	Acceleration of inflammatory response Destruction of invading organisms
Monocyte	Interleukin-1	Acceleration of inflammatory response Destruction of invading organisms
	Colony stimulation factor	Formation of colony forming blastocytes
	Platelet-activating factor	Aggregation of platelets
	Chemokines	Chemotaxis
T lymphocytes	Interleukin-2, 4 and 5	Acceleration of inflammatory response Destruction of invading organisms Activation of T cells
	Gamma interferon	Stimulation of phagocytic actions of cytotoxic cells, macrophages and natural killer cells
	Lysosomal enzymes	Destruction of invading organisms
	Tumor necrosis factor	Necrosis of tumor Activation of immune system Promotion of inflammation
	Chemokines	Chemotaxis

Contd...

	Immunoglobulins	Destruction of invading organisms
B lymphocytes	Tumor necrosis factor	Necrosis of tumor Activation of immune system Acceleration of inflammatory response
	Chemokines	Chemotaxis

released over the invading parasites from the granules, these substances become lethal and destroy the parasites. The lethal substances present in the granules of eosinophils and released at the time of exposure to parasites or foreign proteins are:

1. *Eosinophil peroxidase*: This enzyme is capable of destroying helminths (parasitic worms), bacteria and tumor cells.
2. *Major basic protein (MBP):* It is very active against helminths. It destroys the parasitic worms by causing distension (ballooning) and detachment of the tegumental sheath (skin-like covering) of these organisms.
3. *Eosinophil cationic protein (ECP):* This substance is the major destroyer of helminths and it is about 10 times more toxic than MBP. It destroys the parasites by means of complete disintegration. It is also a neurotoxin.
4. *Eosinophil-derived neurotoxin:* It destroys the nerve fibers particularly, the myelinated nerve fibers.
5. *Cytokines:* Cytokines such as interleukin-4 and interleukin-5 accelerate inflammatory responses by activating eosinophils. These cytokines also kill the invading organisms.

■ BASOPHILS

Basophils play an important role in healing processes. So their number increases during healing process.

Basophils also play an important role in allergy or acute hypersensitivity reactions (allergy). This is because of the presence of receptors for IgE in basophil membrane.

Mechanism of Action of Basophils

Functions of basophils are executed by the release of some important substances from their granules such as:

1. *Heparin:* Heparin is essential to prevent the intravascular blood clotting.
2. *Histamine, slow-reacting substances of anaphylaxis, bradykinin and serotonin:* Theses substances produce the acute hypersensitivity reactions by causing vascular and tissue responses.
3. *Proteases and myeloperoxidase:* These enzymes destroy the microorganisms.

4. *Cytokine:* Cytokine such as interleukin-4 accelerates inflammatory responses and kill the invading organisms.

Mast Cell

Mast cell is a large tissue cell resembling the basophil. Generally, mast cells are found along with the blood vessels and are prominently seen in the areas such as skin, mucosa of the lungs and digestive tract, mouth, conjunctiva and nose. These cells usually do not enter the bloodstream.

Origin

Mast cells are developed in the bone marrow, but their precursor cells are different. After differentiation, the immature mast cells enter the tissues. Maturation of mast cells takes place only after entering the tissue.

Functions

Mast cell plays an important role in producing the hypersensitivity reactions like allergy and anaphylaxis (Chapter 17). When activated, the mast cell immediately releases various chemical mediators from its granules into the interstitium. Two types of substances are secreted by mast cell:

1. *Preformed mediators:* These substances are already formed and stored in secretory granules. These substances are histamine, heparin, serotonin, hydrolytic enzymes, proteoglycans and chondroitin sulfates.
2. *Newly generated mediators:* These substances are absent in the mast cell during resting conditions and are produced only during activation. These substances are **arachidonic acid** derivatives such as leukotriene C (LTC), prostaglandin and cytokines.

■ MONOCYTES

Monocytes are the largest cells among the leukocytes. Like neutrophils, monocytes also are motile and phagocytic in nature. These cells wander freely through all tissues of the body.

Monocytes play an important role in defense of the body. Along with neutrophils, these leukocytes provide the first line of defense.

Monocytes secrete:

1. Interleukin-1 (IL-1).
2. Colony stimulating factor (M-CSF).
3. Platelet-activating factor (PAF).

Monocytes are the precursors of the tissue macrophages. Matured monocytes stay in the blood only for few hours. Afterwards, these cells enter the tissues from the blood and become tissue macrophages. Examples of tissue macrophages are Kupffer cells in liver, alveolar macrophages in lungs and macrophages in spleen. Functions of macrophages are discussed in Chapter 24.

■ LYMPHOCYTES

Lymphocytes play an important role in immunity. Functionally, the lymphocytes are classified into two categories, namely T lymphocytes and B lymphocytes. T lymphocytes are responsible for the development of cellular immunity and B lymphocytes are responsible for the development of humoral immunity. The functions of these two types of lymphocytes are explained in detail in Chapter 17.

■ LEUKOPOIESIS

Leukopoiesis is the development and maturation of leukocytes (Fig. 16.2).

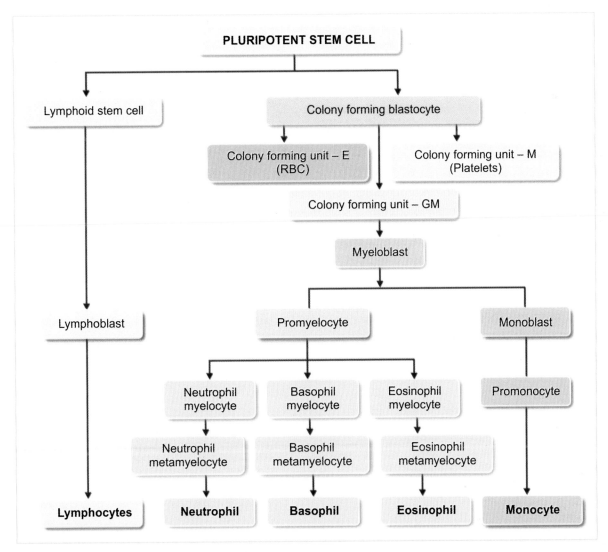

FIGURE 16.2: Leukopoiesis

■ STEM CELLS

Committed pluripotent stem cell gives rise to leukocytes through various stages. Details are given in Chapter 10.

■ FACTORS NECESSARY FOR LEUKOPOIESIS

Leukopoiesis is influenced by hemopoietic growth factors and colony stimulating factors. Hemopoietic growth factors are discussed in Chapter 10.

Colony stimulating Factors

Colony stimulating factors (CSF) are proteins which cause the formation of colony forming blastocytes. Colony stimulating factors are of three types:

1. Granulocyte-CSF (G-CSF) secreted by monocytes and endothelial cells
2. Granulocyte-monocyte-CSF (GM-CSF) secreted by monocytes, endothelial cells and T lymphocytes
3. Monocyte-CSF (M-CSF) secreted by monocytes and endothelial cells.

Immunity

Chapter 17

- ■ DEFINITION AND TYPES OF IMMUNITY
- ■ DEVELOPMENT AND PROCESSING OF LYMPHOCYTES
- ■ ANTIGENS
- ■ DEVELOPMENT OF CELL-MEDIATED IMMUNITY
- ■ DEVELOPMENT OF HUMORAL IMMUNITY
- ■ NATURAL KILLER CELL
- ■ CYTOKINES
- ■ IMMUNIZATION
- ■ IMMUNE DEFICIENCY DISEASES
- ■ AUTOIMMUNE DISEASES
- ■ ALLERGY AND IMMUNOLOGICAL HYPERSENSITIVITY REACTIONS

■ DEFINITION AND TYPES OF IMMUNITY

Immunity is defined as the capacity of the body to resist pathogenic agents. It is the ability of body to resist the entry of different types of foreign bodies like bacteria, virus, toxic substances, etc.

Immunity is of two types:
I. Innate immunity.
II. Acquired immunity.

■ INNATE IMMUNITY OR NON-SPECIFIC IMMUNITY

Innate immunity is the inborn capacity of the body to resist pathogens. By chance, if the organisms enter the body, innate immunity eliminates them before the development of any disease. It is otherwise called the natural or non-specific immunity.

This type of immunity represents the first line of defense against any type of pathogens. Therefore, it is also called non-specific immunity.

Mechanisms of Innate Immunity

Various mechanisms of innate immunity are given in Table 17.1.

■ ACQUIRED IMMUNITY OR SPECIFIC IMMUNITY

Acquired immunity is the resistance developed in the body against any specific foreign body like bacteria, viruses, toxins, vaccines or transplanted tissues. So, this type of immunity is also known as specific immunity.

It is the most powerful immune mechanism that protects the body from the invading organisms or toxic substances. Lymphocytes are responsible for acquired immunity (Fig. 17.1).

Types of Acquired Immunity

Two types of acquired immunity develop in the body:
1. Cellular immunity
2. Humoral immunity.

Lymphocytes are responsible for the development of these two types of immunity.

■ DEVELOPMENT AND PROCESSING OF LYMPHOCYTES

In fetus, lymphocytes develop from the bone marrow (Chapter 10). All lymphocytes are released in the circulation and are differentiated into two categories.

TABLE 17.1: Mechanisms of innate immunity

Structures and Mediators	Mechanism
Gastrointestinal tract	Enzymes in digestive juices and the acid in stomach destroy the toxic substances or organisms entering digestive tract through food Lysozyme present in saliva destroys bacteria
Respiratory system	Defensins and cathelicidins in epithelial cells of air passage are antimicrobial peptides Neutrophils, lymphocytes, macrophages and natural killer cells present in lungs act against bacteria and virus
Urinogenital system	Acidity in urine and vaginal fluid destroy the bacteria
Skin	The keratinized stratum corneum of epidermis protects the skin against toxic chemicals The β-defensins in skin are antimicrobial peptides Lysozyme secreted in skin destroys bacteria
Phagocytic cells	Neutrophils, monocytes and macrophages ingest and destroy the microorganisms and foreign bodies by phagocytosis
Interferons	Inhibit multiplication of viruses, parasites and cancer cells
Complement proteins	Accelerate the destruction of microorganisms

The two categories are:
1. T lymphocytes or T cells, which are responsible for the development of cellular immunity
2. B lymphocytes or B cells, which are responsible for humoral immunity.

■ T LYMPHOCYTES

T lymphocytes are processed in thymus. The processing occurs mostly during the period between just before birth and few months after birth.

Thymus secretes a hormone called thymosin, which plays an important role in immunity. It accelerates the proliferation and activation of lymphocytes in thymus. It also increases the activity of lymphocytes in lymphoid tissues.

Types of T Lymphocytes

During the processing, T lymphocytes are transformed into four types:
1. Helper T cells or inducer T cells. These cells are also called **CD4 cells** because of the presence of molecules called CD4 on their surface.
2. Cytotoxic T cells or killer T cells. These cells are also called **CD8 cells** because of the presence of molecules called CD8 on their surface.
3. Suppressor T cells.
4. Memory T cells.

Storage of T Lymphocytes

After the transformation, all the types of T lymphocytes leave the thymus and are stored in lymphoid tissues of lymph nodes, spleen, bone marrow and GI tract.

■ B LYMPHOCYTES

B lymphocytes were first discovered in the bursa of Fabricius in birds, hence the name B lymphocytes. **Bursa of Fabricius** is a lymphoid organ situated near the cloaca of birds. Bursa is absent in mammals and the processing of B lymphocytes takes place in liver (during fetal life) and bone marrow (after birth).

Types of B Lymphocytes

After processing, the B lymphocytes are transformed into two types:
1. Plasma cells.
2. Memory cells.

Storage of B Lymphocytes

After transformation, the B lymphocytes are stored in the lymphoid tissues of lymph nodes, spleen, bone marrow and the GI tract.

■ ANTIGENS

■ DEFINITION AND TYPES

Antigens are the substances which induce specific immune reactions in the body.

Antigens are of two types:
1. Autoantigens or self antigens present on the body's own cells such as 'A' antigen and 'B' antigen in RBCs.
2. Foreign antigen s or non-self antigens that enter the body from outside.

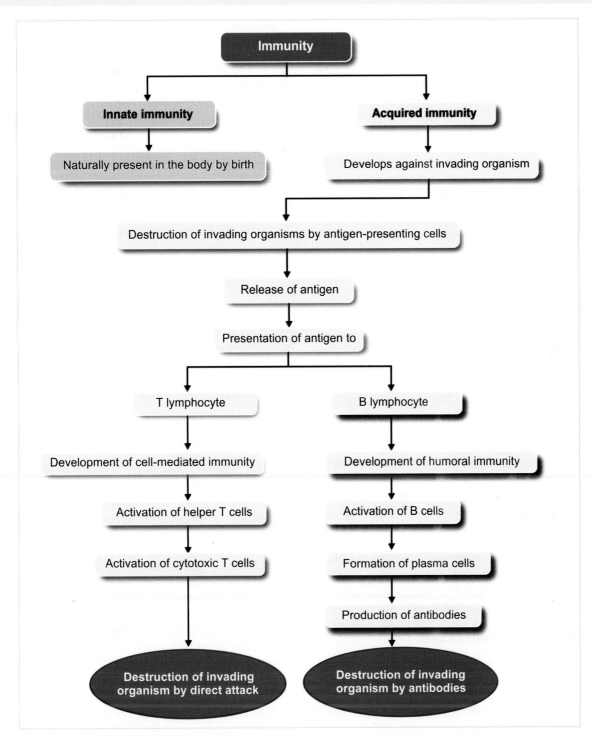

FIGURE 17.1: Schematic diagram showing development of immunity

■ NON-SELF ANTIGENS

Following are non-self antigens:

1. Receptors on the cell membrane of microbial organisms such as bacteria, viruses and fungi.

2. Toxins from microbial organisms.

3. Materials from transplanted organs or incompatible blood cells.

4. **Allergens** or allergic substances like pollen grains.

Types of Non-self Antigens

Non-self antigens are classified into two types, depending upon the response developed against them in the body:
1. Antigens, which induce the development of immunity or production of antibodies (**immunogenicity**).
2. Antigens, which react with specific antibodies and produce allergic reactions (**allergic reactivity**). (The allergic reaction is explained in the later part of this chapter).

■ CHEMICAL NATURE OF THE ANTIGENS

Antigens are mostly the conjugated proteins like lipoproteins, glycoproteins and nucleoproteins.

■ DEVELOPMENT OF CELL-MEDIATED IMMUNITY

■ INTRODUCTION

Cell-mediated immunity is defined as the immunity developed by cell-mediated response. It is also called cellular immunity or T cell immunity. It involves several types of cells such as T lymphocytes, macrophages and natural killer cells and hence the name cell mediated immunity. Cell-mediated immunity does not involve antibodies.

Cellular immunity is the major defense mechanism against infections by viruses, fungi and few bacteria like tubercle bacillus. It is also responsible for delayed allergic reactions and the rejection of transplanted tissues.

Cell-mediated immunity is offered by T lymphocytes and it starts developing when T cells come in contact with the antigens. Usually, the invading microbial or non-microbial organisms carry the antigenic materials. These antigenic materials are released from invading organisms and are presented to the helper T cells by antigen-presenting cells.

■ ANTIGEN-PRESENTING CELLS

Antigen-presenting cells are the special type of cells in the body, which induce the release of antigenic materials from invading organisms and later present these materials to the helper T cells.

Types of Antigen-Presenting Cells

Antigen-presenting cells are of three types:
1. Macrophages
2. Dendritic cells
3. B lymphocytes.
Among these cells, macrophages are the major antigen-presenting cells.

1. Macrophages

Macrophages are the large phagocytic cells, which digest the invading organisms to release the antigen. The macrophages are present along with lymphocytes in almost all the lymphoid tissues.

2. Dendritic Cells

Dendritic cells are nonphagocytic in nature. Based on the location, dendritic cells are classified into three categories:
   i. Dendritic cells of spleen, which trap the antigen in blood.
   ii. Follicular dendritic cells in lymph nodes, which trap the antigen in the lymph.
   iii. Langerhans dendritic cells in skin, which trap the organisms coming in contact with body surface.

3. B Lymphocytes

Recently, it is found that B lymphocytes also act as antigen-presenting cells. Thus, the B cells function as both antigen-presenting cells and antigen receiving cells. However, B cells are the least efficient antigen-presenting cells and need to be activated by helper T cells.

Role of Antigen-presenting Cells

Invading foreign organisms are either engulfed by macrophages through phagocytosis or trapped by dendritic cells. Later, the antigen from these organisms is digested into small peptide products. These antigenic peptide products move towards the surface of the antigen-presenting cells and bind with human leukocyte antigen (HLA). HLA is a genetic matter present in the molecule of class II major histocompatiblility complex (MHC), which is situated on the surface of the antigen-presenting cells.

B-cells ingest the foreign bodies by means of pinocytosis. Role of B cells as antigen-presenting cells in the body is not fully understood.

MHC and HLA

Major histocompatibility complex (MHC) is a large molecule present in the short arm of chromosome 6. It is made up of a group of genes which are involved in immune system. It has more than 200 genes including HLA genes. HLA is made up of genes with small molecules. It encodes antigen-presenting proteins on the cell surface.

Though MHC molecules and HLA genes are distinct terms, both are used interchangeably. Particularly in human, the MHC molecules are often referred as HLA molecules. MHC molecules in human beings are divided into two types:

1. Class I MHC molecule: It is found on every cell in human body. It is specifically responsible for presentation of endogenous antigens (antigens produced intracellularly such as viral proteins and tumor antigens) to cytotoxic T cells.
2. Class II MHC molecule: It is found on B cells, macrophages and other antigen-presenting cells. It is responsible for presenting the exogenous antigens (antigens of bacteria or viruses which are engulfed by antigen-presenting cells) to helper T cells.

Presentation of Antigen

Antigen-presenting cells present their class II MHC molecules together with antigen-bound HLA to the helper T cells. This activates the helper T cells through series of events (Fig. 17.2).

Sequence of Events during Activation of Helper T cells

1. Helper T cell recognizes the antigen displayed on the surface of the antigen-presenting cell with the help of its own surface receptor protein called T cell receptor.
2. Recognition of the antigen by the helper T cell initiates a complex interaction between the helper T cell receptor and the antigen. This reaction activates helper T cells.
3. At the same time, macrophages (the antigen-presenting cells) release interleukin-1, which facilitates the activation and proliferation of helper T cells.
4. Activated helper T cells proliferate and the proliferated cells enter the circulation for further actions.

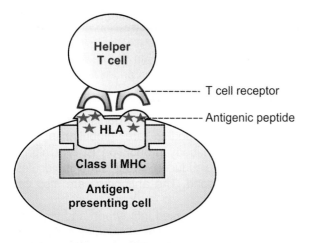

FIGURE 17.2: Antigen presentation. The antigen-presenting cells present their class II MHC molecules together with antigen-bound HLA to the helper T cells. MHC = Major histocompatiblility complex. HLA = Human leukocyte antigen.

5. Simultaneously, the antigen which is bound to class II MHC molecules activates the B cells also, resulting in the development of humoral immunity (see below).

■ ROLE OF HELPER T CELLS

Helper T cells (CD4 cells) which enter the circulation activate all the other T cells and B cells. Normal, CD4 count in healthy adults varies between 500 and 1500 per cubic millimeter of blood.

Helper T cells are of two types:
1. Helper-1 (TH1) cells
2. Helper-2 (TH2) cells.

Role of TH1 Cells

TH1 cells are concerned with cellular immunity and secrete two substances:
   i. Interleukin-2, which activates the other T cells.
   ii. Gamma interferon, which stimulates the phagocytic activity of cytotoxic cells, macrophages and natural killer (NK) cells.

Role of TH2 Cells

TH2 cells are concerned with humoral immunity and secrete interleukin-4 and interleukin-5, which are concerned with:
   i. Activation of B cells.
   ii. Proliferation of plasma cells.
   iii. Production of antibodies by plasma cell.

■ ROLE OF CYTOTOXIC T CELLS

Cytotoxic T cells that are activated by helper T cells, circulate through blood, lymph and lymphatic tissues and destroy the invading organisms by attacking them directly.

Mechanism of Action of Cytotoxic T Cells

1. Receptors situated on the outer membrane of cytotoxic T cells bind the antigens or organisms tightly with cytotoxic T cells.
2. Then, the cytotoxic T cells enlarge and release cytotoxic substances like the lysosomal enzymes.
3. These substances destroy the invading organisms.
4. Like this, each cytotoxic T cell can destroy a large number of microorganisms one after another.

Other Actions of Cytotoxic T Cells

1. Cytotoxic T cells also destroy cancer cells, transplanted cells, such as those of transplanted heart or kidney or any other cells, which are foreign bodies.

2. Cytotoxic T cells destroy even body's own tissues which are affected by the foreign bodies, particularly the viruses. Many viruses are entrapped in the membrane of affected cells. The antigen of the viruses attracts the T cells. And the cytotoxic T cells kill the affected cells also along with viruses. Because of this, the cytotoxic T cell is called killer cell.

■ ROLE OF SUPPRESSOR T CELLS

Suppressor T cells are also called regulatory T cells. These T cells suppress the activities of the killer T cells. Thus, the suppressor T cells play an important role in preventing the killer T cells from destroying the body's own tissues along with invaded organisms. Suppressor cells suppress the activities of helper T cells also.

■ ROLE OF MEMORY T CELLS

Some of the T cells activated by an antigen do not enter the circulation but remain in lymphoid tissue. These T cells are called memory T cells.

In later periods, the memory cells migrate to various lymphoid tissues throughout the body. When the body is exposed to the same organism for the second time, the memory cells identify the organism and immediately activate the other T cells. So, the invading organism is destroyed very quickly. The response of the T cells is also more powerful this time.

■ SPECIFICITY OF T CELLS

Each T cell is designed to be activated only by one type of antigen. It is capable of developing immunity against that antigen only. This property is called the specificity of T cells.

■ DEVELOPMENT OF HUMORAL IMMUNITY

■ INTRODUCTION

Humoral immunity is defined as the immunity mediated by antibodies, which are secreted by B lymphocytes. B lymphocytes secrete the antibodies into the blood and lymph. The blood and lymph are the body fluids (**humours** or **humors** in Latin). Since the B lymphocytes provide immunity through humors, this type of immunity is called humoral immunity or B cell immunity.

Antibodies are the gamma globulins produced by B lymphocytes. These antibodies fight against the invading organisms. The humoral immunity is the major defense mechanism against the bacterial infection.

As in the case of cell-mediated immunity, the macrophages and other antigen-presenting cells play an important role in the development of humoral immunity also.

■ ROLE OF ANTIGEN-PRESENTING CELLS

The ingestion of foreign organisms and digestion of their antigen by the antigen-presenting cells are already explained.

Presentation of Antigen

Antigen-presenting cells present the antigenic products bound with HLA (which is present in class II MHC molecule) to B cells. This activates the B cells through series of events.

Sequence of Events during Activation of B Cells

1. B cell recognizes the antigen displayed on the surface of the antigen-presenting cell, with the help of its own surface receptor protein called B cell receptor.
2. Recognition of the antigen by the B cell initiates a complex interaction between the B cell receptor and the antigen. This reaction activates B cells.
3. At the same time, macrophages (the antigen-presenting cells) release interleukin-1, which facilitates the activation and proliferation of B cells.
4. Activated B cells proliferate and the proliferated cells carry out the further actions.
5. Simultaneously, the antigen bound to class II MHC molecules activates the helper T cells, also resulting in development of cell-mediated immunity (already explained).

Transformation B Cells

Proliferated B cells are transformed into two types of cells:
1. Plasma cells
2. Memory cells.

■ ROLE OF PLASMA CELLS

Plasma cells destroy the foreign organisms by producing the antibodies. Antibodies are globulin in nature. The rate of the antibody production is very high, i.e. each plasma cell produces about 2000 molecules of antibodies per second. The antibodies are also called immunoglobulins.

Antibodies are released into lymph and then transported into the circulation. The antibodies are produced until the end of lifespan of each plasma cell, which may be from several days to several weeks.

■ ROLE OF MEMORY B CELLS

Memory B cells occupy the lymphoid tissues throughout the body. The memory cells are in inactive condition until the body is exposed to the same organism for the second time.

During the second exposure, the memory cells are stimulated by the antigen and produce more quantity of antibodies at a faster rate, than in the first exposure. The antibodies produced during the second exposure to the foreign antigen are also more potent than those produced during first exposure. This phenomenon forms the basic principle of vaccination against the infections.

■ ROLE OF HELPER T CELLS

Helper T cells are simultaneously activated by antigen. Activated helper T cells secrete two substances called interleukin-2 and B cell growth factor, which promote:
1. Activation of more number of B lymphocytes.
2. Proliferation of plasma cells.
3. Production of antibodies.

■ ANTIBODIES OR IMMUNOGLOBULINS

An antibody is defined as a protein that is produced by B lymphocytes in response to the presence of an antigen. Antibody is gamma globulin in nature and it is also called immunoglobulin (Ig). Immunoglobulins form 20% of the total plasma proteins. Antibodies enter almost all the tissues of the body.

Types of Antibodies

Five types of antibodies are identified:
1. IgA (Ig alpha)
2. IgD (Ig delta)
3. IgE (Ig epsilon)
4. IgG (Ig gamma)
5. IgM (Ig mu).
    Among these antibodies, IgG forms 75% of the antibodies in the body.

Structure of Antibodies

Antibodies are gamma globulins with a molecular weight of 1,50,000 to 9,00,000. The antibodies are formed by two pairs of chains, namely one pair of heavy or long chains and one pair of light or short chains. Each heavy chain consists of about 400 amino acids and each light chain consists of about 200 amino acids.

Actually, each antibody has two halves, which are identical. The two halves are held together by disulfide bonds (S–S). Each half of the antibody consists of one

heavy chain (H) and one light chain (L). The two chains in each half are also joined by disulfide bonds (S – S). The disulfide bonds allow the movement of amino acid chains. In each antibody, the light chain is parallel to one end of the heavy chain. The light chain and the part of heavy chain parallel to it form one arm. The remaining part of the heavy chain forms another arm. A hinge joins both the arms (Fig. 17.3).

Each chain of the antibody includes two regions:
1. Constant region
2. Variable region.

1. Constant Region

Amino acids present in this region are similar in number and placement (sequence) in all the antibodies of each type. So, this region is called constant region or **Fc** (Fragment crystallizable) region. Thus, the identification and the functions of different types of immunoglobulins depend upon the constant region. This region binds to the antibody receptor situated on the surface of the cell membrane. It also causes complement fixation. So, this region is also called the complement binding region.

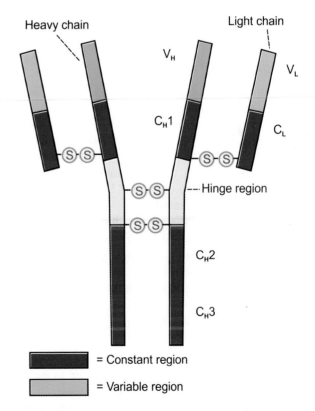

FIGURE 17.3: Structure of antibody (IgG) molecule. V_L = Variable region of light chain, V_H = Variable region of heavy chain, C_L = Constant region of light chain, C_H1, C_H2 and C_H3 = Constant regions of heavy chains.

2. *Variable Region*

Variable region is smaller compared to constant region. Amino acids occupying this region are different in number and placement (sequence) in each antibody. So, it is called the variable region. This region enables the antibody to recognize the specific antigen and to bind itself with the antigen. So, this region of the chain is called antigen-binding region or **Fab** (Fragment antigen binding) region.

Functions of Different Antibodies

1. IgA plays a role in localized defense mechanism in external secretions like tear
2. IgD is involved in recognition of the antigen by B lymphocytes
3. IgE is involved in allergic reactions
4. IgG is responsible for complement fixation
5. IgM is also responsible for complement fixation.

Mechanism of Actions of Antibodies

Antibodies protect the body from invading organisms in two ways (Fig. 17.4):
1. By direct actions
2. Through complement system.

1. Direct Actions of Antibodies

Antibodies directly inactivate the invading organism by any one of the following methods:
  i. Agglutination: In this, the foreign bodies like RBCs or bacteria with antigens on their surfaces are held together in a clump by the antibodies.
  ii. Precipitation: In this, the soluble antigens like tetanus toxin are converted into insoluble forms and then precipitated.
  iii. Neutralization: During this, the antibodies cover the toxic sites of antigenic products.
  iv. Lysis: It is done by the most potent antibodies. These antibodies rupture the cell membrane of the organisms and then destroy them.

2. Actions of Antibodies through Complement System

The indirect actions of antibodies are stronger than the direct actions and play more important role in defense mechanism of the body than the direct actions.

Complement system is the one that enhances or accelerates various activities during the fight against the invading organisms. It is a system of plasma enzymes, which are identified by numbers from C_1 to

C_9. Including the three subunits of C_1 (C_{1q} C_{1r} C_{1s}), there are 11 enzymes in total. Normally, these enzymes are in inactive form and are activated in three ways:
    a. Classical pathway
    b. Lectin pathway
    c. Alternate pathway.

a. Classical pathway

In this the C_1 binds with the antibodies and triggers a series of events in which other enzymes are activated in sequence. These enzymes or the byproducts formed during these events produce the following activities:
  i. *Opsonization:* Activation of neutrophils and macrophages to engulf the bacteria, which are bound with a protein in the plasma called opsonin.
  ii. *Lysis:* Destruction of bacteria by rupturing the cell membrane.
  iii. *Chemotaxis*: Attraction of leukocytes to the site of antigen-antibody reaction.
  iv. *Agglutination:* Clumping of foreign bodies like RBCs or bacteria.
  v. *Neutralization:* Covering the toxic sites of antigenic products.
  vi. *Activation of mast cells and basophils, which liberate histamine:* Histamine dilates the blood vessels and increases capillary permeability. So, plasma proteins from blood enter the tissues and inactivate the antigenic products.

b. Lectin pathway

Lectin pathway occurs when mannose-binding lectin (MBL), which is a serum protein binds with mannose or fructose group on wall of bacteria, fungi or virus.

c. Alternate pathway

Complementary system is also activated by another way, which is called alternate pathway. It is due to a protein in circulation called factor I. It binds with polysaccharides present in the cell membrane of the invading organisms. This binding activates C_3 and C_5, which ultimately attack the antigenic products of invading organism.

Specificity of B Lymphocytes

Each B lymphocyte is designed to be activated only by one type of antigen. It is also capable of producing antibodies against that antigen only. This property of B lymphocyte is called specificity. In lymphoid tissues, the lymphocytes, which produce a specific antibody, are together called the clone of lymphocytes.

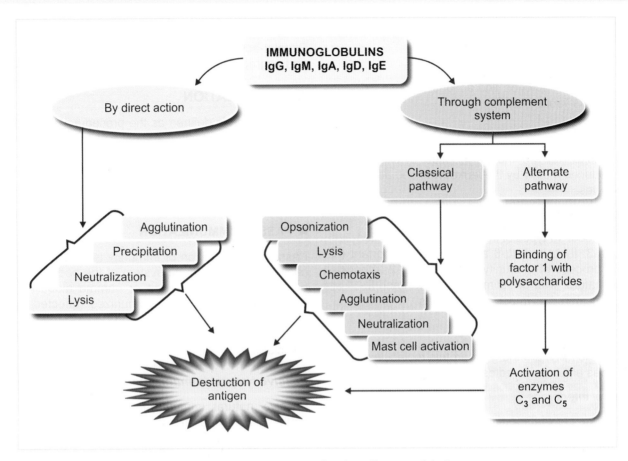

FIGURE 17.4: Mechanism of action of immunoglobulins

■ NATURAL KILLER CELL

Natural killer (NK) cell is a large granular cell that plays an important role in defense mechanism of the body. It has an indented nucleus. Considered as the third type of lymphocyte, it is often called the non-T, non-B cell. It is derived from bone marrow. NK cell is said to be the first line of defense in specific immunity, particularly against viruses.

NK cell kills the invading organisms or the cells of the body without prior sensitization. It is not a phagocytic cell but its granules contain hydrolytic enzymes such as perforins and granzymes. These hydrolytic enzymes play an important role in the lysis of cells of invading organisms.

Functions of Natural Killer (NK) Cell

Natural killer cell:
1. Destroys the viruses
2. Destroys the viral infected or damaged cells, which might form tumors
3. Destroys the malignant cells and prevents develop- ment of cancerous tumors

4. Secretes cytokines such as interleukin-2, interferons, colony stimulating factor (GM-CSF) and tumor necrosis factor-α. Cytokines are explained later in this chapter.

■ CYTOKINES

Cytokines are the hormone-like small proteins acting as intercellular messengers (cell signaling molecules) by binding to specific receptors of target cells. These non-antibody proteins are secreted by WBCs and some other types of cells. Their major function is the activation and regulation of general immune system of the body.

Cytokines are distinct from the other cell-signaling molecules such as growth factors (Chapter 1) and hormones (Chapter 65).

■ TYPES OF CYTOKINES

Depending upon the source of secretion and effects, cytokines are classified into several types:
1. Interleukins
2. Interferons
3. Tumor necrosis factors

4. Chemokines
5. Defensins
6. Cathelicidins
7. Platelet-activating factor.

Source of secretion and actions of these cytokines are given in Table 17.2.

1. Interleukins

Interleukins (IL) are the polypeptide cytokines which are produced mainly by the leukocytes and act on other leukocytes.

Types of interleukins

So far, about 16 types of interleukins are identified. IL-1, IL-2, IL-3, IL-4, IL-5, IL-6 and IL-8 play important role in the process of immunity. Recently IL-12 (otherwise called natural killer cell stimulatory factor) and IL-11 are also considered as important cytokines.

2. Interferons

Interferons (IFN) are the glycoprotein molecules. These cytokines are considered as antiviral agents.

Types of interferons

Interferons are of three types namely, INF-α, INF-β and INF-γ.

3. Tumor Necrosis Factors

Tumor necrosis factors (TNF) are of three types, TNF-α (cachectin), TNF-β (lymphotoxin) and TNF-γ.

4. Chemokines

Cytokines having chemoattractant action are called chemokines.

5. Defensins

Defensins are the antimicrobial peptides.

Types of defensins

Two types of defensins are identified in human:
  i. α-defensins, secreted by neutrophils, macrophages and paneth cells in small intestine.
  ii. β-defensins, secreted by airway epithelial cells (respiratory tract), salivary glands and cutaneous cells.

6. Cathelicidins

Cathelicidins are also the antimicrobial peptides which play an important role in a wide range of antimicrobial activity in air passage and lungs.

7. Platelet-activating Factor

Platelet-activating factor (PAF) accelerates agglutination and aggregation of platelets.

■ IMMUNIZATION

Immunization is defined as the procedure by which the body is prepared to fight against a specific disease. It is used to induce the immune resistance of the body to a specific disease. Immunization is of two types:
  1. Passive immunization
  2. Active immunization.

■ PASSIVE IMMUNIZATION

Passive immunization or immunity is produced without challenging the immune system of the body. It is done by administration of serum or gamma globulins from a person who is already immunized (affected by the disease) to a non-immune person.

Passive immunization is acquired either naturally or artificially.

Passive Natural Immunization

Passive natural immunization is acquired from the mother before and after birth. Before birth, immunity is transferred from mother to the fetus in the form of maternal antibodies (mainly IgG) through placenta. After birth, the antibodies (IgA) are transferred through breast milk.

Lymphocytes of the child are not activated. In addition, the antibodies received from the mother are metabolized soon. Therefore, the passive immunity is short lived. The significance of passive immunity that is obtained before birth is the prevention of Rh incompatibility in pregnancy.

Passive Artificial Immunization

Passive artificial immunization is developed by injecting previously prepared antibodies using serum from humans or animals. Antibodies are obtained from the persons affected by the disease or from animals, particularly horses which have been immunized artificially. The serum containing the antibody (antiserum) is administered to people who have developed the disease (therapeutic). It is also used as a prophylactic measure. Prophylaxis refers to medical or public health procedures to prevent a disease in people who may be exposed to the disease in a later period.

This type of immunity is useful for providing immediate protection against acute infections like tetanus, measles, diphtheria, etc. and for poisoning by insects, snakes and venom from other animals. It is also used as a prophylactic measure. However, this may result

TABLE 17.2: Cytokines

Cytokine	Source of secretion	Action
Interleukins	1. T cells 2. B cells 3. Eosinophils 4. Basophils 5. Monocytes 6. Mast cells 7. Macrophages 8. NK cells	1. Activation of T cells, macrophages and natural killer (NK) cells 2. Promotion of growth of hemopoietic cells and B cells 3. Acceleration of inflammatory response by activating eosinophils 4. Chemotaxis of neutrophils, eosinophils, basophils and T cells 5. Destruction of invading organisms
Interferons	1. WBCs 2. NK cells 3. Fibroblasts	1. Fighting against viral infection by suppressing virus multiplication in target cells 2. Inhibition of multiplication of parasites and cancer cells 3. Promotion of phagocytosis by monocytes and macrophages 4. Activation of NK cells
Tumor necrosis factors	1. T cells 2. B cells 3. Mast cells 4. Macrophages 5. NK cells 6. Platelets	1. Causing necrosis of tumor 2. Activation of general immune system 3. Production of vascular effects 4. Promotion of inflammation
Chemokines	1. T cells 2. B cells 3. Monocytes 4. Macrophages	Attraction of WBCs by chemotaxis
Defensins	1. Neutrophils 2. Macrophages 3. Paneth cells in small intestine 4. Airway epithelial cells 5. Salivary glands 6. Cutaneous cells	1. Role in innate immunity in airway surface and lungs 2. Killing the phagocytozed bacteria 3. Antiinflammatory actions 4. Promotion of wound healing 5. Attraction of monocytes and T cells by chemotaxis
Cathelicidins	1. Neutrophils 2. Macrophages 3. Airway epithelial cells 4. Macrophages	Antimicrobial activity in air passage and lungs
Platelet-activating factor	1. Neutrophils 2. Monocytes	Acceleration of agglutination and aggregation of platelets

in complications and anaphylaxis. There is a risk of transmitting HIV and hepatitis.

■ ACTIVE IMMUNIZATION

Active immunization or immunity is acquired by activating immune system of the body. Body develops resistance against disease by producing antibodies following the exposure to antigens. Active immunity is acquired either naturally or artificially.

Active Natural Immunization

Naturally acquired active immunity involves activation of immune system in the body to produce antibodies. It is achieved in both clinical and subclinical infections.

Clinical infection

Clinical infection is defined as the invasion of the body tissues by pathogenic microorganisms which reproduce, multiply and cause disease by injuring the cells, secreting a toxin or antigen-antibody reaction. During infection, the plasma cells produce immunoglobulins to destroy the invading antigens. Later, due to the activity of memory cells, body retains the ability to produce the antibodies against the specific antigens invaded previously.

Subclinical infection

Subclinical infection is defined as an infection in which symptoms are very mild and do not alert the affected subject. The disease thus produced may not be severe to develop any manifestations. However, it causes the activation of B lymphocytes, resulting in production of antibodies.

Active Artificial Immunization

Active artificial immunization is a type of immunization is achieved by the administration of vaccines or toxoids.

Vaccines

Vaccine is a substance that is introduced into the body to prevent the disease produced by certain pathogens. Vaccine consists of dead pathogens or live but attenuated (artificially weakened) organisms. The vaccine induces immunity against the pathogen, either by production of antibodies or by activation of T lymphocytes.

Edward Jenner produced first live vaccine. He produced the vaccine for **smallpox** from **cowpox virus.** Nowadays, vaccines are used to prevent many diseases like measles, mumps, poliomyelitis, tuberculosis, smallpox, rubella, yellow fever, rabies, typhoid, influenza, hepatitis B, etc.

Toxoids

Toxoid is a substance which is normally toxic and has been processed to destroy its toxicity but retains its capacity to induce antibody production by immune system. Toxoid consists of weakened components or toxins secreted by the pathogens. Toxoids are used to develop immunity against diseases like diphtheria, tetanus, cholera, etc.

The active artificial immunity may be effective life-long or for short period. It is effective lifelong against the diseases such as mumps, measles, smallpox, tuberculosis and yellow fever. It is effective only for short period against some diseases like cholera (about 6 months) and tetanus (about 1 year).

■ IMMUNE DEFICIENCY DISEASES

Immune deficiency diseases are a group of diseases in which some components of immune system is missing or defective. Normally, the defense mechanism protects the body from invading pathogenic organism. When the defense mechanism fails or becomes faulty (defective), the organisms of even low virulence produce severe disease. The organisms, which take advantage of defective defense mechanism, are called opportunists.

Immune deficiency diseases caused by such opportunists are of two types:
1. Congenital immune deficiency diseases
2. Acquired immune deficiency diseases.

■ CONGENITAL IMMUNE DEFICIENCY DISEASES

Congenital diseases are inherited and occur due to the defects in B cell or T cell or both. The common examples are **DiGeorge syndrome** (due to absence of thymus) and severe combined immune deficiency (due to lymphopenia or the absence of lymphoid tissue).

■ ACQUIRED IMMUNE DEFICIENCY DISEASES

Acquired immune deficiency diseases occur due to infection by some organisms. The most common disease of this type is acquired immune deficiency syndrome (AIDS).

Acquired Immune Deficiency Syndrome (AIDS)

AIDS is an infectious disease caused by immune deficiency virus (HIV). A person is diagnosed with AIDS when the CD4 count is below 200 cells per cubic millimeter of blood.

AIDS is the most common problem throughout the world because of rapid increase in the number of victims. Infection occurs when a glycoprotein from HIV binds to surface receptors of T lymphocytes, monocytes, macrophages and dendritic cells leading to the destruction of these cells. It causes slow progressive decrease in immune function, resulting in opportunistic infections of various types. The common opportunistic infections, which kill the AIDS patient are **pneumonia (Pneumocystis carinii)** and malignant skin cancer **(Kaposi sarcoma).** These diseases are also called AIDS-related diseases.

After entering the body of the host, the HIV activates the enzyme called **reverse transcriptase.** HIV utilizes this enzyme and converts its own viral RNA into viral DNA with the help of host cell DNA itself. Now, the viral DNA gets incorporated into the host cell DNA and prevents the normal activities of the host cell DNA. At the same time, the HIV increases in number inside the host's body. The infected host cell ruptures and releases more number of HIV into the bloodstream. After exposure to HIV, no symptoms develop for several weeks. This is the incubation period. The patient develops symptoms only when sufficient number of infected cells is ruptured. The common symptoms are fatigue, loss of weight, chronic diarrhea, low-grade fever, night sweats, oral ulcers, vaginal ulcers, etc. This phase prolongs for about three years before the disease is diagnosed.

Mode of transmission

The HIV infection spreads when secretions from the body of infected individual come in contact with blood of the recipient through the damaged skin or mucous membrane. The most common ways of infection are contaminated blood transfusion, contaminated needles or other invasive instruments, transmission from mother to fetus during pregnancy, transmission from mother to child during delivery or breastfeeding and vaginal sexual intercourse.

Prevention

Prevention of AIDS is essential because the authentic treatment for this disease has not been established so far. Progress in the development of effective treatment is very slow. Moreover, the maximum duration of survival after initial infection is only about 10 to 15 years. So, it is necessary to prevent this disease.

Following safety measures should be followed to prevent AIDS:
1. Public must be educated about the seriousness and prevention of the disease.
2. HIV infected persons should be educated to avoid spreading the disease to others.
3. Blood should be screened for HIV before transfusion.
4. Intravenous drug users should not share the needles.
5. Pregnant women should get the blood tested for HIV. If the mother is infected, the treatment with zidovudine may reduce incidence of infection in infants. The baby must be given zidovudine for 6 weeks after birth.
6. Young adults and teenagers must be informed about the safer sex techniques and use of condoms. The need for limitation of sexual partners must be emphasized.

■ AUTOIMMUNE DISEASES

Autoimmune disease is defined as a condition in which the immune system mistakenly attacks body's own cells and tissues. Normally, an antigen induces the immune response in the body. The condition in which the immune system fails to give response to an antigen is called tolerance. This is true with respect to body's own antigens that are called self antigens or autoantigens. Normally, body has the **tolerance** against self antigen. However, in some occasions, the tolerance fails or becomes incomplete against self antigen. This state is called autoimmunity and it leads to the activation of T lymphocytes or production of autoantibodies from B lymphocytes. The T lymphocytes (cytotoxic T cells) or autoantibodies attack the body's normal cells whose surface contains the self antigen or autoantigen.

Thus, the autoimmune disease is produced when body's normal tolerance decreases and the immune system fails to recognize the body's own tissues as 'self'.

Autoimmune diseases are of two types:
1. Organ specific diseases which affect only one organ
2. Organ nonspecific or multisystemic diseases, which affect many organs or systems.

■ HUMAN LEUKOCYTE ANTIGEN SYSTEM AND AUTOIMMUNE DISEASES

Human leukocyte antigen (HLA) is a group of genes on human chromosome 6. These genes encode the proteins which function in the cells to transport the antigens from within the cell towards the cell surface. HLA is the product of major histocompatilility complex.

HLA system monitors the immune system in the body (see above). The HLA molecules are recognized by the T and B lymphocytes and hence the name called antigens. HLA is distributed in almost all the tissues of the body. Antibodies are directed against the tissues possessing the HLA, leading to autoimmune diseases. Most of the autoimmune diseases are HLA linked.

■ COMMON AUTOIMMUNE DISEASES

Common autoimmune diseases are:
1. Insulin-dependent diabetes mellitus
2. Myasthenia gravis
3. Hashimoto thyroiditis
4. Graves disease
5. Rheumatoid arthritis.

1. *Insulin-dependent Diabetes Mellitus*

Insulin-dependent diabetes mellitus (IDDM) is very common in childhood and it is due to HLA-linked autoimmunity.

Common causes for IDDM

   i. Development of islet cell autoantibody against β-cells in the islets of Langerhans in pancreas.
   ii. Development of antibody against insulin and glutamic acid decarboxylase.
   iii. Activation of T cells against islets.

Other details of IDDM are given in Chapter 69.

2. *Myasthenia Gravis*

This neuromuscular disease occurs due to the development of autoantibodies against the receptors acetylcholine in neuromuscular junction. Details of myasthenia gravis are given in Chapter 34.

3. *Hashimoto Thyroiditis*

Hashimoto thyroiditis is common in the late middle-aged women. The autoantibodies impair the activity of thyroid follicles leading to hypothyroidism. Hypothyroidism is explained in detail in Chapter 67.

4. Graves Disease

In some cases, the autoantibodies activate thyroid-stimulating hormone (TSH) receptors leading to hyperthyroidism. The details of this disease are given in Chapter 67.

5. Rheumatoid Arthritis

Rheumatiod arthritis is the disease due to chronic inflammation of synovial lining of joints (synovitis). The synovium becomes thick, leading to the development of swelling around joint and tendons. The characteristic symptoms are pain and stiffness of joints. The chronic inflammation occurs due to the continuous production of autoantibodies called rheumatoid arthritis factors (RA factors).

■ ALLERGY AND IMMUNOLOGICAL HYPERSENSITIVITY REACTIONS

The term allergy means hypersensitivity. It is defined as abnormal immune response to a chemical or physical agent (allergen). During the first exposure to an allergen, the immune response does not normally produce any reaction in the body. Sensitization or an initial exposure to the allergen is required for the reaction. So, the subsequent exposure to the allergen causes variety of inflammatory responses. These responses are called allergic reactions or immunological hypersensitivity reactions.

Immunological hypersensitivity reactions may be innate or acquired. These reactions are mediated mostly by antibodies. In some conditions, T cells are involved. Common symptoms include sneezing, itching and skin rashes. However, in some persons the symptoms may be severe.

Common allergic conditions are:
1. Food allergy
2. Allergic rhinitis
3. Bronchial asthma
4. Urticaria.

■ ALLERGENS

Any substance that produces the manifestations of allergy is called an allergen. It may be an antigen or a protein or any other type of substance. Even physical agents can develop allergy.

Allergens are introduced by:
1. Contact (e.g.: chemical substance)
2. Inhalation (e.g.: pollen)
3. Ingestion (e.g.: food)
4. Injection (e.g.: drug).

Common Allergens

1. *Food substances:* Wheat, egg, milk and chocolate.
2. *Inhalants:* Pollen grains, fungi, dust, smoke, perfumes and disagreeable odor.
3. *Contactants:* Chemical substances, metals, animals and plants.
4. *Infectious agents:* Parasites, bacteria, viruses and fungi.
5. *Drugs:* Aspirin and antibiotics.
6. *Physical agents:* Cold, heat, light, pressure and radiation.

■ IMMUNOLOGICAL HYPERSENSITIVE REACTIONS

Immunological hypersensitive reactions to an agent give rise to several allergic conditions and autoimmune diseases.

Hypersensitive reactions are classified into five types:

Type I or anaphylactic reactions.
Type II or cytotoxic reactions.
Type III or antibody-mediated reactions.
Type IV or cell-mediated reactions.
Type V or stimulatory/blocking reactions.

Type I or Anaphylactic Reactions

Anaphylaxis means exaggerated reactions of the body to an antigen or other agents to which the body is sensitized already. It is also called immediate hypersensitive reaction because it develops within few minutes of exposure to an allergen. Anaphylactic reactions are mediated by IgE and other factors involved in inflammation (inflammation means the protective response of the tissues to the damage or destruction of cells).

When the body is exposed to an allergen, the IgE immunoglobulins are produced. Also called reagins or sensitizing antibodies, these immunoglobulins bind with the surface receptors of mast cells and circulating basophils. Mast cells are the granulated wandering cells found in connective tissue and beneath the mucous membrane in the throat, lungs and eyes.

During subsequent exposure of the body to the same allergen, the allergen IgE antibody reaction takes place. This leads to degranulation of mast cells and basophils, with the release of some chemical mediators such histamine. The chemical mediators produce the hypersensitivity reactions. Most serious reactions are fall in blood pressure (due to vasodilatation),obstruction of air passage and difficulty in breathing (due to bronchoconstriction) and shock (Chapter 116).

Type II or Cytotoxic Reactions

Cytotoxic reactions involve mainly the IgG antibodies, which bind with antigens on the surface of the cells, particularly the blood cells. The affected cells are destroyed. Sometimes, IgM and IgA antibodies are also involved. The diseases developed due to cytotoxic reactions are hemolytic diseases of newborn in case of Rh incompatibility and **autoimmune hemolytic anemia.**

Type III or Antibody-mediated Reactions

Excess amounts of antibodies like IgG or IgM are produced in this type. The antigen-antibody complexes are precipitated and deposited in localized areas like joints causing **arthritis,** heart causing **myocarditis** and glomeruli of kidney producing **glomerulonephritis.**

Type IV or Cell-mediated Reactions

This type of hypersensitivity is also called delayed or slow type of hypersensitivity. It is found in allergic reactions due to the bacteria, viruses and fungi. It is also seen in contact dermatitis caused by chemical allergens and during rejection of transplanted tissues. An example of type IV reaction is the delayed reaction after intradermal injection of tuberculin in persons who are previously affected by tuberculosis (tuberculosis skin test or **Mantoux test**). The important feature of delayed type of hypersensitivity is the involvement of T lymphocytes rather than the antibodies.

Type V or Stimulatory/Blocking Reactions

It is seen in autoimmune diseases like Graves' disease (stimulatory reactions) and myasthenia gravis (blocking reactions).

Graves' disease: Normally, TSH combines with surface receptors of thyroid cells and causes synthesis and secretion of thyroid hormones. The secretion of thyroid hormones can be increased by thyroid-stimulating antibodies (TSAB) produced by plasma cells (B lymphocytes). The excess secretion of thyroid hormone leads to Graves' disease.

Myasthenia gravis: It is due to the development of IgG autoantibodies (see above).

Platelets

Chapter
18

```
■  INTRODUCTION
■  STRUCTURE AND COMPOSITION
■  NORMAL COUNT AND VARIATIONS
■  PROPERTIES
■  FUNCTIONS
■  ACTIVATORS AND INHIBITORS
■  DEVELOPMENT
■  LIFESPAN AND FATE
■  APPLIED PHYSIOLOGY – PLATELET DISORDERS
```

■ INTRODUCTION

Platelets or thrombocytes are the formed elements of blood. Platelets are small colorless, non-nucleated and moderately refractive bodies. These formed elements of blood are considered to be the fragments of cytoplasm.

Size of Platelets

Diameter : 2.5 µ (2 to 4 µ)
Volume   : 7.5 cu µ (7 to 8 cu µ).

Shape of Platelets

Normally, platelets are of several shapes, viz. spherical or rod-shaped and become oval or disk-shaped when inactivated. Sometimes, the platelets have dumbbell shape, comma shape, cigar shape or any other unusual shape. Inactivated platelets are without processes or filopodia and the activated platelets develop processes or filopodia (see below).

■ STRUCTURE AND COMPOSITION

Platelet is constituted by:
1. Cell membrane or surface membrane
2. Microtubules
3. Cytoplasm.

■ CELL MEMBRANE

Cell membrane of platelet is 6 nm thick. Extensive invagination of cell membrane forms an open **canalicular system** (Fig. 18.1). This canalicular system is a delicate tunnel system through which the platelet granules extrude their contents.

Cell membrane of platelet contains lipids in the form of phospholipids, cholesterol and glycolipids, carbohydrates as glycocalyx and glycoproteins and proteins. Of these substances, glycoproteins and phospholipids are functionally important.

Glycoproteins

Glycoproteins prevent the adherence of platelets to normal endothelium, but accelerate the adherence of platelets to collagen and damaged endothelium in ruptured blood vessels. Glycoproteins also form the receptors for adenosine diphosphate (ADP) and thrombin.

Phospholipids

Phospholipids accelerate the clotting reactions. The phospholipids form the precursors of thromboxane A_2 and other prostaglandin-related substances.

■ MICROTUBULES

Microtubules form a ring around cytoplasm below the cell membrane. Microtubules are made up of polymerized proteins called **tubulin.** These tubules provide structural support for the inactivated platelets to maintain the disk-like shape.

■ CYTOPLASM

Cytoplasm of platelets contains the cellular organelles, Golgi apparatus, endoplasmic reticulum, mitochondria, microtubule, microvessels, filaments and granules.

Cytoplasm also contains some chemical substances such as proteins, enzymes, hormonal substances, etc.

Proteins

1. *Contractile proteins*
   i. Actin and myosin: Contractile proteins, which are responsible for contraction of platelets.
   ii. Thrombosthenin: Third contractile protein, which is responsible for clot retraction.
2. *von Willebrand factor:* Responsible for adherence of platelets and regulation of plasma level of factor VIII.
3. *Fibrin-stabilizing factor:* A clotting factor.
4. *Platelet-derived growth factor (PDGF):* Responsible for repair of damaged blood vessels and wound healing. It is a potent mytogen (chemical agent that promotes mitosis) for smooth muscle fibers of blood vessels.
5. *Platelet-activating factor (PAF):* Causes aggregation of platelets during the injury of blood vessels, resulting in prevention of excess loss of blood.
6. *Vitronectin (serum spreading factor):* Promotes adhesion of platelets and spreading of tissue cells in culture.
7. *Thrombospondin:* Inhibits angiogenesis (formation of new blood vessels from pre-existing vessels).

Enzymes

1. Adensosine triphosphatase (ATPase)
2. Enzymes necessary for synthesis of prostaglandins.

Hormonal Substances

1. Adrenaline
2. 5-hydroxytryptamine (5-HT; serotonin)
3. Histamine.

Other Chemical Substances

1. Glycogen
2. Substances like blood group antigens

3. Inorganic substances such as calcium, copper, magnesium and iron.

Platelet Granules

Granules present in cytoplasm of platelets are of two types:
1. Alpha granules
2. Dense granules.
   Substances present in these granules are given in Table 18.1.

Alpha granules

Alpha granules contain:
1. Clotting factors – fibrinogen, V and XIII
2. Platelet-derived growth factor
3. Vascular endothelial growth factor (VEGF)
4. Basic fibroblast growth factor (FGF)
5. Endostatin
6. Thrombospondin.

Dense granules

Dense granules contain:
1. Nucleotides
2. Serotonin
3. Phospholipid
4. Calcium
5. Lysosomes.

■ NORMAL COUNT AND VARIATIONS

Normal platelet count is 2,50,000/cu mm of blood. It ranges between 2,00,000 and 4,00,000/cu mm of blood.

■ PHYSIOLOGICAL VARIATIONS

1. *Age:* Platelets are less in infants (1,50,000 to 2,00,000/cu mm) and reaches normal level at 3rd month after birth.
2. *Sex:* There is no difference in the platelet count between males and females. In females, it is reduced during menstruation.
3. *High altitude:* Platelet count increases.
4. *After meals:* After taking food, the platelet count increases.

TABLE 18.1: Substances present in platelet granules

Alpha granules	Dense granules
Clotting factors: fibrinogen, V and XIII Platelet-derived growth factor Vascular endothelial growth factor Basic fibroblast growth factor Endostatin Thrombospondin	Nucleotides Serotonin Phospholipid Calcium Lysosomes

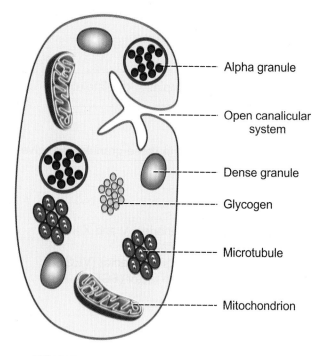

FIGURE 18.1: Platelet under electron microscope

■ PATHOLOGICAL VARIATIONS

Refer applied physiology of this chapter.

■ PROPERTIES OF PLATELETS

Platelets have three important properties (three 'A's):
1. Adhesiveness
2. Aggregation
3. Agglutination.

■ ADHESIVENESS

Adhesiveness is the property of sticking to a rough surface. During injury of blood vessel, endothelium is damaged and the subendothelial collagen is exposed. While coming in contact with collagen, platelets are activated and adhere to collagen. Adhesion of platelets involves interaction between **von Willebrand factor** secreted by damaged endothelium and a receptor protein called glycoprotein Ib situated on the surface of platelet membrane. Other factors which accelerate adhesiveness are collagen, thrombin, ADP, Thromboxane A_2, calcium ions, P-selectin and vitronectin.

■ AGGREGATION (GROUPING OF PLATELETS)

Aggregation is the grouping of platelets. Adhesion is followed by activation of more number of platelets by substances released from dense granules of platelets.

During activation, the platelets change their shape with elongation of long filamentous pseudopodia which are called processes or filopodia (Fig. 18.2).

Filopodia help the platelets aggregate together. Activation and aggregation of platelets is accelerated by ADP, thromboxane A_2 and platelet-activating factor (PTA: cytokine secreted by neutrophils and monocytes; Chapter 16).

■ AGGLUTINATION

Agglutination is the clumping together of platelets. Aggregated platelets are agglutinated by the actions of some platelet agglutinins and platelet-activating factor.

■ FUNCTIONS OF PLATELETS

Normally, platelets are inactive and execute their actions only when activated. Activated platelets immediately release many substances. This process is known as platelet release reaction. Functions of platelets are carried out by these substances.

Functions of platelets are:

■ 1. ROLE IN BLOOD CLOTTING

Platelets are responsible for the formation of intrinsic prothrombin activator. This substance is responsible for the onset of blood clotting (Chapter 20).

■ 2. ROLE IN CLOT RETRACTION

In the blood clot, blood cells including platelets are entrapped in between the fibrin threads. Cytoplasm of platelets contains the **contractile proteins,** namely actin, myosin and thrombosthenin, which are responsible for clot retraction (Chapter 20).

■ 3. ROLE IN PREVENTION OF BLOOD LOSS (HEMOSTASIS)

Platelets accelerate the hemostasis by three ways:
  i. Platelets secrete 5-HT, which causes the constriction of blood vessels.
 ii. Due to the adhesive property, the platelets seal the damage in blood vessels like capillaries.
iii. By formation of temporary plug, the platelets seal the damage in blood vessels (Chapter 19).

■ 4. ROLE IN REPAIR OF RUPTURED BLOOD VESSEL

Platelet-derived growth factor (PDGF) formed in cytoplasm of platelets is useful for the repair of the endothelium and other structures of the ruptured blood vessels.

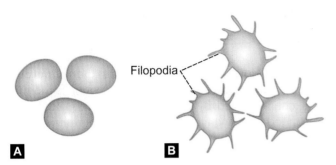

FIGURE 18.2: A. Inactive platelets. B. Activated platelets.

■ 5. ROLE IN DEFENSE MECHANISM

By the property of agglutination, platelets encircle the foreign bodies and destroy them.

■ ACTIVATORS AND INHIBITORS OF PLATELETS

■ ACTIVATORS OF PLATELETS

1. Collagen, which is exposed during damage of blood vessels
2. von Willebrand factor
3. Thromboxane A_2
4. Platelet-activating factor
5. Thrombin
6. ADP
7. Calcium ions
8. P-selectin: Cell adhesion molecule secreted from endothelial cells
9. Convulxin: Purified protein from snake venom.

■ INHIBITORS OF PLATELETS

1. Nitric oxide
2. Clotting factors: II, IX, X, XI and XII
3. Prostacyclin
4. Nucleotidases which breakdown the ADP.

■ DEVELOPMENT OF PLATELETS

Platelets are formed from bone marrow. Pluripotent stem cell gives rise to the colony forming unit-megakaryocyte (CFU-M). This develops into megakaryocyte. Cytoplasm of megakaryocyte form **pseudopodium.** A portion of pseudopodium is detached to form platelet, which enters the circulation (Fig. 10.2).

Production of platelets is influenced by colony-stimulating factors and **thrombopoietin.** Colony-stimulating factors are secreted by monocytes and T lymphocytes. Thrombopoietin is a glycoprotein like erythropoietin. It is secreted by liver and kidneys.

■ LIFESPAN AND FATE OF PLATELETS

Average lifespan of platelets is 10 days. It varies between 8 and 11 days. Platelets are destroyed by tissue macrophage system in spleen. So, **splenomegaly** (enlargement of spleen) decreases platelet count and **splenectomy** (removal of spleen) increases platelet count.

■ APPLIED PHYSIOLOGY – PLATELET DISORDERS

Platelet disorders occur because of pathological variation in platelet count and dysfunction of platelets.
  Platelet disorders are:
1. Thrombocytopenia
2. Thrombocytosis
3. Thrombocythemia
4. Glanzmann's thrombasthenia.

1. *Thrombocytopenia*

Decrease in platelet count is called thrombocytopenia. It leads to thrombocytopenic purpura (Chapter 20).
  Thrombocytopenia occurs in the following conditions:
  i. Acute infections
  ii. Acute leukemia
  iii. Aplastic and pernicious anemia
  iv. Chickenpox
  v. Smallpox
  vi. Splenomegaly
  vii. Scarlet fever
  viii. Typhoid
  ix. Tuberculosis
  x. Purpura
  xi. Gaucher's disease.

2. *Thrombocytosis*

Increase in platelet count is called thrombocytosis.
  Thrombocytosis occurs in the following conditions:
  i. Allergic conditions
  ii. Asphyxia
  iii. Hemorrhage
  iv. Bone fractures
  v. Surgical operations
  vi. Splenectomy
  vii. Rheumatic fever
  viii. Trauma (wound or injury or damage caused by external force).

3. *Thrombocythemia*

Thrombocythemia is the condition with persistent and abnormal increase in platelet count. Thrombocythemia occurs in the following conditions:

   i. Carcinoma
   ii. Chronic leukemia
   iii. Hodgkin's disease.

4. *Glanzmann's Thrombasthenia*

Glanzmann's thrombasthenia is an inherited hemorrhagic disorder, caused by structural or functional abnormality of platelets. It leads to **thrombasthenic purpura** (Chapter 20). However, the platelet count is normal. It is characterized by normal clotting time, normal or prolonged bleeding time but defective clot retraction.

Hemostasis

Chapter 19

- **DEFINITION**
- **STAGES OF HEMOSTASIS**
  - **VASOCONSTRICTION**
  - **PLATELET PLUG FORMATION**
  - **COAGULATION OF BLOOD**

■ DEFINITION

Hemostasis is defined as arrest or stoppage of bleeding.

■ STAGES OF HEMOSTASIS

When a blood vessel is injured, the injury initiates a series of reactions, resulting in hemostasis. It occurs in three stages (Fig. 19.1):
1. Vasoconstriction
2. Platelet plug formation
3. Coagulation of blood.

■ VASOCONSTRICTION

Immediately after injury, the blood vessel constricts and decreases the loss of blood from damaged portion. Usually, arterioles and small arteries constrict. Vasoconstriction is purely a local phenomenon. When the blood vessels are cut, the endothelium is damaged and the collagen is exposed. Platelets adhere to this collagen and get activated. The activated platelets secrete serotonin and other vasoconstrictor substances which cause constriction of the blood vessels. Adherence of platelets to the collagen is accelerated by von Willebrand factor. This factor acts as a bridge between a specific glycoprotein present on the surface of platelet and collagen fibrils.

■ PLATELET PLUG FORMATION

Platelets get adhered to the collagen of ruptured blood vessel and secrete adenosine diphosphate (ADP) and thromboxane A_2. These two substances attract more and more platelets and activate them. All these platelets aggregate together and form a loose temporary platelet plug or temporary hemostatic plug, which closes the ruptured vessel and prevents further blood loss. Platelet aggregation is accelerated by platelet-activating factor (PAF).

■ COAGULATION OF BLOOD

During this process, the fibrinogen is converted into fibrin. Fibrin threads get attached to the loose platelet plug, which blocks the ruptured part of blood vessels and prevents further blood loss completely. Mechanism of blood coagulation is explained in the next chapter.

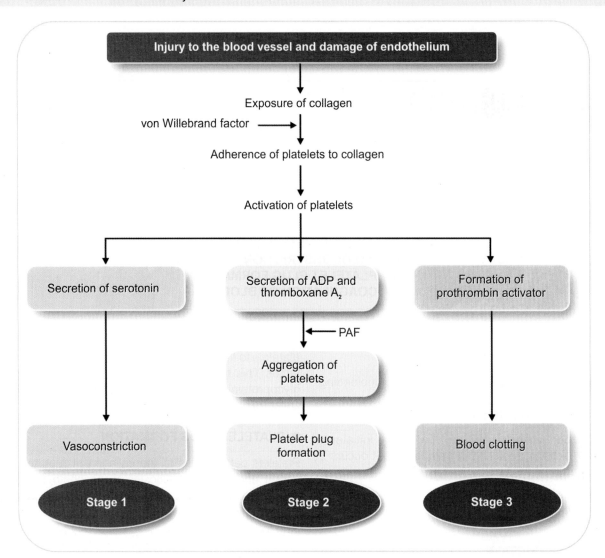

FIGURE 19.1: States of hemostasis. ADP = Adenosine diphosphate; PAF = Platelet-activating factor.

Coagulation of Blood

20

- ■ **DEFINITION**
- ■ **FACTORS INVOLVED IN BLOOD CLOTTING**
- ■ **SEQUENCE OF CLOTTING MECHANISM**
- ■ **BLOOD CLOT**
- ■ **ANTICLOTTING MECHANISM IN THE BODY**
- ■ **ANTICOAGULANTS**
- ■ **PHYSICAL METHODS TO PREVENT BLOOD CLOTTING**
- ■ **PROCOAGULANTS**
- ■ **TESTS FOR BLOOD CLOTTING**
- ■ **APPLIED PHYSIOLOGY**

■ DEFINITION

Coagulation or clotting is defined as the process in which blood loses its fluidity and becomes a jelly-like mass few minutes after it is shed out or collected in a container.

■ FACTORS INVOLVED IN BLOOD CLOTTING

Coagulation of blood occurs through a series of reactions due to the activation of a group of substances. Substances necessary for clotting are called clotting factors.

Thirteen clotting factors are identified:

Factor I	Fibrinogen
Factor II	Prothrombin
Factor III	Thromboplastin (Tissue factor)
Factor IV	Calcium
Factor V	Labile factor (Proaccelerin or accelerator globulin)
Factor VI	Presence has not been proved
Factor VII	Stable factor
Factor VIII	Antihemophilic factor (Antihemophilic globulin)
Factor IX	Christmas factor
Factor X	Stuart-Prower factor
Factor XI	Plasma thromboplastin antecedent

Factor XII	Hageman factor (Contact factor)
Factor XIII	Fibrin-stabilizing factor (Fibrinase).

Clotting factors were named after the scientists who discovered them or as per the activity, except factor IX. Factor IX or Christmas factor was named after the patient in whom it was discovered.

■ SEQUENCE OF CLOTTING MECHANISM

■ ENZYME CASCADE THEORY

Most of the clotting factors are proteins in the form of enzymes. Normally, all the factors are present in the form of inactive **proenzyme.** These proenzymes must be activated into enzymes to enforce clot formation. It is carried out by a series of proenzyme-enzyme conversion reactions. First one of the series is converted into an active enzyme that activates the second one, which activates the third one; this continues till the final active enzyme thrombin is formed.

Enzyme cascade theory explains how various reactions, involved in the conversion of proenzymes to active enzymes take place in the form of a cascade. Cascade refers to a process that occurs through a series of steps, each step initiating the next, until the final step is reached.

Stages of Blood Clotting

In general, blood clotting occurs in three stages:
1. Formation of prothrombin activator
2. Conversion of prothrombin into thrombin
3. Conversion of fibrinogen into fibrin.

■ STAGE 1: FORMATION OF PROTHROMBIN ACTIVATOR

Blood clotting commences with the formation of a substance called prothrombin activator, which converts prothrombin into thrombin. Its formation is initiated by substances produced either within the blood or outside the blood.

Thus, formation of prothrombin activator occurs through two pathways:
i. Intrinsic pathway
ii. Extrinsic pathway.

i. *Intrinsic Pathway for the Formation of Prothrombin Activator*

In this pathway, the formation of prothrombin activator is initiated by platelets, which are within the blood itself (Fig. 20.1).

Sequence of Events in Intrinsic pathway

i. During the injury, the blood vessel is ruptured. Endothelium is damaged and collagen beneath the endothelium is exposed.
ii. When factor XII (Hageman factor) comes in contact with collagen, it is converted into activated factor XII in the presence of **kallikrein** and high molecular weight (HMW) **kinogen.**
iii. The activated factor XII converts factor XI into activated factor XI in the presence of HMW kinogen.
iv. The activated factor XI activates factor IX in the presence of factor IV (calcium).
v. Activated factor IX activates factor X in the presence of factor VIII and calcium.
vi. When platelet comes in contact with collagen of damaged blood vessel, it gets activated and releases phospholipids.
vii. Now the activated factor X reacts with platelet phospholipid and factor V to form prothrombin activator. This needs the presence of calcium ions.
viii. Factor V is also activated by positive feedback effect of thrombin (see below).

ii. *Extrinsic Pathway for the Formation of Prothrombin Activator*

In this pathway, the formation of prothrombin activator is initiated by the tissue thromboplastin, which is formed from the injured tissues.

Sequence of Events in Extrinsic Pathway

i. Tissues that are damaged during injury release tissue thromboplastin (factor III). Thromboplastin contains proteins, phospholipid and glycoprotein, which act as proteolytic enzymes.
ii. Glycoprotein and phospholipid components of thromboplastin convert factor X into activated factor X, in the presence of factor VII.
iii. Activated factor X reacts with factor V and phospholipid component of tissue thromboplastin to form prothrombin activator. This reaction requires the presence of calcium ions.

■ STAGE 2: CONVERSION OF PROTHROMBIN INTO THROMBIN

Blood clotting is all about thrombin formation. Once thrombin is formed, it definitely leads to clot formation.

Sequence of Events in Stage 2

i. Prothrombin activator that is formed in intrinsic and extrinsic pathways converts prothrombin into thrombin in the presence of calcium (factor IV).
ii. Once formed thrombin initiates the formation of more thrombin molecules. The initially formed thrombin activates Factor V. Factor V in turn accelerates formation of both extrinsic and intrinsic prothrombin activator, which converts prothrombin into thrombin. This effect of thrombin is called **positive feedback** effect (Fig. 20.1).

■ STAGE 3: CONVERSION OF FIBRINOGEN INTO FIBRIN

The final stage of blood clotting involves the conversion of fibrinogen into fibrin by thrombin.

Sequence of Events in Stage 3

i. Thrombin converts inactive fibrinogen into activated fibrinogen due to loss of 2 pairs of

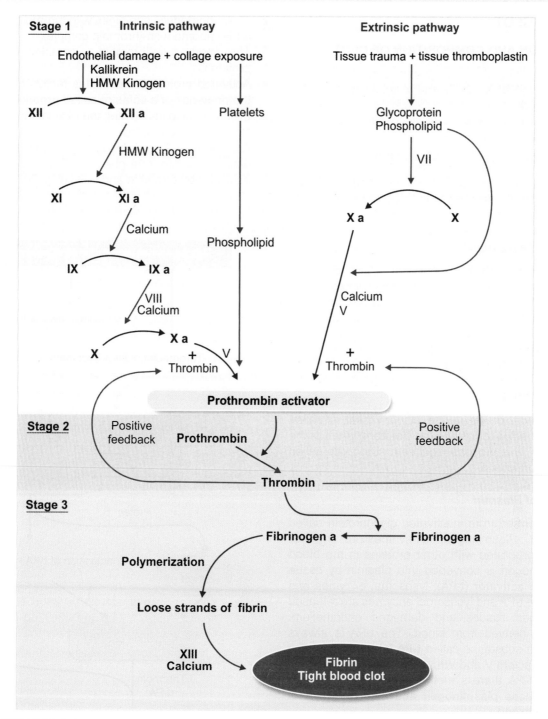

FIGURE 20.1: Stages of blood coagulation. a = Activated, + = Thrombin induces formation of more thrombin (positive feedback); HMW = High molecular weight.

polypeptides from each fibrinogen molecule. The activated fibrinogen is called **fibrin monomer.**

ii. Fibrin monomer polymerizes with other monomer molecules and form loosely arranged strands of fibrin.

iii. Later these loose strands are modified into dense and tight fibrin threads by fibrin-stabilizing factor (factor XIII) in the presence of calcium ions (Fig. 20.1). All the tight fibrin threads are aggregated to form a meshwork of **stable clot.**

■ BLOOD CLOT

■ DEFINITION AND COMPOSITION OF CLOT

Blood clot is defined as the mass of coagulated blood which contains RBCs, WBCs and platelets entrapped in fibrin meshwork.

RBCs and WBCs are not necessary for clotting process. However, when clot is formed, these cells are trapped in it along with platelets. The trapped RBCs are responsible for the red color of the clot.

The external blood clot is also called scab. It adheres to the opening of damaged blood vessel and prevents blood loss.

■ CLOT RETRACTION

After the formation, the blood clot starts contracting. And after about 30 to 45 minutes, the straw-colored serum oozes out of the clot. The process involving the contraction of blood clot and oozing of serum is called clot retraction.

Contractile proteins, namely actin, myosin and thrombosthenin in the cytoplasm of platelets are responsible for clot retraction.

■ FIBRINOLYSIS

Lysis of blood clot inside the blood vessel is called fibrinolysis. It helps to remove the clot from lumen of the blood vessel. This process requires a substance called plasmin or fibrinolysin.

Formation of Plasmin

Plasmin is formed from inactivated glycoprotein called plasminogen. Plasminogen is synthesized in liver and it is incorporated with other proteins in the blood clot. Plasminogen is converted into plasmin by tissue **plasminogen activator (t-PA)**, lysosomal enzymes and thrombin. The t-PA and lysosomal enzymes are released from damaged tissues and damaged endothelium. Thrombin is derived from blood. The t-PA is always inhibited by a substance called **t-PA inhibitor.** It is also inhibited by factors V and VIII.

Besides t-PA, there is another plasminogen activator called **urokinase plasminogen activator (u-PA).** It is derived from blood.

Sequence of Events Involved in the Activation of Plasminogen

1. During intravascular clotting, the endothelium of the blood vessel secretes a thrombin-binding protein, the **thrombomodulin.** It is secreted by the endothelium of all the blood vessels, except the minute vessels of brain.

2. Thrombomodulin combines with thrombin and forms a thrombomodulin-thrombin complex
3. Thrombomodulin-thrombin complex activates protein C
4. Activated protein C inactivates factor V and VIII in the presence of a cofactor called **protein S**
5. Protein C also inactivates the t-PA inhibitor
6. Now, the t-PA becomes active
7. Activated t-PA and lysosomal enzymes activate plasminogen to form plasmin. Plasminogen is also activated by thrombin and u-PA (Fig. 20.2).

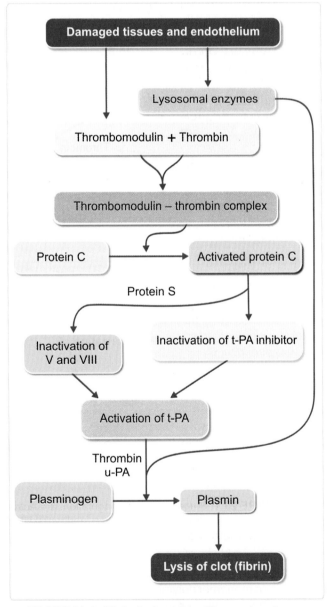

FIGURE 20.2: Fibrinolysis. t-PA = Tissue plasminogen activator, u-PA = Urokinase plasminogen activator.

■ ANTICLOTTING MECHANISM IN THE BODY

Under physiological conditions, intravascular clotting does not occur. It is because of the presence of some physicochemical factors in the body.

1. *Physical Factors*

i. Continuous circulation of blood.
ii. Smooth endothelial lining of the blood vessels.

2. *Chemical Factors – Natural Anticoagulants*

i. Presence of natural anticoagulant called heparin that is produced by the liver
ii. Production of thrombomodulin by endothelium of the blood vessels (except in brain capillaries). Thrombomodulin is a thrombin-binding protein. It binds with thrombin and forms a thrombomo-dulin-thrombin complex. This complex activates protein C. Activated protein C along with its cofactor protein S inactivates Factor V and Factor VIII. Inactivation of these two clotting factors prevents clot formation
iii. All the clotting factors are in inactive state.

■ ANTICOAGULANTS

Substances which prevent or postpone coagulation of blood are called anticoagulants.

Anticoagulants are of three types:

1. Anticoagulants used to prevent blood clotting inside the body, i.e. *in vivo*.
2. Anticoagulants used to prevent clotting of blood that is collected from the body, i.e. *in vitro*.
3. Anticoagulants used to prevent blood clotting both *in vivo* and *in vitro*.

■ 1. HEPARIN

Heparin is a naturally produced anticoagulant in the body. It is produced by **mast cells** which are the wandering cells present immediately outside the capillaries in many tissues or organs that contain more connective tissue. These cells are abundant in liver and lungs. Basophils also secrete heparin.

Heparin is a conjugated polysaccharide. Commercial heparin is prepared from the liver and other organs of animals. Commercial preparation is available in liquid form or dry form as sodium, calcium, ammonium or lithium salts.

Mechanism of Action of Heparin

Heparin:

i.   Prevents blood clotting by its antithrombin activity. It directly suppresses the activity of thrombin
ii. Combines with antithrombin III (a protease inhibitor present in circulation) and removes thrombin from circulation
iii. Activates antithrombin III
iv. Inactivates the active form of other clotting factors like IX, X, XI and XII (Fig. 20.3).

Uses of Heparin

Heparin is used as an anticoagulant both *in vivo* and *in vitro*.

Clinical use

Intravenous injection of heparin (0.5 to 1 mg/kg body weight) postpones clotting for 3 to 4 hours (until it is destroyed by the enzyme **heparinase**). So, it is widely used as an anticoagulant in clinical practice. In clinics, heparin is used for many purposes such as:

i.   To prevent intravascular blood clotting during surgery.
ii. While passing the blood through artificial kidney for dialysis.
iii. During cardiac surgery, which involves heart-lung machine.
iv. To preserve the blood before transfusion.

Use in the laboratory

Heparin is also used as anticoagulant *in vitro* while collecting blood for various investigations. About 0.1 to 0.2 mg is sufficient for 1 mL of blood. It is effective for 8 to 12 hours. After that, blood will clot because heparin only delays clotting and does not prevent it.

Heparin is the most expensive anticoagulant.

■ 2. COUMARIN DERIVATIVES

Warfarin and dicoumoral are the derivatives of coumarin.

Mechanism of Action

Coumarin derivatives prevent blood clotting by inhibiting the action of vitamin K. Vitamin K is essential for the formation of various clotting factors, namely II, VII, IX and X.

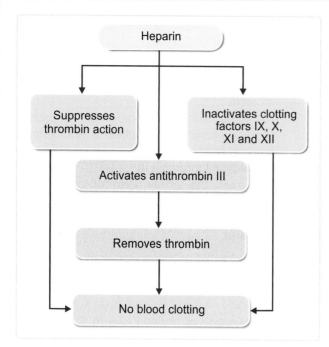

FIGURE 20.3: Mechanism of action of heparin

Uses

Dicoumoral and warfarin are the commonly used **oral anticoagulants** (*in vivo*). Warfarin is used to prevent myocardial infarction (heart attack), strokes and thrombosis.

■ 3. EDTA

Ethylenediaminetetraacetic acid (EDTA) is a strong anticoagulant. It is available in two forms:
  i. Disodium salt (Na_2 EDTA).
  ii. Tripotassium salt (K_3 EDTA).

Mechanism of Action

These substances prevent blood clotting by removing calcium from blood.

Uses

EDTA is used as an anticoagulant both *in vivo* and *in vitro*. It is:
  i. Commonly administered intravenously, in cases of lead poisoning.
  ii. Used as an anticoagulant in the laboratory (*in vitro*). 0.5 to 2.0 mg of EDTA per mL of blood is sufficient to preserve the blood for at least 6 hours. On refrigeration, it can preserve the blood up to 24 hours.

■ 4. OXALATE COMPOUNDS

Oxalate compounds prevent coagulation by forming calcium oxalate, which is precipitated later. Thus, these compounds reduce the blood calcium level.

Earlier sodium and potassium oxalates were used. Nowadays, mixture of ammonium oxalate and potassium oxalate in the ratio of 3 : 2 is used. Each salt is an anticoagulant by itself. But potassium oxalate alone causes shrinkage of RBCs. Ammonium oxalate alone causes swelling of RBCs. But together, these substances do not alter the cellular activity.

Mechanism of Action

Oxalate combines with calcium and forms insoluble calcium oxalate. Thus, oxalate removes calcium from blood and lack of calcium prevents coagulation.

Uses

Oxalate compounds are used only as *in vitro* anticoagulants. 2 mg of mixture is necessary for 1 ml of blood. Since oxalate is poisonous, it cannot be used *in vivo*.

■ 5. CITRATES

Sodium, ammonium and potassium citrates are used as anticoagulants.

Mechanism of Action

Citrate combines with calcium in blood to form insoluble calcium citrate. Like oxalate, citrate also removes calcium from blood and lack of calcium prevents coagulation.

Uses

Citrate is used as in vitro anticoagulant.
  i. It is used to store blood in the **blood bank** as:
      a. Acid citrate dextrose (ACD): 1 part of ACD with 4 parts of blood
      b. Citrate phosphate dextrose (CPD): 1 part of CPD with 4 parts of blood
  ii. Citrate is also used in laboratory in the form of formol-citrate solution (Dacie's solution) for RBC and platelet counts.

■ OTHER SUBSTANCES WHICH PREVENT BLOOD CLOTTING

Peptone, C-type lectin (proteins from venom of viper snake) and **hirudin** (from the leach Hirudinaria manillensis) are the known anticoagulants.

■ PHYSICAL METHODS TO PREVENT BLOOD CLOTTING

Coagulation of blood is postponed or prevented by the following physical methods:

■ COLD

Reducing the temperature to about 5°C postpones the coagulation of blood.

■ COLLECTING BLOOD IN A CONTAINER WITH SMOOTH SURFACE

Collecting the blood in a container with smooth surface like a **silicon-coated** container prevents clotting. The smooth surface inhibits the activation of factor XII and platelets. So, the formation of prothrombin activator is prevented.

■ PROCOAGULANTS

Procoagulants or hemostatic agents are the substances which accelerate the process of blood coagulation. Procoagulants are:

■ THROMBIN

Thrombin is sprayed upon the bleeding surface to arrest bleeding by hastening blood clotting.

■ SNAKE VENOM

Venom of some snakes (vipers, cobras and rattle snakes) contains proteolytic enzymes which enhance blood clotting by activating the clotting factors.

■ EXTRACTS OF LUNGS AND THYMUS

Extract obtained from the lungs and thymus has thromboplastin, which causes rapid blood coagulation.

■ SODIUM OR CALCIUM ALGINATE

Sosium or calcium alginate substances enhance blood clotting process by activating the Hageman factor.

■ OXIDIZED CELLULOSE

Oxidized cellulose causes clotting of blood by activating the Hageman factor.

■ TESTS FOR BLOOD CLOTTING

Blood clotting tests are used to diagnose blood disorders. Some tests are also used to monitor the patients treated with anticoagulant drugs such as heparin and warfarin.

1. Bleeding time
2. Clotting time
3. Prothrombin time
4. Partial prothrombin time
5. International normalized ratio
6. Thrombin time.

■ BLEEDING TIME

Bleeding time (BT) is the time interval from oozing of blood after a cut or injury till arrest of bleeding. Usually, it is determined by Duke method using blotting paper or filter paper method. Its normal duration is 3 to 6 minutes. It is prolonged in purpura.

■ CLOTTING TIME

Clotting time (CT) is the time interval from oozing of blood after a cut or injury till the formation of clot. It is usually determined by capillary tube method. Its normal duration is 3 to 8 minutes. It is prolonged in hemophilia.

■ PROTHROMBIN TIME

Prothrombin time (PT) is the time taken by blood to clot after adding tissue thromboplastin to it. Blood is collected and oxalated so that, the calcium is precipitated and prothrombin is not converted into thrombin. Thus, the blood clotting is prevented. Then a large quantity of tissue thromboplastin with calcium is added to this blood. Calcium nullifies the effect of oxalate. The tissue thromboplastin activates prothrombin and blood clotting occurs.

During this procedure, the time taken by blood to clot after adding tissue thromboplastin is determined. Prothrombin time indicates the total quantity of prothrombin present in the blood.

Normal duration of prothrombin time is 10 to 12 seconds. It is prolonged in deficiency of prothrombin and other factors like factors I, V, VII and X. However, it is normal in hemophilia.

■ PARTIAL PROTHROMBIN TIME OR ACTIVATED PROTHROMBIN TIME

Partial prothrombin time (PPT) is the time taken for the blood to clot after adding an activator such as phospholipid, along with calcium to it. It is also called activated partial prothrombin time (APTT). This test is useful in monitoring the patients taking anticoagulant drugs.

It is carried out by observing clotting time after adding phospholipid, a **surface activator** and calcium to a patient's plasma. Phospholipid serves as **platelet substitute.** Commonly used surface activator is **kaolin.**

Normal duration of partial prothrombin time is 30 to 45 seconds. It is prolonged in **heparin or warfarin therapy** (since heparin and warfarin inhibit clotting) and deficiency or inhibition of factors II, V, VIII, IX, X, XI and XII.

■ INTERNATIONAL NORMALIZED RATIO

International normalized ratio (INR) is the rating of a patient's prothrombin time when compared to an average. It measures extrinsic clotting pathway system.

INR is useful in monitoring impact of anticoagulant drugs such as warfarin and to adjust the dosage of anticoagulants. Patients with atrial fibrillation are usually treated with warfarin to protect against blood clot, which may cause strokes. These patients should have regular blood tests to know their INR in order to adjust warfarin dosage.

Blood takes longer time to clot if INR is higher. Normal INR is about 1. In patients taking anticoagulant therapy for atrial fibrillation, INR should be between 2 and 3. For patients with heart valve disorders, INR should be between 3 and 4. But, INR greater than 4 indicates that blood is clotting too slowly and there is a risk of uncontrolled blood clotting.

■ THROMBIN TIME

Thrombin time (TT) is the time taken for the blood to clot after adding thrombin to it. It is done to investigate the presence of heparin in plasma or to detect fibrinogen abnormalities. This test involves observation of clotting time after adding thrombin to patient's plasma. Normal duration of thrombin time is 12 to 20 seconds. It is prolonged in heparin therapy and during dysfibrinogenimia (abnormal function of fibrinogen with normal fibrinogen level).

■ APPLIED PHYSIOLOGY

■ BLEEDING DISORDERS

Bleeding disorders are the conditions characterized by prolonged bleeding time or clotting time.

Bleeding disorders are of three types:
1. Hemophilia.
2. Purpura.
3. von Willebrand disease.

1. *Hemophilia*

Hemophilia is a group of sex-linked inherited blood disorders, characterized by prolonged clotting time. However, the bleeding time is normal. Usually, it affects the males, with the females being the carriers.

Because of prolonged clotting time, even a mild trauma causes excess bleeding which can lead to death. Damage of skin while falling or extraction of a tooth may cause excess bleeding for few weeks. Easy bruising and hemorrhage in muscles and joints are also common in this disease.

Causes of hemophilia

Hemophilia occurs due to lack of formation of prothrombin activator. That is why the coagulation time is prolonged. The formation of prothrombin activator is affected due to the deficiency of factor VIII, IX or XI.

Types of hemophilia

Depending upon the deficiency of the factor involved, hemophilia is classified into three types:
 i. Hemophilia A or **classic hemophilia:** Due to the deficiency of factor VIII. 85% of people with hemophilia are affected by hemophilia A.
 ii. Hemophilia B or **Christmas disease:** Due to the deficiency of factor IX. 15% of people with hemophilia are affected by hemophilia B.
 iii. Hemophilia C or factor XI deficiency: Due to the deficiency of factor XI. It is a very rare bleeding disorder.

Symptoms of hemophilia

 i. Spontaneous bleeding.
 ii. Prolonged bleeding due to cuts, tooth extraction and surgery.
 iii. Hemorrhage in gastrointestinal and urinary tracts.
 iv. Bleeding in joints followed by swelling and pain
 v. Appearance of blood in urine.

Treatment for hemophilia

Effective therapy for classical hemophilia involves replacement of missing clotting factor.

2. *Purpura*

Purpura is a disorder characterized by prolonged bleeding time. However, the clotting time is normal. Characteristic feature of this disease is spontaneous bleeding under the skin from ruptured capillaries. It causes small tiny **hemorrhagic spots** in many areas of the body. The hemorrhagic spots under the skin are called **purpuric spots** (purple colored patch like appearance). That is why this disease is called purpura. Blood also sometimes collects in large areas beneath the skin which are called **ecchymoses.**

Types and causes of purpura

Purpura is classified into three types depending upon the causes:

i. *Thrombocytopenic purpura*

Thrombocytopenic purpura is due to the deficiency of platelets (thrombocytopenia). In bone marrow disease, platelet production is affected leading to the deficiency of platelets.

ii. *Idiopathic thrombocytopenic purpura*

Purpura due to some unknown cause is called idiopathic thrombocytopenic purpura. It is believed that platelet count decreases due to the development of antibodies against platelets, which occurs after blood transfusion.

iii. *Thrombasthenic purpura*

Thrombasthenic purpura is due to structural or functional abnormality of platelets. However, the platelet count is normal. It is characterized by normal clotting time, normal or prolonged bleeding time but defective clot retraction.

3. von Willebrand Disease

von Willebrand disease is a bleeding disorder, characterized by excess bleeding even with a mild injury. It is due to deficiency of von Willebrand factor, which is a protein secreted by endothelium of damaged blood vessels and platelets. This protein is responsible for adherence of platelets to endothelium of blood vessels during hemostasis after an injury. It is also responsible for the survival and maintenance of factor VIII in plasma.

Deficiency of von Willebrand factor suppresses platelet adhesion. It also causes deficiency of factor VIII. This results in excess bleeding, which resembles the bleeding that occurs during platelet dysfunction or hemophilia.

■ THROMBOSIS

Thrombosis or intravascular blood clotting refers to coagulation of blood inside the blood vessels. Normally, blood does not clot in the blood vessel because of some factors which are already explained. But some abnormal conditions cause thrombosis.

Causes of Thrombosis

1. *Injury to blood vessels*

During infection or mechanical obstruction, the endothelial lining of the blood vessel is damaged and it initiates thrombosis.

2. *Roughened endothelial lining*

In infection, damage or arteriosclerosis, the endothelium becomes rough and this initiates clotting.

3. *Sluggishness of blood flow*

Decreased rate of blood flow causes aggregation of platelets and formation of thrombus. Slowness of blood flow occurs in reduced cardiac action, hypotension, low metabolic rate, prolonged confinement to bed and immobility of limbs.

4. *Agglutination of RBCs*

Agglutination of the RBCs leads to thrombosis. Agglutination of RBCs occurs by the foreign antigens or toxic substances.

5. *Toxic thrombosis*

Thrombosis is common due to the action of chemical poisons like arsenic compounds, mercury, poisonous mushrooms and snake venom.

6. *Congenital absence of protein C*

Protein C is a circulating anticoagulant, which inactivates factors V and VIII. Thrombosis occurs in the absence of this protein. Congenital absence of protein C causes thrombosis and death in infancy.

Complications of Thrombosis

1. *Thrombus*

During thrombosis, lumen of blood vessels is occluded. The solid mass of platelets, red cells and/or clot, which obstructs the blood vessel, is called thrombus. The thrombus formed due to agglutination of RBC is called agglutinative thrombus.

2. *Embolism and embolus*

Embolism is the process in which the thrombus or a part of it is detached and carried in bloodstream and occludes the small blood vessels, resulting in arrests of blood flow to any organ or region of the body. Embolus is the thrombus or part of it, which arrests the blood flow. The obstruction of blood flow by embolism is common in lungs (**pulmonary embolism**), brain (**cerebral embolism**) or heart (**coronary embolism**).

3. *Ischemia*

Insufficient blood supply to an organ or area of the body by the obstruction of blood vessels is called ischemia. Ischemia results in tissue damage because of hypoxia (lack of oxygen). Ischemia also causes discomfort, pain and tissue death. Death of body tissue is called necrosis.

4. Necrosis and infarction

Necrosis is a general term that refers to tissue death caused by loss of blood supply, injury, infection, inflammation, physical agents or chemical substances.

Infarction means the tissue death due to loss of blood supply. Loss of blood supply is usually caused by occlusion of an artery by thrombus or embolus and sometimes by atherosclerosis (Chapter 67).

Area of tissue that undergoes infarction is called infarct. Infarction commonly occurs in heart, brain, lungs, kidneys and spleen.

Blood Groups

■ INTRODUCTION

When blood from two individuals is mixed, sometimes clumping (agglutination) of RBCs occurs. This clumping is because of the immunological reactions. But, why clumping occurs in some cases and not in other cases remained a mystery until the discovery of blood groups by the Austrian Scientist **Karl Landsteiner,** in 1901. He was honored with Nobel Prize in 1930 for this discovery.

■ ABO BLOOD GROUPS

Determination of ABO blood groups depends upon the immunological reaction between antigen and antibody. Landsteiner found two antigens on the surface of RBCs and named them as A antigen and B antigen. These antigens are also called agglutinogens because of their capacity to cause agglutination of RBCs. He noticed the corresponding antibodies or agglutinins in the plasma and named them anti-A or α-antibody and anti-B or β-antibody. However, a particular agglutinogen and the corresponding agglutinin cannot be present together. If present, it causes clumping of the blood. Based on this, Karl Landsteiner classified the blood groups. Later it became the 'Landsteiner Law' for grouping the blood.

■ LANDSTEINER LAW

Landsteiner law states that:
1. If a particular **agglutinogen** (antigen) is present in the RBCs, corresponding **agglutinin** (antibody) must be absent in the serum.
2. If a particular agglutinogen is absent in the RBCs, the corresponding agglutinin must be present in the serum.

Though the second part of Landsteiner law is a fact, it is not applicable to Rh factor.

■ BLOOD GROUP SYSTEMS

More than 20 genetically determined blood group systems are known today. But, Landsteiner discovered two blood group systems called the ABO system and the Rh system. These two blood group systems are the most important ones that are determined before blood transfusions.

■ ABO SYSTEM

Based on the presence or absence of antigen A and antigen B, blood is divided into four groups:
1. 'A' group
2. 'B' group
3. 'AB' group
4. 'O' group.

Blood having antigen A belongs to 'A' group. This blood has β-antibody in the serum. Blood with antigen B and α-antibody belongs to 'B' group. If both the antigens are present, blood group is called 'AB' group and serum of this group does not contain any antibody. If both antigens are absent, the blood group is called 'O' group and both α and β antibodies are present in the serum. Antigens and antibodies present in different groups of ABO system are given in Table 21.1. Percentage of people among Asian and European population belonging to different blood group is given in Table 21.2.

'A' group has two subgroups namely 'A$_1$' and 'A$_2$'. Similarly 'AB' group has two subgroups namely 'A$_1$B' and 'A$_2$B'.

■ DETERMINATION OF ABO GROUP

Determination of the ABO group is also called blood grouping, blood typing or blood matching.

Principle of Blood Typing – Agglutination

Blood typing is done on the basis of agglutination. Agglutination means the collection of separate particles like RBCs into clumps or masses. Agglutination occurs if an antigen is mixed with its corresponding antibody which is called **isoagglutinin.** Agglutination occurs when

TABLE 21.1: Antigen and antibody present in ABO blood groups

Group	Antigen in RBC	Antibody in serum
A	A	Anti-B (β)
B	B	Anti-A (α)
AB	A and B	No antibody
O	No antigen	Anti-A and Anti-B

TABLE 21.2: Percentage of people having different blood groups

Population	A	B	AB	O
Indians	23	33	7	37
Asians	25	25	5	45
Europeans	42	9	3	46

A antigen is mixed with anti-A or when B antigen is mixed with anti-B.

Requisites for Blood Typing

To determine the blood group of a person, a suspension of his RBC and testing antisera are required. Suspension of RBC is prepared by mixing blood drops with isotonic saline (0.9%).

Test sera are:
1. Antiserum A, containing anti-A or α-antibody.
2. Antiserum B, containing anti-B or β-antibody.

Procedure

1. One drop of antiserum A is placed on one end of a glass slide (or a tile) and one drop of antiserum B on the other end.
2. One drop of RBC suspension is mixed with each antiserum. The slide is slightly rocked for 2 minutes. The presence or absence of agglutination is observed by naked eyes and if necessary, it is confirmed by using microscope.
3. Presence of agglutination is confirmed by the presence of thick masses (clumping) of RBCs
4. Absence of agglutination is confirmed by clear mixture with dispersed RBCs.

Results

1. *If agglutination occurs with antiserum A:* The antiserum A contains α-antibody. The agglutination occurs if the RBC contains A antigen. So, the blood group is A (Fig. 21.1).
2. *If agglutination occurs with antiserum B:* The antiserum B contains β-antibody. The agglutination occurs if the RBC contains B antigen. So, the blood group is B.
3. *If agglutination occurs with both antisera A and B:* The RBC contains both A and B antigens to cause agglutination. And, the blood group is AB.
4. If agglutination does not occur either with antiserum A or antiserum B: The agglutination does not occur because RBC does not contain any antigen. The blood group is O.

Anti-A	Anti-B	Reaction

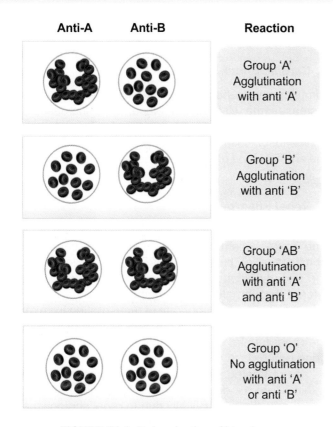

Group 'A'
Agglutination
with anti 'A'

Group 'B'
Agglutination
with anti 'B'

Group 'AB'
Agglutination
with anti 'A'
and anti 'B'

Group 'O'
No agglutination
with anti 'A'
or anti 'B'

FIGURE 21.1: Determination of blood group

■ IMPORTANCE OF ABO GROUPS IN BLOOD TRANSFUSION

During blood transfusion, only compatible blood must be used. The one who gives blood is called the **'donor'** and the one who receives the blood is called **'recipient'.**

While transfusing the blood, antigen of the donor and the antibody of the recipient are considered. The antibody of the donor and antigen of the recipient are ignored mostly.

Thus, RBC of 'O' group has no antigen and so agglutination does not occur with any other group of blood. So, 'O' group blood can be given to any blood group persons and the people with this blood group are called **'universal donors'.**

Plasma of AB group blood has no antibody. This does not cause agglutination of RBC from any other group of blood. People with AB group can receive blood from any blood group persons. So, people with this blood group are called **'universal recipients'.**

■ MATCHING AND CROSS-MATCHING

Blood matching (typing) is a laboratory test done to determine the blood group of a person. When the

person needs blood transfusion, another test called cross-matching is done after the blood is typed. It is done to find out whether the person's body will accept the donor's blood or not.

For blood matching, RBC of the individual (recipient) and test sera are used. Cross-matching is done by mixing the serum of the recipient and the RBCs of donor. Cross-matching is always done before blood transfusion. If agglutination of RBCs from a donor occurs during cross-matching, the blood from that person is not used for transfusion.

Matching   = Recipient's RBC + Test sera.

Cross-matching = Recipient's serum + Donor's RBC.

■ INHERITANCE OF ABO AGGLUTINOGENS AND AGGLUTININS

Blood group of a person depends upon the two genes inherited from each parent. Gene A and gene B are dominant by themselves and gene O is recessive. Inheritance of blood group is represented schematically as given in Table 21.3.

Agglutinogens appear during the 6th month of fetal life. Concentration at birth is 1/5 of the adult concentration. It rises to the adult level at puberty. Agglutinogens are present not only in RBCs but also present in many organs like salivary glands, pancreas, kidney, liver, lungs, etc. The A and B agglutinogens are inherited from the parents as Mendelian phenotypes.

Agglutinin α or β is not produced during fetal life. It starts appearing only 2 or 3 months after birth. Agglutinin is produced in response to A or B agglutinogens which enter the body through respiratory system or digestive system along with bacteria.

Agglutinins are the gamma-globulins which are mainly IgG and IgM immunoglobulins.

■ TRANSFUSION REACTIONS DUE TO ABO INCOMPATIBILITY

Transfusion reactions are the adverse reactions in the body, which occur due to transfusion error that involves transfusion of incompatible **(mismatched)** blood. The reactions may be mild causing only fever and hives (skin disorder characterized by itching) or may be severe leading to renal failure, shock and death.

In mismatched transfusion, the transfusion reactions occur between donor's RBC and recipient's plasma. So, if the donor's plasma contains agglutinins against recipient's RBC, agglutination does not occur because these antibodies are diluted in the recipient's blood.

But, if recipient's plasma contains agglutinins against donor's RBCs, the immune system launches a response

TABLE 21.3: Inheritance of ABO group

Gene from parents	Group of offspring	Genotype
A + A A + O	A	AA or AO
B + B B + O	B	BB or BO
A + B O + O	AB O	AB OO

against the new blood cells. Donor RBCs are agglutinated resulting in transfusion reactions.

Severity of Transfusion Reactions

Severity of transfusion reactions varies from mild (fever and chills) to severe (acute kidney failure, shock and death). Severity depends upon the amount of blood transfused, type of reaction and general health of the patient.

Cause for Transfusion Reactions

Transfusion of incompatible blood produces hemolytic reactions. The recipient's antibodies (IgG or IgM) adhere to the donor RBCs, which are agglutinated and destroyed. Large amount of free hemoglobin is liberated into plasma. This leads to transfusion reactions.

Signs and Symptoms of Transfusion Reactions

Non-hemolytic transfusion reaction

Non-hemolytic transfusion reaction develops within a few minutes to hours after the commencement of blood transfusion. Common symptoms are fever, difficulty in breathing and itching.

Hemolytic transfusion reaction

Hemolytic transfusion reaction may be acute or delayed. The acute hemolytic reaction occurs within few minutes of transfusion. It develops because of rapid hemolysis of donor's RBCs. Symptoms include fever, chills, increased heart rate, low blood pressure, shortness of breath, bronchospasm, nausea, vomiting, red urine, chest pain, back pain and rigor. Some patients may develop pulmonary edema and congestive cardiac failure.

Delayed hemolytic reaction occurs from 1 to 5 days after transfusion. The hemolysis of RBCs results in release of large amount of hemoglobin into the plasma. This leads to the following complications.

1. Jaundice

Normally, hemoglobin released from destroyed RBC is degraded and bilirubin is formed from it. When the serum bilirubin level increases above 2 mg/dL, jaundice occurs (Chapter 40).

2. Cardiac Shock

Simultaneously, hemoglobin released into the plasma increases the viscosity of blood. This increases the workload on the heart leading to **heart failure.** Moreover, toxic substances released from hemolyzed cells reduce the arterial blood pressure and develop circulatory shock (Fig. 21.2).

3. Renal Shutdown

Dysfunction of kidneys is called renal shutdown. The toxic substances from hemolyzed cells cause constriction of blood vessels in kidney. In addition, the toxic substances along with free hemoglobin are filtered through glomerular membrane and enter renal tubules. Because of poor rate of reabsorption from renal tubules, all these substances precipitate and obstruct the renal tubule. This suddenly stops the formation of urine (anuria).

If not treated with artificial kidney, the person dies within 10 to 12 days because of jaundice, circulatory shock and more specifically due to renal shutdown and anuria.

■ Rh FACTOR

Rh factor is an antigen present in RBC. This antigen was discovered by Landsteiner and Wiener. It was first discovered in **Rhesus monkey** and hence the name 'Rh factor'. There are many Rh antigens but only the D antigen is more antigenic in human.

The persons having D antigen are called 'Rh positive' and those without D antigen are called 'Rh negative'. Among Indian population, 85% of people are Rh positive and 15% are Rh negative. Percentage of Rh positive people is more among black people.

Rh group system is different from ABO group system because, the antigen D does not have corresponding natural antibody (anti-D). However, if Rh positive blood is transfused to a Rh negative person anti-D is developed in that person. On the other hand, there is no risk of complications if the Rh positive person receives Rh negative blood.

■ INHERITANCE OF Rh ANTIGEN

Rhesus factor is an inherited dominant factor. It may be homozygous Rhesus positive with DD or heterozygous Rhesus positive with Dd (Fig. 21.3). Rhesus negative occurs only with complete absence of D (i.e. with homozygous dd).

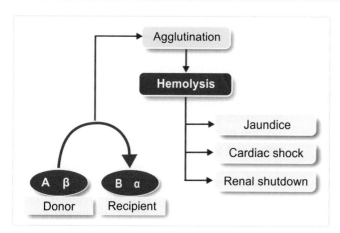

FIGURE 21.2: Complications of mismatched blood transfusion

■ TRANSFUSION REACTIONS DUE TO Rh INCOMPATIBILITY

When a Rh negative person receives Rh positive blood for the first time, he is not affected much, since the reactions do not occur immediately. But, the Rh antibodies develop within one month. The transfused RBCs, which are still present in the recipient's blood, are agglutinated. These agglutinated cells are lysed by macrophages. So, a delayed transfusion reaction occurs. But, it is usually mild and does not affect the recipient. However, antibodies developed in the recipient remain in the body forever. So, when this person receives Rh positive blood for the second time, the donor RBCs are agglutinated and severe transfusion reactions occur immediately (Fig. 21.4). These reactions are similar to the reactions of ABO incompatibility (see above).

■ HEMOLYTIC DISEASE OF FETUS AND NEWBORN – ERYTHROBLASTOSIS FETALIS

Hemolytic disease is the disease in fetus and newborn, characterized by abnormal hemolysis of RBCs. It is due to Rh incompatibility, i.e. the difference between the Rh blood group of the mother and baby. Hemolytic disease leads to erythroblastosis fetalis.

Erythroblastosis fetalis is a disorder in fetus, characterized by the presence of erythroblasts in blood. When a mother is Rh negative and fetus is Rh positive (the Rh factor being inherited from the father), usually the first child escapes the complications of Rh incompatibility. This is because the Rh antigen cannot pass from fetal blood into the mother's blood through the **placental barrier.**

However, at the time of parturition (delivery of the child), the Rh antigen from fetal blood may leak into mother's blood because of **placental detachment.** During

postpartum period, i.e. within a month after delivery, the mother develops Rh antibody in her blood.

When the mother conceives for the second time and if the fetus happens to be Rh positive again, the Rh antibody from mother's blood crosses placental barrier and enters the fetal blood. Thus, the Rh antigen cannot cross the placental barrier, whereas Rh antibody can cross it.

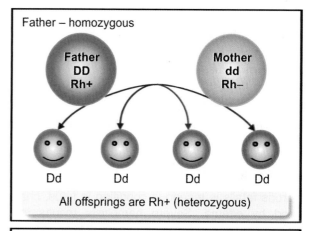

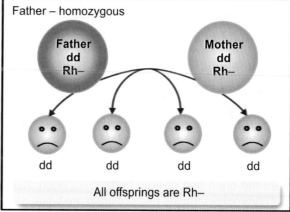

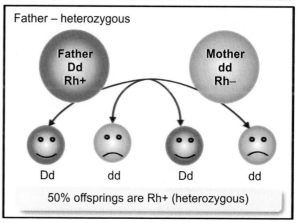

FIGURE 21.3: Inheritance of Rh antigen

Rh antibody which enters the fetus causes agglutination of fetal RBCs resulting in hemolysis.

Severe hemolysis in the fetus causes jaundice. To compensate the hemolysis of more and more number of RBCs, there is rapid production of RBCs, not only from bone marrow, but also from spleen and liver. Now, many large and immature cells in proerythroblastic stage are released into circulation. Because of this, the disease is called erythroblastosis fetalis.

Ultimately due to excessive hemolysis severe complications develop, viz.
1. Severe anemia
2. Hydrops fetalis
3. Kernicterus.

1. *Severe Anemia*

Excessive hemolysis results in anemia and the infant dies when anemia becomes severe.

2. *Hydrops Fetalis*

Hydrops fetails is a serious condition in fetus, characterized by edema. Severe hemolysis results in the development of edema, enlargement of liver and spleen and cardiac failure. When this condition becomes more severe, it may lead to **intrauterine death** of fetus.

3. *Kernicterus*

Kernicterus is the form of **brain damage** in infants caused by severe jaundice. If the baby survives anemia in erythroblastosis fetalis (see above), then kernicterus develops because of high bilirubin content.

The blood-brain barrier is not well developed in infants as in the adults (Chapter 163). So, the bilirubin enters the brain and causes permanent brain damage. Most commonly affected parts of brain are basal ganglia, hippocampus, geniculate bodies, cerebellum and cranial nerve nuclei. The features of this disease are:
i. When brain damage starts, the babies become lethargic and sleepy. They have high-pitched cry, hypotonia and arching of head backwards.
ii. As the disease progresses, they develop hypertonia and opisthotonus (Chapter 155).
iii. Advanced signs of the disease are inability to suckle milk, irritability and crying, bicycling movements, choreoathetosis (Chapter 151), spasticity, (Chapter 34) seizures (Chapter 161), fever and coma.

Prevention or treatment for erythroblastosis fetalis
i. If mother is found to be Rh negative and fetus is Rh positive, anti D (antibody against D antigen) should be administered to the mother at 28th and 34th weeks of gestation, as prophylactic measure. If Rh negative mother delivers Rh positive baby, then anti D should be administered to the mother within 48 hours of delivery. This develops passive immunity and prevents the formation of Rh antibodies in mother's blood. So, the hemolytic disease of newborn does not occur in a subsequent pregnancy.
ii. If the baby is born with erythroblastosis fetalis, the treatment is given by means of exchange transfusion (Chapter 22). Rh negative blood is transfused into the infant, replacing infant's own Rh positive blood. It will now take at least 6 months for the infant's new Rh positive blood to replace the transfused Rh negative blood. By this time, all the molecules of Rh antibody derived from the mother get destroyed.

■ OTHER BLOOD GROUPS

In addition to ABO blood groups and Rh factor, many more blood group systems were found, such as Lewis blood group and MNS blood groups. However, these systems of blood groups do not have much clinical importance.

■ LEWIS BLOOD GROUP

Lewis blood group was first found in a subject named Mrs Lewis. The antibody that was found in this lady reacted with the antigens found on RBCs and in body

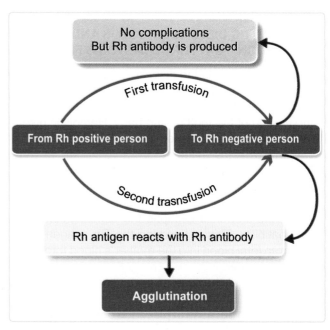

FIGURE 21.4: Rh incompatibility

fluids such as saliva, gastric juice, etc. The antigens, which are named Lewis antigens are formed in the tissues, released in the body secretions and then absorbed by the RBC membrane. Because of secretion along with body secretions, these antigens are also known as secretor antigens. Presence of Lewis antigens in children leads to some complications such as retarded growth. Sometimes, it causes transfusion reactions also.

■ MNS BLOOD GROUPS

MNS blood groups are determined by their reactions with anti-M, anti-N and anti-S. However, these blood groups rarely cause any trouble like hemolysis following transfusion.

■ OTHER BLOOD GROUPS

Other blood groups include:
   i. Auberger groups
  ii. Diego group
 iii. Bombay group
 iv. Duffy group
  v. Lutheran group
 vi. P group
 vii. Kell group
viii. I group
 ix. Kidd group
  x. Sulter Xg group.

■ IMPORTANCE OF KNOWING BLOOD GROUP

Nowadays, knowledge of blood group is very essential medically, socially and judicially. The importance of knowing blood group is:
1. Medically, it is important during blood transfusions and in tissue transplants.
2. Socially, one should know his or her own blood group and become a member of the Blood Donor's Club so that he or she can be approached for blood donation during emergency conditions.
3. It general among the couples, knowledge of blood groups helps to prevent the complications due to Rh incompatibility and save the child from the disorders like erythroblastosis fetalis.
4. Judicially, it is helpful in medico-legal cases to sort out parental disputes.

Blood Transfusion

- ■ INTRODUCTION
- ■ PRECAUTIONS
- ■ HAZARDS OF BLOOD TRANSFUSION
- ■ BLOOD SUBSTITUTES
- ■ EXCHANGE TRANSFUSION
- ■ AUTOLOGOUS BLOOD TRANSFUSION

■ INTRODUCTION

Blood transfusion is the process of transferring blood or blood components from one person (the donor) into the bloodstream of another person (the recipient). Transfusion is done as a **life-saving procedure** to replace blood cells or blood products lost through bleeding.

■ CONDITIONS WHEN BLOOD TRANSFUSION IS NECESSARY

Blood transfusion is essential in the following conditions:
1. Anemia
2. Hemorrhage
3. Trauma
4. Burns
5. Surgery.

■ PRECAUTIONS

Certain precautions must be followed before and during the transfusion of blood to a patient.

■ PRECAUTIONS TO BE TAKEN BEFORE THE TRANSFUSION OF BLOOD

1. Donor must be healthy, without any diseases like:
   a. Sexually transmitted diseases such as syphilis
   b. Diseases caused by virus like hepatitis, AIDS, etc.
2. Only compatible blood must be transfused
3. Both matching and cross-matching must be done
4. Rh compatibility must be confirmed.

■ PRECAUTIONS TO BE TAKEN WHILE TRANSFUSING BLOOD

1. Apparatus for transfusion must be sterile
2. Temperature of blood to be transfused must be same as the body temperature
3. Transfusion of blood must be slow. The sudden rapid infusion of blood into the body increases the load on the heart, resulting in many complications.

■ HAZARDS OF BLOOD TRANSFUSION

Hazards of blood transfusion are of four types:
1. Reactions due to mismatched (incompatible) blood transfusion – transfusion reactions
2. Reactions due to massive blood transfusion
3. Reactions due to faulty techniques during blood transfusion
4. Transmission of infections.

■ REACTIONS DUE TO MISMATCHED BLOOD TRANSFUSION – TRANSFUSION REACTIONS

Transfusion reactions due to ABO incompatibility and Rh incompatibility are explained in the Chapter 21.

■ REACTIONS DUE TO MASSIVE BLOOD TRANSFUSION

Massive transfusion is the transfusion of blood equivalent or more than the patient's own blood volume. It leads to

   i. Circulatory shock, particularly in patients suffering from chronic anemia, cardiac diseases or renal diseases
  ii. Hyperkalemia due to increased potassium concentration in stored blood
 iii. Hypocalcemia leading to tetany due to massive transfusion of citrated blood
  iv. Hemosiderosis (increased deposition of ion in the form of **hemosiderin,** in organs such as endocrine glands, heart and liver) due to iron overload after repeated transfusions.

■ REACTIONS DUE TO FAULTY TECHNIQUES DURING BLOOD TRANSFUSION

Faulty techniques adapted during blood transfusion leads to:

   i. **Thrombophlebitis** (inflammation of vein, associated with formation of thrombus).
  ii. **Air embolism** (obstruction of blood vessel due to entrance of air into the bloodstream).

■ TRANSMISSION OF INFECTIONS

Blood transfusion without precaution leads to transmission of blood-borne infections such as:

   i. HIV
  ii. Hepatitis B and A
 iii. **Glandular fever** or infectious mononucleosis (acute infectious disease caused by **Epstein-Barr virus** and characterized by fever, swollen lymph nodes, sore throat and abnormal lymphocytes)
  iv. **Herpes** (viral disease with eruption of small blister-like vesicles on skin or membranes)
   v. Bacterial infections.

■ BLOOD SUBSTITUTES

Fluids infused into the body instead of whole blood are known as blood substitutes.

   Commonly used blood substitutes are:
1. Human plasma
2. 0.9% sodium chloride solution (saline) and 5% glucose
3. Colloids like gum acacia, isinglass, albumin and animal gelatin.

■ EXCHANGE TRANSFUSION

Exchange transfusion is the procedure which involves removal of patient's blood completely and replacement with fresh blood or plasma of the donor. It is otherwise known as **replacement transfusion.** It is an important life-saving procedure carried out in conditions such as severe jaundice, sickle cell anemia, erythroblastosis fetalis, etc.

■ PROCEDURE

Procedure involves both removal and replacement of affected blood in stages. Exchange transfusion is carried out in short cycles of few minutes duration, as follows:

1. Affected person's blood is slowly drawn out in small quantities of 5 to 20 mL, depending upon the age and size of the person and the severity of the condition.
2. Equal quantity of fresh, prewarmed blood or plasma is infused through intravenous catheter. This is carried out for few minutes.
3. Catheter is left in place and the transfusion is repeated within few hours.
4. This procedure is continued till the whole or predetermined volume of blood is exchanged.

■ CONDITIONS WHICH NEED EXCHANGE TRANSFUSION

1. Hemolytic disease of the newborn (erythroblastosis fetalis).
2. Severe sickle cell anemia.
3. Severe polycythemia (replacement with saline, plasma or albumin).
4. Toxicity of certain drugs.
5. Severe jaundice in newborn babies, which does not respond to **ultraviolet light therapy.** Normally, neonatal jaundice is treated by exposure to ultraviolet rays. It breaks down the bilirubin which is excreted by liver.

■ AUTOLOGOUS BLOOD TRANSFUSION

Autologous blood transfusion is the collection and reinfusion of patient's own blood. It is also called **self blood donation.** The conventional transfusion of blood that is collected from persons other than the patient is called **allogeneic** or **heterologous blood transfusion.**

Autologous blood transfusion is used for planned surgical procedures. Patient's blood is withdrawn in advance and stored. Later, it is infused if necessary during surgery.

This type of blood transfusion prevents the transmission of viruses such as HIV or hepatitis B. It also eliminates transfusion reactions.

Blood Volume

■ NORMAL BLOOD VOLUME
■ VARIATIONS
■ MEASUREMENT
■ REGULATION
■ APPLIED PHYSIOLOGY

■ NORMAL BLOOD VOLUME

Total amount of blood present in the circulatory system, blood reservoirs, organs and tissues together constitute blood volume. In a normal young healthy adult male weighing about 70 kg, the blood volume is about 5 L. It is about 7% of total body weight. It ranges between 6% and 8% of body weight. In relation to body surface area, blood volume is 2.8 to 3.1 L/sq M.

■ VARIATIONS IN BLOOD VOLUME

■ PHYSIOLOGICAL VARIATIONS

1. Age

Absolute blood volume is less at birth and it increases steadily as the age advances. However, at birth, the blood volume is more when compared to body weight and less when compared to the body surface area. At birth and at 24 hours after birth, the blood volume is about 80 mL/kg body weight. At the end of 6 months, it increases to about 86 mL/kg. At the end of one year, it is about 80 mL/kg. It remains at this level until 6 years of age. At 10 years, it is about 75 mL/kg. At the age of 15 years, the blood volume is about 70 mL/kg body weight, which is almost the adult volume.

2. Sex

In males, the blood volume is slightly more than in females because of the increase in erythropoietic activity, body weight and surface area of the body. In females, it is slightly less because of loss of blood through menstruation, more fats and less body surface area.

3. Surface Area of the Body

Blood volume is directly proportional to the surface area of the body.

4. Body Weight

Blood volume is directly proportional to body weight.

5. Atmospheric Temperature

Exposure to cold environment reduces the blood volume and exposure to warm environment increases the blood volume.

6. Pregnancy

During early stage of pregnancy, blood volume increases by 20% to 30% due to the increased fetal mass and sodium retention. However, it reduces in later stages.

7. Exercise

Exercise increases the blood volume by increasing the release of erythropoietin and production of more RBCs.

8. Posture

Standing (erect posture) for long time reduces the blood volume by about 15%. It is because the pooling of blood in lower limbs while standing increases the hydrostatic pressure. This pressure pushes fluid from blood vessels into the tissue spaces; so blood volume decreases.

9. *High Altitude*

Blood volume increases in high altitude. It is because of hypoxia, which stimulates the secretion of erythropoietin. It induces the production of more RBCs, which leads to increase in blood volume.

10. *Emotion*

Excitement increases blood volume. It is because of sympathetic stimulation, which causes splenic contraction and release of stored blood into circulation.

■ PATHOLOGICAL VARIATIONS

Abnormal increase in blood volume is called hypervolemia and abnormal decrease in blood volume is called hypovolemia. Refer applied physiology for details.

■ MEASUREMENT OF BLOOD VOLUME

Blood volume is measured by two methods, direct method and indirect method.

■ DIRECT METHOD

Direct method is employed only in animals because it involves sacrificing the life. The animal is killed by decapitation and the blood is collected. The blood vessels and the tissues are washed thoroughly with known quantity of water or saline. And, this is added to the blood collected already. The total volume is measured. From this, the volume of water or saline used for washing the tissues is deducted to obtain the volume of the blood in the animal.

This method was first employed by Welcker, in 1854. Later, B'Schoff employed the same method on decapitated criminals, to determine the blood volume in human beings.

■ INDIRECT METHOD

Indirect method is advantageous because, it is used to measure the blood volume in human beings without causing any discomfort or any difficulty to the subject.

Measurement of total blood volume involves two steps:
1. Determination of plasma volume
2. Determination of blood cell volume.

Determination of Plasma Volume

Plasma volume is determined by two methods:
  i. Indicator or dye dilution technique
  ii. Radioisotope method.

i. Determination of plasma volume by indicator or dye dilution technique

Principles and other details of this technique are explained in Chapter 6. The dye which is used to measure plasma volume is Evans blue or T-1824.

Procedure

10 mL of blood is drawn from the subject. This is divided into 2 equal portions. To one part, a known quantity of the dye is added. This is used as control sample in the procedure. The other portion is used to determine the hematocrit value.

Then, a known volume of the dye is injected intravenously. After 10 minutes, a sample of blood is drawn. Then, another 4 samples of blood are collected at the interval of 10 minutes. All the 5 samples are centrifuged and plasma is separated from the samples. In each sample of plasma, the concentration of the dye is measured by colorimetric method and the average concentration is found.

The subject's urine is collected and the amount of dye excreted in the urine is measured.

Calculation

Plasma volume is determined by using the formula,

$$\text{Volume} = \frac{\text{Amount of dye injected} - \text{Amount excreted}}{\text{Average concentration of dye in plasma}}$$

ii. Determination of plasma volume by radioisotope method

Radioactive iodine (^{131}I or ^{132}I) is injected. After sometime, a sample of blood is collected. The radioactivity is determined by using appropriate counter. From this, the plasma volume is determined.

Determination of Blood Cell Volume

Blood cell volume is determined by two methods:
  i. By hematocrit value
  ii. By radioisotope method.

i. Determination of blood cell volume by hematocrit value

This is usually done by centrifuging the blood and measuring the packed cell volume (Chapter 13). Packed cell volume (PCV) is expressed in percentage. If this is deducted from 100, the percentage of plasma is known. From this and from the volume of plasma, the amount of total blood is calculated by using the formula.

$$\text{Blood volume} = \frac{100 \times \text{Amount of plasma}}{100 - \text{PCV}}$$

ii. Determination of blood cell volume by radioisotope method

Volume of blood cell is measured by radioisotope method also. Radioactive chromium (Cr^{52}) is added with heparinized blood and incubated for 2 hours at 37°C. During this time, all the red cells in the blood are 'tagged' with Cr^{52}. Then, this is injected intravenously. After giving sufficient time for mixing, a sample of blood is drawn. Hematocrit value is determined by measuring the radioactivity in the blood sample. Radioactive iron (Fe^{59}, Fe^{55}) or radioactive phosphorus (P^{32}) is also used for determining the hematocrit value.

■ REGULATION OF BLOOD VOLUME

Various mechanisms are involved in the regulation of blood volume. The important ones are the renal and hormonal mechanisms. Hypothalamus plays a vital role in the activation of these two mechanisms during the regulation of blood volume.

When blood volume increases, hypothalamus causes loss of fluid from the body. When the blood volume reduces, hypothalamus induces retention of water. Hypothalamus regulates the extracellular fluid (ECF) volume and blood volume by acting mainly through kidneys and sweat glands and by inducing thirst. This function of hypothalamus is described in Chapter 149.

Hormones also are involved in the regulation of blood volume through the regulation of ECF volume. Hormones which are involved in the maintenance of ECF volume are:
1. Antidiuretic hormone (Chapter 66)
2. Aldosterone (Chapter 70)
3. Cortisol (Chapter 70)
4. Atrial natriuretic peptide (Chapter 72).

■ APPLIED PHYSIOLOGY

■ HYPERVOLEMIA

Increase in blood volume is called hypervolemia. It occurs in the following pathological conditions:

1. *Hyperthyroidism*

Blood volume increases because thyroxine increases the RBC count and plasma volume.

2. *Hyperaldosteronism*

In hyperaldosteronism, excess retention of sodium and water leads to increase in the ECF volume and blood volume.

3. *Cirrhosis of the Liver*

In this condition, the blood volume is more because of increase in the plasma volume.

4. *Congestive Cardiac Failure*

Retention of sodium occurs in this condition. Sodium retention leads to water retention and increase in ECF volume, plasma volume and blood volume.

■ HYPOVOLEMIA

Decrease in blood volume is called hypovolemia. It occurs in the following pathological conditions:

1. *Hemorrhage or Blood Loss*

Acute hemorrhage occurs due to cuts or accidents. The chronic hemorrhage occurs in ulcers, bleeding piles and excessive uterine bleeding in females during menstruation.

2. *Fluid Loss*

Fluid loss occurs in burns, vomiting, diarrhea, excessive sweating and polyuria.

3. *Hemolysis*

Excessive destruction of RBCs occurs because of the presence of various hemolytic agents and other factors such as, hypotonic solution, snake venom, acidity or alkalinity, mismatched blood transfusion, hemorrhagic smallpox and measles.

4. *Anemia*

Blood volume decreases in various types of anemia because of decrease in RBC count. In some cases, the quantity (volume) of blood remains the same but the quality of the blood alters. Blood becomes dilute (hemodilution) because of the entrance of fluid into the blood vessel.

5. *Hypothyroidism*

During hypothyroidism, the blood volume is decreased because of reduction in plasma volume and RBC count.

Reticuloendothelial System and Tissue Macrophage

Chapter

24

- ■ **DEFINITION AND DISTRIBUTION**
  - ■ **RETICULOENDOTHELIAL SYSTEM OR MACROPHAGE SYSTEM**
  - ■ **MACROPHAGE**
- ■ **CLASSIFICATION OF RETICULOENDOTHELIAL CELLS**
  - ■ **FIXED RETICULOENDOTHELIAL CELLS – TISSUE MACROPHAGES**
  - ■ **WANDERING RETICULOENDOTHELIAL CELLS AND TISSUE MACROPHAGES**
- ■ **FUNCTIONS OF RETICULOENDOTHELIAL SYSTEM**

■ DEFINITION AND DISTRIBUTION

■ RETICULOENDOTHELIAL SYSTEM OR MACROPHAGE SYSTEM

Reticuloendothelial system or tissue macrophage system is the system of primitive phagocytic cells, which play an important role in defense mechanism of the body. The reticuloendothelial cells are found in the following structures:
1. Endothelial lining of vascular and lymph channels.
2. Connective tissue and some organs like spleen, liver, lungs, lymph nodes, bone marrow, etc.

Reticular cells in these tissues form the tissue macrophage system.

■ MACROPHAGE

Macrophage is a large phagocytic cell, derived from monocyte (Chapter 17).

■ CLASSIFICATION OF RETICULOENDOTHELIAL CELLS

Reticuloendothelial cells are classified into two types:
1. Fixed reticuloendothelial cells or tissue macrophages.
2. Wandering reticuloendothelial cells.

■ FIXED RETICULOENDOTHELIAL CELLS – TISSUE MACROPHAGES

Fixed reticuloendothelial cells are also called the tissue macrophages or fixed histiocytes because, these cells are usually located in the tissues.

Tissue macrophages are present in the following areas:

1. *Connective Tissue*

Reticuloendothelial cells in connective tissues and in serous membranes like pleura, omentum and mesentery are called the fixed macrophages of connective tissue.

2. *Endothelium of Blood Sinusoid*

Endothelium of the blood sinusoid in bone marrow, liver, spleen, lymph nodes, adrenal glands and pituitary glands also contain fixed cells. Kupffer cells present in liver belong to this category.

3. *Reticulum*

Reticulum of spleen, lymph node and bone marrow contain fixed reticuloendothelial cells.

4. *Central Nervous System*

Meningocytes of meninges and microglia form the tissue macrophages of brain.

5. *Lungs*

Tissue macrophages are present in the alveoli of lungs.

6. *Subcutaneous Tissue*

Fixed reticuloendothelial cells are present in subcutaneous tissue also.

■ **WANDERING RETICULOENDOTHELIAL CELLS AND TISSUE MACROPHAGES**

Wandering reticuloendothelial cells are also called free histiocytes. There are two types of wandering reticuloendothelial cells:

1. Free Histiocytes of Blood

 i. Neutrophils
 ii. Monocytes, which become macrophages and migrate to the site of injury or infection.

2. Free Histiocytes of Solid Tissue

During emergency, the fixed histiocytes from connective tissue and other organs become wandering cells and enter the circulation.

■ **FUNCTIONS OF RETICULOENDOTHELIAL SYSTEM**

Reticuloendothelial system plays an important role in the defense mechanism of the body. Most of the functions of the reticuloendothelial system are carried out by the tissue macrophages.

Functions of tissue macrophages:

1. Phagocytic Function

Macrophages are the large phagocytic cells, which play an important role in defense of the body by phagocytosis.

When any foreign body invades, macrophages ingest them by phagocytosis and liberate the antigenic products of the organism. The antigens activate the helper T lymphocytes and B lymphocytes. (Refer Chapter 17 for details).

Lysosomes of macrophages contain proteolytic enzymes and lipases, which digest the bacteria and other foreign bodies.

2. Secretion of Bactericidal Agents

Tissue macrophages secrete many bactericidal agents which kill the bacteria. The important bactericidal agents of macrophages are the **oxidants.** An oxidant is a substance that oxidizes another substance.

Oxidants secreted by macrophages are:

 i. Superoxide (O_2^-)
 ii. Hydrogen peroxide (H_2O_2)
 iii. Hydroxyl ions (OH^-).

These oxidants are the most potent bactericidal agents. So, even the bacteria which cannot be digested by lysosomal enzymes are degraded by these oxidants.

3. Secretion of Interleukins

Tissue macrophages secrete the following interleukins, which help in immunity:

 i. Interleukin-1 (IL-1): Accelerates the maturation and proliferation of specific B lymphocytes and T lymphocytes.
 ii. Interleukin-6 (IL-6): Causes the growth of B lymphocytes and production of antibodies.
 iii. Interleukin-12 (IL-12): Influences the T helper cells.

4. Secretion of Tumor Necrosis Factors

Two types of tumor necrosis factors (TNF) are secreted by tissue macrophages:

 i. TNF-α: Causes necrosis of tumor and activates the immune responses in the body
 ii. TNF-β: Stimulates immune system and vascular response, in addition to causing necrosis of tumor.

5. Secretion of Transforming Growth Factor

Tissue macrophages secrete transforming growth factor, which plays an important role in preventing rejection of transplanted tissues or organs by immunosuppression.

6. Secretion of Colony-stimulation Factor

Colony-stimulation factor (CSF) secreted by macrophages is M-CSF. It accelerates the growth of granulocytes, monocytes and macrophages.

7. Secretion of Platelet-derived Growth Factor

Tissue macrophages secrete the platelet-derived growth factor (PDGF), which accelerates repair of damaged blood vessel and wound healing.

8. Removal of Carbon Particles and Silicon

Macrophages ingest the substances like carbon dust particles and silicon, which enter the body.

9. Destruction of Senile RBC

Reticuloendothelial cells, particularly those in spleen destroy the senile RBCs and release hemoglobin (Chapter 9).

10. Destruction of Hemoglobin

Hemoglobin released from broken senile RBCs is degraded by the reticuloendothelial cells (Chapter 11).

Spleen

- ■ **STRUCTURE**
  - ■ RED PULP
  - ■ WHITE PULP
- ■ **FUNCTIONS**
  - ■ FORMATION OF BLOOD CELLS
  - ■ DESTRUCTION OF BLOOD CELLS
  - ■ BLOOD RESERVOIR FUNCTION
  - ■ ROLE IN DEFENSE OF BODY
- ■ **APPLIED PHYSIOLOGY**
  - ■ SPLENOMEGALY AND HYPERSPLENISM
  - ■ HYPOSPLENISM AND ASPLENIA

■ STRUCTURE OF SPLEEN

Spleen is the largest **lymphoid organ** in the body and it is highly vascular. It is situated in left hypochondrial region, i.e. upper left part of the abdomen, behind the stomach and just below the diaphragm. About 10% of people have one or more **accessory spleens** which are situated near the main spleen.

Spleen is covered by an outer serous coat and an inner fibromuscular capsule. From the capsule, the trabeculae and trabecular network arise. All the three structures, viz. capsule, trabeculae and trabecular network contain collagen fibers, elastic fibers, smooth muscle fibers and reticular cells. The parenchyma of spleen is divided into red and white pulp.

■ RED PULP

Red pulp consists of venous sinus and cords of structures like blood cells, macrophages and mesenchymal cells.

■ WHITE PULP

The structure of white pulp is similar to that of lymphoid tissue. It has a central artery, which is surrounded by splenic corpuscles or **Malpighian corpuscles.** These corpuscles are formed by lymphatic sheath containing lymphocytes and macrophages.

■ FUNCTIONS OF SPLEEN

■ 1. FORMATION OF BLOOD CELLS

Spleen plays an important role in the hemopoietic function in embryo. During the hepatic stage, spleen produces blood cells along with liver. In myeloid stage, it produces the blood cells along with liver and bone marrow.

■ 2. DESTRUCTION OF BLOOD CELLS

Older RBCs, lymphocytes and thrombocytes are destroyed in the spleen. When the RBCs become old (120 days), the cell membrane becomes more fragile. Diameter of most of the capillaries is less or equal to that of RBC. The fragile old cells are destroyed while trying to squeeze through the capillaries because, these cells cannot withstand the stress of squeezing.

Destruction occurs mostly in the capillaries of spleen because the splenic capillaries have a thin lumen. So, the spleen is known as 'graveyard of RBCs'.

■ 3. BLOOD RESERVOIR FUNCTION

In animals, spleen stores large amount of blood. However, this function is not significant in humans. But, a large number of RBCs are stored in spleen. The RBCs are released from spleen into circulation during the emergency conditions like hypoxia and hemorrhage.

■ 4. ROLE IN DEFENSE OF BODY

Spleen filters the blood by removing the microorganisms. The macrophages in splenic pulp destroy the microorganisms and other foreign bodies by phagocytosis. Spleen contains about 25% of T lymphocytes and 15% of B lymphocytes and forms the site of antibody production.

■ APPLIED PHYSIOLOGY

■ SPLENOMEGALY AND HYPERSPLENISM

Splenomegaly refers to enlargement of spleen. Increase in the activities of spleen is called hypersplenism. Some diseases cause splenomegaly resulting in hypersplenism.

Diseases which cause splenomegaly:
1. Infectious diseases such as malaria, typhoid and tuberculosis
2. Inflammatory diseases like rheumatoid arthritis
3. Pernicious anemia
4. Liver diseases
5. Hematological disorders like spherocytosis
6. Cysts in spleen
7. Hodgkin's disease
8. Glandular fever.

Effects of Splenomegaly

1. Hemolysis resulting in anemia
2. Leukopenia
3. Thrombocytopenia
4. Increase in plasma volume.

■ HYPOSPLENISM AND ASPLENIA

Hyposplenism or hyposplenia refers to diminished functioning of spleen. It occurs after partial removal of spleen due to trauma or cyst. Asplenia means absence of spleen. Functional asplenia means normal functions of spleen. It occurs in the following conditions:

1. Congenital absence of spleen function (congenital asplenia).
2. Acquired through surgical removal of spleen (splenectomy).
3. Acquired through some diseases, which destroy spleen to such an extent that it becomes non-functional. This process is called autosplenectomy. The diseases which cause autosplenectomy are sickle cell anemia and spherocytosis.

Lymphatic System and Lymph

- ■ **LYMPHATIC SYSTEM**
  - ■ ORGANIZATION
  - ■ DRAINAGE
  - ■ SITUATION
- ■ **LYMPH NODES**
  - ■ STRUCTURE
  - ■ FUNCTIONS
  - ■ APPLIED PHYSIOLOGY – SWELLING OF LYMPH NODES
- ■ **LYMPH**
  - ■ FORMATION
  - ■ RATE OF FLOW
  - ■ COMPOSITION
  - ■ FUNCTIONS

■ LYMPHATIC SYSTEM

Lymphatic system is a closed system of lymph channels or lymph vessels, through which lymph flows. It is a **one-way system** and allows the lymph flow from tissue spaces toward the blood.

■ ORGANIZATION OF LYMPHATIC SYSTEM

Lymphatic system arises from tissue spaces as a meshwork of delicate vessels. These vessels are called **lymph capillaries.**

Lymph capillaries start from tissue spaces as enlarged blind-ended terminals called **capillary bulbs.** These bulbs contain valves, which allow flow of lymph in only one direction. There are some muscle fibers around these bulbs. These muscle fibers cause contraction of bulbs so that, lymph is pushed through the vessels.

Lymph capillaries are lined by endothelial cells. Capillaries unite to form large lymphatic vessels. Lymphatic vessels become larger and larger because of the joining of many tributaries along their course.

The structure of lymph capillaries is slightly different from that of the blood capillaries. Lymph capillaries are

more porous and the cells lie overlapping on one another. This allows the fluid to move into the lymph capillaries and not in the opposite direction.

■ DRAINAGE OF LYMPHATIC SYSTEM

Larger lymph vessels ultimately form the **right lymphatic duct** and **thoracic duct.** Right lymphatic duct opens into right subclavian vein and the thoracic duct opens into left subclavian vein. Thoracic duct drains the lymph from more than two third of the tissue spaces in the body (Fig. 26.1).

■ SITUATION OF LYMPH VESSELS

Lymph vessels are situated in the following regions:
1. Deeper layers of skin
2. Subcutaneous tissues
3. Diaphragm
4. Wall of abdominal cavity
5. Omentum
6. Linings of respiratory tract except alveoli
7. Linings of digestive tract
8. Linings of urinary tract

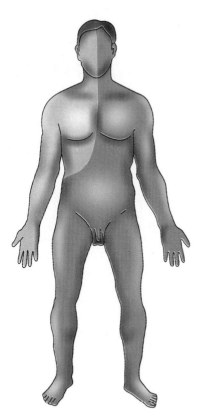

FIGURE 26.1: Lymph drainage. Blue area = Drained by right lymphatic duct; Pink area = Drained by thoracic duct.

9. Linings of genital tract
10. Liver
11. Heart.
    Lymph vessels are not present in the following structures:
1. Superficial layers of skin
2. Central nervous system
3. Cornea
4. Bones
5. Alveoli of lungs.

■ LYMPH NODES

Lymph nodes are small glandular structures located in the course of lymph vessels. The lymph nodes are also called lymph glands or lymphatic nodes.

■ STRUCTUTRE OF LYMPH NODES

Each lymph node constitutes masses of lymphatic tissue, covered by a dense connective tissue capsule. The structures are arranged in three layers namely cortex, paracortex and medulla (Fig. 26.2).

Cortex

Cortex of lymph node consists of primary and secondary **lymphoid follicles.** Primary follicle develops first. When some antigens enter the body and reach the lymph nodes, the cells of primary follicle proliferate. The active proliferation of the cells occurs in a particular area of the follicle called the germinal center. After proliferation of cells, the primary follicles become the secondary follicle. Cortex also contains some B lymphocytes, which are usually aggregated into the primary follicles. Macrophages are also found in the cortex.

Paracortex

Paracortex is in between the cortex and medulla. Paracortex contains T lymphocytes.

Medulla

Medulla contains B and T lymphocytes and macrophages. Blood vessels of lymph node pass through medulla.

Lymphatic Vessels to Lymph Node

Lymph node receives lymph by one or two lymphatic vessels called **afferent vessels.** Afferent vessels divide into small channels. Lymph passes through afferent vessels and small channels and reaches the cortex. It circulates through cortex, paracortex and medulla of the lymph node. From medulla, the lymph leaves the node via one or two **efferent vessels.**

Distribution of Lymph Nodes

Lymph nodes are present along the course of lymphatic vessels in elbow, axilla, knee and groin. Lymph nodes

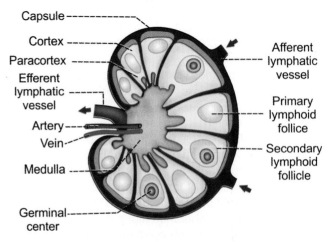

FIGURE 26.2: Structure of a lymph node

are also present in certain points in abdomen, thorax and neck, where many lymph vessels join.

■ FUNCTIONS OF LYMPH NODES

Lymph nodes serve as filters which filter bacteria and toxic substances from the lymph.

Functions of the lymph nodes are:

1. When lymph passes through the lymph nodes, it is filtered, i.e. the water and electrolytes are removed. But, the proteins and lipids are retained in the lymph.
2. Bacteria and other toxic substances are destroyed by macrophages of lymph nodes. Because of this, lymph nodes are called defense barriers.

■ APPLIED PHYSIOLOGY – SWELLING OF LYMPH NODES

During infection or any other processes in a particular region of the body, activities of the lymph nodes in that region increase. This causes swelling of the lymph nodes. Sometimes, the swollen lymph nodes cause pain.

Most common cause of swollen lymph nodes is infection. Lymph nodes situated near an infected area swell immediately. When the body recovers from infection, the lymph nodes restore their original size gradually, in one or two weeks.

Causes for Lymph Node Swelling

1. Skin infection of arm causes swelling of lymph nodes in armpit.
2. **Tonsillitis** or throat infection causes swelling of lymph nodes in neck.
3. Infection of genital organs or leg results in swelling of lymph nodes in groin.
4. Viral infections such as **glandular fever** which affect the whole body cause swelling of lymph nodes in various parts of the body.
5. Cancer in a particular region may spread into the nearby lymph nodes causing the swelling.
   Examples:
   i. **Throat cancer** may spread into lymph nodes in neck.

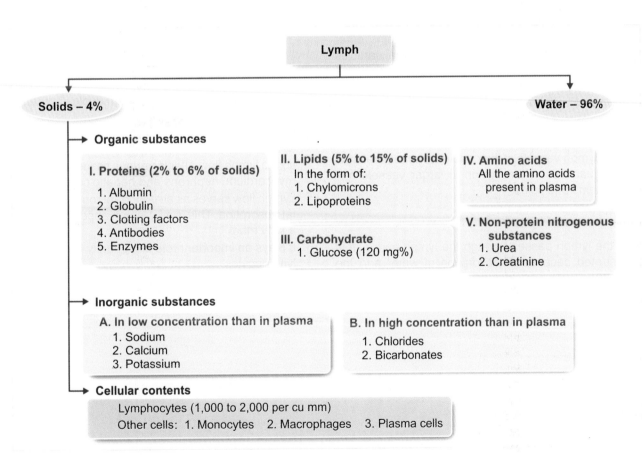

FIGURE 26.3: Composition of lymph

ii. **Lung cancer** may spread into lymph nodes in chest.
iii. **Breast cancer** may spread into lymph nodes in armpit.
iv. **Intestinal cancer** may spread into lymph nodes in abdomen.
v.. **Lymphomas** (cancer of lymphatic system) and leukemia cause swelling of lymph nodes in many parts of the body.

■ LYMPH

■ FORMATION OF LYMPH

Lymph is formed from interstitial fluid, due to the permeability of lymph capillaries. When blood passes via blood capillaries in the tissues, 9/10th of fluid passes into venous end of capillaries from the arterial end. And, the remaining 1/10th of the fluid passes into lymph capillaries, which have more permeability than blood capillaries.

So, when lymph passes through lymph capillaries, the composition of lymph is more or less similar to that of interstitial fluid including protein content. Proteins present in the interstitial fluid cannot enter the blood capillaries because of their larger size. So, these proteins enter lymph vessels, which are permeable to large particles also.

Addition of Proteins and Fats

Tissue fluid in liver and gastrointestinal tract contains more protein and lipid substances. So, proteins and lipids enter the lymph vessels of liver and gastrointestinal tract in large quantities. Thus, lymph in larger vessels has more proteins and lipids.

Concentration of Lymph

When the lymph passes through the lymph nodes, it is concentrated because of absorption of water and the electrolytes. However, the proteins and lipids are not absorbed.

■ RATE OF LYMPH FLOW

About 120 mL of lymph flows into blood per hour. Out of this, about 100 mL/hour flows through thoracic duct and 20 mL/ hour flows through the right lymphatic duct.

Factors Increasing the Flow of Lymph

Flow of lymph is promoted by the increase in:
1. Interstitial fluid pressure.
2. Blood capillary pressure.
3. Surface area of lymph capillary by means of dilatation.
4. Permeability of lymph capillaries.
5. Functional activities of tissues.

■ COMPOSITION OF LYMPH

Usually, lymph is a clear and colorless fluid. It is formed by 96% water and 4% solids. Some blood cells are also present in lymph (Fig. 26.3).

■ FUNCTIONS OF LYMPH

1. Important function of lymph is to return the proteins from tissue spaces into blood.
2. It is responsible for redistribution of fluid in the body.
3. Bacteria, toxins and other foreign bodies are removed from tissues via lymph.
4. Lymph flow is responsible for the maintenance of structural and functional integrity of tissue. Obstruction to lymph flow affects various tissues, particularly myocardium, nephrons and hepatic cells.
5. Lymph flow serves as an important route for intestinal fat absorption. This is why lymph appears milky after a fatty meal.
6. It plays an important role in immunity by transport of lymphocytes.

Tissue Fluid and Edema

Chapter 27

> ■ DEFINITION
> ■ FUNCTIONS
> ■ FORMATION
>   ■ FILTRATION
>   ■ REABSORPTION
> ■ APPLIED PHYSIOLOGY – EDEMA
>   ■ DEFINITION
>   ■ TYPES
>   ■ INTRACELLULAR EDEMA
>   ■ EXTRACELLULAR EDEMA
>   ■ PITTING AND NON-PITTING EDEMA

■ DEFINITION

Tissue fluid is the medium in which cells are bathed. It is otherwise known as **interstitial fluid.** It forms about 20% of extracellular fluid (ECF).

■ FUNCTIONS OF TISSUE FLUID

Because of the capillary membrane, there is no direct contact between blood and cells. And, tissue fluid acts as a medium for exchange of various substances between the cells and blood in the capillary loop. Oxygen and nutritive substances diffuse from the arterial end of capillary through the tissue fluid and reach the cells. Carbon dioxide and waste materials diffuse from the cells into the venous end of capillary through this fluid.

■ FORMATION OF TISSUE FLUID

Formation of tissue fluid involves two processes:
1. Filtration.
2. Reabsorption.

■ FILTRATION

Tissue fluid is formed by the process of filtration. Normally, the blood pressure (also called **hydrostatic** **pressure**) in arterial end of the capillary is about 30 mm Hg. This hydrostatic pressure is the driving force for filtration of water and other substances from blood into tissue spaces. Along the course of the capillary, the pressure falls gradually and it is about 15 mm Hg at the venous end.

Capillary membrane is not permeable to the large molecules, particularly the plasma proteins. So, these proteins remain in the blood and exert a pressure called **oncotic pressure** or **colloidal osmotic pressure.** It is about 25 mm Hg.

Osmotic pressure is constant throughout the circulatory system and it is an opposing force for the filtration of water and other materials from capillary blood into the tissue space. However, the hydrostatic pressure in the arterial end of the capillary (30 mm Hg) is greater than the osmotic pressure. And, the net filtration pressure of 5 mm Hg is responsible for continuous filtration (Fig. 27.1).

Starling Hypothesis

Determination of net filtration pressure is based on Starling hypothesis. Starling hypothesis states that the net filtration through capillary membrane is proportional to the hydrostatic pressure difference across the membrane minus the oncotic pressure difference. These pressures are called **Starling forces** (Refer Chapter 52 for more details).

■ REABSORPTION

Fluid filtered at the arterial end of capillaries is reabsorbed back into the blood at the venous end of capillaries. Here also, the pressure gradient plays an important role. At the venous end of capillaries, the hydrostatic pressure is less (15 mm Hg) and the oncotic pressure is more (25 mm Hg). Due to the pressure gradient of 10 mm Hg, the fluid is reabsorbed along with waste materials from the tissue fluid into the capillaries. About 10% of filtered fluid enters the lymphatic vessels.

Thus, the process of filtration at the arterial end of the capillaries helps in the formation of tissue fluids and the process of reabsorption at the venous end helps to maintain the volume of tissue fluid.

■ APPLIED PHYSIOLOGY – EDEMA

■ DEFINITION

Edema is defined as the swelling caused by excessive accumulation of fluid in the tissues. It may be generalized or local. Edema that involves the entire body is called generalized edema. Local edema is the one that occurs is specific areas of the body such as abdomen, lungs and extremities like feet, ankles and legs. Accumulation of fluid may be inside or outside the cell.

■ TYPES OF EDEMA

Edema is classified into two types, depending upon the body fluid compartment where accumulation of excess fluid occurs:
1. Intracellular edema
2. Extracellular edema.

■ INTRACELLULAR EDEMA

Intracellular edema is the accumulation of fluid inside the cell. It occurs because of three reasons:
1. Malnutrition
2. Poor metabolism
3. Inflammation of the tissues.

1. *Edema due to Malnutrition*

Malnutrition occurs because of poor intake of food or poor circulatory system, through which the nutritive substances are supplied. Due to the lack of nutrition, the ionic pumps of the cell membrane are depressed leading to poor exchange of ions. Especially, the sodium ions leaking into the cells cannot be pumped out. Excess

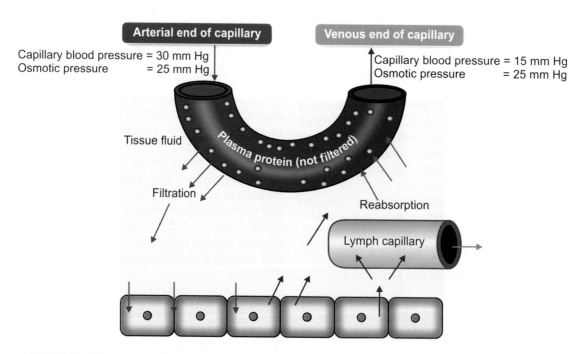

FIGURE 27.1: Formation of tissue fluid. Plasma proteins remain inside the blood capillary as the capillary membrane is not permeable to plasma proteins.

sodium inside the cells causes endosmosis, resulting in intracellular edema.

2. Edema due to Poor Metabolism

Poor metabolism is caused by poor blood supply. Poor blood supply leads to lack of oxygen. It results in poor function of cell membrane and edema, as explained above.

3. Edema due to Inflammation of Tissues

During inflammation of the tissues, usually the permeability of cell membrane increases. This causes the movement of many ions, including sodium into the cells resulting in endosmosis and intracellular edema.

■ EXTRACELLULAR EDEMA

Extracellular edema is defined as the accumulation of fluid outside the cell.

Causes for extracellular edema

1. Abnormal leakage of fluid from capillaries into interstitial space.
2. Obstruction of lymphatic vessels that prevents fluid return from interstitium to blood.

Conditions which lead to extracellular edema

1. Heart failure.
2. Renal disease.
3. Decreased amount of plasma proteins.
4. Lymphatic obstruction.
5. Increased endothelial permeability.

1. Edema due to Heart Failure

Edema occurs in heart failure because of various reasons such as:
 i. Failure of heart to pump blood: Failure of the heart to pump blood from veins to arteries increases venous pressure and capillary pressure. This leads to increased capillary permeability and leakage of fluid from blood into interstitial fluid, causing extracellular edema.
 ii. Fall in blood pressure during heart failure: It decreases the glomerular filtration rate in the kidneys, resulting in sodium and water retention. So, the volume of blood and body fluid increases. This in turn increases the capillary hydrostatic pressure. These two factors together increase the accumulation of fluid causing extracellular edema.
 iii. Low blood supply to kidneys during heart failure: It increases renin secretion, which in turn

increases aldosterone secretion. Aldosterone increases the reabsorption of sodium and water from renal tubules into ECF resulting in the development of extracellular edema.

Pulmonary Edema

Pulmonary edema is the accumulation of fluid in pulmonary interstitium. In left heart failure, the blood is easily pumped into pulmonary circulation by right ventricle. However, the blood cannot return from lungs to left side of the heart because of weakness of this side of the heart. This increases pulmonary vascular pressure leading to leakage of fluid from capillaries into pulmonary interstitium. It causes pulmonary edema which can be life threatening.

2. Edema due to Renal Diseases – Generalized Edema

In renal disease, the kidneys fail to excrete water and electrolytes particularly sodium, leading to retention of water and electrolytes. So, the fluid leaks from blood into interstitial space causing extracellular edema. Initially, the edema develops in the legs, but later it progresses to the entire body (generalized edema).

3. Edema due to Decreased Amount of Plasma Proteins

When the amount of plasma proteins decreases, the colloidal osmotic pressure decreases. Because of this, the permeability of the capillary increases, resulting in increased capillary filtration. So, more amount of water leaks out of the capillary. It accumulates in the tissue spaces resulting in extracellular edema.
 Amount of plasma proteins decreases during the conditions like malnutrition, liver diseases, renal diseases, burns and inflammation.

4. Edema due to Lymphatic Obstruction – Lymphedema

Lymphedema is the edema caused by lymphatic obstruction. It is common in filariasis. During this disease, the parasitic worms live in the lymphatics and obstruct the drainage of lymph. Accumulation of lymph along with cellular reactions leads to swelling that is very prominent in legs and scrotum. Repeated obstruction of lymphatic drainage in these regions results in fibrosis and development of elephantiasis.

Elephantiasis

Elephantiasis is a disorder of lymphatic system, characterized by thickening of skin and extreme enlargement of the affected area, most commonly limbs (legs), genitals, certain areas of trunk and parts of head.

5. *Edema due to Increased Endothelial Permeability*

The permeability of the capillary endothelium increases in conditions like burns, inflammation, trauma, allergic reactions and immunologic reactions, which lead to oozing out of fluid. This fluid accumulates leading to development of edema.

■ PITTING AND NON-PITTING EDEMA

Interstitial fluid is present in the form of a gel that is almost like a semisolid substance. It is because the interstitial fluid is not present as fluid but is bound in a proteoglycan meshwork. It does not allow any free space for the fluid movement except for a diameter of about a few hundredths of a micron.

Normal volume of interstitial fluid is 12 L and it exerts a negative pressure of about 3 mm Hg. It applies a slight suction effect and holds the tissues together. However, in abnormal conditions, where the interstitial fluid volume increases enormously, the pressure becomes positive. Most of the fluid becomes free fluid that is not bound to proteoglycan meshwork. It flows freely through tissue spaces, producing a swelling called edema. This type of edema is known as pitting edema because, when this area is pressed with the finger, displacement of fluid occurs producing a depression or pit. When the finger is removed, the pit remains for few seconds, sometimes as long as one minute, till the fluid flows back into that area.

Edema also develops due to swelling of the cells or clotting of interstitial fluid in the presence of fibrinogen. This is called non-pitting edema because, it is hard and a pit is not formed by pressing.

QUESTIONS IN BLOOD AND BODY FLUIDS

■ LONG QUESTIONS

1. What are the compartments of body fluid? Enumerate the differences between ECF and ICF and explain the measurement of ECF volume.
2. What is indicator dilution technique? How is it applied in the measurement of total body water? Describe dehydration briefly.
3. Give a detailed account of erythropoiesis.
4. Define erythropoiesis. List the different stages of erythropoiesis. Describe the changes which take place in each stage and the factors necessary for erythropoiesis.
5. Describe the morphology, development and functions of leukocytes.
6. Describe the development of cell-mediated immunity.
7. Describe the development of humoral immunity.
8. Define blood coagulation. Describe the mechanisms involved in coagulation. Add a note on anticoagulants.
9. Enumerate the factors involved in blood coagulation and describe the intrinsic mechanism of coagulation.
10. Give an account of extrinsic mechanism of coagulation of blood. Give a brief description of bleeding disorders.
11. What is normal blood volume and what are the factors regulating blood volume? Describe the measurement of blood volume and give a brief account of edema.
12. Give an account of tissue fluid. Add a note on edema.

■ SHORT QUESTIONS

1. Dye or indicator dilution technique.
2. Measurement of total body water.
3. Measurement of ECF volume.
4. Measurement of ICF volume.
5. Measurement of blood volume.
6. Measurement of plasma volume.
7. Dehydration.
8. Water intoxication.
9. Functions of blood.
10. Plasma proteins.
11. Plasmapheresis.
12. Functions of RBCs.
13. Fate of RBCs.
14. Lifespan of RBCs.
15. Physiological variations of RBC count.
16. Polycythemia.
17. Stem cells.
18. Factors necessary for erythropoiesis.
19. Destruction of hemoglobin.
20. Abnormal hemoglobin.
21. Abnormal hemoglobin derivatives.
22. Iron metabolism.
23. Pernicious anemia.
24. Erythrocyte sedimentation rate.
25. Packed cell volume or hematocrit.
26. Anemia.
27. Blood indices.
28. Hemolysins.
29. Types and morphology WBCs.
30. Functions of WBCs.
31. T lymphocytes.
32. B lymphocytes.
33. Role of macrophages/antigen-presenting cells in immunity.
34. Immunoglobulins or antibodies.
35. Immune deficiency diseases.
36. Autoimmune diseases.
37. Immunization.
38. Cytokines.
39. Platelets.
40. Hemostasis.
41. Fibrinolysis.
42. Tests for coagulation.
43. Anticoagulants.
44. Procoagulants.
45. Bleeding disorders.
46. Hemophilia.
47. Purpura.
48. Thrombosis.
49. ABO blood groups.
50. Rh factor.
51. Transfusion reactions.
52. Hemolytic disease of the newborn/ erythroblastosis fetalis.
53. Exchange transfusion
54. Blood volume.
55. Reticuloendothelial system or tissue macrophage.
56. Functions of spleen.
57. Lymph.
58. Lymph nodes.
59. Tissue fluid.
60. Edema.

Section
3
Muscle Physiology

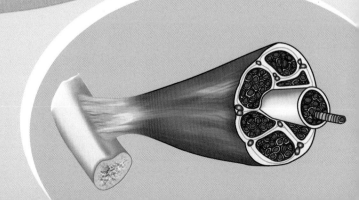

Classification of Muscles

Chapter 28

> ■ **DEPENDING UPON STRIATIONS**
> ■ **DEPENDING UPON CONTROL**
> ■ **DEPENDING UPON SITUATION**

Human body has more than 600 muscles. Muscles perform many useful functions and help us in doing everything in day-to-day life. Muscles are classified by three different methods, based on different factors:

I. Depending upon the presence or absence of striations
II. Depending upon the control
III. Depending upon the situation.

■ DEPENDING UPON STRIATIONS

Depending upon the presence or absence of cross striations, the muscles are divided into two groups:

1. Striated muscle
2. Non-striated muscle.

1. *Striated Muscle*

Striated muscle is the muscle which has a large number of cross-striations (transverse lines). Skeletal muscle and cardiac muscle belong to this category.

2. *Non-striated Muscle*

Muscle which does not have cross-striations is called non-striated muscle. It is also called plain muscle or smooth muscle. It is found in the wall of the visceral organs.

■ DEPENDING UPON CONTROL

Depending upon control, the muscles are classified into two types:

1. Voluntary muscle
2. Involuntary muscle.

1. *Voluntary Muscle*

Voluntary muscle is the muscle that is controlled by the will. Skeletal muscles are the voluntary muscles. These muscles are innervated by somatic nerves.

2. *Involuntary Muscle*

Muscle that cannot be controlled by the will is called involuntary muscle. Cardiac muscle and smooth muscle are involuntary muscles. These muscles are innervated by autonomic nerves.

■ DEPENDING UPON SITUATION

Depending upon situation, the muscles are classified into three types:

1. Skeletal muscle
2. Cardiac muscle
3. Smooth muscle.
   Features of these muscles are given in Table 28.1.

1. *Skeletal Muscle*

Skeletal muscle is situated in association with bones forming the skeletal system. The skeletal muscles form 40% to 50% of body mass and are voluntary and striated. These muscles are supplied by somatic nerves.

TABLE 28.1: Features of skeletal, cardiac and smooth muscle fibers

Features	Skeletal muscle	Cardiac muscle	Smooth muscle
Location	In association with bones	In the heart	In the visceral organs
Shape	Cylindrical and unbranched	Branched	Spindle-shaped, unbranched
Length	1 cm to 4 cm	80 μ to 100 μ	50 μ to 200 μ
Diameter	10 μ to 100 μ	15 μ to 20 μ	2 μ to 5 μ
Number of nucleus	More than one	One	One
Cross-striations	Present	Present	Absent
Myofibrils	Present	Present	Absent
Sarcomere	Present	Present	Absent
Troponin	Present	Present	Absent
Sarcotubular system	Well developed	Well developed	Poorly developed
'T' tubules	Long and thin	Short and broad	Absent
Depolarization	Upon stimulation	Spontaneous	Spontaneous
Fatigue	Possible	Not possible	Not possible
Summation	Possible	Not possible	Possible
Tetanus	Possible	Not possible	Possible
Resting membrane potential	Stable	Stable	Unstable
For trigger of contraction, calcium binds with	Troponin	Troponin	Calmodulin
Source of calcium	Sarcoplasmic reticulum	Sarcoplasmic reticulum	Extracellular
Speed of contraction	Fast	Intermediate	Slow
Neuromuscular junction	Well defined	Not well defined	Not well defined
Action	Voluntary action	Involuntary action	Involuntary action
Control	Only neurogenic	Myogenic	Neurogenic and myogenic
Nerve supply	Somatic nerves	Autonomic nerves	Autonomic nerves

Fibers of the skeletal muscles are arranged in parallel. In most of the skeletal muscles, muscle fibers are attached to tendons on either end. Skeletal muscles are anchored to the bones by the tendons.

2. Cardiac Muscle

Cardiac muscle forms the musculature of the heart. These muscles are striated and involuntary. Cardiac muscles are supplied by autonomic nerve fibers.

3. Smooth Muscle

Smooth muscle is situated in association with viscera. It is also called visceral muscle. It is different from skeletal and cardiac muscles because of the absence of cross-striations, hence the name smooth muscle. Smooth muscle is supplied by autonomic nerve fibers. Smooth muscles form the main contractile units of wall of the various visceral organs.

Structure of Skeletal Muscle

Chapter 29

- ■ **MUSCLE MASS**
- ■ **MUSCLE FIBER**
- ■ **MYOFIBRIL**
  - ■ MICROSCOPIC STRUCTURE
- ■ **SARCOMERE**
  - ■ ELECTRON MICROSCOPIC STUDY
- ■ **CONTRACTILE ELEMENTS (PROTEINS) OF MUSCLE**
  - ■ MYOSIN MOLECULE
  - ■ ACTIN MOLECULE
  - ■ TROPOMYOSIN
  - ■ TROPONIN
- ■ **OTHER PROTEINS OF THE MUSCLE**
- ■ **SARCOTUBULAR SYSTEM**
  - ■ STRUCTURES
  - ■ FUNCTIONS
- ■ **COMPOSITION OF MUSCLE**

■ MUSCLE MASS

Muscle mass or muscle tissue is made up of a large number of individual **muscle cells** or **myocytes**. The muscle cells are commonly called muscle fibers because these cells are long and slender in appearance. Skeletal muscle fibers are multinucleated and are arranged parallel to one another with some connective tissue in between (Fig. 29.1).

Muscle mass is separated from the neighboring tissues by a thick fibrous tissue layer known as **fascia.** Beneath the fascia, muscle is covered by a connective tissue sheath called **epimysium.** In the muscle, the muscle fibers are arranged in various groups called bundles or **fasciculi.** Connective tissue sheath that covers each fasciculus is called **perimysium.** Each muscle fiber is covered by a connective tissue layer called the **endomysium** (Fig. 29.2).

■ MUSCLE FIBER

Each muscle cell or muscle fiber is cylindrical in shape. Average length of the fiber is 3 cm. It varies between 1 cm and 4 cm, depending upon the length of the muscle. The diameter of the muscle fiber varies from 10 μ to 100 μ. The diameter varies in a single muscle.

Muscle fibers are attached to a tough cord of connective tissue called **tendon.** Tendon is in turn attached to the bone. Tendon of some muscles is thin, flat and stretched but tough. Such type of tendon is called **aponeurosis.**

Each muscle fiber is enclosed by a cell membrane called plasma membrane, that lies beneath the endomysium. It is also called **sarcolemma** (Fig. 29.3). Cytoplasm of the muscle is known as **sarcoplasm.**

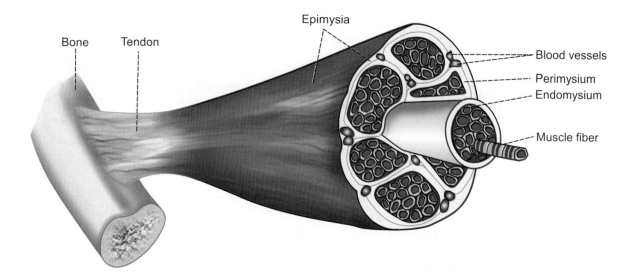

FIGURE 29.1: Structure of a skeletal muscle

Structures embedded within the sarcoplasm are:

1. Nuclei
2. Myofibril
3. Golgi apparatus
4. Mitochondria
5. Sarcoplasmic reticulum
6. Ribosomes
7. Glycogen droplets
8. Occasional lipid droplets.

Each muscle fiber has got one or more nuclei. In long muscle fibers, many nuclei are seen. Nuclei are oval or elongated and situated just beneath the sarcolemma. Usually in other cells, the nucleus is in the interior of the cell.

All the organelles of muscle fiber have the same functions as those of other cells.

■ MYOFIBRIL

Myofibrils or myofibrillae are the fine parallel filaments present in sarcoplasm of the muscle cell. Myofibrils run through the entire length of the muscle fiber.

In the cross-section of a muscle fiber, the myofibrils appear like small distinct dots within the sarcoplasm. Diameter of the myofibril is 0.2 to 2 μ. The length of a myofibril varies between 1 cm and 4 cm, depending upon the length of the muscle fiber (Table 29.1).

In some muscle fibers, some of the myofibrils are arranged in groups called **Cohnheim's areas** or fields.

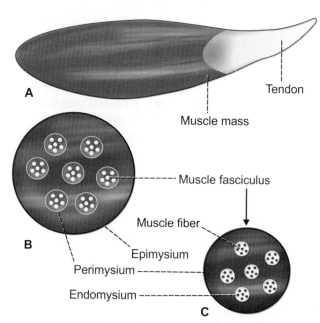

FIGURE 29.2: Diagram showing. **A.** Skeletal muscle mass; **B.** Cross-section of muscle; **C.** One muscle fasciculus.

■ MICROSCOPIC STRUCTURE OF A MYOFIBRIL

Light microscopic studies show that, each myofibril consists of a number of two alternating bands which are also called the sections, segments or disks. These bands are formed by muscle proteins.

The two bands are:

1. Light band or 'I' band.
2. Dark band or 'A' band.

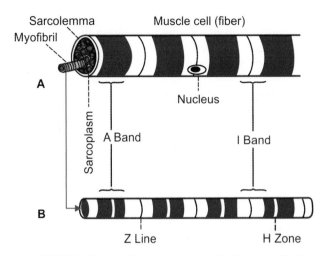

FIGURE 29.3: A. One muscle cell; **B.** One myofibril.

Light Band or 'I' Band

Light band is called 'I' **(isotropic)** band because it is isotropic to **polarized light.** When polarized light is passed through the muscle fiber at this area, light rays are refracted at the same angle.

Dark Band or 'A' Band

Dark band is called 'A' **(anisotropic)** band because it is anisotropic to polarized light. When polarized light is passed through the muscle fiber at this area, the light rays are refracted at different directions (An = not; iso = it; trops = turning). Dark band is also called **'Q' disk** (Querscheibe = cross disk).

In an intact muscle fiber, 'I' band and 'A' band of the adjacent myofibrils are placed side-by-side. It gives the appearance of characteristic cross-striations in the muscle fiber.

I band is divided into two portions, by means of a narrow and dark line called **'Z' line** or **'Z' disk** (in German, zwischenscheibe = between disks). The 'Z' line is formed by a protein disk, which does not permit passage of light. The portion of myofibril in between two 'Z' lines is called sarcomere.

TABLE 29.1: Dimensions of structures in skeletal muscle

Structure	Length	Diameter
Muscle fiber	1 cm to 4 cm	10 µ to 100 µ
Myofibril	1 cm to 4 cm	0.2 µ to 2 µ
Actin filament	1 µ	20 Å
Myosin filament	1.5 µ	115 Å

■ SARCOMERE

Definition

Sarcomere is defined as the structural and functional unit of a skeletal muscle. It is also called the basic contractile unit of the muscle.

Extent

Each sarcomere extends between two 'Z' lines of myofibril. Thus, each myofibril contains many sarcomeres arranged in series throughout its length. When the muscle is in relaxed state, the average length of each sarcomere is 2 to 3 µ.

Components

Each myofibril consists of an alternate dark 'A' band and light 'I' band (Fig. 29.4). In the middle of 'A' band, there is a light area called **'H' zone** (H = hell = light – in German, H = Henson – discoverer). In the middle of 'H' zone lies the middle part of myosin filament. This is called **'M' line** (in German-mittel = middle). 'M' line is formed by myosin binding proteins.

■ ELECTRON MICROSCOPIC STUDY OF SARCOMERE

Electron microscopic studies reveal that the sarcomere consists of many thread-like structures called **myofilaments.**

Myofilaments are of two types:
1. Actin filaments
2. Myosin filaments.

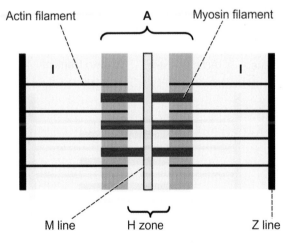

FIGURE 29.4: Sarcomere. A = A band, I = I band.

Actin Filaments

Actin filaments are the thin filaments with a diameter of 20 Å and a length of 1 μ. These filaments extend from either side of the 'Z' lines, run across 'I' band and enter into 'A' band up to 'H' zone.

Myosin Filaments

Myosin filaments are thick filaments with a diameter of 115 Å and a length of 1.5 μ. These filaments are situated in 'A' band.

Cross-bridges

Some lateral processes (projections) called cross-bridges arise from each myosin filament. These bridges have enlarged structures called myosin heads at their tips. Myosin heads attach themselves to actin filaments. These heads pull the actin filaments during contraction of the muscle, by means of a mechanism called sliding mechanism or ratchet mechanism.

During the contraction of the muscle, the actin filaments glide down between the myosin filaments towards the center of 'H' zone and approach the corresponding actin filaments from the next 'Z' line (Fig. 29.5). The 'Z' lines also approach the ends of myosin filaments, so that the 'H' zone and 'I' bands are shortened during contraction of the muscle. During the relaxation of the muscle, the actin filaments and 'Z' lines come back to the original position.

■ CONTRACTILE ELEMENTS (PROTEINS) OF MUSCLE

Myosin filaments are formed by myosin molecules. Actin filaments are formed by three types of proteins called actin, tropomyosin and troponin. These four proteins together constitute the contractile proteins or the contractile elements of the muscle.

■ MYOSIN MOLECULE

Each myosin filament consists of about 200 myosin molecules. Though about 18 classes of myosin are identified, only myosin II is present in the sarcomere.

Myosin II is a globulin with a molecular weight of 480,000. Each myosin molecule is made up of 6 polypeptide chains, of which two are heavy chains and four are light chains (Fig. 29.5). Molecular weight of each heavy chain is 200,000 (2 × 200,000 = 400,000). Molecular weight of each light chain is 20,000 (4 × 20,000 = 80,000). Thus, total molecular weight of each myosin molecule is 480,000 (400,000 + 80,000).

Portions of Myosin Molecule

Each myosin molecule has two portions:
1. Tail portion
2. Head portion.

Tail portion of myosin molecule

It is made up of two heavy chains, which twist around each other in the form of a double helix (Fig. 29.6).

Head portion of myosin molecule

At one end of the double helix, both the heavy chains turn away in opposite directions and form the globular head portion. Thus the head portion has two parts. Two light chains are attached to each part of the head portion of myosin molecule (Fig. 29.6).

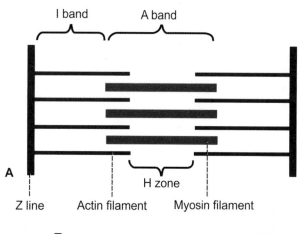
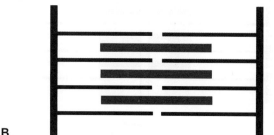

FIGURE 29.5: Sarcomere in resting muscle **A.** Contracted muscle; **B.** During contraction; Z lines come close, H zone and I band are reduced and no change in A band.

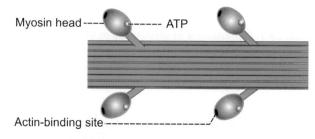

FIGURE 29.6: Diagram showing myosin filament. ATP = Adenosine triphosphate.

Each myosin head has two attachment sites. One site is for actin filament and the other one is for one ATP molecule (Fig. 29.7). Myosin head is absent in the central part of myosin filament, i.e. in the 'H' zone.

■ ACTIN MOLECULE

Actin molecules are the major constituents of the thin actin filaments. Each actin molecule is called **F-actin** and it is the polymer of a small protein known as **G-actin.** There are about 300 to 400 actin molecules in each actin filament. The molecular weight of each molecule is 42,000. The actin molecules in the actin filament are also arranged in the form of a double helix.

Each F-actin molecule has an active site to which the myosin head is attached (Fig. 29.8).

■ TROPOMYOSIN

About 40 to 60 tropomyosin molecules are situated along the double helix strand of actin filament. Each tropomyosin molecule has the molecular weight of 70,000. In relaxed condition of the muscle, the tropomyosin molecules cover all the active sites of F-actin molecules.

■ TROPONIN

It is formed by three subunits:
1. Troponin I, which is attached to F-actin
2. Troponin T, which is attached to tropomyosin
3. Troponin C, which is attached to calcium ions.

■ OTHER PROTEINS OF THE MUSCLE

In addition to the contractile proteins, the sarcomere contains several other proteins such as:
1. **Actinin,** which attaches actin filament to 'Z' line.
2. **Desmin,** which binds 'Z' line with sarcolemma.
3. **Nebulin,** which runs in close association with and parallel to actin filaments.
4. **Titin,** a large protein connecting 'M' line and 'Z' line. Each titin molecule forms **scaffolding** (framework) for sarcomere and provides elasticity to the muscle.

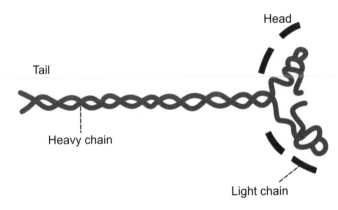

FIGURE 29.7: Myosin molecule formed by two heavy chains and four light chains of polypeptides

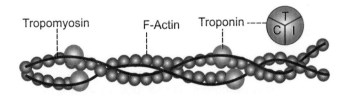

FIGURE 29.8: Part of actin filament. Troponin has three subunits, T, C and I.

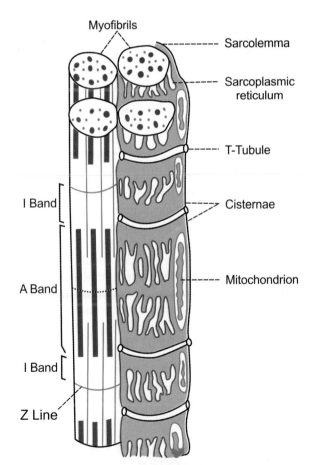

FIGURE 29.9: Diagram showing the relation between sarcotubular system and parts of sarcomere. Only few myofilaments are shown in the myofibril drawn on the right side of the diagram.

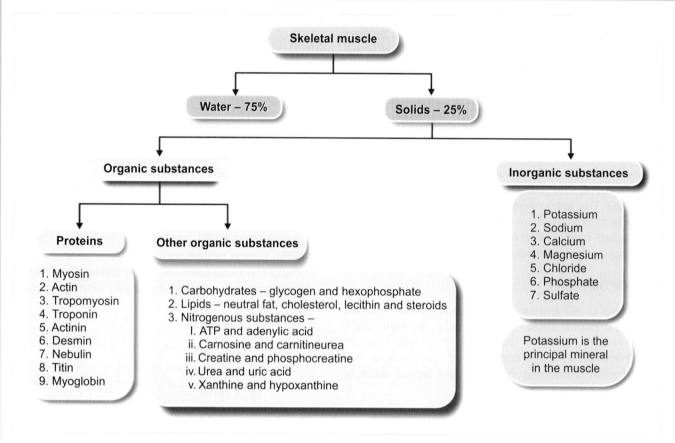

FIGURE 29.10: Composition of skeletal muscle

When the muscle is stretched, the titin unfolds itself. However, if the stretching is more, it offers resistance and protects the sarcomere from overstretching.

5. **Dystrophin,** a rod-shaped large protein that connects actin filament to **dystroglycan.** Dystroglycan is a transmembrane protein, present in the sarcolemma. Dystrophin and dystroglycan form dystrophin-dystroglycan or dystrophin-glycoprotein complex.

■ SARCOTUBULAR SYSTEM

Sarcotubular system is a system of membranous structures in the form of vesicles and tubules in the sarcoplasm of the muscle fiber. It surrounds the myofibrils embedded in the sarcoplasm (Fig. 29.9).

■ STRUCTURES CONSTITUTING THE SARCOTUBULAR SYSTEM

Sarcotubular system is formed mainly by two types of structures:

1. T-tubules
2. L-tubules or sarcoplasmic reticulum.

T-Tubules

T-tubules or transverse tubules are narrow tubules formed by the invagination of the sarcolemma. These tubules penetrate all the way from one side of the muscle fiber to an another side. That is, these tubules penetrate the muscle cell through and through. Because of their origin from sarcolemma, the T-tubules open to the exterior of the muscle cell. Therefore, the ECF runs through their lumen.

L-Tubules or Sarcoplasmic Reticulum

L-tubules or longitudinal tubules are the closed tubules that run in long axis of the muscle fiber, forming **sarcoplasmic reticulum.** These tubules form a closed tubular system around each myofibril and do not open to exterior like T-tubules.

L-tubules correspond to the endoplasmic reticulum of other cells. At regular intervals, throughout the length of the myofibrils, the L-tubules dilate to form a pair of lateral sacs called terminal **cisternae.** Each pair of terminal cisternae is in close contact with T-tubule. The T-tubule along with the cisternae on either side is called the triad of skeletal muscle.

In human skeletal muscle, the triads are situated at the junction between 'A' band and 'I' band. Calcium ions are stored in L-tubule and the amount of calcium ions is more in cisternae.

■ FUNCTIONS OF SARCOTUBULAR SYSTEM

Function of T-Tubules

T-tubules are responsible for rapid transmission of impulse in the form of action potential from sarcolemma to the myofibrils. When muscle is stimulated, the action potential develops in sarcolemma and spreads through it. Since T-tubules are the continuation of sarcolemma, the action potential passes through them and reaches the interior of the muscle fiber rapidly.

Function of L-Tubules

L-tubules store a large quantity of calcium ions. When action potential reaches the cisternae of L-tubule, the calcium ions are released into the sarcoplasm. Calcium ions trigger the processes involved in contraction of the muscle. The process by which the calcium ions cause contraction of muscle is called excitation-contraction coupling (Chapter 31).

■ COMPOSITION OF MUSCLE

Skeletal muscle is formed by 75% of water and 25% of solids. Solids are 20% of proteins and 5% of organic substances other than proteins and inorganic substances (Fig. 29.10).

Among the proteins, the first eight proteins are already described in this chapter. **Myoglobin** is present in sarcoplasm. It is also called myohemoglobin. Its function is similar to that of hemoglobin, that is, to carry oxygen. It is a conjugated protein with a molecular weight of 17,000.

Properties of Skeletal Muscle

```
■ EXCITABILITY
    ■ DEFINITIONS
    ■ TYPES OF STIMULUS
    ■ QUALITIES OF STIMULUS
    ■ EXCITABILITY CURVE OR STRENGTH-DURATION CURVE
■ CONTRACTILITY
    ■ TYPES OF CONTRACTION
    ■ SIMPLE MUSCLE CONTRACTION OR TWITCH OR CURVE
    ■ CONTRACTION TIME – RED MUSCLE AND PALE MUSCLE
    ■ FACTORS AFFECTING FORCE OF CONTRACTION
    ■ LENGTH-TENSION RELATIONSHIP
    ■ REFRACTORY PERIOD
■ MUSCLE TONE
    ■ DEFINITION
    ■ MAINTENANCE OF MUSCLE TONE
    ■ APPLIED PHYSIOLOGY – ABNORMALITIES OF MUSCLE TONE
```

■ EXCITABILITY

■ DEFINITIONS

Excitability

Excitability is defined as the reaction or response of a tissue to irritation or stimulatiosn. It is a physicochemical change.

Stimulus

Stimulus is the change in environment. It is defined as an agent or influence or act, which causes the response in an excitable tissue.

■ TYPES OF STIMULUS

Stimuli, which can excite the tissue are of four types :
1. Mechanical stimulus (pinching)
2. Electrical stimulus (electric shock)
3. Thermal stimulus (applying heated glass rod or ice piece)
4. Chemical stimulus (applying chemical substances like acids).

Electrical stimulus is commonly used for experimental purposes because of the following reasons:
  i. It can be handled easily
  ii. Intensity (strength) of stimulus can be easily adjusted
  iii. Duration of stimulus can be easily adjusted
  iv. Stimulus can be applied to limited (small) area on the tissues
  v. Damage caused to tissues is nil or least.

■ QUALITIES OF STIMULUS

To excite a tissue, the stimulus must possess two characters:
1. Intensity or strength
2. Duration.

1. Intensity

Intensity or strength of a stimulus is of five types:
  i. Subminimal stimulus
  ii. Minimal stimulus
  iii. Submaximal stimulus
  iv. Maximal stimulus
  v. Supramaximal stimulus.
   Stimulus whose strength (or voltage) is sufficient to excite the tissue is called threshold or liminal or minimal stimulus. Other details are given under the heading 'Factors affecting force of contraction' in this chapter.

2. Duration

Whatever may be the strength of the stimulus, it must be applied for a minimum duration to excite the tissue. However, the duration of a stimulus depends upon the strength of the stimulus. For a weak stimulus, the duration is longer and for a stronger stimulus, the duration is shorter. The relationship between the strength and duration of stimulus is demonstrated by means of excitability curve or strength-duration curve.

■ EXCITABILITY CURVE OR STRENGTH-DURATION CURVE

Excitability curve is the graph that demonstrates the exact relationship between the strength and the duration of a stimulus. So, it is also called the strength-duration curve (Fig. 30.1).

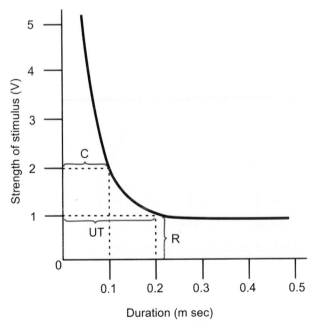

FIGURE 30.1: Strength–duration curve. R = Rheobase, UT = Utilization time, C = Chronaxie.

Method to Obtain the Curve

In this curve, the strength of the stimulus is plotted (in volts) vertically and the duration (in milliseconds) horizontally.
   To start with, a stimulus with higher strength or voltage (4 or 5 volt) is applied. The minimum duration, taken by the stimulus with particular strength to excite the tissue is noted. The strength and duration are plotted in the graph. Then, the strength of the stimulus is decreased and the duration is determined. Like this, the voltage is decreased gradually and the duration is determined every time. All the results are plotted and the curve is obtained.

Characteristic Features of the Curve

The shape of the curve is similar in almost all the excitable tissues. Following are the important points to be observed in the excitability curve:
  1. Rheobase
  2. Utilization time
  3. Chronaxie.

1. Rheobase

Rheobase is the minimum strength (voltage) of stimulus, which can excite the tissue. The voltage below this cannot excite the tissue, whatever may be the duration of the stimulus.

2. Utilization Time

Utilization time is the minimum time required for rheobasic strength of stimulus (threshold strength) to excite the tissue.

3. Chronaxie

Chronaxie is the minimum time required for a stimulus with double the rheobasic strength (voltage) to excite the tissue.

Importance of chronaxie

Measurement of chronaxie determines the excitability of the tissues. It is used to compare the excitability in different tissues. Longer the chronaxie, lesser is the excitability.

Normal chronaxie

In human skeletal muscles : 0.08 to 0.32 milliseconds.
In frog skeletal muscle : 3 milliseconds.

Variations in chronaxie

Chronaxie is:
  1. Ten times more in skeletal muscles of infants than in the skeletal muscles of adults

2. Shorter in red muscles than in pale muscles
3. Shorter in **warm-blooded (homeothermic)** animals than in **cold-blooded (poikilothermic)** animals
4. Shortened during increased temperature and prolonged during cold temperature
5. Longer in paralyzed muscles than in normal muscle
6. Prolonged gradually during progressive neural diseases.

■ CONTRACTILITY

Contractility is the response of the muscle to a stimulus. Contraction is defined as the internal events of muscle with change in either length or tension of the muscle fibers.

■ TYPES OF CONTRACTION

Muscular contraction is classified into two types based on change in the length of muscle fibers or tension of the muscle:
1. Isotonic contraction
2. Isometric contraction.

1. Isotonic Contraction

Isotonic contraction is the type of muscular contraction in which the tension remains the same and the length of the muscle fiber is altered (iso = same: tonic = tension).

Example: Simple flexion of arm, where shortening of muscle fibers occurs but the tension does not change.

2. Isometric Contraction

Isometric contraction is the type of muscular contraction in which the length of muscle fibers remains the same and the tension is increased.

Example: Pulling any heavy object when muscles become stiff and strained with increased tension but the length does not change.

■ SIMPLE MUSCLE CONTRACTION OR TWITCH OR CURVE

The contractile property of the muscle is studied by using **gastrocnemius-sciatic preparation** from frog. It is also called muscle-nerve preparation.

When the stimulus with threshold strength is applied, the muscle contracts and then relaxes. These activities are recorded graphically by using suitable instruments. The contraction is recorded as upward deflection from the base line. And, relaxation is recorded as downward deflection back to the base line (Fig. 30.2).

Simple contraction of the muscle is called simple muscle twitch and the graphical recording of this is called simple muscle curve.

Important Points in Simple Muscle Curve

Four points are to be observed in simple muscle curve:
1. Point of stimulus (PS): The time when the stimulus is applied.
2. Point of contraction (PC): The time when muscle begins to contract.
3. Point of maximum contraction (PMC): The point up to which the muscle contracts. It also indicates the beginning of relaxation of the muscle.
4. Point of maximum relaxation (PMR): The point when muscle relaxes completely.

Periods of Simple Muscle Curve

All the four points mentioned above divide the entire simple muscle curve into three periods:
1. Latent period (LP)
2. Contraction period (CP)
3. Relaxation period (RP).

1. Latent period

Latent period is the time interval between the point of stimulus and point of contraction. The muscle does not show any mechanical activity during this period.

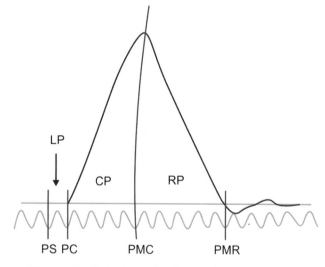

FIGURE 30-2: Isotonic simple muscle curve
PS   = Point of stimulus
PC   = Point of contraction
PMC = Point of maximum contraction
PMR = Point of maximum relaxation
LP   = Latent period (0.01 sec)
CP   = Contraction period (0.04 sec)
RP   = Relaxation period (0.05 sec)

2. *Contraction period*

Contraction period is the interval between point of contraction and point of maximum contraction. Muscle contracts during this period.

3. *Relaxation period*

Relaxation period is the interval between point of maximum contraction and point of maximum relaxation. The muscle relaxes during this period.

Duration of different periods in a typical simple muscle curve:

Latent period	:	0.01 second
Contraction period	:	0.04 second
Relaxation period	:	0.05 second
		——————
Total twitch period	:	0.10 second

Contraction period is always shorter than relaxation period. It is because, the contraction is an active process and relaxation is a passive process.

Causes of Latent Period

1. Latent period is the time taken by the impulse to travel along the nerve from place of stimulation to muscle.
2. It is the time taken for the onset of initial chemical changes in the muscle.
3. It is due to the delay in the conduction of impulse at the neuromuscular junction.
4. It is due to the resistance offered by viscosity of the muscle.
5. It is also due to the inertia of the recording instrument.

Variations in Latent Period

Latent period is not constant. It varies even in physiological conditions. It decreases in high temperature. It increases in low temperature, during fatigue and with increase in weight.

■ CONTRACTION TIME – RED MUSCLE AND PALE MUSCLE

Contraction time or total twitch period varies from species to species. It is less in homeothermic animals than in poikilothermic animals. In the same animal, it varies in different groups of muscles.

Based on contraction time, the skeletal muscles are classified into two types:
1. Red muscles
2. Pale muscles.

Similarly, depending upon contraction time and myosin ATPase activity the muscle fibers are also divided into two types:
1. Type I fibers or slow fibers or slow twitch fibers, which have small diameter.
2. Type II fibers or fast fibers or fast twitch fibers, which have large diameter.

Most of the skeletal muscles in human beings contain both the types of fibers.

Red Muscles

Muscles, which contain large quantity of myoglobin are called red muscles. These muscles are also called **slow muscles** or slow twitch muscles. Red muscles have large number of type I fibers. The contraction time is longer in this type of muscles.

Example: Back muscles and gastrocnemius muscles.

Pale Muscles

Muscles, which contain less quantity of myoglobin are called pale muscles or white muscles. These muscles are also called **fast muscles** or fast twitch muscles. Pale muscles have large number of type II fibers. Contraction time is shorter in this type of muscles.

Examples: Hand muscles and ocular muscles.

Characteristic features of red and pale muscles are given in Table 30.1.

■ FACTORS AFFECTING FORCE OF CONTRACTION

Force of contraction of the skeletal muscle is affected by the following factors:
1. Strength of stimulus
2. Number of stimulus
3. Temperature
4. Load.

1. Effect of Strength of Stimulus

When the muscle is stimulated by stimuli with different strength (voltage of current), the force of contraction also differs.

Types of strength of stimulus

Strength of stimulus is of five types:
  i. *Subminimal or subliminal stimulus:* It is less than minimal strength and does not produce any response in the muscle if applied once.

TABLE 30.1: Features of red and pale muscles

	Red (slow) muscle	Pale (fast) muscle
1.	Type I fibers are more	Type II fibers are more
2.	Myoglobin content is high. So, it is red	Myoglobin content is less. So, it is pale
3.	Sarcoplasmic reticulum is less extensive	Sarcoplasmic reticulum is more extensive
4.	Blood vessels are more extensive	Blood vessels are less extensive
5.	Mitochondria are more in number	Mitochondria are less in number
6.	Response is slow with long latent period	Response is rapid with short latent period
7.	Contraction is less powerful	Contraction is more powerful
8.	This muscle is involved in prolonged and continued activity as it undergoes sustained contraction	This muscle is not involved in prolonged and continued activity as it relaxes immediately
9.	Fatigue occurs slowly	Fatigue occurs quickly
10.	Depends upon cellular respiration for ATP production	Depends upon glycolysis for ATP production

ii. *Minimal stimulus, threshold stimulus or liminal stimulus:* It is the least strength of stimulus at which minimum force of contraction is produced.
iii. *Submaximal stimulus:* It is more than minimal and less than maximal strength of stimulus. It produces more force of contraction than minimal stimulus.
iv. *Maximal stimulus:* It produces almost the maximum force of contraction.
v. *Supramaximal stimulus:* It produces the maximum force of contraction. Beyond this, the force of contraction cannot be increased.

2. Effect of Number of Stimulus

Contractility of the muscle varies, depending upon the number of stimuli. If a single stimulus is applied, muscle contracts once (simple muscle twitch). Two or more than two (multiple) stimuli produce two different effects.

Effects of two successive stimuli

When two stimuli are applied successively to a muscle, three different effects are noticed depending upon the interval between the two stimuli (Fig. 30.3):
  i. Beneficial effect
 ii. Superposition or wave summation
iii. Summation effect.

i. Beneficial Effect

When two successive stimuli are applied to the muscle in such a way that the second stimulus falls after the relaxation period of the first curve, two separate curves are obtained and the force of second contraction is greater than that of first one. This is called beneficial effect.

Cause for beneficial effect

During first contraction, the temperature increases. It decreases the viscosity of muscle. So, the force of second contraction is more.

ii. Superposition

While applying two successive stimuli, if the second stimulus falls during relaxation period of first twitch, two curves are obtained. However, the first curve is superimposed by the second curve. This is called superposition or superimposition or **incomplete summation.** Here also, the second curve is bigger than the first curve because of beneficial effect.

iii. Summation

If second stimulus is applied during contraction period, or during second half of latent period, the two contractions are summed up and a single curve is obtained. This is called summation curve or complete summation curve.

Summation curve is different from the simple muscle curve because, the amplitude of the summation curve is greater than that of simple muscle curve. This is due to the summation of two contractions to give rise to one single curve. Base of the summation curve is also broader than that of the simple muscle curve.

Effects of multiple stimuli

In a muscle-nerve preparation, the multiple stimuli cause two types of effects depending upon the frequency of stimuli:
  i. Fatigue
 ii. Tetanus.

i. *Fatigue*

Definition

Fatigue is defined as the decrease in muscular activity due to repeated stimuli. When stimuli are applied repeatedly, after some time, the muscle does not show any response to the stimulus. This condition is called fatigue.

Fatigue curve

When the effect of repeated stimuli is recorded continuously, the amplitude of first two or three contractions increases. It is due to the beneficial effect. Afterwards, the force of contraction decreases gradually. It is shown by gradual decrease in the amplitude of the curves. All the periods are gradually prolonged. Just before fatigue occurs, the muscle does not relax completely. It remains in a partially contracted state. This state is called **contracture** or **contraction remainder** (Fig. 30.4).

Causes for fatigue

a. Exhaustion of acetylcholine in motor endplate
b. Accumulation of metabolites like lactic acid and phosphoric acid
c. Lack of nutrients like glycogen
d. Lack of oxygen.

Site (seat) of fatigue

In the muscle-nerve preparation of frog, neuromuscular junction is the first seat of fatigue. It is proved by direct stimulation of fatigued muscle. Fatigued muscle gives response if stimulated directly. However, the force of contraction is less and the contraction is very slow. Second seat of fatigue is the muscle. And the nerve cannot be fatigued.

In the intact body, the sites of fatigue are in the following order:

a. Betz (pyramidal) cells in cerebral cortex
b. Anterior gray horn cells (motor neurons) of spinal cord
c. Neuromuscular junction
d. Muscle.

Recovery of the muscle after fatigue

Fatigue is a reversible phenomenon. Fatigued muscle recovers (Fig. 30.5) if given rest and nutrition. For this, the muscle is washed with saline.

Causes of recovery

a. Removal of metabolites
b. Formation of acetylcholine at the neuromuscular junction
c. Re-establishment of normal polarized state of the muscle
d. Availability of nutrients
e. Availability of oxygen.

The recovered muscle differs from the fresh resting muscle by having acid reaction. The fresh resting muscle is alkaline. But the muscle, recovered from fatigue is acidic. So it relaxes slowly.

In the intact body, all the processes involved in recovery are achieved by circulation itself. In human beings, fatigue is recorded by using Mosso's ergograph.

ii. *Tetanus*

Definition

Tetanus is defined as the sustained contraction of muscle due to repeated stimuli with high frequency. When the multiple stimuli are applied at a higher frequency in such a way that the successive stimuli fall during contraction period of previous twitch, the muscle remains in state of tetanus. It relaxes only after the stoppage of stimulus or when the muscle is fatigued.

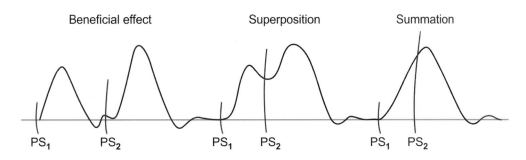

Beneficial effect   Superposition   Summation

PS₁   PS₂   PS₁   PS₂   PS₁   PS₂

FIGURE 30.3: Effects of two successive stimuli. PS$_1$ = Point of first stimulus, PS$_2$ = Point of second stimulus.

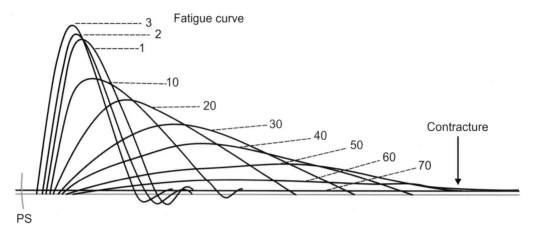

FIGURE 30.4: Fatigue curve. PS = Point of stimulus.

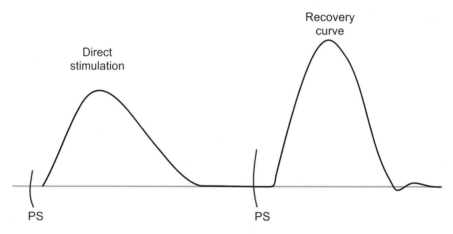

FIGURE 30.5: Recovery curve. PS = Point of stimulus.

Tetanus and genesis of tetanus curves

Genesis of tetanus and tetanus in frog's muscle is recorded by using the instrument called vibrating interruptor. It is used to adjust the frequency of stimuli as 5, 10, 15, 20, 25, 30 and 35/second. While increasing the frequency, fusion of contractions increases every time and finally complete tetanus occurs (Fig. 30.6). Nowadays, electronic stimulator is used. By using this instrument, the stimuli with different strength and frequency are obtained.

When the frequency of stimuli is not sufficient to cause tetanus, the fusion of contractions is not complete. It is called incomplete tetanus or clonus.

Frequency of stimuli necessary to cause tetanus and clonus

In frog gastrocnemius-sciatic preparation, the frequency of stimuli required to cause tetanus is 40/second and for clonus it is 35/second.

In gastrocnemius muscle of human being, the frequency required to cause tetanus is 60/second. And for clonus, the frequency of stimuli necessary is 55/second.

Pathological Tetanus

Sustained contraction of muscle due to repeated stimuli of high frequency is usually called **physiological tetanus.** It is distinct from pathological tetanus, which refers to the spastic contraction of the different muscle groups in pathological conditions. This disease is caused by bacillus ***Clostridium tetani*** found in the soil, dust and manure. The bacillus enters the body through a cut, wound or puncture caused by objects like metal pieces, metal nails, pins, wood splinters, etc.

This disease affects the nervous system and its common features are **muscle spasm** and **paralysis.** The first appearing symptom is the spasm of the jaw muscles resulting in locking of jaw. Therefore, tetanus is also called **lockjaw disease.** The manifestations of tetanus are due to a toxin secreted by the bacteria. If timely treatment is not provided, the condition becomes serious and it may even lead to death.

Treppe or Staircase Phenomenon

Treppe or staircase phenomenon is the gradual increase in force of contraction of muscle when it is stimulated repeatedly with a maximal strength at a low frequency. It is due to beneficial effect. Treppe is distinct from summation of contractions and tetanus.

3. Effect of Variations in Temperature

If the temperature of muscle is altered, the force of contraction is also affected (Fig. 30.7).

Warm temperature

At warm temperature of about 40°C, the force of muscle contraction increases and all the periods are shortened because of the following reasons:
  i. Excitability of muscle increases
  ii. Chemical processes involved in muscular contraction are accelerated
  iii. Viscosity of muscle decreases.

Cold temperature

At cold temperature of about 10°C, the force of contraction decreases and all the periods are prolonged because of the following reasons:

  i. Excitability of muscle decreases
  ii. Chemical processes are slowed or delayed
  iii. Viscosity of the muscle increases.

High or hot temperature – Heat rigor

At high temperature above 60°C, the muscle develops heat rigor. Rigor refers to shortening and stiffening of muscle fibers. Heat rigor is the rigor that occurs due to increased temperature. It is an irreversible phenomenon.

Cause of heat rigor is the coagulation of muscle proteins, actin and myosin.

Other types of rigors

  i. *Cold rigor:* Due to the exposure to severe cold. It is a reversible phenomenon.
  ii. *Calcium rigor:* Due to increased calcium content. It is also reversible.
  iii. *Rigor mortis:* Develops after death.

Rigor mortis

Rigor mortis refers to a condition of the body after death, which is characterized by stiffness of muscles and joints (Latin word 'rigor' means stiff). It occurs due to stoppage of aerobic respiration, which causes changes in the muscles.

Cause of rigor mortis

Soon after death, the cell membrane becomes highly permeable to calcium. So a large number of calcium ions

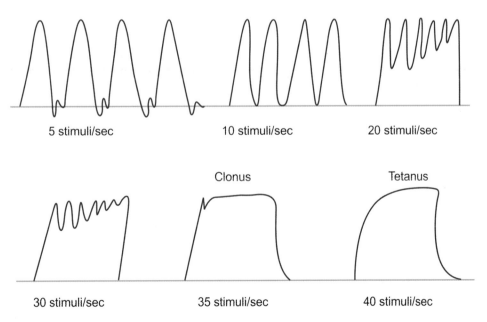

5 stimuli/sec   10 stimuli/sec   20 stimuli/sec

30 stimuli/sec   Clonus   Tetanus

30 stimuli/sec   35 stimuli/sec   40 stimuli/sec

FIGURE 30.6: Genesis of tetanus and tetanus curves

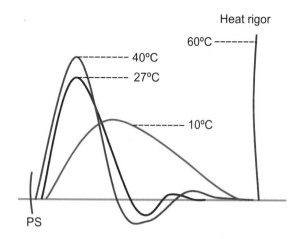

FIGURE 30.7: Effects of variations of temperature

enters the muscle fibers and promotes the formation of actomyosin complex resulting in contraction of the muscles.

Few hours after death, all the muscles of body undergo severe contraction and become rigid. The joints also become stiff and locked.

Normally for relaxation, the muscle needs to drive out the calcium, which requires ATP. But during continuous muscular contraction and other cellular processes after death, the ATP molecules are completely exhausted. New ATP molecules cannot be produced because of lack of oxygen. So in the absence of ATP, the muscles remain in contracted state until the onset of decomposition.

Medicolegal importance of rigor mortis

Rigor mortis is useful in determining the time of death. Onset of stiffness starts between 10 minutes and 3 hours after death depending upon condition of the body and environmental temperature at the time of death. If the body is active or the environmental temperature is high at the time of death, the stiffness sets in quickly.

The stiffness develops first in facial muscles and then spreads to other muscles. The maximum stiffness occurs around 12 to 24 hours after death. The stiffness of muscles and joints continues for 1 to 3 days.

Afterwards, the decomposition of the general tissues starts. Now the lysosomal intracellular hydrolytic enzymes like **cathepsins** and **calpains** are released. These enzymes hydrolyze the muscle proteins, actin and myosin resulting in breakdown of actomyosin complex. It relieves the stiffness of the muscles. This process is known as **resolution of rigor.**

4. *Effect of Load*

Load acting on muscle is of two types:
  i. After load
  ii. Free load.

After load

After load is the load, that acts on the muscle after the beginning of muscular contraction. Example of after load is lifting any object from the ground. The load acts on muscles of arm only after lifting the object off the ground, i.e. only after beginning of the muscular contraction.

Free load

Free load is the load, which acts on the muscle freely, even before the onset of contraction of the muscle. It is otherwise called fore load. Example of free load is filling water from a tap by holding the bucket in hand.

Free load Vs after load

Free load is more beneficial (advantageous) since force of contraction and work done by the muscles are greater in free-loaded condition than in after-loaded condition. It is because, in free-loaded condition, the muscle fibers are stretched and the initial length of muscle fibers is increased. It facilitates the force of contraction. This is in accordance with Frank-Starling law.

Frank-Starling law

Frank-Starling law states that the force of contraction is directly proportional to the initial length of muscle fibers within physiological limits.

Experiment to prove Frank-Starling law

Frank-Starling law can be proved by using the muscle-nerve preparation of frog. First, one simple muscle curve is recorded with 10 g weight in after-loaded condition of the muscle (Fig. 30.8). Then, many contractions are recorded by increasing the weight everytime, until the muscle fails to lift the weight or till the curve becomes almost flat near the base line. The work done by the muscle is calculated for every weight (Fig. 30.9).

Effects of increasing the weight in after-loaded condition are:
  i. Force of contraction decreases gradually
  ii. Latent period prolongs
  iii. Contraction and relaxation periods shorten (Fig. 30.8).

Afterwards, the muscle (with weight added for last contraction) in after-loaded condition, is brought to the free-loaded condition and stimulated. Now, the muscle contracts and a curve is recorded. The work done by the muscle is calculated.

Work done in free-loaded condition is more than in after-loaded condition. This proves Frank-Starling law, i.e. the force of contraction is directly proportional to the initial length of muscle fiber.

Work done by the muscle

Work done is calculated by the formula:

Work done = W × h

Where, W = Weight lifted by the muscle
　　　　h = Height up to which the weight is lifted
'h' is determined by the formula

$$h = \frac{l \times H}{L}$$

This formula is derived as follows:

$$\Delta ABC = \Delta DEC$$

$$\frac{BC}{EC} = \frac{AB}{DE} \quad or \quad \frac{L}{l} = \frac{H}{h}$$

$$h \times L = l \times H$$

$$h = \frac{l \times H}{L}$$

L = Length between fulcrum and writing point
l = Length between fulcrum and point where weight is added
H = Height of the curve
h = Height up to which the weight is lifted

So work done by the muscle =

$$W \times \frac{l \times H}{L} \; g\,cm$$

Work done is expressed as ergs or g cm.

Optimum load

Optimum load is the load at which the work done by the muscle is maximum.

■ LENGTH-TENSION RELATIONSHIP

Tension or force developed in the muscle during resting condition and during contraction varies with the length of the muscle.

Tension developed in the muscle during resting condition is known as **passive tension.** Tension developed in the muscle during isometric contraction is called **total tension.**

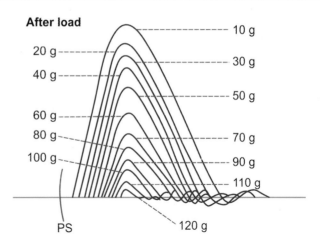
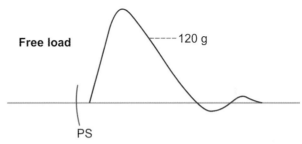

FIGURE 30.8: Effect of after load and free load. PS = Point of stimulus. In free-loaded condition, the force of contraction is greater than in after-loaded condition with the same weight.

Active Tension

Difference between the passive tension and total tension at a particular length of the muscle is called **active tension.** Active tension is considered as the real tension that is generated in the muscle during contractile process. It can be determined by the length-tension curve.

Length-Tension Curve

Length-tension curve is the curve that determines the relationship between length of muscle fibers and the tension developed by the muscle. It is also called **length-force curve.** The curve is obtained by using frog gastrocnemius-sciatic preparation. Muscle is attached to micrometer on one end and to a force transducer on other end. Muscle is not allowed to shorten because of its attachment on both the ends (Fig. 30.10).

A micrometer is used to set length of the muscle fibers. Force transducer is connected to a polygraph. Polygraph is used to measure the tension developed by the muscle during isometric contraction.

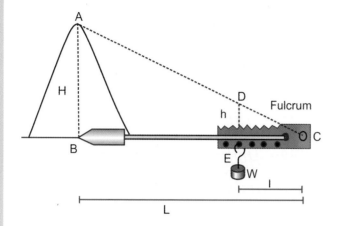

FIGURE 30.9: Work done by the muscle

L = Length between fulcrum and writing point
l = Length between fulcrum and point where weight is added
H = Height of the curve
h = Height up to which the weight is lifted
W = Weight

To begin with, the minimum length of the muscle is set by using the micrometer. The passive tension is determined by using force transducer. Then the muscle is stimulated and total tension is determined. From these two values the active tension is calculated. Then the length of muscle is increased gradually. At every length, both passive tension and total tension are determined followed by calculation of active tension. All the values of active tension at different lengths are plotted to obtain the length-tension curve (Fig. 30.11). From the curve the resting length is determined.

Resting Length

Resting length is the length of the muscle at which the active tension is maximum. Active tension is proportional to the length of the muscle up to resting length. Beyond resting length, the active tension decreases.

Tension Vs Overlap of Myofilaments

Length-tension relationship is explained on the basis of sliding of actin filaments over the myosin filaments during muscular contraction. The active tension is proportional to overlap between actin and myosin filaments in the sarcomere and the number of cross bridges formed between actin and myosin filaments. When the length of the muscle is less than the resting length, there is increase in the overlap between the actin and myosin filaments and the number of cross bridges. The active

tension gradually increases up to the resting length. During stretching of the muscle beyond resting length, there is reduction in the overlap between the actin and myosin filaments and the number of cross bridges. And the active tension starts declining beyond resting length.

■ REFRACTORY PERIOD

Refractory period is the period at which the muscle does not show any response to a stimulus. It is because already one action potential is in progress in the muscle during this period. The muscle is unexcitable to further stimulation until it is repolarized.

Refractory period is of two types.
1. Absolute refractory period
2. Relative refractory period

1. *Absolute Refractory Period*

Absolute refractory period is the period during which the muscle does not show any response at all, whatever may be the strength of stimulus.

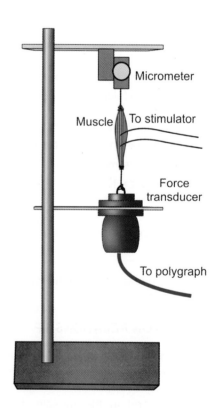

FIGURE 30.10: Experimental setup to measure the tension developed in the muscle

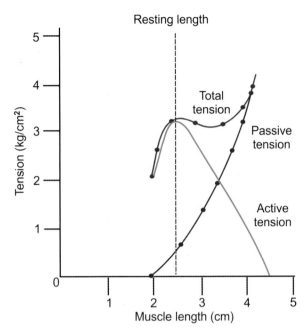

FIGURE 30.11: Length-tension curve

2. *Relative Refractory Period*

Relative refractory period is the period, during which the muscle shows some response if the strength of stimulus is increased to maximum.

Refractory Period in Skeletal Muscle

In skeletal muscle, whole of the latent period is refractory period. The absolute refractory period falls during first half of latent period (0.005 sec). And, relative refractory period extends during second half of latent period (0.005 sec). Totally, it is 0.01 sec.

Refractory Period in Cardiac Muscle

In cardiac muscle, absolute refractory period extends throughout contraction period (0.27 sec). And, relative refractory period extends during first half of relaxation period (about 0.26 sec). Totally it is about 0.53 sec. Thus, the refractory period in cardiac muscle is very long compared to that of skeletal muscle.

Significance of long refractory period in cardiac muscle

Because of the long refractory period, cardiac muscle does not show:

   i. Complete summation of contractions
  ii. Fatigue
 iii. Tetanus.

■ MUSCLE TONE

■ DEFINITION

Muscle tone is defined as continuous and partial contraction of the muscles with certain degree of vigor and tension. More details on muscle tone are given in Chapter 157.

■ MAINTENANCE OF MUSCLE TONE

In Skeletal Muscle

Maintenance of tone in skeletal muscle is neurogenic. It is due to continuous discharge of impulses from gamma motor neurons in anterior gray horn of spinal cord. The gamma motor neurons in spinal cord are controlled by higher centers in brain (Chapter 157).

In Cardiac Muscle

In cardiac muscle, maintenance of tone is purely myogenic, i.e. the muscles themselves control the tone. The tone is not under nervous control in cardiac muscle.

In Smooth Muscle

In smooth muscle, tone is myogenic. It depends upon calcium level and number of cross bridges.

■ APPLIED PHYSIOLOGY – ABNORMALITIES OF MUSCLE TONE

Abnormalities of muscle tone are:
1. Hypertonia
2. Hypotonia
3. Myotonia.
   Refer Chapter 34 for details.

Changes during Muscular Contraction

■ INTRODUCTION

The muscle contracts when it is stimulated. Contraction of the muscle is a physical or mechanical event. In addition, several other changes occur in the muscle.

Changes taking place during muscular contraction:
1. Electrical changes
2. Physical changes
3. Histological (molecular) changes
4. Chemical changes
5. Thermal changes.

■ ELECTRICAL CHANGES DURING MUSCULAR CONTRACTION

Electrical events occur in the muscle during resting condition as well as active conditions. Electrical potential in the muscle during resting condition is called resting membrane potential.

Electrical changes that occur in active conditions, i.e. when the muscle is stimulated are together called action potential.

Electrical potentials in a muscle (or any living tissue) are measured by using a cathode ray oscilloscope or computerized polygraph.

■ RESTING MEMBRANE POTENTIAL

Resting membrane potential is defined as the electrical potential difference (voltage) across the cell membrane (between inside and outside of the cell) under resting condition.

It is also called membrane potential, transmembrane potential, transmembrane potential difference or transmembrane potential gradient.

When two electrodes are connected to a cathode ray oscilloscope through a suitable amplifier and placed over the surface of the muscle fiber, there is no potential difference, i.e. there is zero potential difference. But, if one of the electrodes is inserted into the interior of muscle fiber, potential difference is observed across the sarcolemma (cell membrane). There is negativity inside and positivity outside the muscle fiber. This potential difference is constant and is called resting membrane potential. The condition of the muscle during resting membrane potential is called **polarized state.** In human skeletal muscle, the resting membrane potential is −90 mV.

Ionic Basis of Resting Membrane Potential

Development and maintenance of resting membrane potential in a muscle fiber or a neuron are carried out by movement of ions, which produce ionic imbalance across the cell membrane. This results in the development of more positivity outside and more negativity inside the cell.

Ionic imbalance is produced by two factors:
1. Sodium-potassium pump
2. Selective permeability of cell membrane.

1. Sodium-potassium pump

Sodium and potassium ions are actively transported in opposite directions across the cell membrane by means of an electrogenic pump called sodium-potassium pump. It moves three sodium ions out of the cell and two potassium ions inside the cell by using energy from ATP. Since more positive ions (cations) are pumped outside than inside, a net deficit of positive ions occurs inside the cell. It leads to negativity inside and positivity outside the cell (Fig. 31.1). More details of this pump are given in Chapter 3.

2. Selective permeability of cell membrane

Permeability of cell membrane depends largely on the transport channels. The transport channels are selective for the movement of some specific ions. Their permeability to these ions also varies. Most of the channels are **gated channels** and the specific ions can move across the membrane only when these gated channels are opened.

Two types of channels are involved:
  i. Channels for major anions like proteins
  ii. Leak channels.

i. Channels for major anions (negatively charged substances) like proteins

Channels for some of the negatively charged large substances such as proteins, organic phosphate and sulfate compounds are absent or closed. So, such substances remain inside the cell and play a major role in the

development and maintenance of negativity inside the cell (resting membrane potential).

ii. Leak channels

Leak channels are the passive channels, which maintain the resting membrane potential by allowing movement of positive ions (Na^+ and K^+) across the cell membrane.

Three important ions, sodium, chloride and potassium are unequally distributed across the cell membrane. Na^+ and Cl^- are more outside and K^+ is more inside.

Since, Cl^- channels are mostly closed in resting conditions Cl^- are retained outside the cell. Thus, only the positive ions, Na^+ and K^+ can move across the cell membrane.

Na^+ is actively transported (against the concentration gradient) out of cell and K^+ is actively transported (against the concentration gradient) into the cell. However, because of concentration gradient, Na^+ diffuses back into the cell through Na^+ leak channels and K^+ diffuses out of the cell through K^+ leak channels.

In resting conditions, almost all the K^+ leak channels are opened but most of the Na^+ leak channels are closed. Because of this, K^+, which are transported actively into the cell, can diffuse back out of the cell in an attempt to maintain the **concentration equilibrium.** But among the $Na+$, which are transported actively out of the cell, only a small amount can diffuse back into the cell. That means, in resting conditions, the passive K^+ efflux is much greater than the passive Na^+ influx. It helps in establishing and maintaining the resting membrane potential.

After establishment of the resting membrane potential (i.e. inside negativity and outside positivity), the efflux of K^+ stops in spite of concentration gradient.

It is because of two reasons:
  i. Positivity outside the cell repels positive $K+$ and prevents further efflux of these ions
  ii. Negativity inside the cell attracts positive $K+$ and prevents further leakage of these ions outside.

Importance of intracellular potassium ions

Concentration of K^+ inside the cell is about 140 mEq/L. It is almost equal to that of Na^+ outside. The high concentration of K^+ inside the cell is essential to check the negativity. Normally, the negativity (resting membrane potential) inside the muscle fiber is −90 mV and in a nerve fiber, it is −70 mV. It is because of the presence of negatively charged proteins, organic phosphates and sulfates, which cannot move out normally. Suppose if the K^+ is not present or decreased, the negativity increases

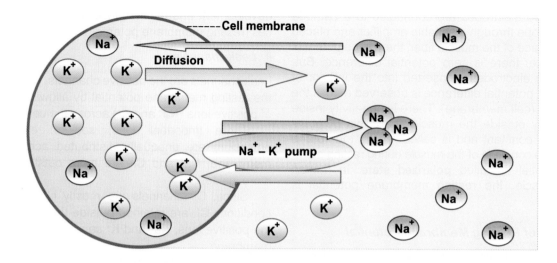

FIGURE 31.1: Development of resting membrane potential by sodium-potassium (Na⁺-K⁺) pump and diffusion of ions. Na⁺-K⁺ pump actively pumps three Na⁺ outside and two K⁺ into the cell. However, the diffusion of K⁺ out of the cell is many times greater than the diffusion of Na⁺ inside the cell because many of the K⁺ leak channels are opened and many of the Na⁺ leak channels are closed.

beyond −120 mV, which is called hyperpolarization. At this stage, the development of action potential is either delayed or does not occur.

■ ACTION POTENTIAL

Action potential is defined as a series of electrical changes that occur in the membrane potential when the muscle or nerve is stimulated.

Action potential occurs in two phases:
1. Depolarization
2. Repolarization.

Depolarization

Depolarization is the initial phase of action potential in which inside of the muscle becomes positive and outside becomes negative. That is, the polarized state (resting membrane potential) is abolished resulting in depolarization.

Repolarization

Repolarization is the phase of action potential in which the muscle reverses back to the resting membrane potential. That is, within a short time after depolarization the inside of muscle becomes negative and outside becomes positive. So, the polarized state of the muscle is re-established.

Properties of Action Potential

Properties of action potential are listed in Table 31.1.

■ ACTION POTENTIAL CURVE

Action potential curve is the graphical registration of electrical activity that occurs in an excitable tissue such as muscle after stimulation. It shows three major parts:
1. Latent period
2. Depolarization
3. Repolarization.

Resting membrane potential in skeletal muscle is −90 mV and it is recorded as a straight baseline (Fig. 31.2).

1. *Latent Period*

Latent period is the period when no change occurs in the electrical potential immediately after applying the stimulus. It is a very short period with duration of 0.5 to 1 millisecond.

Stimulus artifact

When a stimulus is applied, there is a slight irregular deflection of baseline for a very short period. This is called stimulus artifact. The artifact occurs because of the disturbance in the muscle due to leakage of current from stimulating electrode to the recording electrode. The stimulus artifact is followed by latent period.

2. *Depolarization*

Depolarization starts after the latent period. Initially, it is very slow and the muscle is depolarized for about 15 mV.

Firing level and depolarization

After the initial slow depolarization for 15 mV (up to –75 mV), the rate of depolarization increases suddenly. The point at which, the depolarization increases suddenly is called firing level.

Overshoot

From firing level, the curve reaches **isoelectric potential (zero potential)** rapidly and then shoots up (overshoots) beyond the zero potential **(isoelectric base)** up to +55 mV. It is called overshoot.

3. *Repolarization*

When depolarization is completed (+55 mV), the repolarization starts. Initially, the repolarization occurs rapidly and then it becomes slow.

Spike potential

Rapid rise in depolarization and the rapid fall in repolarization are together called spike potential. It lasts for 0.4 millisecond.

After depolarization or negative after potential

Rapid fall in repolarization is followed by a slow re-polarization. It is called after depolarization or negative after potential. Its duration is 2 to 4 milliseconds.

After hyperpolarization or positive after potential

After reaching the resting level (–90 mV), it becomes more negative beyond resting level. This is called after hyperpolarization or positive after potential. This lasts for more than 50 milliseconds. After this, the normal resting membrane potential is restored slowly.

Ionic Basis of Action Potential

Voltage gated Na^+ channels and the voltage gated K^+ channels play important role in the development of action potential.

During the onset of depolarization, voltage gated sodium channels open and there is slow influx of Na^+. When depolarization reaches 7 to 10 mV, the voltage gated Na^+ channels start opening at a faster rate. It is called Na^+ channel activation. When the firing level is reached, the influx of Na^+ is very great and it leads to overshoot.

But the Na^+ transport is short lived. It is because of rapid inactivation of Na^+ channels. Thus, the Na^+ channels open and close quickly. At the same time, the K^+ channels start opening. This leads to efflux of K^+ out of the cell, causing repolarization.

Unlike the Na^+ channels, the K^+ channels remain open for longer duration. These channels remain opened for few more milliseconds after completion of repolarization. It causes efflux of more number of K^+ producing more negativity inside. It is the cause for hyperpolarization.

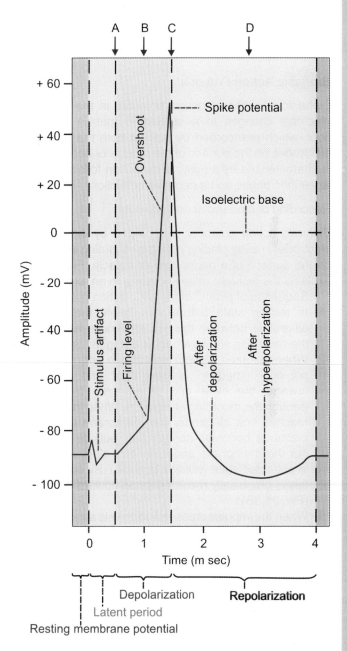

FIGURE 31.2: Action potential in a skeletal muscle
A = Opening of few Na^+ channels
B = Opening of many Na^+ channels
C = Closure of Na^+ channels and opening
       of K^+ channels
D = Closure of K^+ channels

■ MONOPHASIC, BIPHASIC AND COMPOUND ACTION POTENTIALS

Monophasic Action Potential

Monophasic action potential is the series of electrical changes that occur in a stimulated muscle or nerve fiber, which is recorded by placing one electrode on its surface and the other inside. It is characterized by a positive deflection. The action potential in the muscle discussed above belongs to this category.

Biphasic Action Potential

Biphasic or diphasic action potential is the series of electrical changes in a stimulated muscle or nerve fiber, which is recorded by placing both the recording electrodes on the surface of the muscle or nerve fiber. It is characterized by a positive deflection followed by an isoelectric pause and a negative deflection.

Recording of biphasic action potential

Biphasic action potential is recorded by extracellular electrodes, i.e. by placing both the recording electrodes on the surface of a nerve fiber or muscle. Figure 31.3 explains the biphasic action potential in an axon.

Sequence of events of biphasic action potential:
1. In resting state before stimulation, the potential difference between the two electrodes is zero. So the recording shows a baseline (Fig. 31.3A).
2. When the axon is stimulated at one end, the action potential (impulse) is generated and it travels towards the other end of an axon by passing through the recording electrodes. When the impulse reaches first electrode, the membrane under this electrode becomes depolarized (outside negative) but the membrane under second electrode is still in polarized state (outside positive). By convention, this is graphically recorded as an upward deflection (Fig. 31.3B).
3. When the impulse crosses and travels away from the first electrode, the membrane under this electrode is repolarized. Later when the impulse just travels in between the two electrodes (before reaching the second electrode) the potential difference between both the electrode falls to zero and the baseline is recorded (Fig. 31.3C)
4. When the impulse reaches the second electrode, the membrane under this electrode is depolarized (outside negative) and a negative deflection is recorded (Fig. 31.3D).
5. When the impulse travels away from second electrode, the membrane under this gets repolarized. Once again the potential difference between the two

electrodes becomes zero and the graph shows the baseline (Fig. 31.3E). Since this recording shows both positive and negative components it is called biphasic action potential.

Effect of crushing or local anesthetics

When a small portion of axon between the two electrodes is affected by crushing or local anesthetics, the action potential cannot travel through this part of the axon. So, while recording the potential only a single deflection (monophasic) action potential is recorded (Fig. 31.4).

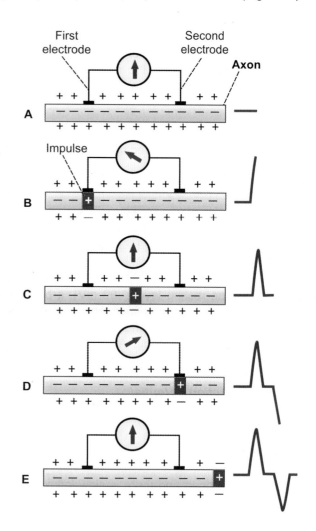

FIGURE 31.3: Biphasic action potential in an axon recorded by placing both the electrodes outside the axon
A = Resting state – zero potential
B = Depolarization of membrane under first electrode
C = Repolarization of membrane under first electrode followed by zero potential
D = Depolarization of membrane under second electrode
E = Repolarization of membrane under second electrode

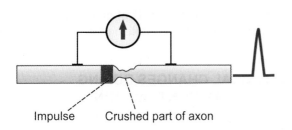

Impulse   Crushed part of axon

FIGURE 31.4: Monophasic action potential in a crushed axon

Compound Action Potential

Compound action potential (CAP) is the algebraic summation of all the action potentials produced by all the nerve fibers. Each nerve is made up of thousands of axons. While stimulating the whole nerve, all the nerve fibers are activated and produce action potential. The compound action potential is obtained by recording all the action potentials simultaneously.

■ GRADED POTENTIAL

Graded potential is a mild local change in the membrane potential that develops in receptors, synapse or neuro-muscular junction when stimulated. It is also called graded membrane potential, graded depolarization or local potential. It is non-propagative and characterized by mild depolarization or **hyperpolarization.** Graded potential is distinct from the action potential and the properties of these two potentials are given in table 31.1.

In most of the cases, the graded potential is responsible for the generation of action potential. However, in some cases the graded potential hyperpolarizes the membrane potential (more negativity than resting membrane potential) and inhibits the generation of action potential (as in inhibitory synapses: Chapter 140).

Different Graded potentials

1. End plate potential in neuromuscular junction (Chapter 32)
2. Electronic potential in nerve fibers (Chapter 136)
3. Receptor potential (Chapter 139)
4. Excitatory postsynaptic potential (Chapter 140)
5. Inhibitory postsynaptic potential (Chapter 140).

■ PATCH-CLAMP TECHNIQUE

Patch-clamp technique or patch clamping is the method to measure the ion currents across the biological membranes. This advanced technique in modern electrophysiology was established by Erwin Neher in 1992. Patch clamp is modified as voltage clamp to

TABLE 31.1: Properties of action potential and graded potential

Action Potential	Graded potential
Propagative	Non-propagative
Long-distance signal	Short-distance signal
Both depolarization and repolarization	Only depolarization or hyperpolarization
Obeys all-or-none law	Does not obey all-or-none law
Summation is not possible	Summation is possible
Has refractory period	No refractory period

study the ion currents across the membrane of neuron (Chapter 136).

Procedure

Patch-clamp experiments use mostly the cultured cells. The cells isolated from the body are placed in dishes containing culture media and kept in an incubator.

Probing a single cell

The dish with tissue culture cells is mounted on a microscope. A micropipette with an opening of about 0.5 µ is also mounted by means of a pipette holder. The pipette is filled with saline solution. An electrode is fitted to the pipette and connected to a recording device called patch-clamp amplifier. The micropipette is pressed firmly against the membrane of an intact cell. A gentle suction applied to the inside of the pipette forms a tight seal of giga ohms (GΩ) resistance between the membrane and the pipette.

This patch (minute part) of the cell membrane under the pipette is studied by means of various approaches called patch-clamp configurations (Fig. 31.5).

Patch-clamp Configurations

1. Cell-attached patch

The cell is left intact with its membrane. This allows measurement of current flow through ion channel or channels under the micropipette (Fig. 31.5 A).

2. Inside-out patch

From the cell-attached configuration, the pipette is gently pulled away from the cell. It causes the detachment of a small portion of membrane from the cell. The external surface of the membrane patch faces pipette solution. But internal surface of the membrane patch is exposed out hence the name inside-out patch (Fig. 31.5 B).

Pipette with membrane patch is inserted into a container with free solution. Concentration of ions can

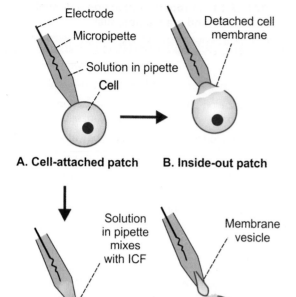

A. Cell-attached patch

B. Inside-out patch

C. Whole-cell patch

D. Outside-out patch

FIGURE 31.5: Patch-clamp configurations

be altered in the free solution. It is used to study the effect of alterations in the ion concentrations on the ion channels.

3. *Whole-cell patch*

From the cell-attached configuration, further suction is applied to the inside of the pipette. It causes rupture of the membrane and the pipette solution starts mixing with intracellular fluid. When the mixing is complete, the equilibrium is obtained between the pipette solution and the intracellular fluid (Fig. 31.5 C).

Whole-cell patch is used to record the current flow through all the ion channels in the cell. The cellular activity also can be studied directly.

4. *Outside-out patch*

From the whole-cell configuration the pipette is gently pulled away from the cell. A portion of membrane is torn away from the cell. Immediately, the free ends of the torn membrane fuse and reseal forming a membrane vesicle at tip of the pipette. The pipette solution enters the membrane vesicle and forms the intracellular fluid. The vesicle is placed inside a bath solution, which forms the extracellular environment (Fig. 31.5D).

This patch is used to study the effect of changes in the extracellular environment on the ion channels. It

also helps to study the effects of neurotransmitters and compounds like ozone, G-protein regulators, etc. on the ion channels.

■ PHYSICAL CHANGES DURING MUSCULAR CONTRACTION

Physical change, which takes place during muscular contraction, is the change in length of the muscle fibers or change in tension developed in the muscle. Depending upon this, the muscular contraction is classified into two types namely isotonic contraction and isometric contraction (refer previous chapter).

■ HISTOLOGICAL CHANGES DURING MUSCULAR CONTRACTION

■ ACTOMYOSIN COMPLEX

In relaxed state of the muscle, the thin actin filaments from opposite ends of sarcomere are away from each other leaving a broad 'H' zone.

During contraction of the muscle, actin (thin) filaments glide over myosin (thick) filaments and form actomyosin complex.

■ MOLECULAR BASIS OF MUSCULAR CONTRACTION

Molecular mechanism is responsible for formation of actomyosin complex that results in muscular contraction. It includes three stages:
1. Excitation-contraction coupling.
2. Role of troponin and tropomyosin.
3. Sliding mechanism.

1. *Excitation-contraction Coupling*

Excitation-contraction coupling is the process that occurs in between the excitation and contraction of the muscle. This process involves series of activities, which are responsible for the contraction of excited muscle.

Stages of excitation-contraction coupling

When a muscle is excited (stimulated) by the impulses passing through motor nerve and neuromuscular junction, action potential is generated in the muscle fiber.

Action potential spreads over sarcolemma and also into the muscle fiber through the 'T' tubules. The 'T' tubules are responsible for the rapid spread of action potential into the muscle fiber. When the action potential reaches the cisternae of 'L' tubules, these cisternae are excited. Now, the calcium ions stored in the cisternae are released into the sarcoplasm (Fig. 31.6). The calcium ions from the sarcoplasm move towards the actin filaments to produce the contraction.

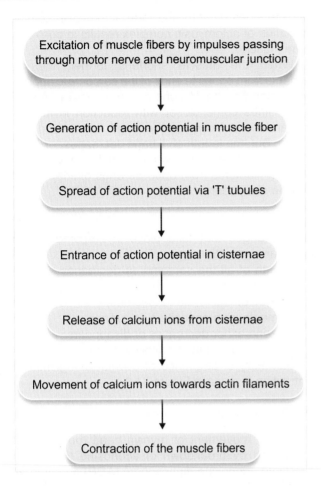

FIGURE 31.6: Excitation-contraction coupling

Thus, the calcium ion forms the link or coupling material between the excitation and the contraction of muscle. Hence, the calcium ions are said to form the basis of excitation-contraction coupling.

2. *Role of Troponin and Tropomyosin*

Normally, the head of myosin molecules has a strong tendency to get attached with active site of F actin. However, in relaxed condition, the active site of F actin is covered by the tropomyosin. Therefore, the myosin head cannot combine with actin molecule.

Large number of calcium ions, which are released from 'L' tubules during the excitation of the muscle, bind with troponin C. The loading of troponin C with calcium ions produces some change in the position of troponin molecule. It in turn, pulls tropomyosin molecule away from F actin. Due to the movement of tropomyosin, the active site of F actin is uncovered and exposed. Immediately the head of myosin gets attached to the actin.

3. *Sliding Mechanism and Formation of Actomyosin Complex – Sliding Theory*

Sliding theory explains how the actin filaments slide over myosin filaments and form the actomyosin complex during muscular contraction. It is also called **ratchet theory** or **walk along theory.**

Each cross bridge from the myosin filaments has got three components namely, a hinge, an arm and a head.

After binding with active site of F actin, the myosin head is tilted towards the arm so that the actin filament is dragged along with it (Fig. 31.7). This tilting of head is called power stroke. After tilting, the head immediately breaks away from the active site and returns to the original position. Now, it combines with a new active site on the actin molecule. And, tilting movement occurs again. Thus, the head of cross bridge bends back and forth and pulls the actin filament towards the center of sarcomere. In this way, all the actin filaments of both the ends of sarcomere are pulled. So, the actin filaments of

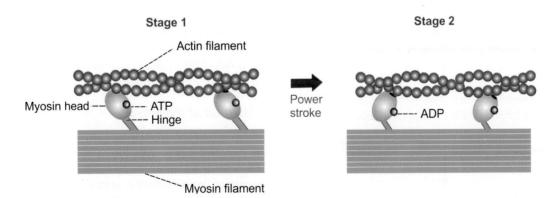

FIGURE 31.7: Diagram showing power stroke by myosin head.
Stage 1: Myosin head binds with actin; Stage 2: Tilting of myosin head (power stroke) drags the actin filament.

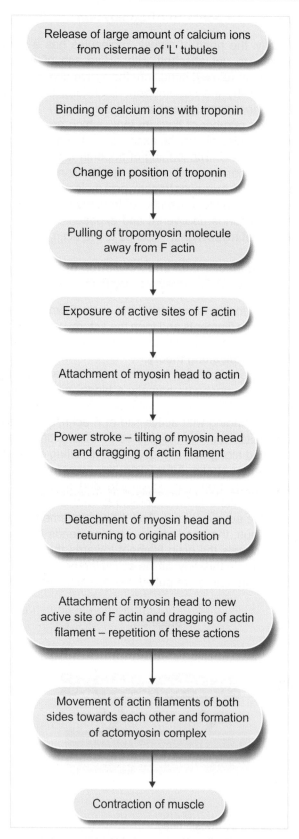

Release of large amount of calcium ions from cisternae of 'L' tubules

↓

Binding of calcium ions with troponin

↓

Change in position of troponin

↓

Pulling of tropomyosin molecule away from F actin

↓

Exposure of active sites of F actin

↓

Attachment of myosin head to actin

↓

Power stroke – tilting of myosin head and dragging of actin filament

↓

Detachment of myosin head and returning to original position

↓

Attachment of myosin head to new active site of F actin and dragging of actin filament – repetition of these actions

↓

Movement of actin filaments of both sides towards each other and formation of actomyosin complex

↓

Contraction of muscle

FIGURE 31.8: Sliding mechanism

opposite sides overlap and form actomyosin complex. Formation of actomyosin complex results in contraction of the muscle.

When the muscle shortens further, the actin filaments from opposite ends of the sarcomere approach each other. So, the 'H' zone becomes narrow. And, the two 'Z' lines come closer with reduction in length of the sarcomere. However, the length of 'A' band is not altered. But, the length of 'I' band decreases.

When the muscular contraction becomes severe, the actin filaments from opposite ends overlap and the 'H' zone disappears.

Changes in sarcomere during muscular contraction

Thus, changes that take place in sarcomere during muscular contraction are:

1. Length of all the sarcomeres decreases as the 'Z' lines come close to each other
2. Length of the 'I' band decreases since the actin filaments from opposite side overlap
3. 'H' zone either decreases or disappears
4. Length of 'A' band remains the same.

Summary of sequence of events during muscular contraction is given in Figure 31.8.

Energy for Muscular Contraction

Energy for movement of myosin head (power stroke) is obtained by breakdown of adenosine triphosphate (ATP) into adenosine diphosphate (ADP) and inorganic phosphate (Pi).

Head of myosin has a site for ATP. Actually the head itself can act as the enzyme ATPase and catalyze the breakdown of ATP. Even before the onset of contraction, an ATP molecule binds with myosin head.

When tropomyosin moves to expose the active sites, the head is attached to the active site. Now ATPase cleaves ATP into ADP and Pi, which remains in head itself. The energy released during this process is utilized for contraction.

When head is tilted, the ADP and Pi are released and a new ATP molecule binds with head. This process is repeated until the muscular contraction is completed.

Relaxation of the Muscle

Relaxation of the muscle occurs when the calcium ions are pumped back into the L tubules. When calcium ions enter the L tubules, calcium content in sarcoplasm decreases leading to the release of calcium ions from the troponin. It causes detachment of myosin from actin followed by relaxation of the muscle (Fig. 31.9). The detachment of myosin from actin obtains energy from breakdown of ATP. Thus, the chemical process of

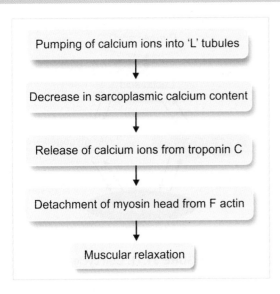

FIGURE 31.9: Sequence of events during muscular relaxation

muscular relaxation is an active process although the physical process is said to be passive.

Molecular Motors

Along with other proteins and some enzymes, actin and myosin form the molecular motors, which are involved in movements. Refer Chapter 3 for details.

■ CHEMICAL CHANGES DURING MUSCULAR CONTRACTION

■ LIBERATION OF ENERGY

Energy necessary for muscular contraction is liberated during the processes of breakdown and resynthesis of ATP.

Breakdown of ATP

During muscular contraction, the supply of energy is from the breakdown of ATP. This is broken into ADP and inorganic phosphate (Pi) and energy is liberated.

$$ATP \rightarrow ADP + Pi$$
$$\downarrow$$
$$Energy$$

Energy liberated by breakdown of ATP is responsible for the following activities during muscular contraction:
1. Spread of action potential into the muscle
2. Liberation of calcium ions from cisternae of 'L' tubules into the sarcoplasm
3. Movements of myosin head
4. Sliding mechanism.

Energy liberated during ATP breakdown is sufficient for maintaining full contraction of the muscle for a short duration of less than one second.

Resynthesis of ATP

Adenosine diphosphate, which is formed during ATP breakdown, is immediately utilized for the resynthesis of ATP. But, for the resynthesis of ATP, the ADP cannot combine with Pi. It should combine with a high-energy phosphate radical. There are two sources from which the high-energy phosphate is obtained namely, creatine phosphate and carbohydrate metabolism.

Resynthesis of ATP from creatine phosphate

Immediate supply of **high-energy phosphate** radical is from the creatine phosphate (CP). Plenty of CP is available in resting muscle. In the presence of the enzyme creatine phosphotransferase, high-energy phosphate is released from creatine phosphate. The reaction is called **Lohmann's reaction.**

$$ADP + CP \rightarrow ATP + Creatine$$

Energy produced in this reaction is sufficient to maintain muscular contraction only for few seconds. Creatine should be resynthesized into creatine phosphate and this requires the presence of high-energy phosphate. So, the required amount of high-energy phosphate radicals is provided by the carbohydrate metabolism in the muscle.

Resynthesis of ATP by carbohydrate metabolism

Carbohydrate metabolism starts with catabolic reactions of glycogen in the muscle. In resting muscle, an adequate amount of glycogen is stored in sarcoplasm.

Each molecule of glycogen undergoes catabolism, to produce ATP. The energy liberated during the catabolism of glycogen can cause muscular contraction for a longer period. The first stage of catabolism of glycogen is via glycolysis. It is called **glycolytic pathway** or **Embden-Meyerhof pathway** (Fig. 31.10).

Glycolysis

Each glycogen molecule is converted into 2 pyruvic acid molecules. Only small amount of ATP (2 molecules) is synthesized in this pathway.

This pathway has 10 steps. Each step is catalyzed by one or two enzymes as shown in Figure 31.10.

During glycolysis, 4 hydrogen atoms are released which are also utilized for formation of additional molecules of ATP. Formation of ATP by the utilization of hydrogen is explained later.

Further changes in pyruvic acid depend upon the availability of oxygen. In the absence of oxygen, the pyruvic acid is converted into lactic acid that enters the **Cori cycle**. It is known as **anaerobic glycolysis**. If oxygen is available, the pyruvic acid enters into **Krebs cycle**. It is known as **aerobic glycolysis.**

Cori cycle

Lactic acid is transported to liver where it is converted into glycogen and stored there. If necessary, glycogen breaks into glucose, which is carried by blood to muscle. Here, the glucose is converted into glycogen, which enters the Embden-Meyerhof pathway (Figs 31.11 and 31.12).

Krebs cycle

Krebs cycle is otherwise known as **tricarboxylic acid cycle** (TCA cycle) or **citric acid cycle.** A greater amount of energy is liberated through this cycle. The pyruvic acid derived from glycolysis is taken into mitochondria where it is converted into acetyl coenzyme A with release of 4 hydrogen atoms. The acetyl coenzyme A enters the Krebs cycle.

Krebs cycle is a series of reactions by which acetyl coenzyme A is degraded in various steps to form carbon

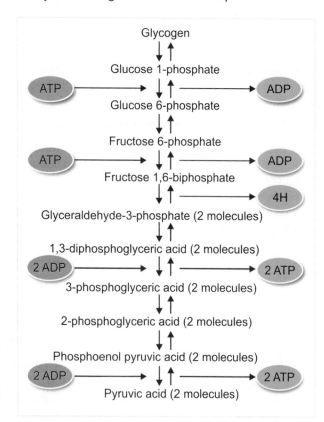

FIGURE 31.10: Glycolysis/Embden-Meyerhof pathway
Number of ATP molecules formed in this pathway:
Total ATP formed   = 4 molecules
Loss of ATP during phosphorylation = 2 molecules
Net ATP formed during glycolysis   = 2 molecules

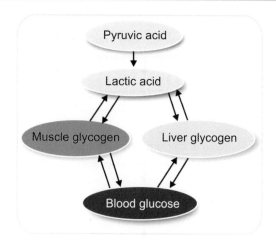

FIGURE 31.11: Cori cycle

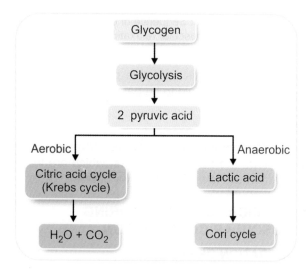

FIGURE 31.12: Schematic diagram showing carbohydrate metabolism in muscle

dioxide and hydrogen atoms. All these reactions occur in the matrix of mitochondrion. During Krebs cycle, 2 molecules of ATP and 16 atoms of hydrogen are released. Hydrogen atoms are also utilized for the formation of ATP (see below).

Significance of Hydrogen Atoms Released during Carbohydrate Metabolism

Altogether 24 hydrogen atoms are released during glycolysis and Krebs cycle:

4H : During breakdown of glycogen into pyruvic acid

4H : During formation of acetyl coenzyme A from pyruvic acid

16H : During degradation of acetyl coenzyme A in Krebs cycle.

Hydrogen atoms are released in the form of two pockets into intracellular fluid and it is catalyzed by the enzyme dehydrogenase. Once released, 20 hydrogen atoms combine with nicotinamide adenine dinucleotide (NAD), which acts as hydrogen carrier. NAD transfers the hydrogen atoms to the cytochrome system where oxidative phosphorylation takes place. Oxidative phosphorylation is the process during which the ATP molecules are formed by utilizing hydrogen atoms.

For every 2 hydrogen atoms 3 molecules of ATP are formed. So, from 20 hydrogen atoms 30 molecules of ATP are formed. Remaining 4 hydrogen atoms enter the oxidative phosphorylation processes directly without combining with NAD. Only 2 ATP molecules are formed for every 2 hydrogen atoms. So, 4 hydrogen atoms give rise to 4 ATP molecules. Thus, 34 ATP molecules are formed from the hydrogen atoms released during glycolysis and Krebs cycle.

Summary of Resynthesis of ATP during Carbohydrate Metabolism

A total of 38 ATP molecules are formed during breakdown of each glycogen molecule in the muscle as summarized below:

During glycolysis	: 2 molecules of ATP
During Krebs cycle	: 2 molecules of ATP
By utilization of hydrogen	: 34 molecules of ATP
Total	: 38 molecules of ATP

■ CHANGES IN pH DURING MUSCULAR CONTRACTION

Reaction and the pH of muscle are altered in different stages of muscular contraction.

In Resting Condition

During resting condition, the reaction of muscle is alkaline with a pH of 7.3.

During Onset of Contraction

At the beginning of the muscular contraction, the reaction becomes acidic. The acidity is due to dephosphorylation of ATP into ADP and Pi.

During Later Part of Contraction

During the later part of contraction, the muscle becomes alkaline. It is due to the resynthesis of ATP from CP.

At the End of Contraction

At the end of contraction, the muscle becomes once again acidic. This acidity is due to the formation of pyruvic acid and/or lactic acid.

■ THERMAL CHANGES DURING MUSCULAR CONTRACTION

During muscular contraction, heat is produced. Not all the heat is liberated at a time. It is released in different stages:

1. Resting heat
2. Initial heat
3. Recovery heat.

■ RESTING HEAT

Heat produced in the muscle at rest is called the resting heat. It is due to the basal metabolic process in the muscle.

■ INITIAL HEAT

During muscular activity, heat production occurs in three stages:

    i. Heat of activation
    ii. Heat of shortening
    iii. Heat of relaxation.

i. Heat of Activation

Heat of activation is the heat produced before the actual shortening of the muscle fibers. Most of this heat is produced during the release of calcium ions from 'L' tubules. It is also called **maintenance heat.**

ii. Heat of Shortening

Heat of shortening is the heat produced during contraction of muscle. The heat is produced due to various structural changes in the muscle fiber like movements of cross bridges and myosin heads and breakdown of glycogen.

iii. Heat of Relaxation

Heat released during relaxation of the muscle is known as the heat of relaxation. In fact, it is the heat produced during the contraction of muscle due to breakdown of ATP molecule. It is released when the muscle lengthens during relaxation.

■ RECOVERY HEAT

Recovery heat is the heat produced in the muscle after the end of activities. After the end of muscular activities, some amount of heat is produced due to the chemical processes involved in resynthesis of chemical substances broken down during contraction.

Neuromuscular Junction

- DEFINITION AND STRUCTURE
  - DEFINITION
  - STRUCTURE
- NEUROMUSCULAR TRANSMISSION
  - RELEASE OF ACETYLCHOLINE
  - ACTION OF ACETYLCHOLINE
  - ENDPLATE POTENTIAL
  - MINIATURE ENDPLATE POTENTIAL
  - FATE OF ACETYLCHOLINE
- NEUROMUSCULAR BLOCKERS
- DRUGS STIMULATING NEUROMUSCULAR JUNCTION
- MOTOR UNIT
  - DEFINITION
  - NUMBER OF MUSCLE FIBERS IN MOTOR UNIT
  - RECRUITMENT OF MOTOR UNITS
- APPLIED PHYSIOLOGY – DISORDERS OF NEUROMUSCULAR JUNCTION
  - MYASTHENIA GRAVIS
  - EATON-LAMBERT SYNDROME

■ DEFINITION AND STRUCTURE

■ DEFINITION

Neuromuscular junction is the junction between terminal branch of the nerve fiber and muscle fiber.

■ STRUCTURE

Skeletal muscle fibers are innervated by the motor nerve fibers. Each nerve fiber (axon) divides into many terminal branches. Each terminal branch innervates one muscle fiber through the neuromuscular junction (Fig. 32.1).

Axon Terminal and Motor Endplate

Terminal branch of nerve fiber is called axon terminal. When the axon comes close to muscle fiber, it loses the myelin sheath. So, the axis cylinder is exposed.

This portion of the axis cylinder is expanded like a bulb, which is called motor endplate.

Axon terminal contains **mitochondria** and **synaptic vesicles.** Synaptic vesicles contain the neurotransmitter

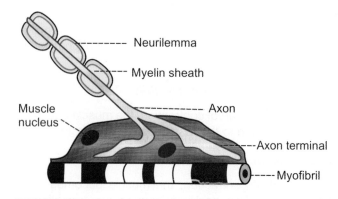

FIGURE 32.1: Longitudinal section of neuromuscular junction

substance, acetylcholine (Ach). The Ach is synthesized by mitochondria present in the axon terminal and stored in the vesicles. Mitochondria contain ATP, which is the source of energy for the synthesis of acetylcholine.

Synaptic Trough or Gutter

Motor endplate invaginates inside the muscle fiber and forms a depression, which is known as **synaptic trough** or **synaptic gutter.** The membrane of the muscle fiber below the motor endplate is thickened.

Synaptic Cleft

Membrane of the nerve ending is called the **presynaptic membrane.** Membrane of the muscle fiber is called **postsynaptic membrane.** Space between these two membranes is called **synaptic cleft.**

Synaptic cleft contains **basal lamina.** It is a thin layer of spongy reticular matrix through which, the extracellular fluid diffuses. An enzyme called acetylcholinesterase (AchE) is attached to the matrix of basal lamina, in large quantities.

Subneural Clefts

Postsynaptic membrane is the membrane of the muscle fiber. It is thrown into numerous folds called **subneural clefts.** Postsynaptic membrane contains the receptors called nicotinic **acetylcholine receptors** (Fig. 32.2).

■ NEUROMUSCULAR TRANSMISSION

Definition

Neuromuscular transmission is defined as the transfer of information from motor nerve ending to the muscle fiber through neuromuscular junction. It is the mechanism

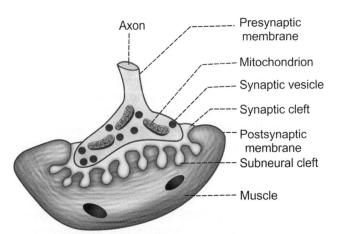

Axon
Presynaptic membrane
Mitochondrion
Synaptic vesicle
Synaptic cleft
Postsynaptic membrane
Subneural cleft
Muscle

FIGURE 32.2: Structure of neuromuscular junction

by which the motor nerve impulses initiate muscle contraction.

Events of Neuromuscular Transmission

A series of events take place in the neuromuscular junction during this process (Fig. 32.3). The events are:
1. Release of acetylcholine
2. Action of acetylcholine
3. Development of endplate potential
4. Development of miniature endplate potential
5. Destruction of acetylcholine.

■ 1. RELEASE OF ACETYLCHOLINE

When action potential reaches axon terminal, it opens the voltage-gated calcium channels in the membrane of axon terminal. Calcium ions from extracellular fluid (ECF) enter the axon terminal. These cause bursting of the vesicles by forcing the synaptic vesicles move and fuse with presynaptic membrane. Now, acetylcholine is released from the ruptured vesicles. By **exocytosis,** acetylcholine diffuses through the presynaptic membrane and enters the synaptic cleft.

Each vesicle contains about 10,000 acetylcholine molecules. And, at a time, about 300 vesicles open and release acetylcholine.

■ 2. ACTION OF ACETYLCHOLINE

After entering the synaptic cleft, acetylcholine molecules bind with nicotinic receptors present in the postsynaptic membrane and form acetylcholine-receptor complex. It increases the permeability of postsynaptic membrane for sodium by opening the ligand-gated sodium channels. Now, sodium ions from ECF enter the neuromuscular junction through these channels. And there, sodium ions alter the resting membrane potential and develops the electrical potential called the endplate potential.

■ 3. DEVELOPMENT OF ENDPLATE POTENTIAL

Endplate potential is the change in resting membrane potential when an impulse reaches the neuromuscular junction. Resting membrane potential at neuromuscular junction is –90 mV. When sodium ions enter inside, slight depolarization occurs up to –60 mV, which is called endplate potential.

Properties of Endplate Potential

Endplate potential is a graded potential (Chapter 31) and it is not action potential. Refer Table 31.1 for the properties of graded potential.

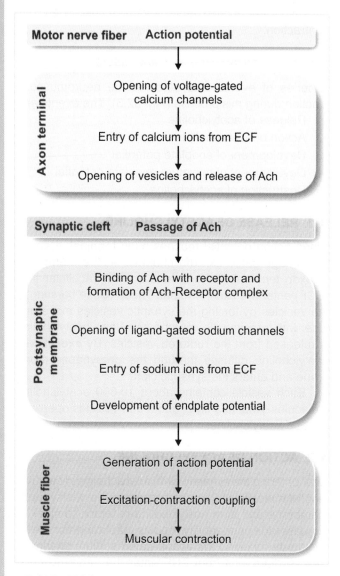

FIGURE 32.3: Sequence of events during neuromuscular transmission. Ach = Acetylcholine, ECF = Extracellular fluid.

Significance of Endplate Potential

Endplate potential is non-propagative. But it causes the development of action potential in the muscle fiber.

■ 4. DEVELOPMENT OF MINIATURE ENDPLATE POTENTIAL

Miniature endplate potential is a weak endplate potential in neuromuscular junction that is developed by the release of a small quantity of acetylcholine from axon terminal. And, each quantum of this neurotransmitter produces a weak miniature endplate potential. The amplitude of this potential is only up to 0.5 mV.

Miniature endplate potential cannot produce action potential in the muscle. When more and more quanta of acetylcholine are released continuously, the miniature endplate potentials are added together and finally produce endplate potential resulting in action potential in the muscle.

■ 5. DESTRUCTION OF ACETYLCHOLINE

Acetylcholine released into the synaptic cleft is destroyed very quickly, within one millisecond by the enzyme, acetylcholinesterase. However, the acetylcholine is so potent, that even this short duration of 1 millisecond is sufficient to excite the muscle fiber. Rapid destruction of acetylcholine has got some important functional significance. It prevents the repeated excitation of the muscle fiber and allows the muscle to relax.

Reuptake Process

Reuptake is a process in neuromuscular junction, by which a degraded product of neurotransmitter re-enters the presynaptic axon terminal where it is reused. Acetylcholinesterase splits (degrades) acetylcholine into inactive choline and acetate. Choline is taken back into axon terminal from synaptic cleft by reuptake process. There, it is reused in synaptic vesicle to form new acetylcholine molecule.

■ NEUROMUSCULAR BLOCKERS

Neuromuscular blockers are the drugs, which prevent transmission of impulses from nerve fiber to the muscle fiber through the neuromuscular junctions. These drugs are used widely during surgery and trauma care. Neuromuscular blockers used during anesthesia relax the skeletal muscles and induce paralysis so that surgery can be conducted with less complication.

Following are important neuromuscular blockers, which are commonly used in clinics and research.

1. Curare

Curare prevents the neuromuscular transmission by combining with acetylcholine receptors. So, the acetylcholine cannot combine with the receptors. And, the endplate potential cannot develop. Since curare blocks the neuromuscular transmission by acting on the acetylcholine receptors, it is called receptor blocker.

2. Bungarotoxin

Bungarotoxin is a toxin from the venom of deadly snakes. It affects the neuromuscular transmission by blocking the acetylcholine receptors.

3. *Succinylcholine and Carbamylcholine*

These drugs block the neuromuscular transmission by acting like acetylcholine and keeping the muscle in a depolarized state. But, these drugs are not destroyed by cholinesterase. So, the muscle remains in a depolarized state for a long time.

4. *Botulinum Toxin*

Botulinum toxin is derived from the bacteria *Clostridium botulinum*. It prevents release of acetylcholine from axon terminal into the neuromuscular junction.

■ DRUGS STIMULATING NEUROMUSCULAR JUNCTION

Neuromuscular junction can be stimulated by some drugs like neostigmine, physostigmine and diisopropyl fluorophosphate. These drugs inactivate the enzyme, acetylcholinesterase. So, the acetylcholine is not hydrolyzed. It leads to repeated stimulation and continuous contraction of the muscle.

■ MOTOR UNIT

■ DEFINITION

Single motor neuron, its axon terminals and the muscle fibers innervated by it are together called motor unit. Each motor neuron activates a group of muscle fibers through the axon terminals. Stimulation of a motor neuron causes contraction of all the muscle fibers innervated by that neuron.

■ NUMBER OF MUSCLE FIBERS IN MOTOR UNIT

Number of muscle fiber in each motor unit varies. The motor units of the muscles concerned with fine, graded and precise movements have smaller number of muscle fibers.

For example,

Laryngeal muscles : 2 to 3 muscle fibers per motor unit
Pharyngeal muscles : 2 to 6 muscle fibers per motor unit
Ocular muscles : 3 to 6 muscle fibers per motor unit

Muscles concerned with crude or coarse movements have motor units with large number of muscle fibers. There are about 120 to 165 muscle fibers in each motor unit in these muscles. Examples are the muscles of leg and back.

■ RECRUITMENT OF MOTOR UNITS

While stimulating the muscle with weak strength, only a few motor units are involved. When the strength of stimulus is increased, many motor units are put into action. So, the force of contraction increases. The process by which more and more motor units are put into action is called recruitment of motor unit. Thus, the graded response in the muscle is directly proportional to the number of motor units activated.

Activation of motor units can be studied by electromyography.

■ APPLIED PHYSIOLOGY – DISORDERS OF NEUROMUSCULAR JUNCTION

■ MYASTHENIA GRAVIS

Myasthenia gravis is an autoimmune disorder of neuromuscular junction caused by antibodies to cholinergic receptors. Refer Chapter 34 for details.

■ EATON-LAMBERT SYNDROME

Eaton-Lambert syndrome is also an autoimmune disorder of neuromuscular junction. It is caused by antibodies to calcium channels in axon terminal. Refer Chapter 34 for details.

Smooth Muscle

Chapter 33

- ■ DISTRIBUTION
- ■ FUNCTIONS
- ■ STRUCTURE
- ■ TYPES
- ■ ELECTRICAL ACTIVITY IN SINGLE-UNIT SMOOTH MUSCLE
- ■ ELECTRICAL ACTIVITY IN MULTIUNIT SMOOTH MUSCLE
- ■ CONTRACTILE PROCESS
- ■ NEUROMUSCULAR JUNCTION
- ■ CONTROL OF SMOOTH MUSCLE

■ DISTRIBUTION OF SMOOTH MUSCLE

Smooth muscles are **non-striated** (plain) and involuntary muscles. These muscles are present in almost all the organs in the form of sheets, bundles or sheaths around other tissues. Smooth muscles form the major contractile tissues of various organs.

Structures in which smooth muscle fibers are present:

1. Wall of organs like esophagus, stomach and intestine in the gastrointestinal tract
2. Ducts of digestive glands
3. Trachea, bronchial tube and alveolar ducts of respiratory tract
4. Ureter, urinary bladder and urethra in excretory system
5. Wall of the blood vessels in circulatory system
6. Arrector pilorum of skin
7. Mammary glands, uterus, genital ducts, prostate gland and scrotum in the reproductive system
8. Iris and ciliary body of the eye.

■ FUNCTIONS OF SMOOTH MUSCLE

Smooth muscles are concerned with very important functions in different parts of the body.

■ IN CARDIOVASCULAR SYSTEM

Smooth muscle fibers around the blood vessels regulate blood pressure and blood flow through different organs and regions of the body.

■ IN RESPIRATORY SYSTEM

Contraction and relaxation of smooth muscle fibers of the air passage alter the diameter of air passage and regulate the inflow and outflow of air.

■ IN DIGESTIVE SYSTEM

Smooth muscle fibers in digestive tract help in movement of food substances, mixing of food substance with digestive juices, absorption of digested material and elimination of unwanted substances. Sphincters along the digestive tract regulate the flow of materials.

■ IN RENAL SYSTEM

Smooth muscle fibers in renal blood vessels regulate renal blood flow and glomerular filtration. Smooth muscles in the ureters propel urine from kidneys to urinary bladder through ureters. Smooth muscles present in urinary bladder help voiding urine to the exterior.

■ IN REPRODUCTIVE SYSTEM

In males, smooth muscle fibers facilitate the movement of sperms and secretions from accessory glands along the reproductive tract. In females, these muscles accelerate the movement of sperms through genital tract after sexual act, movement of ovum into uterus through fallopian tube, expulsion of menstrual fluid and delivery of the baby.

■ STRUCTURE OF SMOOTH MUSCLE

Smooth muscle fibers are **fusiform** or elongated cells. These fibers are generally very small, measuring 2 to 5 microns in diameter and 50 to 200 microns in length. Nucleus is single and elongated and it is centrally placed. Normally, two or more nucleoli are present in the nucleus (Fig. 33.1).

Myofibrils and Sarcomere

Well-defined myofibrils and sarcomere are absent in smooth muscles. So the alternate dark and light bands are absent. Absence of dark and light bands gives the non-striated appearance to the smooth muscle.

Myofilaments and Contractile Proteins

Contractile proteins in smooth muscle fiber are actin, myosin and tropomyosin. But troponin or troponin-like substance is absent.

Thick and thin filaments are present in smooth muscle. However, these filaments are not arranged in orderly fashion as in skeletal muscle. Thick filaments are formed by myosin molecules and are scattered in sarcoplasm. These thick filaments contain more number of cross bridges than in skeletal muscle. Thin filaments are formed by actin and tropomyosin molecules.

Dense Bodies

Dense bodies are the special structures of smooth muscle fibers to which the actin and tropomyosin molecules of thin filaments are attached. The dense bodies are scattered all over the sarcoplasm in the network of intermediate filaments, which is formed by the protein **desmin**. Some of the dense bodies are firmly attached with sarcolemma. The anchoring of the dense bodies, intermediate filaments and thin filaments make the smooth muscle fiber shorten when sliding occurs between thick and thin filaments.

Another interesting feature is that the dense bodies are not arranged in straight line. Because of this, smooth muscle fibers twist like corkscrew during contraction. Adjacent smooth muscle fibers are bound together at

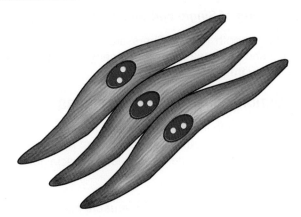

FIGURE 33.1: Smooth muscle fibers

dense bodies. It helps to transmit the contraction from one cell to another throughout the tissue.

Covering and Tendons

Smooth muscle fibers are covered by connective tissue. But the tendons and aponeurosis are absent.

Sarcotubular System

Sarcotubular system in smooth muscle fibers is in the form of network. 'T' tubules are absent and 'L' tubules are poorly developed (see Table 28.1).

■ TYPES OF SMOOTH MUSCLE FIBERS

Smooth muscle fibers are of two types:
1. Single-unit or visceral smooth muscle fibers
2. Multiunit smooth muscle fibers.

■ SINGLE-UNIT OR VISCERAL SMOOTH MUSCLE FIBERS

Single-unit smooth muscle fibers are the fibers with interconnecting gap junctions. The gap junctions allow rapid spread of action potential throughout the tissue so that all the muscle fibers show synchronous contraction as a single unit. Single unit smooth muscle fibers are also called **visceral smooth muscle fibers.**

Features of single-unit smooth muscle fibers:

1. Muscle fibers are arranged in sheets or bundles
2. Cell membrane of adjacent fibers fuses at many points to form gap junctions. Through the gap junctions, ions move freely from one cell to the other. Thus a **functional syncytium** is developed. The syncytium contracts as a single unit. In this way, the visceral smooth muscle resembles cardiac muscle more than the skeletal muscle.

Distribution of Single-unit Smooth Muscle Fibers

Visceral smooth muscle fibers are in the walls of the organs such as gastrointestinal organs, uterus, ureters, respiratory tract, etc.

■ MULTIUNIT SMOOTH MUSCLE FIBERS

Multiunit smooth muscle fibers are the muscle fibers without **interconnecting gap junctions**. These smooth muscle fibers resemble the skeletal muscle fibers in many ways.

Features of multiunit smooth muscle fibers:

1. Muscle fibers are individual fibers
2. Each muscle fiber is innervated by a single nerve ending
3. Each muscle fiber has got an outer membrane made up of glycoprotein, which helps to insulate and separate the muscle fibers from one another
4. Control of these muscle fibers is mainly by nerve signals
5. These smooth muscle fibers do not exhibit spontaneous contractions.

Distribution of Multiunit Smooth Muscle Fibers

Multiunit muscle fibers are in ciliary muscles of the eye, iris of the eye, **nictitating membrane** (in cat), **arrector pili** and smooth muscles of the blood vessels and urinary bladder.

■ ELECTRICAL ACTIVITY IN SINGLE-UNIT SMOOTH MUSCLE

Usually 30 to 40 smooth muscle fibers are simultaneously depolarized, which leads to development of self-propagating action potential. It is possible because of gap junctions and syncytial arrangements of single-unit smooth muscles.

■ RESTING MEMBRANE POTENTIAL

Resting membrane potential in visceral smooth muscle is very **unstable** and ranges between –50 and –75 mV. Sometimes, it reaches the low level of –25 mV.

■ CAUSE FOR UNSTABLE RESTING MEMBRANE POTENTIAL – SLOW-WAVE POTENTIAL

The unstable resting membrane potential is caused by the appearance of some wave-like fluctuations called slow waves. The slow waves occur in a rhythmic fashion at a frequency of 4 to 10 per minute with the amplitude of 10 to 15 mV (Fig. 33.2). The cause of the slow-wave rhythm is not known. It is suggested that it may be due to the rhythmic modulations in the activities of sodium-potassium pump. The slow wave is not action potential and it cannot cause contraction of the muscle. But it initiates the action potential (see below).

■ ACTION POTENTIAL

Three types of action potential occur in visceral smooth muscle fibers:

1. Spike potential
2. Spike potential initiated by slow-wave rhythm
3. Action potential with plateau.

1. Spike Potential

Spike potential in visceral smooth muscle appears similar to that of skeletal muscle. However, it is different from the spike potential in skeletal muscles in many ways. In smooth muscle, the average duration of spike potential varies between 30 and 50 milliseconds. Its amplitude is very low and it does not reach the isoelectric base. Sometimes, the spike potential rises above the isoelectric base (overshoot). The spike potential is due to nervous and other stimuli and it leads to contraction of the muscle.

2. Spike Potential Initiated by Slow-wave Rhythm

Sometimes the slow-wave rhythm of resting membrane potential initiates the spike potentials, which lead to contraction of the muscle. The spike potentials appear rhythmically at a rate of about one or two spikes at the peak of each slow wave. The spike potentials initiated by the slow-wave rhythm cause rhythmic contractions of smooth muscles. This type of potentials appears mostly in smooth muscles, which are self-excitatory and contract themselves without any external stimuli. So, the spike potentials initiated by slow-wave rhythm are otherwise called **pacemaker waves**. The smooth muscles showing rhythmic contractions are present in some of the visceral organs such as intestine.

3. Action Potential with Plateau

This type of action potential starts with rapid depolarization as in the case of skeletal muscle. But, repolarization does not occur immediately. The muscle remains depolarized for long periods of about 100 to 1,000 milliseconds. This type of action potential is responsible for sustained contraction of smooth muscle fibers. After the long depolarized state, slow repolarization occurs.

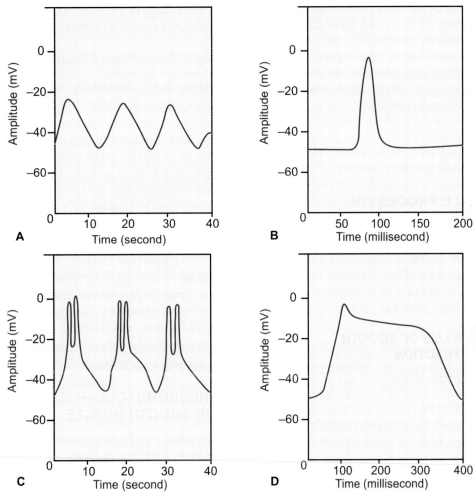

FIGURE 33.2: Electrical activities in smooth muscle
A = Slow-wave rhythm of resting membrane potential
B = Spike potential
C = Spike potential initiated by slow wave rhythm
D = Action potential with plateau

■ TONIC CONTRACTION OF SMOOTH MUSCLE WITHOUT ACTION POTENTIAL

Smooth muscles of some visceral organs maintain a state of partial contraction called **tonus** or **tone.** It is due to the tonic contraction of the muscle that occurs without any action potential or any stimulus. Sometimes, the tonic contraction occurs due to the action of some hormones.

■ IONIC BASIS OF ACTION POTENTIAL

The important difference between action potential in skeletal muscle and smooth muscle lies in the ionic basis of depolarization. In skeletal muscle, the depolarization occurs due to opening of sodium channels and entry of sodium ions from extracellular fluid into the muscle fiber. But in smooth muscle, the depolarization is due to entry of calcium ions rather than sodium ions. Unlike the fast sodium channels, the calcium channels open and close slowly. It is responsible for the prolonged action potential with plateau in smooth muscles. The calcium ions play an important role during the contraction of the muscle.

■ ELECTRICAL ACTIVITY IN MULTIUNIT SMOOTH MUSCLE

Electrical activity in multiunit smooth muscle is different from that in the single unit smooth muscle. Electrical changes leading to contraction of multiunit smooth muscle are triggered by nervous stimuli. Nerve endings secrete the neurotransmitters like acetylcholine and noradrenaline. Neurotransmitters depolarize the membrane of smooth muscle fiber slightly leading to contraction. The action potential does not develop. This type of depolarization is called **local depolarization** or **excitatory junctional potential** (EJP). This local depolarization travels throughout the entire smooth muscle fiber and causes contraction. Local depolarization is developed because the multiunit smooth muscle fibers are too small to develop action potential.

■ CONTRACTILE PROCESS IN SMOOTH MUSCLE

Compared to skeletal muscles, in smooth muscles, the contraction and relaxation processes are slow. The latent period is also long. Thus, the total twitch period is very long and it is about 1 to 3 seconds. In skeletal muscle, the total twitch period is 0.1 sec.

■ MOLECULAR BASIS OF SMOOTH MUSCLE CONTRACTION

The process of excitation and contraction is very slow in smooth muscles because of poor development of 'L' tubules (sarcoplasmic reticulum). So, the calcium ions, which are responsible for excitation-contraction coupling, must be obtained from the extracellular fluid. It makes the process of excitation-contraction coupling slow.

Calcium-calmodulin Complex

Stimulation of ATPase activity of myosin in smooth muscle is different from that in the skeletal muscle. In smooth muscle, the myosin has to be phosphorylated for the activation of myosin ATPase.

Phosphorylation of myosin occurs in the following manner:

1. Calcium, which enters the sarcoplasm from the extracellular fluid combines with a protein called calmodulin and forms calcium-calmodulin complex (Fig. 33.3)
2. It activates calmodulin-dependent myosin light chain kinase
3. This enzyme in turn causes phosphorylation of myosin followed by activation of myosin ATPase
4. Now, the sliding of actin filaments starts.

Phosphorylated myosin gets attached to the actin molecule for longer period. It is called **latch-bridge mechanism** and it is responsible for the sustained contraction of the muscle with expenditure of little energy.

Relaxation of the muscle occurs due to dissociation of calcium-calmodulin complex.

Length-Tension Relationship – Plasticity

Plasticity is the adaptability of smooth muscle fibers to a wide range of lengths. If the smooth muscle fiber is stretched, it adapts to this new length and contracts when stimulated. Because of this property, tension produced in the muscle fiber is not directly proportional to resting length of the muscle fiber. In other words, Starling's law is not applicable to smooth muscle. Starling's law is applicable in skeletal and cardiac muscles and the tension or force of contraction is directly proportional to initial length of fibers in these muscles.

The property of plasticity in smooth muscle fibers is especially important in digestive organs such as stomach, which undergo remarkable changes in volume.

In spite of plasticity, smooth muscle fibers contract powerfully like the skeletal muscle fibers. Smooth muscle fibers also show sustained tetanic contractions like skeletal muscle fibers.

■ NEUROMUSCULAR JUNCTION IN SMOOTH MUSCLE

Well-defined neuromuscular junctions are absent in smooth muscle. The nerve fibers (axons) do not end in the

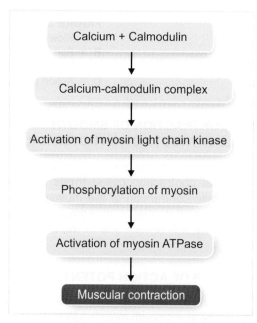

FIGURE 33.3: Molecular basis of smooth muscle contraction

form of endplate. Instead, these nerve fibers end on smooth muscle fibers in three different ways:

1. Nerve fibers diffuse on the sheet of smooth muscle fibers without making any direct contact with the muscle. The diffused nerve fibers form diffuse junctions, which contain neurotransmitters. Neurotransmitters are released into the matrix, which coats the smooth muscle fiber. From here the neurotransmitters enter the muscle fibers

2. In some smooth muscle fibers, the axon terminal ends in the form of many **varicosities.** The varicosities have vesicles, which contain the neurotransmitter. Neurotransmitter is released from varicosities through their wall into the muscle fiber

3. In some of the multiunit smooth muscle fibers, a gap is present between varicosities and the membrane of smooth muscle fibers, which resembles the synaptic cleft in skeletal muscle. The width of this gap is 30 to 40 nm. This gap is called contact junction and it functions as neuromuscular junction of skeletal muscle.

■ CONTROL OF SMOOTH MUSCLE

Smooth muscle fibers are controlled by:
1. Nervous factors
2. Humoral factors.

■ NERVOUS FACTORS

Smooth muscles are supplied by both sympathetic and parasympathetic nerves, which antagonize (act opposite to) each other and control the activities of smooth muscles. However, these nerves are not responsible for the initiation of any activity in smooth muscle. The tonus of smooth muscles is also independent of nervous control.

■ HUMORAL FACTORS

Activity of smooth muscle is also controlled by humoral factors, which include hormones, neurotransmitters and other humoral factors.

Hormones and Neurotransmitters

Action of the hormones and neurotransmitters depends upon the type of receptors present in membrane of smooth muscle fibers in particular area. The receptors are of two types, excitatory receptors and inhibitory receptors.

If excitatory receptors are present, the hormones or the neurotransmitters contract the muscle by producing depolarization. If inhibitory receptors are present, the hormones or the neurotransmitters relax the muscles by producing hyperpolarization.

Hormones and neurotransmitters, which act on smooth muscles are:
1. Acetylcholine
2. Antidiuretic hormone (ADH)
3. Adrenaline
4. Angiotensin II, III and IV
5. Endothelin
6. Histamine
7. Noradrenaline
8. Oxytocin
9. Serotonin.

Other Humoral Factors

Humoral factors other than the hormones cause relaxation of smooth muscle fibers.

Humoral factors which relax the smooth muscles:
1. Lack of oxygen
2. Excess of carbon dioxide
3. Increase in hydrogen ion concentration
4. Adenosine
5. Lactic acid
6. Excess of potassium ion
7. Decrease in calcium ion
8. Nitric oxide (NO), the **endothelium-derived relaxing factor** (EDRF).

Electromyogram and Disorders of Skeletal Muscle

Chapter 34

- ■ **DEFINITION**
- ■ **ELECTROMYOGRAPHIC TECHNIQUE**
- ■ **ELECTROMYOGRAM**
- ■ **DISORDERS OF SKELETAL MUSCLE – MYOPATHY**
  - ■ MUSCULAR DYSTROPHY
  - ■ DISEASES INVOLVING MUSCLE TONE
  - ■ FIBRILLATION AND DENERVATION HYPERSENSITIVITY
  - ■ MYASTHENIA GRAVIS
  - ■ LAMBERT-EATON SYNDROME
  - ■ McARDLE DISEASE
  - ■ MITOCHONDRIAL MYOPATHY
  - ■ NEMALINE MYOPATHY

■ DEFINITION

Electromyography is the study of electrical activity of the muscle. Electromyogram (EMG) is the graphical registration of the electrical activity of the muscle.

■ ELECTROMYOGRAPHIC TECHNIQUE

Cathode ray oscilloscope or a polygraph is used to record the electromyogram. Two types of electrodes are used for recording the electrical activities of the muscle:

1. Surface electrode or skin electrode for studying the activity of a muscle.
2. Needle electrodes for studying the electrical activity of a single motor unit.

■ ELECTROMYOGRAM

Structural basis for electromyogram is the motor unit. Electrical potential developed by the activation of one motor unit is called motor unit potential. It lasts for 5 to 8 milliseconds and has an amplitude of 0.5 mV. Mostly it is monophasic (Fig. 34.1).

Electrical potential recorded from the whole muscle shows smaller potentials if the force of contraction is less. When the force increases, larger potentials are obtained due to the recruitment of more and more number of motor neurons.

Uses of Electromyogram

Electromyogram is useful in the diagnosis of neuro-muscular diseases such as motor neuron lesions, peripheral nerve injury and myopathies.

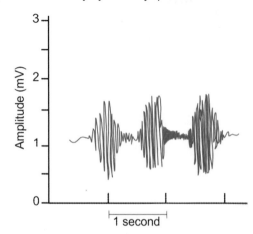

FIGURE 34.1: Electromyogram during alternate contraction and relaxation of biceps muscle

■ DISORDERS OF SKELETAL MUSCLES – MYOPATHY

Myopathy is a muscular disorder in which the dysfunction of muscle fiber leads to muscular weakness. Myopathies may be acquired or genetically derived. These diseases may or may not involve the nervous system.

Common diseases of skeletal muscles are:
1. Muscular dystrophy
2. Diseases involving muscle tone
3. Fibrillation and denervation hypersensitivity
4. Myasthenia gravis
5. Lambert-Eaton syndrome
6. McArdle disease
7. Mitochondrial myopathy
8. Nemaline myopathy.

■ 1. MUSCULAR DYSTROPHY

Muscular dystrophy is a disease characterized by progressive degeneration of muscle fibers, without the involvement of nervous system. Mostly it has a hereditary origin. The muscles fail to regenerate, resulting in progressive weakness and confinement to a wheelchair. Eventually, death occurs. Common types of muscular dystrophy are Duchenne muscular dystrophy and Becker muscular dystrophy.

Duchenne Muscular Dystrophy

Duchenne muscular dystrophy is a sex-linked recessive disorder. It is due to the absence of a gene product called **dystrophin** in the X chromosome. Dystrophin is necessary for the stability of sarcolemma. This disease is characterized by degeneration and necrosis of muscle fibers. The degenerated muscle fibers are replaced by fat and fibrous tissue. Common symptom is the muscular weakness. Sometimes, there is **enlargement of muscles (pseudohypertrophy).** In severe conditions, the respiratory muscles become weak, resulting in difficulty in breathing and death.

Becker Muscular Dystrophy

Becker muscular dystrophy is also a sex-linked disorder. It occurs due to the reduction in quantity or alteration of dystrophin. Common features of this disorder are slow progressive weakness of legs and pelvis, pseudohypertrophy of calf muscles, difficulty in walking, fatigue and mental retardation.

■ 2. DISEASES INVOLVING MUSCLE TONE

Hypertonia

Hypertonia or hypertonicity is a muscular disease characterized by increased muscle tone and inability of the muscle to stretch.

Causes

Hypertonia occurs in upper motor neuron lesion (Chapter 144). During the lesion of upper motor neuron, inhibition of lower motor neurons (gamma-motor-neurons in the spinal cord) is lost. It causes exaggeration of lower motor neuron activity, resulting in hypertonia.

In children, hypertonia is associated with cerebral palsy (permanent disorder caused by brain damage, which occurs at or before birth and is characterized by muscular impairment). Here also, the motor pathway is affected. Such children usually have speech and language delays, with lack of communication skills.

Hypertonia and spasticity

Hypertonia may be related to spasticity, but it is present with or without spasticity. Spasticity is a motor disorder characterized by stiffness of the certain muscles due to continuous contraction. Hypertonicity is one of the major symptoms of spasticity. **Paralysis** (complete loss of function) of the muscle due to hypertonicity is called spastic paralysis.

In hypertonia, there is a resistance to passive movement and it does not depend on velocity (the speed at which the movement occurs), where as in spasticity there is an increase in resistance to sudden passive movement. It is velocity dependent, i.e. faster the passive movement stronger the resistance.

Hypotonia

Hypotonia is the muscular disease characterized by decreased muscle tone. The tone of the muscle is decreased or lost. Muscle offers very little resistance to stretch. Muscle becomes flaccid (lack of firmness) and the condition is called flaccidity.

Causes

Major cause for hypotonia is lower motor neuron lesion (Chapter 144). The paralysis of muscle with hypotonicity is called flaccid paralysis and it results in wastage of muscles.

Hypotonia may also occur because of central nervous system dysfunction, genetic disorders or muscular disorders.

Clinical conditions associated with hypotonia are:
i. **Down syndrome** (chromosomal disorder, characterized by physical and learning disabilities)
ii. **Myasthenia gravis** (see below)
iii. **Kernicterus** (brain damage caused by jaundice in infants; Chapter 163)
iv. Congenital **cerebellar ataxia** (incoordination)
v. Muscular dystrophy

vi. Congenital hypothyroidism
vii. Hypervitaminosis D
viii. Rickets (Chapter 68)
ix. Infant botulism (paralysis due to *botulinum* toxin).

Myotonia

Myotonia is a congenital disease characterized by continuous contraction of muscle and slow relaxation even after the cessation of voluntary act. The main feature of this disease is the muscle stiffness, which is sometimes referred as cramps. Muscle relaxation is delayed.

This type of muscular stiffness with delayed relaxation causes discomfort during simple actions like walking, grasping and chewing. The muscles are enlarged (hypertrophy) because of the continuous contraction. Myotonia sets in during early to late childhood and it is not progressive.

Cause

Myotonia is caused by mutation in the genes of channel proteins in sarcolemma. Such disorders are called channelopathies.

Types

Myotonia is of two types:
   i. **Becker-type myotonia** or **generalized myotonia,** which is more common than Thomsen-type myotonia. It is an autosomal recessive disorder produced by defective genes contributed by both the parents
   ii. **Thomsen-type myotonia** is relatively rare and it is an autosomal recessive disorder produced by defective gene contributed by one parent.

■ 3. FIBRILLATION AND DENERVATION HYPERSENSITIVITY

Denervation of a skeletal muscle (lower motor neuron lesion) causes fibrillation with flaccid paralysis and denervation hypersensitivity.

Fibrillation

Fibrillation means fine irregular contractions of individual muscle fibers.

Denervation Hypersensitivity

After denervation, the muscle becomes highly sensitive to acetylcholine, which is released from neuromuscular junction. It is called denervation hypersensitivity.

■ 4. MYASTHENIA GRAVIS

Myasthenia gravis is an autoimmune disease of neuromuscular junction caused by antibodies to cholinergic receptors. It is characterized by grave weakness of the muscle due to the inability of neuromuscular junction to transmit impulses from nerve to the muscle. It is a serious and sometimes a fatal disease.

Causes

Myasthenia gravis is caused due to the development of **autoantibodies** (IgG autoantibodies) against the receptors of acetylcholine (Chapter 17). That is, the body develops antibodies against its own acetylcholine receptors. These antibodies prevent binging of acetylcholine with it receptors or destroy the receptors. So, though the acetylcholine release is normal, it cannot execute its action.

Symptoms

Muscles which are more susceptible for myasthenia gravis are muscles of neck, limbs, eyeballs and the muscle responsible for eyelid movements, chewing, swallowing, speech and respiration.
   Common symptoms are:
   i. Slow and weak muscular contraction because of the defective neuromuscular activity
   ii. Inability to maintain the prolonged contraction of skeletal muscle
   iii. Quick fatigability when the patient attempts repeated muscular contractions
   iv. Weakness and fatigability of arms and legs
   v. Double vision and droopy eyelids due to the weakness of ocular muscles
   vi. Difficulty in swallowing due to weakness of throat muscles
   vii. Difficulty in speech due to weakness of muscles of speech.
   In severe conditions, there is paralysis of muscles. Patient dies mostly due to the paralysis of respiratory muscles.

Treatment

Myasthenia gravis is treated by administration of cholinesterase inhibitors such as **neostigmine** and **pyridostigmine.** These drugs inhibit cholinesterase, which degrades acetylcholine. So acetylcholine remaining in the synaptic cleft for long period can bind with its receptors.

■ 5. LAMBERT-EATON SYNDROME

Lambert-eaton syndrome is a disorder of neuromuscular junction caused by development of antibodies against **calcium channel** in the nerve terminal, resulting in reduction in the release of quanta of acetylcholine. This disease is commonly associated with carcinoma. So, it is also called **carcinomatous myopathy.** This disease is characterized by several features of myasthenia gravis. In addition, the patients have blurred vision and dry mouth.

■ 6. McARDLE DISEASE

McArdle disease is a glycogen storage disease (accumulation of glycogen in muscles) due to the mutation of genes involving the **muscle glycogen phosphorylase,** necessary for the breakdown of glycogen in muscles. Muscular pain and stiffness are the common features of this disease.

■ 7. MITOCHONDRIAL MYOPATHY

Mitochondrial myopathy is an inherited disease due to the defects in the mitochondria (which provide critical source of energy) of muscle fibers.

■ 8. NEMALINE MYOPATHY

Nemaline myopathy is a congenital myopathy characterized by microscopic changes and formation of small rod-like structures in the muscle fibers. It is also called **nemaline-rod myopathy.** The features are delayed development of motor activities and weakness of muscles.

Endurance of Muscle

Chapter 35

- ■ STRENGTH OF THE MUSCLE
  - ■ TYPES OF MUSCLE STRENGTH
- ■ POWER OF THE MUSCLE
- ■ ENDURANCE OF THE MUSCLE

Three factors are essential for the contraction of skeletal muscle:

1. Strength of the muscle
2. Power of the muscle
3. Endurance of the muscle.

Strength and power of the muscle are the two factors which determine the endurance of the muscle. Power of the muscle is developed by strength of the muscle

■ STRENGTH OF THE MUSCLE

Maximum force that can be developed during contraction is known as strength of the muscle. It is defined as the maximal contractile force produced per square centimeter of the cross-sectional area of a skeletal muscle. The normal force produced by a muscle is about 3 to 4 kg/cm^2 area of muscle. If the size of the muscle is more, the strength developed also will be more.

The size of the muscle can be increased either by exercise or by some hormones like androgens. For example, weight lifters will have the quadriceps muscle with cross-sectional area of about 150 cm^2. So, the total strength of the quadriceps muscles is between 500 and 550 kg/cm^2.

■ TYPES OF MUSCLE STRENGTH

Strength of the muscle is of two types:

1. Contractile strength
2. Holding strength.

1. *Contractile Strength*

Contractile strength is the strength of the muscle during the actual contraction or shortening of muscle fibers. For example, while jumping, when a person takes his body off the ground, there is contraction of the leg muscles. This is called the contractile strength.

2. *Holding Strength*

Holding strength is the force produced while stretching the contracted muscles. For example, while landing after jumping, the leg muscles are stretched. The force developed by the muscles at that time is called the holding strength. The holding strength is greater than the contractile strength.

■ POWER OF THE MUSCLE

Amount of work done by the muscle in a given unit of time is called the power. Power of the muscle depends upon three factors. Muscle power is directly proportional to these factors:

1. Strength of the muscle.
2. Force of contraction.
3. Frequency of contraction.

Muscle power is generally expressed in kilogram-meter per min (kg-m/min), i.e. the weight lifted by a muscle to a height of 1 meter for one minute. The maximum power achieved by all the muscles in the body of a highly trained athlete, with all the muscles working together is approximately,

First 8 to 10 seconds	: 7,000 kg-m/min
Next 1 minute	: 4,000 kg-m/min
Next 30 minute	: 1,700 kg-m/min

This shows that the maximum power is developed only for a short period of time.

■ ENDURANCE OF THE MUSCLE

Capacity of the muscle to withstand the power produced during activity is called endurance. It depends mostly on the supply of nutrition to the muscle.

Most important nutritive substance for the muscle is glycogen. This is actually stored in the muscle before the beginning of the activity. More amount of glycogen can be stored in the muscles if a person takes diet containing more carbohydrates than the diet containing fat or a mixed diet. Following is the amount of glycogen stored in the muscle in persons taking different diets.

High carbohydrate diet : 40 gm/kg muscle
Mixed diet : 20 gm/kg muscle
High fat diet : 6 gm/kg muscle.

QUESTIONS IN MUSCLE PHYSIOLOGY

■ LONG QUESTIONS

1. Enumerate the properties of muscles and give an account on contractile property of the skeletal muscle.
2. List the various changes taking place during muscular contraction and explain the molecular basis of contraction.
3. Write about the electrical changes during muscular contraction.
4. Explain the ionic basis of electrical events during contraction of skeletal muscle.
5. Describe the neuromuscular junction with a suitable diagram. Add a note on neuromuscular transmission

■ SHORT QUESTIONS

1. Compare skeletal muscle and cardiac muscle.
2. Compare skeletal muscle and smooth muscle.
3. Sarcomere.
4. Contractile elements of the muscle.
5. Muscle proteins.
6. Sarcotubular system.
7. Sarcoplasmic reticulum.
8. Composition of muscle.
9. Excitability or strength-duration curve.
10. Factors affecting force of muscular contraction.
11. Simple muscle curve.
12. Latent period.
13. Differences between pale and red muscles.
14. Effects of two successive stimuli on muscle.
15. Effects of temperature variation on muscle.
16. Rigor.
17. Effects of repeated stimuli on skeletal muscle.
18. Fatigue.
19. Tetanus.
20. Starling's law of muscle.
21. Refractory period.
22. Muscle tone.
23. Resting membrane potential.
24. Action potential.
25. Graded potential.
26. Patch clamp.
27. Actomyosin complex.
28. Excitation-contraction coupling.
29. Sliding theory of muscular contraction.
30. Chemical changes during muscular contraction.
31. Liberation of energy for muscular contraction.
32. Thermal changes during muscular contraction.
33. Electrical activity in smooth muscle.
34. Molecular basis of smooth muscular contraction.
35. Neuromuscular junction.
36. Neuromuscular transmission.
37. Endplate potential.
38. Neuromuscular blockers.
39. Motor unit.
40. Electromyogram.
41. Myopathy.
42. Muscular dystrophy.
43. Myasthenia gravis.
44. Hypertonia.
45. Hypotonia.

Section
4

Digestive System

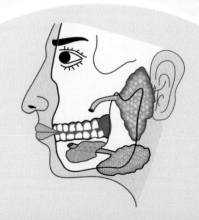

Section

7

Digestive System

Introduction to Digestive System

```
■ INTRODUCTION
■ FUNCTIONAL ANATOMY
■ WALL OF GASTROINTESTINAL TRACT
    ■ MUCUS LAYER
    ■ SUBMUCUS LAYER
    ■ MUSCULAR LAYER
    ■ SEROUS OR FIBROUS LAYER
■ NERVE SUPPLY TO GASTROINTESTINAL TRACT
    ■ INTRINSIC NERVE SUPPLY
    ■ EXTRINSIC NERVE SUPPLY
```

■ INTRODUCTION

Digestion is defined as the process by which food is broken down into simple chemical substances that can be absorbed and used as nutrients by the body. Most of the substances in the diet cannot be utilized as such. These substances must be broken into smaller particles, so that they can be absorbed into blood and distributed to various parts of the body for utilization. Digestive system is responsible for these functions.

Digestive process is accomplished by mechanical and enzymatic breakdown of food into simpler chemical compounds. A normal young healthy adult consumes about 1 kg of solid diet and about 1 to 2 liter of liquid diet every day. All these food materials are subjected to digestive process, before being absorbed into blood and distributed to the tissues of the body. Digestive system plays the major role in the digestion and absorption of food substances.

Thus, the functions of digestive system include:
1. Ingestion or consumption of food substances
2. Breaking them into small particles
3. Transport of small particles to different areas of the digestive tract
4. Secretion of necessary enzymes and other substances for digestion
5. Digestion of the food particles
6. Absorption of the digestive products (nutrients)
7. Removal of unwanted substances from the body.

■ FUNCTIONAL ANATOMY OF DIGESTIVE SYSTEM

Digestive system is made up of **gastrointestinal tract** (GI tract) or alimentary canal and accessory organs, which help in the process of digestion and absorption (Fig. 36.1). GI tract is a tubular structure extending from the mouth up to anus, with a length of about 30 feet. It opens to the external environment on both ends.

GI tract is formed by two types of organs:
1. Primary digestive organs.
2. Accessory digestive organs.

1. *Primary Digestive Organs*

Primary digestive organs are the organs where actual digestion takes place.

Primary digestive organs are:
i. Mouth
ii. Pharynx
iii. Esophagus
iv. Stomach

v. Small intestine
vi. Large intestine.

2. *Accessory Digestive Organs*

Accessory digestive organs are those which help primary digestive organs in the process of digestion.

Accessory digestive organs are:

i. Teeth
ii. Tongue
iii. Salivary glands
iv. Exocrine part of pancreas
v. Liver
vi. Gallbladder.

■ WALL OF GASTROINTESTINAL TRACT

In general, wall of the GI tract is formed by four layers which are from inside out:

1. Mucus layer
2. Submucus layer
3. Muscular layer
4. Serous or fibrous layer.

■ 1. MUCUS LAYER

Mucus layer is the innermost layer of the wall of GI tract. It is also called gastrointestinal mucosa or mucus membrane. It faces the cavity of GI tract.

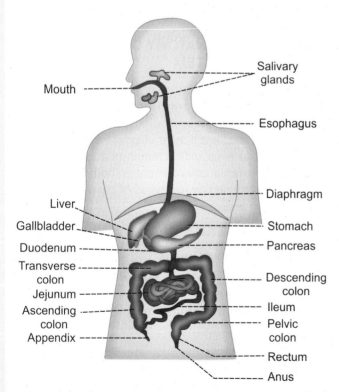

Mouth
Salivary glands
Esophagus
Diaphragm
Liver
Gallbladder
Stomach
Duodenum
Pancreas
Transverse colon
Jejunum
Descending colon
Ascending colon
Ileum
Appendix
Pelvic colon
Rectum
Anus

FIGURE 36.1: Gastrointestinal tract

Mucosa has three layer of structures:

i. Epithelial lining
ii. Lamina propria
iii. Muscularis mucosa.

Epithelial Lining

Epithelial lining is in contact with the contents of GI tract. The type of cells in this layer varies in different parts of GI tract. The inner surface of mouth, surface of tongue, inner surface of pharynx and esophagus have stratified squamous epithelial cells. However, mucus membrane lining the other parts such as stomach, small intestine and large intestine has columnar epithelial cells.

Lamina Propria

Lamina propria is formed by connective tissues, which contain fibroblasts, macrophages, lymphocytes and eosinophils.

Muscularis Mucosa

Muscularis mucosa layer consists of a thin layer of smooth muscle fibers. It is absent in mouth and pharynx. It is present from esophagus onwards.

■ 2. SUBMUCUS LAYER

Submucus layer is also present in all parts of GI tract, except the mouth and pharynx. It contains loose collagen fibers, elastic fibers, reticular fibers and few cells of connective tissue. Blood vessels, lymphatic vessels and nerve plexus are present in this layer.

■ 3. MUSCULAR LAYER

Muscular layer in lips, cheeks and wall of pharynx contains skeletal muscle fibers. The esophagus has both skeletal and smooth muscle fibers. Wall of the stomach and intestine is formed by smooth muscle fibers.

Smooth muscle fibers in stomach are arranged in three layers:

i. Inner oblique layer
ii. Middle circular layer
iii. Outer longitudinal layer.

Smooth muscle fibers in the intestine are arranged in two layers:

i. Inner circular layer
ii. Outer longitudinal layer.

Auerbach nerve plexus is present in between the circular and longitudinal muscle fibers. The smooth muscle fibers present in inner circular layer of anal canal constitute **internal anal sphincter.** The **external anal sphincter** is formed by skeletal muscle fibers.

■ 4. SEROUS OR FIBROUS LAYER

Outermost layer of the wall of GI tract is either serous or fibrous in nature. The serous layer is also called **serosa** or **serous membrane** and it is formed by connective tissue and mesoepithelial cells. It covers stomach, small intestine and large intestine.

The fibrous layer is otherwise called **fibrosa** and it is formed by connective tissue. It covers pharynx and esophagus.

■ NERVE SUPPLY TO GASTROINTESTINAL TRACT

GI tract has two types of nerve supply:
    I. Intrinsic nerve supply
    II. Extrinsic nerve supply.

■ INTRINSIC NERVE SUPPLY – ENTERIC NERVOUS SYSTEM

Intrinsic nerves to GI tract form the enteric nervous system that controls all the secretions and movements of GI tract. Enteric nervous system is present within the wall of GI tract from esophagus to anus. Nerve fibers of this system are interconnected and form two major networks called
1. Auerbach plexus
2. Meissner plexus.

These nerve plexus contain nerve cell bodies, processes of nerve cells and the receptors. The receptors in the GI tract are stretch receptors and chemoreceptors. Enteric nervous system is controlled by extrinsic nerves.

1. *Auerbach Plexus*

Auerbach plexus is also known as **myenteric nerve plexus.** It is present in between the inner circular muscle layer and the outer longitudinal muscle layer (Fig. 36.2).

Functions of Auerbach plexus

Major function of this plexus is to regulate the movements of GI tract. Some nerve fibers of this plexus accelerate the movements by secreting the excitatory neurotransmitter substances like acetylcholine, serotonin and substance P. Other fibers of this plexus inhibit the GI motility by secreting the inhibitory neurotransmitters such as vasoactive intestinal polypeptide (VIP), neurotensin and enkephalin.

2. *Meissner Nerve Plexus*

Meissner plexus is otherwise called submucus nerve plexus. It is situated in between the muscular layer and submucosal layer of GI tract.

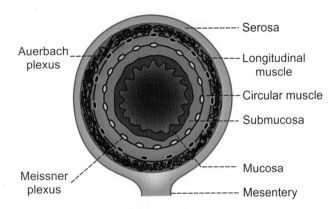

FIGURE 36.2: Structure of intestinal wall with intrinsic nerve plexus

Functions of Meissner plexus

Function of Meissner plexus is the regulation of secretory functions of GI tract. These nerve fibers cause constriction of blood vessels of GI tract.

■ EXTRINSIC NERVE SUPPLY

Extrinsic nerves that control the enteric nervous system are from autonomic nervous system. Both sympathetic and parasympathetic divisions of autonomic nervous system innervate the GI tract (Fig. 36.3).

Sympathetic Nerve Fibers

Preganglionic sympathetic nerve fibers to GI tract arise from lateral horns of spinal cord between fifth thoracic and second lumbar segments (T5 to L2). From here, the fibers leave the spinal cord, pass through the ganglia of sympathetic chain without having any synapse and then terminate in the **celiac** and **mesenteric ganglia.** The postganglionic fibers from these ganglia are distributed throughout the GI tract.

Functions of sympathetic nerve fibers

Sympathetic nerve fibers inhibit the movements and decrease the secretions of GI tract by secreting the neurotransmitter noradrenaline. It also causes constriction of sphincters.

Parasympathetic Nerve Fibers

Parasympathetic nerve fibers to GI tract pass through some of the **cranial nerves** and **sacral nerves.** The preganglionic and postganglionic parasympathetic nerve fibers to mouth and salivary glands pass through facial and glossopharyngeal nerves.

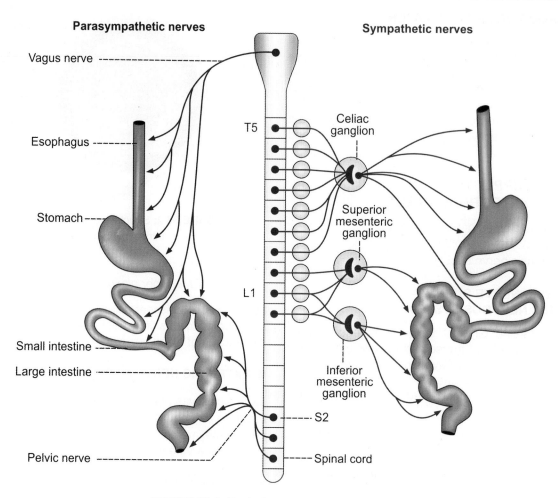

Parasympathetic nerves

Sympathetic nerves

Vagus nerve

Esophagus

Stomach

Small intestine

Large intestine

Pelvic nerve

T5

L1

Celiac ganglion

Superior mesenteric ganglion

Inferior mesenteric ganglion

S2

Spinal cord

FIGURE 36.3: Extrinsic nerve supply to GI tract.
T5 = 5th thoracic segment of spinal cord
L1 = 1st lumbar segment of spinal cord
S2 = 2nd sacral segment of spinal cord

Preganglionic parasympathetic nerve fibers to esophagus, stomach, small intestine and upper part of large intestine pass through vagus nerve. Preganglionic nerve fibers to lower part of large intestine arise from second, third and fourth sacral segments (S2, S3 and S4) of spinal cord and pass through pelvic nerve. All these preganglionic parasympathetic nerve fibers synapse with the postganglionic nerve cells in the myenteric and submucus plexus.

Functions of parasympathetic nerve fibers

Parasympathetic nerve fibers accelerate the movements and increase the secretions of GI tract. The neurotransmitter secreted by the parasympathetic nerve fibers is acetylcholine (Ach).

Mouth and Salivary Glands

Chapter 37

- ■ FUNCTIONAL ANATOMY OF MOUTH
- ■ FUNCTIONS OF MOUTH
- ■ SALIVARY GLANDS
- ■ PROPERTIES AND COMPOSITION OF SALIVA
- ■ FUNCTIONS OF SALIVA
- ■ REGULATION OF SALIVARY SECRETION
- ■ EFFECT OF DRUGS AND CHEMICALS ON SALIVARY SECRETION
- ■ APPLIED PHYSIOLOGY

■ FUNCTIONAL ANATOMY OF MOUTH

Mouth is otherwise known as oral cavity or **buccal cavity.** It is formed by cheeks, lips and palate. It encloses the teeth, tongue and salivary glands. Mouth opens anteriorly to the exterior through lips and posteriorly through fauces into the pharynx.

Digestive juice present in the mouth is saliva, which is secreted by the salivary glands.

■ FUNCTIONS OF MOUTH

Primary function of mouth is eating and it has few other important functions also.

Functions of mouth include:
1. Ingestion of food materials
2. Chewing the food and mixing it with saliva
3. Appreciation of taste of the food
4. Transfer of food (bolus) to the esophagus by swallowing
5. Role in speech
6. Social functions such as smiling and other expressions.

■ SALIVARY GLANDS

In humans, the saliva is secreted by three pairs of major (larger) salivary glands and some minor (small) salivary glands.

■ MAJOR SALIVARY GLANDS

Major glands are:
1. Parotid glands
2. Submaxillary or submandibular glands
3. Sublingual glands.

1. *Parotid Glands*

Parotid glands are the largest of all salivary glands, situated at the side of the face just below and in front of the ear. Each gland weighs about 20 to 30 g in adults. Secretions from these glands are emptied into the oral cavity by **Stensen duct.** This duct is about 35 mm to 40 mm long and opens inside the cheek against the upper second molar tooth (Fig. 37.1).

2. *Submaxillary Glands*

Submaxillary glands or submandibular glands are located in submaxillary triangle, medial to mandible. Each gland weighs about 8 to 10 g. Saliva from these glands is emptied into the oral cavity by **Wharton duct,** which is about 40 mm long. The duct opens at the side of **frenulum** of tongue, by means of a small opening on the summit of papilla called **caruncula sublingualis.**

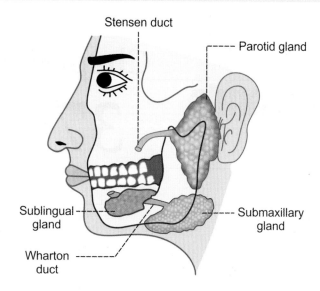

FIGURE 37.1: Major salivary glands

TABLE 37.1: Ducts of major salivary glands

Gland	Duct
Parotid gland	Stensen duct
Submaxillary gland	Wharton duct
Sublingual gland	Ducts of Rivinus/Bartholin duct

5. *Palatal Glands*

Palatal glands are found beneath the mucus membrane of the soft palate.

■ CLASSIFICATION OF SALIVARY GLANDS

Salivary glands are classified into three types, based on the type of secretion:

1. *Serous Glands*

Serous glands are mainly made up of serous cells. These glands secrete thin and watery saliva. Parotid glands and lingual serous glands are the serous glands.

2. *Mucus Glands*

Mucus glands are mainly made up of mucus cells. These glands secrete thick, viscous saliva with high mucin content. Lingual mucus glands, buccal glands and palatal glands belong to this type.

3. *Mixed Glands*

Mixed glands are made up of both serous and mucus cells. Submandibular, sublingual and labial glands are the mixed glands.

■ STRUCTURE AND DUCT SYSTEM OF SALIVARY GLANDS

Salivary glands are formed by **acini** or **alveoli.** Each acinus is formed by a small group of cells which surround a central globular cavity. Central cavity of each acinus is continuous with the lumen of the duct. The fine duct draining each acinus is called **intercalated duct.** Many intercalated ducts join together to form **intralobular duct.** Few intralobular ducts join to form **interlobular ducts,** which unite to form the main duct of the gland (Fig. 37.2). A gland with this type of structure and duct system is called **racemose type** (racemose = bunch of grapes).

■ PROPERTIES AND COMPOSITION OF SALIVA

■ PROPERTIES OF SALIVA

1. *Volume:* 1000 mL to 1500 mL of saliva is secreted per day and it is approximately about 1 mL/minute.

3. *Sublingual Glands*

Sublingual glands are the smallest salivary glands situated in the mucosa at the floor of the mouth. Each gland weighs about 2 to 3 g. Saliva from these glands is poured into 5 to 15 small ducts called **ducts of Rivinus.** These ducts open on small papillae beneath the tongue. One of the ducts is larger and it is called **Bartholin duct** (Table 37.1). It drains the anterior part of the gland and opens on caruncula sublingualis near the opening of submaxillary duct.

■ MINOR SALIVARY GLANDS

1. *Lingual Mucus Glands*

Lingual mucus glands are situated in posterior one third of the tongue, behind **circumvallate papillae** and at the tip and margins of tongue.

2. *Lingual Serous Glands*

Lingual serous glands are located near circumvallate papillae and **filiform papillae.**

3. *Buccal Glands*

Buccal glands or molar glands are present between the mucus membrane and buccinator muscle. Four to five of these are larger and situated outside buccinator, around the terminal part of parotid duct.

4. *Labial Glands*

Labial glands are situated beneath the mucus membrane around the orifice of mouth.

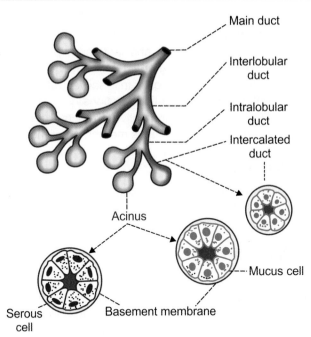

FIGURE 37.2: Diagram showing acini and duct system in salivary glands

Contribution by each major salivary gland is:
i.   Parotid glands   : 25%
ii. Submaxillary glands : 70%
iii. Sublingual glands   : 5%.

2. *Reaction:* Mixed saliva from all the glands is slightly acidic with pH of 6.35 to 6.85
3. *Specific gravity:* It ranges between 1.002 and 1.012
4. *Tonicity:* Saliva is hypotonic to plasma.

■ COMPOSITION OF SALIVA

Mixed saliva contains 99.5% water and 0.5% solids. Composition of saliva is given in Figure 37.3.

■ FUNCTIONS OF SALIVA

Saliva is a very essential digestive juice. Since it has many functions, its absence leads to many inconveniences.

■ 1. PREPARATION OF FOOD FOR SWALLOWING

When food is taken into the mouth, it is moistened and dissolved by saliva. The mucus membrane of mouth is also moistened by saliva. It facilitates chewing. By the movement of tongue, the moistened and masticated food is rolled into a bolus. **Mucin** of saliva lubricates the bolus and facilitates swallowing.

■ 2. APPRECIATION OF TASTE

Taste is a chemical sensation. By its solvent action, saliva dissolves the solid food substances, so that the

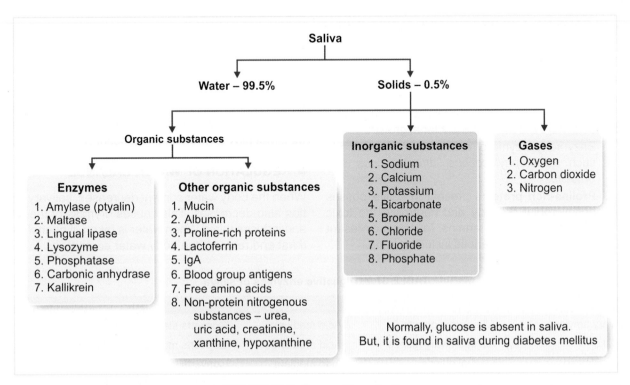

FIGURE 37.3: Composition of saliva

dissolved substances can stimulate the taste buds. The stimulated taste buds recognize the taste.

■ 3. DIGESTIVE FUNCTION

Saliva has three digestive enzymes, namely salivary amylase, maltase and lingual lipase (Table 37.1).

Salivary Amylase

Salivary amylase is a carbohydrate-digesting (amylolytic) enzyme. It acts on cooked or boiled starch and converts it into **dextrin** and **maltose.** Though starch digestion starts in the mouth, major part of it occurs in stomach because, food stays only for a short time in the mouth.

Optimum pH necessary for the activation of salivary amylase is 6. Salivary amylase cannot act on **cellulose.**

Maltase

Maltase is present only in traces in human saliva and it converts maltose into glucose.

Lingual Lipase

Lingual lipase is a lipid-digesting **(lipolytic)** enzyme. It is secreted from serous glands situated on the posterior aspect of tongue. It digests milk fats **(pre-emulsified fats).** It hydrolyzes triglycerides into fatty acids and diacylglycerol (Table 37.2).

■ 4. CLEANSING AND PROTECTIVE FUNCTIONS

i. Due to the constant secretion of saliva, the mouth and teeth are rinsed and kept free off food debris, shed epithelial cells and foreign particles. In this way, saliva prevents bacterial growth by removing materials, which may serve as culture media for the bacterial growth.

ii. Enzyme lysozyme of saliva kills some bacteria such as *staphylococcus, streptococcus* and *brucella.*

iii. **Proline-rich proteins** present in saliva posses antimicrobial property and neutralize the toxic substances such as tannins. Tannins are present in many food substances including fruits.

iv. Lactoferrin of saliva also has antimicrobial property.

v. Proline-rich proteins and lactoferrin protect the teeth by stimulating enamel formation.

vi. Immunoglobulin IgA in saliva also has antibacterial and antiviral actions.

vii. Mucin present in the saliva protects the mouth by lubricating the mucus membrane of mouth.

■ ROLE IN SPEECH

By moistening and lubricating soft parts of mouth and lips, saliva helps in speech. If the mouth becomes dry, articulation and pronunciation becomes difficult.

■ EXCRETORY FUNCTION

Many substances, both organic and inorganic, are excreted in saliva. It excretes substances like mercury, potassium iodide, lead, and thiocyanate. Saliva also excretes some viruses such as those causing rabies and mumps.

In some pathological conditions, saliva excretes certain substances, which are not found in saliva under normal conditions. Example is glucose in diabetes mellitus. In certain conditions, some of the normal constituents of saliva are excreted in large quantities. For example, excess urea is excreted in saliva during nephritis and excess calcium is excreted during hyperparathyroidism.

■ REGULATION OF BODY TEMPERATURE

In dogs and cattle, excessive dripping of saliva during panting helps in the loss of heat and regulation of body temperature. However, in human beings, sweat glands play a major role in temperature regulation and saliva does not play any role in this function.

■ REGULATION OF WATER BALANCE

When the body water content decreases, salivary secretion also decreases. This causes dryness of the mouth and induces thirst. When water is taken, it quenches the thirst and restores the body water content.

TABLE 37.2: Digestive enzymes of saliva

Enzyme	Source of secretion	Activator	Action
Salivary amylase	All salivary glands	Acid medium	Converts starch into maltose
Maltase	Major salivary glands	Acid medium	Converts maltose into glucose
Lingual lipase	Lingual glands	Acid medium	Converts triglycerides of milk fat into fatty acids and diacylglycerol

■ REGULATION OF SALIVARY SECRETION

Salivary secretion is regulated only by nervous mechanism. Autonomic nervous system is involved in the regulation of salivary secretion.

■ NERVE SUPPLY TO SALIVARY GLANDS

Salivary glands are supplied by both parasympathetic and sympathetic divisions of autonomic nervous system.

■ PARASYMPATHETIC FIBERS

Parasympathetic Fibers to Submandibular and Sublingual Glands

Parasympathetic preganglionic fibers to submandibular and sublingual glands arise from the superior salivatory nucleus, situated in pons. After taking origin from this nucleus, the preganglionic fibers run through nervus intermedius of Wrisberg, geniculate ganglion, the motor fibers of facial nerve, chorda tympani branch of facial nerve and lingual branch of trigeminal nerve and finally reach the submaxillary ganglion (Fig. 37.4).

Postganglionic fibers arising from this ganglion supply the submaxillary and sublingual glands.

Parasympathetic Fibers to Parotid Gland

Parasympathetic preganglionic fibers to parotid gland arise from inferior salivatory nucleus situated in the upper part of medulla oblongata. From here, the fibers

pass through the tympanic branch of glossopharyngeal nerve, tympanic plexus and lesser petrosal nerve and end in otic ganglion (Fig. 37.5).

Postganglionic fibers arise from this ganglion and supply the parotid gland by passing through auriculotemporal branch in mandibular division of trigeminal nerve.

Function of Parasympathetic Fibers

Stimulation of parasympathetic fibers of salivary glands causes secretion of saliva with large quantity of water. It is because the parasympathetic fibers activate the acinar cells and dilate the blood vessels of salivary glands. However, the amount of organic constituents in saliva is less. The neurotransmitter is acetylcholine.

■ SYMPATHETIC FIBERS

Sympathetic preganglionic fibers to salivary glands arise from the lateral horns of first and second thoracic segments of spinal cord. The fibers leave the cord through the anterior nerve roots and end in superior cervical ganglion of the sympathetic chain.

Postganglionic fibers arise from this ganglion and are distributed to the salivary glands along the nerve plexus, around the arteries supplying the glands.

Function of Sympathetic Fibers

Stimulation of sympathetic fibers causes secretion of saliva, which is thick and rich in organic constituents such

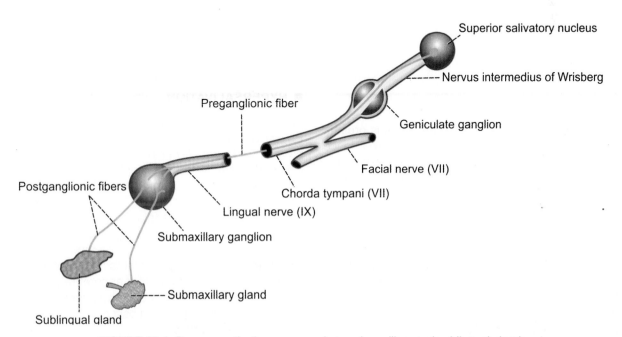

FIGURE 37.4: Parasympathetic nerve supply to submaxillary and sublingual glands

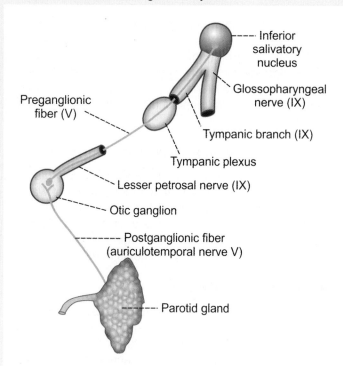

FIGURE 37.5: Parasympathetic nerve supply to parotid gland

as mucus. It is because, these fibers activate the acinar cells and cause vasoconstriction. The neurotransmitter is noradrenaline.

■ REFLEX REGULATION OF SALIVARY SECRETION

Salivary secretion is regulated by nervous mechanism through reflex action.

Salivary reflexes are of two types:

1. Unconditioned reflex.
2. Conditioned reflex.

1. *Unconditioned Reflex*

Unconditioned reflex is the inborn reflex that is present since birth. It does not need any previous experience (Chapter 162). This reflex induces salivary secretion when any substance is placed in the mouth. It is due to the stimulation of nerve endings in the mucus membrane of the oral cavity.

2. *Conditioned Reflex*

Conditioned reflex is the one that is acquired by experience and it needs previous experience (Chapter 162). Presence of food in the mouth is not necessary to elicit this reflex. The stimuli for this reflex are the sight, smell, hearing or thought of food.

■ EFFECT OF DRUGS AND CHEMICALS ON SALIVARY SECRETION

Substances which increase salivary secretion

1. Sympathomimetic drugs like adrenaline and ephedrine.
2. Parasympathomimetic drugs like acetylcholine, pilocarpine, muscarine and physostigmine.
3. Histamine.

Substances which decrease salivary secretion

1. Sympathetic depressants like ergotamine and dibenamine.
2. Parasympathetic depressants like atropine and scopolamine.
3. Anesthetics such as chloroform and ether stimulate the secretion of saliva. However, deep anesthesia decreases the secretion due to central inhibition.

■ APPLIED PHYSIOLOGY

■ HYPOSALIVATION

Reduction in the secretion of saliva is called hyposalivation. It is of two types, namely temporary hyposalivation and permanent hyposalivation.

1. Temporary hyposalivation occurs in:
   i. Emotional conditions like fear.
   ii. Fever.
   iii. Dehydration.
2. Permanent hyposalivation occurs in:
   i. Sialolithiasis (obstruction of salivary duct).
   ii. Congenital absence or hypoplasia of salivary glands.
   iii. Bell palsy (paralysis of facial nerve).

■ HYPERSALIVATION

Excess secretion of saliva is known as hypersalivation. Physiological condition when hypersalivation occurs is pregnancy. Hypersalivation in pathological conditions is called ptyalism, sialorrhea, sialism or sialosis.

Hypersalivation occurs in the following pathological conditions:

1. Decay of tooth or neoplasm (abnormal new growth or tumor) in mouth or tongue due to continuous irritation of nerve endings in the mouth.
2. Disease of esophagus, stomach and intestine.
3. Neurological disorders such as cerebral palsy, mental retardation, cerebral stroke and parkinsonism.
4. Some psychological and psychiatric conditions.
5. Nausea and vomiting.

■ OTHER DISORDERS

In addition to hyposalivation and hypersalivation, salivary secretion is affected by other disorders also, which include:
1. Xerostomia
2. Drooling
3. Chorda tympani syndrome
4. Paralytic secretion of saliva
5. Augmented secretion of saliva
6. Mumps
7. Sjögren syndrome.

1. *Xerostomia*

Xerostomia means dry mouth. It is also called pasties or cottonmouth. It is due to hyposalivation or absence of salivary secretion (aptyalism).

Causes

i. Dehydration or renal failure.
ii. Sjögren syndrome (see below).
iii. Radiotherapy.
iv. Trauma to salivary gland or their ducts.
v. Side effect of some drugs like antihistamines, antidepressants, monoamine oxidase inhibitors, antiparkinsonian drugs and antimuscarinic drugs.
vi. Shock.
vii. After smoking marijuana (psychoactive compound from the plant *Cannabis*).

Xerostomia causes difficulties in mastication, swallowing and speech. It also causes halitosis (bad breath; exhalation of unpleasant odors).

2. *Drooling*

Uncontrolled flow of saliva outside the mouth is called drooling. It is often called ptyalism.

Causes

Drooling occurs because of excess production of saliva, in association with inability to retain saliva within the mouth.
Drooling occurs in the following conditions:
i. During teeth eruption in children.
ii. Upper respiratory tract infection or nasal allergies in children.
iii. Difficulty in swallowing.
iv. Tonsillitis.
v. Peritonsillar abscess.

3. *Chorda Tympani Syndrome*

Chorda tympani syndrome is the condition characterized by sweating while eating. During trauma or surgical procedure, some of the parasympathetic nerve fibers to salivary glands may be severed. During the regeneration, some of these nerve fibers, which run along with chorda tympani branch of facial nerve may deviate and join with the nerve fibers supplying sweat glands. When the food is placed in the mouth, salivary secretion is associated with sweat secretion.

4. *Paralytic Secretion of Saliva*

When the parasympathetic nerve to salivary gland is cut in experimental animals, salivary secretion increases for first three weeks and later diminishes; finally it stops at about sixth week. The increased secretion of saliva after cutting the parasympathetic nerve fibers is called paralytic secretion. It is because of hyperactivity of sympathetic nerve fibers to salivary glands after cutting the parasympathetic fibers. These hyperactive sympathetic fibers release large amount of catecholamines, which induce paralytic secretion. Moreover, the acinar cells of the salivary glands become hypersensitive to catecholamines after denervation. The paralytic secretion does not occur after the sympathetic nerve fibers to salivary glands are cut.

5. *Augmented Secretion of Saliva*

If the nerves supplying salivary glands are stimulated twice, the amount of saliva secreted by the second stimulus is more than the amount secreted by the first stimulus. It is because, the first stimulus increases excitability of acinar cells, so that when the second stimulus is applied, the salivary secretion is augmented.

6. *Mumps*

Mumps is the acute viral infection affecting the parotid glands. The virus causing this disease is paramyxovirus. It is common in children who are not immunized. It occurs in adults also. Features of mumps are puffiness of cheeks (due to swelling of parotid glands), fever, sore throat and weakness. Mumps affects meninges, gonads and pancreas also.

7. *Sjögren Syndrome*

Sjögren syndrome is an autoimmune disorder in which the immune cells destroy exocrine glands such as lacrimal glands and salivary glands. It is named after Henrik Sjögren who discovered it. Common symptoms of this syndrome are dryness of the mouth due to lack of saliva (xerostomia), persistent cough and dryness of eyes. In some cases, it causes dryness of skin, nose and vagina. In severe conditions, the organs like kidneys, lungs, liver, pancreas, thyroid, blood vessels and brain are affected.

Stomach

Chapter 38

- ■ FUNCTIONAL ANATOMY OF STOMACH
- ■ GLANDS OF STOMACH – GASTRIC GLANDS
- ■ FUNCTIONS OF STOMACH
- ■ PROPERTIES AND COMPOSITION OF GASTRIC JUICE
- ■ FUNCTIONS OF GASTRIC JUICE
- ■ SECRETION OF GASTRIC JUICE
- ■ REGULATION OF GASTRIC SECRETION
- ■ COLLECTION OF GASTRIC JUICE
- ■ GASTRIC ANALYSIS
- ■ APPLIED PHYSIOLOGY

■ FUNCTIONAL ANATOMY OF STOMACH

Stomach is a hollow organ situated just below the diaphragm on the left side in the abdominal cavity. Volume of empty stomach is 50 mL. Under normal conditions, it can expand to accommodate 1 L to 1.5 L of solids and liquids. However, it is capable of expanding still further up to 4 L.

■ PARTS OF STOMACH

In humans, stomach has four parts:
1. Cardiac region
2. Fundus
3. Body or corpus
4. Pyloric region.

1. Cardiac Region

Cardiac region is the upper part of the stomach where esophagus opens. The opening is guarded by a sphincter called **cardiac sphincter,** which opens only towards stomach. This portion is also known as **cardiac end.**

2. Fundus

Fundus is a small dome-shaped structure. It is elevated above the level of esophageal opening.

3. Body or Corpus

Body is the largest part of stomach forming about 75% to 80% of the whole stomach. It extends from just below the fundus up to the pyloric region (Fig. 38.1).

4. Pyloric Region

Pyloric region has two parts, antrum and pyloric canal. The body of stomach ends in **antrum**. Junction between body and antrum is marked by an angular notch called **incisura angularis.** Antrum is continued as the narrow canal, which is called **pyloric canal** or pyloric end. Pyloric canal opens into first part of small intestine called duodenum. The opening of pyloric canal is guarded by a sphincter called pyloric sphincter. It opens towards duodenum.

Stomach has two curvatures. One on the right side is **lesser curvature** and the other on left side is **greater curvature.**

■ STRUCTURE OF STOMACH WALL

Stomach wall is formed by four layers of structures:
1. *Outer serous layer:* Formed by **peritoneum**
2. *Muscular layer:* Made up of three layers of smooth muscle fibers, namely inner oblique, middle circular and outer longitudinal layers

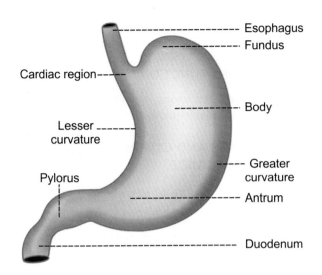

FIGURE 38.1: Parts of stomach

3. *Submucus layer:* Formed by areolar tissue, blood vessels, lymph vessels and **Meissner nerve plexus.**
4. *Inner mucus layer:* Lined by mucus-secreting columnar epithelial cells. The gastric glands are situated in this layer. Under resting conditions, the mucosa of the stomach is thrown into many folds. These folds are called rugae. The rugae disappear when the stomach is distended after meals. Throughout the inner mucus layer, small depressions called **gastric pits** are present. Glands of the stomach open into these pits. Inner surface of mucus layer is covered by 2 mm thick mucus.

■ GLANDS OF STOMACH – GASTRIC GLANDS

Glands of the stomach or gastric glands are tubular structures made up of different types of cells. These glands open into the stomach cavity via gastric pits.

■ CLASSIFICATION OF GLANDS OF THE STOMACH

Gastric glands are classified into three types, on the basis of their location in the stomach:
1. *Fundic glands or main gastric glands or oxyntic glands:* Situated in body and fundus of stomach
2. *Pyloric glands:* Present in the pyloric part of the stomach
3. *Cardiac glands:* Located in the cardiac region of the stomach.

■ STRUCTURE OF GASTRIC GLANDS

1. *Fundic Glands*

Fundic glands are considered as the typical gastric glands (Fig. 38.2). These glands are long and tubular. Each gland has three parts, viz. body, neck and isthmus.

Cells of fundic glands

1. Chief cells or pepsinogen cells
2. Parietal cells or oxyntic cells
3. Mucus neck cells
4. Enterochromaffin (EC) cells or Kulchitsky cells
5. Enterochromaffin-like (ECL) cells.
    Parietal cells are different from other cells of the gland because of the presence of **canaliculi** (singular = canaliculus). Parietal cells empty their secretions into the lumen of the gland through the canaliculi. But, other cells empty their secretions directly into lumen of the gland.

2. *Pyloric Glands*

Pyloric glands are short and tortuous in nature. These glands are formed by G cells, mucus cells, EC cells and ECL cells.

3. *Cardiac Glands*

Cardiac glands are also short and tortuous in structure, with many mucus cells. EC cells, ECL cells and chief cells are also present in the cardiac glands

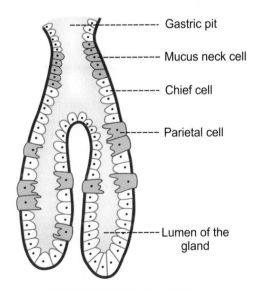

FIGURE 38.2: Gastric glands

Enteroendocrine Cells

Enteroendocrine cells are the hormone-secreting cells present in the glands or mucosa of gastrointestinal tract, particularly stomach and intestine. The enteroendocrine cells present in gastric glands are G cells, EC cells and ECL cells (Table 38.1).

◼ FUNCTIONS OF GASTRIC GLANDS

Function of the gastric gland is to secrete gastric juice. Secretory activities of different cells of gastric glands and enteroendocrine cells are listed in Table 38.1.

◼ FUNCTIONS OF STOMACH

◼ 1. MECHANICAL FUNCTION

i. *Storage Function*

Food is stored in the stomach for a long period, i.e. for 3 to 4 hours and emptied into the intestine slowly. The maximum capacity of stomach is up to 1.5 L. Slow emptying of stomach provides enough time for proper digestion and absorption of food substances in the small intestine.

ii. *Formation of Chyme*

Peristaltic movements of stomach mix the bolus with gastric juice and convert it into the semisolid material known as chyme.

◼ 2. DIGESTIVE FUNCTION

Refer functions of gastric juice.

◼ 3. PROTECTIVE FUNCTION

Refer functions of gastric juice.

TABLE 38.1: Secretory function of cells in gastric glands

Cell	Secretory products
Chief cells	Pepsinogen Rennin Lipase Gelatinase Urase
Parietal cells	Hydrochloric acid Intrinsic factor of Castle
Mucus neck cells	Mucin
G cells	Gastrin
Enterochromaffin (EC) cells	Serotonin
Enterochromaffin-like (ECL) cells	Histamine

◼ 4. HEMOPOIETIC FUNCTION

Refer functions of gastric juice.

◼ 5. EXCRETORY FUNCTION

Many substances like toxins, alkaloids and metals are excreted through gastric juice.

◼ PROPERTIES AND COMPOSITION OF GASTRIC JUICE

Gastric juice is a mixture of secretions from different gastric glands.

◼ PROPERTIES OF GASTRIC JUICE

Volume : 1200 mL/day to 1500 mL/day.
Reaction : Gastric juice is highly acidic with a pH of 0.9 to 1.2. Acidity of gastric juice is due to the presence of hydrochloric acid.
Specific gravity : 1.002 to 1.004

◼ COMPOSITION OF GASTRIC JUICE

Gastric juice contains 99.5% of water and 0.5% solids. Solids are organic and inorganic substances. Refer Fig. 38.3 for composition of gastric juice.

◼ FUNCTIONS OF GASTRIC JUICE

◼ 1. DIGESTIVE FUNCTION

Gastric juice acts mainly on proteins. Proteolytic enzymes of the gastric juice are pepsin and rennin (Table 38.2). Gastric juice also contains some other enzymes like gastric lipase, gelatinase, urase and gastric amylase.

Pepsin

Pepsin is secreted as inactive pepsinogen. Pepsinogen is converted into pepsin by hydrochloric acid. Optimum pH for activation of pepsinogen is below 6.

Action of pepsin

Pepsin converts proteins into proteoses, peptones and polypeptides. Pepsin also causes curdling and digestion of milk (casein).

Gastric Lipase

Gastric lipase is a weak lipolytic enzyme when compared to pancreatic lipase. It is active only when the pH is between 4 and 5 and becomes inactive at a pH below

2.5. Gastric lipase is a tributyrase and it hydrolyzes tributyrin (butter fat) into fatty acids and glycerols.

Actions of Other Enzymes of Gastric Juice

i. Gelatinase: Degrades type I and type V gelatin and type IV and V collagen (which are proteoglycans in meat) into peptides
ii. Urase: Acts on urea and produces ammonia
iii. Gastric amylase: Degrades starch (but its action is insignificant)
iv. Rennin: Curdles milk (present in animals only).

■ 2. HEMOPOIETIC FUNCTION

Intrinsic factor of **Castle,** secreted by parietal cells of gastric glands plays an important role in erythropoiesis. It is necessary for the absorption of vitamin B12 (which is called extrinsic factor) from GI tract into the blood.

Vitamin B12 is an important maturation factor during erythropoiesis. Absence of **intrinsic factor** in gastric juice causes deficiency of vitamin B12, leading to **pernicious anemia** (Chapter 14).

■ PROTECTIVE FUNCTION – FUNCTION OF MUCUS

Mucus is a mucoprotein, secreted by mucus neck cells of the gastric glands and surface mucus cells in fundus, body and other parts of stomach. It protects the gastric wall by the following ways:

Mucus:

i. Protects the stomach wall from irritation or mechanical injury, by virtue of its high viscosity.
ii. Prevents the digestive action of pepsin on the wall of the stomach, particularly gastric mucosa.

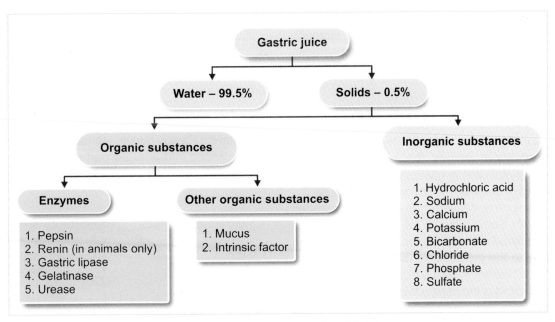

FIGURE 38.3: Composition of gastric juice

TABLE 38.2: Digestive enzymes of gastric juice

Enzyme	Activator	Substrate	End products
Pepsin	Hydrochloric acid	Proteins	Proteoses, peptones and polypeptides
Gastric lipase	Acid medium	Triglycerides of butter	Fatty acids and glycerols
Gastric amylase	Acid medium	Starch	Dextrin and maltose (negligible action)
Gelatinase	Acid medium	Gelatin and collagen of meat	Peptides
Urase	Acid medium	Urea	Ammonia

iii. Protects the gastric mucosa from hydrochloric acid of gastric juice because of its alkaline nature and its acid-combining power.

■ 4. FUNCTIONS OF HYDROCHLORIC ACID

Hydrochloric acid is present in the gastric juice:
  i.   Activates pepsinogen into pepsin
  ii. Kills some of the bacteria entering the stomach along with food substances. This action is called bacteriolytic action
  iii. Provides acid medium, which is necessary for the action of hormones.

■ SECRETION OF GASTRIC JUICE

■ SECRETION OF PEPSINOGEN

Pepsinogen is synthesized from amino acids in the ribosomes attached to **endoplasmic reticulum** in chief cells. Pepsinogen molecules are packed into **zymogen granules** by Golgi apparatus.

When zymogen granule is secreted into stomach from chief cells, the granule is dissolved and pepsinogen is released into gastric juice. Pepsinogen is activated into pepsin by hydrochloric acid.

■ SECRETION OF HYDROCHLORIC ACID

According to **Davenport theory,** hydrochloric acid secretion is an active process that takes place in the canaliculi of parietal cells in gastric glands. The energy for this process is derived from oxidation of glucose.

Carbon dioxide is derived from metabolic activities of parietal cell. Some amount of carbon dioxide is obtained from blood also. It combines with water to form **carbonic acid** in the presence of **carbonic anhydrase.** This enzyme is present in high concentration in parietal cells. Carbonic acid is the most unstable compound and immediately splits into hydrogen ion and bicarbonate ion. The hydrogen ion is actively pumped into the canaliculus of parietal cell.

Simultaneously, the chloride ion is also pumped into canaliculus actively. The chloride is derived from sodium chloride in the blood. Now, the hydrogen ion combines with chloride ion to form hydrochloric acid. To compensate the loss of chloride ion, the bicarbonate ion from parietal cell enters the blood and combines with sodium to form sodium bicarbonate. Thus, the entire process is summarized as (Fig. 38.4):

$$CO_2 + H_2O + NaCl \rightarrow HCl + NaHCO_3$$

Factors Stimulating the Secretion of Hydrochloric Acid

1. Gastrin
2. Histamine
3. Vagal stimulation.

Factors Inhibiting the Secretion of Hydrochloric Acid

1. Secretin
2. Gastric inhibitory polypeptide
3. Peptide YY.

■ REGULATION OF GASTRIC SECRETION

Regulation of gastric secretion and intestinal secretion is studied by some experimental procedures.

■ METHODS OF STUDY

1. Pavlov Pouch

Pavlov pouch is a small part of the stomach that is incompletely separated from the main portion and made into a small bag-like pouch (Fig. 38.5). Pavlov pouch was designed by the Russian scientist Pavlov, in a dog during his studies on conditioned reflexes.

Procedure

To prepare a Pavlov pouch, stomach of an anesthetized dog is divided into a larger part and a smaller part by making an incomplete incision. The mucus membrane

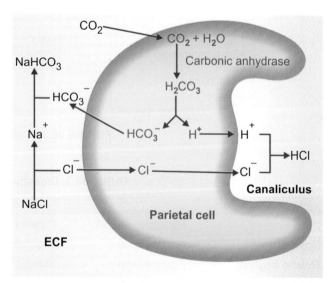

FIGURE 38.4: Secretion of hydrochloric acid in the parietal cell of gastric gland

is completely divided. A small part of muscular coat called **isthmus** is retained. Isthmus connects the two parts.

The cut edges of major portions are stitched. Smaller part is also stitched, leaving a small outlet. This outlet is brought out through the abdominal wall and used to drain the pouch.

Nerve supply of Pavlov pouch

Pavlov pouch receives parasympathetic (vagus) nerve fibers through isthmus and sympathetic fibers through blood vessels.

Use of Pavlov pouch

Pavlov pouch is used to demonstrate the different phases of gastric secretion, particularly the cephalic phase and used to demonstrate the role of vagus in cephalic phase.

2. Heidenhain Pouch

Heidenhain pouch is the modified Pavlov pouch. It is completely separated from main portion of stomach by cutting the isthmus without damaging blood vessels. So, the blood vessels are intact. Thus, Heidenhain pouch does not have parasympathetic supply, but the sympathetic fibers remain intact through the blood vessels.

Uses of Heidenhain pouch

Heidenhain pouch is useful to demonstrate the role of sympathetic nerve and the hormonal regulation of gastric secretion after vagotomy (cutting the vagus nerve).

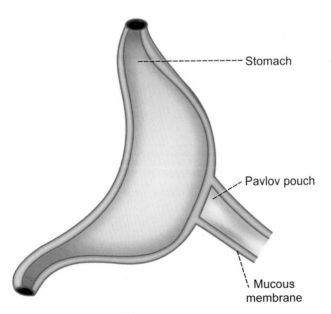

FIGURE 38.5: Pavlov pouch

3. Bickel Pouch

In this, even the sympathetic nerve fibers are cut by removing the blood vessels. So, Bickel pouch is a totally denervated pouch.

Uses of Bickel pouch

Bickel pouch is used to demonstrate the role of hormones in gastric secretion.

4. Farrel and Ivy Pouch

Farrel and Ivy pouch is prepared by completely removing the Bickel pouch from the stomach and transplanting it in the subcutaneous tissue of abdominal wall or thoracic wall in the same animal. New blood vessels develop after some days. It is used for experimental purpose, when the new blood vessels are developed.

Uses of Farrel and Ivy pouch

This pouch is useful to study the role of hormones during gastric and intestinal phases of gastric secretion.

5. Sham Feeding

Sham feeding means the false feeding. It is another experimental procedure devised by Pavlov to demonstrate the regulation of gastric secretion.

Procedure

   i. A hole is made in the neck of an anesthetized dog
  ii. Esophagus is transversely cut and the cut ends are drawn out through the hole in the neck
 iii. When the dog eats food, it comes out through the cut end of the esophagus
  iv. But the dog has the satisfaction of eating the food. Hence it is called sham feeding.

This experimental procedure is supported by the preparation of Pavlov pouch with a **fistula** from the stomach. The fistula opens to exterior and it is used to observe the gastric secretion. The animal is used for experimental purpose after a week, when healing is completed.

Advantage of sham feeding

Sham feeding is useful to demonstrate the secretion of gastric juice during cephalic phase. In the same animal after **vagotomy,** sham feeding does not induce gastric secretion. It proves the role of vagus nerve during cephalic phase.

■ PHASES OF GASTRIC SECRETION

Secretion of gastric juice is a continuous process. But the quantity varies, depending upon time and stimulus.

Accordingly, gastric secretion occurs in three different phases:

    I. Cephalic phase
   II. Gastric phase
  III. Intestinal phase.

In human beings, a fourth phase called **interdigestive phase** exists. Each phase is regulated by neural mechanism or hormonal mechanism or both.

■ CEPHALIC PHASE

Secretion of gastric juice by the stimuli arising from head region (cephalus) is called cephalic phase (Fig. 38.6). This phase of gastric secretion is regulated by nervous mechanism. The gastric juice secreted during this phase is called appetite juice.

During this phase, gastric secretion occurs even without the presence of food in stomach. The quantity of the juice is less but it is rich in enzymes and hydrochloric acid.

Nervous mechanism regulates cephalic phase through reflex action. Two types of reflexes occur:

1. Unconditioned reflex
2. Conditioned reflex.

1. *Unconditioned Reflex*

Unconditioned reflex is the inborn reflex. When food is placed in the mouth, salivary secretion is induced (Chapter 37). Simultaneously, gastric secretion also occurs.

Stages of reflex action:

   i. Presence of food in the mouth stimulates the taste buds and other receptors in the mouth
  ii. Sensory (afferent) impulses from mouth pass via afferent nerve fibers of glossopharyngeal and facial nerves to **amygdala** and **appetite center** present in hypothalamus

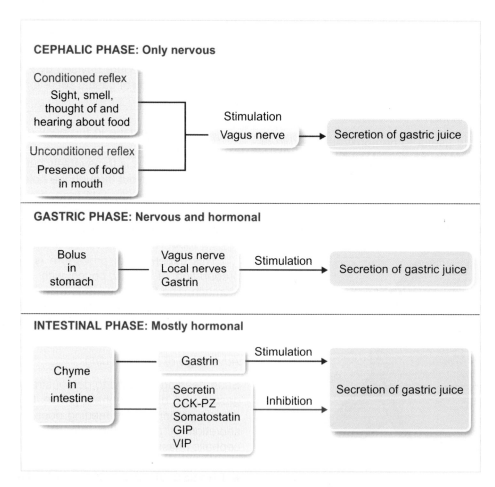

FIGURE 38.6: Schematic diagram showing the regulation of gastric secretion
CCK-PZ = Cholecystokinin-pancreozymin, GIP = Gastric inhibitory peptide, VIP = Vasoactive intestinal peptide.

iii. From here, the efferent impulses pass through dorsal nucleus of vagus and vagal efferent nerve fibers to the wall of the stomach

iv. Vagal efferent nerve endings secrete acetylcholine, which stimulates gastric secretion.

2. Conditioned Reflex

Conditioned reflex is the reflex response acquired by previous experience (Chapter 162). Presence of food in the mouth is not necessary to elicit this reflex. The sight, smell, hearing or thought of food, which induce salivary secretion induce gastric secretion also.

Stages of reflex action:

i. Impulses from the special sensory organs (eye, ear and nose) pass through afferent fibers of neural circuits to the cerebral cortex. Thinking of food stimulates the cerebral cortex directly

ii. From cerebral cortex, the impulses pass through dorsal nucleus of vagus and vagal efferents and reach the stomach wall

iii. Vagal nerve endings secrete acetylcholine, which stimulates the gastric secretion.

Experimental evidences to prove cephalic phase

i. Unconditioned reflex of gastric secretion is proved by sham feeding along with Pavlov pouch (see above). After vagotomy, sham feeding does not cause gastric secretion. It proves the importance of vagus nerve in this phase.

ii. Conditioned reflex of gastric secretion is proved by Pavlov pouch and **belldog experiment** (Chapter 162).

■ GASTRIC PHASE

Secretion of gastric juice when food enters the stomach is called gastric phase. This phase is regulated by both nervous and hormonal control. Gastric juice secreted during this phase is rich in pepsinogen and hydrochloric acid.

Mechanisms involved in gastric phase are:
1. Nervous mechanism through local myenteric reflex and vagovagal reflex
2. Hormonal mechanism through gastrin

Stimuli, which initiate these two mechanisms are:
1. Distention of stomach
2. Mechanical stimulation of gastric mucosa by bulk of food
3. Chemical stimulation of gastric mucosa by the food contents.

1. Nervous Mechanism

Local myenteric reflex

Local myenteric reflex is the reflex elicited by stimulation of myenteric nerve plexus in stomach wall. After entering stomach, the food particles stimulate the local nerve plexus (Chapter 36) present in the wall of the stomach. These nerve fibers release acetylcholine, which stimulates the gastric glands to secrete a large quantity of gastric juice. Simultaneously, acetylcholine stimulates G cells to secrete gastrin (see below).

Vagovagal reflex

Vagovagal reflex is the reflex which involves both afferent and efferent vagal fibers. Entrance of bolus into the stomach stimulates the sensory (afferent) nerve endings of vagus and generates sensory impulses. These sensory impulses are transmitted by sensory fibers of vagus to dorsal nucleus of vagus, located in medulla of brainstem. This nucleus in turn, sends efferent impulses through the motor (efferent) fibers of vagus, back to stomach and cause secretion of gastric juice. Since, both afferent and efferent impulses pass through vagus, this reflex is called vagovagal reflex (Fig. 38.7).

2. Hormonal Mechanism – Gastrin

Gastrin is a gastrointestinal hormone secreted by the G cells which are present in the pyloric glands of stomach. Small amount of gastrin is also secreted in mucosa of upper small intestine. In fetus, it is also secreted by islets of Langerhans in pancreas. Gastrin is a polypeptide containing G14, G17 or G34 amino acids.

Gastrin is released when food enters stomach. Mechanism involved in the release of gastrin may be the local nervous reflex or vagovagal reflex. Nerve endings release the neurotransmitter called gastrin-releasing peptide, which stimulates the G cells to secrete gastrin.

Actions of gastrin on gastric secretion

Gastrin stimulates the secretion of pepsinogen and hydrochloric acid by the gastric glands. Refer Chapter 44 for other actions of gastrin.

Experimental evidences of gastric phase

Nervous mechanism of gastric secretion during gastric phase is proved by Pavlov pouch. Hormonal mechanism of gastric secretion is proved by Heidenhain pouch, Bickel pouch and Farrel and Ivy pouch.

■ INTESTINAL PHASE

Intestinal phase is the secretion of gastric juice when chyme enters the intestine. When chyme enters the

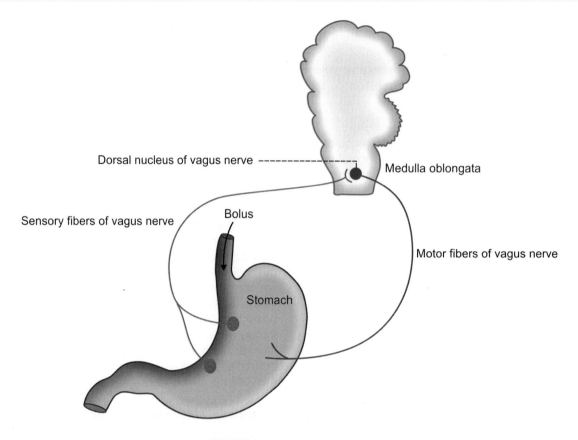

FIGURE 38.7: Vagovagal reflex

intestine, initially, the gastric secretion increases but later it stops. Intestinal phase of gastric secretion is regulated by nervous and hormonal control.

Initial Stage of Intestinal Phase

Chyme that enters the intestine stimulates the duodenal mucosa to release gastrin, which is transported to stomach by blood. There it increases gastric secretion.

Later Stage of Intestinal Phase

After the initial increase, there is a decrease or complete stoppage of gastric secretion. Gastric secretion is inhibited by two factors:
1. Enterogastric reflex
2. Gastrointestinal (GI) hormones.

1. Enterogastric reflex

Enterogastric reflex inhibits the gastric secretion and motility. It is due to the distention of intestinal mucosa by chyme or chemical or osmotic irritation of intestinal mucosa by chemical substances in the chyme. It is mediated by myenteric nerve (Auerbach) plexus and vagus.

2. Gastrointestinal hormones

Presence of chyme in the intestine stimulates the secretion of many GI hormones from intestinal mucosa and other structures. All these hormones inhibit the gastric secretion. Some of these hormones inhibit the gastric motility also.

GI hormones which inhibit gastric secretion:

  i. *Secretin:* Secreted by the presence of acid chyme in the intestine
 ii. *Cholecystokinin:* Secreted by the presence of chyme containing fats and amino acids in intestine
iii. *Gastric inhibitory peptide (GIP):* Secreted by the presence of chyme containing glucose and fats in the intestine
 iv. *Vasoactive intestinal polypeptide (VIP):* Secreted by the presence of acidic chyme in intestine
  v. *Peptide YY:* Secreted by the presence of fatty chyme in intestine.

In addition to these hormones, pancreas also secretes a hormone called **somatostatin** during intestinal phase. It also inhibits gastric secretion. Refer Chapter 44 for details of GI hormones.

Thus, enterogastric reflex and intestinal hormones collectively apply a strong brake on the secretion and motility of stomach during intestinal phase.

Experimental evidences for intestinal phase

Intestinal phase of gastric secretion is demonstrated by Bickel pouch and Farrel and Ivy pouch.

■ INTERDIGESTIVE PHASE

Secretion of small amount of gastric juice in between meals (or during period of fasting) is called interdigestive phase. Gastric secretion during this phase is mainly due to the hormones like gastrin. This phase of gastric secretion is demonstrated by Farrel and Ivy pouch.

■ FACTORS INFLUENCING GASTRIC SECRETION

Gastric secretion is also influenced by some factors which increase the gastric secretion by stimulating gastric mucosa such as:
1. Alcohol
2. Caffeine.

■ COLLECTION OF GASTRIC JUICE

In human beings, the gastric juice is collected by using Ryle tube. The tube is made out of rubber or plastic. It is passed through nostril or mouth and through esophagus into the stomach. A line is marked in the tube. The entrance of the tip of the tube into stomach is indicated when this line comes near the mouth. Then, the contents of stomach are collected by means of aspiration.

■ GASTRIC ANALYSIS

For analysis, the gastric juice is collected from patient only in the morning. Analysis of the gastric juice is done for the diagnosis of ulcer and other disorders of stomach.

Gastric juice is analyzed for the following:
1. Measurement of peptic activity
2. Measurement of gastric acidity: Total acid, free acid (hydrochloric acid) and combined acid.

■ METHODS OF GASTRIC ANALYSIS

1. *Fractional Test Meal (FTM)*

After overnight fasting, the gastric juice is collected. Then, the patient takes a small test meal called fractional test meal (FTM).

Typical test meals are:

i. A piece of bread and a cup of tea
ii. Wheat biscuit and 400 mL of water
iii. 300 mL of oatmeal gruel.

Fractional gastric analysis

After the ingestion of a test meal, gastric juice is collected at every 15th minute for a period of two and a half hours. All these samples are analyzed for peptic activity and acidity.

2. *Nocturnal Gastric Analysis*

Patient is given a clear liquid diet at noon and at 5 pm. At 7.30 pm, the tube is introduced into the patients's stomach. Then from 8 pm to 8 am, hourly samples of gastric juice are collected and analyzed.

3. *Histamine Test*

After overnight fasting, the stomach is emptied in the morning by aspiration. Then histamine is injected subcutaneously (0.01 mg/kg). Histamine stimulates secretion of hydrochloric acid in the stomach. After 30 minutes, 4 samples of gastric juice are collected over a period of 1 hour at 15 minutes interval and analyzed.

■ APPLIED PHYSIOLOGY

Gastric secretion is affected by the following disorders:

■ 1. GASTRITIS

Inflammation of gastric mucosa is called gastritis. It may be acute or chronic. Acute gastritis is characterized by inflammation of superficial layers of mucus membrane and infiltration with leukocytes, mostly neutrophils. Chronic gastritis involves inflammation of even the deeper layers and infiltration with more lymphocytes. It results in the atrophy of the gastric mucosa, with loss of chief cells and parietal cells of glands. Therefore, the secretion of gastric juice decreases.

Causes of Acute Gastritis

i. Infection with bacterium *Helicobacter pylori*
ii. Excess consumption of alcohol
iii. Excess administration of Aspirin and other non-steroidal antiinflammatory drugs (NSAIDs)
iv. Trauma by nasogastric tubes
v. Repeated exposure to radiation (rare).

Causes of Chronic Gastritis

i. Chronic infection with *Helicobacter pylori*

    ii. Long-term intake of excess alcohol
    iii. Long-term use of NSAIDs
    iv. Autoimmune disease.

Features

Features of gastritis are nonspecific. Common feature is abdominal upset or pain felt as a diffused burning sensation. It is often referred to **epigastric pain.** Other features are:

    i. Nausea
    ii. Vomiting
    iii. **Anorexia** (loss of appetite)
    iv. Indigestion
    v. Discomfort or feeling of fullness in the epigastric region
    vi. **Belching** (process to relieve swallowed air that is accumulated in stomach).

■ 2. GASTRIC ATROPHY

Gastric atrophy is the condition in which the muscles of the stomach shrink and become weak. Gastric glands also shrink, resulting in the deficiency of gastric juice.

Cause

Gastric atrophy is caused by chronic gastritis called chronic atrophic gastritis. There is atrophy of gastric mucosa including loss of gastric glands. **Autoimmune atrophic gastritis** also causes gastric atrophy.

Features

Generally, gastric atrophy does not cause any noticeable symptom. However, it may lead to **achlorhydria** (absence of hydrochloric acid in gastric juice) and pernicious anemia. Some patients develop gastric cancer.

■ 3. PEPTIC ULCER

Ulcer means the erosion of the surface of any organ due to shedding or sloughing of inflamed **necrotic tissue** that lines the organ. Peptic ulcer means an ulcer in the wall of stomach or duodenum, caused by digestive action of gastric juice. If peptic ulcer is found in stomach, it is called **gastric ulcer** and if found in duodenum, it is called **duodenal ulcer.**

Causes

    i. Increased peptic activity due to excessive secretion of pepsin in gastric juice
    ii. Hyperacidity of gastric juice
    iii. Reduced alkalinity of duodenal content
    iv. Decreased mucin content in gastric juice or decreased protective activity in stomach or duodenum
    v. Constant physical or emotional stress
    vi. Food with excess spices or smoking (classical causes of ulcers)
    vii. Long-term use of NSAIDs (see above) such as Aspirin, Ibuprofen and Naproxen
    viii. Chronic inflammation due to *Helicobacter pylori.*

Features

Most common feature of peptic ulcer is severe burning pain in epigastric region. In gastric ulcer, pain occurs while eating or drinking. In duodenal ulcer, pain is felt 1 or 2 hours after food intake and during night.

    Other symptoms accompanying pain are:
    i. Nausea
    ii. Vomiting
    iii. **Hematemesis** (vomiting blood)
    iv. **Heartburn** (burning pain in chest due to regurgitation of acid from stomach into esophagus)
    v. Anorexia (loss of appetite)
    vi. Loss of weight.

■ 4. ZOLLINGER-ELLISON SYNDROME

Zollinger-Ellison syndrome is characterized by secretion of excess hydrochloric acid in the stomach.

Cause

This disorder is caused by tumor of pancreas. Pancreatic tumor produces a large quantity of gastrin. Gastrin increases the hydrochloric acid secretion in stomach by stimulating the parietal cells of gastric glands.

Features

    i. Abdominal pain
    ii. Diarrhea (frequent and watery, loose bowel movements)
    iii. Difficulty in eating
    iv. Occasional hematemesis (see above).

Pancreas

Chapter 39

- ■ **FUNCTIONAL ANATOMY AND NERVE SUPPLY OF PANCREAS**
- ■ **PROPERTIES AND COMPOSITION OF PANCREATIC JUICE**
- ■ **FUNCTIONS OF PANCREATIC JUICE**
  - ■ **DIGESTIVE FUNCTIONS**
  - ■ **DIGESTION OF PROTEINS**
  - ■ **DIGESTION OF LIPIDS**
  - ■ **DIGESTION OF CARBOHYDRATES**
  - ■ **NEUTRALIZING ACTION**
- ■ **MECHANISM OF PANCREATIC SECRETION**
  - ■ **SECRETION OF PANCREATIC ENZYMES**
  - ■ **SECRETION OF BICARBONATE IONS**
- ■ **REGULATION OF PANCREATIC SECRETION**
  - ■ **STAGES OF PANCREATIC SECRETION**
  - ■ **CEPHALIC PHASE**
  - ■ **GASTRIC PHASE**
  - ■ **INTESTINAL PHASE**
- ■ **COLLECTION OF PANCREATIC JUICE**
  - ■ **IN ANIMALS**
  - ■ **IN HUMAN**
- ■ **APPLIED PHYSIOLOGY**
  - ■ **PANCREATITIS**
  - ■ **STEATORRHEA**

■ FUNCTIONAL ANATOMY AND NERVE SUPPLY OF PANCREAS

Pancreas is a dual organ having two functions, namely **endocrine function** and **exocrine function**. Endocrine function is concerned with the production of hormones (Chapter 69). The exocrine function is concerned with the secretion of digestive juice called pancreatic juice.

■ FUNCTIONAL ANATOMY OF EXOCRINE PART OF PANCREAS

Exocrine part of pancreas resembles salivary gland in structure. It is made up of **acini** or **alveoli**. Each acinus has a single layer of acinar cells with a lumen in the center. Acinar cells contain zymogen granules, which possess digestive enzymes.

A small duct arises from lumen of each alveolus. Some of these ducts from neighboring alveoli unite to form **intralobular duct.** All the intralobular ducts unite to form the main duct of pancreas called **Wirsung duct.** Wirsung duct joins common bile duct to form **ampulla of Vater,** which opens into duodenum (see Fig. 40.3).

In some persons, an accessory duct called **duct of Santorini** exists. It also opens into duodenum, proximal to the opening of ampulla of Vater.

■ NERVE SUPPLY TO PANCREAS

Pancreas is supplied by both sympathetic and parasympathetic fibers. Sympathetic fibers are supplied through splanchnic nerve and parasympathetic fibers are supplied through vagus nerve.

■ PROPERTIES AND COMPOSITION OF PANCREATIC JUICE

■ PROPERTIES OF PANCREATIC JUICE

Volume   : 500 to 800 mL/day
Reaction   : Highly alkaline with a pH of 8 to 8.3
Specific gravity : 1.010 to 1.018

■ COMPOSITION OF PANCREATIC JUICE

Pancreatic juice contains 99.5% of water and 0.5% of solids. The solids are the organic and inorganic substances. Composition of pancreatic juice is given in Fig. 39.1.

Bicarbonate content is very high in pancreatic juice. It is about 110 to 150 mEq/ L, against the plasma level of 24 mEq/L. High bicarbonate content of pancreatic juice is important because of two reasons:

i. High bicarbonate content makes the pancreatic juice **highly alkaline,** so that it protects the intestinal mucosa from acid chyme by neutralizing it
ii. Bicarbonate ions provide the required pH (7 to 9) for the activation of pancreatic enzymes.

■ FUNCTIONS OF PANCREATIC JUICE

Pancreatic juice has digestive functions and neutralizing action.

■ DIGESTIVE FUNCTIONS OF PANCREATIC JUICE

Pancreatic juice plays an important role in the digestion of proteins and lipids. It also has mild digestive action on carbohydrates.

■ DIGESTION OF PROTEINS

Major proteolytic enzymes of pancreatic juice are trypsin and chymotrypsin. Other proteolytic enzymes are carboxypeptidases, nuclease, elastase and collagenase.

1. *Trypsin*

Trypsin is a single polypeptide with a molecular weight of 25,000. It contains 229 amino acids.

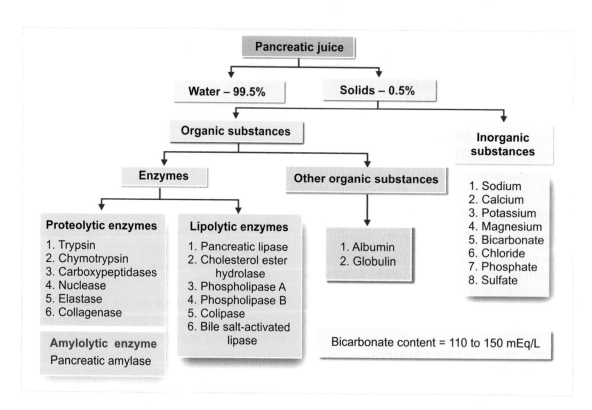

FIGURE 39.1: Composition of pancreatic juice

It is secreted as inactive trypsinogen, which is converted into active trypsin by **enterokinase.** Enterokinase is also called **enteropeptidase** and it is secreted by the brush-bordered cells of duodenal mucus membrane. Once formed, trypsin itself activates trypsinogen by means of **autocatalytic** or **autoactive action.**

Trypsin inhibitor

Trypsinogen is activated only when it reaches the small intestine. If trypsin is activated when it is in pancreas, it may hydrolyze the pancreatic tissue proteins, resulting in pancreatic damage. But its activation in the secretory cells, acini and ducts of pancreas is prevented by an inhibitor protein called trypsin inhibitor. Any abnormality or deficiency of the trypsin inhibitor will result in unopposed trypsin activity, which damages the pancreas.

Actions of trypsin

i. Digestion of proteins: Trypsin is the most powerful proteolytic enzyme. It is an **endopeptidase** and breaks the interior bonds of the protein molecules and converts proteins into proteoses and polypeptides

ii. Curdling of milk: It converts **caseinogen** in the milk into **casein**

iii. Blood clotting: It accelerates blood clotting

iv. It activates the other enzymes of pancreatic juice, viz.

   a. Chymotrypsinogen into chymotrypsin

   b. Procarboxypeptidases into carboxypeptidases

   c. Proelastase into elastase

   d. Procolipase into colipase

v. Trypsin also activates collagenase, phospholipase A and phospholipase B

vi. Autocatalytic action: Once formed, trypsin itself converts trypsinogen into trypsin.

2. Chymotrypsin

Chymotrypsin is a polypeptide with a molecular weight of 25,700 and 246 amino acids. It is secreted as inactive chymotrypsinogen, which is activated into chymotrypsin by trypsin.

Actions of chymotrypsin

i. *Digestion of proteins:* Chymotrypsin is also an endopeptidase and it converts proteins into polypeptides

ii. *Digestion of milk:* Chymotrypsin digests caseinogen faster than trypsin. Combination of both enzymes causes rapid digestion of milk

iii. *On blood clotting:* No action.

3. Carboxypeptidases

Carboxypeptidases are carboxypeptidase A and carboxypeptidase B. Carboxypeptidase A is derived from the precursor procarboxypeptidase A. Carboxypeptidase B is derived from procarboxypeptidase B. Procarboxypeptidases are activated into carboxypeptidases by trypsin.

Actions of carboxypeptidases

Carboxypeptidases are **exopeptidases** and break the terminal bond of protein molecules. Exopeptidases split the polypeptides and other proteins into amino acids.

Carboxypeptidase A splits the proteins into amino acids having aromatic or aliphatic side chains. Carboxypeptidase B converts the proteins into amino acids having basic side chains.

4. Nucleases

Nucleases of pancreatic juice are ribonuclease and deoxyribonuclease, which are responsible for the digestion of nucleic acids. These enzymes convert the ribonucleic acid (RNA) and deoxyribonucleic acid (DNA) into mononucleotides.

5. Elastase

Elastase is secreted as inactive proelastase, which is activated into elastase by trypsin. Elastase digests the elastic fibers.

6. Collagenase

Collagenase is secreted as inactive procollagenase, which is activated into collagenase by trypsin. It digests collagen.

■ DIGESTION OF LIPIDS

Lipolytic enzymes present in pancreatic juice are pancreatic lipase, cholesterol ester hydrolase, phospholipase A, phospholipase B, colipase and bile-salt-activated lipase.

1. Pancreatic lipase

Pancreatic lipase is a powerful lipolytic enzyme. It digests triglycerides into monoglycerides and fatty acids. Activity of pancreatic lipase is accelerated in the presence of bile. Optimum pH required for activity of this enzyme is 7 to 9.

Digestion of fat by pancreatic lipase requires two more factors:

i. Bile salts, which are responsible for the emulsification of fat, prior to their digestion

ii. Colipase, which is a coenzyme necessary for the pancreatic lipase to digest the dietary lipids.

About 80% of the fat is digested by pancreatic lipase. Deficiency or absence of this enzyme leads to excretion of undigested fat in feces (steatorrhea; see below).

2. *Cholesterol ester hydrolase*

Cholesterol ester hydrolase or cholesterol esterase converts cholesterol ester into free cholesterol and fatty acid by hydrolysis.

3. *Phospholipase A*

Phospholipase A is activated by trypsin. Phospholipase A digests phospholipids, namely **lecithin** and **cephalin** and converts them into **lysophospholipids.** It converts lecithin into lysolecithin and **cephalin** into **lysocephalin.**

4. *Phospholipase B*

Phospholipase B is also activated by trypsin. It converts lysophospholipids (lysolecithin and lysocephalin) to **phosphoryl choline** and free fatty acids.

5. *Colipase*

Colipase is a small coenzyme, secreted as inactive procolipase. Procolipase is activated into colipase by trypsin. Colipase facilitates digestive action of pancreatic lipase on fats.

6. *Bile-salt-activated lipase*

Bile-salt-activated lipase is the lipolytic enzyme activated by bile salt. It is also called **carboxyl ester lipase** or **cholesterol esterase.** This enzyme has a weak lipolytic action than pancreatic lipase. But it hydrolyses a variety of lipids such as phospholipids, cholesterol esters and triglycerides. **Human milk** contains an enzyme similar to bile-salt-activated lipase (Table 39.1).

■ DIGESTION OF CARBOHYDRATES

Pancreatic amylase is the amylolytic enzyme present in pancreatic juice. Like salivary amylase, the pancreatic amylase also converts starch into dextrin and maltose.

■ NEUTRALIZING ACTION OF PANCREATIC JUICE

When acid chyme enters intestine from stomach, pancreatic juice with large quantity of bicarbonate is released into intestine. Presence of large quantity of bicarbonate ions makes the pancreatic juice highly alkaline. This alkaline pancreatic juice neutralizes acidity of chyme in the intestine.

Neutralizing action is an important function of pancreatic juice because it protects the intestine from the destructive action of acid in the chyme.

■ MECHANISM OF PANCREATIC SECRETION

■ SECRETION OF PANCREATIC ENZYMES

Pancreatic enzymes are synthesized in ribosomes, which are attached to the endoplasmic reticulum of acinar cells in pancreas. The raw materials for the synthesis of pancreatic enzymes are the amino acids, which are derived from the blood. After synthesis, the enzymes are packed into different zymogen granules by Golgi apparatus and stored in cytoplasm. When stimulated, the acinar cells release zymogen granules into the pancreatic duct. From the granules, the enzymes are liberated into intestine.

■ SECRETION OF BICARBONATE IONS

Bicarbonate ions of pancreatic juice are secreted from the cells of pancreatic ductules and released into the pancreatic duct.

Mechanism of bicarbonate secretion

1. Carbon dioxide derived from blood or metabolic process combines with water inside the cell to form carbonic acid in the presence of carbonic anhydrase
2. Carbonic acid dissociates into hydrogen and bicarbonate ions
3. Bicarbonate ions are actively transported out of the cell into the lumen
4. Hydrogen ion is actively transported into blood in exchange for sodium ion
5. Sodium ion from the cell is transported into the lumen, where it combines with bicarbonate to form sodium bicarbonate
6. Because of the loss of sodium and bicarbonate ions from the blood, there is some disturbance in the **osmotic equilibrium** of the blood. To maintain

TABLE 39.1: Digestive enzymes of pancreatic juice

Enzyme	Activator	Acts on (substrate)	End products
Trypsin	Enterokinase Trypsin	Proteins	Proteoses and polypeptides
Chymotrypsin	Trypsin	Proteins	Polypeptides
Carboxypeptidases	Trypsin	Polypeptides	Amino acids
Nucleases	Trypsin	RNA and DNA	Mononucleotides
Elastase	Trypsin	Elastin	Amino acids
Collagenase	Trypsin	Collagen	Amino acids
Pancreatic lipase	Alkaline medium	Triglycerides	Monoglycerides and fatty acids
Cholesterol ester hydrolase	Alkaline medium	Cholesterol ester	Cholesterol and fatty acids
Phospholipase A	Trypsin	Phospholipids	Lysophospholipids
Phospholipase B	Trypsin	Lysophospholipids	Phosphoryl choline and free fatty acids
Colipase	Trypsin	Facilitates action of pancreatic lipase	–
Bile-salt-activated lipase	Trypsin	Phospholipids	Lysophospholipids
		Cholesterol esters	Cholesterol and fatty acids
		Triglycerides	Monoglycerides and fatty acids
Pancreatic amylase	–	Starch	Dextrin and maltose

the osmotic equilibrium, water leaves the blood and enters the lumen of pancreatic duct by osmosis

7. In the lumen, bicarbonate combines with water forming the solution of bicarbonate.

■ REGULATION OF PANCREATIC SECRETION

Secretion of pancreatic juice is regulated by both nervous and hormonal factors.

■ STAGES OF PANCREATIC SECRETION

Pancreatic juice is secreted in three stages (Fig. 39.2) like the gastric juice:

1. Cephalic phase
2. Gastric phase
3. Intestinal phase.

These three phases of pancreatic secretion correspond with the three phases of gastric secretion.

■ 1. CEPHALIC PHASE

As in case of gastric secretion, cephalic phase is regulated by nervous mechanism through reflex action.

Two types of reflexes occur:

1. Unconditioned reflex
2. Conditioned reflex.

Unconditioned Reflex

Unconditioned reflex is the inborn reflex. When food is placed in the mouth, salivary secretion (Chapter 37) and gastric secretion (Chapter 38) are induced. Simultaneously, pancreatic secretion also occurs.

Stages of reflex action:

i. Presence of food in the mouth stimulates the **taste buds** and other receptors in the mouth
ii. Sensory (afferent) impulses from mouth reach dorsal nucleus of vagus and efferent impulses reach pancreatic acini via vagal efferent nerve fibers
iii. Vagal efferent nerve endings secrete acetylcholine, which stimulates pancreatic secretion.

Conditioned Reflex

Conditioned reflex is the reflex response acquired by previous experience (Chapter 162). Presence of food in the mouth is not necessary to elicit this reflex. The sight, smell, hearing or thought of food, which induce salivary secretion and gastric secretion induce pancreatic secretion also.

Stages of reflex action:

i. Impulses from the special sensory organs (eye, ear and nose) pass through afferent fibers of neural circuits to the cerebral cortex. Thinking of food stimulates the cerebral cortex directly

ii. From cerebral cortex, the impulses pass through dorsal nucleus of vagus and vagal efferents and reach pancreatic acini

iii. Vagal nerve endings secrete acetylcholine, which stimulates pancreatic secretion.

■ 2. GASTRIC PHASE

Secretion of pancreatic juice when food enters the stomach is known as gastric phase. This phase of pancreatic secretion is under hormonal control. The hormone involved is gastrin.

When food enters the stomach, gastrin is secreted from stomach (Chapter 39). When gastrin is transported to pancreas through blood, it stimulates the pancreatic secretion. The pancreatic juice secreted during gastric phase is rich in enzymes.

■ 3. INTESTINAL PHASE

Intestinal phase is the secretion of pancreatic juice when the chyme enters the intestine. This phase is also under hormonal control.

When chyme enters the intestine, many hormones are released. Some hormones stimulate the pancreatic secretion and some hormones inhibit the pancreatic secretion.

Hormones Stimulating Pancreatic Secretion

i. Secretin

ii. Cholecystokinin.

Secretin

Secretin is produced by S cells of mucous membrane in duodenum and jejunum. It is secreted as inactive prosecretin, which is activated into secretin by acid chyme.

The stimulant for the release and activation of prosecretin is the acid chyme entering intestine. Products of protein digestion also stimulate the hormonal secretion.

Action of secretin

Secretin stimulates the secretion of watery juice which is rich in of bicarbonate ion and high in volume. It increases the pancreactic secretion by acting on pancreatic ductules via cyclic AMP (messenger). Other actions of secretin are explained in Chapter 44.

Cholecystokinin

Cholecystokinin (CCK) is also called cholecystokinin-pancreozymin (CCK-PZ). It is secreted by I cells in duodenal and jejunal mucosa. The stimulant for the

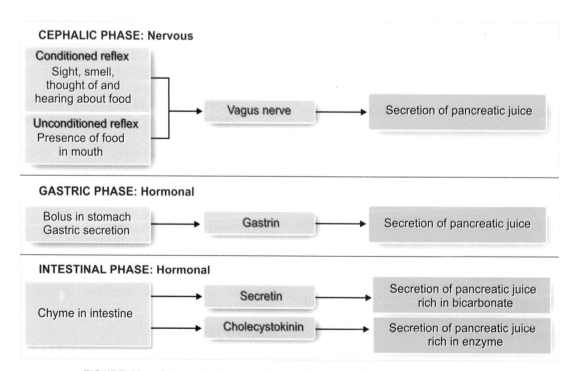

FIGURE 39.2: Schematic diagram showing the regulation of pancreatic secretion

release of this hormone is the chyme containing digestive products such as fatty acids, peptides and amino acids.

Action of cholecystokinin

Cholecystokinin stimulates the secretion of pancreatic juice which is rich in enzyme and low in volume, by acting on pancreatic acinar cells via inosine triphosphate (second messenger). The other actions of cholecystokinin are described in Chapter 44.

Hormones Inhibiting Pancreatic Secretion

    i. Pancreatic polypeptide (PP) secreted by PP cells in islets of Langerhans of pancreas
    ii. Somatostatin secreted by D cells in islets of Langerhans of pancreas
    iii. Peptide YY secreted by intestinal mucosa
    iv. Peptides like ghrelin and leptin
    Refer Chapter 44 for details of these hormones.

■ COLLECTION OF PANCREATIC JUICE

■ IN ANIMALS

In animals, the pancreatic juice is collected by connecting a fistula between the pancreatic duct and the opening in the abdominal wall.

■ IN HUMAN

In human beings, a multilumen tube is inserted through nose or mouth, till the tip of this tube reaches the intestine near the ampulla of Vater. The tube has a marking. The entrance of the tip of the tube into the intestine near the ampulla is indicated when this line comes near the mouth. The tube has three lumens. Small balloons are attached to the two outer lumens. When balloons are inflated by air, the intestine near the ampulla is enlarged. Now, the pancreatic juice is collected through the middle lumen by means of aspiration.

■ APPLIED PHYSIOLOGY

■ PANCREATITIS

Pancreatitis is the inflammation of pancreatic acini. It is a rare but dangerous disease.
    Pancreatitis is of two types:
1. Acute pancreatitis
2. Chronic pancreatitis.

1. *Acute Pancreatitis*

Acute pancreatitis is more severe and it occurs because of heavy alcohol intake or gallstones.

Features of acute pancreatitis:

    i. Severe upper abdominal pain
    ii. Nausea and vomiting
    iii. Loss of appetite and weight
    iv. Fever
    v. Shock.

2. *Chronic Pancreatitis*

Chronic pancreatitis develops due to repeated acute inflammation or chronic damage to pancreas.

Causes of chronic pancreatitis

    i. Long-time consumption of alcohol
    ii. Chronic obstruction of ampulla of Vater by gallstone
    iii. Hereditary cause (passed on genetically from one generation to another)
    iv. Congenital abnormalities of pancreatic duct
    v. **Cystic fibrosis,** a generalized disorder affecting the functions of many organs such as lungs (due to excessive mucus), exocrine glands like pancreas, biliary system and immune system
    vi. Malnutrition (poor nutrition; mal = bad)
    vii. Idiopathic pancreatitis (due to unknown cause).

Features of chronic pancreatitis

    i. *Complete destruction of pancreas:* During the obstruction of biliary ducts, more amount of trypsinogen and other enzymes are accumulated. In spite of the presence of trypsin inhibitor in acini, some trypsinogen is activated. Trypsin in turn activates other proteolytic enzymes. All these enzymes destroy the pancreatic tissues completely
    ii. *Absence of pancreatic enzymes:* Pancreatitis is more dangerous because the destruction of acinar cells in pancreas leads to deficiency or total absence of pancreatic enzymes. So the digestive processes are affected; worst affected

is fat digestion that results in steatorrhea (see below)

iii. Severe pain in upper abdominal region, which radiates to the back

iv. Fever, nausea and vomiting

v. Tender and swollen abdomen

vi. Weight loss.

■ STEATORRHEA

Steatorrhea is the formation of bulky, foul-smelling, frothy and clay-colored stools with large quantity of undigested fat because of impaired digestion and absorption of fat.

Causes of Steatorrhea

Any condition that causes indigestion or malabsorption of fat leads to steatorrhea. Various causes of steatorrhea are:

1. *Lack of pancreatic lipase:* Since most of the fat is digested only by pancreatic lipase, its deficiency leads to steatorrhea

2. *Liver disease affecting secretion of bile:* Bile salts are essential for the digestion of fat by lipase and absorption of fat from intestine. Absence of bile salts results in excretion of fatty stool

3. *Celiac disease:* Atrophy of intestinal villi leads to malabsorption, resulting in steatorrhea

4. Cystic fibrosis (see above).

- ■ FUNCTIONAL ANATOMY OF LIVER AND BILIARY SYSTEM
- ■ BLOOD SUPPLY TO LIVER
- ■ PROPERTIES AND COMPOSITION OF BILE
- ■ SECRETION OF BILE
- ■ STORAGE OF BILE
- ■ BILE SALTS
- ■ BILE PIGMENTS
- ■ FUNCTIONS OF BILE
- ■ FUNCTIONS OF LIVER
- ■ GALLBLADDER
- ■ REGULATION OF BILE SECRETION
- ■ APPLIED PHYSIOLOGY

■ FUNCTIONAL ANATOMY OF LIVER AND BILIARY SYSTEM

Liver is a dual organ having both secretory and excretory functions. It is the largest gland in the body, weighing about 1.5 kg in man. It is located in the upper and right side of the abdominal cavity, immediately beneath diaphragm.

■ LIVER

Hepatic Lobes

Liver is made up of many lobes called hepatic lobes (Fig. 40.1). Each lobe consists of many lobules called hepatic lobules.

Hepatic Lobules

Hepatic lobule is the structural and functional unit of liver. There are about 50,000 to 100,000 lobules in the liver. The lobule is a **honeycomb-like structure** and it is made up of liver cells called hepatocytes.

Hepatocytes and Hepatic Plates

Hepatocytes are arranged in columns, which form the hepatic plates. Each plate is made up of two columns of cells. In between the two columns of each plate lies a bile canaliculus (Fig. 40.2).

In between the neighboring plates, a blood space called **sinusoid** is present. Sinusoid is lined by the endothelial cells. In between the endothelial cells some special macrophages called **Kupffer cells** are present.

Portal Triads

Each lobule is surrounded by many portal triads. Each portal triad consists of three vessels:
1. A branch of hepatic artery
2. A branch of portal vein
3. A tributary of bile duct.

Branches of hepatic artery and portal vein open into the sinusoid. Sinusoid opens into the central vein. Central vein empties into hepatic vein.

Bile is secreted by hepatic cells and emptied into **bile canaliculus.** From canaliculus, the bile enters the

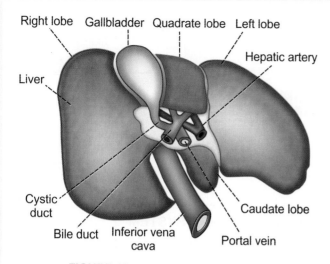

FIGURE 40.1: Posterior surface of liver

Right lobe · Gallbladder · Quadrate lobe · Left lobe · Hepatic artery · Liver · Cystic duct · Bile duct · Inferior vena cava · Portal vein · Caudate lobe

tributary of bile duct. Tributaries of bile duct from canaliculi of neighboring lobules unite to form small bile ducts. These small bile ducts join together and finally form left and right hepatic ducts, which emerge out of liver.

■ BILIARY SYSTEM

Biliary system or **extrahepatic biliary apparatus** is formed by gallbladder and **extrahepatic bile ducts** (bile ducts outside the liver). Right and left **hepatic bile ducts** which come out of liver join to form **common hepatic duct.** It unites with the **cystic duct** from gallbladder to form **common bile duct** (Fig. 40.3). All these ducts have similar structures.

Common bile duct unites with pancreatic duct to form the **common hepatopancreatic duct** or **ampulla of Vater,** which opens into the duodenum.

There is a sphincter called **sphincter of Oddi** at the lower part of common bile duct, before it joins the pancreatic duct. It is formed by smooth muscle fibers of common bile duct. It is normally kept closed; so the bile secreted from liver enters gallbladder where it is stored. Upon appropriate stimulation, the sphincter opens and allows flow of bile from gallbladder into the intestine.

■ BLOOD SUPPLY TO LIVER

Liver receives maximum blood supply of about 1,500 mL/minute. It receives blood from two sources, namely the hepatic artery and portal vein (Fig. 40.4).

■ HEPATIC ARTERY

Hepatic artery arises directly from aorta and supplies **oxygenated blood** to liver. After entering the liver, the

hepatic artery divides into many branches. Each branch enters a portal triad.

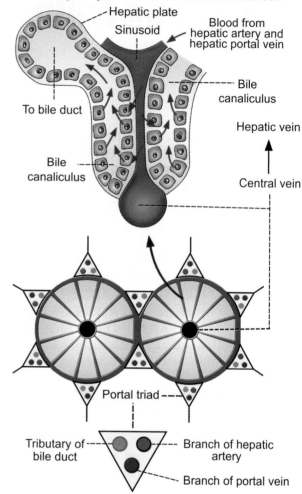

Two hepatic plates with a sinusoid in between

Hepatic plate · Sinusoid · Blood from hepatic artery and hepatic portal vein · Bile canaliculus · Hepatic vein · To bile duct · Bile canaliculus · Central vein

Portal triad · Tributary of bile duct · Branch of hepatic artery · Branch of portal vein

FIGURE 40.2: Hepatic lobule

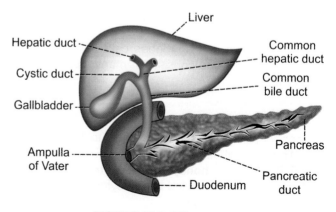

Liver · Hepatic duct · Cystic duct · Gallbladder · Ampulla of Vater · Common hepatic duct · Common bile duct · Pancreas · Duodenum · Pancreatic duct

FIGURE 40.3: Biliary system

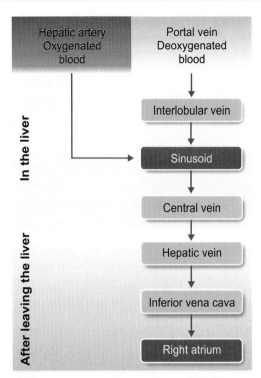

FIGURE 40.4: Schematic diagram of blood flow through liver

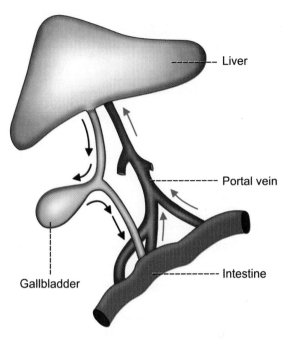

FIGURE 40.5: Enterohepatic circulation

■ PORTAL VEIN

Portal vein is formed by superior mesenteric vein and splenic vein. It brings **deoxygenated blood** from stomach, intestine, spleen and pancreas. Portal blood is rich in monosaccharides and amino acids. It also contains bile salts, bilirubin, urobilinogen and GI hormones. However, the oxygen content is less in portal blood.

Flow of blood from intestine to liver through portal vein is known as **enterohepatic circulation** (Fig. 40.5).

The blood from hepatic artery mixes with blood from portal vein in **hepatic sinusoids.** Hepatic cells obtain oxygen and nutrients from the sinusoid.

■ HEPATIC VEIN

Substances synthesized by hepatic cells, waste products and carbon dioxide are discharged into **sinusoids.** Sinusoids drain them into **central vein** of the lobule. Central veins from many lobules unite to form bigger veins, which ultimately form hepatic veins (right and left) which open into **inferior vena cava.**

■ PROPERTIES AND COMPOSITION OF BILE

■ PROPERTIES OF BILE

Volume   : 800 to 1,200 mL/day
Reaction   : Alkaline
pH   : 8 to 8.6
Specific gravity : 1.010 to 1.011
Color   : Golden yellow or green.

■ COMPOSITION OF BILE

Bile contains 97.6% of water and 2.4% of solids. Solids include organic and inorganic substances. Refer Fig. 40.6 for details.

■ SECRETION OF BILE

Bile is secreted by hepatocytes. The initial bile secreted by hepatocytes contains large quantity of bile acids, bile pigments, cholesterol, lecithin and fatty acids. From hepatocytes, bile is released into canaliculi. From here, it passes through small ducts and hepatic ducts and reaches the common hepatic duct. From common hepatic duct, bile is diverted either directly into the intestine or into the gallbladder.

Sodium, bicarbonate and water are added to bile when it passes through the ducts. These substances are secreted by the epithelial cells of the ducts. Addition of sodium, bicarbonate and water increases the total quantity of bile.

■ STORAGE OF BILE

Most of the bile from liver enters the gallbladder, where it is stored. It is released from gallbladder into the intestine whenever it is required. When bile is stored in gallbladder,

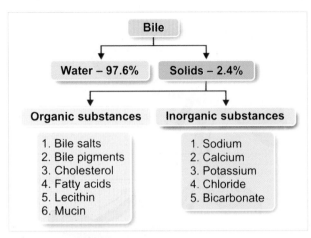

FIGURE 40.6: Composition of bile

TABLE 40.1: Differences between liver bile and gallbladder bile

Types of entities	Liver bile	Gallbladder bile
pH	8 to 8.6	7 to 7.6
Specific gravity	1010 to 1011	1026 to 1032
Water content	97.6%	89%
Solids	2.4%	11%
Organic substances		
Bile Salts	0.5 g/dL	6.0 g/dL
Bile Pigments	0.05 g/dL	0.3 g/dL
Cholesterol	0.1 g/dL	0.5 g/dL
Fatty Acids	0.2 g/dL	1.2 g/dL
Lecithin	0.05 g/dL	0.4 g/dL
Mucin	Absent	Present
Inorganic substances		
Sodium	150 mEq/L	135 mEq/L
Calcium	4 mEq/L	22 mEq/L
Potassium	5 mEq/L	12 mEq/L
Chloride	100 mEq/L	10 mEq/L
Bicarbonate	30 mEq/L	10 mEq/L

it undergoes many changes both in quality and quantity such as:
1. Volume is decreased because of absorption of a large amount of water and electrolytes (except calcium and potassium)
2. Concentration of bile salts, bile pigments, cholesterol, fatty acids and lecithin is increased because of absorption of water and electrolytes
3. The pH is decreased slightly
4. Specific gravity is increased
5. Mucin is added to bile (Table 40.1).

■ BILE SALTS

Bile salts are the sodium and potassium salts of bile acids, which are conjugated with glycine or taurine.

■ FORMATION OF BILE SALTS

Bile salts are formed from bile acids. There are two **primary bile** acids in human, namely **cholic acid** and **chenodeoxycholic acid,** which are formed in liver and enter the intestine through bile. Due to the bacterial action in the intestine, the primary bile acids are converted into **secondary bile acids:**

Cholic acid → deoxycholic acid
Chenodeoxycholic acid → lithocholic acid

Secondary bile acids from intestine are transported back to liver through enterohepatic circulation. In liver, the secondary bile acids are conjugated with **glycine** (amino acid) or **taurin** (derivative of an amino acid) and form conjugated bile acids, namely **glycocholic acid** and **taurocholic acids.** These bile acids combine with sodium or potassium ions to form the salts, sodium or potassium **glycocholate** and sodium or potassium **taurocholate** (Fig. 40.7).

■ ENTEROHEPATIC CIRCULATION OF BILE SALTS

Enterohepatic circulation is the transport of substances from small intestine to liver through portal vein. About 90% to 95% of bile salts from intestine are transported to liver through enterohepatic circulation. Remaining 5% to 10% of the bile salts enter large intestine. Here, the bile salts are converted into deoxycholate and lithocholate, which are excreted in feces.

■ FUNCTIONS OF BILE SALTS

Bile salts are required for digestion and absorption of fats in the intestine. The functions of bile salts are:

1. *Emulsification of Fats*

Emulsification is the process by which the fat globules are broken down into minute droplets and made in the form of a milky fluid called **emulsion** in small intestine, by the action of bile salts.

Lipolytic enzymes of GI tract cannot digest the fats directly because the fats are insoluble in water due to the surface tension. Bile salts emulsify the fats by reducing the surface tension due to their **detergent action.** Now the fats can be easily digested by lipolytic enzymes.

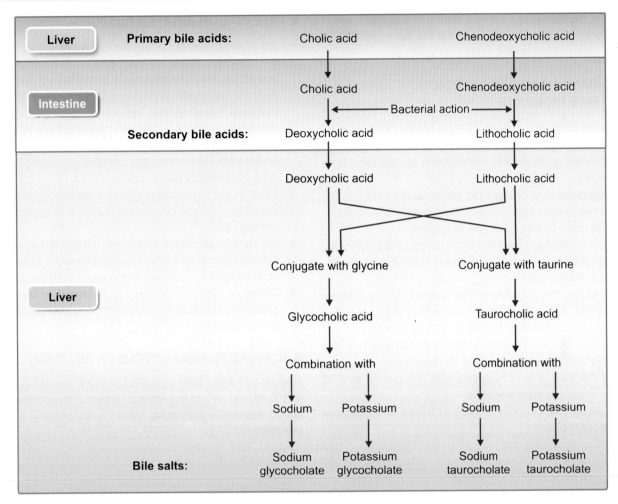

FIGURE 40.7: Formation of bile salts

Unemulsified fat usually passes through the intestine and then it is eliminated in feces.

Emulsification of fats by bile salts needs the presence of lecithin from bile.

2. *Absorption of Fats*

Bile salts help in the absorption of digested fats from intestine into blood. Bile salts combine with fats and make complexes of fats called **micelles**. The fats in the form of micelles can be absorbed easily.

3. *Choleretic Action*

Bile salts stimulate the secretion of bile from liver. This action is called choleretic action.

4. *Cholagogue Action*

Cholagogue is an agent which causes contraction of gallbladder and release of bile into the intestine. Bile salts act as cholagogues indirectly by stimulating the secretion of hormone cholecystokinin. This hormone causes contraction of gallbladder, resulting in release of bile.

5. *Laxative Action*

Laxative is an agent which induces defecation. Bile salts act as laxatives by stimulating peristaltic movements of the intestine.

6. *Prevention of Gallstone Formation*

Bile salts prevent the formation of gallstone by keeping the cholesterol and lecithin in solution. In the absence of bile salts, cholesterol precipitates along with lecithin and forms gallstone.

■ BILE PIGMENTS

Bile pigments are the excretory products in bile. **Bilirubin** and **biliverdin** are the two bile pigments and bilirubin is the major bile pigment in human beings.

Bile pigments are formed during the breakdown of hemoglobin, which is released from the destroyed RBCs in the reticuloendothelial system (Fig. 40.8).

■ FORMATION AND EXCRETION OF BILE PIGMENTS

Stages of formation and circulation of bile pigments:
1. Senile erythrocytes are destroyed in reticuloendothelial system and hemoglobin is released from them
2. Hemoglobin is broken into globin and heme
3. Heme is split into iron and the pigment biliverdin
4. Iron goes to iron pool and is reused
5. First formed pigment biliverdin is reduced to bilirubin.
6. Bilirubin is released into blood from the reticuloendothelial cells
7. In blood, the bilirubin is transported by the plasma protein, albumin. Bilirubin circulating in the blood is called free bilirubin or unconjugated bilirubin
8. Within few hours after entering the circulation, the free bilirubin is taken up by the liver cells
9. In the liver, it is conjugated with glucuronic acid to form **conjugated bilirubin**
10. Conjugated bilirubin is then excreted into intestine through bile.

■ FATE OF CONJUGATED BILIRUBIN

Stages of excretion of conjugated bilirubin:
1. In intestine, 50% of the conjugated bilirubin is converted into **urobilinogen** by intestinal bacteria. First the conjugated bilirubin is deconjugated into **free bilirubin**, which is later reduced into urobilinogen.
2. Remaining 50% of conjugated bilirubin from intestine is absorbed into blood and enters the liver through portal vein (enterohepatic circulation). From liver, it is re-excreted in bile
3. Most of the urobilinogen from intestine enters liver via enterohepatic circulation. Later, it is re-excreted through bile
4. About 5% of urobilinogen is excreted by kidney through urine. In urine, due to exposure to air, the urobilinogen is converted into urobilin by oxidation
5. Some of the urobilinogen is excreted in feces as stercobilinogen. In feces, stercobilinogen is oxidized to stercobilin.

■ NORMAL PLASMA LEVELS OF BILIRUBIN

Normal bilirubin (Total bilirubin) content in plasma is 0.5 to 1.5 mg/dL. When it exceeds 1mg/dL, the condition is called **hyperbilirubinemia.** When it exceeds 2 mg/dL, **jaundice** occurs.

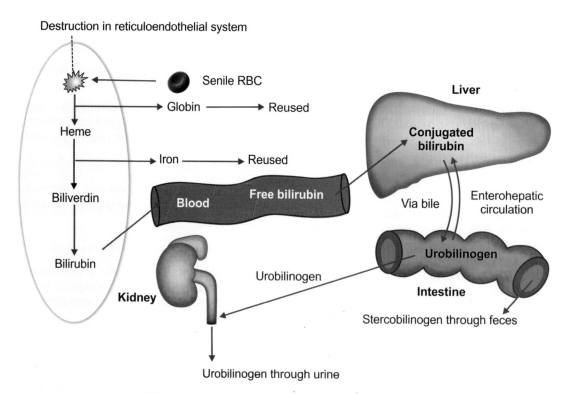

FIGURE 40.8: Formation and circulation of bile pigments

■ FUNCTIONS OF BILE

Most of the functions of bile are due to the bile salts.

■ 1. DIGESTIVE FUNCTION

Refer functions of bile salts.

■ 2. ABSORPTIVE FUNCTIONS

Refer functions of bile salts.

■ 3. EXCRETORY FUNCTIONS

Bile pigments are the major excretory products of the bile. Other substances excreted in bile are:

   i. Heavy metals like copper and iron
   ii. Some bacteria like typhoid bacteria
   iii. Some toxins
   iv. Cholesterol
   v. Lecithin
   vi. Alkaline phosphatase.

■ 4. LAXATIVE ACTION

Bile salts act as laxatives (see above).

■ 5. ANTISEPTIC ACTION

Bile inhibits the growth of certain bacteria in the lumen of intestine by its **natural detergent action.**

■ 6. CHOLERETIC ACTION

Bile salts have the choleretic action (see above).

■ 7. MAINTENANCE OF pH IN GASTROINTESTINAL TRACT

As bile is highly alkaline, it neutralizes the acid chyme which enters the intestine from stomach. Thus, an optimum pH is maintained for the action of digestive enzymes.

■ 8. PREVENTION OF GALLSTONE FORMATION

Refer function of bile salts.

■ 9. LUBRICATION FUNCTION

The mucin in bile acts as a lubricant for the chyme in intestine.

■ 10. CHOLAGOGUE ACTION

Bile salts act as cholagogues (see above).

■ FUNCTIONS OF LIVER

Liver is the largest gland and one of the vital organs of the body. It performs many vital metabolic and homeostatic functions, which are summarized below.

■ 1. METABOLIC FUNCTION

Liver is the organ where maximum metabolic reactions such as metabolism of carbohydrates, proteins, fats, vitamins and many hormones are carried out.

■ 2. STORAGE FUNCTION

Many substances like glycogen, amino acids, iron, folic acid and vitamins A, B12 and D are stored in liver.

■ 3. SYNTHETIC FUNCTION

Liver produces glucose by gluconeogenesis. It synthesizes all the plasma proteins and other proteins (except immunoglobulins) such as clotting factors, complement factors and hormone-binding proteins. It also synthesizes steroids, somatomedin and heparin.

■ 4. SECRETION OF BILE

Liver secretes bile which contains bile salts, bile pigments, cholesterol, fatty acids and lecithin.

    The functions of bile are mainly due to bile salts. Bile salts are required for digestion and absorption of fats in the intestine. Bile helps to carry away waste products and breakdown fats, which are excreted through feces or urine.

■ 5. EXCRETORY FUNCTION

Liver excretes cholesterol, bile pigments, heavy metals (like lead, arsenic and bismuth), toxins, bacteria and virus (like that of yellow fever) through bile.

■ 6. HEAT PRODUCTION

Enormous amount of heat is produced in the liver because of metabolic reactions. Liver is the organ where maximum heat is produced.

■ 7. HEMOPOIETIC FUNCTION

In fetus (hepatic stage), liver produces the blood cells (Chapter 10). It stores vitamin B12 necessary for erythropoiesis and iron necessary for synthesis of hemoglobin. Liver produces thrombopoietin that promotes production of thrombocytes.

■ 8. HEMOLYTIC FUNCTION

The senile RBCs after a lifespan of 120 days are destroyed by reticuloendothelial cells (Kupffer cells) of liver.

■ 9. INACTIVATION OF HORMONES AND DRUGS

Liver catabolizes the hormones such as growth hormone, parathormone, cortisol, insulin, glucagon and estrogen. It also inactivates the drugs, particularly the fat-soluble drugs. The fat-soluble drugs are converted into water-soluble substances, which are excreted through bile or urine.

■ 10. DEFENSIVE AND DETOXIFICATION FUNCTIONS

Reticuloendothelial cells (Kupffer cells) of the liver play an important role in the defense of the body. Liver is also involved in the detoxification of the foreign bodies.

  i. Foreign bodies such as bacteria or antigens are swallowed and digested by reticuloendothelial cells of liver by means of **phagocytosis.**
  ii. Reticuloendothelial cells of liver also produce substances like interleukins and tumor necrosis factors, which activate the immune system of the body (Chapter 17).
  iii. Liver cells are involved in the removal of toxic property of various harmful substances. Removal of toxic property of the harmful agent is known as detoxification.

Detoxification in liver occurs in two ways:

  a. Total destruction of the substances by means of metabolic degradation.
  b. Conversion of toxic substances into non-toxic materials by means of conjugation with glucuronic acid or sulfates.

■ GALLBLADDER

Bile secreted from liver is stored in gallbladder. The capacity of gallbladder is approximately 50 mL. Gallbladder is not essential for life and it is removed **(cholecystectomy)** in patients suffering from gallbladder dysfunction. After cholecystectomy, patients do not suffer from any major disadvantage. In some species, gallbladder is absent.

■ FUNCTIONS OF GALLBLADDER

Major functions of gallbladder are the storage and concentration of bile.

1. *Storage of Bile*

Bile is continuously secreted from liver. But it is released into intestine only intermittently and most of the bile is stored in gallbladder till it is required.

2. *Concentration of Bile*

Bile is concentrated while it is stored in gallbladder. The mucosa of gallbladder rapidly reabsorbs water and electrolytes, except calcium and potassium. But the bile salts, bile pigments, cholesterol and lecithin are not reabsorbed. So, the concentration of these substances in bile increases 5 to 10 times (Fig. 40.9).

3. *Alteration of pH of Bile*

The pH of bile decreases from 8 – 8.6 to 7 – 7.6 and it becomes less alkaline when it is stored in gallbladder.

4. *Secretion of Mucin*

Gallbladder secretes mucin and adds it to bile. When bile is released into the intestine, mucin acts as a lubricant for movement of chyme in the intestine.

5. *Maintenance of Pressure in Biliary System*

Due to the concentrating capacity, gallbladder maintains a pressure of about 7 cm H_2O in biliary system. This pressure in the biliary system is essential for the release of bile into the intestine.

■ FILLING AND EMPTYING OF GALLBLADDER

Usually, the sphincter of Oddi is closed during fasting and the pressure in the biliary system is only 7 cm H_2O. Because of this pressure, the bile from liver enters the gallbladder.

While taking food or when chyme enters the intestine, gallbladder contracts along with relaxation of sphincter of Oddi. Now, the pressure increases to about 20 cm H_2O. Because of the increase in pressure, the bile from gallbladder enters the intestine. Contraction of gallbladder is influenced by neural and hormonal factors.

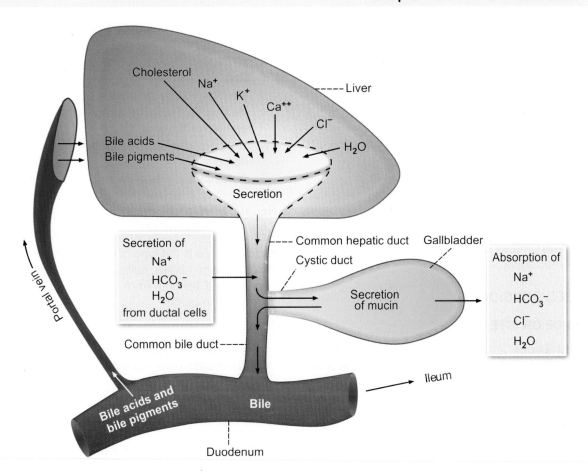

FIGURE 40.9: Diagram showing the formation of bile from liver and changes taking place in the composition of gallbladder bile

1. Neural Factor

Stimulation of parasympathetic nerve (vagus) causes contraction of gallbladder by releasing acetylcholine. The vagal stimulation occurs during the cephalic phase and gastric phase of gastric secretion.

2. Hormonal Factor

When a fatty chyme enters the intestine from stomach, the intestine secretes the cholecystokinin, which causes contraction of the gallbladder.

■ REGULATION OF BILE SECRETION

Bile secretion is a continuous process though the amount is less during fasting. It starts increasing after meals and continues for three hours. Secretion of bile from liver and release of bile from the gallbladder are influenced by some chemical factors, which are categorized into three groups:

1. Choleretics
2. Cholagogue
3. Hydrocholeretic agents.

1. Choleretics

Substances which increase the secretion of bile from liver are known as choleretics.
   Effective choleretic agents are:
   i. Acetylcholine
   ii. Secretin
   iii. Cholecystokinin
   iv. Acid chyme in intestine
   v. Bile salts.

2. Cholagogues

Cholagogue is an agent which increases the release of bile into the intestine by contracting gallbladder.

Common cholagogues are:
  i. Bile salts
  ii. Calcium
  iii. Fatty acids
  iv. Amino acids
  v. Inorganic acids

All these substances stimulate the secretion of cholecystokinin, which in turn causes contraction of gallbladder and flow of bile into intestine.

3. Hydrocholeretic Agents

Hydrocholeretic agent is a substance which causes the secretion of bile from liver, with large amount of water and less amount of solids. Hydrochloric acid is a hydrocholeretic agent.

■ APPLIED PHYSIOLOGY

■ JAUNDICE OR ICTERUS

Jaundice or icterus is the condition characterized by yellow coloration of the skin, mucous membrane and deeper tissues due to increased bilirubin level in blood. The word jaundice is derived from the French word **'jaune'** meaning yellow.

The normal serum bilirubin level is 0.5 to 1.5 mg/dL. Jaundice occurs when bilirubin level exceeds 2 mg/dL.

Types of Jaundice

Jaundice is classified into three types:
  1. Prehepatic or hemolytic jaundice
  2. Hepatic or hepatocellular jaundice
  3. Posthepatic or obstructive jaundice.

1. Prehepatic or Hemolytic Jaundice

Hemolytic jaundice is the type of jaundice that occurs because of excessive destruction of RBCs resulting in increased blood level of free (unconjugated) bilirubin. In this condition, the excretory function of liver is normal. But the quantity of bilirubin increases enormously. The liver cells cannot excrete that much excess bilirubin rapidly. Unconjugated bilirubin is insoluble in water and is not excreted in urine. So, it accumulates in the blood resulting in jaundice.

Formation of urobilinogen also increases resulting in the excretion of more amount of urobilinogen in urine.

Causes

Any condition that causes hemolytic anemia can lead to hemolytic jaundice.

Common causes of hemolytic jaundice are:
  i. Renal disorder
  ii. Hypersplenism
  iii. Burns
  iv. Infections such as malaria
  v. Hemoglobin abnormalities such as sickle cell anemia or thalassemia
  vi. Drugs or chemical substances causing red cell damage
  vii. Autoimmune diseases.

2. Hepatic or Hepatocellular or Cholestatic Jaundice

Hepatic jaundice is the type of jaundice that occurs due to the damage of hepatic cells. Because of the damage, the conjugated bilirubin from liver cannot be excreted and it returns to blood.

Causes

  i. Infection (infective jaundice) by virus, resulting in hepatitis (viral hepatitis)
  ii. Alcoholic hepatitis
  iii. Cirrhosis of liver
  iv. Exposure to toxic materials.

3. Posthepatic or Obstructive or Extrahepatic Jaundice

Posthepatic type of jaundice occurs because of the obstruction of bile flow at any level of the biliary system. The bile cannot be excreted into small intestine. So, bile salts and bile pigments enter the circulation. The blood contains more amount of conjugated bilirubin (Table 40.2).

Causes

  i. Gallstones
  ii. Cancer of biliary system or pancreas.

■ HEPATITIS

Hepatitis is the liver damage caused by many agents. It is characterized by swelling and inadequate functioning of liver. Hepatitis may be acute or chronic. In severe conditions, it may lead to liver failure and death.

Causes and Types

  1. Viral infection (viral hepatitis: see below)
  2. Bacterial infection like leptospirosis and Q fever
  3. Excess consumption of alcohol

TABLE 40.2: Features of different types of jaundice

Features	Prehepatic jaundice (Hemolytic)	Hepatic jaundice (hepatocellular)	Posthepatic jaundice (Obstructive)
Cause	Excess breakdown of RBCs	Liver damage	Obstruction of bile ducts
Type of bilirubin in blood	Unconjucated	Conjugated and unconjugated	Conjugated
Urinary excretion of urobilinogen	Increases	Decreases	Decreases Absent in severe obstruction
Fecal excretion of stercobilinogen	Increases	Decreases (pale feces)	Absent (clay-colored feces)
van den Bergh reaction	Indirect – positive	Biphasic	Direct – positive
Liver functions	Normal	Abnormal	Exaggerated
Blood picture	Anemia Reticulocytosis Abnormal RBC	Normal	Normal
Plasma albumin and globulin	Normal	Albumin – increases Globulin – increases A : G ratio – decreases	Normal
Hemorrhagic tendency	Absent	Present due to lack of vitamin K	Present due to lack of vitamin K

4. Excess administration of drugs like paracetamol
5. Poisons like carbon tetrachloride and aflatoxin
6. Wilson disease (Chapter 151)
7. Circulatory insufficiency
8. Inheritance from mother during parturition.

Viral Hepatitis

Viral hepatitis is the type of hepatitis caused by viruses. It is caused by two types of viruses, hepatitis A and hepatitis B.

Causes of viral hepatitis

i. Mainly by intake of water and food contaminated with hepatitis virus
ii. Sharing needles with infected persons
iii. Accidental prick by infected needle
iv. Having unprotected sex with infected persons
v. Inheritance from mother during parturition
vi. Blood transfusion from infected donors.

Hepatitis caused by hepatitis B virus is more common and considered more serious because it may lead to cirrhosis and cancer of liver.

Features of Hepatitis

1. Fever
2. Nausea
3. Vomiting, diarrhea and loss of appetite
4. Headache and weakness
5. In addition, chronic hepatitis is characterized by

i. Stomach pain
ii. Paleness of skin
iii. Dark-colored urine and pale stool
iv. Jaundice
v. Personality changes.

■ **CIRRHOSIS OF LIVER**

Cirrhosis of liver refers to inflammation and damage of parenchyma of liver. It results in degeneration of hepatic cells and dysfunction of liver.

Causes

1. Infection
2. Retention of bile in liver due to obstruction of ducts of biliary system
3. Enlargement of liver due to intoxication
4. Inflammation around liver (perihepatitis)
5. Infiltration of fat in hepatic cells.

Features

1. Fever, nausea and vomiting
2. Jaundice
3. Increased heart rate and cardiac output
4. Portal hypertension
5. Muscular weakness and wasting of muscles
6. Drowsiness
7. Lack of concentration and confused state of mind
8. Coma in advanced stages.

■ GALLSTONES

Definitions

Gallstone is a solid crystal deposit that is formed by cholesterol, calcium ions and bile pigments in the gallbladder or bile duct. **Cholelithiasis** is the presence of gallstones in gallbladder. **Choledocholithiasis** is the presence of gallstones in the bile ducts.

Formation of Gallstones

Normally, cholesterol present in the bile combines with bile salts and lecithin, which make the cholesterol soluble in water. Under some abnormal conditions, this water-soluble cholesterol precipitates resulting in the formation of gallstone.

Initially, small quantity of cholesterol begins to precipitate forming many small crystals of cholesterol in the mucosa of gallbladder. This stimulates further formation of crystals and the crystals grow larger and larger. Later, bile pigments and calcium are attached to these crystals, resulting in formation of gallstones.

Causes for Gallstone Formation

1. Reduction in bile salts and/or lecithin
2. Excess of cholesterol
3. Disturbed cholesterol metabolism
4. Excess of calcium ions due to increased concentration of bile
5. Damage or infection of gallbladder epithelium. It alters the absorptive function of the mucous membrane of the gallbladder. Sometimes, there is excessive absorption of water or even bile salts, leading to increased concentration of cholesterol, bile pigments and calcium ions
6. Obstruction of bile flow from the gallbladder.

Diagnosis of Gallstone

Presence of gallstone is diagnosed by ultrasound scanning and **cholangiography.** Cholangiography is the radiological study of biliary ducts after the administration of a contrast medium.

Features

Common feature of gallstone is the pain in stomach area or in upper right part of the belly under the ribs. Other features include nausea, vomiting, abdominal bloating and indigestion.

Treatment for Gallstone

Simple cholesterol gallstones can be dissolved over a period of one or two years by giving 1 to 1.5 gm of chemodeoxycholic acid daily. This increases the concentration of bile acids. So, excessive concentration of bile does not occur.

In severe conditions, the gallbladder has to be removed **(cholecystectomy).** Laparoscopic surgery is the common method.

Small Intestine

Chapter 41

- ■ FUNCTIONAL ANATOMY
- ■ INTESTINAL VILLI AND GLANDS
- ■ PROPERTIES AND COMPOSITION OF SUCCUS ENTERICUS
- ■ FUNCTIONS OF SUCCUS ENTERICUS
- ■ FUNCTIONS OF SMALL INTESTINE
- ■ REGULATION OF SECRETION OF SUCCUS ENTERICUS
- ■ METHODS OF COLLECTION OF SUCCUS ENTERICUS
- ■ APPLIED PHYSIOLOGY

■ FUNCTIONAL ANATOMY

Small intestine is the part of gastrointestinal (GI) tract, extending between the **pyloric sphincter** of stomach and **ileocecal valve,** which opens into large intestine. It is called small intestine because of its small diameter, compared to that of the large intestine. But it is longer than large intestine. Its length is about 6 meter.

Important function of small intestine is absorption. Maximum absorption of digested food products takes place in small intestine.

Small intestine consists of three portions:
1. Proximal part known as duodenum
2. Middle part known as jejunum
3. Distal part known as ileum.

Wall of the small intestine has all the four layers as in stomach (Chapter 36).

■ INTESTINAL VILLI AND GLANDS OF SMALL INTESTINE

■ INTESTINAL VILLI

Mucous membrane of small intestine is covered by minute projections called villi. The height of villi is about 1 mm and the diameter is less than 1 mm.

Villi are lined by columnar cells, which are called **enterocytes.** Each enterocyte gives rise to hair-like projections called **microvilli.** Villi and microvilli increase the surface area of mucous membrane by many folds. Within each villus, there is a central channel called lacteal, which opens into lymphatic vessels. It contains blood vessels also.

■ CRYPTS OF LIEBERKÜHN OR INTESTINAL GLANDS

Crypts of Lieberkühn or intestinal glands are simple tubular glands of intestine. Intestinal glands do not penetrate the muscularis mucosa of the intestinal wall, but open into the lumen of intestine between the villi. Intestinal glands are lined by columnar cells. Lining of each gland is continuous with epithelial lining of the villi (Fig. 41.1).

Epithelial cells lining the intestinal glands undergo division by mitosis at a faster rate. Newly formed cells push the older cells upward over the lining of villi. These cells which move to villi are called enterocytes. Enterocytes secrete the enzymes. Old enterocytes are continuously shed into lumen along with enzymes.

Types of cells interposed between columnar cells of intestinal glands:
1. **Argentaffin cells** or **enterochromaffin cells,** which secrete **intrinsic factor of Castle**
2. **Goblet cells,** which secrete mucus
3. **Paneth cells,** which secrete the cytokines called **defensins.**

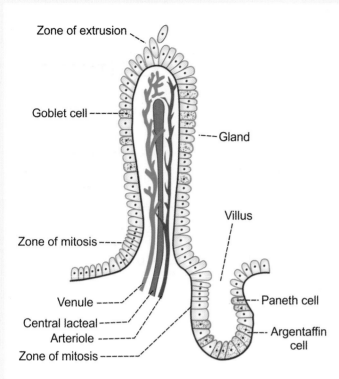

FIGURE 41.1: Intestinal gland and villus

■ BRUNNER GLANDS

In addition to intestinal glands, the first part of duodenum contains some mucus glands, which are called Brunner glands. These glands penetrate muscularis mucosa and extend up to the submucus coat of the intestinal wall. Brunner glands open into the lumen of intestine directly. Brunner gland secretes mucus and traces of enzymes.

■ PROPERTIES AND COMPOSITION OF SUCCUS ENTERICUS

Secretion from small intestine is called succus entericus.

■ PROPERTIES OF SUCCUS ENTERICUS

Volume   : 1800 mL/day
Reaction : Alkaline
pH   : 8.3

■ COMPOSITION OF SUCCUS ENTERICUS

Succus entericus contains water (99.5%) and solids (0.5%). Solids include organic and inorganic substances (Fig. 41.2). Bicarbonate concentration is slightly high in succus entericus.

■ FUNCTIONS OF SUCCUS ENTERICUS

■ 1. DIGESTIVE FUNCTION

Enzymes of succus entericus act on the partially digested food and convert them into final digestive products. Enzymes are produced and released into succus entericus by enterocytes of the villi.

Proteolytic Enzymes

Proteolytic enzymes present in succus entericus are the peptidases, which are given in Fig. 41.2. These peptidases convert peptides into amino acids.

Amylolytic Enzymes

Amylolytic enzymes of succus entericus are listed in Fig. 41.2.

Lactase, sucrase and maltase convert the disaccharides (lactose, sucrose and maltose) into two molecules of monosaccharides (Table 41.1).

Dextrinase converts dextrin, maltose and maltriose into glucose. Trehalase or trehalose glucohydrolase causes hydrolysis of trehalose (carbohydrate present in mushrooms and yeast) and converts it into glucose.

Lipolytic Enzyme

Intestinal lipase acts on triglycerides and converts them into fatty acids.

■ 2. PROTECTIVE FUNCTION

i. Mucus present in the succus entericus protects the intestinal wall from the acid chyme, which enters the intestine from stomach; thereby it prevents the **intestinal ulcer.**
ii. **Defensins** secreted by paneth cells of intestinal glands are the **antimicrobial peptides.**

These peptides are called natural peptide antibiotics because of their role in killing the phagocytosed bacteria.

■ 3. ACTIVATOR FUNCTION

Enterokinase present in intestinal juice activates trypsinogen into trypsin. Trypsin, in turn activates other enzymes (Chapter 39).

■ 4. HEMOPOIETIC FUNCTION

Intrinsic factor of Castle present in the intestine plays an important role in erythropoiesis (Chapter 10). It is necessary for the absorption of vitamin B12.

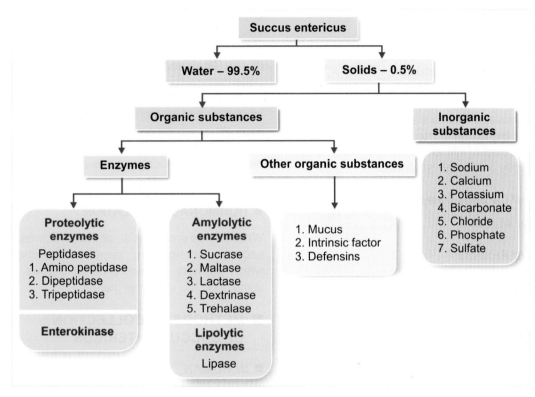

FIGURE 41.2: Composition of succus entericus

■ 5. HYDROLYTIC PROCESS

Intestinal juice helps in all the enzymatic reactions of digestion.

■ FUNCTIONS OF SMALL INTESTINE

■ 1. MECHANICAL FUNCTION

Mixing movements of small intestine help in the thorough mixing of chyme with the digestive juices like succus entericus, pancreatic juice and bile.

■ 2. SECRETORY FUNCTION

Small intestine secretes succus entericus, enterokinase and the GI hormones.

■ 3. HORMONAL FUNCTION

Small intestine secretes many GI hormones such as secretin, cholecystokinin, etc. These hormones regulate the movement of GI tract and secretory activities of small intestine and pancreas (Chapter 44).

■ 4. DIGESTIVE FUNCTION

Refer functions of succus entericus.

■ 5. ACTIVATOR FUNCTION

Refer functions of succus entericus.

■ 6. HEMOPOIETIC FUNCTION

Refer functions of succus entericus.

■ 7. HYDROLYTIC FUNCTION

Refer functions of succus entericus.

TABLE 41.1: Digestive enzymes of succus entericus

Enzyme	Substrate	End products
Peptidases	Peptides	Amino acids
Sucrase	Sucrose	Fructose and glucose
Maltase	Maltose and maltriose	Glucose
Lactase	Lactose	Galactose and glucose
Dextrinase	Dextrin, maltose and maltriose	Glucose
Trehalase	Trehalose	Glucose
Intestinal lipase	Triglycerides	Fatty acids

■ 8. ABSORPTIVE FUNCTIONS

Presence of villi and microvilli in small intestinal mucosa increases the surface area of mucosa. This facilitates the absorptive function of intestine.

Digested products of foodstuffs, proteins, carbohydrates, fats and other nutritive substances such as vitamins, minerals and water are absorbed mostly in small intestine. From the lumen of intestine, these substances pass through lacteal of villi, cross the mucosa and enter the blood directly or through lymphatics.

Absorption of Carbohydrates

Refer Chapter 45.

Absorption of Proteins

Refer Chapter 46.

Absorption of Fats

Refer Chapter 47.

Absorption of Water and Minerals

i. In small intestine, sodium is absorbed actively. It is responsible for absorption of glucose, amino acids and other substances by means of sodium cotransport.
ii. Water moves in or out of the intestinal lumen until the osmotic pressure of intestinal contents becomes equal to that of plasma.
iii. In ileum, chloride ion is actively absorbed in exchange for bicarbonate. The significance of this exchange is not known.
iv. Calcium is actively absorbed mostly in upper part of small intestine.

Absorption of Vitamins

Most of the vitamins are absorbed in upper part of small intestine and vitamin B_{12} is absorbed in ileum. Absorption of water-soluble vitamins is faster than fat-soluble vitamins.

■ REGULATION OF SECRETION OF SUCCUS ENTERICUS

Secretion of succus entericus is regulated by both nervous and hormonal mechanisms.

■ NERVOUS REGULATION

Stimulation of parasympathetic nerves causes vasodilatation and increases the secretion of succus entericus. Stimulation of sympathetic nerves causes vasoconstriction and decreases the secretion of succus entericus. But, the role of these nerves in the regulation of intestinal secretion in physiological conditions is uncertain.

However, the local nervous reflexes play an important role in increasing the secretion of intestinal juice. When chyme enters the small intestine, the mucosa is stimulated by tactile stimuli or irritation. It causes the development of local nervous reflexes, which stimulate the glands of intestine.

■ HORMONAL REGULATION

When chyme enters the small intestine, intestinal mucosa secretes enterocrinin, secretin and cholecystokinin, which promote the secretion of succus entericus by stimulating the intestinal glands.

■ METHODS OF COLLECTION OF SUCCUS ENTERICUS

■ IN HUMAN

In human beings, the intestinal juice is collected by using multilumen tube. The multilumen tube is inserted through nose or mouth, until the tip of this tube reaches the intestine. A line is marked on the tube. Entrance of tip of the tube into small intestine is indicated when this line comes near the mouth. This tube has three lumens. To the outer two lumens, small balloons are attached. When these balloons are inflated, the intestine is enlarged. Now, the intestinal juice is collected through the middle lumen, by means of aspiration.

■ IN ANIMALS

Thiry Loop

A portion of intestine is separated from the gut by incising at both ends. The cut ends of the main gut are connected and the continuity is re-established. One end of isolated segment is closed and the other end is brought out through abdominal wall. It is called Thiry loop or **Thiry fistula.**

Thiry-Vella Loop

Thiry-Vella loop is the modified Thiry loop. In this, a long segment of intestine is cut and separated from the main gut. Both the ends of this segment are brought out through the abdominal wall. The cut ends of the main gut are joined.

■ APPLIED PHYSIOLOGY

■ 1. MALABSORPTION

Malabsorption is the failure to absorb nutrients such as proteins, carbohydrates, fats and vitamins.

Malabsorption affects growth and development of the body. It also causes specific diseases (see below).

■ 2. MALABSORPTION SYNDROME

Malabsorption syndrome is the condition characterized by the failure of digestion and absorption in small intestine. Malabsorption syndrome is generally caused by **Crohn's disease, tropical sprue, steatorrhea** and **celiac disease.**

■ 3. CROHN'S DISEASE OR ENTERITIS

Enteritis is an inflammatory bowel disease (IBD), characterized by inflammation of small intestine. Usually, it affects the lower part of small intestine, the ileum. The inflammation causes malabsorption and diarrhea.

Causes

Crohn's disease develops because of abnormalities of the immune system. The immune system reacts to a virus or a bacterium, resulting in inflammation of the intestine.

Features

   i. Malabsorption of vitamin
   ii. Weight loss
  iii. Abdominal pain
  iv. Diarrhea
   v. Rectal bleeding, anemia and fever
  vi. Delayed or stunted growth in children.

■ 4. TROPICAL SPRUE

Tropical sprue is a malabsorption syndrome, affecting the residents of or the visitors to tropical areas where the disease is epidemic.

Cause

The cause of this disease is not known and it may be related to infectious organisms.

Features

   i. Indigestion
   ii. Diarrhea
  iii. Anorexia and weight loss
  iv. Abdominal and muscle cramps.

■ 5. STEATORRHEA

Steatorrhea is the condition caused by deficiency of pancreatic lipase, resulting in malabsorption of fat. Refer Chapter 39 for details.

■ 6. CELIAC DISEASE

Celiac disease is an autoimmune disorder characterized by the damage of mucosa and atrophy of villi in small intestine, resulting in impaired digestion and absorption. It is also known as **gluten-sensitive enteropathy,** celiac sprue and non-tropical sprue.

Cause

Celiac disease is caused by gluten. It is a protein present in wheat, oats, rye, barley and other grains. **Gluten** is like a poison to individuals with celiac disease, because it damages the intestine severely.

Features

   i. Diarrhea
   ii. Steatorrhea
  iii. Abdominal pain
  iv. Weight loss
   v. Irritability
  vi. Depression.

Large Intestine

Chapter

42

- ■ **FUNCTIONAL ANATOMY**
  - ■ PARTS OF LARGE INTESTINE
  - ■ STRUCTURE OF WALL OF LARGE INTESTINE
- ■ **SECRETIONS OF LARGE INTESTINE**
  - ■ COMPOSITION OF LARGE INTESTINAL JUICE
  - ■ FUNCTIONS OF LARGE INTESTINAL JUICE
- ■ **FUNCTIONS OF LARGE INTESTINE**
  - ■ ABSORPTIVE FUNCTION
  - ■ FORMATION OF FECES
  - ■ EXCRETORY FUNCTION
  - ■ SECRETORY FUNCTION
  - ■ SYNTHETIC FUNCTION
- ■ **DIETARY FIBER**
- ■ **APPLIED PHYSIOLOGY**
  - ■ DIARRHEA
  - ■ CONSTIPATION
  - ■ APPENDICITIS
  - ■ ULCERATIVE COLITIS

■ FUNCTIONAL ANATOMY OF LARGE INTESTINE

Large intestine or colon extends from ileocecal valve up to anus (Fig. 36.1).

■ PARTS OF LARGE INTESTINE

Large intestine is made up of the following parts:
1. Cecum with appendix
2. Ascending colon
3. Transverse colon
4. Descending colon
5. Sigmoid colon or pelvic colon
6. Rectum
7. Anal canal.

■ STRUCTURE OF WALL OF LARGE INTESTINE

Wall of large intestine is formed by four layers of structures like any other part of the gut.
1. *Serous layer:* It is formed by peritoneum
2. *Muscular layer:* Smooth muscles of large intestine are distributed in two layers, namely the outer longitudinal layer and inner circular layer. The longitudinal muscle fibers of large intestine are arranged in the form of three long bands called **tenia coli.** The length of the tenia coli is less when compared to the length of large intestine. Because of this, the large intestine is made into series of pouches called **haustra**

3. *Submucus layer:* It is not well developed in large intestine

4. *Mucus layer:* The crypts of Leiberkühn are present in mucosa of large intestine. But the villi, which are present in mucus membrane of small intestine, are absent in the large intestine. Only mucus-secreting glands are present in the mucosa of large intestine.

■ SECRETIONS OF LARGE INTESTINE

Large intestinal juice is a watery fluid with pH of 8.0.

■ COMPOSITION OF LARGE INTESTINAL JUICE

Large intestinal juice contains 99.5% of water and 0.5% of solids (Fig. 42.1). Digestive enzymes are absent and concentration of bicarbonate is high in large intestinal juice.

■ FUNCTIONS OF LARGE INTESTINAL JUICE

Neutralization of Acids

Strong acids formed by bacterial action in large intestine are neutralized by the alkaline nature of large intestinal juice. The alkalinity of this juice is mainly due to the presence of large quantity of bicarbonate.

Lubrication Activity

Mucin present in the secretion of large intestine lubricates the mucosa of large intestine and the bowel contents, so that, the movement of bowel is facilitated.

Mucin also protects the mucus membrane of large intestine by preventing the damage caused by mechanical injury or chemical substances.

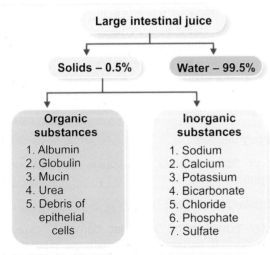

FIGURE 42.1: Composition of large intestinal juice

■ FUNCTIONS OF LARGE INTESTINE

■ 1. ABSORPTIVE FUNCTION

Large intestine plays an important role in the absorption of various substances such as:

i. Water
ii. Electrolytes
iii. Organic substances like glucose
iv. Alcohol
v. Drugs like anesthetic agents, sedatives and steroids.

■ 2. FORMATION OF FECES

After the absorption of nutrients, water and other substances, the unwanted substances in the large intestine form feces. This is excreted out.

■ 3. EXCRETORY FUNCTION

Large intestine excretes heavy metals like mercury, lead, bismuth and arsenic through feces.

■ 4. SECRETORY FUNCTION

Large intestine secretes mucin and inorganic substances like chlorides and bicarbonates.

■ 5. SYNTHETIC FUNCTION

Bacterial flora of large intestine synthesizes folic acid, vitamin B12 and vitamin K. By this function, large intestine contributes in **erythropoietic activity** and blood clotting mechanism.

■ DIETARY FIBER

Dietary fiber or roughage is a group of food particles which pass through stomach and small intestine without being digested and reach the large intestine unchanged. Other nutritive substances of food are digested and absorbed before reaching large intestine.

Characteristic feature of dietary fiber is that it is not hydrolyzed by digestive enzymes. So, it escapes digestion in small intestine and passes to large intestine. It provides substrate for **microflora** of large intestine and increases the bacterial mass. The anaerobic bacteria, in turn, degrade the **fermentable components** of the fiber. Thus, in large intestine, some of the components of fiber are broken down and absorbed and remaining components are excreted through feces.

Components of Dietary Fiber

Major components of dietary fiber are cellulose, hemicelluloses, D-glucans, pectin, lignin and gums. Cellulose, hemicelluloses and pectin are partially degradable, while other components are indigestible. Dietary fiber also contains minerals, antioxidants and other chemicals that are useful for health.

Sources of Dietary Fiber

Sources of dietary fiber are fruits, vegetables, cereals, bread and wheat grain (particularly its outer layer).

Significance of Dietary Fiber

Diet with high dietary fiber has health benefits since dietary fiber:
1. Delays emptying of stomach
2. Increases formation of bulk and soft feces and eases defecation
3. Contains substances such as antioxidants and other useful substances.

When high dietary fiber food is taken, other foods, which may cause some diseases may be decreased in quantity or completely excluded from diet. Diet with high fiber content tends to be low in energy and it may be useful in reducing the body weight. Some components of dietary fiber also reduce blood cholesterol level and thereby decrease the risk for **coronary heart disease** and **gallstones.**

Dietary fiber is suggested for treating or to prevent **constipation** and **bowel syndrome.** It is also useful in treatment of some disorders such as diabetics, cancer, ulcer, etc.

■ APPLIED PHYSIOLOGY

■ DIARRHEA

Diarrhea is the frequent and profuse discharge of intestinal contents in loose and fluid form. It occurs due to the increased movement of intestine. It may be acute or chronic.

Causes

Normally, when digested food passes through colon, large portion of fluid is absorbed and only a semisolid stool remains. In diarrhea, the fluid is not absorbed sufficiently, resulting in watery bowel discharge. Acute diarrhea may be caused by temporary problems like infection and chronic diarrhea may be due to disorders of intestinal mucosa. Thus, the general causes of diarrhea are:

1. *Dietary abuse:* Diarrhea is caused by intake of contaminated water or food, artificial sweeteners found in food, spicy food, etc.
2. *Food intolerance:* Acute diarrhea is caused mainly by indigestion of food substances, particularly lactose, a sugar present in milk and milk products may not be digested easily
3. *Infections by:*
   i. Bacteria such as *Escherichia coli, Salmonella, Shigella,* etc.
   ii. Viruses like rotavirus, hepatitis virus, etc.
   iii. Parasites like *Entamoeba histolytica, Giardia lamblia,* etc.
4. *Reaction to medicines such as:*
   i. Antibiotics
   ii. Antihypertensive drugs
   iii. Antacids containing magnesium
   iv. Laxatives
5. *Intestinal diseases:* Chronic diarrhea occurs during inflammation of intestine, irritable bowel syndrome and abnormal motility of the intestine.

Features

Severe diarrhea results in loss of excess water and electrolytes. This leads to **dehydration** and electrolyte imbalance. Chronic diarrhea results in **hypokalemia** and **metabolic acidosis.** Other features of diarrhea are abdominal pain, nausea and **bloating** (a condition in which the subject feels the abdomen full and tight due to excess intestinal gas).

■ CONSTIPATION

Failure of voiding of feces, which produces discomfort is known as constipation. It is due to the lack of movements necessary for defecation (Chapter 43). Due to the absence of mass movement in colon, feces remain in the large intestine for a long time, resulting in absorption of fluid. So the feces become hard and dry.

Causes

1. *Dietary causes*

Lack of fiber or lack of liquids in diet causes constipation.

2. *Irregular bowel habit*

Irregular bowel habit is most common cause for constipation. It causes constipation by inhibiting the normal defecation reflexes.

3. *Spasm of sigmoid colon*

Spasm in the sigmoid colon **(spastic colon)** prevents its motility, resulting in constipation.

4. *Diseases*

Constipation is common in many types of diseases.

5. *Dysfunction of myenteric plexus in large intestine – megacolon*

Megacolon is the condition characterized by distension and hypertrophy of colon, associated with constipation. It is caused by the absence or damage of ganglionic cells in myenteric plexus, which causes dysfunction of myenteric plexus. It leads to accumulation of large quantity of feces in colon. The colon is distended to a diameter of 4 to 5 inch. It also results in hypertrophy of colon. Congenital development of megacolon is called **Hirschsprung disease.**

6. *Drugs*

The drugs like diuretics, pain relievers (narcotics), antihypertensive drugs (calcium channel blockers), antiparkinson drugs, antidepressants and the anticonvulsants cause constipation.

■ APPENDICITIS

Inflammation of appendix is known as appendicitis. Appendix is a small, worm-like appendage, projecting from cecum of ascending colon. It is situated on the lower right side of the abdomen.

Appendix does not have any function in human beings. But, it can create major problems when diseased. Appendicitis can develop at any age. However, it is very common between 10 and 30 years of age.

Causes

The cause for appendicitis is not known. It may occur by bacterial or viral infection. It also occurs during blockage of connection between appendix and large intestine by feces, foreign body or tumor.

Features

1. Main symptom of appendicitis is the pain, which starts around the umbilicus and then spreads to the lower right side of the abdomen. It becomes severe within 6 to 12 hours
2. Nausea
3. Vomiting
4. Constipation or diarrhea
5. Difficulty in passing gas
6. Low fever
7. Abdominal swelling
8. Loss of appetite.

If not treated immediately, the appendix may rupture and the inflammation will spread to the whole body, leading to severe complications, sometimes even death. Therefore, the treatment of appendicitis is considered as an emergency.

Usual standard treatment for appendicitis is **appendectomy** (surgical removal of appendix).

■ ULCERATIVE COLITIS

Ulcerative colitis is an inflammatory bowel disease (IBD), characterized by the inflammation and ulcerative aberrations in the wall of the large intestine. It is also known as **colitis** or **proctitis.** Rectum and lower part of the colon are commonly affected. Sometimes, the entire colon is affected.

Ulcerative colitis can occur at any age. More commonly, it affects people in the age group of 15 to 30 years. Rarely it affects 50 to 70 years old people.

Cause

Exact cause for ulcerative colitis is not known. However, it is believed that the interaction between the immune system and viral or bacterial infection causes this disease.

Features

1. Abdominal pain
2. Diarrhea with blood in the stools
3. Early fatigue
4. Loss of appetite and weight
5. Arthritis and osteoporosis
6. Eye inflammation
7. Liver diseases like hepatitis, cirrhosis, etc.
8. Skin rashes
9. Anemia.

Movements of Gastrointestinal Tract

Chapter

43

- ■ MASTICATION
- ■ DEGLUTITION
- ■ MOVEMENTS OF STOMACH
- ■ FILLING AND EMPTYING OF STOMACH
- ■ VOMITING
- ■ MOVEMENTS OF SMALL INTESTINE
- ■ MOVEMENTS OF LARGE INTESTINE
- ■ DEFECATION
- ■ EVACUATION OF GASES FROM GASTROINTESTINAL TRACT

■ MASTICATION

Mastication or **chewing** is the first mechanical process in the gastrointestinal (GI) tract, by which the food substances are torn or cut into small particles and crushed or ground into a soft **bolus.**

Significances of mastication

1. Breakdown of foodstuffs into smaller particles
2. Mixing of saliva with food substances thoroughly
3. Lubrication and moistening of dry food by saliva, so that the bolus can be easily swallowed
4. Appreciation of taste of the food.

■ MUSCLES AND THE MOVEMENTS OF MASTICATION

Muscles of Mastication

1. Masseter muscle
2. Temporal muscle
3. Pterygoid muscles
4. Buccinator muscle.

Movements of Mastication

1. Opening and closure of mouth
2. Rotational movements of jaw
3. Protraction and retraction of jaw.

■ CONTROL OF MASTICATION

Action of mastication is mostly a reflex process. It is carried out voluntarily also. The center for mastication is situated in medulla and cerebral cortex. Muscles of mastication are supplied by mandibular division of 5th cranial (trigeminal) nerve.

■ DEGLUTITION

Definition

Deglutition or swallowing is the process by which food moves from mouth into stomach.

Stages of Deglutition

Deglutition occurs in three stages:
- I. Oral stage, when food moves from mouth to pharynx
- II. Pharyngeal stage, when food moves from pharynx to esophagus
- III. Esophageal stage, when food moves from esophagus to stomach.

■ ORAL STAGE OR FIRST STAGE

Oral stage of deglutition is a voluntary stage. In this stage, the bolus from mouth passes into pharynx by means of series of actions.

Sequence of Events during Oral Stage

1. Bolus is placed over postero-dorsal surface of the tongue. It is called the preparatory position
2. Anterior part of tongue is retracted and depressed.
3. Posterior part of tongue is elevated and retracted against the hard palate. This pushes the bolus backwards into the pharynx
4. Forceful contraction of tongue against the palate produces a positive pressure in the posterior part of oral cavity. This also pushes the food into pharynx (Fig. 43.1).

■ **PHARYNGEAL STAGE OR SECOND STAGE**

Pharyngeal stage is an involuntary stage. In this stage, the bolus is pushed from pharynx into the esophagus.

Pharynx is a common passage for food and air. It divides into larynx and esophagus. Larynx lies anteriorly and continues as respiratory passage. Esophagus lies behind the larynx and continues as GI tract. Since pharynx communicates with mouth, nose, larynx and esophagus, during this stage of deglutition, bolus from the pharynx can enter into four paths:

1. Back into mouth
2. Upward into nasopharynx
3. Forward into larynx
4. Downward into esophagus.

However, due to various coordinated movements, bolus is made to enter only the esophagus. Entrance of bolus through other paths is prevented as follows:

1. *Back into Mouth*

Return of bolus back into the mouth is prevented by:
   i. Position of tongue against the soft palate (roof of the mouth)
   ii. High intraoral pressure, developed by the movement of tongue.

2. *Upward into Nasopharynx*

Movement of bolus into the nasopharynx from pharynx is prevented by elevation of soft palate along with its extension called uvula.

3. *Forward into Larynx*

Movement of bolus into the larynx is prevented by the following actions:
   i. Approximation of the vocal cords
   ii. Forward and upward movement of larynx
   iii. Backward movement of epiglottis to seal the opening of the larynx (glottis)

iv. All these movements arrest respiration for a few seconds. It is called deglutition apnea.

Deglutition apnea

Apnea refers to temporary arrest of breathing. Deglutition apnea or **swallowing apnea** is the arrest of breathing during pharyngeal stage of deglutition.

4. *Entrance of Bolus into Esophagus*

As the other three paths are closed, the bolus has to pass only through the esophagus. This occurs by the combined effects of various factors:
   i. Upward movement of larynx stretches the opening of esophagus
   ii. Simultaneously, upper 3 to 4 cm of esophagus relaxes. This part of esophagus is formed by the cricopharyngeal muscle and it is called **upper esophageal sphincter** or **pharyngoesophageal sphincter**
   iii. At the same time, peristaltic contractions start in the pharynx due to the contraction of pharyngeal muscles
   iv. Elevation of larynx also lifts the glottis away from the food passage.

All the factors mentioned above act together so that, bolus moves easily into the esophagus. The whole process takes place within 1 to 2 seconds and this process is purely involuntary.

■ **ESOPHAGEAL STAGE OR THIRD STAGE**

Esophageal stage is also an involuntary stage. In this stage, food from esophagus enters the stomach. Esophagus forms the passage for movement of bolus from pharynx to the stomach. Movements of esophagus are specifically organized for this function and the movements are called peristaltic waves. Peristalsis means a wave of contraction, followed by the wave of relaxation of muscle fibers of GI tract, which travel in aboral direction (away from mouth). By this type of movement, the contents are propelled down along the GI tract.

When bolus reaches the esophagus, the peristaltic waves are initiated. Usually, two types of peristaltic contractions are produced in esophagus.

1. Primary peristaltic contractions
2. Secondary peristaltic contractions.

1. *Primary Peristaltic Contractions*

When bolus reaches the upper part of esophagus, the peristalsis starts. This is known as primary peristalsis.

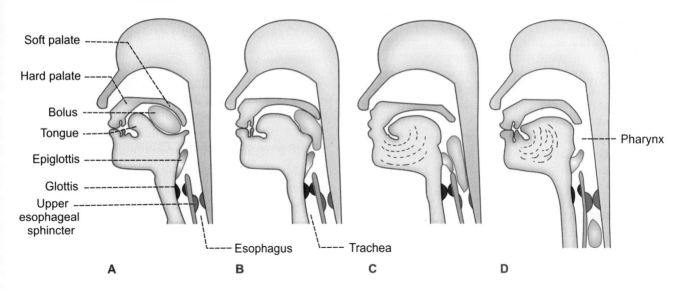

FIGURE 43.1: Stages of deglutition. **A.** Preparatory stage; **B.** Oral stage; **C.** Pharyngeal stage; **D.** Esophageal stage.

After origin, the peristaltic contractions pass down through the rest of the esophagus, propelling the bolus towards stomach.

Pressure developed during the primary peristaltic contractions is important to propel the bolus. Initially, the pressure becomes negative in the upper part of esophagus. This is due to the stretching of the closed esophagus by the elevation of larynx. But immediately, the pressure becomes positive and increases up to 10 to 15 cm of H_2O.

2. Secondary Peristaltic Contractions

If the primary peristaltic contractions are unable to propel the bolus into the stomach, the secondary peristaltic contractions appear and push the bolus into stomach.

Secondary peristaltic contractions are induced by the distention of upper esophagus by the bolus. After origin, these contractions pass down like the primary contractions, producing a positive pressure.

Role of Lower Esophageal Sphincter

Distal 2 to 5 cm of esophagus acts like a sphincter and it is called lower esophageal sphincter. It is constricted always. When bolus enters this part of the esophagus, this sphincter relaxes so that the contents enter the stomach. After the entry of bolus into the stomach, the sphincter constricts and closes the lower end of esophagus. The relaxation and constriction of sphincter occur in sequence with the arrival of peristaltic contractions of esophagus.

■ DEGLUTITION REFLEX

Though the beginning of swallowing is a voluntary act, later it becomes involuntary and is carried out by a reflex action called deglutition reflex. It occurs during the pharyngeal and esophageal stages.

Stimulus

When the bolus enters the oropharyngeal region, the receptors present in this region are stimulated.

Afferent Fibers

Afferent impulses from the **oropharyngeal receptors** pass via the glossopharyngeal nerve fibers to the deglutition center.

Center

Deglutition center is at the floor of the fourth ventricle in medulla oblongata of brain.

Efferent Fibers

Impulses from deglutition center travel through glossopharyngeal and vagus nerves (parasympathetic motor fibers) and reach soft palate, pharynx and esophagus. The glossopharyngeal nerve is concerned with pharyngeal stage of swallowing. The vagus nerve is concerned with esophageal stage.

Response

The reflex causes upward movement of soft palate, to close nasopharynx and upward movement of larynx, to close respiratory passage so that bolus enters the esophagus. Now the peristalsis occurs in esophagus, pushing the bolus into stomach.

■ APPLIED PHYSIOLOGY

1. *Dysphagia*

Dysphagia means difficulty in swallowing.

Causes of dysphagia

  i. Mechanical obstruction of esophagus due to tumor, strictures, diverticular hernia (out pouching of the wall), etc.
 ii. Decreased movement of esophagus due to neurological disorders such as **parkinsonism**
iii. Muscular disorders leading to difficulty in swallowing during oral stage or esophageal stage.

2. *Esophageal Achalasia or Achalasia Cardia*

Esophageal achalasia or achalasia cardia is a neuromuscular disease, characterized by accumulation of food substances in the esophagus preventing normal swallowing. It is due to the failure of lower **esophageal (cardiac) sphincter** to relax during swallowing. The accumulated food substances cause dilatation of esophagus.

Features of esophageal achalasia

  i. Dysphagia
 ii. Chest pain
iii. Weight loss
 iv. Cough.

3. *Gastroesophageal Reflux Disease (GERD)*

GERD is a disorder characterized by regurgitation of acidic gastric content through esophagus. The regurgitated gastric content flows into pharynx or mouth. Regurgitation is due to the weakness or **incompetence** (failure to constrict) of **lower esophageal sphincter.**

Features of GERD

  i. Heart burn or pyrosis (painful burning sensation in chest due to regurgitation of acidic gastric content into esophagus)
 ii. Esophagitis (inflammation of esophagus)
iii. Dysphagia
 iv. Cough and change of voice
  v. Esophageal ulcers or cancer (in chronic cases).

■ MOVEMENTS OF STOMACH

Activities of smooth muscles of stomach increase during gastric digestion (when stomach is filled with food) and when the stomach is empty.

Types of movements in stomach

1. Hunger contractions
2. Receptive relaxation
3. Peristalsis.

■ 1. HUNGER CONTRACTIONS

Hunger contractions are the movements of empty stomach. These contractions are related to the sensations of hunger.

Hunger contractions are the peristaltic waves superimposed over the contractions of gastric smooth muscle as a whole. This type of peristaltic waves is different from the digestive peristaltic contractions. The digestive peristaltic contractions usually occur in body and pyloric parts of the stomach. But, peristaltic contractions of empty stomach involve the entire stomach. Hunger contractions are of three types:

Type I Hunger Contractions

Type I hunger contractions are the first contractions to appear in the empty stomach, when the tone of the gastric muscles is low. Each contraction lasts for about 20 seconds. The interval between contractions is about 3 to 4 seconds. Tone of the muscles does not increase between contractions. Pressure produced by these contractions is about 5 cm of H_2O.

Type II Hunger Contractions

Type II hunger contractions appear when the tone of stomach is stronger. Tone increases in stomach if food intake is postponed, even after the appearance of the type I contractions. Each of the type II contractions lasts for 20 seconds like type I contractions. But the pause between the contractions is decreased. Pressure produced by these contractions is 10 to 15 cm of H_2O.

Type III Hunger Contractions

Type III hunger contractions are like incomplete tetanus. These contractions appear when the hunger becomes severe and the tone increases to a great extent. Type III hunger contractions are rare in man as the food is taken usually before the appearance of these contractions. These contractions last for 1 to 5 minutes. The pressure produced by these contractions increases to 10 to 20 cm of H_2O.

When the stomach is empty, the type I contractions occur first, followed by type II contractions. If food intake is still postponed, then type III contractions appear and as soon as food is consumed, hunger contractions disappear.

■ 2. RECEPTIVE RELAXATION

Receptive relaxation is the relaxation of the upper portion of the stomach when bolus enters the stomach from esophagus. It involves the fundus and upper part of the body of stomach. Its significance is to accommodate the food easily, without much increase in pressure inside the stomach. This process is called **accommodation** of stomach.

■ 3. PERISTALSIS

When food enters the stomach, the peristaltic contraction or peristaltic wave appears with a frequency of 3 per minute. It starts from the lower part of the body of stomach, passes through the pylorus till the **pyloric sphincter.**

Initially, the contraction appears as a slight indentation on the greater and lesser curvatures and travels towards pylorus. The contraction becomes deeper while traveling. Finally, it ends with the constriction of pyloric sphincter. Some of the waves disappear before reaching the sphincter. Each peristaltic wave takes about one minute to travel from the point of origin to the point of ending.

This type of peristaltic contraction is called **digestive peristalsis** because it is responsible for the grinding of food particles and mixing them with gastric juice for digestive activities.

■ FILLING AND EMPTYING OF STOMACH

■ FILLING OF STOMACH

While taking food, it arranges itself in the stomach in different layers. The first eaten food is placed against the greater curvature in the fundus and body of the stomach. The successive layers of food particles lie nearer, the lesser curvature, until the last portion of food eaten lies near the upper end of lesser curvature, adjacent to cardiac sphincter.

The liquid remains near the lesser curvature and flows towards the pyloric end of the stomach along a V-shaped groove. This groove is formed by the smooth muscle and it is called **magenstrasse.** But, if a large quantity of fluid is taken, it flows around the entire food mass and is distributed over the interior part of stomach, between wall of the stomach and food mass.

■ EMPTYING OF STOMACH

Gastric emptying is the process by which the chyme from stomach is emptied into intestine. Food that is swallowed enters the stomach and remains there for about 3 hours. During this period, digestion takes place. Partly digested food in stomach becomes the chyme.

Chyme

Chyme is the semisolid mass of partially digested food that is formed in the stomach. It is acidic in nature. Acid chyme is emptied from stomach into the intestine slowly, with the help of peristaltic contractions. It takes about 3 to 4 hours for emptying of the chyme. This slow emptying is necessary to facilitate the final digestion and maximum (about 80%) absorption of the digested food materials from small intestine. Gastric emptying occurs due to the peristaltic waves in the body and pyloric part of the stomach and simultaneous relaxation of pyloric sphincter.

Gastric emptying is influenced by various factors of the gastric content and food.

Factors Affecting Gastric Emptying

1. *Volume of gastric content*

For any type of meal, gastric emptying is directly proportional to the volume. If the content of stomach is more, a large amount is emptied into the intestine rapidly.

2. *Consistency of gastric content*

Emptying of the stomach depends upon consistency (degree of density) of the contents. Liquids, particularly the inert liquids like water leave the stomach rapidly. Solids leave the stomach only after being converted into fluid or semifluid. Undigested solid particles are not easily emptied.

3. *Chemical composition*

Chemical composition of the food also plays an important role in the emptying of the stomach. Carbohydrates are emptied faster than the proteins. Proteins are emptied faster than the fats. Thus, the fats are emptied very slowly.

4. *pH of the gastric content*

Gastric emptying is directly proportional to pH of the chyme.

5. *Osmolar concentration of gastric content*

Gastric content which is isotonic to blood, leaves the stomach rapidly than the hypotonic or hypertonic content.

■ REGULATION OF GASTRIC EMPTYING

Gastric emptying is regulated by nervous and hormonal factors.

Nervous Factor

Nervous factor which regulates the emptying of stomach is the enterogastric reflex.

Enterogastric Reflex

Enterogastric reflex is the reflex that inhibits gastric emptying. It is elicited by the presence of chyme in the duodenum, which prevents further emptying of stomach.

Mechanism of enterogastric reflex

1. Presence of chyme in duodenum causes generation of nerve impulses which are transmitted to stomach by the intrinsic nerve fibers of GI tract. After reaching the stomach, these impulses inhibit emptying.
2. Impulses from duodenum pass via extrinsic sympathetic fibers to stomach and inhibit emptying.
3. Some impulses from duodenum travel through afferent vagal fibers to the brainstem. Normally, brainstem neurons send excitatory impulses to stomach through efferent vagal fibers and stimulate gastric emptying. However, the impulses from duodenum inhibit these brainstem neurons and thereby inhibit gastric emptying.

Factors which initiate enterogastric reflex

1. Duodenal distension
2. Irritation of the duodenal mucosa
3. Acidity of the chyme
4. Osmolality of the chyme
5. Breakdown products of proteins and fats.

Hormonal Factors

When an acid chyme enters the duodenum, the duodenal mucosa releases some hormones which enter the stomach through blood and inhibit the motility of stomach.

Hormones inhibiting gastric motility and emptying

1. Vasoactive intestinal peptide (VIP)
2. Gastric inhibitory peptide (GIP)
3. Secretin
4. Cholecystokinin
5. Somatostatin
6. Peptide YY.

■ APPLIED PHYSIOLOGY – ABNORMAL GASTRIC EMPTYING

1. Gastric Dumping Syndrome

Gastric dumping syndrome or rapid gastric emptying is the condition characterized by series of upper abdominal symptoms. It is due to the rapid or quick dumping of undigested food from stomach into the jejunum. It occurs in patients following partial **gastrectomy** (removal of stomach) or **gastroenterostomy** (gastric bypass surgery). The rapid gastric emptying may begin immediately after taking meals **(early dumping)** or about few hours after taking meals **(late dumping).**

Causes

  i. Gastric surgery.
 ii. Zollinger-Ellison syndrome (rare disorder due to severe peptic ulcer and gastrin-secreting tumor in pancreas).

Symptoms of early dumping

  i. Nausea and vomiting
 ii. Bloating (increase in abdominal volume with feeling of abdominal fullness and tightness)
iii. Diarrhea
 iv. Sweating and weakness
  v. Fatigue and dizziness
 vi. Fainting and palpitations (sensation of heart beat).

Symptoms of late dumping

  i. Hypoglycemia
 ii. Sweating and weakness
iii. Dizziness.

2. Gastroparesis

Gastroparesis is a chronic disorder characterized by delayed gastric emptying. It usually occurs as a secondary disorder, precipitated by a primary cause.

Causes

  i. Diabetes mellitus
 ii. Postsurgical complications
iii. Motility disorder
 iv. Gastric infection
  v. Metabolic and endocrine disorder
 vi. Decrease in myenteric ganglia (rare).

Symptoms

  i. Early satiety (feeling full with small quantity of food)
 ii. Nausea
iii. Vomiting
 iv. Bloating
  v. Upper abdominal discomfort.

■ VOMITING

Vomiting or **emesis** is the abnormal emptying of stomach and upper part of intestine through esophagus and mouth.

■ CAUSES OF VOMITING

1. Presence of irritating contents in GI tract
2. Mechanical stimulation of pharynx
3. Pregnancy
4. Excess intake of alcohol
5. Nauseating sight, odor or taste
6. Unusual stimulation of labyrinthine apparatus, as in the case of sea sickness, air sickness, car sickness or swinging
7. Abnormal stimulation of sensory receptors in other organs like kidney, heart, semicircular canals or uterus
8. Drugs like antibiotics, opiates, etc.
9. Any GI disorder
10. Acute infection like urinary tract infection, influenza, etc.
11. Metabolic disturbances like carbohydrate starvation and ketosis (pregnancy), uremia, ketoacidosis (diabetes) and hypercalcemia.

■ MECHANISM OF VOMITING

Nausea

Vomiting is always preceded by nausea. Nausea is unpleasant sensation which induces the desire for vomiting. It is characterized by secretion of large amount of saliva containing more amount of mucus.

Retching

Strong involuntary movements in the GI tract which start even before actual vomiting. These movements intensify the feeling of vomiting. This condition is called retching **(try to vomit)** and vomiting occurs few minutes after this.

Act of Vomiting

Act of vomiting involves series of movements that takes place in GI tract.

Sequence of events:

1. Beginning of **antiperistalsis,** which runs from ileum towards the mouth through the intestine, pushing the intestinal contents into the stomach within few minutes. Velocity of the antiperistalsis is about 2 to 3 cm/second
2. Deep inspiration followed by temporary cessation of breathing

3. Closure of glottis
4. Upward and forward movement of larynx and hyoid bone
5. Elevation of soft palate
6. Contraction of diaphragm and abdominal muscles with a characteristic jerk, resulting in elevation of intra-abdominal pressure
7. Compression of the stomach between diaphragm and abdominal wall leading to rise in intragastric pressure
8. Simultaneous relaxation of lower esophageal sphincter, esophagus and upper esophageal sphincter
9. Forceful expulsion of gastric contents **(vomitus)** through esophagus, pharynx and mouth.

Movements during act of vomiting throw the vomitus (materials ejected during vomiting) to the exterior through mouth. Some of the movements play important roles by preventing the entry of vomitus through other routes and thereby prevent the adverse effect of the vomitus on many structures.

Such movements are:

1. Closure of glottis and cessation of breathing prevents entry of vomitus into the lungs
2. Elevation of soft palate prevents entry of vomitus into the nasopharynx
3. Larynx and hyoid bone move upward and forward and are placed in this position rigidly. This causes the dilatation of throat, which allows free exit of vomitus.

■ VOMITING REFLEX

Vomiting is a reflex act. Sensory impulses for vomiting arise from the irritated or distended part of GI tract or other organs and are transmitted to the vomiting center through vagus and sympathetic afferent fibers.

Vomiting center is situated bilaterally in medulla oblongata near the nucleus tractus solitarius.

Motor impulses from the vomiting center are transmitted through V, VII, IX, X and XII cranial nerves to the upper part of GI tract; and through spinal nerves to diaphragm and abdominal muscles.

Center for Vomiting during Motion Sickness and Vomiting Induced by Drugs

Center for vomiting during motion sickness and vomiting induced by drugs such as morphine, apomorphine, etc. is on the floor of fourth ventricle. This area is called **chemoreceptor trigger zone.** During motion sickness, the afferent impulses from vestibular apparatus reach vomiting center through this zone.

Center for Psychic-stimuli-induced Vomiting

Center for vomiting due to psychic stimuli such as nauseating odor, sight or noise is in cerebral cortex.

■ MOVEMENTS OF SMALL INTESTINE

Movements of small intestine are essential for mixing the chyme with digestive juices, propulsion of food and absorption.

Types of Movements of Small Intestine

Movements of small intestine are of four types:
1. Mixing movements:
    i. Segmentation movements
    ii. Pendular movements.
2. Propulsive movements:
    i. Peristaltic movements
    ii. Peristaltic rush.
3. Peristalsis in fasting – migrating motor complex
4. Movements of villi.

■ 1. MIXING MOVEMENTS

Mixing movements of small intestine are responsible for proper mixing of chyme with digestive juices such as pancreatic juice, bile and intestinal juice. The mixing movements of small intestine are segmentation contractions and pendular movements.

i. *Segmentation Contractions*

Segmentation contractions are the common type of movements of small intestine, which occur regularly or irregularly, but in a rhythmic fashion. So, these movements are also called rhythmic segmentation contractions.

The contractions occur at regularly spaced intervals along a section of intestine. The segment of the intestine involved in each contraction is about 1 to 5 cm long. The segments of intestine in between the contracted segments are relaxed. The length of the relaxed segments is same as that of the contracted segments. These alternate segments of contraction and relaxation give appearance of rings, resembling the chain of sausages.

After sometime, the contracted segments are relaxed and the relaxed segments are contracted (Fig. 43.2). Therefore, the segmentation contractions **chop** the chyme many times. This helps in mixing of chyme with digestive juices.

ii. *Pendular Movement*

Pendular movement is the sweeping movement of small intestine, resembling the movements of **pendulum** of

clock. Small portions of intestine (loops) sweep forward and backward or upward and downward. It is a type of mixing movement, noticed only by close observation.

It helps in mixing of chyme with digestive juices.

■ 2. PROPULSIVE MOVEMENTS

Propulsive movements are the movements of small intestine which push the chyme in the aboral direction through intestine. The propulsive movements are peristaltic movements and peristaltic rush.

i. *Peristaltic Movements*

Peristalsis is defined as the wave of contraction followed by wave of relaxation of muscle fibers. In GI tract, it always travels in aboral direction. Stimulation of smooth muscles of intestine initiates the peristalsis. It travels from point of stimulation in both directions. But under normal conditions, the progress of contraction in an oral direction is inhibited quickly and the contractions disappear. Only the contraction that travels in an aboral direction persists.

Starling's law of intestine

Depending upon the direction of the peristalsis, 'Law of intestine' was put forth by Starling.

According to the law of intestine, the response of the intestine for a local stimulus consists of a contraction

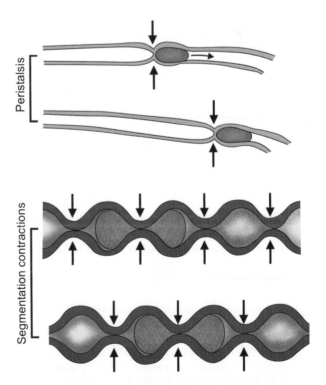

FIGURE 43.2: Movements of small intestine

of smooth muscle above and relaxation below the stimulated area.

Peristaltic contractions start at any part of the intestine and travel towards anal end, at a velocity of 1 to 2 cm/sec. The contractions are always weak and usually disappear after traveling for few centimeter. Because of this, the average movement of chyme through small intestine is very slow and the average velocity of movement of the chyme is less than 1 cm/sec. So, the chyme requires several hours to travel from duodenum to the end of small intestine.

Peristaltic waves in small intestine increase to a great extent immediately after a meal. This is because of **gastroenteric reflex,** which is initiated by the distention of stomach. Impulses for this reflex are transmitted from stomach along the wall of the intestine via myenteric plexus.

ii. *Peristaltic Rush*

Sometimes, the small intestine shows a powerful peristaltic contraction. It is caused by excessive irritation of intestinal mucosa or extreme distention of the intestine. This type of powerful contraction begins in duodenum and passes through entire length of small intestine and reaches the ileocecal valve within few minutes. This is called peristaltic rush or rush waves.

Peristaltic rush sweeps the contents of intestine into the colon. Thus, it relieves the small intestine off either irritants or excessive distention.

■ 3. PERISTALSIS IN FASTING – MIGRATING MOTOR COMPLEX

Migrating motor complex is a type of peristaltic contraction, which occurs in stomach and small intestine during the periods of fasting for several hours. It is also called **migrating myoelectric complex.** It is different from the regular peristalsis because, a large portion of stomach or intestine is involved in the contraction. The contraction extends to about 20 to 30 cm of stomach or intestine. This type of movement occurs once in every 1½ to 2 hours.

It starts as a moderately active peristalsis in the body of stomach and runs through the entire length of small intestine. It travels at a velocity of 6 to 12 cm/min. Thus, it takes about 10 minutes to reach the colon after taking origin from the stomach.

Significance of Peristalsis in Fasting

Migrating motor complex sweeps the excess digestive secretions into the colon and prevents the accumulation of the secretions in stomach and intestine. It also sweeps the residual indigested materials into colon.

■ 4. MOVEMENTS OF VILLI

Intestinal villi also show movements simultaneously along with intestinal movements. It is because of the extension of smooth muscle fibers of the intestinal wall into the villi.

Movements of villi are shortening and elongation, which occur alternatively and help in emptying lymph from the central lacteal into the lymphatic system. The surface area of villi is increased during elongation. This helps absorption of digested food particles from the lumen of intestine.

Movements of villi are caused by local nervous reflexes, which are initiated by the presence of chyme in small intestine. Hormone secreted from the small intestinal mucosa called **villikinin** is also believed to play an important role in increasing the movements of villi.

■ MOVEMENTS OF LARGE INTESTINE

Usually, the large intestine shows sluggish movements. Still, these movements are important for mixing, propulsive and absorptive functions.

Types of Movements of Large Intestine

Movements of large intestine are of two types:
1. Mixing movements: Segmentation contractions
2. Propulsive movements: Mass peristalsis.

■ 1. MIXING MOVEMENTS – SEGMENTATION CONTRACTIONS

Large circular constrictions, which appear in the colon, are called mixing segmentation contractions. These contractions occur at regular distance in colon. Length of the portion of colon involved in each contraction is nearly about 2.5 cm.

■ 2. PROPULSIVE MOVEMENTS – MASS PERISTALSIS

Mass peristalsis or mass movement propels the feces from colon towards anus. Usually, this movement occurs only a few times every day. Duration of mass movement is about 10 minutes in the morning before or after breakfast. This is because of the neurogenic factors like **gastrocolic reflex** (see below) and parasympathetic stimulation.

■ DEFECATION

Voiding of feces is known as defecation. Feces is formed in the large intestine and stored in sigmoid colon. By the influence of an appropriate stimulus, it is expelled out through the anus. This is prevented by tonic constriction of anal sphincters, in the absence of the stimulus.

■ DEFECATION REFLEX

Mass movement drives the feces into sigmoid or pelvic colon. In the sigmoid colon, the feces is stored. The desire for defecation occurs when some feces enters rectum due to the mass movement. Usually, the desire for defecation is elicited by an increase in the intrarectal pressure to about 20 to 25 cm H_2O.

Usual stimulus for defecation is intake of liquid like coffee or tea or water. But it differs from person to person.

Act of Defecation

Act of defecation is preceded by voluntary efforts like assuming an appropriate posture, voluntary relaxation of external sphincter and the compression of abdominal contents by voluntary contraction of abdominal muscles.

Usually, the rectum is empty. During the development of mass movement, the feces is pushed into rectum and the defecation reflex is initiated. The process of defecation involves the contraction of rectum and relaxation of internal and external anal sphincters.

Internal anal sphincter is made up of smooth muscle and it is innervated by parasympathetic nerve fibers via pelvic nerve. **External anal sphincter** is composed of skeletal muscle and it is controlled by somatic nerve fibers, which pass through **pudendal nerve.** Pudendal nerve always keeps the external sphincter constricted and the sphincter can relax only when the pudendal nerve is inhibited.

Gastrocolic Reflex

Gastrocolic reflex is the contraction of rectum, followed by the desire for defecation caused by distention of stomach by food. It is mediated by intrinsic nerve fibers of GI tract.

This reflex causes only a weak contraction of rectum. But, it initiates defecation reflex.

■ PATHWAY FOR DEFECATION REFLEX

When rectum is distended due to the entry of feces by mass movement, sensory nerve endings are stimulated. Impulses from the nerve endings are transmitted via afferent fibers of pelvic nerve to the defecation center, situated in sacral segments (center) of spinal cord.

The center in turn, sends motor impulses to the descending colon, sigmoid colon and rectum via efferent

nerve fibers of pelvic nerve. Motor impulses cause strong contraction of descending colon, sigmoid colon and rectum and relaxation of internal sphincter.

Simultaneously, voluntary relaxation of external sphincter occurs. It is due to the inhibition of pudendal nerve, by impulses arising from cerebral cortex (Fig. 43.3).

■ CONSTIPATION

Constipation is the failure of voiding of feces. Refer Chapter 42 for details.

■ EVACUATION OF GASES FROM GASTROINTESTINAL TRACT

Normally, gas accumulates in the GI tract either because of entrance of outside air or production of gases in the body. Accordingly, the gases accumulated in GI tract are classified into two groups:
1. Exogenous gases
2. Endogenous gases.

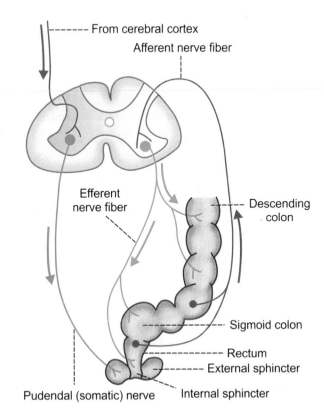

FIGURE 43.3: Defecation reflex. Afferent and efferent fibers of the reflex pass through pelvic (parasympathetic) nerve. Voluntary control of defecation is by pudendal (somatic) nerve. Defecation center is in the sacral segments of spinal cord

1. *Exogenous Gases*

Exogenous gases form about 90% of accumulated gases. These gases enter the GI tract either by swallowing through mouth or drinking carbonated beverages.

2. *Endogenous Gases*

Endogenous gases form about 10% of accumulated gases. These gases are produced by digestion of food stuffs and interaction between bacteria and food stuffs in the intestine.

■ EVACUATION OF ACCUMULATED GASES

Evacuation of accumulated gases usually occurs by two processes:
1. Belching
2. Flatulence.

■ BELCHING

Belching is the process by which the gas accumulated in stomach is expelled through mouth. It is also called **burping.** It occurs because of inflation (distention) of stomach by swallowed air. The distention of the stomach causes abdominal discomfort and the belching expels the air and relieves the discomfort.

Most of the gas accumulated in stomach is expelled through mouth. Only a small amount enters the intestine.

Causes for Accumulation of Gases in Stomach

1. Aerophagia: Swallowing large amounts of air due to gulping the food or drink too rapidly
2. Drinking carbonated beverages
3. During some emotional conditions like anxiety lot of air enters the stomach through mouth.

Act of Belching

Belching is not a simple act and it requires the coordination of several activities such as:
1. Closure of larynx, which prevents entry of liquid or food with the air from stomach into the lungs.
2. Elevation of larynx and relaxation of upper esophageal sphincter. It allows exit of air through esophagus more easily.

3. Opening of lower esophageal sphincter.
4. Descent of diaphragm, which increases abdominal pressure and decreases intrathoracic pressure.

All these activities are responsible for the expulsion of air from stomach to the exterior via esophagus.

■ FLATULENCE

Flatulence is the production of a mixture of intestinal gases. The mixture of gases is known as **flatus** (in Latin, flatus = wind). Expulsion of flatus through anus under pressure is called farting or passing gas. Farting is associated with disagreeable odor (due to odorous gases) and sound (due to vibration of anal sphincter).

Quantity of Flatus

Average flatus released by human is about 500 to 1500 mL per day, with 10 to 25 episodes throughout the day.

Source of Gases in Intestine

Flatulence is the mixture of gases present in the intestine. Flatulence by swallowed air is rare.

Common sources of gases in flatulence are:
1. Bacterial action on undigested sugars and polysaccharides (e.g. starch, cellulose)
2. Digestion of some flatulence producing food stuffs such as cheese, yeast in bread, oats, onion, beans, cabbage, milk, etc.

Constituents of Flatus

Major constituents of flatus:
1. Swallowed non-odorous gases
   i. Nitrogen (major constituent)
   ii. Oxygen
2. Non-odorous gases produced by microbes
   i. Methane
   ii. Carbon dioxide
   iii. Hydrogen
3. Odorous materials such as
   i. Low molecular weight fatty acids like butyric acid
   ii. Reduced sulfur compounds (hydrogen sulfide and carbonyl sulfide).

Gastrointestinal Hormones

```
■ INTRODUCTION
■ CELLS SECRETING THE HORMONES
■ DESCRIPTION OF GASTROINTESTINAL HORMONES
    ■ GASTRIN
    ■ SECRETIN
    ■ CHOLECYSTOKININ
    ■ GLUCOSE-DEPENDENT INSULINOTROPIC HORMONE
    ■ VASOACTIVE INTESTINAL POLYPEPTIDE
    ■ GLUCAGON
    ■ GLICENTIN
    ■ GLUCAGON-LIKE POLYPEPTIDE-1
    ■ GLUCAGON-LIKE POLYPEPTIDE-2
    ■ SOMATOSTATIN
    ■ PANCREATIC POLYPEPTIDE
    ■ PEPTIDE YY
    ■ NEUROPEPTIDE Y
    ■ MOTILIN
    ■ SUBSTANCE P
    ■ GHRELIN
    ■ OTHER GASTROINTESTINAL HORMONES
```

■ INTRODUCTION

Gastrointestinal (GI) hormones are the hormones secreted in GI tract. These hormones are polypeptides in nature and belong to the family of **local hormones** (Chapter 73). Major function of these hormones is to regulate the secretory activities and motility of the GI tract.

■ CELLS SECRETING THE HORMONES

Enteroendocrine Cells

Enteroendocrine cells are the **hormone-secreting cells** in GI tract. These are the nerve cells and glandular cells which are present in the gastric mucosa, intestinal mucosa and the pancreatic cells.

Neuroendocrine Cells or APUD Cells

Enteroendocrine cells which secrete hormones from amines are known as **amine precursor uptake and decarboxylation cells** (APUD cells) or neuroendocrine cells. For the synthesis of a GI hormone, first a precursor substance of an amine is taken up by these cells. Later, this precursor substance is decarboxylated to form the amine. From this amine, the hormone is synthesized. Because of the uptake of the amine precursor and decarboxylation of this precursor substance, these cells are called APUD cells. This type of cells is also present in other parts of the body, particularly the brain, lungs and the endocrine glands.

Enterochromaffin Cells

Enteroendocrine cells which secrete serotonin are called enterochromaffin cells.

■ DESCRIPTION OF GASTROINTESTINAL HORMONES

■ 1. GASTRIN

Gastrin is a peptide with 34 amino acid residues. It is secreted mainly by the **G cells** of pyloric glands of stomach. It is also secreted by **TG cells** in **stomach, duodenum** and **jejunum**. In fetus, the islets of Langerhans also secrete this hormone (Table 44.1).

Gastrin is secreted from stomach during the gastric (second) phase of gastric secretion and from small intestine during the intestinal (third) phase of gastric secretion.

Stimulant for Secretion

Stimulants for secretion of gastrin are:
  i. Presence of food in the stomach.
  ii. Stimulation of local nervous plexus in stomach and small intestine.
  iii. **Vagovagal reflex** during the gastric phase of gastric secretion: **Gastrin-releasing polypeptide** is released at the vagal nerve ending. It causes the secretion of gastrin by stimulating the G cells or TG cells.

TABLE 44.1: Gastrointestinal hormones

Hormone	Source of secretion	Actions
Gastrin	G cells in stomach TG cells in GI tract Islets in fetal pancreas Anterior pituitary Brain	Stimulates gastric secretion and motility Promotes growth of gastric mucosa Stimulates release of pancreatic hormones Stimulates secretion of pancreatic juice Stimulates secretion of pancreatic hormones
Secretin	S cells of small intestine	Stimulates secretion of watery and alkaline pancreatic secretion Inhibits gastric secretion and motility Constricts pyloric sphincter Increases potency of cholecystokinin action
Cholecystokinin	I cells of small intestine	Contracts gallbladder Stimulates pancreatic secretion with enzymes Accelerates secretin activity Increases enterokinase secretion Inhibits gastric motility Increases intestinal motility Augments contraction of pyloric sphincter Suppresses hunger Induces drug tolerance to opioids
Gastric inhibitory peptide (GIP)	K cells in duodenum and jejunum Antrum of stomach	Stimulates insulin secretion Inhibits gastric secretion and motility
Vasoactive intestinal polypeptide (VIP)	Stomach Small and large intestines	Dilates splanchnic (peripheral) blood vessels Inhibits Hcl secretion in gastric juice Stimulates secretion of succus entericus Relaxes smooth muscles of intestine Augments acetylcholine action on salivary glands Stimulates insulin secretion
Glucagon	α-cells in pancreas A cells in stomach L cells in intestine	Increases blood sugar level
Glicentin	L cells in duodenum and jejunum	Increases blood sugar level
Glucagon-like polypeptide-1 (GLP-1)	α-cells in pancreas Brain	Stimulates insulin secretion Inhibits gastric motility
GLP-2	L cells in ileum and colon	Suppresses appetite

Contd...

Contd...

Hormone	Source of secretion	Actions
Somatostatin	Hypothalamus D cells in pancreas D cells in stomach and small intestine	Inhibits secretion of growth hormone Inhibits gastric secretion and motility Inhibits secretion of pancreatic juice Inhibits secretion of GI hormones
Pancreatic polypeptide	PP cells in pancreas Small intestine	Increases secretion of glucagons Decreases pancreatic secretion
Peptide YY	L cells of ileum and colon	Inhibits gastric secretion and motility Reduces secretion of pancreatic juice Inhibits intestinal motility and bowel passage Suppresses appetite and food intake
Neuropeptide Y	Ileum and colon Brain and autonomic nervous system (ANS)	Increases blood flow in enteric blood vessels
Motilin	Mo cells in stomach and intestine Enterochromoffin cells in intestine	Accelerates gastric emptying Increases movements of small intestine Increases peristalsis in colon
Substance P	Brain Small intestine	Increases movements of small intestine
Ghrelin	Stomach Hypothalamus Pituitary Kidney Placenta	Promotes growth hormone (GH) release Induces appetite and food intake Stimulates gastric emptying

Actions

Gastrin:

   i. Stimulates gastric glands to secrete gastric juice with more pepsin and hydrochloric acid.
   ii. Accelerates gastric motility.
   iii. Promotes growth of gastric mucosa.
   iv. Stimulates secretion of pancreatic juice, which is rich in enzymes.
   v. Stimulates islets of Langerhans in pancreas to release pancreatic hormones.

■ 2. SECRETIN

Secretin is a peptide hormone with 27 amino acid residues. Historical importance of secretin is that, it was the first ever hormone discovered. It was discovered in 1902 by Bayliss and Starling. It is secreted by the **S cells** of **duodenum, jejunum** and **ileum.**

Secretin is first produced in an inactive form called **prosecretin.** It is converted into secretin by the acidity of chyme.

Stimulant for Secretion

Stimulant for the release and activation of prosecretin is the **acid chyme** entering the duodenum from stomach.

Products of protein digestion also stimulate secretin secretion.

Actions

Major actions

Secretin stimulates exocrine pancreatic secretion. It acts on the cells of pancreatic ductule via cyclic AMP and causes secretion of large amount of watery juice with high content of bicarbonate ion. Bicarbonate content of pancreatic juice (released by secretin) has functional significance (Chapter 39).

Other actions

Secretin:

   i. Inhibits secretion of gastric juice
   ii. Inhibits motility of stomach
   iii. Causes constriction of pyloric sphincter
   iv. Increases the potency of action of cholecystokinin on pancreatic secretion.

■ 3. CHOLECYSTOKININ

Cholecystokinin is made up of 39 amino acid residues. Previously it was thought that there were two separate hormones, namely pancreozymin and cholecystokinin. It was thought that pancreozymin stimulated the secretion of pancreatic juice with large amount of enzymes and the cholecystokinin stimulated the contraction of gallbladder. But now it is established that the same hormone has actions on both pancreas and gallbladder. So, it is named as **cholecystokinin-pancreozymin** (CCK-PZ) or cholecystokinin (CCK).

Cholecystokinin is secreted by **I cells** in mucosa of **duodenum** and **jejunum**. A small quantity of the hormone is secreted in the **ileum** also.

Stimulant for Secretion

Stimulant for the release of this hormone is the presence of chyme-containing digestive products of fats and proteins, viz. fatty acids, peptides and amino acids in the upper part of small intestine.

Actions

Major actions

Cholecystokinin:
  i.   Contracts gallbladder.
  ii. Stimulates exocrine pancreatic secretion: It activates the pancreatic acinar cells via the second messenger inositol triphosphate. Cholecystokinin causes secretion of pancreatic juice with large amount of enzymes.

Other actions

Cholecystokinin:
  i.   Accelerates the activity of secretin to produce alkaline pancreatic juice, with large amount of bicarbonate ions.
  ii. Increases the secretion of enterokinase.
  iii. Inhibits the gastric motility.
  iv. Increases the motility of intestine.
  v.   Augments contraction of pyloric sphincter.
  vi. Plays an important role in satiety by suppressing hunger.
  vii. Induces drug tolerance to opioids.

■ 4. GLUCOSE-DEPENDENT INSULINOTROPIC HORMONE

Earlier it was called **gastric inhibitory peptide** (GIP). It is a peptide hormone, formed by 42 amino acid residues. It is secreted by **K cells** in **duodenum** and in **jejunum**. It is also secreted in antrum of **stomach.**

Stimulant for Secretion

GIP is secreted when chyme containing **glucose** and **fat** enters the duodenum.

Actions

Gastric inhibitory peptide (GIP):
  i.   Stimulates the beta cells in the islets of Langerhans in pancreas to release insulin. It causes insulin secretion, whenever chyme with glucose enters the small intestine. Hence it is called glucose-dependent insulinotropic hormone.
  ii. Inhibits the secretion of gastric juice.
  iii. Inhibits gastric motility.

Recent studies reveal that GIP does not show significant action on gastric secretion.

■ 5. VASOACTIVE INTESTINAL POLYPEPTIDE

Vasoactive intestinal polypeptide (VIP) contains 28 amino acid residues. This polypeptide is secreted in the **stomach** and **small intestine**. A small amount of this hormone is also secreted in large intestine.

Stimulant for Secretion

Presence of **acid chyme** in the stomach and intestine causes secretion of VIP.

Actions

Vasoactive intestinal polypeptide (VIP):
  i.   Dilates splanchnic (peripheral) blood vessels.
  ii. Inhibits hydrochloric acid secretion in gastric juice.
  iii. Stimulates secretion of succus entericus with large amounts of electrolytes and water.
  iv. Relaxes smooth muscles of intestine.
  v.   Augments action of acetylcholine on salivary glands.
  vi. Stimulates insulin secretion.

■ 6. GLUCAGON

Glucagon has 29 amino acid residues. It is secreted mainly by **alpha cells** of islets of Langerhans in pancreas. It is also secreted by **A cells** in the **stomach** and **L cells** in the **intestine**. In intestine, it is secreted as **preproglucagon.**

Stimulant for Secretion

Presence of food with more **fat** and **protein** in the stomach is the stimulant for glucagon secretion in stomach and duodenum. **Hypoglycemia** is the stimulant for secretion of pancreatic glucagon.

Action

Glucagon increases blood sugar level (Chapter 69).

■ 7. GLICENTIN

Glicentin polypeptide is secreted by L cells in duodenum and jejunum and **α-cells** of pancreatic islets. It is also secreted in **brain.**

Precursor of this hormone is the **preproglucagon.** In intestine, the preproglucagon is converted into glicentin and glucagon-like polypeptide-2 (GLP-2). In pancreas, it is converted into glucagon, glucagon-like polypeptide-1 (GLP-1) and major proglucagon fragment.

Stimulant for Secretion

Glicentin is secreted when chyme with **fat** and **protein** enters the intestine.

Action

Like glucagon, glicentin also increases the blood sugar level.

■ 8. GLUCAGON-LIKE POLYPEPTIDE-1

Glucagon-like polypeptide-1 (GLP-1) is secreted in **α-cells** of pancreatic islets (see above). Structurally, it is similar to GLP-2 and glucagon. It is found in brain also.

Stimulant for Secretion

Presence of food with **glucose** in the small intestine stimulates the release of GLP-1.

Actions

Glucagon-like polypeptide-1 (GLP-1):
   i.   Stimulates the insulin secretion from β-cells of islets in pancreas
   ii. Inhibits gastric motility.

■ 9. GLUCAGON-LIKE POLYPEPTIDE-2

Glucagon-like polypeptide-2 (GLP-2) is secreted by **L cells** in **ileum** and **colon** (see above). Structurally, it is similar to GLP-1 and glucagons. Like GLP-1, it is also found in brain.

Stimulant for Secretion

Presence of food with **glucose** in the small intestine stimulates the release of GLP-2 also.

Action

GLP-2 is believed to suppress appetite.

■ 10. SOMATOSTATIN

Somatostatin was first found in **hypothalamus** and named as **growth hormone-inhibiting hormone.** Now it is found in **D cells** of **stomach** and upper part of **small intestine** and **D cells** of **pancreatic** islets also. Somatostatin is secreted in two forms, one with 14 amino acids and the other one with 28 amino acids.

Stimulant for Secretion

Presence of chyme with **glucose** and **proteins** in stomach and small intestine causes release of somatostatin.

Actions

Somatostatin:
   i.   Inhibits the secretion of growth hormone (GH) and thyroid-stimulating hormone (TSH) from anterior pituitary
   ii. Inhibits gastric secretion and motility
   iii. Inhibits secretion of pancreatic juice
   iv. Inhibits secretion of GI hormones such as:
        a. Gastrin
        b. Cholecystokinin (CCK)
        c. Vasoactive intestinal polypeptide (VIP)
        d. Gastric inhibitory peptide (GIP).

■ 11. PANCREATIC POLYPEPTIDE

Source of Secretion

Pancreatic polypeptide is a polypeptide with 36 amino acid residues. It is secreted mainly by the **PP cells** of the islets of Langerhans in **pancreas.** It is also found in **small intestine** (Table 44.1).

Stimulant for Secretion

Pancreatic polypeptide is secreted by the presence of chyme with **proteins** in the small intestine. It is also secreted in conditions like **hypoglycemia, fasting** and **exercise.**

Actions

Pancreatic polypeptide:
   i.   Increases the secretion of glucagon from α-cells of islets of Langerhans in pancreas.
   ii. Decreases the secretion of pancreatic juice from exocrine part of pancreas.

■ 12. PEPTIDE YY

Polypeptide YY with 36 amino acid residues, is structurally related to pancreatic polypeptide and neuropeptide Y. It is secreted in **L cells** of **ileum** and **colon.**

Stimulant for Secretion

Presence of **fat**-containing chyme stimulates the release of peptide YY.

Actions

Peptide YY:

   i. Inhibits gastric secretion and motility
   ii. Reduces secretion of pancreatic juice
   iii. Inhibits the intestinal motility and stops passage of bowel beyond ileum (ileal brake)
   iv. Suppresses appetite and food intake.

■ 13. NEUROPEPTIDE Y

Neuropeptide Y contains 36 amino acid residues. It is structurally related to pancreatic polypeptide and peptide YY. It is secreted by **enteric nerve endings** particularly in **ileum** and **colon**. It is also secreted in medulla, hypothalamus and neurons of autonomic nervous system (ANS).

Stimulant for Secretion

Secretion of neuropeptide Y is stimulated by **fat-containing chyme.**

Action

Neuropeptide Y increases the blood flow in enteric blood vessels and stimulates food intake (Chapter 141).

■ 14. MOTILIN

Motilin is built by 22 amino acid residues. It is secreted by **Mo cells,** which are present in **stomach** and **intestine.** It is also believed to be secreted by enterochromoffin cells of intestine.

Stimulant for Secretion

Motilin is secreted when the **chyme** from stomach enters the duodenum.

Actions

Motilin:

   i. Accelerates gastric emptying
   ii. Increases the mixing and propulsive movements of small intestine
   iii. Increases the peristalsis in colon.

■ 15. SUBSTANCE P

Source of Secretion

Substance P is a neurotransmitter with 11 amino acid residues. It is secreted at the **pain nerve endings** in **brain** and **enteric nerve endings** in **small intestine.**

Stimulant for Secretion

Secretion of substance P in intestine is caused by the presence of **chyme.**

Actions

In GI tract, substance P increases the mixing and propulsive movements of small intestine (refer Chapter 141 for its actions in brain).

■ 16. GHRELIN

Ghrelin is a recently discovered hormone. This 28 amino acid polypeptide is synthesized by **epithelial cells** in the fundus of **stomach.** It is also produced in smaller amounts in hypothalamus, pituitary, kidney and placenta.

Stimulant for Secretion

Secretion of ghrelin increases during **fasting** and decreases when stomach is full.

Actions

Ghrelin:

   i. Promotes the secretion of growth hormone (GH) by stimulating somatotropes (growth hormone synthesizing cells) in anterior pituitary. Receptors for this hormone called growth hormone secretogogues receptor (GHS-R) were identified in the somatotropes before the discovery of the hormone itself. These receptors are also found in adipose tissue, heart and hypothalamus.
   ii. Induces appetite and food intake by acting via feeding center in hypothalamus (Chapter 149).
   iii. Stimulates gastric emptying.

■ OTHER GASTROINTESTINAL HORMONES

Mucosa of GI tract secretes many other hormones such as:
1. Enkephalins
2. Dynorphin
3. Neurotensin
4. Serotonin
5. Urogastrone
6. Enterocrinin
7. Villikinin
8. Guanylin
9. Bombesin.

   However, the significant biological actions of these hormones on GI tract are not clear.

Digestion, Absorption and Metabolism of Carbohydrates

- ■ CARBOHYDRATES IN DIET
- ■ DIGESTION
- ■ ABSORPTION
- ■ METABOLISM
- ■ DIETARY FIBER

■ CARBOHYDRATES IN DIET

Human diet contains three types of carbohydrates:

■ 1. POLYSACCHARIDES

Large polysaccharides are glycogen, amylose and amylopectin, which are in the form of starch (glucose polymers). Glycogen is available in **non-vegetarian diet.** Amylose and amylopectin are available in **vegetarian diet** because of their plant origin.

■ 2. DISACCHARIDES

Two types of disaccharides are available in the diet.
  i. Sucrose (Glucose + Fructose), which is called table sugar or cane sugar
  ii. Lactose (Glucose + Galactose), which is the sugar available in milk.

■ 3. MONOSACCHARIDES

Monosaccharides consumed in human diet are mostly glucose and fructose.

Other carbohydrates in the diet include
  i. Alcohol
  ii. Lactic acid
  iii. Pyruvic acid
  iv. Pectins
  v. Dextrins
  vi. Carbohydrates in meat.

Diet also contains large amount of **cellulose,** which cannot be digested in the human GI tract so it is not considered as a food for human beings.

■ DIGESTION OF CARBOHYDRATES

■ IN THE MOUTH

Enzymes involved in the digestion of carbohydrates are known as **amylolytic enzymes.** The only amylolytic enzyme present in saliva is the salivary amylase or ptyalin (Chapter 37).

■ IN THE STOMACH

Gastric juice contains a **weak amylase,** which plays a minor role in digestion of carbohydrates.

■ IN THE INTESTINE

Amylolytic enzymes present in the small intestine are derived from pancreatic juice and succus entericus (Table 45.1).

Amylolytic Enzyme in Pancreatic Juice

Pancreatic juice contains **pancreatic amylase** (Chapter 39).

Amylolytic Enzymes in Succus Entericus

Amylolytic enzymes present in succus entericus are **maltase, sucrase, lactase, dextrinase** and **trehalase** (Chapter 41).

■ FINAL PRODUCTS OF CARBOHYDRATE DIGESTION

Final products of carbohydrate digestion are monosaccharides, which are glucose, fructose and galactose.

TABLE 45.1: Digestion of carbohydrates

Area	Juice	Enzyme	Substrate	End product
Mouth	Saliva	Salivary amylase	Polysaccharides – cooked starch	Disaccharides – dextrin and maltose
Stomach	Gastric juice	Gastric amylase	Weak amylase	The action is negligible
Small intestine	Pancreatic juice	Pancreatic amylase	Polysaccharides	Disaccharides – Dextrin, maltose and maltriose
	Succus entericus	Sucrase	Sucrose	Glucose and fructose
		Maltase	Maltose and maltriose	Glucose
		Lactase	Lactose	Glucose and galactose
		Dextrinase	Dextrin, maltose and maltriose	Glucose
		Trehalase	Trehalose	Glucose

Glucose represents 80% of the final product of carbohydrate digestion. Galactose and fructose represent the remaining 20%.

■ ABSORPTION OF CARBOHYDRATES

Carbohydrates are absorbed from the small intestine mainly as monosaccharides, viz. glucose, galactose and fructose.

■ ABSORPTION OF GLUCOSE

Glucose is transported from the lumen of small intestine into the epithelial cells in the mucus membrane of small intestine, by means of sodium cotransport. Energy for this is obtained by the binding process of sodium ion and glucose molecule to carrier protein.

From the epithelial cell, glucose is absorbed into the portal vein by **facilitated diffusion.** However, sodium ion moves laterally into the intercellular space. From here, it is transported into blood by active transport, utilizing the energy liberated by breakdown of ATP.

■ ABSORPTION OF GALACTOSE

Galactose is also absorbed from the small intestine in the same mechanism as that of glucose.

■ ABSORPTION OF FRUCTOSE

Fructose is absorbed into blood by means of **facilitated diffusion.** Some molecules of fructose are converted into glucose. Glucose is absorbed as described above.

■ METABOLISM OF CARBOHYDRATES

Metabolism is the process in which food substances undergo chemical and energy transformation. After digestion and absorption, food substances must be utilized by the body. The utilization occurs mainly by oxidative process in which the carbohydrates, proteins and lipids are burnt slowly to release energy. This process is known as catabolism.

Part of the released energy is utilized by tissues for physiological actions and rest of the energy is stored as rich energy phosphate bonds and in the form of proteins, carbohydrates and lipids in the tissues. This process is called anabolism.

Metabolism of carbohydrates is given in the form of schematic diagram (Fig. 45.1).

■ DIETARY FIBER

Dietary fiber or roughage is a group of food particles which pass through stomach and small intestine, without being digested and reach the large intestine unchanged. Other nutritive substances of food are digested and absorbed before reaching large intestine.

Characteristic feature of dietary fiber is that it is not digestible by digestive enzymes. So it escapes digestion in small intestine and passes to large intestine. It provides substrate for microflora of large intestine and increases the bacterial mass. The anaerobic bacteria in turn, degrade the fermentable components of the fiber. Thus, in large intestine, some of the components of fiber are broken down and absorbed and remaining components are excreted through feces.

Components of Dietary Fiber

Major components of dietary fiber are cellulose, hemicelluloses, D-glucans, pectin, lignin and gums. Cellulose, hemicelluloses and pectin are partially degradable, while other components are indigestible. Dietary fiber also contains minerals, antioxidants and other chemicals that are useful for health.

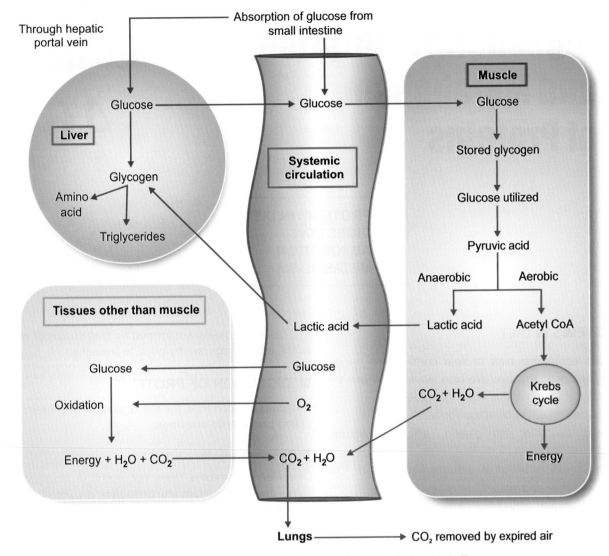

FIGURE 45.1: Schematic diagram of carbohydrate metabolism

Source of Dietary Fiber

Source of dietary fiber are fruits, vegetables, cereals, bread and wheat grain (particularly its outer layer).

Health Benefits of Dietary Fiber

1. By intake of high dietary fiber food, some disease-producing food substances may be decreased in quantity or completely excluded in diet
2. Dietary fiber helps in weight maintenance because it requires more chewing and promotes **hunger satisfaction** by delaying the emptying of stomach and by giving the person a sense of fullness of stomach

3. Diet with high fiber content tends to be low in energy and it is also useful in reducing the body weight
4. Dietary fiber increases the formation of bulk and soft feces and eases defecation
5. It contains some useful substances such as antioxidants
6. Some components of dietary fiber also reduce blood cholesterol level and thereby, decrease the risk of some diseases such as **coronary heart disease** and **gallstones**
7. Dietary fiber is also suggested to prevent or to treat some disorders such as **constipation, bowel syndrome, diabetics, ulcer** and **cancer.**

Digestion, Absorption and Metabolism of Proteins

Chapter 46

- ■ PROTEINS IN DIET
- ■ DIGESTION
- ■ ABSORPTION
- ■ METABOLISM

■ PROTEINS IN DIET

Foodstuffs containing high protein content are meat, fish, egg and milk. Proteins are also available in wheat, soybeans, oats and various types of pulses.

Proteins present in common foodstuffs are:

1. *Wheat:* Glutenin and gliadin, which constitute gluten
2. *Milk:* Casein, lactalbumin, albumin and myosin
3. *Egg:* Albumin and vitellin
4. *Meat:* Collagen, albumin and myosin.

Dietary proteins are formed by long chains of amino acids, bound together by peptide linkages.

■ DIGESTION OF PROTEINS

Enzymes responsible for the digestion of proteins are called **proteolytic enzymes.**

■ IN THE MOUTH

Digestion of proteins does not occur in mouth, since saliva does not contain any proteolytic enzymes. So, the digestion of proteins starts only in stomach (Table 46.1).

TABLE 46.1: Digestion of proteins

Area	Juice	Enzyme	Substrate	End product
Mouth	Saliva	No proteolytic enzyme	Polysaccharides – cooked starch	Disaccharides – dextrin and maltose
Stomach	Gastric juice	Pepsin	Proteins	Proteoses, peptones, large polypeptides
Small intestine	Pancreatic juice	Trypsin	Proteoses Peptones	Dipeptides Tripeptides Polypeptides
		Chymotrypsin		
		Carboxypeptidases A and B	Dipeptides Tripeptides Polypeptides	Amino acids
	Succus entericus	Dipeptidases	Dipeptides	Amino acids
		Tripeptidases	Tripeptides	
		Amino peptidases	Large polypeptides	

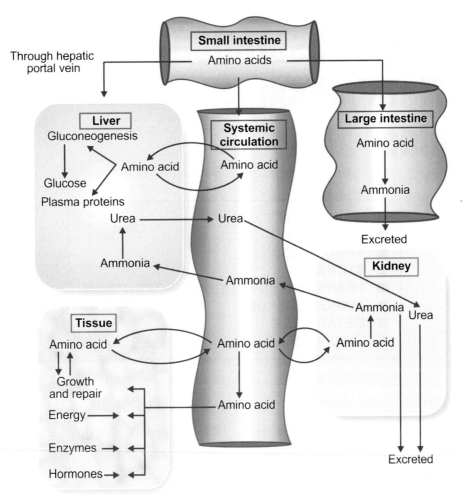

FIGURE 46.1: Schematic diagram of protein metabolism

■ IN THE STOMACH

Pepsin is the only proteolytic enzyme in gastric juice (Chapter 38). **Rennin** is also present in gastric juice. But it is absent in human.

■ IN THE SMALL INTESTINE

Most of the proteins are digested in the duodenum and jejunum by the proteolytic enzymes of the pancreatic juice and succus entericus.

Proteolytic Enzymes in Pancreatic Juice

Pancreatic juice contains **trypsin, chymotrypsin** and **carboxypeptidases.** Trypsin and chymotrypsin are called **endopeptidases,** as these two enzymes break the interior bonds of the protein molecules (Chapter 39).

Proteolytic Enzymes in Succus Entericus

Final digestion of proteins is by the proteolytic enzymes present in the succus entericus. It contains **dipeptidases, tripeptidases** and **aminopeptidases** (Chapter 41).

■ FINAL PRODUCTS OF PROTEIN DIGESTION

Final products of protein digestion are the amino acids, which are absorbed into blood from intestine.

■ ABSORPTION OF PROTEINS

Proteins are absorbed in the form of amino acids from small intestine. The levo amino acids are actively absorbed by means of **sodium cotransport,** whereas, the dextro amino acids are absorbed by means of **facilitated diffusion.**

Absorption of amino acids is faster in duodenum and jejunum and slower in ileum.

■ METABOLISM OF PROTEINS

Metabolism of proteins is given in the form of a schematic diagram (Fig. 46.1).

Digestion, Absorption and Metabolism of Lipids

Chapter 47

- **LIPIDS IN DIET**
- **DIGESTION**
- **ABSORPTION**
- **STORAGE**
- **TRANSPORT IN BLOOD – LIPOPROTEINS**
- **ADIPOSE TISSUE**
- **METABOLISM**
- **LIPID PROFILE**

■ LIPIDS IN DIET

Lipids are mostly consumed in the form of **neutral fats,** which are also known as **triglycerides.** Triglycerides are made up of glycerol nucleus and free fatty acids. Triglycerides form the major constituent in foods of animal origin and much less in foods of plant origin. Apart from triglycerides, usual diet also contains small quantities of **cholesterol** and **cholesterol esters.**

Dietary fats are classified into two types:
1. Saturated fats
2. Unsaturated fats.

■ SATURATED FATS

Saturated fats are the fats which contain triglycerides formed from only saturated fatty acids. The fatty acids having maximum amount of hydrogen ions without any double bonds between carbon atoms are called saturated fatty acids.

■ UNSATURATED FATS

Fats containing unsaturated fatty acids are known as unsaturated fats. Unsaturated fatty acids are fatty acids formed by dehydrogenation of saturated fatty acids.

Unsaturated fats are classified into three types:
1. Monounsaturated fats
2. Polyunsaturated fats
3. Trans fats.

1. *Monounsaturated Fats*

Unsaturated fats which contain one double bond between the carbon atoms are called monounsaturated fats.

2. *Polyunsaturated Fats*

Unsaturated fats with more than one double bond between the carbon atoms are called polyunsaturated fats. Polyunsaturated fats belong to the family of essential fatty acids (fatty acids required in diet).

Polyunsaturated fats are of two types:
1. **Omega-3** fats or omega-3 fatty acids having double bond in the third space from the end of the carbon chain
2. **Omega-6** fats or omega-6 fatty acids having double bond in the sixth space from the end of the carbon chain.

Both omega-3 and omega-6 fatty acids are beneficial to the body. However, consuming too much of omega-6 fatty acids results in hazards than benefits. So, the diet containing 3 : 1 ratio of omega-6 to omega-3 fatty acids is often recommended by experts.

3. *Trans Fats*

Trans fats or trans fatty acids are unsaturated fatty acids, with molecules containing trans (across or opposite side) double bonds between carbon atoms.

Sources and the functions of the different types of dietary fats are listed in Table 47.1.

■ DIGESTION OF LIPIDS

Lipids are digested by **lipolytic enzymes.**

■ IN THE MOUTH

Saliva contains **lingual lipase.** This enzyme is secreted by lingual glands of mouth and swallowed along with saliva. So, the lipid digestion does not commence in the mouth (Table 47.2) (Chapter 37).

■ IN THE STOMACH

Gastric lipase or **tributyrase** is the lipolytic enzyme present in gastric juice (Chapter 38).

■ IN THE INTESTINE

Almost all the lipids are digested in the small intestine because of the availability of bile salts, **pancreatic lipolytic enzymes** and **intestinal lipase.**

Role of Bile Salts

Bile salts play an important role in the digestion of lipids (Chapter 40).

Lipolytic Enzymes in Pancreatic Juice

Pancreatic lipase is the most important enzyme for the digestion of fats. Other lipolytic enzymes of pancreatic juice are cholesterol ester hydrolase, phospholipase A and phospholipase B (Chapter 39).

Lipolytic Enzyme in Succus Entericus

Intestinal lipase is the only lipolytic enzyme present in succus entericus (Chapter 41).

■ FINAL PRODUCTS OF FAT DIGESTION

Fatty acids, cholesterol and monoglycerides are the final products of lipid digestion.

■ ABSORPTION OF LIPIDS

Monoglycerides, cholesterol and fatty acids from the micelles enter the cells of intestinal mucosa by simple diffusion.

From here, further transport occurs as follows:

1. In the mucosal cells, most of the monoglycerides are converted into triglycerides. Triglycerides are also formed by **re-esterification** of fatty acids with more than 10 to 12 carbon atoms. Some of the cholesterol is also esterified.

TABLE 47.1: Sources and functions of dietary fats

Type of fat	Sources	Functions
Saturated fats	Full fat milk, cheese, cream, butter. Commercially baked biscuits and pastries Deep-fried fast food Coconut oil and palm oil Fatty meat	Increase blood cholesterol and thereby increase the risk of atherosclerosis and coronary heart diseases
Monounsaturated fats	Oils (canola, olive and peanut oils) Nuts (cashews, almonds, hazelnuts and peanuts) Margarine	Decrease blood cholesterol and thereby decrease the risk of coronary heart diseases
Polyunsaturated fats	*Fruits and vegetables* Vegetable oils (sunflower, safflower, corn or soy oils) Nuts (walnuts) Flax seeds Polyunsaturated margarines Lean meat Fish and sea foods Egg	*Decrease* Blood cholesterol and triglycerides and thereby reduces blood pressure Risk of coronary heart diseases Risk of obesity Platelet aggregation and prevents excess blood clotting Inflammation throughout body *Increase* Disease-countering actions in the body
Trans fats	Milk Cheese and table margarines Lamb and beef	Increase low density lipoproteins and thereby increase the risk of atherosclerosis and coronary heart diseases

TABLE 47.2: Digestion of lipids

Area	Juice	Enzyme	Substrate	End product
Mouth	Saliva	Lingual lipase	Triglycerides	Fatty acid 1, 2-diacylglycerol
Stomach	Gastric juice	Gastric lipase (weak lipase)	Triglycerides	Fatty acids Glycerol
Small intestine	Pancreatic juice	Pancreatic lipase	Triglycerides	Monoglycerides Fatty acid
		Cholesterol ester hydrolase	Cholesterol ester	Free cholesterol Fatty acid
		Phospholipase A	Phospholipids	Lysophospholipids
		Phospholipase B	Lysophospholipids	Phosphoryl choline Free fatty acids
		Colipase	Facilitates action of pancreatic lipase	–
		Bile-salt-activated lipase	Phospholipids	Lysophospholipids
			Cholesterol esters	Cholesterol and fatty acids
	Succus entericus	Intestinal lipase	Triglycerides	Fatty acids Glycerol (weak action)

Triglycerides and cholesterol esters are coated with a layer of protein, cholesterol and phospholipids to form the particles called **chylomicrons.**

Chylomicrons cannot pass through the membrane of the blood capillaries because of the larger size. So, these lipid particles enter the lymph vessels and then are transferred into blood from lymph.

2. Fatty acids containing less than 10 to 12 carbon atoms enter the portal blood from mucosal cells and are transported as free fatty acids or unesterified fatty acids. Most of the fats are absorbed in the upper part of small intestine. Presence of bile is essential for fat absorption.

■ STORAGE OF LIPIDS

Lipids are stored in adipose tissue and liver. Fat stored in adipose tissue is called **neutral fat** or **tissue fat.** When chylomicrons are traveling through capillaries of adipose tissue or liver, the enzyme called **lipoprotein lipase** present in the capillary endothelium hydrolyzes triglycerides of chylomicrons into free fatty acids (FFA) and glycerol. FFA and glycerol enter the **fat cells** (adipocytes or lipocytes) of the adipose tissue or liver cells. Then, the FFA and glycerol are again converted into triglycerides and stored in these cells. Other contents of chylomicrons such as cholesterol and phospholipids, which are released into the blood combine with proteins to form lipoproteins.

When other tissues of the body need energy, triglycerides stored in adipose tissue is hydrolyzed into FFA and glycerol. FFA is transported to the body tissues through blood.

■ TRANSPORT OF LIPIDS IN BLOOD – LIPOPROTEINS

Free fatty acids are transported in the blood in combination with albumin. Other lipids are transported in the blood, in the form of lipoproteins.

■ LIPOPROTEINS

Lipoproteins are the small particles in the blood which contain cholesterol, phospholipids, triglycerides and proteins. Proteins are beta-globulins called **apoproteins.**

Classification of Lipoproteins

Lipoproteins are classified into four types on the basis of their density:

1. *Very-low-density lipoproteins (VLDL):* Contain high concentration of triglycerides (formed from FFA and glycerol) and moderate concentration of cholesterol and phospholipids
2. *Intermediate-density lipoproteins (IDL):* Formed by the removal of large portion of triglycerides from VLDL by lipoprotein lipase. Concentration of

cholesterol and phospholipids increases because of removal of triglycerides

3. *Low-density lipoproteins (LDL):* Formed from IDL by the complete removal of triglycerides. These lipoproteins contain only cholesterol and phospholipids
4. *High-density lipoproteins (HDL):* Contain high concentrations of proteins with low concentration of cholesterol and phospholipids.

All the lipoproteins are synthesized in liver. HDL is synthesized in intestine also.

Functions of Lipoproteins

Primary function of lipoproteins is to transport the lipids via blood to and from the tissues. Functions of each type of lipoproteins are given in Table 47.3.

Importance of Lipoproteins

High-density lipoprotein

High-denisty lipoprotein (HDL) is referred as the **'good cholesterol'** because it carries cholesterol and phospholipids from tissues and organs back to the liver for degradation and elimination. It prevents the deposition of cholesterol on the walls of arteries, by carrying cholesterol away from arteries to the liver.

High level of HDL is a good indicator of a healthy heart, because it reduces the blood cholesterol level. HDL also helps in the normal functioning of some hormones and certain tissues of the body. It is also used for the formation of bile in liver.

Low-density lipoprotein

Low-density lipoprotein (LDL) is considered as the **'bad cholesterol'** because it carries cholesterol and phospholipids from the liver to different areas of the body, viz. muscles, other tissues and organs such as heart. It is responsible for deposition of cholesterol on walls of arteries causing **atherosclerosis** (blockage and hardening of the arteries). High level of LDL increases the **risk of heart disease.**

TABLE 47.3: Functions of lipoproteins

Lipoproteins	Functions
VLDL	Transports triglycerides from liver to adipose tissue
IDL	Transports triglycerides, cholesterol and phospholipids from liver to peripheral tissues
LDL	Transports cholesterol and phospholipids from liver to tissues and organs like heart
HDL	Transports cholesterol and phospholipids from tissues and organs like heart back to liver

Very-low-density lipoprotein

Very-low-density lipoprotein (VLDL) carries cholesterol from liver to organs and tissues in the body. It is also associated with **atherosclerosis** and **heart disease.**

■ ADIPOSE TISSUE

Adipose tissue or fat is a loose connective tissue that forms the storage site of fat in the form of triglycerides. It is composed of **adipocytes,** which are also called **fat cells** or **lipocytes.** Obesity does not depend on the body weight, but on the amount of body fat, specifically adipose tissue.

Adipose tissue is of two types, white adipose tissue and brown adipose tissue.

■ WHITE ADIPOSE TISSUE OR WHITE FAT

White adipose tissue is distributed through the body beneath the skin, forming **subcutaneous fat.** It also surrounds the internal organs. This adipose tissue is formed by fat cells which are **unilocular,** i.e. these cells contain one large vacuole filled with fat.

Functions of White Adipose Tissue

White adipose tissue has three functions:

1. Storage of energy: Main function of white adipose tissue is the storage of lipids. Utilization or storage of fat is regulated by hormones, particularly insulin, depending upon the blood glucose level. If the blood glucose level increases, insulin stimulates synthesis and storage of fat in white adipose tissue (Chapter 69). On the other hand, if blood glucose level decreases insulin causes release of fat from adipose tissue. Released fat is utilized for energy
2. Heat insulation: **Insulation function** is due to the presence of adipose tissue beneath the skin (subcutaneous adipose tissue)
3. Protection of internal organs: White adipose tissue protects the body and internal organs by surrounding them and by acting like a **mechanical cushion.**

■ BROWN ADIPOSE TISSUE OR BROWN FAT

Brown adipose tissue is a specialized form of adipose tissue, having the function opposite to that of white adipose tissue. It is present only in certain areas of the body such as back of neck and intrascapular region. It is abundant in infants forming about 5% of total adipose tissue. After infancy, brown adipose tissue disappears gradually and forms only about 1% of total adipose tissue in adults. It is formed by fat cells which are **multilocular,** i.e. these cells contain many small

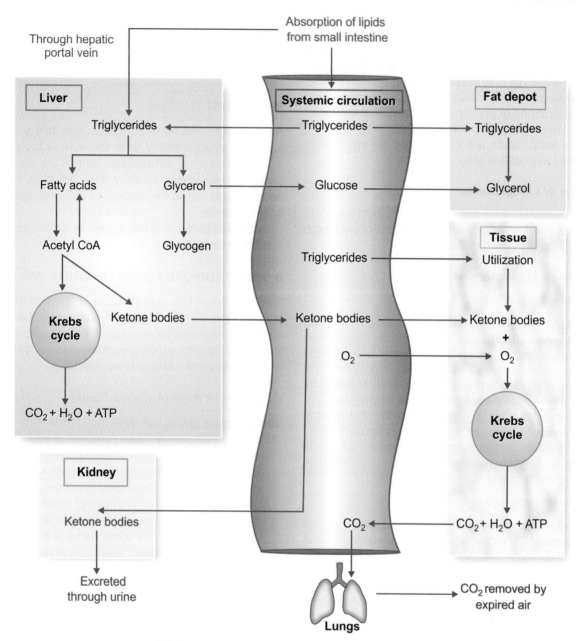

FIGURE 47.1: Schematic diagram of lipid metabolism

vacuoles filled with fat. The coloration of this adipose tissue is due to high vascularization and large number of **iron-rich mitochondria.**

Functions of Brown Adipose Tissue

Brown adipose tissue does not store lipids but generates heat by burning lipids. In infants and hibernating animals, brown adipose tissue plays an important role in regulating body temperature via **non-shivering thermogenesis.** Heat production in brown fat is very essential for survival of infants and small animals in cold environment. It is because, the lipid in this tissue releases energy directly as heat.

The mitochondria found in brown adipose tissue contain a unique uncoupling protein called **mitochondrial uncoupling protein 1** (UCP1). Also called **thermogenin,** this protein allows the controlled entry of protons without adenosine triphosphate (ATP) synthesis, in order to generate heat.

TABLE 47.4: Values of lipid profile

Lipids	Desirable optimal level	Borderline range	High-risk level
Total cholesterol	< 200 mg/dL	200 to 240 mg/dL	> 240 mg/dL
Triglycerides	< 150 mg/dL	150 to 200 mg/dL	> 200 mg/dL
HDL	> 60 mg/dL	40 to 60 mg/dL	< 40 mg/dL
LDL	< 60 mg/dL	60 to 100 mg/dL	> 100 mg/dL
Total cholesterol – HDL ratio	< 2	2 to 6	> 6

■ METABOLISM OF LIPIDS

Metabolism of lipids is given in the form of schematic diagram (Fig. 47.1).

■ LIPID PROFILE

Lipid profile is a group of **blood tests** which are carried out to determine the risk of **coronary artery diseases** (CAD). Results of lipid profile are considered as good indicators of whether someone is prone to develop **stroke** or **heart attack,** caused by **atherosclerosis.** In order to plan the course of treatment, the results of the lipid profile are correlated with age, sex and other risk factors of heart disease.

Tests included in lipid profile are total cholesterol, triglyceride, HDL, LDL, VLDL and total cholesterol – HDL ratio.

Total cholesterol to HDL ratio is helpful in predicting atherosclerosis and CAD. It is obtained by dividing total cholesterol by HDL. High total cholesterol and low HDL increases the ratio. The increase in the ratio is undesirable. Conversely, high HDL and low total cholesterol lowers the ratio and the decrease in the ratio is desirable. The values of lipid profile are given in Table 47.4.

QUESTIONS IN DIGESTIVE SYSTEM

■ LONG QUESTIONS

1. What are the different types of salivary glands? Describe the composition, functions and regulation of secretion of saliva.
2. Explain the composition and functions of gastric juice and give an account of hormonal regulation of gastric secretion.
3. Describe the different phases of gastric secretion with experimental evidences.
4. Explain the composition, functions and regulation of secretion of pancreatic juice.
5. Describe the composition, functions and regulation of secretion of bile. Enumerate the differences between the liver bile and gallbladder bile. Add a note on enterohepatic circulation.
6. Give an account of succus entericus.
7. Write an essay on gastric motility. What are the factors influencing gastric emptying?
8. Describe in detail, the gastrointestinal movements.

■ SHORT QUESTIONS

1. Properties and composition of saliva.
2. Functions of saliva.
3. Nerve supply to salivary glands.
4. Glands of stomach.
5. Functions of stomach.
6. Properties and composition of gastric juice.
7. Functions of gastric juice.
8. Mechanism of secretion of hydrochloric acid in stomach.
9. Pavlov's pouch.
10. Sham feeding.
11. Cephalic phase of gastric secretion.
12. Gastrin.
13. Hormones acting on stomach.
14. FTM.
15. Peptic ulcer.
16. Exocrine function of pancreas.
17. Properties and composition of pancreatic juice.
18. Functions of pancreatic juice.
19. Regulation of exocrine function of pancreas.
20. Steatorrhea.
21. Secretin.
22. Cholecystokinin.
23. Composition of bile.
24. Functions of bile.
25. Bile salts.
26. Bile pigments.
27. Enterohepatic circulation.
28. Functions of liver.
29. Differences between liver bile and gallbladder bile.
30. Functions of gallbladder.
31. Jaundice.
32. Hepatitis.
33. Gallstones.
34. Succus entericus.
35. Functions of small intestine.
36. Functions of large intestine.
37. Mastication.
38. Swallowing.
39. Dysphagia.
40. Movements of stomach.
41. Filling and emptying of stomach.
42. Hunger contractions.
43. Vomiting.
44. Movements of small intestine.
45. Peristalsis.
46. Movements of large intestine.
47. Defecation.
48. Constipation.
49. Diarrhea.
50. Gastrointestinal hormones.
51. Digestion and absorption of carbohydrates.
52. Dietary fiber.
53. Digestion and absorption of proteins.
54. Digestion and absorption of lipids.
55. Lipoproteins.
56. Brown fat.

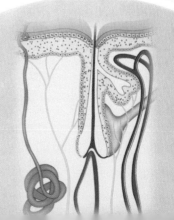

Section
5

Renal Physiology and Skin

Kidney

- ■ **INTRODUCTION**
- ■ **FUNCTIONS OF KIDNEY**
  - ■ ROLE IN HOMEOSTASIS
  - ■ HEMOPOIETIC FUNCTION
  - ■ ENDOCRINE FUNCTION
  - ■ REGULATION OF BLOOD PRESSURE
  - ■ REGULATION OF BLOOD CALCIUM LEVEL
- ■ **FUNCTIONAL ANATOMY OF KIDNEY**
  - ■ DIFFERENT LAYERS OF KIDNEY
  - ■ TUBULAR STRUCTURES OF KIDNEY

■ INTRODUCTION

Excretion is the process by which the unwanted substances and metabolic wastes are eliminated from the body.

A large amount of waste materials and carbon dioxide are produced in the tissues during metabolic process. In addition, residue of undigested food, heavy metals, drugs, toxic substances and pathogenic organisms like bacteria are also present in the body.

All these substances must be removed to keep the body in healthy condition. Various systems/organs in the body are involved in performing the excretory function, viz.

1. **Digestive system** excretes food residues in the form of feces. Some bacteria and toxic substances also are excreted through feces
2. **Lungs** remove carbon dioxide and water vapor
3. **Skin** excretes water, salts and some wastes. It also removes heat from the body
4. **Liver** excretes many substances like bile pigments, heavy metals, drugs, toxins, bacteria, etc. through bile.

Although various organs are involved in removal of wastes from the body, their excretory capacity is limited. But renal system or urinary system has maximum excretory capacity and so it plays a major role in homeostasis.

Renal system includes:

1. A pair of kidneys
2. Ureters
3. Urinary bladder
4. Urethra.

Kidneys produce the urine. Ureters transport the urine to urinary bladder. Urinary bladder stores the urine until it is voided (emptied). Urine is voided from bladder through urethra (Fig. 48.1).

■ FUNCTIONS OF KIDNEY

Kidneys perform several vital functions besides formation of urine. By excreting urine, kidneys play the principal role in homeostasis. Thus, the functions of kidney are:

■ 1. ROLE IN HOMEOSTASIS

Primary function of kidneys is **homeostasis.** It is accomplished by the formation of urine. During the formation of urine, kidneys regulate various activities in the body, which are concerned with homeostasis such as:

i. *Excretion of Waste Products*

Kidneys excrete the unwanted waste products, which are formed during metabolic activities:

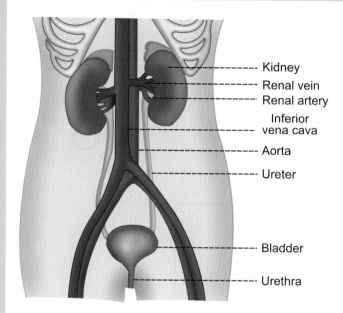

FIGURE 48.1: Urinary system

a. Urea (end product of amino acid metabolism)
b. Uric acid (end product of nucleic acid metabolism)
c. Creatinine (end product of metabolism in muscles)
d. Bilirubin (end product of hemoglobin degradation)
e. Products of metabolism of other substances.

Kidneys also excrete harmful foreign chemical substances such as toxins, drugs, heavy metals pesticides, etc.

ii. *Maintenance of Water Balance*

Kidneys maintain the water balance in the body by conserving water when it is decreased and excreting water when it is excess in the body. This is an important process for homeostasis (Refer Chapter 4 for details).

iii. *Maintenance of Electrolyte Balance*

Maintenance of electrolyte balance, especially sodium is in relation to water balance. Kidneys retain sodium if the **osmolarity** of body water decreases and eliminate sodium when osmolarity increases.

iv. *Maintenance of Acid–Base Balance*

The pH of the blood and body fluids should be maintained within narrow range for healthy living. It is achieved by the function of kidneys (Chapter 54). Body is under constant threat to develop **acidosis**, because of production of lot of acids during metabolic activities. However, it is prevented by kidneys, lungs and blood buffers, which eliminate these acids. Among these organs, kidneys play major role in preventing acidosis. In fact, kidneys are the only organs, which are capable of eliminating certain metabolic acids like sulfuric and phosphoric acids.

■ 2. HEMOPOIETIC FUNCTION

Kidneys stimulate the production of erythrocytes by secreting **erythropoietin.** Erythropoietin is the important stimulating factor for erythropoiesis (Chapter 10). Kidney also secretes another factor called **thrombopoietin,** which stimulates the production of thrombocytes (Chapter 18).

■ 3. ENDOCRINE FUNCTION

Kidneys secrete many hormonal substances in addition to erythropoietin and thrombopoietin (Chapter 72).

Hormones secreted by kidneys

   i. Erythropoietin
  ii. Thrombopoietin
 iii. Renin
 iv. 1,25-dihydroxycholecalciferol (calcitriol)
  v. Prostaglandins.

■ 4. REGULATION OF BLOOD PRESSURE

Kidneys play an important role in the long-term regulation of arterial blood pressure (Chapter 103) by two ways:
   i. By regulating the volume of extracellular fluid
  ii. Through **renin-angiotensin** mechanism.

■ 5. REGULATION OF BLOOD CALCIUM LEVEL

Kidneys play a role in the regulation of blood calcium level by activating 1,25-dihydroxycholecalciferol into **vitamin D.** Vitamin D is necessary for the absorption of calcium from intestine (Chapter 68).

■ FUNCTIONAL ANATOMY OF KIDNEY

Kidney is a compound tubular gland covered by a connective tissue capsule. There is a depression on the medial border of kidney called hilum, through which renal artery, renal veins, nerves and ureter pass.

■ DIFFERENT LAYERS OF KIDNEY

Components of kidney are arranged in three layers (Fig. 48.2):
1. Outer cortex
2. Inner medulla
3. Renal sinus.

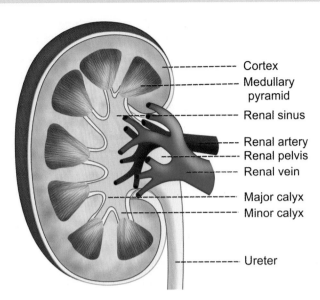

FIGURE 48.2: Longitudinal section of kidney

Cortex
Medullary pyramid
Renal sinus
Renal artery
Renal pelvis
Renal vein
Major calyx
Minor calyx
Ureter

1. *Outer Cortex*

Cortex is dark and granular in appearance. It contains renal corpuscles and convoluted tubules. At intervals, cortical tissue penetrates medulla in the form of columns, which are called renal columns or **columns of Bertini.**

2. *Inner Medulla*

Medulla contains tubular and vascular structures arranged in parallel radial lines. Medullary mass is divided into 8 to 18 **medullary** or **Malpighian pyramids.** Broad base of each pyramid is in contact with cortex and the apex projects into **minor calyx.**

3. *Renal Sinus*

Renal sinus consists of the following structures:
  i. Upper expanded part of ureter called **renal pelvis**
  ii. Subdivisions of pelvis: 2 or 3 **major calyces** and about 8 minor calyces
  iii. Branches of nerves, arteries and tributaries of veins
  iv. Loose connective tissues and fat.

■ TUBULAR STRUCTURES OF KIDNEY

Kidney is made up of closely arranged tubular structures called **uriniferous tubules.** Blood vessels and interstitial connective tissues are interposed between these tubules.

Uriniferous tubules include:
1. Terminal or secretary tubules called **nephrons,** which are concerned with formation of urine
2. **Collecting ducts** or tubules, which are concerned with transport of urine from nephrons to pelvis of ureter.

Collecting ducts unite to form **ducts of Bellini,** which open into minor calyces through **papilla.** Other details are given in Chapter 49.

Nephron

- ■ INTRODUCTION
- ■ RENAL CORPUSCLE
  - ■ SITUATION – TYPES OF NEPHRON
  - ■ STRUCTURE
- ■ TUBULAR PORTION OF NEPHRON
  - ■ PROXIMAL CONVOLUTED TUBULE
  - ■ LOOP OF HENLE
  - ■ DISTAL CONVOLUTED TUBULE
- ■ COLLECTING DUCT
- ■ PASSAGE OF URINE

■ INTRODUCTION

Nephron is defined as the structural and functional unit of kidney. Each kidney consists of 1 to 1.3 millions of nephrons. The number of nephrons starts decreasing after about 45 to 50 years of age at the rate of 0.8% to 1% every year.

Each nephron is formed by two parts (Fig. 49.1):
1. A blind end called renal corpuscle or **Malpighian corpuscle**
2. A tubular portion called **renal tubule.**

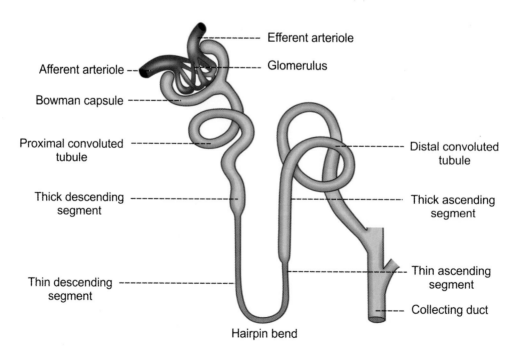

Afferent arteriole
Bowman capsule
Proximal convoluted tubule
Thick descending segment
Thin descending segment
Hairpin bend
Efferent arteriole
Glomerulus
Distal convoluted tubule
Thick ascending segment
Thin ascending segment
Collecting duct

FIGURE 49.1: Structure of nephron

■ RENAL CORPUSCLE

Renal corpuscle or Malpighian corpuscle is a spheroidal and slightly flattened structure with a diameter of about 200 μ.

Function of the renal corpuscle is the filtration of blood which forms the first phase of urine formation.

■ SITUATION OF RENAL CORPUSCLE AND TYPES OF NEPHRON

Renal corpuscle is situated in the cortex of the kidney either near the periphery or near the medulla.

Classification of Nephrons

Based on the situation of renal corpuscle, the nephrons are classified into two types:

1. **Cortical nephrons** or superficial nephrons: Nephrons having the corpuscles in outer cortex of the kidney near the periphery (Fig. 49.2). In human kidneys, 85% nephrons are cortical nephrons.

2. **Juxtamedullary nephrons:** Nephrons having the corpuscles in inner cortex near medulla or corticomedullary junction.

Features of the two types of nephrons are given in Table 49.1.

■ STRUCTURE OF RENAL CORPUSCLE

Renal corpuscle is formed by two portions:
1. Glomerulus
2. Bowman capsule.

Glomerulus

Glomerulus is a tuft of capillaries enclosed by Bowman capsule. It consists of glomerular capillaries interposed between afferent arteriole on one end and efferent arteriole on the other end. Thus, the vascular system in the glomerulus is purely arterial (Fig. 49.3).

Glomerular capillaries arise from the afferent arteriole. After entering the Bowman capsule, the afferent

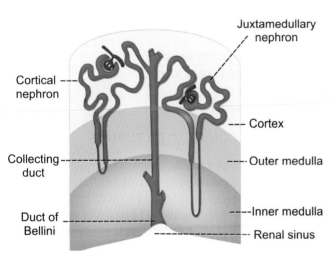

FIGURE 49.2: Types of nephron

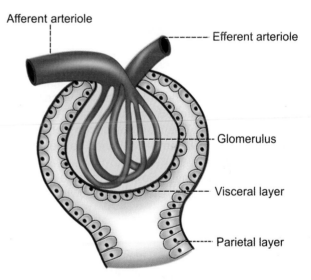

FIGURE 49.3: Renal corpuscle

TABLE 49.1: Features of two types of nephron

Features	Cortical nephron	Juxtamedullary nephron
Percentage	85%	15%
Situation of renal corpuscle	Outer cortex near the periphery	Inner cortex near medulla
Loop of Henle	Short	Long
	Hairpin bend penetrates only up to outer zone of medulla	Hairpin bend penetrates up to the tip of papilla
Blood supply to tubule	Peritubular capillaries	Vasa recta
Function	Formation of urine	Mainly the concentration of urine and also formation of urine

arteriole divides into 4 or 5 large capillaries. Each large capillary subdivides into many small capillaries. These small capillaries are arranged in irregular loops and form anastomosis. All the smaller capillaries finally reunite to form the efferent arteriole, which leaves the Bowman capsule.

Diameter of the efferent arteriole is less than that of afferent arteriole. This difference in diameter has got functional significance.

Functional histology

Glomerular capillaries are made up of single layer of endothelial cells, which are attached to a basement membrane. Endothelium has many pores called **fenestrae** or **filtration pores.** Diameter of each pore is 0.1 μ. Presence of the fenestra is the evidence of the filtration function of the glomerulus.

Bowman Capsule

Bowman capsule is a capsular structure, which encloses the glomerulus.

It is formed by two layers:
  i. Inner visceral layer
  ii. Outer parietal layer.

Visceral layer covers the glomerular capillaries. It is continued as the parietal layer at the visceral pole. Parietal layer is continued with the wall of the tubular portion of nephron. The cleft-like space between the visceral and parietal layers is continued as the lumen of the tubular portion.

Functional anatomy of Bowman capsule resembles a funnel with filter paper. Diameter of Bowman capsule is 200 μ.

Functional histology

Both the layers of Bowman capsule are composed of a single layer of flattened epithelial cells resting on a basement membrane. Basement membrane of the visceral layer fuses with the basement membrane of glomerular capillaries on which the capillary endothelial cells are arranged. Thus, the basement membranes, which are fused together, form the separation between the glomerular capillary endothelium and the epithelium of visceral layer of Bowman capsule.

Epithelial cells of the visceral layer fuse with the basement membrane but the fusion is not complete. Each cell is connected with basement membrane by cytoplasmic extensions of epithelial cells called **pedicles** or feet. These pedicles are arranged in an interdigitating manner leaving small cleft-like spaces in between. The cleft-like space is called **slit pore.** Epithelial cells with pedicles are called **podocytes** (Fig. 49.4).

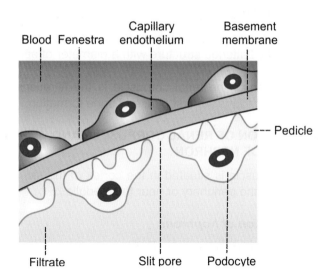

FIGURE 49.4: Filtering membrane in renal corpuscle. It is formed by capillary endothelium on one side (red) and visceral layer of Bowman capsule (yellow) on the other side.

■ TUBULAR PORTION OF NEPHRON

Tubular portion of nephron is the continuation of Bowman capsule.

It is made up of three parts:
1. Proximal convoluted tubule
2. Loop of Henle
3. Distal convoluted tubule.

■ PROXIMAL CONVOLUTED TUBULE

Proximal convoluted tubule is the coiled portion arising from Bowman capsule. It is situated in the cortex. It is continued as descending limb of loop of Henle. Length of proximal convoluted tubule is 14 mm and the diameter is 55 μ. Proximal convoluted tubule is continued as loop of Henle.

Functional histology

Proximal convoluted tubule is formed by single layer of cuboidal epithelial cells. Characteristic feature of these cells is the presence of hair-like projections directed towards the lumen of the tubule. Because of the presence of these projections, the epithelial cells are called **brush-bordered cells.**

■ LOOP OF HENLE

Loop of Henle consists of:
  i.   Descending limb
  ii. Hairpin bend
  iii. Ascending limb.

i. Descending Limb

Descending limb of loop of Henle is made up of two segments:
   a. Thick descending segment
   b. Thin descending segment.

Thick descending segment

Thick descending segment is the direct continuation of the proximal convoluted tubule. It descends down into medulla. It has a length of 6 mm and a diameter of 55 μ. It is formed by brush-bordered cuboidal epithelial cells.

Thin descending segment

Thick descending segment is continued as thin descending segment (Fig. 49.5). It is formed by flattened epithelial cells without brush border and it is continued as hairpin bend of the loop.

ii. Hairpin Bend

Hairpin bend formed by flattened epithelial cells without brush border and it is continued as the ascending limb of loop of Henle.

iii. Ascending Limb

Ascending limb or segment of Henle loop has two parts:
   a. Thin ascending segment
   b. Thick ascending segment.

Thin ascending segment

Thin ascending segment is the continuation of hairpin bend. It is also lined by flattened epithelial cells without brush border.

Total length of thin descending segment, hairpin bend and thin ascending segment of Henle loop is 10 mm to 15 mm and the diameter is 15 μ.

Thin ascending segment is continued as thick ascending segment.

Thick ascending segment

Thick ascending segment is about 9 mm long with a diameter of 30 μ. Thick ascending segment is lined by cuboidal epithelial cells without brush border.

The terminal portion of thick ascending segment, which runs between the afferent and efferent arterioles of the same nephrons forms the **macula densa**. Macula densa is the part of juxtaglomerular apparatus (Chapter 50).

Thick ascending segment ascends to the cortex and continues as distal convoluted tubule.

Length and Extent of Loop of Henle

Length and the extent of the loop of Henle vary in different nephrons:
   i. In cortical nephrons, it is short and the hairpin bend penetrates only up to outer medulla

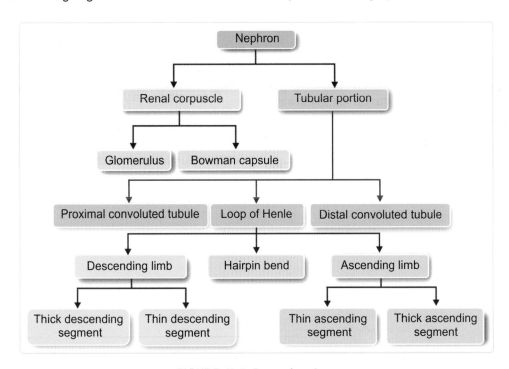

FIGURE 49.5: Parts of nephron

TABLE 49.2: Size and cells of different parts of nephron and collecting duct

Segment	Epithelium	Length (mm)	Diameter (μ)
Bowman Capsule	Flattened epithelium	-	200
Proximal convoluted tubule	Cuboidal cells with brush border	14	55
Thick descending segment	Cuboidal cells with brush border	6	55
Thin descending segment, hairpin bend and thin ascending segment	Flattened epithelium	10 to 15	15
Thick ascending segment	Cuboidal epithelium without brush border	9	30
Distal convoluted tubule	Cuboidal epithelium without brush border	14.5 to 15	22 to 50
Collecting duct	Cuboidal epithelium without brush border	20 to 22	40 to 200

ii. In juxtamedullary nephrons, this is long and the hairpin bend extends deep into the inner medulla. In some nephrons it even runs up to the papilla.

■ **DISTAL CONVOLUTED TUBULE**

Distal convoluted tubule is the continuation of thick ascending segment and occupies the cortex of kidney. It is continued as collecting duct. The length of the distal convoluted tubule is 14.5 to 15 mm. It has a diameter of 22 to 50 μ (Table 49.2).

Functional histology

Distal convoluted tubule is lined by single layer of cuboidal epithelial cells without brush border. Epithelial cells in distal convoluted tubule are called intercalated cells (I cells).

■ **COLLECTING DUCT**

Distal convoluted tubule continues as the initial or arched collecting duct, which is in cortex. The lower part of the collecting duct lies in medulla. Seven to ten initial collecting ducts unite to form the straight collecting duct, which passes through medulla.

Length of the collecting duct is 20 to 22 mm and its diameter varies between 40 and 200 μ. Collecting duct is formed by cuboidal or columnar epithelial cells.

Functional histology

Collecting duct is formed by two types of epithelial cells:
1. Principal or **P cells**
2. Intercalated or **I cells.**

These two types of cells have some functional significance (Chapters 53 and 54).

■ **PASSAGE OF URINE**

At the inner zone of medulla, the straight collecting ducts from each medullary pyramid unite to form **papillary ducts** or **ducts of Bellini,** which open into a 'V' shaped area called **papilla.** Urine from each medullary pyramid is collected in the papilla. From here it is drained into a **minor calyx.** Three or four minor calyces unite to form one **major calyx.** Each kidney has got about 8 minor calyces and 2 to 3 major calyces.

From minor calyces urine passes through major calyces, which open into the **pelvis** of the **ureter.** Pelvis is the expanded portion of ureter present in the renal sinus.

From renal pelvis, urine passes through remaining portion of ureter and reaches urinary bladder.

Juxtaglomerular Apparatus

Chapter 50

- ■ **DEFINITION**
- ■ **STRUCTURE**
  - ■ MACULA DENSA
  - ■ EXTRAGLOMERULAR MESANGIAL CELLS
  - ■ JUXTAGLOMERULAR CELLS
- ■ **FUNCTIONS**
  - ■ SECRETION OF HORMONES
  - ■ SECRETION OF OTHER SUBSTANCES
  - ■ REGULATION OF GLOMERULAR BLOOD FLOW AND GLOMERULAR FILTRATION RATE

■ DEFINITION

Juxtaglomerular apparatus is a specialized organ situated near the glomerulus of each nephron (juxta = near).

■ STRUCTURE OF JUXTAGLOMERULAR APPARATUS

Juxtaglomerular apparatus is formed by three different structures (Fig. 50.1):
1. Macula densa
2. Extraglomerular mesangial cells
3. Juxtaglomerular cells.

■ MACULA DENSA

Macula densa is the end portion of thick ascending segment before it opens into distal convoluted tubule. It is situated between afferent and efferent arterioles of the same nephron. It is very close to afferent arteriole.

Macula densa is formed by tightly packed cuboidal epithelial cells.

■ EXTRAGLOMERULAR MESANGIAL CELLS

Extraglomerular mesangial cells are situated in the triangular region bound by afferent arteriole, efferent arteriole and macula densa. These cells are also called **agranular cells, lacis cells** or **Goormaghtigh cells.**

Glomerular Mesangial Cells

Besides extraglomerular mesangial cells there is another type of mesangial cells situated in between glomerular capillaries called **glomerular mesangial** or **intraglomerular mesangial cells.**

Glomerular mesangial cells support the glomerular capillary loops by surrounding the capillaries in the form of a cellular network.

These cells play an important role in regulating the glomerular filtration by their contractile property.

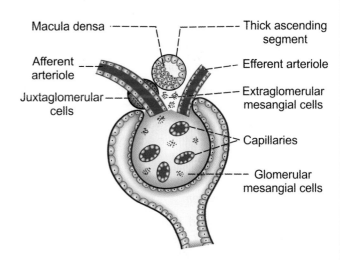

FIGURE 50.1: Juxtaglomerular apparatus

Glomerular mesangial cells are phagocytic in nature. These cells also secrete glomerular **interstitial matrix,** prostaglandins and cytokines.

■ JUXTAGLOMERULAR CELLS

Juxtaglomerular cells are specialized smooth muscle cells situated in the wall of afferent arteriole just before it enters the Bowman capsule. These smooth muscle cells are mostly present in tunica media and tunica adventitia of the wall of the afferent arteriole.

Juxtaglomerular cells are also called **granular cells** because of the presence of secretary granules in their cytoplasm.

Polar Cushion or Polkissen

Juxtaglomerular cells form a thick cuff called **polar cushion** or **polkissen** around the afferent arteriole before it enters the Bowman capsule.

■ FUNCTIONS OF JUXTAGLOMERULAR APPARATUS

Primary function of juxtaglomerular apparatus is the secretion of hormones. It also regulates the glomerular blood flow and glomerular filtration rate.

■ SECRETION OF HORMONES

Juxtaglomerular apparatus secretes two hormones:
1. Renin
2. Prostaglandin.

1. Renin

Juxtaglomerular cells secrete renin. Renin is a peptide with 340 amino acids. Along with angiotensins, renin forms the renin-angiotensin system, which is a hormone system that plays an important role in the maintenance of blood pressure (Chapter 103).

Stimulants for renin secretion

Secretion of renin is stimulated by four factors:
i.   Fall in arterial blood pressure
ii. Reduction in the ECF volume
iii. Increased sympathetic activity
iv. Decreased load of sodium and chloride in macula densa.

Renin-angiotensin system

When renin is released into the blood, it acts on a specific plasma protein called **angiotensinogen** or **renin substrate.** It is the α_2-globulin. By the activity of renin, the angiotensinogen is converted into a **decapeptide** called angiotensin I. Angiotensin I is converted into angiotensin II, which is an **octapeptide** by the activity of **angiotensin-converting enzyme** (ACE) secreted from lungs. Most of the conversion of angiotensin I into angiotensin II takes place in lungs.

Angiotensin II has a short half-life of about 1 to 2 minutes. Then it is rapidly degraded into a **heptapeptide** called angiotensin III by **angiotensinases,** which are present in RBCs and vascular beds in many tissues. Angiotensin III is converted into angiotensin IV, which is a **hexapeptide** (Fig. 50.2).

Actions of Angiotensins

Angiotensin I

Angiotensin I is physiologically inactive and serves only as the precursor of angiotensin II.

Angiotensin II

Angiotensin II is the most active form. Its actions are:

On blood vessels:
i. Angiotensin II increases arterial blood pressure by directly acting on the blood vessels and causing vasoconstriction. It is a potent constrictor of arterioles. Earlier, when its other actions were not found it was called **hypertensin.**
ii. It increases blood pressure indirectly by increasing the release of noradrenaline from postganglionic sympathetic fibers. Noradrenaline is a general vasoconstrictor (Chapter 71).

On adrenal cortex:

It stimulates zona glomerulosa of adrenal cortex to secrete aldosterone. Aldosterone acts on renal tubules and increases retention of sodium, which is also responsible for elevation of blood pressure.

On kidney:
i. Angiotensin II regulates glomerular filtration rate by two ways:
    a. It constricts the efferent arteriole, which causes decrease in filtration after an initial increase (Chapter 52)
    b. It contracts the glomerular mesangial cells leading to decrease in surface area of glomerular capillaries and filtration (see above)
ii. It increases sodium reabsorption from renal tubules. This action is more predominant on proximal tubules.

On brain:
i. Angiotensin II inhibits the **baroreceptor reflex** and thereby indirectly increases the blood pressure. Baroreceptor reflex is responsible for decreasing the blood pressure (Chapter 103)

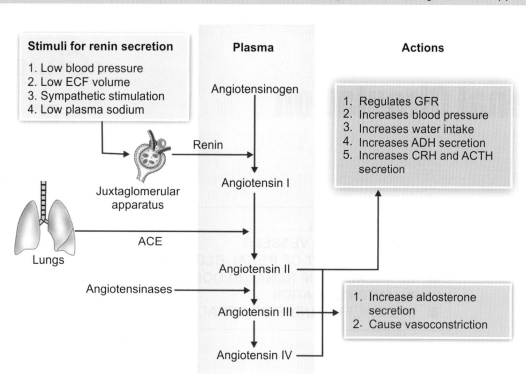

Stimuli for renin secretion

1. Low blood pressure
2. Low ECF volume
3. Sympathetic stimulation
4. Low plasma sodium

Plasma

Angiotensinogen

Renin

Juxtaglomerular apparatus

Lungs

ACE

Angiotensin I

Angiotensinases

Angiotensin II

Angiotensin III

Angiotensin IV

Actions

1. Regulates GFR
2. Increases blood pressure
3. Increases water intake
4. Increases ADH secretion
5. Increases CRH and ACTH secretion

1. Increase aldosterone secretion
2. Cause vasoconstriction

FIGURE 50.2: Renin-angiotensin system. ECF = Extracellular fluid, ACE = Angiotensin-converting enzyme, GFR = Glomerular filtration rate, ADH = Antidiuretic hormone, CRH = Corticotropin-releasing hormone, ACTH = Adrenocorticotropic hormone.

ii. It increases water intake by stimulating the thirst center

iii. It increases the secretion of orticotropin-releasing hormone (CRH) from hypothalamus. CRH in turn increases secretion of adrenocorticotropic hormone (ACTH) from pituitary

iv. It increases secretion of antidiuretic hormone (ADH) from hypothalamus.

Other actions:

Angiotensin II acts as a growth factor in heart and it is thought to cause muscular hypertrophy and cardiac enlargement.

Angiotensin III

Angiotensin III increases the blood pressure and stimulates aldosterone secretion from adrenal cortex. It has 100% adrenocortical stimulating activity and 40% vasopressor activity of angiotensin II.

Angiotensin IV

It also has adrenocortical stimulating and vasopressor activities.

2. Prostaglandin

Extraglomerular mesangial cells of juxtaglomerular apparatus secrete prostaglandin. Prostaglandin is also secreted by interstitial cells of medulla called type I medullary interstitial cells. Refer Chapter 72 for details.

■ SECRETION OF OTHER SUBSTANCES

1. Extraglomerular mesangial cells of juxtaglomerular apparatus secrete cytokines like interleukin-2 and tumor necrosis factor (Chapter 17)
2. Macula densa secretes thromboxane A_2.

■ REGULATION OF GLOMERULAR BLOOD FLOW AND GLOMERULAR FILTRATION RATE

Macula densa of juxtaglomerular apparatus plays an important role in the feedback mechanism called **tubuloglomerular feedback** mechanism, which regulates the renal blood flow and glomerular filtration rate (Refer Chapter 52 for details).

Renal Circulation

Chapter 51

- ■ INTRODUCTION
- ■ RENAL BLOOD VESSELS
- ■ MEASUREMENT OF RENAL BLOOD FLOW
- ■ REGULATION OF RENAL BLOOD FLOW
  - ■ AUTOREGULATION
- ■ SPECIAL FEATURES OF RENAL CIRCULATION

■ INTRODUCTION

Blood vessels of kidneys are highly specialized to facilitate the functions of nephrons in the formation of urine. In the adults, during resting conditions both the kidneys receive 1,300 mL of blood per minute or about 26% of the cardiac output.

Maximum blood supply to kidneys has got the functional significance. Renal arteries supply blood to the kidneys.

■ RENAL BLOOD VESSELS

Renal Artery

Renal artery arises directly from abdominal aorta and enters the kidney through the hilus. While passing through renal sinus, the renal artery divides into many segmental arteries.

Segmental Artery

Segmental artery subdivides into interlobar arteries (Fig. 51.1).

Interlobar Artery

Interlobar artery passes in between the medullary pyramids. At the base of the pyramid, it turns and runs parallel to the base of pyramid forming arcuate artery.

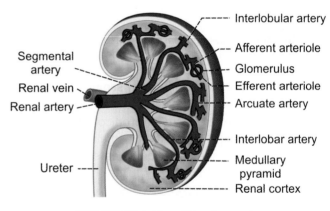

FIGURE 51.1: Renal blood vessels

Arcuate Artery

Each arcuate artery gives rise to interlobular arteries.

Interlobular Artery

Interlobular arteries run through the renal cortex perpendicular to arcuate artery. From each interlobular artery, numerous afferent arterioles arise.

Afferent Arteriole

Afferent arteriole enters the Bowman capsule and forms glomerular capillary tuft. After entering the Bowman capsule, the afferent arteriole divides into 4 or 5 large capillaries.

Glomerular Capillaries

Each large capillary divides into small glomerular capillaries, which form the loops. And, the **capillary loops** unite to form the efferent arteriole, which leaves the Bowman capsule.

Efferent Arteriole

Efferent arterioles form a second capillary network called peritubular capillaries, which surround the tubular portions of the nephrons. Thus, the renal circulation forms a portal system by the presence of two sets of capillaries namely glomerular capillaries and peritubular capillaries.

Peritubular Capillaries and Vasa Recta

Peritubular capillaries are found around the tubular portion of cortical nephrons only. The tubular portion of juxtamedullary nephrons is supplied by some specialized capillaries called vasa recta. These capillaries are straight blood vessels hence the name vasa recta. Vasa recta arise directly from the efferent arteriole of the juxtamedullary nephrons and run parallel to the renal tubule into the medulla and ascend up towards the cortex (Fig. 51.2).

Venous System

Peritubular capillaries and vasa recta drain into the venous system. Venous system starts with peritubular venules and continues as interlobular veins, arcuate

veins, interlobar veins, segmental veins and finally the renal vein (Fig. 51.3).

Renal vein leaves the kidney through the hilus and joins inferior vena cava.

■ MEASUREMENT OF RENAL BLOOD FLOW

Blood flow to kidneys is measured by using plasma clearance of para-aminohippuric acid (Refer Chapter 55).

■ REGULATION OF RENAL BLOOD FLOW

Renal blood flow is regulated mainly by autoregulation. The nerves innervating renal blood vessels do not have any significant role in this.

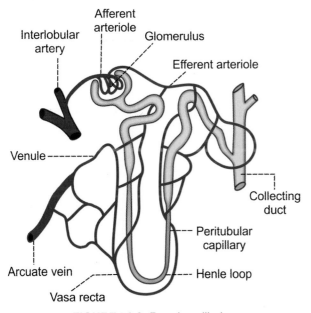

FIGURE 51.2: Renal capillaries

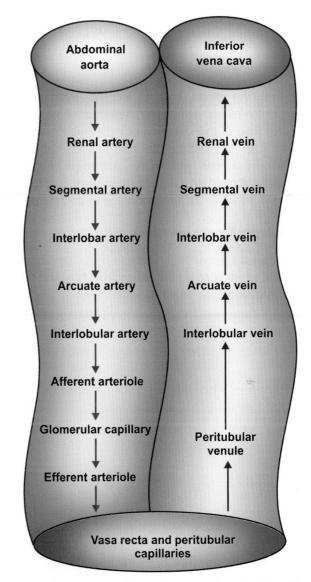

FIGURE 51.3: Schematic diagram showing renal blood flow

■ AUTOREGULATION

Autoregulation is the intrinsic ability of an organ to regulate its own blood flow (Chapter 102). Autoregulation is present in some vital organs in the body such as brain, heart and kidneys. It is highly significant and more efficient in kidneys.

Renal Autoregulation

Renal autoregulation is important to maintain the glomerular filtration rate (GFR). Blood flow to kidneys remains normal even when the mean arterial blood pressure vary widely between 60 mm Hg and 180 mm Hg. This helps to maintain normal GFR.

Two mechanisms are involved in renal autoregulation:
1. Myogenic response
2. Tubuloglomerular feedback.

1. Myogenic Response

Whenever the blood flow to kidneys increases, it stretches the elastic wall of the afferent arteriole.

Stretching of the vessel wall increases the flow of calcium ions from extracellular fluid into the cells. The influx of calcium ions leads to the contraction of smooth muscles in afferent arteriole, which causes constriction of afferent arteriole. So, the blood flow is decreased.

2. Tubuloglomerular Feedback

Macula densa plays an important role in tubuloglomerular feedback, which controls the renal blood flow and GFR. Refer Chapter 52 for details.

■ SPECIAL FEATURES OF RENAL CIRCULATION

Renal circulation has some special features to cope up with the functions of the kidneys. Such special features are:
1. Renal arteries arise directly from the aorta. So, the high pressure in aorta facilitates the high blood flow to the kidneys.
2. Both the kidneys receive about 1,300 mL of blood per minute, i.e. about 26% of cardiac output. Kidneys are the second organs to receive maximum blood flow, the first organ being the liver, which receives 1,500 mL per minute, i.e. about 30% of cardiac output.
3. Whole amount of blood, which flows to kidney has to pass through the glomerular capillaries before entering the venous system. Because of this, the blood is completely filtered at the renal glomeruli.
4. Renal circulation has a **portal system,** i.e. a double network of capillaries, the glomerular capillaries and peritubular capillaries.
5. Renal glomerular capillaries form **high pressure bed** with a pressure of 60 mm Hg to 70 mm Hg. It is much greater than the capillary pressure elsewhere in the body, which is only about 25 mm Hg to 30 mm Hg. High pressure is maintained in the glomerular capillaries because the diameter of afferent arteriole is more than that of efferent arteriole. The high capillary pressure augments glomerular filtration.
6. Peritubular capillaries form a **low pressure bed** with a pressure of 8 mm Hg to 10 mm Hg. This low pressure helps tubular reabsorption.
7. Autoregulation of renal blood flow is well established.

Urine Formation

■ INTRODUCTION

Urine formation is a blood cleansing function. Normally, about 1,300 mL of blood (26% of cardiac output) enters the kidneys. Kidneys excrete the unwanted substances along with water from the blood as urine. Normal **urinary output** is 1 L/day to 1.5 L/day.

Processes of Urine Formation

When blood passes through glomerular capillaries, the plasma is filtered into the Bowman capsule. This process is called glomerular filtration.

Filtrate from Bowman capsule passes through the tubular portion of the nephron. While passing through the tubule, the filtrate undergoes various changes both in quality and in quantity. Many wanted substances like glucose, amino acids, water and electrolytes are reabsorbed from the tubules. This process is called tubular reabsorption.

And, some unwanted substances are secreted into the tubule from peritubular blood vessels. This process is called tubular secretion or excretion (Fig. 52.1).

Thus, the urine formation includes three processes:

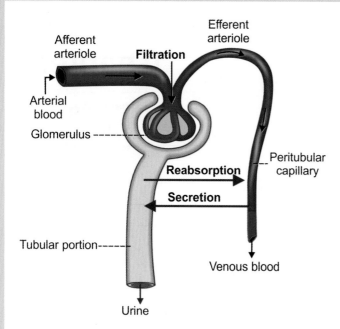

FIGURE 52.1: Events of urine formation

A. Glomerular filtration
B. Tubular reabsorption
C. Tubular secretion.

Among these three processes filtration is the function of the glomerulus. Reabsorption and secretion are the functions of tubular portion of the nephron.

■ GLOMERULAR FILTRATION

■ INTRODUCTION

Glomerular filtration is the process by which the blood is filtered while passing through the glomerular capillaries by filtration membrane. It is the first process of urine formation. The structure of filtration membrane is well suited for filtration.

Filtration Membrane

Filtration membrane is formed by three layers:
1. Glomerular capillary membrane
2. Basement membrane
3. Visceral layer of Bowman capsule.

1. Glomerular capillary membrane

Glomerular capillary membrane is formed by single layer of endothelial cells, which are attached to the basement membrane. The capillary membrane has many pores called **fenestrae** or **filtration pores** with a diameter of 0.1 μ.

2. Basement membrane

Basement membrane of glomerular capillaries and the basement membrane of visceral layer of Bowman capsule fuse together. The fused basement membrane separates the endothelium of glomerular capillary and the epithelium of visceral layer of Bowman capsule.

3. Visceral layer of Bowman capsule

This layer is formed by a single layer of flattened epithelial cells resting on a basement membrane. Each cell is connected with the basement membrane by cytoplasmic extensions called **pedicles** or **feet.** Epithelial cells with pedicles are called **podocytes** (Refer to Fig. 49.4). Pedicles interdigitate leaving small cleft-like spaces in between. The cleft-like space is called **slit pore** or **filtration slit.** Filtration takes place through these slit pores.

Process of Glomerular Filtration

When blood passes through glomerular capillaries, the plasma is filtered into the Bowman capsule. All the substances of plasma are filtered except the plasma proteins. The filtered fluid is called **glomerular filtrate.**

Ultrafiltration

Glomerular filtration is called ultrafiltration because even the minute particles are filtered. But, the plasma proteins are not filtered due to their large molecular size. The protein molecules are larger than the slit pores present in the endothelium of capillaries. Thus, the glomerular filtrate contains all the substances present in plasma except the plasma proteins.

■ METHOD OF COLLECTION OF GLOMERULAR FILTRATE

Glomerular filtrate is collected in experimental animals by micropuncture technique. This technique involves insertion of a **micropipette** into the Bowman capsule and aspiration of filtrate.

■ GLOMERULAR FILTRATION RATE

Glomerular filtration rate (GFR) is defined as the total quantity of filtrate formed in all the nephrons of both the kidneys in the given unit of time.

Normal GFR is 125 mL/minute or about 180 L/day.

■ FILTRATION FRACTION

Filtration fraction is the fraction (portion) of the renal plasma, which becomes the filtrate. It is the ratio between renal plasma flow and glomerular filtration rate. It is expressed in percentage.

$$\text{Filtration fraction} = \frac{\text{GFR}}{\text{Renal plasma flow}} \times 100$$

$$= \frac{125 \text{ mL/min}}{650 \text{ mL/min}} \times 100$$

$$= 19.2\%.$$

Normal filtration fraction varies from 15% to 20%.

■ PRESSURES DETERMINING FILTRATION

Pressures, which determine the GFR are:
1. Glomerular capillary pressure
2. Colloidal osmotic pressure in the glomeruli
3. Hydrostatic pressure in the Bowman capsule.

These pressures determine the GFR by either favoring or opposing the filtration.

1. Glomerular Capillary Pressure

Glomerular capillary pressure is the pressure exerted by the blood in glomerular capillaries. It is about 60 mm Hg and, varies between 45 and 70 mm Hg. Glomerular capillary pressure is the highest capillary pressure in the body. This pressure favors glomerular filtration.

2. Colloidal Osmotic Pressure

It is the pressure exerted by plasma proteins in the glomeruli. The plasma proteins are not filtered through the glomerular capillaries and remain in the glomerular capillaries. These proteins develop the colloidal osmotic pressure, which is about 25 mm Hg. It opposes glomerular filtration.

3. Hydrostatic Pressure in Bowman Capsule

It is the pressure exerted by the filtrate in Bowman capsule. It is also called **capsular pressure.** It is about 15 mm Hg. It also opposes glomerular filtration.

Net Filtration Pressure

Net filtration pressure is the balance between pressure favoring filtration and pressures opposing filtration. It is otherwise known as **effective filtration pressure** or **essential filtration pressure.**

Net filtration pressure =

$$\begin{cases} \text{Glomerular} & \text{Colloidal} & \text{Hydrostatic} \\ \text{capillary} & - \text{ osmotic } + & \text{pressure in} \\ \text{pressure} & \text{pressure} & \text{Bowman capsule} \end{cases}$$

$$= 60 - (25 + 15) = 20 \text{ mm Hg.}$$

Net filtration pressure is about 20 mm Hg and, it varies between 15 and 20 mm Hg.

Starling Hypothesis and Starling Forces

Determination of net filtration pressure is based on Starling hypothesis. Starling hypothesis states that the net filtration through capillary membrane is proportional to hydrostatic pressure difference across the membrane minus oncotic pressure difference. Hydrostatic pressure within the glomerular capillaries is the glomerular capillary pressure.

All the pressures involved in determination of filtration are called **Starling forces.**

■ FILTRATION COEFFICIENT

Filtration coefficient is the GFR in terms of net filtration pressure. It is the GFR per mm Hg of net filtration pressure. For example, when GFR is 125 mL/min and net filtration pressure is 20 mm Hg.

$$\text{Filtration coefficient} = \frac{125 \text{ mL}}{20 \text{ mm Hg}}$$

$$= 6.25 \text{ mL/mm Hg}$$

■ FACTORS REGULATING (AFFECTING) GFR

1. Renal Blood Flow

It is the most important factor that is necessary for glomerular filtration. GFR is directly proportional to renal blood flow. Normal blood flow to both the kidneys is 1,300 mL/minute. The renal blood flow itself is controlled by **autoregulation.** Refer previous chapter for details.

2. Tubuloglomerular Feedback

Tubuloglomerular feedback is the mechanism that regulates GFR through renal tubule and macula densa (Fig. 52.2). **Macula densa** of juxtaglomerular apparatus in the terminal portion of thick ascending limb is sensitive to the sodium chloride in the tubular fluid.

When the glomerular filtrate passes through the terminal portion of thick ascending segment, macula densa acts like a sensor. It detects the concentration of sodium chloride in the tubular fluid and accordingly alters the glomerular blood flow and GFR. Macula densa detects the sodium chloride concentration via Na^+-K^+-$2Cl^-$ cotransporter (NKCC2).

When the concentration of sodium chloride increases in the filtrate

When GFR increases, concentration of sodium chloride increases in the filtrate. Macula densa releases **adenosine**

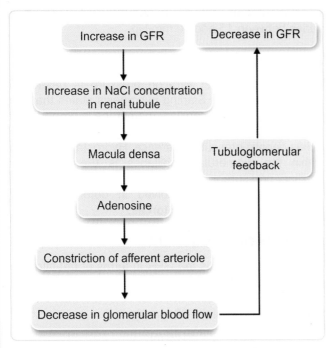

FIGURE 52.2: Tubuloglomerular feedback.
NaCl = Sodium chloride, GFR = Glomerular filtration rate.

from ATP. Adenosine causes constriction of afferent arteriole. So the blood flow through glomerulus decreases leading to decrease in GFR. Adenosine acts on afferent arteriole via adenosine A_1 receptors.

There are several other factors, which increase or decrease the sensitivity of tubuloglomerular feedback.

Factors increasing the sensitivity of tubuloglomerular feedback:

i. Adenosine
ii. Thromboxane
iii. Prostaglandin E_2
iv. Hydroxyeicosatetranoic acid.

Factors decreasing the sensitivity of tubuloglomerular feedback:

i. Atrial natriuretic peptide
ii. Prostaglandin I_2
iii. Cyclic AMP (cAMP)
iv. Nitrous oxide.

When the concentration of sodium chloride decreases in the filtrate

When GFR decreases, concentration of sodium chloride decreases in the filtrate. Macula densa secretes prostaglandin (PGE_2), bradykinin and renin.

PGE_2 and bradykinin cause dilatation of afferent arteriole. Renin induces the formation of angiotensin II, which causes constriction of efferent arteriole. The dilatation of afferent arteriole and constriction of efferent arteriole leads to increase in glomerular blood flow and GFR.

3. *Glomerular Capillary Pressure*

Glomerular filtration rate is directly proportional to glomerular capillary pressure. Normal glomerular capillary pressure is 60 mm Hg. When glomerular capillary pressure increases, the GFR also increases. Capillary pressure, in turn depends upon the renal blood flow and arterial blood pressure.

4. *Colloidal Osmotic Pressure*

Glomerular filtration rate is inversely proportional to colloidal osmotic pressure, which is exerted by plasma proteins in the glomerular capillary blood. Normal colloidal osmotic pressure is 25 mm Hg. When colloidal osmotic pressure increases as in the case of **dehydration** or increased plasma protein level GFR decreases. When colloidal osmotic pressure is low as in **hypoproteinemia,** GFR increases.

5. *Hydrostatic Pressure in Bowman Capsule*

GFR is inversely proportional to this. Normally, it is 15 mm Hg. When the hydrostatic pressure increases in the Bowman capsule, it decreases GFR. Hydrostatic pressure in Bowman capsule increases in conditions like obstruction of urethra and edema of kidney beneath renal capsule.

6. *Constriction of Afferent Arteriole*

Constriction of afferent arteriole reduces the blood flow to the glomerular capillaries, which in turn reduces GFR.

7. *Constriction of Efferent Arteriole*

If efferent arteriole is constricted, initially the GFR increases because of stagnation of blood in the capillaries. Later when all the substances are filtered from this blood, further filtration does not occur. It is because, the efferent arteriolar constriction prevents outflow of blood from glomerulus and no fresh blood enters the glomerulus for filtration.

8. *Systemic Arterial Pressure*

Renal blood flow and GFR are not affected as long as the mean arterial blood pressure is in between 60 and 180 mm Hg due to the autoregulatory mechanism (Chapter 51). Variation in pressure above 180 mm Hg or below 60 mm Hg affects the renal blood flow and GFR accordingly, because the autoregulatory mechanism fails beyond this range.

9. Sympathetic Stimulation

Afferent and efferent arterioles are supplied by sympathetic nerves. The mild or moderate stimulation of sympathetic nerves does not cause any significant change either in renal blood flow or GFR.

Strong sympathetic stimulation causes severe constriction of the blood vessels by releasing the neurotransmitter substance, noradrenaline. The effect is more severe on the efferent arterioles than on the afferent arterioles. So, initially there is increase in filtration but later it decreases. However, if the stimulation is continued for more than 30 minutes, there is recovery of both renal blood flow and GFR. It is because of reduction in sympathetic neurotransmitter.

10. Surface Area of Capillary Membrane

GFR is directly proportional to the surface area of the capillary membrane.

If the glomerular capillary membrane is affected as in the cases of some renal diseases, the surface area for filtration decreases. So there is reduction in GFR.

11. Permeability of Capillary Membrane

GFR is directly proportional to the permeability of glomerular capillary membrane. In many abnormal conditions like hypoxia, lack of blood supply, presence of toxic agents, etc. the permeability of the capillary membrane increases. In such conditions, even plasma proteins are filtered and excreted in urine.

12. Contraction of Glomerular Mesangial Cells

Glomerular mesangial cells are situated in between the glomerular capillaries. Contraction of these cells decreases surface area of capillaries resulting in reduction in GFR (refer Chapter 51 for details).

13. Hormonal and Other Factors

Many hormones and other secretory factors alter GFR by affecting the blood flow through glomerulus.

Factors increasing GFR by vasodilatation

  i. Atrial natriuretic peptide
 ii. Brain natriuretic peptide
iii. cAMP
 iv. Dopamine
  v. Endothelial-derived nitric oxide
 vi. Prostaglandin (PGE_2).

Factors decreasing GFR by vasoconstriction

  i. Angiotensin II
 ii. Endothelins
iii. Noradrenaline
 iv. Platelet-activating factor
  v. Platelet-derived growth factor
 vi. Prostaglandin (PGF_2).

■ TUBULAR REABSORPTION

■ INTRODUCTION

Tubular reabsorption is the process by which water and other substances are transported from renal tubules back to the blood. When the glomerular filtrate flows through the tubular portion of nephron, both quantitative and qualitative changes occur. Large quantity of water (more than 99%), electrolytes and other substances are reabsorbed by the tubular epithelial cells. The reabsorbed substances move into the interstitial fluid of renal medulla. And, from here, the substances move into the blood in peritubular capillaries.

Since the substances are taken back into the blood from the glomerular filtrate, the entire process is called tubular reabsorption.

■ METHOD OF COLLECTION OF TUBULAR FLUID

There are two methods to collect the tubular fluid for analysis.

1. Micropuncture Technique

A micropipette is inserted into the Bowman capsule and different parts of tubular portion in the nephrons of experimental animals, to collect the fluid. The fluid samples are analyzed and compared with each other to assess the changes in different parts of nephron.

2. Stop-flow Method

Ureter is obstructed so that the back pressure rises and stops the glomerular filtration. The obstruction is continued for 8 minutes. It causes some changes in the fluid present in different parts of the tubular portion.

Later, the obstruction is released and about 30 samples of 0.5 mL of urine are collected separately at regular intervals of 30 seconds. The first sample contains the fluid from collecting duct. Successive samples contain the fluid from distal convoluted tubule, loops of Henle and proximal convoluted tubule respectively. All the samples are analyzed.

■ SELECTIVE REABSORPTION

Tubular reabsorption is known as selective reabsorption because the tubular cells reabsorb only the substances necessary for the body. Essential substances such as glucose, amino acids and vitamins are completely reabsorbed from renal tubule. Whereas the unwanted substances like metabolic waste products are not reabsorbed and excreted through urine.

■ MECHANISM OF REABSORPTION

Basic transport mechanisms involved in tubular reabsorption are of two types:
1. Active reabsorption
2. Passive reabsorption.

1. Active Reabsorption

Active reabsorption is the movement of molecules against the **electrochemical (uphill) gradient.** It needs liberation of energy, which is derived from ATP.

Substances reabsorbed actively

Substances reabsorbed actively from the renal tubule are sodium, calcium, potassium, phosphates, sulfates, bicarbonates, glucose, amino acids, ascorbic acid, uric acid and ketone bodies.

2. Passive Reabsorption

Passive reabsorption is the movement of molecules along the **electrochemical (downhill) gradient.** This process does not need energy.

Substances reabsorbed passively

Substances reabsorbed passively are chloride, urea and water.

■ ROUTES OF REABSORPTION

Reabsorption of substances from tubular lumen into the peritubular capillary occurs by two routes:
1. Trancelluar route
2. Paracellular route.

1. Transcellular Route

In this route the substances move through the cell.
It includes transport of substances from:
a. Tubular lumen into tubular cell through apical (luminal) surface of the cell membrane
b. Tubular cell into interstitial fluid
c. Interstitial fluid into capillary.

2. Paracelluar Route

In this route, the substances move through the intercellular space.
It includes transport of substances from:
i. Tubular lumen into interstitial fluid present in lateral intercellular space through the tight junction between the cells
ii. Interstitial fluid into capillary (Fig. 52.3).

■ SITE OF REABSORPTION

Reabsorption of the substances occurs in almost all the segments of tubular portion of nephron.

1. Substances Reabsorbed from Proximal Convoluted Tubule

About 7/8 of the filtrate (about 88%) is reabsorbed in proximal convoluted tubule. The brush border of epithelial cells in proximal convoluted tubule increases the surface area and facilitates the reabsorption.

Substances reabsorbed from proximal convoluted tubule are glucose, amino acids, sodium, potassium, calcium, bicarbonates, chlorides, phosphates, urea, uric acid and water.

2. Substances Reabsorbed from Loop of Henle

Substances reabsorbed from loop of Henle are sodium and chloride.

3. Substances Reabsorbed from Distal Convoluted Tubule

Sodium, calcium, bicarbonate and water are reabsorbed from distal convoluted tubule.

■ REGULATION OF TUBULAR REABSORPTION

Tubular reabsorption is regulated by three factors:

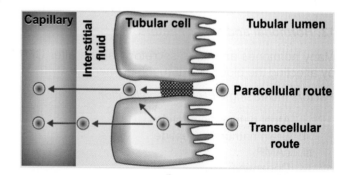

FIGURE 52.3: Routes of reabsorption

1. Glomerulotubular balance
2. Hormonal factors
3. Nervous factors.

1. *Glomerulotubular Balance*

Glomerulotubular balance is the balance between the filtration and reabsorption of solutes and water in kidney. When GFR increases, the tubular load of solutes and water in the proximal convoluted tubule is increased. It is followed by increase in the reabsorption of solutes and water. This process helps in the constant reabsorption of solute particularly sodium and water from renal tubule.

Mechanism of glomerulotubular balance

Glomerulotubular balance occurs because of osmotic pressure in the peritubular capillaries. When GFR increases, more amount of plasma proteins accumulate in the glomerulus. Consequently, the osmotic pressure increases in the blood by the time it reaches efferent arteriole and peritubular capillaries. The elevated osmotic pressure in the peritubular capillaries increases reabsorption of sodium and water from the tubule into the capillary blood.

2. *Hormonal Factors*

Hormones, which regulate GFR are listed in Table 52.1.

3. *Nervous Factor*

Activation of sympathetic nervous system increases the tubular reabsorption (particularly of sodium) from renal tubules. It also increases the tubular reabsorption indirectly by stimulating secretion of renin from juxtaglomerular cells. Renin causes formation of angiotensin II, which increases the sodium reabsorption (Chapter 50).

■ THRESHOLD SUBSTANCES

Depending upon the degree of reabsorption, various substances are classified into three categories:

1. High-threshold substances
2. Low-threshold substances
3. Non-threshold substances.

1. *High-threshold Substances*

High-threshold substances are those substances, which do not appear in urine under normal conditions. The food substances like glucose, amino acids, acetoacetate ions and vitamins are completely reabsorbed from renal tubules and do not appear in urine under normal conditions. These substances can appear in urine, only if their concentration in plasma is abnormally high or in renal diseases when reabsorption is affected. So, these substances are called high-threshold substances.

2. *Low-threshold Substances*

Low-threshold substances are the substances, which appear in urine even under normal conditions. The substances such as urea, uric acid and phosphate are reabsorbed to a little extend. So, these substances appear in urine even under normal conditions.

3. *Non-threshold Substances*

Non-threshold substances are those substances, which are not at all reabsorbed and are excreted in urine irrespective of their plasma level. The metabolic end products such as creatinine are the non-threshold substances.

■ TRANSPORT MAXIMUM – Tm VALUE

Tubular transport maximum or Tm is the rate at which the maximum amount of a substance is reabsorbed from the renal tubule.

So, for every actively reabsorbed substance, there is a maximum rate at which it could be reabsorbed. For example, the transport maximum for glucose (TmG) is 375 mg/minute in adult males and about 300 mg/minute in adult females.

TABLE 52.1: Hormones regulating tubular reabsorption

Hormone	Action
Aldosterone	Increases sodium reabsorption in ascending limb, distal convoluted tubule and collecting duct
Angiotensin II	Increases sodium reabsorption in proximal tubule, thick ascending limb, distal tubule and collecting duct (mainly in proximal convoluted tubule)
Antidiuretic hormone	Increases water reabsorption in distal convoluted tubule and collecting duct
Atrial natriuretic factor	Decreases sodium reabsorption
Brain natriuretic factor	Decreases sodium reabsorption
Parathormone	Increases reabsorption of calcium, magnesium and hydrogen Decreases phosphate reabsorption
Calcitonin	Decreases calcium reabsorption

Threshold Level in Plasma for Substances having Tm Value

Renal threshold is the plasma concentration at which a substance appears in urine. Every substance having Tm value has also a threshold level in plasma or blood. Below that threshold level, the substance is completely reabsorbed and does not appear in urine. When the concentration of that substance reaches the threshold, the excess amount is not reabsorbed and, so it appears in urine. This level is called the renal threshold of that substance.

For example, the renal threshold for glucose is 180 mg/dL. That is, glucose is completely reabsorbed from tubular fluid if its concentration in blood is below 180 mg/dL. So, the glucose does not appear in urine. When the blood level of glucose reaches 180 mg/dL it is not reabsorbed completely; hence it appears in urine.

■ REABSORPTION OF IMPORTANT SUBSTANCES

Reabsorption of Sodium

From the glomerular filtrate, 99% of sodium is reabsorbed. Two thirds of sodium is reabsorbed in proximal convoluted tubule and remaining one third in other segments (except descending limb) and collecting duct.

Sodium reabsorption occurs in three steps:
1. Transport from lumen of renal tubules into the tubular epithelial cells
2. Transport from tubular cells into the interstitial fluid
3. Transport from interstitial fluid to the blood.

1. Transport from Lumen of Renal Tubules into the Tubular Epithelial Cells

Active reabsorption of sodium ions from lumen into the tubular cells occurs by two ways:
  i. In exchange for hydrogen ion by **antiport** (sodium counterport protein) – in proximal convoluted tubules
  ii. Along with other substances like glucose and amino acids by **symport** (sodium co-transport protein) – in other segments and collecting duct.

It is believed that some amount of sodium diffuses along the electrochemical gradient from lumen into tubular cell across the luminar membrane. The electrochemical gradient is developed by sodium-potassium pump (see below).

2. Transport from Tubular Cells into the Interstitial Fluid

Sodium is pumped outside the cells by sodium-potassium pump. This pump moves three sodium ions from the cell into interstitium and two potassium ions from interstitium into the cell.

Tubular epithelial cells are connected with their neighboring cells by tight junctions at their apical luminal edges. But, beyond the tight junction, a small space is left between the adjoining cells along their lateral borders. This space is called **lateral intercellular space.** The interstitium extends into this space.

Most of the sodium ions are pumped into the lateral intercellular space by sodium-potassium pump. The rest of the sodium ions are pumped into the interstitium by the sodium-potassium pump situated at the basal part of the cell membrane.

(Transport of sodium out of the tubular cell by sodium-potassium pump, decreases the sodium concentration within the cell. This develops an electrochemical gradient between the lumen and tubular cell resulting in diffusion of sodium into the cell).

3. Transport from Interstitial Fluid to the Blood

From the interstitial fluid, sodium ions enter the peritubular capillaries by concentration gradient.

In the distal convoluted tubule, the sodium reabsorption is stimulated by the hormone aldosterone secreted by adrenal cortex.

Reabsorption of Water

Reabsorption of water occurs from proximal and distal convoluted tubules and in collecting duct.

Reabsorption of water from proximal convoluted tubule – obligatory water reabsorption

Obligatory reabsorption is the type of water reabsorption in proximal convoluted tubule, which is secondary (obligatory) to sodium reabsorption. When sodium is reabsorbed from the tubule, the osmotic pressure decreases. It causes osmosis of water from renal tubule.

Reabsorption of water from distal convoluted tubule and collecting duct – facultative water reabsorption

Facultative reabsorption is the type of water reabsorption in distal convoluted tubule and collecting duct that occurs by the activity of antidiuretic hormone (ADH). Normally, the distal convoluted tubule and the collecting duct are not permeable to water. But in the presence of ADH, these segments become permeable to water, so it is reabsorbed.

Mechanism of action of ADH – Aquaporins

Antidiuretic hormone increases water reabsorption in distal convoluted tubules and collecting ducts by stimulating the water channels called aquaporins. ADH combines with vasopressin (V2) receptors in the tubular epithelial membrane and activates adenyl cyclase, to form cyclic AMP. This cyclic AMP activates the aquaporins, which increase the water reabsorption.

Aquaporins (AQP) are the membrane proteins, which function as water channels. Though about 10 aquaporins are identified in mammals only 5 are found in humans. Aquaporin-1, 2 and 3 are present in renal tubules. Aquaporin-4 is present in brain and aquaporin-5 is found in salivary glands. Aquaporin-2 forms the water channels in renal tubules.

Reabsorption of Glucose

Glucose is completely reabsorbed in the proximal convoluted tubule. It is transported by secondary active transport (sodium cotransport) mechanism. Glucose and sodium bind to a common carrier protein in the luminal membrane of tubular epithelium and enter the cell. The carrier protein is called **sodium-dependant glucose cotransporter 2** (SGLT2). From tubular cell glucose is transported into medullary interstitium by another carrier protein called **glucose transporter 2** (GLUT2).

Tubular maximum for glucose (TmG)

In adult male, TmG is 375 mg/minute and in adult females it about 300 mg/minute.

Renal threshold for glucose

Renal threshold for glucose is 180 mg/dL in venous blood. When the blood level reaches 180 mg/dL glucose is not reabsorbed completely and appears in urine.

Splay

Splay means deviation. With normal GFR of 125 mL/minute and TmG of 375 mg/minute in an adult male the predicted (expected) renal threshold for glucose should be 300 mg/dL. But actually it is only 180 mg/dL.

When the renal threshold curves are drawn by using these values, the actual curve deviates from the 'should be' or predicted or ideal curve (Fig. 52.4). This type of deviation is called splay. Splay is because of the fact that all the nephrons do not have the same filtering and reabsorbing capacities.

Reabsorption of Amino Acids

Amino acids are also reabsorbed completely in proximal convoluted tubule. Amino acids are reabsorbed actively by the secondary active transport mechanism along with sodium.

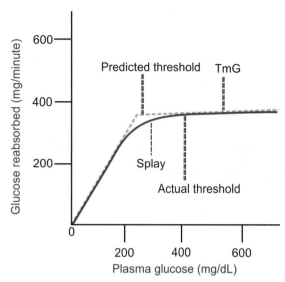

FIGURE 52.4: Splay in renal threshold curve for glucose

Reabsorption of Bicarbonates

Bicarbonate is reabsorbed actively, mostly in proximal tubule (Chapter 54). It is reabsorbed in the form of carbon dioxide.

Bicarbonate is mostly present as sodium bicarbonate in the filtrate. Sodium bicarbonate dissociates into sodium and bicarbonate ions in the tubular lumen. Sodium diffuses into tubular cell in exchange of hydrogen. Bicarbonate combines with hydrogen to form carbonic acid. Carbonic acid dissociates into carbon dioxide and water in the presence of carbonic anhydrase. Carbon dioxide and water enter the tubular cell.

In the tubular cells, carbon dioxide combines with water to form carbonic acid. It immediately dissociates into hydrogen and bicarbonate. Bicarbonate from the tubular cell enters the interstitium. There it combines with sodium to form sodium bicarbonate (Fig. 54.1).

■ TUBULAR SECRETION

■ INTRODUCTION

Tubular secretion is the process by which the substances are transported from blood into renal tubules. It is also called tubular excretion. In addition to reabsorption from renal tubules, some substances are also secreted into the lumen from the peritubular capillaries through the tubular epithelial cells.

Dye phenol red was the first substance found to be secreted in renal tubules in experimental conditions. Later many other substances were found to be secreted.

Such substances are:

1. Para-aminohippuric acid (PAH)
2. Diodrast
3. 5-hydroxyindoleacetic acid (5-HIAA)
4. Amino derivatives
5. Penicillin.

■ SUBSTANCES SECRETED IN DIFFERENT SEGMENTS OF RENAL TUBULES

1. Potassium is secreted actively by sodium-potassium pump in proximal and distal convoluted tubules and collecting ducts
2. Ammonia is secreted in the proximal convoluted tubule
3. Hydrogen ions are secreted in the proximal and distal convoluted tubules. Maximum hydrogen ion secretion occurs in proximal tubule
4. Urea is secreted in loop of Henle.

Thus, urine is formed in nephron by the processes of glomerular filtration, selective reabsorption and tubular secretion.

■ SUMMARY OF URINE FORMATION

Urine formation takes place in three processes (Refer to Fig. 52.1):

1. *Glomerular filtration*

Plasma is filtered in glomeruli and the substances reach the renal tubules along with water as filtrate.

2. *Tubular Reabsorption*

The 99% of filtrate is reabsorbed in different segments of renal tubules.

3. *Tubular Secretion*

Some substances are transported from blood into the renal tubule.

With all these changes, the filtrate becomes urine.

Concentration of Urine

53

```
■ INTRODUCTION
■ MEDULLARY GRADIENT
■ COUNTERCURRENT MECHANISM
■ ROLE OF ADH
■ SUMMARY OF URINE CONCENTRATION
■ APPLIED PHYSIOLOGY
```

■ INTRODUCTION

Every day 180 L of glomerular filtrate is formed with large quantity of water. If this much of water is excreted in urine, body will face serious threats. So the concentration of urine is very essential.

Osmolarity of glomerular filtrate is same as that of plasma and it is 300 mOsm/L. But, normally urine is concentrated and its osmolarity is four times more than that of plasma, i.e. 1,200 mOsm/L.

Osmolarity of urine depends upon two factors:
1. Water content in the body
2. Antidiuretic hormone (ADH).

Mechanism of urine formation is the same for dilute urine and concentrated urine till the fluid reaches the distal convoluted tubule. However, dilution or concentration of urine depends upon water content of the body.

■ FORMATION OF DILUTE URINE

When, water content in the body increases, kidney excretes dilute urine. This is achieved by inhibition of ADH secretion from posterior pituitary (Chapter 66). So water reabsorption from renal tubules does not take place (see Fig. 53.4) leading to excretion of large amount of water. This makes the urine dilute.

■ FORMATION OF CONCENTRATED URINE

When the water content in body decreases, kidney retains water and excretes concentrated urine. Forma-

tion of concentrated urine is not as simple as that of dilute urine.

It involves two processes:
1. Development and maintenance of medullary gradient by countercurrent system
2. Secretion of ADH.

■ MEDULLARY GRADIENT

■ MEDULLARY HYPEROSMOLARITY

Cortical interstitial fluid is isotonic to plasma with the osmolarity of 300 mOsm/L. Osmolarity of medullary interstitial fluid near the cortex is also 300 mOsm/L.

However, while proceeding from outer part towards the inner part of medulla, the osmolarity increases gradually and reaches the maximum at the inner most part of medulla near renal sinus. Here, the interstitial fluid is hypertonic with osmolarity of 1,200 mOsm/L (Fig. 53.1).

This type of gradual increase in the osmolarity of the medullary interstitial fluid is called the medullary gradient. It plays an important role in the concentration of urine.

■ DEVELOPMENT AND MAINTENANCE OF MEDULLARY GRADIENT

Kidney has some unique mechanism called countercurrent mechanism, which is responsible for the development and maintenance of medullary gradient and hyperosmolarity of interstitial fluid in the inner medulla.

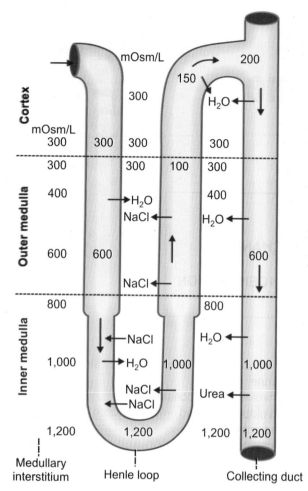

FIGURE 53.1: Countercurrent multiplier.
Numerical indicate osmolarity (mOsm/L)

■ COUNTERCURRENT MECHANISM

■ COUNTERCURRENT FLOW

A countercurrent system is a system of 'U'-shaped tubules (tubes) in which, the flow of fluid is in opposite direction in two limbs of the 'U'-shaped tubules.

Divisions of Countercurrent System

Countercurrent system has two divisions:
1. Countercurrent multiplier formed by loop of Henle
2. Countercurrent exchanger formed by vasa recta.

■ COUNTERCURRENT MULTIPLIER

Loop of Henle

Loop of Henle functions as countercurrent multiplier. It is responsible for development of hyperosmolarity of medullary interstitial fluid and medullary gradient.

Role of Loop of Henle in Development of Medullary Gradient

Loop of Henle of juxtamedullary nephrons plays a major role as countercurrent multiplier because loop of these nephrons is long and extends upto the deeper parts of medulla.

Main reason for the hyperosmolarity of medullary interstitial fluid is the active reabsorption of sodium chloride and other solutes from ascending limb of Henle loop into the medullary interstitium. These solutes accumulate in the medullary interstitium and increase the osmolarity.

Now, due to the concentration gradient, the sodium and chlorine ions diffuse from medullary interstitium into the descending limb of Henle loop and reach the ascending limb again via hairpin bend.

Thus, the sodium and chlorine ions are repeatedly re-circulated between the descending limb and ascending limb of Henle loop through medullary interstitial fluid leaving a small portion to be excreted in the urine.

Apart from this there is regular addition of more and more new sodium and chlorine ions into descending limb by constant filtration. Thus, the reabsorption of sodium chloride from ascending limb and addition of new sodium chlorine ions into the filtrate increase or multiply the osmolarity of medullary interstitial fluid and medullary gradient. Hence, it is called countercurrent multiplier.

Other Factors Responsible for Hyperosmolarity of Medullary Interstitial Fluid

In addition to countercurrent multiplier action provided by the loop of Henle, two more factors are involved in hyperosmolarity of medullary interstitial fluid.

i. Reabsorption of sodium from collecting duct

Reabsorption of sodium from medullary part of collecting duct into the medullary interstitium, adds to the osmolarity of inner medulla.

ii. Recirculation of urea

Fifty percent of urea filtered in glomeruli is reabsorbed in proximal convoluted tubule. Almost an equal amount of urea is secreted in the loop of Henle. So the fluid in distal convoluted tubule has as much urea as amount filtered.

Collecting duct is impermeable to urea. However, due to the water reabsorption from distal convoluted tubule and collecting duct in the presence of ADH, urea concentration increases in collecting duct. Now due to concentration gradient, urea diffuses from inner medullary part of collecting duct into medullary interstitium.

Due to continuous diffusion, the concentration of urea increases in the inner medulla resulting in hyperosmolarity of interstitium in inner medulla.

Again, by concentration gradient, urea enters the ascending limb. From here, it passes through distal convoluted tubule and reaches the collecting duct. Urea enters the medullary interstitium from collecting duct. By this way urea **recirculates** repeatedly and helps to maintain the hyperosmolarity of inner medullary interstitium. Only a small amount of urea is excreted in urine.

Urea recirculation accounts for 50% of hyperosmolarity in inner medulla. Diffusion of urea from collecting duct into medullary interstitium is carried out by **urea transporters,** UT-A1 and UT-A3, which are activated by ADH.

■ COUNTERCURRENT EXCHANGER

Vasa Recta

Vasa recta functions as countercurrent exchanger. It is responsible for the maintenance of medullary gradient, which is developed by countercurrent multiplier (Fig. 53.2).

Role of Vasa Recta in the Maintenance of Medullary Gradient

Vasa recta acts like countercurrent exchanger because of its position. It is also 'U'-shaped tubule with a descending limb, hairpin bend and an ascending limb. Vasa recta runs parallel to loop of Henle. Its descending limb runs along the ascending limb of Henle loop and its ascending limb runs along with descending limb of Henle loop.

The sodium chloride reabsorbed from ascending limb of Henle loop enters the medullary interstitium. From here it enters the descending limb of vasa recta. Simultaneously water diffuses from descending limb of vasa recta into medullary interstitium.

The blood flows very slowly through vasa recta. So, a large quantity of sodium chloride accumulates in descending limb of vasa recta and flows slowly towards ascending limb. By the time the blood reaches the ascending limb of vasa recta, the concentration of sodium chloride increases very much. This causes diffusion of sodium chloride into the medullary interstitium. Simultaneously, water from medullary interstitium enters the ascending limb of vasa recta. And the cycle is repeated.

If the vasa recta would be a straight vessel without hairpin arrangement, blood would leave the kidney quickly at renal papillary level. In that case, the blood would remove all the sodium chloride from medullary

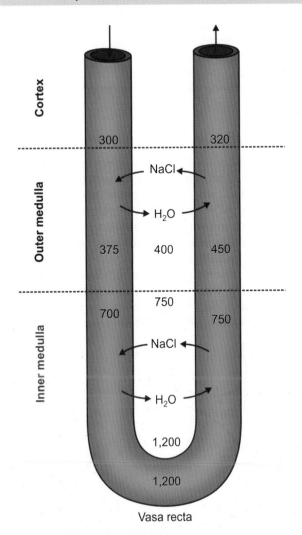

FIGURE 53.2: Countercurrent exchanger. Numerical indicate osmolarity (mOsm/L)

interstitium and thereby the hyperosmolarity will be decreased. However, this does not happen, since the vasa recta has a hairpin bend.

Therefore, when blood passes through the ascending limb of vasa recta, sodium chloride diffuses out of blood and enters the interstitial fluid of medulla and, water diffuses into the blood.

Thus, vasa recta retains sodium chloride in the medullary interstitium and removes water from it. So, the hyperosmolarity of medullary interstitium is maintained. The blood passing through the ascending limb of vasa recta may carry very little amount of sodium chloride from the medulla.

Recycling of urea also occurs through vasa recta. From medullary interstitium, along with sodium chloride, urea also enters the descending limb of vasa recta. When blood passes through ascending limb of vasa recta, urea diffuses back into the medullary interstitium along with sodium chloride.

Thus, sodium chloride and urea are exchanged for water between the ascending and descending limbs of vasa recta, hence this system is called countercurrent exchanger.

■ ROLE OF ADH

Final concentration of urine is achieved by the action of ADH. Normally, the distal convoluted tubule and collecting duct are not permeable to water. But the presence of ADH makes them permeable, resulting in water reabsorption. Water reabsorption induced by ADH is called **facultative reabsorption of water** (Refer Chapter 52 for details).

A large quantity of water is removed from the fluid while passing through distal convoluted tubule and collecting duct. So, the urine becomes hypertonic with an osmolarity of 1,200 mOsm/L (Fig. 53.3).

■ SUMMARY OF URINE CONCENTRATION

When the glomerular filtrate passes through renal tubule, its osmolarity is altered in different segments as described below (Fig. 53.4).

■ 1. BOWMAN CAPSULE

Glomerular filtrate collected at the Bowman capsule is **isotonic to plasma**. This is because it contains all the substances of plasma except proteins. Osmolarity of the filtrate at Bowman capsule is 300 mOsm/L.

■ 2. PROXIMAL CONVOLUTED TUBULE

When the filtrate flows through proximal convoluted tubule, there is active reabsorption of sodium and chloride followed by **obligatory reabsorption of water.**

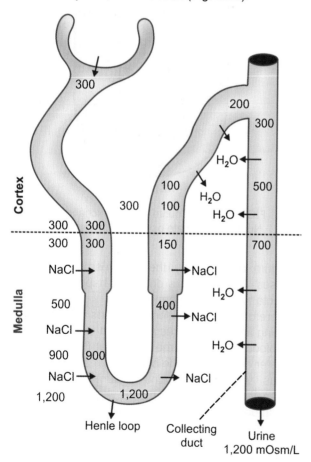

FIGURE 53.3: Role of ADH in the formation of concentrated urine. ADH increases the permeability for water in distal convoluted tubule and collecting duct. Numerical indicate osmolarity (mOsm/L)

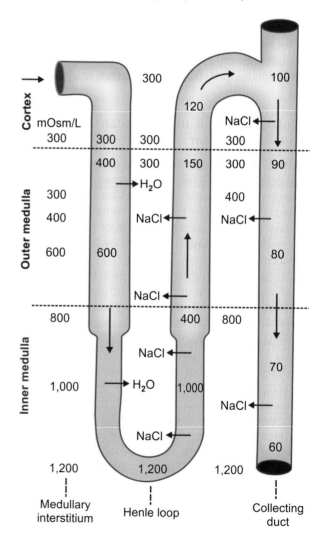

FIGURE 53.4: Mechanism for the formation of dilute urine. Numerical indicate osmolarity (mOsm/L)

So, the osmolarity of fluid remains the same as in the case of Bowman capsule, i.e. 300 mOsm/L. Thus, in proximal convoluted tubules, the fluid is **isotonic to plasma.**

■ 3. THICK DESCENDING SEGMENT

When the fluid passes from proximal convoluted tubule into the thick descending segment, water is reabsorbed from tubule into outer medullary interstitium by means of osmosis. It is due to the increased osmolarity in the medullary interstitium, i.e. outside the thick descending tubule. The osmolarity of the fluid inside this segment is between 450 and 600 mOsm/L. That means the fluid is slightly **hypertonic to plasma.**

■ 4. THIN DESCENDING SEGMENT OF HENLE LOOP

As the thin descending segment of Henle loop passes through the inner medullary interstitium (which is increasingly hypertonic) more water is reabsorbed. This segment is highly permeable to water and so the osmolarity of tubular fluid becomes equal to that of the surrounding medullary interstitium.

In the short loops of cortical nephrons, the osmolarity of fluid at the hairpin bend of loop becomes 600 mOsm/L. And, in the long loops of juxtamedullary nephrons, at the hairpin bend, the osmolarity is 1,200 mOsm/L. Thus in this segment the fluid is **hypertonic to plasma.**

■ 5. THIN ASCENDING SEGMENT OF HENLE LOOP

When the thin ascending segment of the loop ascends upwards through the medullary region, osmolarity decreases gradually.

Due to concentration gradient, sodium chloride diffuses out of tubular fluid and osmolarity decreases to 400 mOsm/L. The fluid in this segment is slightly **hypertonic to plasma.**

■ 6. THICK ASCENDING SEGMENT

This segment is impermeable to water. But there is active reabsorption of sodium and chloride from this. Reabsorption of sodium decreases the osmolarity of tubular fluid to a greater extent. The osmolarity is

between 150 and 200 mOsm/L. The fluid inside becomes **hypotonic to plasma.**

■ 7. DISTAL CONVOLUTED TUBULE AND COLLECTING DUCT

In the presence of ADH, distal convoluted tubule and collecting duct become permeable to water resulting in water reabsorption and final concentration of urine. It is found that in the collecting duct, Principal (P) cells are responsible for ADH induced water reabsorption.

Reabsorption of large quantity of water increases the osmolarity to 1,200 mOsm/L (Fig. 53.3). The urine becomes **hypertonic to plasma.**

■ APPLIED PHYSIOLOGY

1. *Osmotic Diuresis*

Diuresis is the excretion of large quantity of water through urine. Osmotic diuresis is the diuresis induced by the osmotic effects of solutes like glucose. It is common in **diabetes mellitus** (Chapter 69).

2. *Polyuria*

Polyuria is the increased urinary output with frequent voiding. It is common in **diabetes insipidus.** In this disorder, the renal tubules fail to reabsorb water because of ADH deficiency (Chapter 66).

3. *Syndrome of Inappropriate Hypersecretion of ADH (SIADH)*

It is a pituitary disorder characterized by hypersecretion of ADH is the SIADH. Excess ADH causes water retention, which decreases osmolarity of ECF (Chapter 66).

4. *Nephrogenic Diabetes Insipidus*

Sometimes, ADH secretion is normal but the renal tubules fail to give response to ADH resulting in polyuria. This condition is called nephrogenic diabetes insipidus.

5. *Bartter Syndrome*

Bartter syndrome is a genetic disorder characterized by defect in the thick ascending segment. This causes decreased sodium and water reabsorption resulting in loss of sodium and water through urine.

Acidification of Urine and Role of Kidney in Acid-base Balance

- ■ INTRODUCTION
- ■ REABSORPTION OF BICARBONATE IONS
- ■ SECRETION OF HYDROGEN IONS
  - ■ SODIUM-HYDROGEN ANTIPORT PUMP
  - ■ ATP-DRIVEN PROTON PUMP
- ■ REMOVAL OF HYDROGEN IONS AND ACIDIFICATION OF URINE
  - ■ BICARBONATE MECHANISM
  - ■ PHOSPHATE MECHANISM
  - ■ AMMONIA MECHANISM
- ■ APPLIED PHYSIOLOGY

■ INTRODUCTION

Kidney plays an important role in maintenance of acid-base balance by excreting hydrogen ions and retaining bicarbonate ions.

Normally, urine is acidic in nature with a pH of 4.5 to 6. Metabolic activities in the body produce large quantity of acids (with lot of hydrogen ions), which threaten to push the body towards acidosis.

However, kidneys prevent this by two ways:
1. Reabsorption of bicarbonate ions (HCO_3^-)
2. Secretion of hydrogen ions (H^+).

■ REABSORPTION OF BICARBONATE IONS

About 4,320 mEq of HCO_3^- is filtered by the glomeruli everyday. It is called **filtered load** of HCO_3^-. Excretion of this much HCO_3^- in urine will affect the acid-base balance of body fluids. So, HCO_3^- must be taken back from the renal tubule by reabsorption.

■ SECRETION OF HYDROGEN IONS

Reabsorption of filtered HCO_3^- occurs by the secretion of H^+ in the renal tubules. About 4,380 mEq of H^+ appear every day in the renal tubule by means of filtration and secretion. Not all the H^+ are excreted in urine. Out of 4,380 mEq, about 4,280 to 4,330 mEq of H^+ is utilized

for the reabsorption of filtered HCO_3^-. Only the remaining 50 to 100 mEq is excreted. It results in the acidification of urine.

Secretion of H^+ into the renal tubules occurs by the formation of carbonic acid. Carbon dioxide formed in the tubular cells or derived from tubular fluid combines with water to form carbonic acid in the presence of **carbonic anhydrase.** This enzyme is available in large quantities in the epithelial cells of the renal tubules. The carbonic acid immediately dissociates into H^+ and HCO_3^- (Fig. 54.1).

H^+ is secreted into the lumen of proximal convoluted tubule, distal convoluted tubule and collecting duct. Distal convoluted tubule and collecting duct have a special type of cells called **intercalated cells (I cells)** that are involved in handling hydrogen and bicarbonate ions.

Secretion of H^+ occurs by two pumps:
i. Sodium-hydrogen antiport pump
ii. ATP-driven proton pump.

■ SODIUM-HYDROGEN ANTIPORT PUMP

When sodium ion (Na^+) is reabsorbed from the tubular fluid into the tubular cell, H^+ is secreted from the cell into the tubular fluid in exchange for Na^+. The sodium-hydrogen antiport pump present in the tubular cells is responsible for the exchange of Na⁺ and H⁺. This type of sodium-hydrogen counter transport occurs predominantly in distal convoluted tubule (Table 54.1).

■ ATP-DRIVEN PROTON PUMP

This is an additional pump for H⁺ secretion in distal convoluted tubule and collecting duct. This pump operates by energy from ATP.

■ REMOVAL OF HYDROGEN IONS AND ACIDIFICATION OF URINE

Role of Kidney in Preventing Metabolic Acidosis

Kidney plays an important role in preventing metabolic acidosis (Chapter 5) by excreting H⁺.

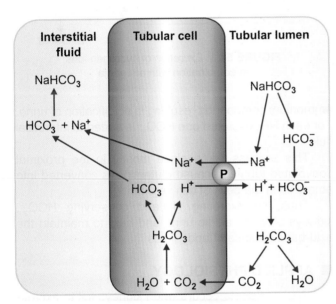

FIGURE 54.1: Reabsorption of bicarbonate ions by secretion of hydrogen ions in renal tubule. P = sodium-hydrogen antiport pump

TABLE 54.1: Mechanisms involved in secretion of hydrogen ions in renal tubule

Mechanism	Segment of renal tubule
Sodium-hydrogen pump	Distal convoluted tubule
ATP-driven proton pump	Distal convoluted tubule Collecting duct
Bicarbonate mechanism	Proximal convoluted tubule Henle loop Distal convoluted tubule
Phosphate mechanism	Distal convoluted tubule Collecting duct
Ammonia mechanism	Proximal convoluted tubule.

Excretion of H⁺ occurs by three mechanisms:
1. Bicarbonate mechanism
2. Phosphate mechanism
3. Ammonia mechanism.

■ BICARBONATE MECHANISM

All the filtered HCO₃⁻ in the renal tubules is reabsorbed. About 80% of it is reabsorbed in proximal convoluted tubule, 15% in Henle loop and 5% in distal convoluted tubule and collecting duct. The reabsorption of HCO₃⁻ utilizes the H⁺ secreted into the renal tubules.

H⁺ secreted into the renal tubule, combines with filtered HCO₃⁻ forming carbonic acid (H₂CO₃). Carbonic acid dissociates into carbon dioxide and water in the presence of carbonic anhydrase. Carbon dioxide and water enter the tubular cell.

In the tubular cells, carbon dioxide combines with water to form carbonic acid. It immediately dissociates into H⁺ and HCO₃⁻. HCO₃⁻ from the tubular cell enters the interstitium. Simultaneously Na⁺ is reabsorbed from the renal tubule under the influence of aldosterone. HCO₃⁻ combines with Na⁺ to form sodium bicarbonate (NaHCO₃). Now, the H⁺ is secreted into the tubular lumen from the cell in exchange for Na⁺ (Fig. 54.1).

Thus, for every hydrogen ion secreted into lumen of tubule, one bicarbonate ion is reabsorbed from the tubule. In this way, kidneys conserve the HCO₃⁻. The reabsorption of filtered HCO₃⁻ is an important factor in maintaining pH of the body fluids.

■ PHOSPHATE MECHANISM

In the tubular cells, carbon dioxide combines with water to form carbonic acid. It immediately dissociates into H⁺ and HCO₃⁻. HCO₃⁻ from the tubular cell enters the interstitium. Simultaneously, Na⁺ is reabsorbed from renal tubule under the influence of aldosterone. Na⁺ enters the interstitium and combines with HCO₃⁻. H⁺ is secreted into the tubular lumen from the cell in exchange for Na⁺ (Fig. 54.2).

H⁺, which is secreted into renal tubules, reacts with phosphate buffer system. It combines with sodium hydrogen phosphate to form sodium dihydrogen phosphate. Sodium dihydrogen phosphate is excreted in urine. The H⁺, which is added to urine in the form of sodium dihydrogen, makes the urine acidic. It happens mainly in distal tubule and collecting duct because of the presence of large quantity of sodium hydrogen phosphate in these segments.

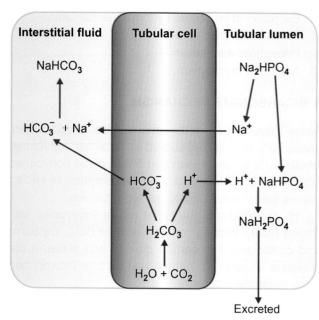

FIGURE 54.2: Excretion of hydrogen ions in combination with phosphate ions

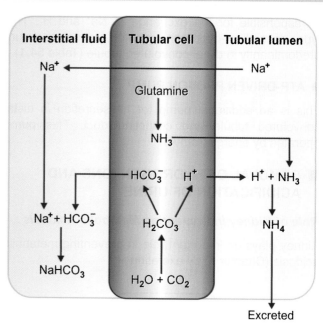

FIGURE 54.3: Excretion of hydrogen ions in combination with ammonia

■ AMMONIA MECHANISM

This is the most important mechanism by which kidneys excrete H$^+$ and make the urine acidic. In the tubular epithelial cells, ammonia is formed when the amino acid **glutamine** is converted into **glutamic acid** in the presence of the enzyme **glutaminase.** Ammonia is also formed by the deamination of some of the amino acids such as **glycine** and **alanine** (Fig. 54.3).

Ammonia (NH$_3$) formed in tubular cells is secreted into tubular lumen in exchange for sodium ion. Here, it combines with H$^+$ to form **ammonium** (NH$_4$). The tubular cell membrane is not permeable to ammonium. Therefore, it remains in the lumen and then excreted into urine. Thus, H$^+$ is added to urine in the form of ammonium compounds resulting in acidification of urine. For each NH$_4$ excreted one HCO$_3^-$ is added to interstitial fluid.

This process takes place mostly in the proximal convoluted tubule because glutamine is converted into ammonia in the cells of this segment.

Thus, by excreting H$^+$ and conserving HCO$_3^-$, kidneys produce acidic urine and help to maintain the acid-base balance of body fluids.

■ APPLIED PHYSIOLOGY

Metabolic acidosis occurs when kidneys fail to excrete metabolic acids. **Metabolic alkalosis** occurs when kidneys excrete large quantity of hydrogen. Refer Chapter 5 for details.

Renal Function Tests

Chapter 55

> ■ **PROPERTIES AND COMPOSITION OF NORMAL URINE**
>   - ■ **PROPERTIES OF URINE**
>   - ■ **COMPOSITION OF URINE**
> ■ **RENAL FUNCTION TESTS**
>   - ■ **EXAMINATION OF URINE – URINALYSIS**
>   - ■ **PHYSICAL EXAMINATION**
>   - ■ **MICROSCOPIC EXAMINATION**
>   - ■ **CHEMICAL ANALYSIS**
> ■ **EXAMINATION OF BLOOD**
> ■ **EXAMINATION OF BLOOD AND URINE**

■ PROPERTIES AND COMPOSITION OF NORMAL URINE

■ PROPERTIES OF URINE

Volume	: 1,000 to 1,500 mL/day
Reaction	: Slightly acidic with pH of 4.5 to 6
Specific gravity	: 1.010 to 1.025
Osmolarity	: 1,200 mOsm/L
Color	: Normally, straw colored
Odor	: Fresh urine has light aromatic odor. If stored for some time, the odor becomes stronger due to bacterial decomposition.

■ COMPOSITION OF URINE

Urine consists of water and solids. Solids include organic and inorganic substances (Fig. 55.1).

■ RENAL FUNCTION TESTS

Renal function tests are the group of tests that are performed to assess the functions of kidney.

Renal function tests are of three types:

A. Examination of urine alone

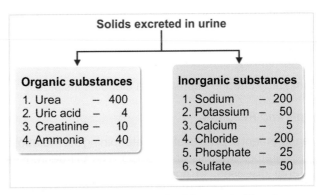

FIGURE 55.1: Quantity of solids excreted in urine (mMols/day)

B. Examination of blood alone
C. Examination of blood and urine.

■ EXAMINATION OF URINE – URINALYSIS

Routine examination of urine or urinalysis is a group of diagnostic tests performed on the sample of urine.

Urinalysis is done by:

i. Physical examination
ii. Microscopic examination
iii. Chemical analysis.

■ PHYSICAL EXAMINATION

1. Volume

Increase in urine volume indicates increase in protein catabolism and renal disorders such as **chronic renal failure, diabetes insipidus** and **glycosuria.**

2. Color

Normally urine is straw colored. Abnormal coloration of urine is due to several causes such as **jaundice, hematuria, hemoglobinuria,** medications, excess urobilinogen, ingestion of beetroot or color added to food.

3. Appearance

Normally urine is clear. It becomes turbid in both physiological and pathological conditions. Physiological conditions causing turbidity of urine are precipitation of crystals, presence of mucus or vaginal discharge. Pathological conditions causing turbidity are presence of blood cells, bacteria or yeast.

4. Specific Gravity

Specific gravity of urine is the measure of dissolved solutes (particles) in urine. It is low in diabetes insipidus and high in **diabetes mellitus, acute renal failure** and excess medications.

5. Osmolarity

Osmolarity of urine decreases in diabetes insipidus.

6. pH and Reaction

Measurement of pH is useful in determining the metabolic or respiratory acidosis or alkalosis. The pH decreases in renal diseases. In normal conditions, pH of urine depends upon diet. It is slightly alkaline in vegetarians and acidic in non-vegetarians.

■ MICROSCOPIC EXAMINATION

Microscopic examination of centrifuged sediment of urine is useful in determining the renal diseases.

1. Red Blood Cells

Presence of red blood cells in urine indicates glomerular disease such as **glomerulonephritis.**

2. White Blood Cells

Normally few white blood cells appear in high power field. The number increases in acute **glomerulonephritis,** infection of urinary tract, vagina or cervix.

3. Epithelial Cells

Normally few tubular epithelial cells slough into urine. Presence of many epithelial cells suggests **nephrotic syndrome** and **tubular necrosis.**

4. Casts

Casts are the cylindrical bodies that are casted (molded) in the shape of renal tubule. Casts may be hyaline, granular or cellular in nature. Hyaline and granular casts, which are formed by precipitation of proteins may appear in urine in small numbers. The number increases in proteinuria due to **glomerulonephritis.**

Cellular casts are formed by sticking together of some cells. Red blood cell casts appear in urine during glomerulonephritis and tubular necrosis. White blood cell casts appear in pyelonephritis. Epithelial casts are formed during acute **tubular necrosis.**

5. Crystals

Several types of crystals are present in normal urine. Common crystals are the crystals of calcium oxalate, calcium phosphate, uric acid and triple phosphate (calcium, ammonium and magnesium).

Abnormal crystals such as crystals of cystine and tyrosine appear in liver diseases.

6. Bacteria

Bacteria are common in urine specimens because of normal microbial flora of urinary tract, urethra and vagina and because of their ability to multiply rapidly in urine. Culture studies are necessary to determine the presence of bacteria in urine.

■ CHEMICAL ANALYSIS

Chemical analysis of urine helps to determine the presence of abnormal constituents of urine or presence of normal constituents in abnormal quantity. Both the findings reveal the presence of renal abnormality. Following are the common chemical tests of urine:

1. Glucose

Glucose appears in urine when the blood glucose level increases above 180 mg/dL. **Glycosuria** (presence of glucose in urine) may be the first indicator of diabetes mellitus.

2. Protein

Presence of excess protein **(proteinuria)** particularly albumin **(albuminuria)** in urine indicates renal diseases. Urinary excretion of albumin in a normal healthy adult is about 30 mg/day. It exceeds this level in glomerulo-nephritis. It also increases in fever and severe exercise.

3. Ketone Bodies

Ketonuria (presence of ketone bodies in urine) occurs in pregnancy, fever, diabetes mellitus, prolonged starvation and glycogen storage diseases.

4. Bilirubin

Bilirubin appears in urine **(bilirubinuria)** during hepatic and posthepatic jaundice.

5. Urobilinogen

Normally, about 1 to 3.5 mg of urobilinogen is excreted in urine daily. Excess of urobilinogen in urine indicates **hemolytic jaundice.**

6. Bile Salts

Presence of bile salts in urine reveals jaundice.

7. Blood

Presence of blood in urine **(hematuria)** indicates glomerulonephritis, renal stones, infection or malignancy of urinary tract. Hematuria must be confirmed by micro-scopic examination since chemical test fails to distinguish the presence of red blood cells or hemoglobin in urine.

8. Hemoglobin

Hemoglobin appears in urine **(hemoglobinuria)** during excess hemolysis.

9. Nitrite

Presence of nitrite in urine indicates presence of bacteria in urine since some bacteria convert nitrate into nitrite in urine.

■ EXAMINATION OF BLOOD

1. Estimation of Plasma Proteins

Normal values of plasma proteins:
Total proteins   : 7.3 g/dL (6.4 to 8.3 g/dL)
Serum albumin : 4.7 g/dL
Serum globulin : 2.3 g/dL
Fibrinogen   : 0.3 g/dL

Level of plasma proteins is altered during renal failure.

2. Estimation of Urea, Uric Acid and Creatinine

Normal values :
Urea   : 25 to 40 mg/dL

Uric acid   : 2.5 mg/dL
Creatinine   : 0.5 to 1.5 mg/dL

The blood level of these substances increases in renal failure.

■ EXAMINATION OF BLOOD AND URINE

Plasma Clearance

Plasma clearance is defined as the amount of plasma that is cleared off a substance in a given unit of time. It is also known as renal clearance. It is based on Fick principle.

Determination of clearance value for certain substances helps in assessing the following renal functions:
1. Glomerular filtration rate
2. Renal plasma flow
3. Renal blood flow.

Value of following factors is required to determine the plasma clearance of a particular substance:
1. Volume of urine excreted
2. Concentration of the substance in urine
3. Concentration of the substance in blood.

Formula to calculate clearance value

$$C = \frac{U V}{P}$$

Where, C = Clearance
   U = Concentration of the substance in urine
   V = Volume of urine flow
   P = Concentration of the substance in plasma.

1. Measurement of Glomerular Filtration Rate

A substance that is completely filtered but neither reabsorbed nor secreted should be used to measure glomerular filtration rate (GFR). Inulin is the ideal substance used to measure GFR. It is completely filtered and neither reabsorbed nor secreted. So, inulin clearance indicates GFR.

Inulin clearance

A known amount of inulin is injected into the body. After sometime, the concentration of inulin in plasma and urine and the volume of urine excreted are estimated.

For example,
   Concentration of inulin in urine   = 125 mg/dL
   Concentration of inulin in plasma = 1 mg/dL
   Volume of urine output   = 1 mL/min

Thus,

$$\text{Glomerular filtration rate} = \frac{U\,V}{P} = \frac{125 \times 1}{1}$$

$$= 125 \text{ mL/min}$$

Creatinine clearance is also used to measure GFR accurately. It is easier than inulin clearance, because, creatinine is already present in body fluids and its plasma concentration is steady throughout the day. It is completely filtered and being a metabolite it is neither reabsorbed nor secreted. The normal value of GFR by this method is approximately the same as determined by inulin clearance.

2. Measurement of Renal Plasma Flow

To measure renal plasma flow, a substance, which is filtered and secreted but not reabsorbed, should be used. Such a substance is **para-aminohippuric acid** (PAH). PAH clearance indicates the amount of plasma passed through kidneys.

A known amount of PAH is injected into the body. After sometime, the concentration of PAH in plasma and urine and the volume of urine excreted are estimated.

For example,

Concentration of PAH in urine = 66 mg/dL
Concentration of PAH in plasma = 0.1 mg/dL
Volume of urine output = 1 mL/min

Thus,

$$\text{Renal plasma flow} = \frac{U\,V}{P}$$

$$= \frac{66 \times 1}{0.1}$$

$$= 660 \text{ mL/min}$$

Diodrast clearance also can be used to measure this.

3. Measurement of Renal Blood Flow

Values of factors necessary to determine renal blood flow are:

i. Renal plasma flow
ii. Percentage of plasma volume in blood.

i. *Renal plasma flow*

Renal plasma flow is measured by using PAH clearance.

ii. *Percentage of plasma volume in blood*

Percentage of plasma volume is indirectly determined by using packed cell volume (PCV).

For example,
If PCV = 45%
Plasma volume in the blood = 100 – 45 = 55%
That is 55 mL of plasma is present in every 100 mL of blood.

Calculation of renal blood blow

Renal blood flow is calculated with the values of renal plasma volume and percentage of plasma in blood by using a formula given below.

$$\text{Renal blood flow} = \frac{\text{Renal plasma flow}}{\text{\% of plasma in blood}}$$

For example,
Renal plasma flow = 660 mL/min
Amount of plasma in blood = 55%

$$\text{Renal blood flow} = \frac{660}{55/100}$$

$$= 1,200 \text{ mL/min}$$

Urea Clearance Test

Urea clearance test is a clinical test to assess renal function by using clearance of urea from plasma by kidney every minute. This test requires a blood sample to determine urea level in blood and two urine sample collected at 1 hour interval to determine the urea cleared by kidneys into urine. Normal value of urea clearance is 70 mL/min.

Urea is a waste product formed during protein metabolism and excreted in urine. So, determination of urea clearance forms a specific test to assess renal function.

Renal Failure

- ■ INTRODUCTION
- ■ ACUTE RENAL FAILURE
  - ■ CAUSES
  - ■ FEATURES
- ■ CHRONIC RENAL FAILURE
  - ■ CAUSES
  - ■ FEATURES

■ INTRODUCTION

Renal failure refers to failure of excretory functions of kidney. It is usually, characterized by decrease in glomerular filtration rate (GFR). So GFR is considered as the best index of renal failure. However, decrease in GFR is not affected much during the initial stages of renal failure. If 50% of the nephrons are affected, GFR decreases only by 20% to 30%. It is because of the compensatory mechanism by the unaffected nephrons. The renal failure may be either acute or chronic.

Renal failure is always accompanied by other complications such as:

1. Deficiency of calcitriol (activated vitamin D) resulting in reduction of calcium absorption from intestine and hypocalcemia (Chapter 72). Deficiency of calcitriol and hypocalcemia may cause secondary hyperparathyroidism in some patients
2. Deficiency of erythropoietin resulting in anemia
3. Disturbances in acid-base balance.

■ ACUTE RENAL FAILURE

Acute renal failure is the abrupt or sudden stoppage of renal functions. It is often reversible within few days to few weeks. Acute renal failure may result in sudden **life-threatening reactions** in the body with the need for emergency treatment.

■ CAUSES

1. Acute **nephritis** (inflammation of kidneys), which usually develops by immune reaction
2. Damage of renal tissues by poisons like lead, mercury and carbon tetrachloride
3. **Renal ischemia,** which develops during circulatory shock
4. Acute **tubular necrosis** (necrosis of tubular cells in kidney) caused by burns, hemorrhage, snake bite, toxins (like insecticides, heavy metals and carbon tetrachloride) and drugs (like diuretics, aminoglycosides and platinum derivatives)
5. Severe **transfusion reactions**
6. Sudden fall in blood pressure during hemorrhage, diarrhea, severe burns and cholera
7. Blockage of ureter due to the formation of calculi (renal stone) or tumor.

■ FEATURES

1. **Oliguria** (decreased urinary output)
2. **Anuria** (cessation of urine formation) in severe cases
3. **Proteinuria** (appearance of proteins in urine) including albuminuria (excretion of albumin in urine)
4. **Hematuria** (presence of blood in urine)

5. **Edema** due to increased volume of extracellular fluid (ECF) caused by retention of sodium and water
6. **Hypertension** within few days because of increased ECF volume
7. **Acidosis** due to the retention of metabolic end products
8. **Coma** due to severe acidosis (if the patient is not treated in time) resulting in death within 10 to 14 days.

CHRONIC RENAL FAILURE

Chronic renal failure is the progressive, long standing and irreversible impairment of renal functions.

When some of the nephrons loose the function, the unaffected nephrons can compensate it. However, when more and more nephrons start losing the function over the months or years, the compensatory mechanism fails and chronic renal failure develops.

CAUSES

1. Chronic nephritis
2. Polycystic kidney disease
3. Renal calculi (kidney stones)
4. Urethral constriction
5. Hypertension
6. Atherosclerosis
7. Tuberculosis
8. Slow poisoning by drugs or metals.

FEATURES

1. Uremia

Uremia is the condition characterized by excess accumulation of end products of protein metabolism such as urea, nitrogen and creatinine in blood. There is also accumulation of some toxic substances like organic acids and phenols. Uremia occurs because of the failure of kidney to excrete the metabolic end products and toxic substances.

Common features of uremia

  i. Anorexia (loss of appetite)
  ii. Lethargy
  iii. Drowsiness
  iv. Nausea and vomiting
  v. Pigmentation of skin
  vi. Muscular twitching, tetany and convulsion
  vii. Confusion and mental deterioration
  viii. Coma.

2. Acidosis

Uremia results in acidosis, which leads to coma and death.

3. Edema

Failure of kidney to excrete sodium and electrolytes causes increase in extracellular fluid volume resulting in development of edema.

4. Blood Loss

Gastrointestinal bleeding accompanied by platelet dysfunction leads to heavy loss of blood.

5. Anemia

Since, erythropoietin is not secreted in the kidney during renal failure, the production of RBC decreases resulting in normocytic normochromic anemia.

6. Hyperparathyroidism

Secondary hyperparathyroidism is developed due to the deficiency of calcitriol (1,25-dihydroxycholecalciferol). It increases the removal of calcium from bones resulting in **osteomalacia.**

Micturition

Chapter 57

- ■ **INTRODUCTION**
- ■ **FUNCTIONAL ANATOMY OF URINARY BLADDER AND URETHRA**
  - ■ **URINARY BLADDER**
  - ■ **URETHRA**
  - ■ **URETHRAL SPHINCTERS**
- ■ **NERVE SUPPLY TO URINARY BLADDER AND SPHINCTERS**
  - ■ **SYMPATHETIC NERVE SUPPLY**
  - ■ **PARASYMPATHETIC NERVE SUPPLY**
  - ■ **SOMATIC NERVE SUPPLY**
- ■ **FILLING OF URINARY BLADDER**
  - ■ **PROCESS OF FILLING**
  - ■ **CYSTOMETROGRAM**
- ■ **MICTURITION REFLEX**
- ■ **APPLIED PHYSIOLOGY – ABNORMALITIES OF MICTURITION**
  - ■ **ATONIC BLADDER – EFFECT OF DESTRUCTION OF SENSORY NERVE FIBERS**
  - ■ **AUTOMATIC BLADDER**
  - ■ **UNINHIBITED NEUROGENIC BLADDER**
  - ■ **NOCTURNAL MICTURITION**

■ INTRODUCTION

Micturition is a process by which urine is voided from the urinary bladder. It is a reflex process. However, in grown up children and adults, it can be controlled voluntarily to some extent. The functional anatomy and nerve supply of urinary bladder are essential for the process of micturition.

■ FUNCTIONAL ANATOMY OF URINARY BLADDER AND URETHRA

■ URINARY BLADDER

Urinary bladder is a triangular hollow organ located in lower abdomen. It consists of a body and neck. Wall of the bladder is formed by smooth muscle. It consists of three ill-defined layers of muscle fibers called **detrusor muscle**, viz. the inner longitudinal layer, middle circular layer and outer longitudinal layer. Inner surface of urinary bladder is lined by mucus membrane. In empty bladder, the **mucosa** falls into many folds called **rugae**.

At the posterior surface of the bladder wall, there is a triangular area called **trigone**. At the upper angles of this trigone, two ureters enter the bladder. Lower part of the bladder is narrow and forms the neck. It opens into urethra via **internal urethral sphincter**.

■ URETHRA

Male urethra has both urinary function and reproductive function. It carries urine and semen. Female urethra has only urinary function and it carries only urine. So, male urethra is structurally different from female urethra.

Male Urethra

Male urethra is about 20 cm long. After origin from bladder it traverses the prostate gland, which lies below the bladder and then runs through the penis (Fig. 57.1).

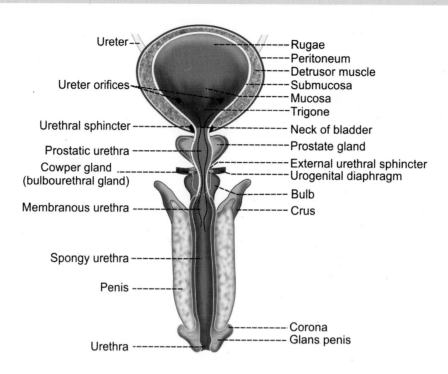

FIGURE 57.1: Male urinary bladder and urethra

Throughout its length, the urethra has mucus glands called glands of Littre.

Male urethra is divided into three parts:
1. Prostatic urethra
2. Membranous urethra
3. Spongy urethra.

1. *Prostatic urethra*

Prostatic urethra is 3 cm long and it runs through prostate gland. The prostatic fluid is emptied into this part of urethra through **prostatic sinuses.** Sperms from vas deferens and the fluid from seminal vesicles are also emptied into prostatic urethra via **ejaculatory ducts** (Chapter 74).

Part of the urethra after taking origin from neck of bladder before entering the prostate gland is known as preprostatic urethra. Its length is about 0.5 to 1.5 cm. This part of urethra is considered as part of prostatic urethra.

2. *Membranous urethra*

Membranous urethra is about 1 to 2 cm long. It runs from base of the prostate gland through **urogenital diaphragm** up to the bulb of urethra.

3. *Spongy urethra*

Spongy urethra is also known as cavernous urethra and its length is about 15 cm. Spongy urethra is surrounded by **corpus spongiosum** of penis. It is divided into a

proximal bulbar urethra and a distal penil urethra. Penile urethra is narrow with a length of about 6 cm. It ends with external urethral meatus or orifice, which is located at the end of penis.

The bilateral bulbourethral glands open into spongy urethra. **Bulbourethral glands** are also called **Cowper glands.**

Female Urethra

Female urethra is narrower and shorter than male urethra. It is about 3.5 to 4 cm long. After origin from bladder it traverses through **urogenital diaphragm** and runs along anterior wall of vagina. Then it terminates at external orifice of urethra, which is located between clitoris and vaginal opening (Fig. 57.2).

■ URETHRAL SPHINCTERS

There are two urethral sphincters in urinary tract:
1. Internal urethral sphincter
2. External urethral sphincter.

1. *Internal Urethral sphincter*

This sphincter is situated between neck of the bladder and upper end of urethra. It is made up of smooth muscle fibers and formed by thickening of detrusor muscle. It is innervated by autonomic nerve fibers. This sphincter closes the urethra when bladder is emptied.

2. *External Urethral sphincter*

External sphincter is located in the urogenital diaphragm. This sphincter is made up of circular skeletal muscle fibers, which are innervated by somatic nerve fibers.

■ NERVE SUPPLY TO URINARY BLADDER AND SPHINCTERS

Urinary bladder and the internal sphincter are supplied by sympathetic and parasympathetic divisions of autonomic nervous system where as, the external sphincter is supplied by the somatic nerve fibers (Fig. 57.3).

■ SYMPATHETIC NERVE SUPPLY

Preganglionic fibers of sympathetic nerve arise from first two lumbar segments (L1 and L2) of spinal cord. After leaving spinal cord, the fibers pass through lateral sympathetic chain without any synapse in the sympathetic ganglia and finally terminate in **hypogastric ganglion.** The postganglionic fibers arising from this ganglion form the **hypogastric nerve,** which supplies the detrusor muscle and internal sphincter.

Function of Sympathetic Nerve

The stimulation of sympathetic (hypogastric) nerve causes relaxation of detrusor muscle and constriction of the internal sphincter. It results in filling of urinary bladder and so, the sympathetic nerve is called **nerve of filling.**

■ PARASYMPATHETIC NERVE SUPPLY

Preganglionic fibers of parasympathetic nerve form the **pelvic nerve** or **nervus erigens.** Pelvic nerve fibers arise from second, third and fourth sacral segments (S1, S2 and S3) of spinal cord. These fibers run through hypogastric ganglion and synapse with postganglionic neurons situated in close relation to urinary bladder and internal sphincter (Table 57.1).

Function of Parasympathetic Nerve

Stimulation of parasympathetic (pelvic) nerve causes contraction of detrusor muscle and relaxation of the internal sphincter leading to emptying of urinary bladder. So, parasympathetic nerve is called the **nerve of emptying** or nerve of micturition.

Pelvic nerve has also the sensory fibers, which carry impulses from stretch receptors present on the wall of the urinary bladder and urethra to the central nervous system.

■ SOMATIC NERVE SUPPLY

External sphincter is innervated by the somatic nerve called **pudendal nerve.** It arises from second, third and fourth sacral segments of the spinal cord.

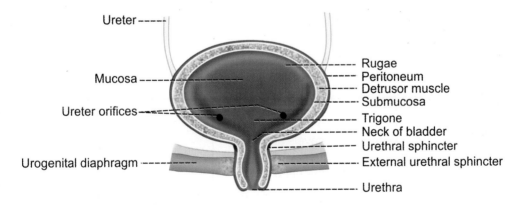

FIGURE 57.2: Female urinary bladder and urethra

TABLE 57.1: Functions of nerves supplying urinary bladder and sphincters

Nerve	On detrusor muscle	On internal sphincter	On external sphincter	Function
Sympathetic nerve	Relaxation	Constriction	Not supplied	Filling of urinary bladder
Parasympathetic nerve	Contraction	Relaxation	Not supplied	Emptying of urinary bladder
Somatic nerve	Not supplied	Not supplied	Constriction	Voluntary control of micturition

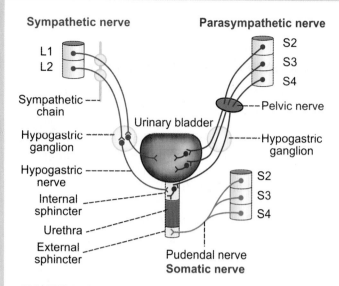

FIGURE 57.3: Nerve supply to urinary bladder and urethra

Function of Pudendal Nerve

Pudendal nerve maintains the **tonic contraction** of the skeletal muscle fibers of the external sphincter and keeps the external sphincter constricted always.

During micturition, this nerve is inhibited. It causes relaxation of external sphincter leading to voiding of urine. Thus, the pudendal nerve is responsible for **voluntary control** of micturition.

■ FILLING OF URINARY BLADDER

■ PROCESS OF FILLING

Urine is continuously formed by nephrons and it flows into urinary bladder drop by drop through ureters. When urine collects in the pelvis of ureter, the contraction sets up in pelvis. This contraction is transmitted through rest of the ureter in the form of peristaltic wave up to trigone of the urinary bladder. **Peristaltic wave** usually travels at a velocity of 3 cm/second. It develops at a frequency of 1 to 5 per minute. The peristaltic wave moves the urine into the bladder.

After leaving the kidney, the direction of the ureter is initially downward and outward. Then, it turns horizontally before entering the bladder. At the entrance of ureters into urinary bladder, a valvular arrangement is present. When peristaltic wave pushes the urine towards bladder, this valve opens towards the bladder. The position of ureter and the valvular arrangement at the end of ureter prevent the back flow of urine from bladder into the ureter when the detrusor muscle contracts. Thus, urine is collected in bladder drop by drop.

A reasonable volume of urine can be stored in urinary bladder without any discomfort and without much increase in pressure inside the bladder **(intravesical pressure)**. It is due to the adaptation of detrusor muscle. This can be explained by cystometrogram.

■ CYSTOMETROGRAM

Definition

Cystometry is the technique used to study the relationship between intravesical pressure and volume of urine in the bladder. Cystometrogram is the graphical registration (recording) of pressure changes in urinary bladder in relation to volume of urine collected in it.

Method of Recording Cystometrogram

A double-lumen catheter is introduced into the urinary bladder. One of the lumen is used to infuse fluid into the bladder and the other one is used to record the pressure changes by connecting it to a suitable recording instrument.

First, the bladder is emptied completely. Then, a known quantity of fluid is introduced into the bladder at regular intervals. The intravesical pressure developed by the fluid is recorded continuously. A graph is obtained by plotting all the values of volume and the pressure. This graph is the cystometrogram (Fig. 57.4).

Description of Cystometrogram

Cystometrogram shows three segments.

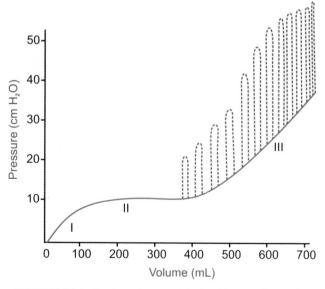

FIGURE 57.4: Cystometrogram. Dotted lines indicate the contraction of detrusor muscle.

Segment I

Initially, when the urinary bladder is empty, the intravesical pressure is 0. When about 100 mL of fluid is collected, the pressure rises sharply to about 10 cm H_2O.

Segment II

Segment II shows the plateau, i.e. no change in intra-vesical pressure. It remains at 10 cm H_2O even after introducing 300 to 400 mL of fluid. It is because of adaptation of urinary bladder by relaxation. It is in accordance with law of Laplace.

Law of Laplace

According to this law, the pressure in a spherical organ is inversely proportional to its radius, the tone remaining constant. That is, if radius is more, the pressure is less and if radius is less the pressure is more, provided the tone remains constant.

$$P = \frac{T}{R}$$

Where, P = Pressure
T = Tension
R = Radius

Accordingly in the bladder, the tension increases as the urine is filled. At the same time, the radius also increases due to relaxation of detrusor muscle. Because of this, the pressure does not change and plateau appears in the graph.

With 100 mL of urine and 10 cm H_2O of intravesical pressure, the desire for micturition occurs. Desire for micturition is associated with a vague feeling in the perineum. But it can be controlled voluntarily.

An additional volume of about 200 to 300 mL of urine can be collected in bladder without much increase in pressure. However, when total volume rises beyond 400 mL, the pressure starts rising sharply.

Segment III

As the pressure increases with collection of 300 to 400 mL of fluid, the contraction of detrusor muscle becomes intense, increasing the consciousness and the urge for micturition. Still, voluntary control is possible up to volume of 600 to 700 mL at which the pressure rises to about 35 to 40 cm H_2O.

When the intravesical pressure rises above 40 cm water, the contraction of detrusor muscle becomes still more intense. And, voluntary control of micturition is not possible. Now, pain sensation develops and micturition is a must at this stage.

■ MICTURITION REFLEX

Micturition reflex is the reflex by which micturition occurs. This reflex is elicited by the stimulation of stretch receptors situated on the wall of urinary bladder and urethra. When about 300 to 400 mL of urine is collected in the bladder, intravesical pressure increases. This stretches the wall of bladder resulting in stimulation of stretch receptors and generation of sensory impulses.

Pathway for Micturition Reflex

Sensory (afferent) impulses from the receptors reach the sacral segments of spinal cord via the sensory fibers of pelvic (parasympathetic) nerve. Motor (efferent) impulses produced in spinal cord, travel through motor fibers of pelvic nerve towards bladder and internal sphincter. Motor impulses cause contraction of detrusor muscle and relaxation of internal sphincter so that, urine enters the urethra from the bladder (Fig. 57.5).

Once urine enters urethra, the **stretch receptors** in the urethra are stimulated and send afferent impulses to spinal cord via pelvic nerve fibers. Now the impulses generated from spinal centers inhibit pudendal nerve. So, the external sphincter relaxes and micturition occurs.

Once a micturition reflex begins, it is **self-regene-rative,** i.e. the initial contraction of bladder further activates the receptors to cause still further increase in sensory impulses from the bladder and urethra. These impulses, in turn cause further increase in reflex contraction of bladder. The cycle continues repeatedly until the force of contraction of bladder reaches the maximum and the urine is voided out completely.

During micturition, the flow of urine is facilitated by the increase in the abdominal pressure due to the voluntary contraction of abdominal muscles.

Higher Centers for Micturition

Spinal centers for micturition are present in sacral and lumbar segments. But, these spinal centers are regulated by higher centers. The higher centers, which control micturition are of two types, inhibitory centers and facilitatory centers.

Inhibitory centers for micturition

Centers in midbrain and cerebral cortex inhibit the micturition by suppressing spinal micturition centers.

Facilitatory centers for micturition

Centers in pons facilitate micturition via spinal centers. Some centers in cerebral cortex also facilitate micturition.

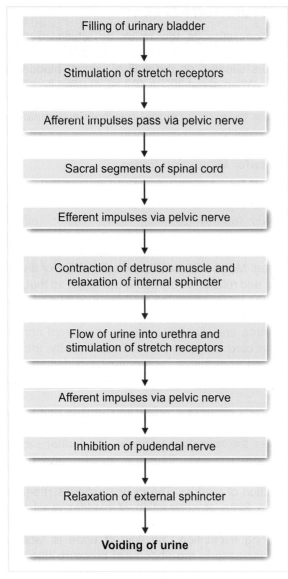

Filling of urinary bladder

↓

Stimulation of stretch receptors

↓

Afferent impulses pass via pelvic nerve

↓

Sacral segments of spinal cord

↓

Efferent impulses via pelvic nerve

↓

Contraction of detrusor muscle and relaxation of internal sphincter

↓

Flow of urine into urethra and stimulation of stretch receptors

↓

Afferent impulses via pelvic nerve

↓

Inhibition of pudendal nerve

↓

Relaxation of external sphincter

↓

Voiding of urine

FIGURE 57.5: Micturition reflex

APPLIED PHYSIOLOGY – ABNORMALITIES OF MICTURITION

■ ATONIC BLADDER – EFFECT OF DESTRUCTION OF SENSORY NERVE FIBERS

Atonic bladder is the urinary bladder with loss of tone in detrusor muscle. It is also called **flaccid neurogenic bladder** or **hypoactive neurogenic bladder.** It is caused by destruction of sensory (pelvic) nerve fibers of urinary bladder.

Due to the destruction of sensory nerve fibers, the bladder is filled without any stretch signals to spinal cord. Due to the absence of stretch signals, detrusor muscle loses the tone and becomes **flaccid.** So the bladder is completely filled with urine without any micturition.

Now, urine overflows in drops as and when it enters the bladder. It is called **overflow incontinence** or **overflow dribbling.**

Conditions of Destruction of Sensory Nerve Fibers

1. *Spinal injury:* During the first stage (stage of spinal shock) after injury to sacral segments of spinal cord (Chapter 143) the bladder becomes atonic
2. *Syphilis:* Syphilis results in the degenerative nervous disorder called **tabes dorsalis,** which is characterized by the degeneration of dorsal (sensory) nerve roots (Chapter 143). Degeneration of sensory nerve roots of sacral region develops **atonic bladder.** The atonic bladder in tabes dorsalis is called **tabetic bladder.**

■ AUTOMATIC BLADDER

Automatic bladder is the urinary bladder characterized by hyperactive micturition reflex with loss of voluntary control. So, even a small amount of urine collected in the bladder elicits the micturition reflex resulting in emptying of bladder.

This occurs during the second stage (stage of recovery) after complete transection of spinal cord above the sacral segments.

During the first stage (stage of spinal shock) after complete transection of spinal cord above sacral segments, the urinary bladder loses the tone and becomes atonic resulting in **overflow incontinence.**

During the second stage after shock period, the micturition reflex returns. However, the voluntary control is lacking because of absence of inhibition or facilitation of micturition by higher centers. There is hypertrophy of detrusor muscles so that the capacity of bladder reduces. Some patients develop hyperactive micturition reflex.

■ UNINHIBITED NEUROGENIC BLADDER

Uninhibited neurogenic bladder is the urinary bladder with frequent and uncontrollable micturition caused by lesion in midbrain. It is also called **spastic neurogenic bladder** or **hyperactive neurogenic bladder.**

The lesion in midbrain causes continuous excitation of spinal micturition centers resulting in frequent and uncontrollable micturition. Even a small quantity of urine collected in bladder will elicit the micturition reflex.

■ NOCTURNAL MICTURITION

Nocturnal micturition is the involuntary voiding of urine during night. It is otherwise known as **enuresis** or

bedwetting. It occurs due to the absence of voluntary control of micturition. It is a common and normal process in infants and children below 3 years. It is because of incomplete myelination of motor nerve fibers of the bladder. When myelination is complete, voluntary control of micturition develops and bedwetting stops.

If nocturnal micturition occurs after 3 years of age it is considered abnormal. It occurs due to neurological disorders like **lumbosacral vertebral defects.** It can also occur due to psychological factors. Loss of voluntary control of micturition occurs even during the impairment of motor area of cerebral cortex.

Dialysis and Artificial Kidney

Chapter 58

- **DIALYSIS**
- **ARTIFICIAL KIDNEY**
  - **MECHANISM OF FUNCTION OF ARTIFICIAL KIDNEY**
- **FREQUENCY AND DURATION OF DIALYSIS**
- **DIALYSATE**
- **PERITONEAL DIALYSIS**
- **UREMIA**
- **COMPLICATIONS OF DIALYSIS**

DIALYSIS

Dialysis is the procedure to remove waste materials and toxic substances and to restore normal volume and composition of body fluid in severe renal failure. It is also called **hemodialysis.**

ARTIFICIAL KIDNEY

Artificial kidney is the machine that is used to carry out dialysis during renal failure. It is used to treat the patients suffering from:
1. Acute renal failure
2. Chronic or permanent renal failure.

MECHANISM OF FUNCTION OF ARTIFICIAL KIDNEY

The term **dialysis** refers to diffusion of solutes from an area of higher concentration to the area of lower concentration, through a semipermeable membrane. This forms the principle of artificial kidney.

Patient's arterial blood is passed continuously or intermittently through the artificial kidney and then back to the body through the vein. Heparin is used as an anticoagulant while passing the blood through the machine.

Inside the artificial kidney, the blood passes through a dialyzer called **hemofilter,** which contains minute channels interposed between two **cellophane membranes** (Fig. 58.1). The cellophane membranes are porous in nature. The outer surface of these membranes is bathed in the dialyzing fluid called **dialysate.** The used dialysate in the artificial kidney is constantly replaced by fresh dialysate.

Urea, creatinine, phosphate and other unwanted substances from the blood pass into the dialysate by concentration gradient. The essential substances required by the body diffuse from dialysate into blood. Almost all the substances, except plasma proteins are exchanged between the blood and dialysate through the cellophane membranes.

In addition to the dialyzer, the dialysis machine has several blood pumps with pressure monitors, which enable easy flow of blood from the patient to the machine and back to the patient. It also has pumps for flow of fresh dialysate and for drainage of used dialysate.

Total amount of blood in the dialysis machine at a time is about 500 mL. The rate of blood flow through the dialysis machine is about 200 to 300 mL/minute. The rate of dialysate flow is about 500 mL/minute.

FREQUENCY AND DURATION OF DIALYSIS

The frequency and duration of dialysis depends upon the severity of renal dysfunction. Dialysis is done usually thrice a week in severe uremia. Each time, the artificial kidney is used for about 6 hours.

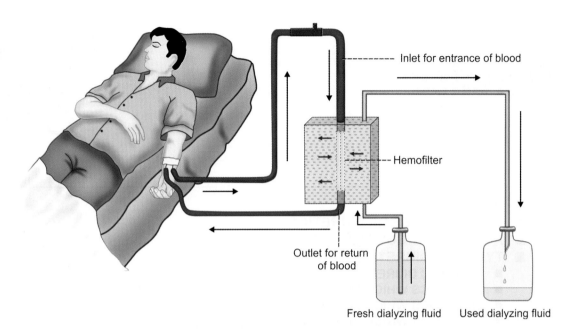

Inlet for entrance of blood

Hemofilter

Outlet for return
of blood

Fresh dialyzing fluid   Used dialyzing fluid

FIGURE 58.1: Principle of dialysis

■ DIALYSATE

The concentration of various substances in the dialysate is adjusted in accordance with the needs of the patient's body. The fluid does not contain urea, urate, sulfate, phosphate or creatinine, so that, these substances move from the blood to the dialysate.

The fluid has low concentration of sodium, potassium and chloride ions than in the uremic blood. But the concentration of glucose, bicarbonate and calcium ions is more in the dialysate than in the uremic blood.

■ PERITONEAL DIALYSIS

Peritoneal dialysis is the technique in which peritoneal membrane is used as a semipermeable membrane. It is also used to treat the patients suffering from renal failure.

A catheter is inserted into the peritoneal cavity through anterior abdominal wall and sutured. The dialysate is passed through this catheter under gravity. The required electrolytes from dialysate pass through vascular perito-neum into blood vessels of abdominal cavity. Urea, creatinine, phosphate and other unwanted substances diffuse from blood vessels into dialysate. Later, dialysate is drained from peritoneal cavity by gravity.

Peritoneal dialysis is a simple, convenient and less-expensive technique, compared to hemodialysis.

Patients themselves can change the fluid on an outpatient basis. However, it has few drawbacks. It is less efficient in removing some of the toxic substances and it may lead to complications by infections.

■ UREMIA

Uremia is explained in Chapter 56. Blood level of urea, nitrogen and creatinine increases during uremia. Toxic substances such as organic acids and phenols also accumulate in blood.

Artificial kidney can excrete more than double the amount of urea that could be excreted by both the normal kidneys. About 200 to 250 mL of plasma could be cleared off urea per minute by the artificial kidney. But, the **urea clearance** by normal kidney is only about 70 mL/minute. Refer Chapter 55 for urea clearance test.

■ COMPLICATIONS OF DIALYSIS

Complications of dialysis depend upon the patient's condition, age, existence of diseases other than renal failure and many other factors.

Common complications of dialysis in individuals having only renal dysfunction are:
1. Sleep disorders
2. Anxiety
3. Depression.

Diuretics

- ■ INTRODUCTION
- ■ GENERAL USES OF DIURETICS
- ■ ABUSES AND COMPLICATIONS OF DIURETICS
- ■ TYPES OF DIURETICS
  - ■ OSMOTIC DIURETICS
  - ■ DIURETICS WHICH INHIBIT ACTIVE REABSORPTION OF ELECTROLYTES
  - ■ DIURETICS WHICH INHIBIT ACTION OF ALDOSTERONE
  - ■ DIURETICS WHICH INHIBIT ACTIVITY OF CARBONIC ANHYDRASE
  - ■ DIURETICS WHICH INCREASE GLOMERULAR FILTRATION RATE
  - ■ DIURETICS WHICH INHIBIT SECRETION OF ADH
  - ■ DIURETICS WHICH INHIBIT ADH RECEPTORS

■ INTRODUCTION

Diuretics or **diuretic agents** are the substances which enhance the urine formation and output. These substances increase the excretion of water, sodium and chloride through urine. Diuretic agents increase the urine formation, by influencing any of the processes involved in urine formation. Diuretics are commonly called **'water pills'**.

■ GENERAL USES OF DIURETICS

Diuretics are generally used for the treatment of disorders involving increase in extracellular fluid volume like:
1. Hypertension
2. Congestive cardiac failure
3. Edema.
   Diuretic agents prevent hypertension, congestive cardiac failure and edema, by increasing the urinary output and reducing extracellular fluid (ECF) volume.

■ ABUSES AND COMPLICATIONS OF DIURETICS

Nowadays, diuretics are misused in order to reduce the body weight and keep the body slim. Even persons suffering from eating disorders attempt to reduce body weight by misusing the diuretics.

However, prolonged use of these substances leads to complications like **syndrome of diuretic-dependent sodium retention,** characterized by edema. The adverse effects depend upon the type of diuretic agents used.

Adverse Effects of Diuretics

1. Dehydration
2. Electrolyte imbalance
3. Potassium deficiency
4. Headache
5. Dizziness
6. Renal damage
7. Cardiac arrhythmia
8. Heart palpitations.

■ TYPES OF DIURETICS

Diuretics are classified into seven types:
1. Osmotic diuretics
2. Diuretics which inhibit active reabsorption of electrolytes
3. Diuretics which inhibit action of aldosterone

4. Diuretics which inhibit activity of carbonic anhydrase
5. Diuretics which increase glomerular filtration rate
6. Diuretics which inhibit secretion of ADH
7. Diuretics which inhibit ADH receptors.

■ **OSMOTIC DIURETICS**

Osmotic diuretics are the substances that induce osmotic diuresis. Osmotic diuresis is the type of diuresis that occurs because of increased osmotic pressure. Some of the osmotically active substances are not reabsorbed from renal tubules. When injected in large quantities into the body, these substances increase the osmotic pressure in the tubular fluid. Increased osmotic pressure in the tubular fluid, in turn reduces water reabsorption. It leads to excretion of excess of water through urine.

Elevated blood sugar level in diabetes can also cause osmotic diuresis in the same manner.

Examples

   i. Urea
   ii. Mannitol
   iii. Sucrose
   iv. Glucose.

■ **DIURETICS WHICH INHIBIT ACTIVE REABSORPTION OF ELECTROLYTES**

Diuretics of this type inhibits the active reabsorption of electrolytes like sodium and potassium from the renal tubular fluid. Inhibition of electrolyte reabsorption causes osmotic diuresis. These diuretic agents are of three types:

1. *Loop Diuretics – Diuretics which Inhibit the Electrolyte Reabsorption in Thick Ascending Limb of Henle Loop*

Loop diuretics are the substances that inhibit electrolyte reabsorption in Henle loop. These diuretics inhibit the sodium and chloride reabsorption from thick ascending limb of Henle loop. So, the osmotic pressure in tubular fluid increases, leading to diuresis. The osmolarity of medullary interstitial fluid also decreases due to inhibition of sodium reabsorption into medullary interstitium. So, the medullary interstitium fails to concentrate the urine, resulting in loss of excess fluid through urine.

Examples

   i. Furosemide
   ii. Torasemide
   iii. Bumetanide.

2. *Diuretics which Inhibit Active Transport of Electrolytes In Proximal Part of Distal Convoluted Tubule*

Diuretics of this type inhibit sodium reabsorption in proximal part of the distal convoluted tubules. These diuretics are usually called **thiazide and related diuretics.**

Examples

   i. Chlorothiazide
   ii. Metolazone
   iii. Chlortalidone.

3. *Diuretics which Inhibit Active Transport of Electrolytes in Distal Part of Distal Convoluted Tubule and Collecting Duct*

Some of the diuretics inhibit reabsorption of sodium and excretion of potassium in distal portion of the distal convoluted tubule and collecting duct. Such substances are called **potassium-retaining diuretics** or **potassium-sparing diuretics.**

Examples

   i. Triamterene
   ii. Amiloride.

■ **DIURETICS WHICH INHIBIT ACTION OF ALDOSTERONE**

Some diuretics inhibit sodium reabsorption and potassium excretion in the distal convoluted tubule and collecting duct, by inhibiting the action of aldosterone. These substances are also called the potassium-retaining diuretics or **aldosterone antagonists.**

Examples

   i. Spironolactone
   ii. Eperenone.

■ **DIURETICS WHICH INHIBIT ACTIVITY OF CARBONIC ANHYDRASE**

Some diuretics inhibit the activity of carbonic anhydrase in proximal convoluted tubules and prevent reabsorption of bicarbonates from renal tubules, resulting in osmotic diuresis. Such diuretic agents are called **carbonic anhydrase inhibitors.** Acetazolamide is a carbonic anhydrase inhibitor.

■ **DIURETICS WHICH INCREASE GLOMERULAR FILTRATION RATE**

Some xanthines (alkaloids, used as mild stimulants) cause diuresis by increasing the glomerular filtration rate and to some extent by decreasing the sodium reabsorption.

Examples

   i. Caffeine

  ii. Theophylline.

■ DIURETICS WHICH INHIBIT SECRETION OF ANTIDIURETIC HORMONE

Some diuretics produce diuresis by inhibiting the secretion of ADH.

Examples

   i. Water

  ii. Ethanol.

■ DIURETICS WHICH INHIBIT ANTIDIURETIC HORMONE RECEPTORS

The antagonists of V2 receptors cause diuresis by inhibiting the receptors of antidiuretic hormone, thereby preventing the activity of this hormone.

Structure of Skin

- ■ **INTRODUCTION**
  - ■ LAYERS OF SKIN
- ■ **EPIDERMIS**
  - ■ STRATUM CORNEUM
  - ■ STRATUM LUCIDUM
  - ■ STRATUM GRANULOSUM
  - ■ STRATUM SPINOSUM
  - ■ STRATUM GERMINATIVUM
- ■ **DERMIS**
  - ■ SUPERFICIAL PAPILLARY LAYER
  - ■ RETICULAR LAYER
- ■ **APPENDAGES OF SKIN**
- ■ **COLOR OF SKIN**
  - ■ PIGMENTATION OF SKIN
  - ■ HEMOGLOBIN IN THE BLOOD

■ INTRODUCTION

Skin is the **largest organ** of the body. It is not uniformly thick. At some places it is thick and at some places it is thin. The average thickness of the skin is about 1 to 2 mm. In the sole of the foot, palm of the hand and in the interscapular region, it is considerably thick, measuring about 5 mm. In other areas of the body, the skin is thin. It is thinnest over eyelids and penis, measuring about 0.5 mm only.

■ LAYERS OF SKIN

Skin is made up of two layers:
  I. Outer epidermis
 II. Inner dermis.

■ EPIDERMIS

Epidermis is the outer layer of skin. It is formed by stratified epithelium. Important feature of epidermis is that, it does not have blood vessels (Fig. 60.1).

Nutrition is provided to the epidermis by the capillaries of dermis.

Layers of Epidermis

Epidermis is formed by five layers:
1. Stratum corneum
2. Stratum lucidum
3. Stratum granulosum
4. Stratum spinosum
5. Stratum germinativum.

■ 1. STRATUM CORNEUM

Stratum corneum is also known as **horny layer.** It is the outermost layer and consists of **dead cells,** which are called **corneocytes.** These cells lose their nucleus due to pressure and become dead cells. The cytoplasm is flattened with fibrous protein known as **keratin.** Apart from this, these cells also contain phospholipids and glycogen.

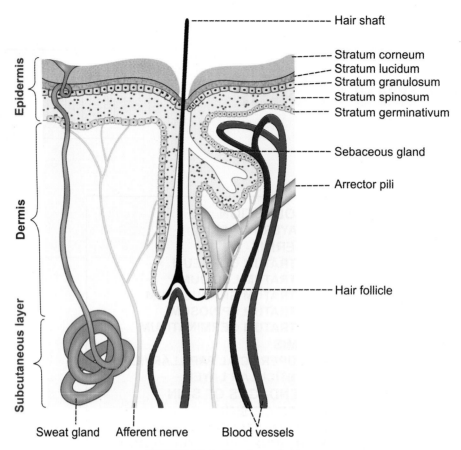

FIGURE 60.1: Structure of skin

■ 2. STRATUM LUCIDUM

Stratum lucidum is made up of flattened epithelial cells. Many cells have degenerated nucleus and in some cells, the nucleus is absent. As these cells exhibit shiny character, the layer looks like a **homogeneous translucent zone.** So, this layer is called stratum lucidum (lucid = clear).

■ 3. STRATUM GRANULOSUM

Stratum granulosum is a thin layer with two to five rows of flattened **rhomboid cells.** Cytoplasm contains granules of a protein called **keratohyalin.** Keratohyalin is the precursor of **keratin.**

■ 4. STRATUM SPINOSUM

Stratum spinosum is also known as **prickle cell layer** because, the cells of this layer possess some spine-like protoplasmic projections. By these projections, the cells are connected to one another.

■ 5. STRATUM GERMINATIVUM

Stratum germinativum is a thick layer made up of polygonal cells, superficially and columnar or cuboidal epithelial cells in the deeper parts. Here, new cells are constantly formed by mitotic division. The newly formed cells move continuously towards the stratum corneum. The stem cells, which give rise to new cells, are known as **keratinocytes.**

Another type of cells called **melanocytes** are scattered between the keratinocytes. Melanocytes produce the pigment called **melanin.** The color of the skin depends upon melanin.

From this layer, some projections called **rete ridges** extend down up to dermis. These projections provide anchoring and nutritional function.

■ DERMIS

Dermis is the inner layer of the skin. It is a connective tissue layer, made up of dense and stout collagen fibers, fibroblasts and histiocytes. Collagen fibers exhibit elastic property and are capable of storing or holding water. Collagen fibers contain the enzyme collagenase, which is responsible for wound healing.

Layers of Dermis

Dermis is made up of two layers:
1. Superficial papillary layer
2. Deeper reticular layer.

■ SUPERFICIAL PAPILLARY LAYER

Superficial papillary layer projects into the epidermis. It contains blood vessels, lymphatics and nerve fibers. This layer also has some pigment-containing cells known as **chromatophores.**

Dermal papillae are finger-like projections, arising from the superficial papillary dermis. Each papilla contains a plexus of capillaries and lymphatics, which are oriented perpendicular to the skin surface. The papillae are surrounded by rete ridges, extending from the epidermis.

■ RETICULAR LAYER

Reticular layer is made up of reticular and elastic fibers. These fibers are found around the hair bulbs, sweat glands and sebaceous glands. The reticular layer also contains mast cells, nerve endings, lymphatics, epidermal appendages and fibroblasts.

Immediately below the dermis, subcutaneous tissue is present. It is a loose connective tissue, which connects the skin with the internal structures of the body. It serves as an insulator to protect the body from excessive heat and cold of the environment. Lot of smooth muscles called **arrector pili** are also found in skin around the hair follicles.

■ APPENDAGES OF SKIN

Hair follicles with hair, nails, sweat glands, sebaceous glands and mammary glands are considered as appendages of the skin.

■ COLOR OF SKIN

Color of skin depends upon two important factors:
1. Pigmentation of skin
2. Hemoglobin in the blood.

■ PIGMENTATION OF SKIN

Cells of the skin contain a brown pigment called **melanin,** which is responsible for the color of the skin. It is synthesized by **melanocytes,** which are present mainly in the stratum germinativum and stratum spinosum of epidermis. After synthesis, this pigment spreads to the cells of the other layers.

Melanin

Melanin is the skin pigment and it forms the major color determinant of human skin. Skin becomes dark when melanin content increases. It is protein in nature and it is synthesized from the amino acid tyrosine via dihydroxyphenylalanine (DOPA).

Deficiency of melanin leads to **albinism** (hypopigmentary congenital disorder).

■ HEMOGLOBIN IN THE BLOOD

Amount and nature of hemoglobin that circulates in the cutaneous blood vessels play an important role in the coloration of the skin.

Skin becomes:
i. Pale, when hemoglobin content decreases
ii. Pink, when blood rushes to skin due to cutaneous vasodilatation (blushing)
iii. Bluish during cyanosis, which is caused by excess amount of reduced hemoglobin.

Functions of Skin

■ **FUNCTIONS OF SKIN**
  ■ **PROTECTIVE FUNCTION**
  ■ **SENSORY FUNCTION**
  ■ **STORAGE FUNCTION**
  ■ **SYNTHETIC FUNCTION**
  ■ **REGULATION OF BODY TEMPERATURE**
  ■ **REGULATION OF WATER AND ELECTROLYTE BALANCE**
  ■ **EXCRETORY FUNCTION**
  ■ **ABSORPTIVE FUNCTION**
  ■ **SECRETORY FUNCTION**

■ FUNCTIONS OF SKIN

Primary function of skin is protection of organs. However, it has many other important functions also.

■ 1. PROTECTIVE FUNCTION

Skin forms the covering of all the organs of the body and protects these organs from the following factors:
  i. Bacteria and toxic substances
  ii. Mechanical blow
  iii. Ultraviolet rays.

i. *Protection from Bacteria and Toxic Substances*

Skin covers the organs of the body and protects the organs from having direct contact with external environment. Thus, it prevents the bacterial infection.

Lysozyme secreted in skin destroys the bacteria. Keratinized stratum corneum of epidermis is responsible for the protective function of skin. This layer also offers resistance against toxic chemicals like acids and alkalis. If the skin is injured, infection occurs due to invasion of bacteria from external environment.

During injury or skin infection, the keratinocytes secrete:
a. **Cytokines** like interleukins, α-tumor necrosis factor and γ-interferon, which play important role in

inflammation, immunological reactions, tissue repair and wound healing
b. Antimicrobial peptides like β-defensins, which prevent invasion of microbes.

ii. *Protection from Mechanical Blow*

Skin is not tightly placed over the underlying organs or tissues. It is somewhat loose and moves over the underlying subcutaneous tissues. So, the mechanical impact of any blow to the skin is not transmitted to the underlying tissues.

iii. *Protection from Ultraviolet Rays*

Skin protects the body from **ultraviolet rays** of sunlight. Exposure to sunlight or to any other source of ultraviolet rays increases the production of **melanin** pigment in skin. Melanin absorbs ultraviolet rays. At the same time, the thickness of stratum corneum increases. This layer of epidermis also absorbs the ultraviolet rays.

■ 2. SENSORY FUNCTION

Skin is considered as the **largest sense organ** in the body. It has many nerve endings, which form the specialized cutaneous receptors (Chapter 139).

These receptors are stimulated by sensations of touch, pain, pressure or temperature sensation and convey these sensations to the brain via afferent nerves. At the brain level, perception of different sensations occurs.

■ 3. STORAGE FUNCTION

Skin stores fat, water, chloride and sugar. It can also store blood by the dilatation of the cutaneous blood vessels.

■ 4. SYNTHETIC FUNCTION

Vitamin D3 is synthesized in skin by the action of ultraviolet rays from sunlight on cholesterol.

■ 5. REGULATION OF BODY TEMPERATURE

Skin plays an important role in the regulation of body temperature. Excess heat is lost from the body through skin by radiation, conduction, convection and evaporation. Sweat glands of the skin play an active part in heat loss, by secreting sweat. The lipid content of sebum prevents loss of heat from the body in cold environment. More details are given in Chapter 63.

■ 6. REGULATION OF WATER AND ELECTROLYTE BALANCE

Skin regulates water balance and electrolyte balance by excreting water and salts through sweat.

■ 7. EXCRETORY FUNCTION

Skin excretes small quantities of waste materials like urea, salts and fatty substance.

■ 8. ABSORPTIVE FUNCTION

Skin absorbs fat-soluble substances and some ointments.

■ 9. SECRETORY FUNCTION

Skin secretes **sweat** through **sweat glands** and **sebum** through **sebaceous glands.** By secreting sweat, skin regulates body temperature and water balance. Sebum keeps the skin smooth and moist.

Glands of Skin

- ■ **GLANDS OF SKIN**
- ■ **SEBACEOUS GLANDS**
- ■ **SWEAT GLANDS**
  - ■ **ECCRINE GLANDS**
  - ■ **APOCRINE GLANDS**

■ GLANDS OF SKIN

Skin contains two types of glands, namely sebaceous glands and sweat glands.

■ SEBACEOUS GLANDS

Sebaceous glands are simple or branched alveolar glands, situated in the dermis of skin.

Structure

Sebaceous glands are ovoid or spherical in shape and are situated at the side of the **hair follicle.** These glands develop from hair follicles. So, the sebaceous glands are absent over the thick skin, which is devoid of hair follicles. Each gland is covered by a connective tissue capsule. The alveoli of the gland are lined by stratified epithelial cells.

Sebaceous glands open into the neck of the hair follicle through a duct. In some areas like face, lips, nipple, glans penis and labia minora, the sebaceous glands open directly into the exterior.

Secretion of Sebaceous Gland – Sebum

Sebaceous glands secrete an oily substance called sebum. Sebum is formed by the liquefaction of the alveolar cells and poured out through the ducts either via the hair follicle or directly into the exterior.

Composition of Sebum

Sebum contains:
1. Free fatty acids
2. Triglycerides
3. Squalene
4. Sterols
5. Waxes
6. Paraffin.

Functions of Sebum

1. Free fatty acid content of the sebum has antibacterial and antifungal actions. Thus, it prevents the infection of skin by bacteria or fungi
2. Lipid nature of sebum keeps the skin smooth and oily. It protects the skin from unnecessary desquamation and injury caused by dryness
3. Lipids of the sebum prevent heat loss from the body. It is particularly useful in cold climate.

Activation of Sebaceous Glands at Puberty

Sebaceous glands are inactive till puberty. At the time of puberty, these glands are activated by sex hormones in both males and females.

At the time of puberty, particularly in males, due to the increased secretion of sex hormones, especially dehydroepiandrosterone, the sebaceous glands are stimulated suddenly. It leads to the development of acne on the face.

Acne

Acne is the localized inflammatory condition of the skin, characterized by pimples on face, chest and back. It occurs because of overactivity of sebaceous glands. Acne vulgaris is the common type of acne that is developed during adolescence. Acne disappears within few years, when the sebaceous glands become adapted to the sex hormones.

◉ SWEAT GLANDS

Sweat glands are of two types:
1. Eccrine glands
2. Apocrine glands.

■ ECCRINE GLANDS

Distribution

Eccrine glands are distributed throughout the body (Table 62.1). There are many eccrine glands over thick skin.

Structure

Eccrine sweat gland is a tubular coiled gland.
  It consists of two parts:
1. A coiled portion lying deeper in dermis, which secretes the sweat
2. A duct portion, which passes through dermis and epidermis.
  Eccrine sweat gland opens out through the sweat pore. The coiled portion is formed by single layer of columnar or cuboidal epithelial cells, which are secretory in nature. Epithelial cells are interposed by the **myoepithelial cells.** Myoepithelial cells support the secretory epithelial cells.
  The duct of eccrine gland is formed by two layers of cuboidal epithelial cells.

Secretory Activity of Eccrine Glands

Eccrine glands function throughout the life since birth. These glands secrete a clear **watery sweat.** The secretion increases during increase in temperature and emotional conditions.
  Eccrine glands play an important role in regulating the body temperature by secreting sweat. Sweat contains water, sodium chloride, urea and lactic acid.

Control of Eccrine Glands

Eccrine glands are under nervous control and are supplied by sympathetic postganglionic cholinergic nerve fibers, which secrete acetylcholine. Stimulation of these nerves causes secretion of sweat.

■ APOCRINE GLANDS

Distribution

Apocrine glands are situated only in certain areas of the body like axilla, pubis, areola and umbilicus.

Structure

Apocrine glands are also tubular coiled glands. The coiled portion lies in deep dermis. But, the duct opens into the hair follicle above the opening of sebaceous gland.

Secretory Activity of Apocrine Glands

Apocrine sweat glands are nonfunctional till puberty and start functioning only at the time of puberty. In old age, the function of these glands gradually declines.
  The secretion of the apocrine glands is thick and milky. At the time of secretion, it is odorless. When microorganisms grow in this secretion, a characteristic odor develops in the regions where apocrine glands are present. Secretion increases only in emotional conditions.

TABLE 62.1: Differences between eccrine and apocrine sweat glands

Features	Eccrine glands	Apocrine glands
1. Distribution	Throughout the body	Only in limited areas like axilla, pubis, areola and umbilicus
2. Opening	Exterior through sweat pore	Into the hair follicle
3. Period of functioning	Function throughout life	Start functioning only at puberty
4. Secretion	Clear and watery	Thick and milky
5. Regulation of body temperature	Play important role in temperature regulation	Do not play any role in temperature regulation
6. Conditions when secretion increases	During increased temperature and emotional conditions	Only during emotional conditions
7. Control of secretory activity	Under nervous control	Under hormonal control
8. Nerve supply	Sympathetic cholinergic fibers	Sympathetic adrenergic fibers

Apocrine glands do not play any role in temperature regulation like eccrine glands.

Control of Apocrine Glands

Apocrine glands are innervated by sympathetic adrenergic nerve fibers. But, the secretory activity is not under nervous control. However, adrenaline from adrenal medulla causes secretion by apocrine glands.

Glands of eyelids, glands of external auditory meatus and mammary glands are the modified apocrine glands.

Pheromones

Pheromones are a group of chemical substances that are secreted by apocrine glands. Some scientists call this substance as **vomeropherins.** When secreted into environment by an organism, pheromones produce some behavioral or physiological changes in other members of the same species. Pheromones are mostly present in urine, vaginal fluid and other secretions of mammals and influence the behavior and reproductive cycle in these animals.

Details of pheromones in lower animals are well documented. However, human pheromones are not fully studied.

Recently, it is found that the pheromones excreted in axilla of a woman affects the menstrual cycle of her room-mate or other woman living with her. These substances stimulate receptors of vomeronasal receptors. **Vomeronasal receptors** are distinct from other olfactory receptors and detect specially the odor of pheromones. Impulses from these receptors are transmitted to hypothalamus, which influences the menstrual cycle via pituitary gonadal axis. This effect of pheromones on the menstrual cycle of other individuals is called **dormitory effect.** Refer Chapter 177 for details of vomeronasal organ and its receptors.

Body Temperature

63

- ■ **INTRODUCTION**
  - ■ HOMEOTHERMIC ANIMALS
  - ■ POIKILOTHERMIC ANIMALS
- ■ **BODY TEMPERATURE**
  - ■ NORMAL BODY TEMPERATURE
  - ■ TEMPERATURE AT DIFFERENT PARTS OF THE BODY
  - ■ VARIATIONS OF BODY TEMPERATURE
- ■ **HEAT BALANCE**
  - ■ HEAT GAIN OR HEAT PRODUCTION IN THE BODY
  - ■ HEAT LOSS FROM THE BODY
- ■ **REGULATION OF BODY TEMPERATURE**
  - ■ HEAT LOSS CENTER
  - ■ HEAT GAIN CENTER
  - ■ MECHANISM OF TEMPERATURE REGULATION
- ■ **APPLIED PHYSIOLOGY**
  - ■ HYPERTHERMIA – FEVER
  - ■ HYPOTHERMIA

■ INTRODUCTION

Living organisms are classified into two groups, depending upon the maintenance (regulation) of body temperature:
1. Homeothermic animals
2. Poikilothermic animals.

■ HOMEOTHERMIC ANIMALS

Homeothermic animals are the animals in which the body temperature is maintained at a constant level, irrespective of the environmental temperature. Birds and mammals including man belong to this category. They are also called **warm-blooded animals.**

■ POIKILOTHERMIC ANIMALS

Poikilothermic animals are the animals in which the body temperature is not constant. It varies according to the environmental temperature. Amphibians and reptiles are the poikilothermic animals. These animals are also called **cold-blooded animals.**

■ BODY TEMPERATURE

Body temperature can be measured by placing the **clinical thermometer** in different parts of the body such as:
1. Mouth (oral temperature)
2. Axilla (axillary temperature)
3. Rectum (rectal temperature)
4. Over the skin (surface temperature).

■ NORMAL BODY TEMPERATURE

Normal body temperature in human is 37°C (98.6°F), when measured by placing the clinical thermometer in the mouth (oral temperature). It varies between 35.8°C and 37.3°C (96.4°F and 99.1°F).

■ TEMPERATURE AT DIFFERENT PARTS OF THE BODY

Axillary temperature is 0.3°C to 0.6°C (0.5°F to 1°F) lower than the **oral temperature.** The **rectal temperature** is 0.3°C to 0.6°C (0.5°F to 1°F) higher than oral temperature.

The superficial temperature (skin or surface temperature) varies between 29.5°C and 33.9°C (85.1°F and 93°F).

Core Temperature

Core temperature is the average temperature of structures present in deeper part of the body. The core temperature is always more than oral or rectal temperature. It is about 37.8°C (100°F).

■ VARIATIONS OF BODY TEMPERATURE

Physiological Variations

1. *Age*

In infants, the body temperature varies in accordance to environmental temperature for the first few days after birth. It is because the temperature regulating system does not function properly during infancy. In children, the temperature is slightly (0.5°C) more than in adults because of more physical activities. In old age, since the heat production is less, the body temperature decreases slightly.

2. *Sex*

In females, the body temperature is less because of low basal metabolic rate, when compared to that of males. During menstrual phase it decreases slightly.

3. *Diurnal variation*

In early morning, the temperature is 1°C less. In the afternoon, it reaches the maximum (about 1°C more than normal).

4. *After meals*

The body temperature rises slightly (0.5°C) after meals.

5. *Exercise*

During exercise, the temperature raises due to production of heat in muscles.

6. *Sleep*

During sleep, the body temperature decreases by 0.5°C.

7. *Emotion*

During emotional conditions, the body temperature increases.

8. *Menstrual cycle*

In females, immediately after ovulation, the temperature rises (0.5°C to 1°C) sharply. It decreases (0.5°C) during menstrual phase.

Pathological Variations

Abnormal increase in body temperature is called **hyperthermia** or **fever** and decreased body temperature

is called **hypothermia** (Refer applied physiology in this Chapter).

■ HEAT BALANCE

Regulation of body temperature depends upon the balance between heat produced in the body and the heat lost from the body.

■ HEAT GAIN OR HEAT PRODUCTION IN THE BODY

Various mechanisms involved in heat production in the body are:

1. Metabolic Activities

Major portion of heat produced in the body is due to the metabolism of foodstuffs. It is called **heat of metabolism.**

Heat production is more during metabolism of fat. About 9 calories of heat is produced during metabolism of fats, when 1 L of oxygen is utilized. For the same amount of oxygen, carbohydrate metabolism produces 4.7 calories of heat. Protein metabolism produces 4.5 calories/L.

Liver is the organ where maximum heat is produced due to metabolic activities.

2. Muscular Activity

Heat is produced in the muscle both at rest and during activities. During rest, heat is produced by muscle tone. Heat produced during muscular activity is called **heat of activity.** About 80% of heat of activity is produced by skeletal muscles.

3. Role of Hormones

Thyroxine and adrenaline increase the heat production by accelerating the metabolic activities.

4. Radiation of Heat from the Environment

Body gains heat by radiation. It occurs when the environmental temperature is higher than the body temperature.

5. Shivering

Shivering refers to shaking of the body caused by rapid involuntary contraction or twitching of the muscles as during exposure to cold. Shivering is a compensatory physiological mechanism in the body, during which enormous heat is produced.

6. Brown Fat Tissue

Brown adipose tissue is one of the two types of adipose tissues, the other being white adipose tissue.

It produces enormous body heat, particularly in infants. Refer Chapter 47 for details.

■ HEAT LOSS FROM THE BODY

Maximum heat is lost from the body through skin and small amount of heat is lost through respiratory system, kidney and GI tract. When environmental temperature is less than body temperature, heat is lost from the body. Heat loss occurs by the following methods:

1. Conduction

Three percent of heat is lost from the surface of the body to other objects such as chair or bed, by means of conduction.

2. Radiation

Sixty percent of heat is lost by means of radiation, i.e. transfer of heat by infrared electromagnetic radiation from body to other objects through the surrounding air.

3. Convection

Fifteen percent of heat is lost from body to the air by convection. First the heat is conducted to the air surrounding the body and then carried away by air currents, i.e. convection.

4. Evaporation – Insensible Perspiration

When water evaporates, heat is lost. Twenty two percent of heat is lost through evaporation of water.

Normally, a small quantity of water is continuously evaporated from skin and lungs. We are not aware of it. So it is called the insensible perspiration or insensible water loss. It is about 50 mL/hour. When body temperature increases, sweat secretion is increased and water evaporation is more with more of heat loss.

5. Panting

Panting is the rapid shallow breathing, associated with dribbling of more saliva. In some animals like dogs which do not have sweat glands, heat is lost by evaporation of water from lungs and saliva by means of panting.

■ REGULATION OF BODY TEMPERATURE

Body temperature is regulated by hypothalamus, which sets the normal range of body temperature. The set point under normal physiological conditions is 37°C.

Hypothalamus has two centers which regulate the body temperature:
1. Heat loss center
2. Heat gain center.

■ HEAT LOSS CENTER

Heat loss center is situated in **preoptic nucleus** of anterior hypothalamus. Neurons in preoptic nucleus are heat-sensitive nerve cells, which are called **thermoreceptors** (Fig. 63.1).

Stimulation of preoptic nucleus results in cutaneous vasodilatation and sweating. Removal or lesion of this nucleus increases the body temperature.

■ HEAT GAIN CENTER

Heat gain is otherwise known as heat production center. It is situated in **posterior hypothalamic nucleus.** Stimulation of posterior hypothalamic nucleus causes shivering. The removal or lesion of this nucleus leads to fall in body temperature.

■ MECHANISM OF TEMPERATURE REGULATION

When Body Temperature Increases

When body temperature increases, blood temperature also increases. When blood with increased temperature passes through hypothalamus, it stimulates the thermoreceptors present in the heat loss center in preoptic nucleus. Now, the heat loss center brings the temperature back to normal by two mechanisms:
1. Promotion of heat loss
2. Prevention of heat production

1. Promotion of heat loss

When body temperature increases, heat loss center promotes heat loss from the body by two ways:
  i. By increasing the secretion of sweat: When sweat secretion increases, more water is lost from skin along with heat
  ii. By inhibiting sympathetic centers in posterior hypothalamus: This causes cutaneous vaso-dilatation. Now, the blood flow through skin increases causing excess sweating. It increases the heat loss through sweat, leading to decrease in body temperature.

2. Prevention of heat production

Heat loss center prevents heat production in the body by inhibiting mechanisms involved in heat production, such as shivering and chemical (metabolic) reactions.

When Body Temperature Decreases

When the body temperature decreases, it is brought back to normal by two mechanisms:
1. Prevention of heat loss
2. Promotion of heat production.

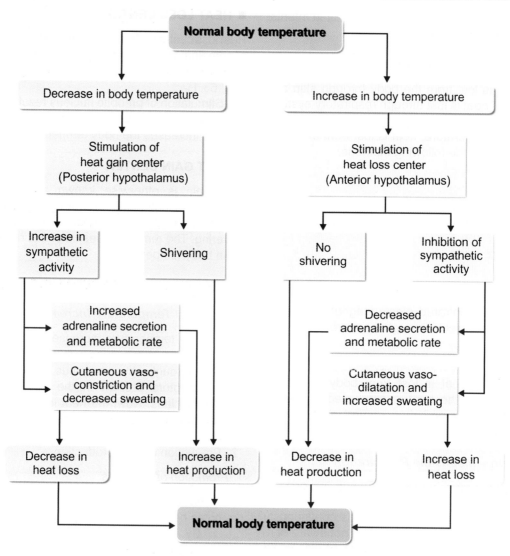

FIGURE 63.1: Regulation of body temperature

1. *Prevention of heat loss*

When body temperature decreases, sympathetic centers in posterior hypothalamus cause cutaneous vasoconstriction. This leads to decrease in blood flow to skin and so the heat loss is prevented.

2. *Promotion of heat production*

Heat production is promoted by two ways:

   i. *Shivering:* When body temperature is low, the heat gain center stimulates the primary motor center for shivering, situated in posterior hypothalamus near the wall of the III ventricle and shivering occurs. During shivering, enormous heat is produced because of severe muscular activities.

   ii. *Increased metabolic reactions:* Sympathetic centers, which are activated by heat gain center, stimulate secretion of adrenaline and

noradrenaline. These hormones, particularly adrenaline increases the heat production by accelerating cellular metabolic activities.

Simultaneously, hypothalamus secretes thyrotropin-releasing hormone. It causes release of thyroid-stimulating hormone from pituitary. It in turn, increases release of thyroxine from thyroid. Thyroxine accelerates the metabolic activities in the body and this increases heat production.

Chemical thermogenesis: It is the process in which heat is produced in the body by metabolic activities induced by hormones.

■ APPLIED PHYSIOLOGY

■ HYPERTHERMIA – FEVER

Elevation of body temperature above the set point is called hyperthermia, fever or **pyrexia.** Fever itself is not an illness. But it is an important sign of something going wrong in the body. It is the part of body's response to disease. Fever may be beneficial to body and on many occasions, it plays an important role in helping the body fight the diseases, particularly the infections.

Classification of Fever

Fever is classified into three categories:
1. *Low-grade fever:* When the body temperature rises to 38°C to 39°C, (100.4°F to 102.2°F)
2. *Moderate-grade fever:* When the temperature rises to 39°C to 40°C (102.2°F to 104°F)
3. *High-grade fever:* When the temperature rises above 40°C to 42°C (104°F to 107.6°F).

Hyperpyrexia

Hyperpyrexia is the rise in body temperature beyond 42°C (107.6°F). Hyperpyrexia results in damage of body tissues. Further increase in temperature becomes life threatening.

Causes of Fever

1. *Infection:* Certain substances (pyrogens) released from bacteria or parasites affect the heat-regulating system in hypothalamus, resulting in the production of excess heat and fever.
2. *Hyperthyroidism:* Increased basal metabolic rate during hyperthyroidism causes fever
3. *Brain lesions:* When lesion involves temperature-regulating centers, fever occurs.
4. *Diabetes insipidus:* In this condition, fever occurs without any apparent cause.

Signs and Symptoms

Signs and symptoms depend upon the cause of fever:
1. Headache
2. Sweating
3. Shivering
4. Muscle pain
5. Dehydration
6. Loss of appetite
7. General weakness.

Hyperpyrexia may result in:
1. Confusion
2. Hallucinations
3. Irritability
4. Convulsions.

■ HYPOTHERMIA

Decrease in body temperature below 35°C (95°F) is called hypothermia. It is considered as the clinical state of subnormal body temperature, when the body fails to produce enough heat to maintain the normal activities. The major setback of this condition is the impairment of metabolic activities of the body. When the temperature drops below 31°C (87.8°F), it becomes fatal. Elderly persons are more susceptible for hypothermia.

Classification of Hypothermia

Hypothermia is classified into three categories:
1. *Mild hypothermia:* When the body temperature falls to 35°C to 33°C (95°F to 91.4°F)
2. *Moderate hypothermia:* When the body temperature falls to 33°C to 31°C (91.4°F to 87.8°F)
3. *Severe hypothermia:* When the body temperature falls below 31° C (87.8°F).

Causes of Hypothermia

1. Exposure to cold temperatures
2. Immersion in cold water
3. Drug abuse
4. Hypothyroidism
5. Hypopituitarism
6. Lesion in hypothalamus
7. Hemorrhage in certain parts of the brainstem, particularly pons.

Signs and Symptoms

1. *Mild hypothermia*

Uncontrolled intense shivering occurs. The affected person can manage by self. But the movements become less coordinated. The chillness causes pain and discomfort.

2. *Moderate hypothermia*

Shivering slows down or stops but the muscles become stiff. Mental confusion and apathy (lack of feeling or emotions) occurs. Respiration becomes shallow, followed by drowsiness. Pulse becomes weak and blood pressure drops. Sometimes a strange behavior develops.

3. *Severe hypothermia*

The person feels very weak and exhausted with incoordination and physical disability. The skin becomes chill and its color changes to bluish gray. Eyes are dilated. The person looses consciousness gradually. Breathing slows down, followed by stiffness of arms and legs. Pulse becomes very weak and blood pressure decreases very much, resulting in unconsciousness.

Further drop in body temperature leads to death.

QUESTIONS IN RENAL PHYSIOLOGY AND SKIN

■ LONG QUESTIONS

1. Describe the process of urine formation.
2. What are the different stages of urine formation? Explain the role of glomerulus of nephron in the formation of urine.
3. Give an account of role of renal tubule in the process of urine formation.
4. What is countercurrent mechanism? Describe the anatomical and physiological basis of counter-current mechanism in kidney.
5. Describe the mechanism involved in the concentration of urine.
6. Describe the role of kidneys in maintaining acid-base balance.
7. Give an account of micturition.
8. What is normal body temperature? Explain heat balance and regulation of body temperature. Add a note on fever.

■ SHORT QUESTIONS

1. Functions of kidney.
2. Structure of nephron.
3. Renal corpuscle.
4. Juxtaglomerular apparatus.
5. Renin-angiotensin system.
6. Peculiarities of renal circulation.
7. Autoregulation of renal circulation.
8. Glomerular filtration rate.
9. Effective filtration pressure in kidney.
10. Tubuloglomerular feedback.
11. Glomerulotubular feedback.
12. Reabsorption of glucose in renal tubule.
13. Reabsorption of water in renal tubule.
14. Reabsorption of sodium in renal tubules.
15. Reabsorption of bicarbonate in renal tubules.
16. Secretion in renal tubule.
17. Renal failure.
18. Renal medullary gradient.
19. Countercurrent multiplier.
20. Countercurrent exchanger.
21. Actions of hormones on renal tubules.
22. Acidification of urine.
23. Role of kidney in maintaining acid-base balance.
24. Plasma clearance.
25. Measurement of glomerular filtration rate.
26. Measurement of renal blood (or plasma) flow.
27. Nerve supply to urinary bladder and sphincters.
28. Cystometrogram.
29. Micturition reflex.
30. Abnormalities of urinary bladder.
31. Dialysis/artificial kidney.
32. Diuretics/loop diuretics.
33. Renal failure.
34. Structure of skin.
35. Functions of skin.
36. Sebaceous glands.
37. Sweat glands.
38. Differences between eccrine glands and apocrine glands.
39. Pheromones.
40. Regulation of body temperature.
41. Role of hypothalamus in temperature regulation.
42. Heat balance.
43. Hyperthermia.
44. Hypothermia.

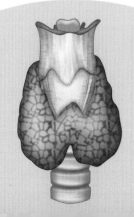

Section 6

Endocrinology

Introduction to Endocrinology

```
■ INTRODUCTION
    ■ CELL-TO-CELL SIGNALING
    ■ CHEMICAL MESSENGERS
    ■ ENDOCRINE GLANDS
■ METHODS OF STUDY
    ■ STUDY OF ENDOCRINE GLANDS
    ■ STUDY OF HORMONES
    ■ STUDY OF ENDOCRINE DISORDERS
```

■ INTRODUCTION

All the physiological activities of the body are regulated by two major systems:
1. Nervous system
2. Endocrine system.

These two systems interact with one another and regulate the body functions. This section deals with endocrine system and Section 10 deals with nervous system. Endocrine system functions by secreting some chemical substances called hormones.

■ CELL-TO-CELL SIGNALING

Cell-to-cell signaling refers to the transfer of information from one cell to another. It is also called **cell signaling** or intercellular communication. The cells of the body communicate with each other through some chemical substances called chemical messengers.

■ CHEMICAL MESSENGERS

Chemical messengers are the substances involved in cell signaling. These messengers are mainly secreted from endocrine glands. Some chemical messengers are secreted by nerve endings and the cells of several other tissues also.

All these chemical messengers carry the message (signal) from the **signaling cells (controlling cells)** to the **target cells.** The messenger substances may be the hormones or hormone-like substances.

Classification of Chemical Messengers

Generally the chemical messengers are classified into two types:
1. Classical hormones secreted by endocrine glands
2. Local hormones secreted from other tissues.

However, recently chemical messengers are classified into four types:
1. Endocrine messengers
2. Paracrine messengers
3. Autocrine messengers
4. Neurocrine messengers.

1. Endocrine Messengers

Endocrine messengers are the classical hormones. A hormone is defined as a chemical messenger, synthesized by endocrine glands and transported by blood to the target organs or tissues (site of action).

Examples are growth hormone and insulin.

2. Paracrine Messengers

Paracrine messengers are the chemical messengers, which diffuse from the control cells to the target cells through the interstitial fluid. Some of these substances directly enter the neighboring target cells through gap junctions. Such substances are also called **juxtacrine messengers** or **local hormones.**

Examples are prostaglandins and histamine.

3. *Autocrine Messengers*

Autocrine messengers are the chemical messengers that control the source cells which secrete them. So, these messengers are also called **intracellular chemical mediators.**

Examples are leukotrienes.

4. *Neurocrine or Neural Messengers*

Neurocrine or neural messengers are neurotransmitters and neurohormones (Fig. 64.1).

Neurotransmitter

Neurotransmitter is an endogenous signaling molecule that carries information form one nerve cell to another nerve cell or muscle or another tissue.

Examples are acetylcholine and dopamine.

Neurohormone

Neurohormone is a chemical substance that is released by the nerve cell directly into the blood and transported to the distant target cells.

Examples are oxytocin, antidiuretic hormone and hypothalamic releasing hormones.

Some of the chemical mediators act as more than one type of chemical messengers. For example, noradrenaline and dopamine function as classical hormones as well as neurotransmitters. Similarly, histamine acts as neurotransmitter and paracrine messenger.

■ ENDOCRINE GLANDS

Endocrine glands are the glands which synthesize and release the classical hormones into the blood. Endocrine glands are also called **ductless glands** because the

Endocrine messenger

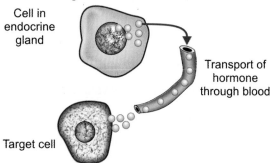

Autocrine messenger

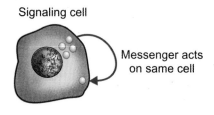

Paracrine messenger

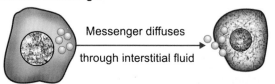

Paracrine messenger – juxtacrine messenger

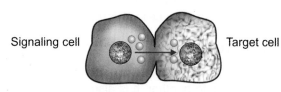

Neurocrine messenger – neurotransmitter

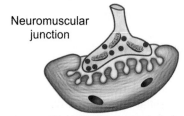

Neurocrine messenger – neurohormone

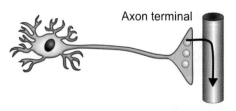

FIGURE 64.1: Chemical messengers

hormones secreted by them are released directly into blood without any duct. Endocrine glands are distinct from exocrine glands which release their secretions through ducts.

Endocrine glands play an important role in homeostasis and control of various other activities in the body through their hormones. Hormones are transported by blood to target organs or tissues in different parts of the body, where the actions are executed.

Major endocrine glands: Fig. 64.2.

Hormones secreted by endocrine glands: Table 64.1.

Hormones secreted by gonads: Table 64.2.

Hormones secreted by other organs: Table 64.3.

Local hormones: Table 64.4.

■ METHODS OF STUDY

■ STUDY OF ENDOCRINE GLANDS

Methods followed to study an endocrine gland:

1. *Functional Anatomy*

  i. Situation
  ii. Divisions or parts
  iii. Histology
  iv. Blood supply
  v. Nerve supply.

2. *Functions*

  i. Hormones secreted by the gland
  ii. Actions of each hormone.

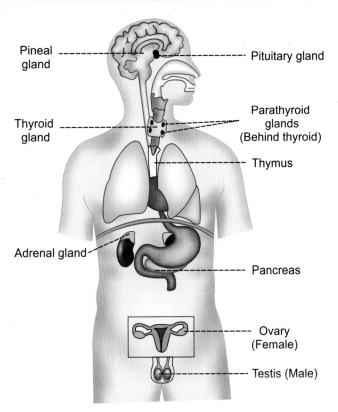

FIGURE 64.2: Diagram showing major endocrine glands

3. *Evidences to Support the Functions of the Gland*

  i. Effects of **extirpation** (removal) of the gland
  ii. Effects of administration of extract or the hormone of the gland
  iii. Clinical observation.

TABLE 64.1: Hormones secreted by major endocrine glands

Anterior pituitary	1. Growth hormone (GH) 2. Thyroid-stimulating hormone (TSH) 3. Adrenocorticotropic hormone (ACTH) 4. Follicle stimulating hormone (FSH) 5. Luteinizing hormone (LH) 6. Prolactin	Adrenal cortex	*Mineralocorticoids* 1. Aldosterone 2. 11-deoxycorticosterone
			Glucocorticoids 1. Cortisol 2. Corticosterone
Posterior pituitary	1. Antidiuretic hormone (ADH) 2. Oxytocin		*Sex hormones* 1. Androgens 2. Estrogen 3. Progesterone
Thyroid gland	1. Thyroxine (T_4) 2. Triiodothyronine (T_3) 3. Calcitonin		
Parathyroid gland	Parathormone	Adrenal medulla	1. Catecholamines 2. Adrenaline (Epinephrine) 3. Noradrenaline (Norepinephrine) 4. Dopamine
Pancreas – Islets of Langerhans	1. Insulin 2. Glucagon 3. Somatostatin 4. Pancreatic polypeptide		

TABLE 64.2: Hormones secreted by gonads

Testis	1. Testosterone 2. Dihydrotestosterone 3. Androstenedion
Ovary	1. Estrogen 2. Progesterone

TABLE 64.3: Hormones secreted by other organs

Pineal gland	Melatonin
Thymus	1. Thymosin 2. Thymin
Kidney	1. Erythropoietin 2. Thrombopoietin 3. Renin 4. 1,25-dihydroxycholecalcifero (calcitriol) 5. Prostaglandins
Heart	1. Atrial natriuretic peptide 2. Brain natriuretic peptide 3. C-type natriuretic peptide
Placenta	1. Human chorionic gonadotropin (HCG) 2. Human chorionic somatomammotropin 3. Estrogen 4. Progesterone

TABLE 64.4: Local hormones

1. Prostaglandins	7. Serotonin
2. Thromboxanes	8. Histamine
3. Prostacyclin	9. Substance P
4. Leukotrienes	10. Heparin
5. Lipoxins	11. Bradykinin
6. Acetylcholine	12. Gastrointestinal hormones

4. *Regulation of Activity of the Gland*
   i.   By other endocrine glands
   ii. By other factors
   iii. By feedback mechanism.

5. *Applied Physiology*
   i. Disorders due to hyperactivity of the gland
   ii. Disorders due to hypoactivity of the gland.

■ STUDY OF HORMONES

A hormone is usually studied as follows:
1. Source of secretion (gland as well as the cell that secretes the hormone)
2. Chemistry
3. Half-life
4. Synthesis and metabolism
5. Actions
6. Mode of action
7. Regulation of secretion

8. Applied physiology
   i. Disorders due to hypersecretion of the hormone
   ii. Disorders due to hyposecretion of the hormone.

Half-life of the Hormones

Half-life is defined as the time during which half the quantity of a hormone, drug or any substance is metabolized or eliminated from circulation by biological process. It is also defined as the time during which the activity or potency of a substance is decreased to half of its initial value.

Half-life is also called biological half-life. Half-life of a hormone denotes the elimination of that hormone from circulation.

■ STUDY OF ENDOCRINE DISORDERS

An endocrine disorder is studied by analyzing:
1. Causes
2. Signs and symptoms
3. Syndrome.

1. *Causes*

Endocrine disorder may be due to the hyperactivity or hypoactivity of the concerned gland. Secretion of hormones increases during hyperactivity and decreases during hypoactivity.

2. *Signs and Symptoms*

A sign is the feature of a disease as detected by the doctor during the physical examination. So, it is the **objective physical evidence** of disease found by the examiner.

Examples of signs are yellow coloration of skin and mucous membrane in jaundice, paleness in anemia, enlargement of liver, etc.

A symptom is the feature of a disease felt by the patient. So, it is the **subjective evidence** perceived by the patient. In simple words, it is a noticeable change in the body, experienced by the patient.

Examples of symptoms are fever, itching, swelling, tremor, etc.

3. *Syndrome*

Syndrome is the combination of signs and symptoms (associated with a disease), which occur together and suggest the presence of a certain disease or the possibility of developing the disease.

Examples are **Stoke-Adams syndrome** and syndrome of inappropriate antidiuretic hormone hypersecretion **(SIADH)**.

Hormones

Chapter 65

- ■ **CHEMISTRY OF HORMONES**
  - ■ **STEROID HORMONES**
  - ■ **PROTEIN HORMONES**
  - ■ **TYROSINE DERIVATIVES**
- ■ **HORMONAL ACTION**
  - ■ **INTRODUCTION**
  - ■ **HORMONE RECEPTORS**
- ■ **MECHANISM OF HORMONAL ACTION**
  - ■ **BY ALTERING PERMEABILITY OF CELL MEMBRANE**
  - ■ **BY ACTIVATING INTRACELLULAR ENZYME**
  - ■ **BY ACTING ON GENES**

■ CHEMISTRY OF HORMONES

Hormones are **chemical messengers,** synthesized by endocrine glands. Based on chemical nature, hormones are classified into three types (Table 65.1):
1. Steroid hormones
2. Protein hormones

3. Derivatives of the amino acid called tyrosine.

■ STEROID HORMONES

Steroid hormones are the hormones synthesized from cholesterol or its derivatives. Steroid hormones are secreted by adrenal cortex, gonads and placenta.

TABLE 65.1: Classification of hormones depending upon chemical nature

Steroids	Proteins	Derivatives of tyrosine
Aldosterone	Growth hormone (GH)	Thyroxine (T_4)
11-deoxycorticosterone	Thyroid-stimulating hormone (TSH)	Triiodothyronine (T_3)
Cortisol	Adrenocorticotropic hormone (ACTH)	Adrenaline (Epinephrine)
Corticosterone	Follicle-stimulating hormone (FSH)	Noradrenaline (Norepinephrine)
Testosterone	Luteinizing hormone (LH)	Dopamine.
Dihydrotestosterone	Prolactin	
Dehydroepiandrosterone	Antidiuretic hormone (ADH)	
Androstenedione	Oxytocin	
Estrogen	Parathormone	
Progesterone	Calcitonin	
	Insulin	
	Glucagon	
	Somatostatin	
	Pancreatic polypeptide	
	Human chorionic gonadotropin (HCG)	
	Human chorionic somatomammotropin.	

■ PROTEIN HORMONES

Protein hormones are large or small peptides. Protein hormones are secreted by pituitary gland, parathyroid glands, pancreas and placenta ('P's).

■ TYROSINE DERIVATIVES

Two types of hormones, namely thyroid hormones and adrenal medullary hormones are derived from the amino acid tyrosine.

■ HORMONAL ACTION

■ INTRODUCTION

Hormone does not act directly on target cells. First it combines with receptor present on the target cells and forms a **hormone-receptor complex.** This hormone-receptor complex induces various changes or reactions in the target cells.

■ HORMONE RECEPTORS

Hormone receptors are the large proteins present in the target cells. Each cell has thousands of receptors. Important characteristic feature of the receptors is that, each receptor is specific for one single hormone, i.e. each receptor can combine with only one hormone.

Thus, a hormone can act on a target cell, only if the target cell has the receptor for that particular hormone.

Situation of the Hormone Receptors

Hormone receptors are situated either in cell membrane or cytoplasm or nucleus of the target cells as follows:
1. *Cell membrane:* Receptors of protein hormones and adrenal medullary hormones (catecholamines) are situated in the cell membrane (Fig. 65.1)
2. *Cytoplasm:* Receptors of steroid hormones are situated in the cytoplasm of target cells
3. *Nucleus:* Receptors of thyroid hormones are in the nucleus of the cell.

Regulation of Hormone Receptors

Receptor proteins are not static components of the cell. Their number increases or decreases in various conditions.

Generally, when a hormone is secreted in excess, the number of receptors of that hormone decreases due to binding of hormone with receptors. This process is called **down regulation.** During the deficiency of the hormone, the number of receptor increases, which is called **upregulation.**

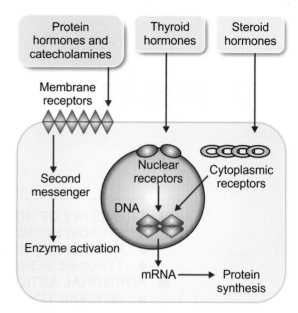

FIGURE 65.1: Situation of hormonal receptors

Hormone in the form of hormone-receptor complex enters the target cell by means of endocytosis and executes the actions. The whole process is called **internalization.**

After internalization, some receptors are recycled, whereas many of them are degraded and new receptors are formed. Formation of new receptors takes a long time. So, the number of receptors decreases when hormone level increases.

■ MECHANISM OF HORMONAL ACTION

Hormone does not act on the target cell directly. It combines with receptor to form hormone-receptor complex. This complex executes the hormonal action by any one of the following mechanisms:
1. By altering permeability of cell membrane
2. By activating intracellular enzyme
3. By acting on genes.

■ BY ALTERING PERMEABILITY OF CELL MEMBRANE

Neurotransmitters in synapse or neuromuscular junction act by changing the permeability of postsynaptic membrane.

For example, in a neuromuscular junction, when an impulse (action potential) reaches the axon terminal of the motor nerve, acetylcholine is released from the vesicles. Acetylcholine increases the permeability of the postsynaptic membrane for sodium, by opening the ligand-gated sodium channels. So, sodium ions enter the neuromuscular junction from ECF through the channels and cause the development of endplate potential. Refer Chapter 32 for details.

■ BY ACTIVATING INTRACELLULAR ENZYME

Protein hormones and the catecholamines act by activating the intracellular enzymes.

First Messenger

The hormone which acts on a target cell, is called first messenger or **chemical mediator.** It combines with the receptor and forms hormone-receptor complex.

Second Messenger

Hormone-receptor complex activates the enzymes of the cell and causes the formation of another substance called the second messenger or **intracellular hormonal mediator.**

Second messenger produces the effects of the hormone inside the cells. Protein hormones and the catecholamines act through second messenger. Most common second messenger is cyclic AMP.

Cyclic AMP

Cyclic AMP, cAMP or cyclic adenosine 3'5'-monophosphate acts as a second messenger for protein hormones and catecholamines.

Formation of cAMP – Role of G proteins

G proteins or **guanosine nucleotide-binding proteins** are the membrane proteins situated on the inner surface of cell membrane. These proteins play an important role in the formation of cAMP

Each G protein molecule is made up of trimeric (three) subunits called α, β and γ subunits. The α-subunit is responsible for most of the biological actions. It is bound with **guanosine diphosphate** (GDP) and forms α-GDP unit. The α-subunit is also having the intrinsic enzyme activity called **GTPase** activity. The β and γ subunits always bind together to form the β-γ dimmer. It can also bring about some actions. In the inactivated G protein, both α-GDP unit and β-γ dimmer are united (Fig. 65.2: Stage 1).

Sequence of events in the formation of cAMP

i. Hormone binds with the receptor in the cell membrane and forms the hormone-receptor complex
ii. It activates the G protein
iii. G protein releases GDP from α-GDP unit

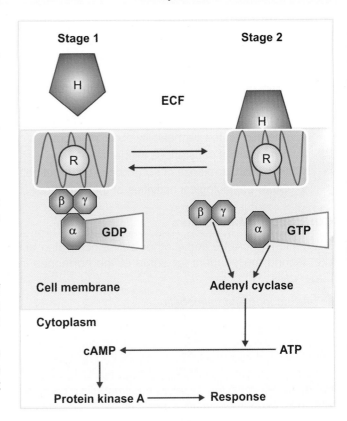

FIGURE 65.2: Mode of action of protein hormones and catecholamines. H = Hormone. R = Receptor, α, β, γ = G protein, GDP = Guanosine diphosphate, GTP = Guanosine triphosphate, ECF = Extracellular fluid, cAMP = Cyclic adenosine 3'5'-monophosphate, ATP = Adenosine triphosphate.

iv. The α-subunit now binds with a new molecule of GTP, i.e. the GDP is exchanged for GTP
v. This exchange triggers the dissociation of α-GTP unit and β-γ dimmer from the receptor
vi. Both α-GTP unit and β-γ dimmer now activate the second messenger pathways (Fig. 65.2: Stage 2)
vii. The α-GTP unit activates the enzyme adenyl cyclase, which is also present in the cell membrane. Most of the adenyl cyclase protrudes into the cytoplasm of the cell from inner surface of the cell membrane
viii. Activated adenyl cyclase converts the adenosine triphosphate of the cytoplasm into cyclic adenosine monophosphate (cAMP)

When the action is over, α-subunit hydrolyzes the attached GTP to GDP by its GTPase activity. This allows the reunion of α-subunit with β-γ dimmer and commencing a new cycle (Fig. 65.2: Stage 1).

Actions of cAMP

Cyclic AMP executes the actions of hormone inside the cell by stimulating the enzymes like protein kinase A.

Cyclic AMP produces the response, depending upon the function of the target cells through these enzymes.

Response produced by cAMP

Cyclic AMP produces one or more of the following responses:
   i. Contraction and relaxation of muscle fibers
   ii. Alteration in the permeability of cell membrane
   iii. Synthesis of substances inside the cell
   iv. Secretion or release of substances by target cell
   v. Other physiological activities of the target cell.

Other Second Messengers

In addition to cAMP, some other substances also act like second messengers for some of the hormones in target cells.

i. Calcium ions and calmodulin

Many hormones act by increasing the calcium ion, which fucntions as second messenger along with another protein called calmodulin or troponin C. Calmodulin is present in smooth muscles and troponin C is present in skeletal muscles. Calcium-calmodulin complex activates various enzymes in the cell, which cause the physiological responses. Common enzyme activated by calcium-calmodulin complex is the **myosin kinase** in smooth muscle. Myosin kinase catalyses the reactions, resulting in muscular contraction (Chapter 33).

In the skeletal muscle, calcium ions bind with troponin C, which is similar to calmodulin (Chapter 31).

ii. Inositol triphosphate

Inositol triphosphate (IP_3) is formed from phosphatidylinositol biphosphate (PIP_2).

Hormone-receptor complex activates the enzyme phospholipase, which converts PIP_2 into IP_3. IP_3 acts on protein kinase C and causes the physiological response by the release of calcium ions into the cytoplasm of target cell.

iii. Diacylglycerol

Diacylglycerol (DAG) is also produced from PIP_2. It acts via protein kinase C.

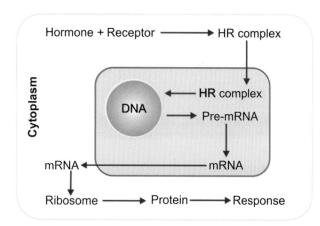

FIGURE 65.3: Mode of action of steroid hormones. Thyroid hormones also act in the similar way but their receptors are in the nucleus. HR = Hormone-receptor complex

iv. Cyclic guanosine monophosphate

Cyclic guanosine monophosphate (cGMP) functions like cAM P by acting on protein kinase A.

■ BY ACTING ON GENES

Thyroid and steroid hormones execute their function by acting on genes in the target cells (Fig. 65.3).

Sequence of Events during Activation of Genes

   i.   Hormone enters the interior of cell and binds with receptor in cytoplasm (steroid hormone) or in nucleus (thyroid hormone) and forms hormone-receptor complex
   ii. Hormone-receptor complex moves towards the DNA and binds with DNA
   iii. This increases transcription of mRNA
   iv. The mRNA moves out of nucleus and reaches ribosomes and activates them
   v.   Activated ribosomes produce large quantities of proteins
   vi. These proteins produce physiological responses in the target cells.

Pituitary Gland

■ INTRODUCTION

Pituitary gland or **hypophysis** is a small endocrine gland with a diameter of 1 cm and weight of 0.5 to 1 g. It is situated in a depression called 'sella turcica', present in the sphenoid bone at the base of skull. It is connected with the hypothalamus by the **pituitary stalk** or **hypophyseal stalk.**

■ DIVISIONS OF PITUITARY GLAND

Pituitary gland is divided into two divisions:
1. Anterior pituitary or adenohypophysis
2. Posterior pituitary or neurohypophysis.

Both the divisions are situated close to each other. Still both are entirely different in their development, structure and function.

Between the two divisions, there is a small and relatively avascular structure called **pars intermedia.** Actually, it forms a part of anterior pituitary.

■ DEVELOPMENT OF PITUITARY GLAND

Both the divisions of pituitary glands develop from different sources.

Anterior pituitary is **ectodermal** in origin and arises from the **pharyngeal epithelium** as an upward growth known as **Rathke pouch.**

Posterior pituitary is **neuroectodermal** in origin and arises from hypothalamus as a downward **diverticulum.** Rathke pouch and the downward diverticulum from hypothalamus grow towards each other and meet in the midway between the roof of the buccal cavity and base of brain. There, the two structures lie close together.

■ REGULATION OF SECRETION

Hypothalamo-hypophyseal Relationship

The relationship between hypothalamus and pituitary gland is called hypothalamo-hypophyseal relationship. Hormones secreted by hypothalamus are transported to anterior pituitary and posterior pituitary. But the mode of transport of these hormones is different.

Hormones from hypothalamus are transported to anterior pituitary through hypothalamo-hypophysial portal blood vessels. But, the hormones from hypothalamus to posterior pituitary are transported by nerve fibers of hypothalamo-hypophyseal tract (see below for details).

■ ANTERIOR PITUITARY OR ADENOHYPOPHYSIS

Anterior pituitary is also known as the **master gland** because it regulates many other endocrine glands through its hormones.

■ PARTS

Anterior pituitary consists of three parts (Fig. 66.1):
1. Pars distalis
2. Pars tuberalis
3. Pars intermedia.

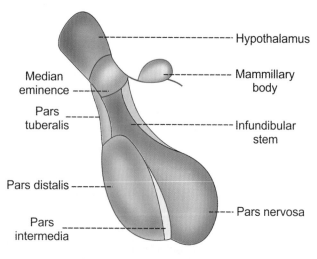

FIGURE 66.1: Parts of pituitary gland
■ Adenohypophysis ■ Neurohypophysis

■ HISTOLOGY

Anterior pituitary has two types of cells, which have different staining properties:
1. Chromophobe cells
2. Chromophil cells.

Chromophobe Cells

Chromophobe cells do not possess granules and stain poorly. These cells form 50% of total cells in anterior pituitary. Chromophobe cells are not secretory in nature, but are the precursors of chromophil cells.

Chromophil Cells

Chromophil cells contain large number of granules and are darkly stained.

Types of chromophil cells

Chromophil cells are classified by two methods.
1. Classification on the basis of staining property: Chromophil cells are divided into two types:
   i. **Acidophilic cells** or **alpha cells,** which form 35%
   ii. **Basophilic cells** or **beta cells,** which form 15%.
2. Classification on the basis of secretory nature: Chromophil cells are classified into five types:
   i. **Somatotropes,** which secrete growth hormone
   ii. **Corticotropes,** which secrete adrenocorticotropic hormone
   iii. **Thyrotropes,** which secrete thyroid-stimulating hormone (TSH)
   iv. **Gonadotropes,** which secrete follicle-stimulating hormone (FSH) and luteinizing hormone (LH)
   v. **Lactotropes,** which secrete prolactin.

Somatotropes and lactotropes are acidophilic cells, whereas others are basophilic cells. Somatotropes form about 30% to 40% of the chromophil cells. So, pituitary tumors that secrete large quantities of human growth hormone are called acidophilic tumors.

■ REGULATION OF ANTERIOR PITUITARY SECRETION

Hypothalamus controls anterior pituitary by secreting the releasing and inhibitory hormones (factors), which are called **neurohormones.** These hormones from hypothalamus are transported anterior pituitary through hypothalamo-hypophyseal **portal vessels.**

Some special nerve cells present in various parts hypothalamus send their nerve fibers (axons) to median eminence and tuber cinereum. These nerve cells synthesize the hormones and release them into median eminence and tuber cinereum. From here, the hormones are transported by blood via hypothalamo-hypophyseal portal vessels to anterior pituitary (Fig. 66.2).

Releasing and Inhibitory Hormones Secreted by Hypothalamus

1. Growth hormone-releasing hormone (GHRH): Stimulates the release of growth hormone
2. Growth hormone-releasing polypeptide (GHRP): Stimulates the release of GHRH and growth hormone
3. Growth hormone-inhibitory hormone (GHIH) or somatostatin: Inhibits the growth hormone release
4. Thyrotropic-releasing hormone (TRH): Stimulates the release of thyroid stimulating hormone
5. Corticotropin-releasing hormone (CRH): Stimulates the release of adrenocorticotropin
6. Gonadotropin-releasing hormone (GnRH): Stimulates the release of gonadotropins, FSH and LH
7. Prolactin-inhibitory hormone (PIH): Inhibits prolactin secretion. It is believed that PIH is dopamine.

■ HORMONES SECRETED BY ANTERIOR PITUITARY

Six hormones are secreted by the anterior pituitary:
1. Growth hormone (GH) or somatotropic hormone (STH)
2. Thyroid-stimulating hormone (TSH) or thyrotropic hormone
3. Adrenocorticotropic hormone (ACTH)
4. Follicle-stimulating hormone (FSH)

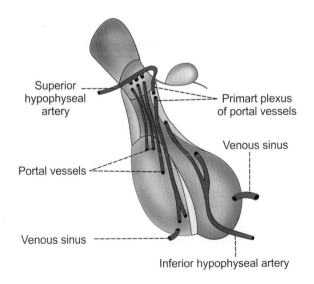

FIGURE 66.2: Blood supply to pituitary gland

5. Luteinizing hormone (LH) in females or interstitial-cell-stimulating hormone (ICSH) in males
6. Prolactin.
    Recently, the hormone β-lipotropin is found to be secreted by anterior pituitary.

Tropic Hormones

First five hormones of anterior pituitary stimulate the other endocrine glands. Growth hormone also stimulates the secretory activity of liver and other tissues. Therefore, these five hormones are called **tropic hormones.** Prolactin is concerned with milk secretion.

Gonadotropic Hormones

Follicle-stimulating hormone and the luteinizing hormone are together called **gonadotropic hormones** or **gonadotropins** because of their action on gonads.

■ GROWTH HORMONE

Source of Secretion

Growth hormone is secreted by somatotropes which are the acidophilic cells of anterior pituitary.

Chemistry, Blood Level and Daily Output

GH is protein in nature, having a single-chain polypeptide with 191 amino acids. Its molecular weight is 21,500.
    Basal level of GH concentration in blood of normal adult is up to 300 g/dL and in children, it is up to 500 ng/dL. Its daily output in adults is 0.5 to1.0 mg.

Transport

Growth hormone is transported in blood by GH-binding proteins (GHBPs).

Half-life and Metabolism

Half-life of circulating growth hormone is about 20 minutes. It is degraded in liver and kidney.

Actions of Growth Hormone

GH is responsible for the general growth of the body. Hypersecretion of GH causes enormous growth of the body, leading to **gigantism.** Deficiency of GH in children causes stunted growth, leading to **dwarfism.**
    GH is responsible for the growth of almost all tissues of the body, which are capable of growing. It increases the size and number of cells by mitotic division. GH also causes specific differentiation of certain types of cells like bone cells and muscle cells.

The labels on the figure read:
- Superior hypophyseal artery
- Primart plexus of portal vessels
- Venous sinus
- Portal vessels
- Venous sinus
- Inferior hypophyseal artery

GH also acts on the metabolism of all the three major types of foodstuffs in the body, viz. proteins, lipids and carbohydrates.

1. *On metabolism*

GH increases the synthesis of proteins, mobilization of lipids and conservation of carbohydrates.

a. *On protein metabolism*

GH accelerates the synthesis of proteins by:

i. *Increasing amino acid transport through cell membrane:* The concentration of amino acids in the cells increases and thus, the synthesis of proteins is accelerated.

ii. *Increasing ribonucleic acid (RNA) translation:* GH increases the translation of RNA in the cells (Refer Chapter 1 for details of translation). Because of this, ribosomes are activated and more proteins are synthesized.

GH can increase the RNA translation even without increasing the amino acid transport into the cells.

iii. *Increasing transcription of DNA to RNA:* It also stimulates the transcription of DNA to RNA. RNA, in turn accelerates the synthesis of proteins in the cells (Refer Chapter 1 for details of transcription).

iv. *Decreasing catabolism of protein:* GH inhibits the breakdown of cellular protein. It helps in the building up of tissues.

v. *Promoting anabolism of proteins indirectly:* GH increases the release of insulin (from β-cells of islets in pancreas), which has anabolic effect on proteins.

b. *On fat metabolism*

GH mobilizes fats from adipose tissue. So, the concentration of fatty acids increases in the body fluids. These fatty acids are used for the production of energy by the cells. Thus, the proteins are spared.

During the utilization of fatty acids for energy production, lot of acetoacetic acid is produced by liver and is released into the body fluids, leading to ketosis. Sometimes, excess mobilization of fat from the adipose tissue causes accumulation of fat in liver, resulting in **fatty liver.**

c. *On carbohydrate metabolism*

Major action of GH on carbohydrates is the conservation of glucose.

Effects of GH on carbohydrate metabolism:

i. Decrease in the **peripheral utilization** of glucose for the production of energy: GH reduces the peripheral utilization of glucose for energy production. It is because of the formation of acetyl-CoA during the metabolism of fat, influenced by GH. The acetyl-CoA inhibits the glycolytic pathway. Moreover, since the GH increases the mobilization of fat, more fatty acid is available for the production of energy. By this way, GH reduces the peripheral utilization of glucose for energy production.

ii. Increase in the deposition of glycogen in the cells: Since glucose is not utilized for energy production by the cells, it is converted into glycogen and deposited in the cells.

iii. Decrease in the uptake of glucose by the cells: As glycogen deposition increases, the cells become saturated with glycogen. Because of this, no more glucose can enter the cells from blood. So, the blood glucose level increases.

iv. Diabetogenic effect of GH: Hypersecretion of GH increases blood glucose level enormously. It causes continuous stimulation of the β-cells in the islets of Langerhans in pancreas and increase in secretion of insulin. In addition to this, the GH also stimulates β-cells directly and causes secretion of insulin. Because of the excess stimulation, β-cells are burnt out at one stage. This causes deficiency of insulin, leading to **true diabetes mellitus** or **full-blown diabetes mellitus.** This effect of GH is called the **diabetogenic effect.**

2. *On bones*

In embryonic stage, GH is responsible for the differentiation and development of bone cells. In later stages, GH increases the growth of the skeleton. It increases both the length as well as the thickness of the bones.

In bones, GH increases:

i. Synthesis and deposition of proteins by chondrocytes and osteogenic cells

ii. Multiplication of **chondrocytes** and **osteogenic cells** by enhancing the intestinal calcium absorption

iii. Formation of new bones by converting chondrocytes into osteogenic cells

iv. Availability of calcium for mineralization of bone matrix.

GH increases the length of the bones, until epiphysis fuses with shaft, which occurs at the time of puberty. After the **epiphyseal fusion,** length of the bones cannot be increased. However, it stimulates the **osteoblasts** strongly. So, the bone continues to grow in thickness throughout the life. Particularly, the membranous bones such as the jaw bone and the skull bones become thicker under the influence of GH.

Hypersecretion of GH before the fusion of epiphysis with the shaft of the bones causes enormous growth of the skeleton, leading to a condition called **gigantism.** Hypersecretion of GH after the fusion of epiphysis with the shaft of the bones leads to a condition called **acromegaly.**

Mode of Action of GH – Somatomedin

GH acts on bones, growth and protein metabolism through somatomedin secreted by liver. GH stimulates the liver to secrete somatomedin. Sometimes, in spite of normal secretion of GH, growth is arrested (dwarfism) due to the absence or deficiency of somatomedin.

Somatomedin

Somatomedin is defined as a substance through which growth hormone acts. It is a polypeptide with the molecular weight of about 7,500.

Types of somatomedin

Somatomedins are of two types:
  i. Insulin-like growth factor-I (IGF-I), which is also called somatomedin C
  ii. Insulin-like growth factor-II.

Somatomedin C (IGF-I) acts on the bones and protein metabolism. Insulin-like growth factor-II plays an important role in the growth of fetus.

Duration of action of GH and somatomedin C

GH is transported in blood by loose binding with plasma protein. So, at the site of action, it is released from plasma protein rapidly. Its action also lasts only for a short duration of 20 minutes. But, the somatomedin C binds with plasma proteins very strongly. Because of this, the molecules of somatomedin C are released slowly from the plasma proteins. Thus, it can act continuously for a longer duration. The action of somatomedin C lasts for about 20 hours.

Mode of action of somatomedin C

Somatomedin C acts through the second messenger called cyclic AMP (refer previous Chapter).

Growth hormone receptor

GH receptor is called **growth hormone secretagogue** (GHS) receptor. It is a transmembrane receptor, belonging to cytokine receptor family. GH binds with the receptor situated mainly in liver cells and forms the hormone-receptor complex. Hormone-receptor complex induces various intracellular enzyme pathways, resulting in somatomedin secretion. Somatomedin in turn, executes the actions of growth hormone.

Regulation of GH Secretion

Growth hormone secretion is altered by various factors. However, hypothalamus and feedback mechanism play an important role in the regulation of GH secretion

GH secretion is stimulated by:
1. Hypoglycemia
2. Fasting
3. Starvation
4. Exercise
5. Stress and trauma
6. Initial stages of sleep.

GH secretion is inhibited by:
1. Hyperglycemia
2. Increase in free fatty acids in blood
3. Later stages of sleep.

Role of hypothalamus in the secretion of GH

Hypothalamus regulates GH secretion via three hormones:
  1. Growth hormone-releasing hormone (GHRH): It increases the GH secretion by stimulating the somatotropes of anterior pituitary
  2. Growth hormone-releasing polypeptide (GHRP): It increases the release of GHRH from hypothalamus and GH from pituitary
  3. Growth hormone-inhibitory hormone (GHIH) or somatostatin: It decreases the GH secretion. Somatostatin is also secreted by delta cells of islets of Langerhans in pancreas.

These three hormones are transported from hypothalamus to anterior pituitary by hypothalamo-hypophyseal portal blood vessels.

Feedback control

GH secretion is under **negative feedback** control (Chapter 4). Hypothalamus releases GHRH and GHRP, which in turn promote the release of GH from anterior pituitary. GH acts on various tissues. It also activates the liver cells to secrete somatomedin C (IGF-I).

Now, the somatomedin C increases the release of GHIH from hypothalamus. GHIH, in turn inhibits the release of GH from pituitary. Somatomedin also inhibits release of GHRP from hypothalamus. It acts on pituitary directly and inhibits the secretion of GH (Fig. 66.3).

GH inhibits its own secretion by stimulating the release of GHIH from hypothalamus. This type of feedback is called **short-loop feedback** control. Similarly, GHRH inhibits its own release by short-loop feedback control.

Whenever, the blood level of GH decreases, the GHRH is secreted from the hypothalamus. It in turn causes secretion of GH from pituitary.

Role of ghrelin in the secretion of GH

Ghrelin is a peptide hormone synthesized by epithelial cells in the fundus of stomach. It is also produced in smaller amount in hypothalamus, pituitary, kidney and placenta (Chapter 44). Ghrelin promotes secretion of GH by stimulating somatotropes directly.

■ OTHER HORMONES OF ANTERIOR PITUITARY

Thyroid-stimulating Hormone (TSH)

TSH is necessary for the growth and secretory activity of the thyroid gland. It has many actions on the thyroid gland. Refer Chapter 67 for details of TSH.

Adrenocorticotropic Hormone (ACTH)

ACTH is necessary for the structural integrity and the secretory activity of adrenal cortex. It has other functions also. Refer Chapter 70 for details of ACTH.

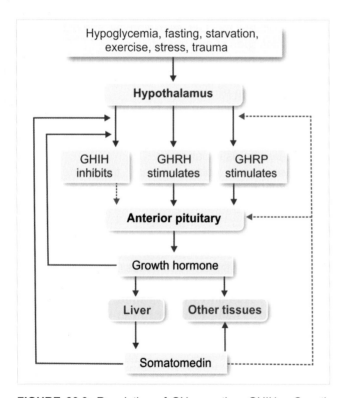

FIGURE 66.3: Regulation of GH secretion. GHIH = Growth hormone-inhibiting hormone, GHRH = Growth hormone-releasing hormone, GHRP = Growth hormone-releasing polypeptide. Growth hormone and somatomedin stimulate hypothalamus to release GHIH . Somatomedin inhibits anterior pituitary directly. Solid green line = Stimulation/secretion, Dashed red line = Inhibition.

Follicle-stimulating Hormone (FSH)

Follicle-stimulating hormone is a glycoprotein made up of one α-subunit and a β-subunit. The α-subunit has 92 amino acids and β-subunit has 118 amino acids. The half-life of FSH is about 3 to 4 hours.

Actions of FSH

In males, FSH acts along with testosterone and accelerates the process of **spermeogenesis** (refer Chapter 74 for details).

In females FSH:

1. Causes the development of **graafian follicle** from primordial follicle
2. Stimulates the theca cells of graafian follicle and causes secretion of estrogen (refer Chapter 79 for details)
3. Promotes the **aromatase activity** in granulosa cells, resulting in conversion of androgens into estrogen (Chapter 80).

Luteinizing Hormone (LH)

LH is a glycoprotein made up of one α-subunit and one β-subunit. The α-subunit has 92 amino acids and β-subunit has 141 amino acids. The half-life of LH is about 60 minutes.

Actions of LH

In males, LH is known as **interstitial cell-stimulating hormone** (ICSH) because it stimulates the interstitial cells of Leydig in testes. This hormone is essential for the secretion of testosterone from Leydig cells (Chapter 74).

In females, LH:

1. Causes maturation of vesicular follicle into graafian follicle along with follicle-stimulating hormone
2. Induces synthesis of androgens from theca cells of growing follicle
3. Is responsible for **ovulation**
4. Is necessary for the formation of corpus luteum
5. Activates the secretory functions of corpus luteum.

Prolactin

Prolactin is a single chain polypeptide with 199 amino acids. Its half-life is about 20 minutes. Prolactin is necessary for the final preparation of mammary glands for the production and secretion of milk.

Prolactin acts directly on the epithelial cells of mammary glands and causes localized **alveolar hyperplasia.** Refer Chapter 87 for details.

β-lipotropin

β-lipotropin is a polypeptide hormone with 31 amino acids. It mobilizes fat from adipose tissue and promotes lipolysis. It also forms the precursor of endorphins. This hormone acts through the adenyl cyclase.

■ POSTERIOR PITUITARY OR NEUROHYPOPHYSIS

■ PARTS

Posterior pituitary consists of three parts:
1. Pars nervosa or infundibular process
2. Neural stalk or infundibular stem
3. Median eminence.
    Pars tuberalis of anterior pituitary and the neural stalk of posterior pituitary together form the **hypophyseal stalk.**

■ HISTOLOGY

Posterior pituitary is made up of neural type of cells called pituicytes and unmyelinated nerve fibers.

Pituicytes

Pituicytes are the fusiform cells derived from glial cells. These cells have several processes and brown pigment granules. Pituicytes act as supporting cells and do not secrete any hormone.

Unmyelinated Nerve Fibers

Unmyelinated nerve fibers come from supraoptic and paraventricular nuclei of the hypothalamus through the pituitary stalk.

Other Structures

Posterior pituitary also has numerous blood vessels, hyaline bodies, neuroglial cells and mast cells.

■ HORMONES OF POSTERIOR PITUITARY

Posterior pituitary hormones are:
1. Antidiuretic hormone (ADH) or vasopressin
2. Oxytocin.

Source of Secretion of Posterior Pituitary Hormones

Actually, the posterior pituitary does not secrete any hormone. ADH and oxytocin are synthesized in the hypothalamus. From hypothalamus, these two hormones are transported to the posterior pituitary through the nerve fibers of **hypothalamo-hypophyseal tract** (Fig. 66.4), by means of axonic flow. Proteins involved in transport of these hormones are called neurophysins (see below).

In the posterior pituitary, these hormones are stored at the nerve endings. Whenever, the impulses from hypothalamus reach the posterior pituitary, these hormones are released from the nerve endings into the circulation. Hence, these two hormones are called **neurohormones.**

Experimental Evidence

Secretion of posterior pituitary hormones in hypothalamus and their transport to posterior pituitary are proved by experimental evidences. When the pituitary stalk is cut above the pituitary gland, by leaving the entire hypothalamus intact, the hormones drip through the cut end of the nerves in the pituitary stalk. This proves the fact that the hormones are secreted by hypothalamus.

Neurophysins

Neurophysins are the binding proteins which transport ADH and oxytocin from hypothalamus to posterior pituitary via hypothalamo-hypophyseal tract and storage of these hormones in posterior pituitary. Neurophysin I or oxytocin-neurophysin is the binding protein for oxytocin and neurophysin II or ADH-neurophysin is the binding protein for ADH.

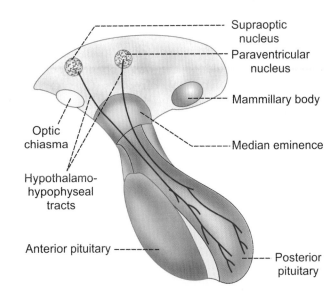

FIGURE 66.4: Hypothalamo-hypophyseal tracts

■ ANTIDIURETIC HORMONE

Source of Secretion

Antidiuretic hormone (ADH) is secreted mainly by **supraoptic nucleus** of hypothalamus. It is also secreted by **paraventricular nucleus** in small quantity. From here, this hormone is transported to posterior pituitary through the nerve fibers of hypothalamo-hypophyseal tract, by means of axonic flow.

Chemistry and Half-life

Antidiuretic hormone is a polypeptide containing 9 amino acids. Its half-life is 18 to 20 minutes.

Actions

Antidiuretic hormone has two actions:
1. Retention of water
2. Vasopressor action.

1. Retention of water

Major function of ADH is retention of water by acting on kidneys. It increases the **facultative reabsorption** of water from distal convoluted tubule and collecting duct in the kidneys (Chapter 52).

In the absence of ADH, the distal convoluted tubule and collecting duct are totally impermeable to water. So, reabsorption of water does not occur in the renal tubules and dilute urine is excreted. This leads to loss of large amount of water through urine. This condition is called **diabetes insipidus** and the excretion of large amount of water is called diuresis.

Mode of action on renal tubules

ADH increases water reabsorption in tubular epithelial membrane by regulating the **water channel proteins** called **aquaporins** through **V2 receptors** (Chapter 52).

2. Vasopressor action

In large amount, ADH shows vasoconstrictor action. Particularly, causes constriction of the arteries in all parts of the body. Due to vasoconstriction, the blood pressure increases. ADH acts on blood vessels through V_{1A} receptors.

However, the amount of ADH required to cause the vasopressor effect is greater than the amount required to cause the **antidiuretic effect.**

Regulation of Secretion

ADH secretion depends upon the volume of body fluid and the osmolarity of the body fluids.

Potent stimulants for ADH secretion are:
1. Decrease in the extracellular fluid (ECF) volume
2. Increase in osmolar concentration in the ECF.

Role of osmoreceptors

Osmoreceptors are the receptors which give response to change in the osmolar concentration of the blood. These receptors are situated in the hypothalamus near supraoptic and paraventricular nuclei. When osmolar concentration of blood increases, the osmoreceptors are activated. In turn, the osmoreceptors stimulate the supraoptic and paraventricular nuclei which send motor impulses to posterior pituitary through the nerve fibers and cause release of ADH. ADH causes reabsorption of water from the renal tubules. This increases ECF volume and restores the normal osmolarity.

■ OXYTOCIN

Source of Secretion

Oxytocin is secreted mainly by **paraventricular nucleus** of hypothalamus. It is also secreted by **supraoptic nucleus** in small quantity and it is transported from hypothalamus to posterior pituitary through the nerve fibers of hypothalamo-hypophyseal tract.

In the posterior pituitary, the oxytocin is stored in the nerve endings of hypothalamo-hypophyseal tract. When suitable stimuli reach the posterior pituitary from hypothalamus, oxytocin is released into the blood. Oxytocin is secreted in both males and females.

Chemistry and Half-life

Oxytocin is a polypeptide having 9 amino acids. It has a half-life of about 6 minutes.

Actions in Females

In females, oxytocin acts on mammary glands and uterus.

Action of oxytocin on mammary glands

Oxytocin causes ejection of milk from the mammary glands. Ducts of the mammary glands are lined by myoepithelial cells. Oxytocin causes contraction of the myoepithelial cells and flow of milk from alveoli of mammary glands to the exterior through duct system and nipple. The process by which the milk is ejected from alveoli of mammary glands is called milk ejection reflex or milk let-down reflex. It is one of the **neuroendocrine reflexes.**

Milk ejection reflex

Plenty of touch receptors are present on the mammary glands, particularly around the nipple. When the infant suckles mother nipple, the touch receptors are stimulated. The impulses discharged from touch receptors are carried by the somatic afferent nerve fibers to paraventricular and supraoptic nuclei of hypothalamus.

Now hypothalamus, in turn sends impulses to the posterior pituitary through hypothalamo-hypophyseal tract. Afferent impulses cause release of oxytocin into the blood. When the hormone reaches the mammary gland, it causes contraction of myoepithelial cells, resulting in ejection of milk from mammary glands (Fig. 66.5).

As this reflex is initiated by the nervous factors and completed by the hormonal action, it is called a **neuroendocrine reflex.** During this reflex, large amount of oxytocin is released by **positive feedback mechanism.**

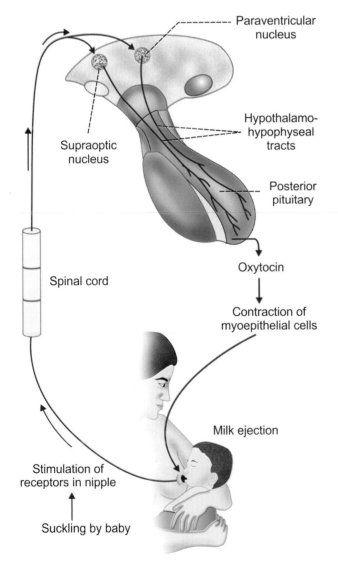

FIGURE 66.5: Milk ejection reflex

Action on uterus

Oxytocin acts on pregnant uterus and also non-pregnant uterus.

On pregnant uterus

Throughout the period of pregnancy, oxytocin secretion is inhibited by estrogen and progesterone. At the end of pregnancy, the secretion of these two hormones decreases suddenly and the secretion of oxytocin increases. Oxytocin causes contraction of uterus and helps in the expulsion of fetus.

During the later stages of pregnancy, the number of receptors for oxytocin increases in the wall of the uterus. Because of this, the uterus becomes more sensitive to oxytocin.

Oxytocin secretion increases during **labor.** At the onset of labor, the cervix dilates and the fetus descends through the birth canal. During the movement of fetus through cervix, the receptors on the cervix are stimulated and start discharging large number of impulses. These impulses are carried to the paraventricular and supraoptic nuclei of hypothalamus by the somatic afferent nerve fibers. Now, these two hypothalamic nuclei secrete large quantity of oxytocin, which enhances labor by causing contraction of uterus (Chapter 84).

Throughout labor, large quantity of oxytocin is released by means of **positive feedback mechanism,** i.e. oxytocin induces contraction of uterus, which in turn causes release of more amount of oxytocin (Fig. 4.5).

The contraction of uterus during labor is also a neuroendocrine reflex. Oxytocin also stimulates the release of prostaglandins in the placenta. Prostaglandins intensify the uterine contraction induced by oxytocin.

On non-pregnant uterus

The action of oxytocin on non-pregnant uterus is to facilitate the transport of sperms through female genital tract up to the fallopian tube, by producing the uterine contraction during sexual intercourse.

During the sexual intercourse, the receptors in the vagina are stimulated. Vaginal receptors generate the impulses, which are transmitted by somatic afferent nerves to the paraventricular and supraoptic nuclei of hypothalamus. When, these two nuclei are stimulated, oxytocin is released and transported by blood. While reaching the female genital tract, the hormone causes antiperistaltic contractions of uterus towards the fallopian tube. It is also a **neuroendocrine reflex.**

Sensitivity of uterus to oxytocin is accelerated by estrogen and decreased by progesterone.

Action in Males

In males, the release of oxytocin increases during ejaculation. It facilitates release of sperm into urethra by causing contraction of smooth muscle fibers in reproductive tract, particularly vas deferens.

Mode of Action of Oxytocin

Oxytocin acts on mammary glands and uterus by activating **G-protein coupled oxytocin receptor.**

■ APPLIED PHYSIOLOGY – DISORDERS OF PITUITARY GLAND

Disorders of pituitary gland are given in Table 66.1.

■ HYPERACTIVITY OF ANTERIOR PITUITARY

1. Gigantism

Gigantism is the pituitary disorder characterized by excess growth of the body. The subjects look like the giants with average height of about 7 to 8 feet.

Causes

Gigantism is due to hypersecretion of GH in childhood or in pre-adult life before the **fusion of epiphysis** of bone with shaft. Hypersecretion of GH is because of tumor of acidophil cells in the anterior pituitary.

Signs and symptoms

i. General overgrowth of the person leads to the development of a huge stature, with a height of more than 7 or 8 feet. The limbs are disproportionately long
ii. Giants are hyperglycemic and they develop glycosuria and pituitary diabetes. Hyperglycemia causes constant stimulation of β-cells of islets of Langerhans in the pancreas and release of insulin. However, the overactivity of β-cells of Langerhans in pancreas leads to degeneration of these cells and deficiency of insulin and ultimately, diabetes mellitus is developed
iii. Tumor of the pituitary gland itself causes constant headache

iv. Pituitary tumor also causes **visual disturbances.** It compresses the lateral fibers of optic chiasma, leading to **bitemporal hemianopia** (Chapter 168)

2. Acromegaly

Acromegaly is the disorder characterized by the enlargement, thickening and broadening of bones, particularly in the extremities of the body.

Causes

Acromegaly is due to hypersecretion of GH in adults after the fusion of epiphysis with shaft of the bone. Hypersecretion of GH is because of tumor of acidophil cells in the anterior pituitary.

Signs and symptoms

i. Acromegalic or **gorilla face:** Face with rough features such as protrusion of supraorbital ridges, broadening of nose, thickening of lips, thickening and wrinkles formation on forehead and **prognathism** (protrusion of lower jaw) (Fig. 66.6)
ii. Enlargement of hands and feet (Fig. 66.7)
iii. Kyphosis (extreme curvature of upper back – thoracic spine)
iv. Thickening of scalp. Scalp is also thrown into folds or wrinkles like **bulldog scalp**
v. Overgrowth of body hair
vi. Enlargement of visceral organs such as lungs, thymus, heart, liver and spleen
vii. Hyperactivity of thyroid, parathyroid and adrenal glands
viii. Hyperglycemia and glucosuria, resulting in diabetes mellitus
ix. Hypertension
x. Headache
xi. Visual disturbance **(bitemporal hemianopia).**

3. Acromegalic Gigantism

Acromegalic gigantism is a rare disorder with symptoms of both gigantism and acromegaly. Hypersecretion of GH

TABLE 66.1: Disorders of pituitary gland

Parts involved	Hyperactivity	Hypoactivity
Anterior pituitary	Gigantism Acromegaly Acromegalic gigantism Cushing disease	Dwarfism Acromicria Simmond disease
Posterior pituitary	Syndrome of inappropriate hypersecretion of ADH (SIADH)	Diabetes insipidus
Anterior and posterior pituitary	–	Dystrophia adiposogenitalis

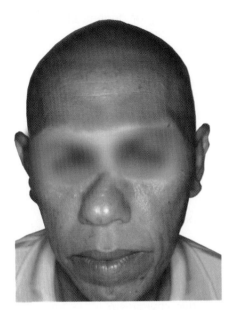
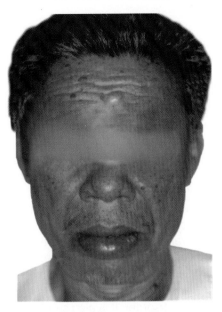

Gorilla face: Protrution of supraorbital ridges, broad nose, thickened lips and protrution of lower jaw.

Wrinkled forehead, with other features of acromegalic face.

FIGURE 66.6: Acromegaly (*Courtesy:* Prof Mafauzy Mohamad)

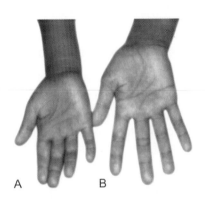

FIGURE 66.7: A. Normal hand; B. Acromegalic hand (*Courtesy:* Prof Mafauzy Mohamad)

in children, before the fusion of epiphysis with shaft of the bones causes gigantism and if hypersecretion of GH is continued even after the fusion of epiphysis, the symptoms of acromegaly also appear.

4. Cushing Disease

It is also a rare disease characterized by obesity.

Causes

Cushing disease develops by basophilic adenoma of adenohypophysis. It increases the secretion of adreno-corticotropic hormone, which in turn stimulates the adrenal cortex to release cortisol. Cushing disease also develops by hyperplasia or tumor of adrenal cortex.

Usually, the disorder due to the pituitary cause is called **Cushing disease** and when it is due to the adrenal cause, it is called **Cushing syndrome.**

Details of this condition are given in Chapter 70.

■ HYPOACTIVITY OF ANTERIOR PITUITARY

1. *Dwarfism*

Dwarfism is a pituitary disorder in children, characterized by the stunted growth.

Causes

Reduction in GH secretion in infancy or early childhood causes dwarfism. It occurs because of the following reasons:

   i. Tumor of chromophobes: It is a non-functioning tumor, which compresses and destroys the normal cells secreting GH. It is the most common cause for hyposecretion of GH, leading to dwarfism

   ii. Deficiency of GH-releasing hormone secreted by hypothalamus

  iii. Deficiency of somatomedin C

  iv. Atrophy or degeneration of acidophilic cells in the anterior pituitary

  iv. **Panhypopituitarism:** In this condition, there is reduction in the secretion of all the hormones of anterior pituitary gland. This type of dwarfism is associated with other symptoms due to the deficiency of other anterior pituitary hormones.

Signs and symptoms

i. Primary symptom of hypopituitarism in children is the stunted skeletal growth. The maximum height of anterior pituitary dwarf at the adult age is only about 3 feet

ii. But the proportions of different parts of the body are almost normal. Only the head becomes slightly larger in relation to the body

iii. Pituitary dwarfs do not show any deformity and their mental activity is normal with no mental retardation

iv. Reproductive function is not affected, if there is only GH deficiency. However, during panhypo-pituitarism, the dwarfs do not obtain puberty due to the deficiency of gonadotropic hormones.

Laron dwarfism

Laron dwarfism is a genetic disorder. It is also called **GH insensitivity.** It occurs due to the presence of abnormal growth hormone **secretagogue** (GHS) receptors in liver. GHS receptors become abnormal because of the mutation of genes for the receptors.

GH secretion is normal or high. But the hormone cannot stimulate growth because of the abnormal GHS receptors. So, dwarfism occurs.

Psychogenic dwarfism

Dwarfism occurs if the child is exposed to extreme emotional deprivation or stress. The short stature is because of deficiency of GH. This type of dwarfism is called psychogenic dwarfism, **psychosocial dwarfism** or **stress dwarfism.**

Dwarfism in dystrophia adiposogenitalis

Dystrophia adiposogenitalis or **Fröhlich syndrome** is a pituitary disorder (see below). Dwarfism occurs if it develops in children.

Dwarfism in panhypopituitarism

Panhypopituitarism is the pituitary disorder due to reduction in secretion of all anterior pituitary hormones. These dwarfs do not attain puberty.

2. Acromicria

Acromicria is a rare disease in adults characterized by the atrophy of the extremities of the body.

Causes

Deficiency of GH in adults causes acromicria. The secretion of GH decreases in the following conditions:

i. Deficiency of GH-releasing hormone from hypothalamus

ii. Atrophy or degeneration of acidophilic cells in the anterior pituitary

iii. Tumor of chromophobes: It is a non-functioning tumor, which compresses and destroys the normal cells secreting the GH. This is the most common cause for hyposecretion of GH leading to acromicria

iv. Panhypopituitarism: In this condition, there is a reduction in secretion of all the hormones of anterior pituitary gland. Acromicria is associated with other symptoms due to the deficiency of other anterior pituitary hormones.

Signs and symptoms

i. Atrophy and thinning of extremities of the body, (hands and feet) are the major symptoms in acromicria

ii. Acromicria is mostly associated with hypothyroidism

iii. Hyposecretion of adrenocortical hormones also is common in acromicria

iv. The person becomes lethargic and obese

v. There is loss of sexual functions.

3. Simmond Disease

Simmond disease is a rare pituitary disease. It is also called **pituitary cachexia.**

Causes

It occurs mostly in panhypopituitarism, i.e. hyposecretion of all the anterior pituitary hormones due to the atrophy or degeneration of anterior pituitary.

Symptoms

i. A major feature of Simmond disease is the rapidly developing **senile decay.** Thus, a 30-years-old person looks like a 60-years-old person. The senile decay is mainly due to deficiency of hormones from target glands of anterior pituitary, i.e. the thyroid gland, adrenal cortex and the gonads

ii. There is loss of hair over the body and loss of teeth

iii. Skin on face becomes dry and wrinkled. So, there is a shrunken appearance of facial features. It is the most common feature of this disease.

■ HYPERACTIVITY OF POSTERIOR PITUITARY

Syndrome of Inappropriate Hypersecretion of Antidiuretic Hormone (SIADH)

SIADH is the disease characterized by loss of sodium through urine due to hypersecretion of ADH.

Causes

SIADH occurs due to cerebral tumors, lung tumors and lung cancers because the **tumor cells** and **cancer cells** secrete ADH.

In normal conditions, ADH decreases the urine output by facultative reabsorption of water in distal convoluted tubule and the collecting duct. Urine that is formed is concentrated with sodium and other ions. Loss of sodium decreases the osmalarity of plasma, making it hypotonic. Hypotonic plasma inhibits ADH secretion resulting in restoration of plasma osmolarity.

However, in SIADH, secretion of ADH from tumor or cancer cells is not inhibited by hypotonic plasma. So there is continuous loss of sodium, resulting in persistent plasma hypotonicity.

Signs and symptoms

1. Loss of appetite
2. Weight loss
3. Nausea and vomiting
4. Headache
5. Muscle weakness, spasm and cramps
6. Fatigue
7. Restlessness and irritability.

In severe conditions, the patients die because of convulsions and coma.

■ HYPOACTIVITY OF POSTERIOR PITUITARY

Diabetes Insipidus

Diabetes insipidus is a posterior pituitary disorder characterized by excess excretion of water through urine.

Causes

This disorder develops due to the deficiency of ADH, which occurs in the following conditions:

i. Lesion (injury) or degeneration of supraoptic and paraventricular nuclei of hypothalamus
ii. Lesion in hypothalamo-hypophyseal tract
iii. Atrophy of posterior pituitary
iv. Inability of renal tubules to give response to ADH hormone. Such condition is called nephrogenic diabetes insipidus (see below).

Signs and symptoms

i. *Polyuria:* Excretion of large quantity of dilute urine, with increased frequency of voiding is called polyuria. Daily output of urine varies between 4 to 12 liter. In the absence of ADH, the epithelial cells of distal convoluted tubule in the nephron and the collecting duct of the kidney become impermeable to water. So, water is not reabsorbed from the renal tubule and collecting duct, leading to loss of water through urine.
ii. *Polydipsia:* Intake of excess water is called polydipsia. Because of polyuria, lot of water is lost from the body. It stimulates the thirst center in hypothalamus, resulting in intake of large quantity of water.
iii. *Dehydration:* In some cases, the thirst center in the hypothalamus is also affected by the lesion. Water intake decreases in these patients and loss of water through urine is not compensated. So, dehydration develops which may lead to death.

Nephrogenic diabetes insipidus

Nephrogenic diabetes insipidus is a genetic disorder due to inability of renal tubules to give response to ADH. It is caused by mutations of genes of V_2 receptors or aquaporin 2.

■ HYPOACTIVITY OF ANTERIOR AND POSTERIOR PITUITARY

Dystrophia Adiposogenitalis

Dystrophia adiposogenitalis is a disease characterized by **obesity** and **hypogonadism,** affecting mainly the adolescent boys. It is also called **Fröhlich syndrome** or **hypothalamic eunuchism.**

Causes

Dystrophia adiposogenitalis is due to hypoactivity of both anterior pituitary and posterior pituitary. Common cause of this disease is the tumor in pituitary gland and hypothalamic regions, concerned with food intake and gonadal development. Other causes are injury or atrophy of pituitary gland and genetic inability of hypothalamus to secrete luteinizing hormone-releasing hormone.

Symptoms

Obesity is the common feature of this disorder. Due to the abnormal stimulation of feeding center, the person overeats and consequently becomes obese. Obesity is accompanied by **sexual infantilism** (failure to develop secondary sexual characters) or eunuchism. **Dwarfism** occurs if the disease starts in growing age. In children, it is called infantile or prepubertal type of Fröhlich syndrome.

This disease develops in adults also. When it occurs in adults, it is called adult type of Fröhlich syndrome. In adults, the major symptoms are obesity and atrophy of sex organs.

Other features of this disorder are behavioral changes and loss of vision. Some patients develop diabetes insipidus.

Thyroid Gland

Chapter 67

- ■ INTRODUCTION
- ■ HISTOLOGY OF THYROID GLAND
- ■ HORMONES OF THYROID GLAND
- ■ SYNTHESIS OF THYROID HORMONES
- ■ STORAGE OF THYROID HORMONES
- ■ RELEASE OF THYROID HORMONES
- ■ TRANSPORT OF THYROID HORMONES IN THE BLOOD
- ■ FUNCTIONS OF THYROID HORMONES
- ■ MODE OF ACTION OF THYROID HORMONES
- ■ APPLIED PHYSIOLOGY – DISORDERS OF THYROID GLAND
- ■ TREATMENT FOR THYROID DISORDERS
- ■ THYROID FUNCTION TESTS

■ INTRODUCTION

Thyroid is an endocrine gland situated at the root of the neck on either side of the trachea. It has two **lobes,** which are connected in the middle by an **isthmus** (Fig. 67.1). It weighs about 20 to 40 g in adults. Thyroid is larger in females than in males. The structure and the function of the thyroid gland change in different stages

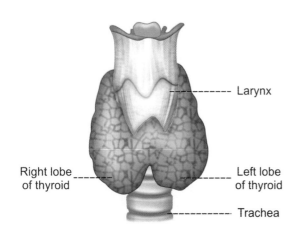

Right lobe of thyroid

Left lobe of thyroid

Larynx

Trachea

FIGURE 67.1: Thyroid gland

of the sexual cycle in females. Its function increases slightly during pregnancy and lactation and decreases during menopause.

■ HISTOLOGY OF THYROID GLAND

Thyroid gland is composed of large number of closed **follicles.** These follicles are lined with cuboidal epithelial cells, which are called the **follicular cells.** Follicular cavity is filled with a colloidal substance known as **thyroglobulin,** which is secreted by the follicular cells. Follicular cells also secrete tetraiodothyronine (T_4 or thyroxine) and tri-iodothyronine (T_3). In between the follicles, the **parafollicular cells** are present (Fig. 67.2). These cells secrete calcitonin.

■ HORMONES OF THYROID GLAND

Thyroid gland secretes three hormones:
1. Tetraiodothyronine or T_4 (thyroxine)
2. Tri-iodothyronine or T_3
3. Calcitonin.

T_4 is otherwise known as **thyroxine** and it forms about 90% of the total secretion, whereas T_3 is only 9% to 10%. Details of calcitonin are given in next chapter.

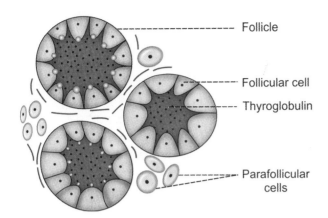

FIGURE 67.2: Histology of thyroid gland

Chemistry

Both T_4 and T_3 are iodine-containing derivatives of amino acid **tyrosine.**

Potency and Duration of Action

The potency of T_3 is four times more than that of T_4. T_4 acts for longer period than T_3. Duration of T_4 action is four times more than T_3 action. This is because of the difference in the affinity of these hormones to plasma proteins. T_3 has less affinity for plasma proteins and combines loosely with them, so that it is released quickly. T_4 has more affinity and strongly binds with plasma proteins, so that it is released slowly. Therefore, T_3 acts on the target cells immediately and T_4 acts slowly.

Half-life

Thyroid hormones have long half-life. T_4 has a long half-life of 7 days. Half-life of T_3 is varying between 10 and 24 hours.

Rate of Secretion

Thyroxine	=	80 to 90 µg/day
Tri-iodothyronine	=	4 to 5 µg/day
Reverse T_3	=	1 to 2 µg/day.

Plasma Level

Total T_3	=	0.12 µg/dL
Total T_4	=	8 µg/dL.

Metabolism of Thyroid Hormones

Degradation of thyroid hormones occurs in muscles, liver and kidney.

■ SYNTHESIS OF THYROID HORMONES

Synthesis of thyroid hormones takes place in thyroglobulin, present in follicular cavity. Iodine and tyrosine are essential for the formation of thyroid hormones. Iodine is consumed through diet. It is converted into iodide and absorbed from GI tract. Tyrosine is also consumed through diet and is absorbed from the GI tract.

For the synthesis of normal quantities of thyroid hormones, approximately 1 mg of iodine is required per week or about 50 mg per year. To prevent iodine deficiency, common table salt is iodized with one part of sodium iodide to every 100,000 parts of sodium chloride.

■ STAGES OF SYNTHESIS OF THYROID HORMONES

Synthesis of thyroid hormones occurs in five stages:
1. Thyroglobulin synthesis
2. Iodide trapping
3. Oxidation of iodide
4. Transport of iodine into follicular cavity
5. Iodination of tyrosine
6. Coupling reactions.

1. Thyroglobulin Synthesis

Endoplasmic reticulum and Golgi apparatus in the follicular cells of thyroid gland synthesize and secrete thyroglobulin continuously. Thyroglobulin molecule is a large glycoprotein containing 140 molecules of amino acid tyrosine. After synthesis, thyroglobulin is stored in the follicle.

2. Iodide Trapping

Iodide is actively transported from blood into follicular cell, against electrochemical gradient. This process is called iodide trapping.

Iodide is transported into the follicular cell along with sodium by sodium-iodide symport pump, which is also called iodide pump. Normally, iodide is 30 times more concentrated in the thyroid gland than in the blood. However, during hyperactivity of the thyroid gland, the concentration of iodide increases 200 times more.

3. Oxidation of Iodide

Iodide must be oxidized to elementary iodine, because only iodine is capable of combining with tyrosine to form thyroid hormones. The oxidation of iodide into iodine occurs inside the follicular cells in the presence of thyroid peroxidase. Absence or inactivity of this enzyme stops the synthesis of thyroid hormones.

4. *Transport of Iodine into Follicular Cavity*

From the follicular cells, iodine is transported into the follicular cavity by an **iodide-chloride pump** called **pendrin.**

5. *Iodination of Tyrosine*

Combination of iodine with tyrosine is known as iodination. It takes place in thyroglobulin. First, iodine is transported from follicular cells into the follicular cavity, where it binds with thyroglobulin. This process is called **organification** of thyroglobulin. Then, iodine (I) combines with tyrosine, which is already present in thyroglobulin (Fig. 67.3). Iodination process is accelerated by the enzyme iodinase, which is secreted by follicular cells.

Iodination of tyrosine occurs in several stages. Tyrosine is iodized first into monoiodotyrosine (MIT) and later into di-iodotyrosine (DIT). MIT and DIT are called the iodotyrosine residues.

6. *Coupling Reactions*

Iodotyrosine residues get coupled with one another. The coupling occurs in different configurations, to give rise to different thyroid hormones.

Coupling reactions are:
i. One molecule of DIT and one molecule of MIT combine to form tri-iodothyronine (T_3)
ii. Sometimes one molecule of MIT and one molecule of DIT combine to produce another form of T_3 called reverse T_3 or rT_3. Reverse T_3 is only 1% of thyroid output
iii. Two molecules of DIT combine to form tetraiodothyronine (T_4), which is thyroxine.

Tyrosine + I = Monoiodotyrosine (MIT)
MIT + I   = Di-iodotyrosine (DIT)
DIT + MIT = Tri-iodothyronine (T_3)
MIT + DIT = Reverse T_3
DIT + DIT = Tetraiodothyronine or Thyroxine (T_4)

■ STORAGE OF THYROID HORMONES

After synthesis, the thyroid hormones remain in the form of vesicles within thyroglobulin and are stored for long period. Each thyroglobulin molecule contains 5 or 6 molecules of thyroxine. There is also an average of 1 tri-iodothyronine molecule for every 10 molecules of thyroxine.

In combination with thyroglobulin, the thyroid hormones can be stored for **several months.** Thyroid gland is unique in this, as it is the only endocrine gland that can store its hormones for a long period of about 4 months. So, when the synthesis of thyroid hormone stops, the signs and symptoms of deficiency do not appear for about 4 months.

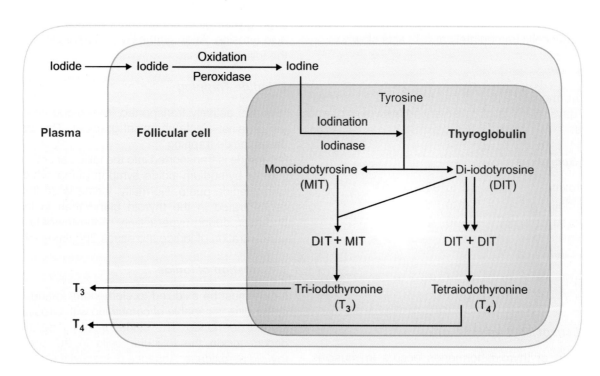

FIGURE 67.3: Synthesis of thyroid hormones

■ RELEASE OF THYROID HORMONES FROM THE THYROID GLAND

Thyroglobulin itself is not released into the bloodstream. On the other hand, the hormones are first cleaved from thyroglobulin and released into the blood.

Sequence of Events

1. Follicular cell sends foot-like extensions called **pseudopods,** which close around the thyroglobulin-hormone complex. This process is mediated by a receptor-like substance called **megalin,** which is present in the membrane of follicular cell
2. Pseudopods convert thyroglobulin-hormone complex into small **pinocytic vesicles**
3. Then, lysosomes of the cell fuse with these vesicles
4. Digestive enzymes such as proteinases present in lysosomes digest (proteolysis) the thyroglobulin and release the hormones
5. Now, the hormones diffuse through base of the follicular cell and enter the capillaries.

Only T_3 and T_4 are released into the blood. In the peripheral tissues, T_4 is converted into T_3. A small amount of inactive reverse T_3 is also formed. It is the biologically inactive form of T_3 and it is produced when T_4 is converted into T_3.

MIT and DIT are not released into blood. These iodotyrosine residues are deiodinated by an enzyme called iodotyrosine deiodinase, resulting in the release of iodine. The iodine is reutilized by the follicular cells for further synthesis of thyroid hormones. During congenital absence of iodotyrosine deiodinase, MIT and DIT are excreted in urine and the symptoms of iodine deficiency develop.

■ TRANSPORT OF THYROID HORMONES IN THE BLOOD

Thyroid hormones are transported in the blood by three types of proteins:
1. Thyroxine-binding globulin (TBG)
2. Thyroxine-binding prealbumin (TBPA)
3. Albumin.

1. Thyroxine-binding Globulin (TBG)

Thyroxine-binding globulin is a glycoprotein and its concentration in the blood is 1 to 1.5 mg/dL. It has a great affinity for thyroxine and about one third of the hormone combines strongly with this protein.

2. Thyroxine-binding Prealbumin (TBPA)

TBPA transports one fourth of the thyroid hormones. It is also called transthyretin (TTR).

3. Albumin

Albumin transports about one tenth of the thyroid hormones.

■ FUNCTIONS OF THYROID HORMONES

Thyroid hormones have two major effects on the body:
   I. To increase basal metabolic rate
  II. To stimulate growth in children.
      The actions of thyroid hormones are:

■ 1. ACTION ON BASAL METABOLIC RATE (BMR)

Thyroxine increases the metabolic activities in most of the body tissues, except brain, retina, spleen, testes and lungs. It increases BMR by increasing the oxygen consumption of the tissues. The action that increases the BMR is called calorigenic action.

In hyperthyroidism, BMR increases by about 60% to 100% above the normal level and in hypothyroidism it falls by 20% to 40% below the normal level.

■ 2. ACTION ON PROTEIN METABOLISM

Thyroid hormone increases the synthesis of proteins in the cells. The protein synthesis is accelerated by the following ways:

i. By Increasing the Translation of RNA

Thyroid hormone increases the translation of RNA in the cells. Because of this, the ribosomes are activated and more proteins are synthesized.

ii. By Increasing the Transcription of DNA to RNA

Thyroid hormone also stimulates the transcription of DNA to RNA. This in turn accelerates the synthesis of proteins in the cells (see above).

iii. By Increasing the Activity of Mitochondria

In addition to acting at nucleus, thyroid hormone acts at mitochondrial level also. It increases the number and the activity of mitochondria in most of the cells of the body. Thyroid hormone accelerates the synthesis of RNA and other substances from mitochondria, by activating series of enzymes. In turn, the mitochondria increase the production of ATP, which is utilized for the energy required for cellular activities.

iv. *By Increasing the Activity of Cellular Enzymes*

Thyroid hormones also increase the activity of at least 100 or more intracellular enzymes such as alpha-glycerophosphate dehydrogenase and oxidative enzymes. These enzymes accelerate the metabolism of proteins and the carbohydrates.

Though thyroxine increases synthesis of protein, it also causes catabolism of proteins.

■ 3. ACTION ON CARBOHYDRATE METABOLISM

Thyroxine stimulates almost all processes involved in the metabolism of carbohydrate.

Thyroxine:
  i. Increases the absorption of glucose from GI tract
  ii. Enhances the glucose uptake by the cells, by accelerating the transport of glucose through the cell membrane
  iii. Increases the breakdown of glycogen into glucose
  iv. Accelerates gluconeogenesis.

■ 4. ACTION ON FAT METABOLISM

Thyroxine decreases the fat storage by mobilizing it from adipose tissues and fat depots. The mobilized fat is converted into free fatty acid and transported by blood. Thus, thyroxine increases the free fatty acid level in blood.

■ 5. ACTION ON PLASMA AND LIVER FATS

Even though there is an increase in the blood level of free fatty acids, thyroxine specifically decreases the cholesterol, phospholipids and triglyceride levels in plasma. So, in hyposecretion of thyroxine, the cholesterol level in plasma increases, resulting in **atherosclerosis.**

Thyroxine also increases deposition of fats in the liver, leading to **fatty liver.** Thyroxine decreases plasma cholesterol level by increasing its excretion from liver cells into bile. Cholesterol enters the intestine through bile and then it is excreted through the feces.

■ 6. ACTION ON VITAMIN METABOLISM

Thyroxine increases the formation of many enzymes. Since vitamins form essential parts of the enzymes, it is believed that the vitamins may be utilized during the formation of the enzymes. Hence, **vitamin deficiency** is possible during hypersecretion of thyroxine.

■ 7. ACTION ON BODY TEMPERATURE

Thyroid hormone increases the heat production in the body, by accelerating various cellular metabolic processes and increasing BMR. It is called **thyroid hormone-induced thermogenesis.** During hypersecretion of thyroxine, the body temperature increases greatly, resulting in excess sweating.

■ 8. ACTION ON GROWTH

Thyroid hormones have general and specific effects on growth. Increase in thyroxine secretion accelerates the growth of the body, especially in growing children. Lack of thyroxine arrests the growth. At the same time, thyroxine causes early closure of epiphysis. So, the height of the individual may be slightly less in hypothyroidism.

Thyroxine is more important to promote growth and development of brain during fetal life and first few years of postnatal life. Deficiency of thyroid hormones during this period leads to **mental retardation.**

■ 9. ACTION ON BODY WEIGHT

Thyroxine is essential for maintaining the body weight. Increase in thyroxine secretion decreases the body weight and fat storage. Decrease in thyroxine secretion increases the body weight because of fat deposition.

■ 10. ACTION ON BLOOD

Thyroxine accelerates erythropoietic activity and increases blood volume. It is one of the important general factors necessary for erythropoiesis. Polycythemia is common in hyperthyroidism.

■ 11. ACTION ON CARDIOVASCULAR SYSTEM

Thyroxine increases the overall activity of cardiovascular system.

i. *On Heart Rate*

Thyroxine acts directly on heart and increases the heart rate. It is an important **clinical investigation** for diagnosis of hypothyroidism and hyperthyroidism.

ii. *On the Force of Contraction of the Heart*

Due to its effect on enzymatic activity, thyroxine generally increases the force of contraction of the heart. But in hyperthyroidism or in thyrotoxicosis, the heart may become weak due to excess activity and protein catabolism. So, the patient may die of **cardiac decompensation.**

Cardiac decompensation refers to failure of the heart to maintain adequate circulation associated with **dyspnea, venous engorgement** (veins overfilled with blood) and edema.

iii. *On Blood Vessels*

Thyroxine causes vasodilatation by increasing the metabolic activities. During increased metabolic activities, a large quantity of metabolites is produced. These metabolites cause vasodilatation.

iv. *On Arterial Blood Pressure*

Because of increase in rate and force of contraction of the heart, increase in blood volume and blood flow by the influence of thyroxine, cardiac output increases. This in turn, increases the blood pressure. But, generally, the mean pressure is not altered. Systolic pressure increases and the diastolic pressure decreases. So, only the pulse pressure increases (Chapter 103).

■ 12. ACTION ON RESPIRATION

Thyroxine increases the rate and force of respiration indirectly. The increased metabolic rate (caused by thyroxine) increases the demand for oxygen and formation of excess carbon dioxide. These two factors stimulate the respiratory centers to increase the rate and force of respiration (Chapter 126).

■ 13. ACTION ON GASTROINTESTINAL TRACT

Generally, thyroxine increases the appetite and food intake. It also increases the secretions and movements of GI tract. So, hypersecretion of thyroxine causes diarrhea and the lack of thyroxine causes constipation.

■ 14. ACTION ON CENTRAL NERVOUS SYSTEM

Thyroxine is very essential for the development and maintenance of normal functioning of central nervous system (CNS).

i. *On Development of Central Nervous System*

Thyroxine is very important to promote growth and development of the brain during fetal life and during the first few years of postnatal life. Thyroid deficiency in infants results in abnormal development of synapses, defective myelination and **mental retardation.**

ii. *On the Normal Function of Central Nervous System*

Thyroxine is a stimulating factor for the central nervous system, particularly the brain. So, the normal functioning of the brain needs the presence of thyroxine. Thyroxine also increases the blood flow to brain.

Thus, during the hypersecretion of thyroxine, there is excess stimulation of the CNS. So, the person is likely to have extreme nervousness and may develop psychoneurotic problems such as **anxiety complexes, excess worries** or **paranoid thoughts** (the persons think without justification that other people are plotting or conspiring against them or harassing them).

Hyposecretion of thyroxine leads to **lethargy** and **somnolence** (excess sleep).

■ 15. ACTION ON SKELETAL MUSCLE

Thyroxine is essential for the normal activity of skeletal muscles. Slight increase in thyroxine level makes the muscles to work with more vigor. But, hypersecretion of thyroxine causes weakness of the muscles due to catabolism of proteins. This condition is called **thyrotoxic myopathy.** The muscles relax very slowly after the contraction. Hyperthyroidism also causes fine muscular **tremor.** Tremor occurs at the frequency of 10 to 15 times per second. It is due to the thyroxine-induced excess neuronal activity, which controls the muscle. The lack of thyroxine makes the muscles more sluggish.

■ 16. ACTION ON SLEEP

Normal thyroxine level is necessary to maintain normal sleep pattern. Hypersecretion of thyroxine causes excessive stimulation of the muscles and central nervous system. So, the person feels tired, exhausted and feels like sleeping. But, the person cannot sleep because of the stimulatory effect of thyroxine on neurons. On the other hand, hyposecretion of thyroxine causes **somnolence.**

■ 17. ACTION ON SEXUAL FUNCTION

Normal thyroxine level is essential for normal sexual function. In men, hypothyroidism leads to complete loss of libido (sexual drive) and hyperthyroidism leads to **impotence.**

In women, hypothyroidism causes menorrhagia and **polymenorrhea** (Chapter 80). In some women, it causes irregular menstruation and occasionally **amenorrhea.** Hyperthyroidism in women leads to **oligomenorrhea** and sometimes **amenorrhea** (Chapter 80).

■ 18. ACTION ON OTHER ENDOCRINE GLANDS

Because of its metabolic effects, thyroxine increases the demand for secretion by other endocrine glands.

■ MODE OF ACTION OF THYROID HORMONES

In the target cells (particularly cells of liver, muscle and kidney), most of the T_4 is deiodinated to form T_3. So, the true intracellular hormone is T_3, rather than T_4. Moreover, T_3 is found freely in the plasma and T_4 is usually bound with plasma proteins. So, at the site of action, T_3 acts more quickly than T_4. T_3 also has got high binding affinity for thyroid hormone receptor.

Thyroid hormones act by activating the genes and increasing the **genetic transcription** (Chapter 65). In addition, the thyroid hormone also acts at mitochondrial level by stimulating the synthesis of proteins and RNA.

Sequence of Events

1. Thyroid hormones enter the nucleus of cell and bind with thyroid hormone receptors (TR), which are either attached to DNA genetic strands or in close proximity to them.
2. TR is always bound to another receptor called **retinoid X receptor** (RXR). Exact role of RXR is not clear. Thyroid hormones bind with receptors and form the hormone-receptor complex
3. This complex initiates the transcription process by activating the enzymes such as RNA polymerase and phosphoprotein kinases
4. It also stimulates the synthesis of nuclear proteins. Thus, a large number of mRNA is formed, which activate the ribosomes to synthesize the new proteins
5. New proteins are involved in many activities including the enzymatic actions.

■ REGULATION OF SECRETION OF THYROID HORMONES

Secretion of thyroid hormones is controlled by anterior pituitary and hypothalamus through feedback mechanism. Many factors are involved in the regulation of thyroid secretion.

■ ROLE OF PITUITARY GLAND

Thyroid-stimulating Hormone

Thyroid-stimulating hormone (TSH) secreted by anterior pituitary is the major factor regulating the synthesis and release of thyroid hormones. It is also necessary for the growth and the secretory activity of the thyroid gland. Thus, TSH influences every stage of formation and release of thyroid hormones.

Chemistry

Thyroid-stimulating hormone is a peptide hormone with one α-chain and one β-chain.

Half-life and Plasma Level

Half-life of TSH is about 60 minutes. The normal plasma level of TSH is approximately 2 U/mL.

Actions of Thyroid-stimulating Hormone

Thyroid-stimulating hormone increases:

1. The number of follicular cells of thyroid
2. The conversion of cuboidal cells in thyroid gland into columnar cells and thereby it causes the development of thyroid follicles
3. Size and secretory activity of follicular cells
4. Iodide pump and iodide trapping in follicular cells
5. Thyroglobulin secretion into follicles
6. Iodination of tyrosine and coupling to form the hormones
7. Proteolysis of the thyroglobulin, by which release of hormone is enhanced and colloidal substance is decreased.

Immediate effect of TSH is proteolysis of the thyroglobulin, by which thyroxine is released within 30 minutes. Effect of TSH on other stages in thyroxine synthesis takes place after some hours, days or weeks.

Mode of Action of TSH

TSH acts through cyclic AMP mechanism.

■ ROLE OF HYPOTHALAMUS

Hypothalamus regulates thyroid secretion by controlling TSH secretion through thyrotropic-releasing hormone (TRH). From hypothalamus, TRH is transported through the hypothalamo-hypophyseal portal vessels to the anterior pituitary. After reaching the pituitary gland, the TRH causes the release of TSH.

■ FEEDBACK CONTROL

Thyroid hormones regulate their own secretion through negative feedback control, by inhibiting the release of TRH from hypothalamus and TSH from anterior pituitary (Fig. 67.4).

■ ROLE OF IODIDE

Iodide is an important factor regulating the synthesis of thyroid hormones. When the dietary level of iodine is moderate, the blood level of thyroid hormones is normal. However, when iodine intake is high, the enzymes necessary for synthesis of thyroid hormones are inhibited by iodide itself, resulting in suppression of hormone synthesis. This effect of iodide is called **Wolff-Chaikoff effect.**

■ ROLE OF OTHER FACTORS

Many other factors are involved in the regulation of thyroid secretion in accordance to the needs of the body.

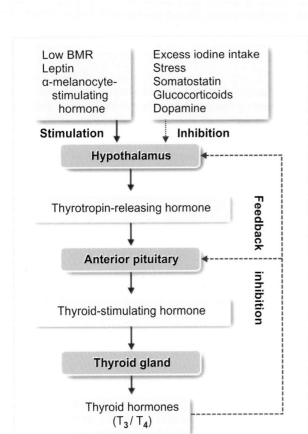

FIGURE 67.4: Regulation of secretion of thyroid hormones

Factors increasing the secretion of thyroid hormones:
1. Low basal metabolic rate
2. Leptin
3. α-melanocyte-stimulating hormone

Leptin (from adipose tissue) and **α-melanocyte-stimulating hormone** (from pituitary) increase the release of TRH and synthesis of T_4. The low body temperature also stimulates the synthesis of thyroid hormones. However, this occurs only in infants.

Factors decreasing the secretion of thyroid hormones:
1. Excess iodide intake
2. Stress
3. Somatostatin
4. Glucocorticoids
5. Dopamine.

These factors decrease the secretion of thyroid hormones, by inhibiting the release of TRH.

■ APPLIED PHYSIOLOGY – DISORDERS OF THYROID GLAND

■ HYPERTHYROIDISM

Increased secretion of thyroid hormones is called hyperthyroidism.

Causes of Hyperthyroidism

Hyperthyroidism is caused by:
1. Graves' disease
2. Thyroid adenoma.

1. *Graves' disease*

Graves' disease is an autoimmune disease and it is the most common cause of hyperthyroidism. Normally, TSH combines with surface receptors of thyroid cells and causes the synthesis and secretion of thyroid hormones. In Graves' disease, the B lymphocytes (plasma cells) produce autoimmune antibodies called **thyroid-stimulating autoantibodies** (TSAbs). These antibodies act like TSH by binding with membrane receptors of TSH and activating cAMP system of the thyroid follicular cells. This results in hypersecretion of thyroid hormones.

Antibodies act for a long time even up to 12 hours in contrast to that of TSH, which lasts only for an hour or so. The high concentration of thyroid hormones caused by the antibodies suppresses the TSH production also. So, the concentration of TSH is low or almost zero in plasma of most of the hyperthyroid patients.

2. *Thyroid adenoma*

Sometimes, a localized tumor develops in the thyroid tissue. It is known as thyroid adenoma and it secretes large quantities of thyroid hormones. It is not associated with autoimmunity. As far as this adenoma remains active, the other parts of thyroid gland cannot secrete the hormone. This is because, the hormone secreted from adenoma depresses the production of TSH.

Signs and Symptoms of Hyperthyroidism

1. Intolerance to heat as the body produces lot of heat due to increased basal metabolic rate caused by excess of thyroxine
2. Increased sweating due to vasodilatation
3. Decreased body weight due to fat mobilization
4. Diarrhea due to increased motility of GI tract
5. Muscular weakness because of excess protein catabolism
6. Nervousness, extreme fatigue, inability to sleep, mild tremor in the hands and psychoneurotic symptoms such as hyperexcitability, extreme anxiety or worry. All these symptoms are due to the excess stimulation of neurons in the central nervous system
7. Toxic goiter (see below)
8. Oligomenorrhea or amenorrhea (Chapter 80)
9. Exophthalmos (see below)
10. Polycythemia
11. Tachycardia and atrial fibrillation

12. Systolic hypertension
13. Cardiac failure.

Exophthalmos

Protrusion of eye balls is called exophthalmos. Most, but not all hyperthyroid patients develop some degree of protrusion of eyeballs.

Causes for exophthalmos

Exophthalmos in hyperthyroidism is due to the edematous swelling of retro-orbital tissues and degenerative changes in the extraocular muscles.

Effect of exophthalmos on vision

Severe exophthalmic condition leads to blindness because of two reasons:

1. Protrusion of the eyeball, which stretches and damages the optic nerve, resulting in **blindness** or
2. Due to the protrusion of eyeballs, the eyelids cannot be closed completely while blinking or during sleep. So, the constant exposure of eyeball to atmosphere causes dryness of the cornea, leading to irritation and infection. It finally results in ulceration of the cornea leading to blindness.

■ HYPOTHYROIDISM

Decreased secretion of thyroid hormones is called hypothyroidism. Hypothyroidism leads to myxedema in adults and cretinism in children.

Myxedema

Myxedema is the hypothyroidism in adults, characterized by generalized edematous appearance.

Causes for myxedema

Myxedema occurs due to diseases of thyroid gland, genetic disorder or iodine deficiency. In addition, it is also caused by deficiency of thyroid-stimulating hormone or thyrotropin-releasing hormone.

Common cause of myxedema is the autoimmune disease called **Hashimoto's thyroiditis,** which is common in late middle-aged women (Chapter 17). In most of the patients, it starts with glandular inflammation called **thyroiditis** caused by autoimmune antibodies. Later it leads to destruction of the glands.

Signs and symptoms of myxedema

Typical feature of this disorder is an edematous appearance throughout the body. It is associated with the following symptoms:

1. Swelling of the face
2. Bagginess under the eyes

3. Non-pitting type of edema, i.e. when pressed, it does not make pits and the edema is hard. It is because of accumulation of proteins with **hyaluronic acid** and **chondroitin sulfate,** which form a hard tissue with increased accumulation of fluid
4. Atherosclerosis: It is the hardening of the walls of arteries because of accumulation of fat deposits and other substances. In myxedema, it occurs because of increased plasma level of cholesterol which leads to deposition of cholesterol on the walls of the arteries.

Atherosclerosis produces **arteriosclerosis,** which refers to thickening and stiffening of arterial wall. Arteriosclerosis causes hypertension.

Other general features of hypothyroidism in adults are:

1. Anemia
2. Fatigue and muscular sluggishness
3. Extreme somnolence with sleeping up to 14 to 16 hours per day
4. Menorrhagia and polymenorrhea
5. Decreased cardiovascular functions such as reduction in rate and force of contraction of the heart, cardiac output and blood volume
6. Increase in body weight
7. Constipation
8. Mental sluggishness
9. Depressed hair growth
10. Scaliness of the skin
11. Frog-like husky voice
12. Cold intolerance.

Cretinism

Cretinism is the hypothyroidism in children, characterized by stunted growth.

Causes for cretinism

Cretinism occurs due to congenital absence of thyroid gland, genetic disorder or lack of iodine in the diet.

Features of cretinism

1. A newborn baby with thyroid deficiency may appear normal at the time of birth because thyroxine might have been supplied from mother. But a few weeks after birth, the baby starts developing the signs like sluggish movements and **croaking sound** while crying. Unless treated immediately, the baby will be mentally retarded permanently.
2. Skeletal growth is more affected than the soft tissues. So, there is stunted growth with bloated

body. The tongue becomes so big that it hangs down with dripping of saliva. The big tongue obstructs swallowing and breathing. The tongue produces characteristic guttural breathing that may sometimes **choke** the baby.

Cretin Vs dwarf

A cretin is different from pituitary dwarf. In cretinism, there is mental retardation and the different parts of the body are disproportionate. Whereas, in dwarfism, the development of nervous system is normal and the parts of the body are proportionate (Fig. 67.5). The reproductive function is affected in cretinism but it may be normal in dwarfism.

■ GOITER

Goiter means enlargement of the thyroid gland. It occurs both in hypothyroidism and hyperthyroidism.

Goiter in Hyperthyroidism – Toxic Goiter

Toxic goiter is the enlargement of thyroid gland with increased secretion of thyroid hormones, caused by thyroid tumor.

Goiter in Hypothyroidism – Non-toxic Goiter

Non-toxic goiter is the enlargement of thyroid gland without increase in hormone secretion. It is also called **hypothyroid goiter** (Fig. 67.6).

Based on the cause, the non-toxic hypothyroid goiter is classified into two types.
1. Endemic colloid goiter
2. Idiopathic non-toxic goiter.

1. Endemic colloid goiter

Endemic colloid goiter is the non-toxic goiter caused by iodine deficiency. It is also called **iodine deficiency goiter.** Iodine deficiency occurs when intake is less than 50 µg/day. Because of lack of iodine, there is no formation of hormones. By feedback mechanism, hypothalamus and anterior pituitary are stimulated. It increases the secretion of TRH and TSH. The TSH then causes the thyroid cells to secrete tremendous amounts of thyroglobulin into the follicle. As there are no hormones to be cleaved, the thyroglobulin remains as it is and gets accumulated in the follicles of the gland. This increases the size of gland.

In certain areas of the world, especially in the Swiss Alps, Andes, Great Lakes region of United States and in India, particularly in Kashmir Valley, the soil does not contain enough iodine. Therefore, the foodstuffs also do not contain iodine. The endemic colloid goiter was very common in these parts of the world before the introduction of iodized salts.

2. Idiopathic non-toxic goiter

Idiopathic non-toxic goiter is the goiter due to unknown cause. Enlargement of thyroid gland occurs even without iodine deficiency. The exact cause is not known. It is suggested that it may be due to thyroiditis and deficiency of enzymes such as **peroxidase, iodinase** and **deiodinase,** which are required for thyroid hormone synthesis.

Some foodstuffs contain **goiterogenic substances** (goitrogens) such as **goitrin.** These substances contain antithyroid substances like propylthiouracil. **Goitrogens** suppress the synthesis of thyroid hormones. Therefore, TSH secretion increases, resulting in enlargement of the gland. Such goitrogens are found in vegetables like turnips and cabbages. Soybean also contains some amount of goitrogens.

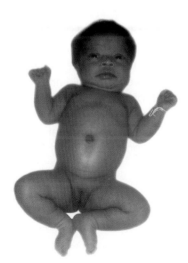

FIGURE 67.5: Cretinism (3-month-old baby)
(*Courtesy:* Prof Mafauzy Mohamad)

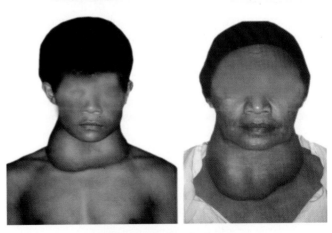

FIGURE 67.6: Non-toxic goiter
(*Courtesy:* Prof Mafauzy Mohamad)

The goitrogens become active only during low iodine intake.

TREATMENT FOR THYROID DISORDERS

TREATMENT FOR HYPERTHYROIDISM

1. By using Antithyroid Substances

Antithyroid substances are the drugs which suppress the secretion of thyroid hormones. Hyperthyroidism in early stage can be treated by antithyroid substances.

Three well-known antithyroid substances are:
  i. Thiocyanate
  ii. Thiourylenes
  iii. High concentration of inorganic iodides.

i. Thiocyanate

Thiocyanate prevents synthesis of thyroxine by inhibiting iodide trapping. The active pump which transports iodide into the thyroid cells, can transport thiocyanate ions also. So, administration of thiocyanate in high concentrations causes competitive inhibition of iodide transport into the cell. So, iodide trapping is inhibited, leading to the inhibition of synthesis of thyroxine.

ii. Thiourylenes

Thiourylenes are the thiourea-related substances such as propylthiouracil and methimazole, which prevent the formation of thyroid hormone from iodides and tyrosine. It is achieved partly by blocking peroxidase enzyme activity and partly by blocking coupling of iodinated tyrosine to form either T_3 or T_4.

During the use of these two antithyroid substances, even though the synthesis of thyroid hormone is inhibited, the formation of thyroglobulin is not stopped. The deficiency of the hormone increases the TSH secretion, which increases the size of thyroid gland with more secretion of thyroglobulin. Thyroglobulin accumulates in the gland and causes enlargement of the gland, resulting in non-toxic goiter.

iii. High concentration of inorganic iodides

Iodides in high concentration decrease all phases of thyroid activity, including the release of hormones. So, the size of the gland is also reduced with decreased blood supply. Because of this, iodides are frequently administered to hyperthyroid patients for 2 or 3 weeks, prior to surgical removal of the thyroid gland.

2. By Surgical Removal

In advanced cases of hyperthyroidism, treatment by using antithyroid substances is not possible. So, thyroid gland of these patients must be removed. Surgical removal of thyroid gland is called **thyroidectomy.** Before surgery, the patient is prepared by reducing the basal metabolic rate. It is done by injecting propylthiouracil for several weeks, until basal metabolic rate reaches almost the basal level. The high concentration of iodides is administered for 2 weeks. It decreases the size of the gland and blood supply to a very great extent. Because of these precautions, the mortality after the operation decreases very much.

TREATMENT FOR HYPOTHYROIDISM

The only treatment for hypothyroidism is the administration of thyroid extract or ingestion of pure thyroxine in the form of tablets, orally.

THYROID FUNCTION TESTS

Functional status of thyroid gland is assessed by the following tests:
  1. Measurement of plasma level of T_3 and T_4: For hyperthyroidism or hypothyroidism, the most accurate diagnostic test is the direct measurement of concentration of "free" thyroid hormones in the plasma, i.e. T_3 and T_4.
  2. Measurement of TRH and TSH: There is almost total absence of these two hormones in hyperthyroidism. It is because of negative feedback mechanism, by the increased level of thyroid hormones.
  3. Measurement of basal metabolic rate: In hyperthyroidism, basal metabolic rate is increased by about 30% to 60%. Basal metabolic rate is decreased in hypothyroidism by 20% to 40%.

Parathyroid Glands and Physiology of Bone

Chapter 68

■ INTRODUCTION

Human beings have four parathyroid glands, which are situated on the posterior surface of upper and lower poles of thyroid gland (Fig. 68.1). Parathyroid glands are very small in size, measuring about 6 mm long, 3 mm wide and 2 mm thick, with dark brown color.

Histology

Each parathyroid gland is made up of **chief cells** and **oxyphil cells.** Chief cells secrete parathormone. Oxyphil cells are the degenerated chief cells and their function is known. However, these cells may secrete parathormone during pathological condition called **parathyroid adenoma.** The number of oxyphil cells increases after puberty.

■ PARATHORMONE

Parathormone secreted by parathyroid gland is essential for the maintenance of blood calcium level within a very narrow critical level. Maintenance of blood calcium level is necessary because calcium is an important inorganic ion for many physiological functions (see below).

Source of Secretion

Parathormone (PTH) is secreted by the chief cells of the parathyroid glands.

Chemistry

Parathormone is protein in nature, having 84 amino acids. Its molecular weight is 9,500.

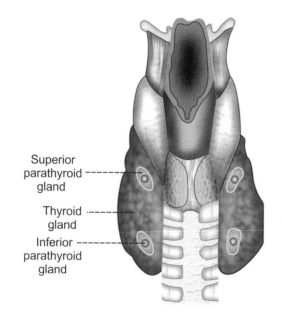

Superior parathyroid gland

Thyroid gland

Inferior parathyroid gland

FIGURE 68.1: Parathyroid glands on the posterior surface of thyroid gland

Half-life and Plasma Level

Parathormone has a half-life of 10 minutes. Normal plasma level of PTH is about 1.5 to 5.5 ng/dL.

Synthesis

Parathormone is synthesized from the precursor called **prepro-PTH** containing 115 amino acids. First, the prepro-PTH enters the endoplasmic reticulum of chief cells of parathyroid glands. There it is converted into a prohormone called **pro-PTH,** which contains 96 amino acids. Pro-PTH enters the Golgi apparatus, where it is converted into PTH.

Metabolism

Sixty to seventy percent of PTH is degraded by **Kupffer cells** of liver, by means of proteolysis. Degradation of about 20% to 30% PTH occurs in kidneys and to a lesser extent in other organs.

■ ACTIONS OF PARATHORMONE

PTH plays an important role in maintaining blood calcium level. It also controls blood phosphate level.

■ ACTIONS OF PARATHORMONE ON BLOOD CALCIUM LEVEL

Primary action of PTH is to maintain the blood calcium level within the critical range of 9 to 11 mg/dL. The blood calcium level has to be maintained critically because, it is very important for many of the activities in the body.

PTH maintains blood calcium level by acting on:
1. Bones
2. Kidney
3. Gastrointestinal tract.

1. On Bone

Parathormone enhances the resorption of calcium from the bones **(osteoclastic activity)** by acting on **osteoblasts** and **osteoclasts** of the bone.

Resorption of calcium from bones occurs in two phases:
   i. Rapid phase
   ii. Slow phase.

Rapid phase

Rapid phase occurs within minutes after the release of PTH from parathyroid glands. Immediately after reaching the bone, PTH gets attached with the receptors on the cell membrane of osteoblasts and osteocytes. The hormone-receptor complex increases the permeability of membranes of these cells for calcium ions. It accelerates the calcium pump mechanism, so that calcium ions move out of these bone cells and enter the blood at a faster rate.

Slow phase

Slow phase of calcium resorption from bone is due to the activation of osteoclasts by PTH. When osteoclasts are activated, some substances such as proteolytic enzymes, citric acid and lactic acid are released from lysosomes of these cells. All these substances digest or dissolve the organic matrix of the bone, releasing the calcium ions. The calcium ions slowly enter the blood.

PTH increases calcium resorption from bone by stimulating the proliferation of osteoclasts also.

2. *On Kidney*

PTH increases the reabsorption of calcium from the renal tubules along with magnesium ions and hydrogen ions. It increases calcium reabsorption mainly from distal convoluted tubule and proximal part of collecting duct.

PTH also increases the formation of **1,25-dihydroxycholecalciferol** (activated form of vitamin D) from 25-hydroxycholecalciferol in kidneys (see below).

3. *On Gastrointestinal Tract*

PTH increases the absorption of calcium ions from the GI tract indirectly. It increases the formation of 1,25-dihydroxycholecalciferol in the kidneys. This vitamin, in turn increases the absorption of calcium from GI tract.

Thus, the activated vitamin D is very essential for the absorption of calcium from the GI tract. And PTH is essential for the formation of activated vitamin D.

Role of PTH in the activation of vitamin D

Vitamin D is very essential for calcium absorption from the GI tract. But vitamin D itself is not an active substance. Instead, vitamin D has to be converted into 1, 25-dihydroxycholecalciferol in the liver and kidney in the presence of PTH. The 1,25-dihydroxycholecalciferol is the active product.

Activation of vitamin D

There are various forms of vitamin D. But, the most important one is vitamin D3. It is also known as chole-calciferol. Vitamin D3 is synthesized in the skin from 7-dehydrocholesterol, by the action of **ultraviolet rays** from the **sunlight.** It is also obtained from dietary sources.

The activation of vitamin D3 occurs in two steps (Fig. 68.2).

First step

Cholecalciferol (vitamin D3) is converted into 25-hydroxycholecalciferol in the liver. This process is limited and is inhibited by 25-hydroxycholecalciferol itself by feedback mechanism. This inhibition is essential for two reasons:

   i. Regulation of the amount of active vitamin D

   ii. Storage of vitamin D for months together.

If vitamin D3 is converted into 25-hydroxycholecalciferol, it remains in the body only for 2 to 5 days. But vitamin D3 is stored in liver for several months.

Second step

25-hydroxycholecalciferol is converted into 1,25-dihydroxycholecalciferol **(calcitriol)** in kidney. It is the active form of vitamin D3. This step needs the presence of PTH.

Role of Calcium Ion in Regulating 1, 25-Dihydroxycholecalciferol

When blood calcium level increases, it inhibits the formation of 1,25-dihydroxycholecalciferol. The mechanism involved in the inhibition of the formation of 1,25-dihydroxycholecalciferol is as follows:

   i. Increase in calcium ion concentration directly suppresses the conversion of 25-hydroxycholecalciferol into 1,25-dihydroxycholecalciferol. This effect is very mild

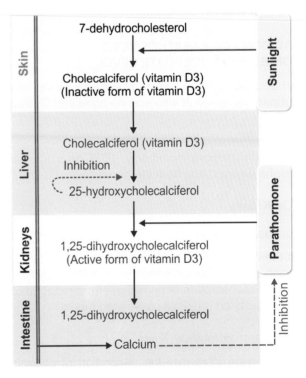

FIGURE 68.2: Schematic diagram showing activation of vitamin D

ii. Increase in calcium ion concentration decreases the PTH secretion, which in turn suppresses the conversion of 25-hydroxycholecalciferol into 1,25-dihydroxycholecalciferol.

This regulates the calcium ion concentration of plasma itself indirectly, i.e. when the PTH synthesis is inhibited, the conversion of 25-hydroxycholecalciferol into 1,25-hydroxycholecalciferol is also inhibited. Lack of 1,25-dihydroxycholecalciferol, decreases the absorption of calcium ions from the intestine, from the bones and from the renal tubules as well. This makes the calcium level in the plasma to fall back to normal.

Actions of 1, 25-Dihydroxycholecalciferol

1. It increases the absorption of calcium from the intestine, by increasing the formation of calcium-binding proteins in the intestinal epithelial cells. These proteins act as carrier proteins for facilitated diffusion, by which the calcium ions are transported. The proteins remain in the cells for several weeks after 1,25-dihydroxycholecalciferol has been removed from the body, thus causing a prolonged effect on calcium absorption
2. It increases the synthesis of calcium-induced ATPase in the intestinal epithelium
3. It increases the synthesis of alkaline phophatase in the intestinal epithelium
4. It increases the absorption of phosphate from intestine along with calcium.

■ ACTIONS OF PARATHORMONE ON BLOOD PHOSPHATE LEVEL

PTH decreases blood level of phosphate by increasing its urinary excretion. It also acts on bone and GI tract.

1. *On Bone*

Along with calcium resorption, PTH also increases phosphate absorption from the bones.

2. *On Kidney*

Phosphaturic action

It is the effect of PTH by which phosphate is excreted through urine. PTH increases phosphate excretion by inhibiting reabsorption of phosphate from renal tubules. It acts mainly on proximal convoluted tubule.

3. *On Gastrointestinal Tract*

Parathormone increases the absorption of phosphate from GI tract through calcitriol.

Sequence of events

i. PTH converts 25-hydroxycholecalciferol into 1,25-dihydroxycholecalciferol (calcitriol: active form of vitamin D3) in kidney
ii. Calcitriol increases the synthesis of calcium induced ATPase in the intestinal epithelium
iii. ATPase increases the synthesis of alkaline phophatase
iv. Alkaline phosphatase increases the absorption of phosphate from intestine along with calcium.

■ MODE OF ACTION OF PARATHORMONE

Parathormone Receptors

Parathormone receptors (PTH receptors) are of three types, PTHR1, PTHR2 and PTHR3, which are G protein-coupled receptors. PTHR1 is physiologically more important than the other two types. PTHR1 mediates the actions of PTH and **PTH-related protein** (see below). Role of PTHR2 and PTHR3 is not known clearly.

On the target cells, PTH binds with PTHR1 which is coupled to G protein and forms hormone-receptor complex. Hormone-receptor complex causes formation of cAMP, which acts as a second messenger for the hormone.

■ REGULATION OF PARATHORMONE SECRETION

Blood level of calcium is the main factor regulating the secretion of PTH. Blood phosphate level also regulates PTH secretion.

Blood Level of Calcium

Parathormone secretion is inversely proportional to blood calcium level. Increase in blood calcium level decreases PTH secretion.

Conditions when PTH secretion decreases are:
1. Excess quantities of calcium in the diet
2. Increased vitamin D in the diet
3. Increased resorption of calcium from the bones, caused by some other factors such as bone diseases.

On the other hand, decrease in calcium ion concentration of blood increases PTH secretion, as in the case of rickets, pregnancy and in lactation.

Blood Level of Phosphate

PTH secretion is directly proportional to blood phosphate level. Whenever the blood level of phosphate increases, it combines with ionized calcium to form calcium hydrogen phosphate. This decreases ionized calcium level in blood which stimulates PTH secretion.

■ APPLIED PHYSIOLOGY – DISORDERS OF PARATHYROID GLANDS

Disorders of parathyroid glands are of two types:
  I. Hypoparathyroidism
  II. Hyperparathyroidism.

■ HYPOPARATHYROIDISM – HYPOCALCEMIA

Hyposecretion of PTH is called hypoparathyroidism. It leads to hypocalcemia (decrease in blood calcium level).

Causes for Hypoparathyroidism

1. Surgical removal of parathyroid glands **(parathyroidectomy)**
2. Removal of parathyroid glands during surgical removal of thyroid gland **(thyroidectomy)**
3. Autoimmune disease
4. Deficiency of receptors for PTH in the target cells. In this, the PTH secretion is normal or increased but the hormone cannot act on the target cells. This condition is called **pseudohypoparathyroidism.**

Hypocalcemia and Tetany

Hypoparathyroidism leads to hypocalcemia, by decreasing the resorption of calcium from bones. Hypocalcemia causes neuromuscular hyperexcitability, resulting in hypocalcemic tetany. Normally, tetany occurs when plasma calcium level falls below 6 mg/dL from its normal value of 9.4 mg/dL.

Hypocalcemic Tetany

Tetany is an abnormal condition characterized by violent and painful **muscular spasm** (spasm = involuntary muscular contraction), particularly in feet and hand. It is because of hyperexcitability of nerves and skeletal muscles due to calcium deficiency.

Signs and symptoms of hypocalcemic tetany:

1. Hyper-reflexia and convulsions

Increase in neural excitability results in hyper-reflexia (overactive reflex actions) and convulsive muscular contractions.

2. Carpopedal spasm

Carpopedal spasm is the spasm in hand and feet that occurs in hypocalcemic tetany. During spasm, the hand shows a peculiar attitude (Fig. 68.3).

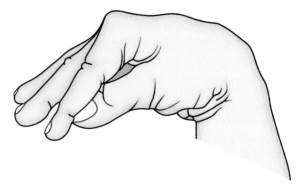

FIGURE 68.3: Carpopedal spasm

Attitude of hand in carpopedal spasm includes:
  i. Flexion at wrist joint
  ii. Flexion at metacarpophalangeal joints
  iii. Extension at interphalangeal joints
  iv. Adduction of thumb.

3. Laryngeal stridor

Stridor means noisy breathing. Laryngeal stridor means a loud crowing sound during inspiration, which occurs mainly due to **laryngospasm** (involuntary contraction of laryngeal muscles). Laryngeal stridor is a common dangerous feature of hypocalcemic tetany.

4. Cardiovascular changes

  i. Dilatation of the heart
  ii. Prolonged duration of ST segment and QT interval in ECG
  iii. Arrhythmias (irregular heartbeat)
  iv. Hypotension
  v. Heart failure.

5. Other features

  i. Decreased permeability of the cell membrane
  ii. Dry skin with brittle nails
  iii. Hair loss
  iv. Grand mal, petit mal or other seizures (Chapter 161)
  v. Signs of mental retardation in children or dementia in adults (Chapter 162).

When the calcium level falls below 4 mg/dL, it becomes fatal. During such severe hypocalcemic conditions, tetany occurs so quickly that a person develops spasm of different groups of muscles in the body. Worst affected are the laryngeal and bronchial muscles which develop respiratory arrest, resulting in death.

Latent Tetany

Latent tetany, also known as **subclinical tetany** is the **neuromuscular hyperexcitability** due to hypocalcemia that develops before the onset of tetany. It is characterized by general weakness and cramps in feet and hand. Hyperexcitability in these patients is detected by some signs, which do not appear in normal persons.

1. *Trousseau sign*

Trousseau sign is the spasm of the hand that is developed after 3 minutes of arresting the blood flow to lower arm and hand. The blood flow to lower arm and hand is arrested by inflating the blood pressure cuff 20 mm Hg above the patient's systolic pressure.

2. *Chvostek sign*

Chvostek sign is the twitch of the facial muscles, caused by a gentle tap over the facial nerve in front of the ear. It is due to the hyperirritability of facial nerve.

3. *Erb sign*

Hyperexcitability of the skeletal muscles even to a mild electrical stimulus is called Erb sign. It is also called **Erb-Westphal sign.**

■ HYPERPARATHYROIDISM – HYPERCALCEMIA

Hypersecretion of PTH is called hyperparathyroidism. It results in hypercalcemia. Hyperparathyroidism is of three types:

1. *Primary hyperparathyroidism*

Primary hyperparathyroidism is due to the development of tumor in one or more parathyroid glands. Sometimes, tumor may develop in all the four glands.

2. *Secondary hyperparathyroidism*

Secondary hyperparathyroidism is due to the physio-logical compensatory hypertrophy of parathyroid glands, in response to hypocalcemia which occurs due to other pathological conditions such as:

   i. Chronic renal failure
   ii. Vitamin D deficiency
   iii. Rickets.

3. *Tertiary hyperparathyroidism*

Tertiary hyperparathyroidism is due to **hyperplasia** (abnormal increase in the number of cells) of all the parathyroid glands that develops due to chronic secondary hyperparathyroidism.

Hypercalcemia

Hypercalcemia is the increase in plasma calcium level. It occurs in hyperparathyroidism because of increased resorption of calcium from bones.

Signs and symptoms of hypercalcemia

   i. Depression of the nervous system
   ii. Sluggishness of reflex activities
   iii. Reduced ST segment and QT interval in ECG
   iv. Lack of appetite
   v. Constipation.

Depressive effects of hypercalcemia are noticed when the blood calcium level increases to 12 mg/dL. The condition becomes severe with 15 mg/dL and it becomes lethal when blood calcium level reaches 17 mg/dL.

Other effects of hypercalcemia:

   i. Development of bone diseases such as osteitis fibrosa cystica
   ii. Development of parathyroid poisoning. It is the condition characterized by severe manifestations that occur when blood calcium level rises above 15 mg/dL. In hyperparathyroidism, the concentration of both calcium and phosphate increases leading to formation of calcium-phosphate crystals. Concentration of phosphate also increases because, kidney cannot excrete the excess amount of phosphate resorbed from the bone
   iii. Deposition of **calcium-phosphate crystals** in renal tubules, thyroid gland, alveoli of lungs, gastric mucosa and in the wall of the arteries, resulting in dysfunction of these organs. **Renal stones** are formed when it is deposited in kidney.

■ PARATHYROID FUNCTION TESTS

  1. Measurement of blood calcium level
  2. Chvostek sign and Trousseau sign for hypo-parathyroidism.

■ CALCITONIN

Source of Secretion

Calcitonin is secreted by the **parafollicular cells** or **clear cells (C cells),** situated amongst the follicles in thyroid gland. In lower animals, the parafollicular cells are derived from ultimobranchial glands, which develop from fifth pharyngeal pouches. In human being, the ultimobranchial glands and fifth pharyngeal pouches are rudimentary and their cells are incorporated with fourth pharyngeal pouches and distributed amongst the follicles of thyroid gland.

Recently, calcitonin is found in brain, prostate and bronchial cells of lungs. However, the physiological role of calcitonin from non-thyroid tissues is not known.

Chemistry and Synthesis

Calcitonin is a polypeptide chain with 32 amino acids. Its molecular weight is about 3,400. It is synthesized from procalcitonin.

Plasma Level and Half-life

Plasma level of calcitonin is 1 to 2 ng/dL. It has a half-life of 5 to 10 minutes.

Metabolism

Calcitonin is degraded and excreted by liver and kidney.

■ ACTIONS OF CALCITONIN

1. On Blood Calcium Level

Calcitonin plays an important role in controlling the blood calcium level. It decreases the blood calcium level and thereby counteracts parathormone.

Calcitonin reduces the blood calcium level by acting on bones, kidneys and intestine.

i. On bones

Calcitonin stimulates **osteoblastic activity** and facilitates the deposition of calcium on bones. At the same time, it suppresses the activity of **osteoclasts** and inhibits the resorption of calcium from bones. It inhibits even the development of new osteoclasts in bones.

ii. On kidney

Calcitonin increases excretion of calcium through urine, by inhibiting the reabsorption from the renal tubules.

iii. On intestine

Calcitonin prevents the absorption of calcium from intestine into the blood.

2. On Blood Phosphate Level

With respect to calcium, calcitonin is an antagonist to PTH. But it has similar actions of PTH, with respect to phosphate. It decreases the blood level of phosphate by acting on bones and kidneys.

i. On bones

Calcitonin inhibits the resorption of phosphate from bone and stimulates the deposition of phosphate on bones.

ii. On kidney

Calcitonin increases the excretion of phosphate through urine, by inhibiting the reabsorption from renal tubules.

■ REGULATION OF CALCITONIN SECRETION

High calcium content in plasma stimulates the calcitonin secretion through a calcium receptor in parafollicular cells. Gastrin also is known to stimulate the release of calcitonin.

■ CALCIUM METABOLISM

■ IMPORTANCE OF CALCIUM

Calcium is very essential for many activities in the body such as:
1. Bone and teeth formation
2. Neuronal activity
3. Skeletal muscle activity
4. Cardiac activity
5. Smooth muscle activity
6. Secretory activity of the glands
7. Cell division and growth
8. Coagulation of blood.

■ NORMAL VALUE

In a normal young healthy adult, there is about 1,100 g of calcium in the body. It forms about 1.5% of total body weight. 99% of calcium is present in the bones and teeth and the rest is present in the plasma. Normal blood calcium level ranges between 9 and 11 mg/dL.

■ TYPES OF CALCIUM

Calcium in Plasma

Calcium is present in three forms in plasma:
  i. Ionized or diffusible calcium: Found freely in plasma and forms about 50% of plasma calcium. It is essential for vital functions such as neuronal activity, muscle contraction, cardiac activity, secretions in the glands, blood coagulation, etc.
 ii. Non-ionized or non-diffusible calcium: Present in non-ionic form such as calcium bicarbonate. It is about 8% to 10% of plasma calcium
iii. Calcium bound to albumin: Forms about 40% to 42% of plasma calcium.

Calcium in Bones

Calcium is constantly removed from bone and deposited in bone. Bone calcium is present in two forms:
  i. Rapidly exchangeable calcium or exchangeable calcium: Available in small quantity in bone and helps to maintain the plasma calcium level
 ii. Slowly exchangeable calcium or stable calcium: Available in large quantity in bones and helps in bone remodeling.

Process of calcium metabolism is explained schematically in Fig. 68.4.

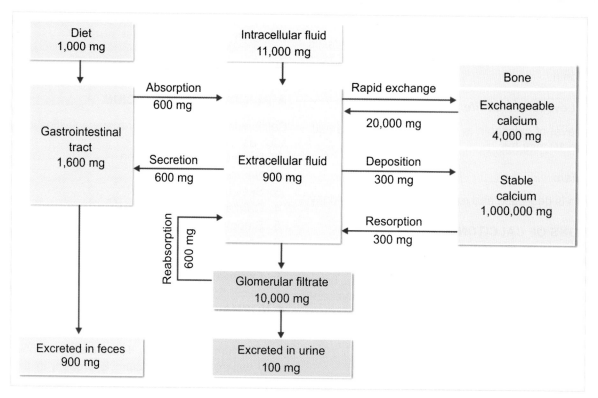

FIGURE 68.4: Schematic diagram showing calcium metabolism. Values belong to adults

■ SOURCE OF CALCIUM

1. Dietary Source

Calcium is available in several foodstuffs. Percentage of calcium in different food substance is:

Whole milk	= 10%
Low fat milk	= 18%
Cheese	= 27%
Other dairy products	= 17%
Vegetables	= 7%
Other substances such as meat, egg, grains, sugar, coffee, tea, chocolate, etc.	= 21%

2. From Bones

Besides dietary calcium, blood also gets calcium from bone by resorption.

■ DAILY REQUIREMENTS OF CALCIUM

1 to 3 years	=	500 mg
4 to 8 years	=	800 mg
9 to 18 years	=	1,300 mg
19 to 50 years	=	1,000 mg
51 years and above	=	1,200 mg
Pregnant ladies and lactating mothers	=	1,300 mg

■ ABSORPTION AND EXCRETION OF CALCIUM

Calcium taken through dietary sources is absorbed from GI tract into blood and distributed to various parts of the body. Depending upon the blood level, the calcium is either deposited in the bone or removed from the bone (resorption). Calcium is excreted from the body through urine and feces.

Absorption from Gastrointestinal Tract

Calcium is absorbed from duodenum by carrier-mediated active transport and from the rest of the small intestine, by facilitated diffusion. Vitamin D is essential for the absorption of calcium from GI tract.

Excretion

While passing through the kidney, large quantity of calcium is filtered in the glomerulus. From the filtrate, 98% to 99% of calcium is reabsorbed from renal tubules into the blood. Only a small quantity is excreted through urine.

Most of the filtered calcium is reabsorbed in the distal convoluted tubules and proximal part of collecting duct. In distal convoluted tubule, parathormone increases the reabsorption. In collecting duct, vitamin D increases the reabsorption and calcitonin decreases reabsorption.

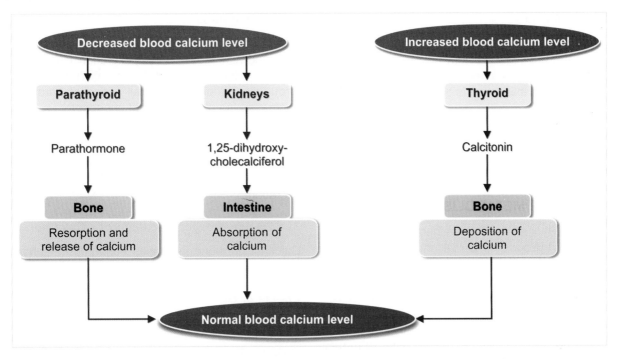

FIGURE 68.5: Schematic diagram showing regulation of blood calcium level

About 1,000 mg of calcium is excreted daily. Out of this, 900 mg is excreted through feces and 100 mg through urine.

■ REGULATION OF BLOOD CALCIUM LEVEL

Blood calcium level is regulated mainly by three hormones (Figs 68.5 and 68.6):
  1. Parathormone
  2. 1,25-dihydroxycholecalciferol (calcitriol)
  3. Calcitonin.

1. *Parathormone*

Parathormone is a protein hormone secreted by parathyroid gland and its main function is to increase the blood calcium level by mobilizing calcium from bone (resorption) (See above for details).

2. *1,25-dihydroxycholecalciferol – Calcitriol*

Calcitriol is a steroid hormone synthesized in kidney. It is the activated form of vitamin D. Its main action is to increase the blood calcium level by increasing the calcium absorption from the small intestine (see above for details).

3. *Calcitonin*

Calcitonin secreted by parafollicular cells of thyroid gland. Thyroid gland is a calcium-lowering hormone. It reduces the blood calcium level mainly by decreasing bone resorption (see above for details).

Effects of Other Hormones

In addition to the above mentioned three hormones, growth hormone and glucocorticoids also influence the calcium level.

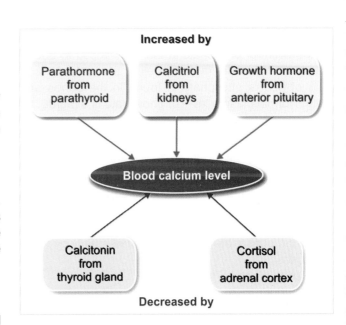

FIGURE 68.6: Effect of hormones on blood calcium level

1. *Growth hormone*

Growth hormone increases the blood calcium level by increasing the intestinal calcium absorption. It is also suggested that it increases the urinary excretion of calcium. However, this action is only transient.

2. *Glucocorticoids*

Glucocorticoids (cortisol) decrease blood calcium by inhibiting intestinal absorption and increasing the renal excretion of calcium.

■ PHOSPHATE METABOLISM

Phosphorus (P) is an essential mineral that is required by every cell in the body for normal function. Phosphorus is present in many food substances, such as peas, dried beans, nuts, milk, cheese and butter. Inorganic phosphorus (Pi) is in the form of the **phosphate** (PO_4). The majority of the phosphorus in the body is found as phosphate. Phosphorus is also the body's source of phosphate. In body, phosphate is the most abundant intracellular anion.

■ IMPORTANCE OF PHOSPHATE

1. Phosphate is an important component of many organic substances such as, ATP, DNA, RNA and many intermediates of metabolic pathways
2. Along with calcium, it forms an important constituent of bone and teeth
3. It forms a buffer in the maintenance of acid-base balance.

■ NORMAL VALUE

Total amount of phosphate in the body is 500 to 800 g. Though it is present in every cell of the body, 85% to 90% of body's phosphate is found in the bones and teeth. Normal plasma level of phosphate is 4 mg/dL.

■ REGULATION OF PHOSPHATE LEVEL

Phosphorus is taken through dietary sources. It is absorbed from GI tract into blood. It is also resorbed from bone. From blood it is distributed to various parts of the body. While passing through the kidney, large quantity of phosphate is excreted through urine.

Blood phosphate level is regulated mainly by three hormones:
1. Parathormone
2. Calcitonin
3. 1,25-dihydroxycholecalciferol (calcitriol).

1. *Parathormone*

Parathormone stimulates resorption of phosphate from bone and increases its urinary excretion. It also increases the absorption of phosphate from gastrointestinal tract through calcitriol. The overall action of parathormone decreases the plasma level of phosphate.

2. *Calcitonin*

Calcitonin also decreases the plasma level of phosphate by inhibiting bone resorption and stimulating the urinary excretion.

3. *1,25-Dihydroxycholecalciferol – Calcitriol*

Calcitriol hormone increases absorption of phosphate from small intestine (Fig. 68.7).

Effects of Other Hormones

In addition to the above mentioned three hormones, growth hormone and glucocorticoids also influence the phosphate level.

1. *Growth hormone*

Growth hormone increases the blood phosphate level by increasing the intestinal phosphate absorption.

2. *Glucocorticoids*

Glucocorticoids (cortisol) decreases blood phosphate by inhibiting intestinal absorption and increasing the renal excretion of phosphate.

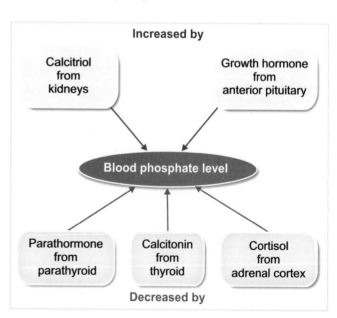

FIGURE 68.7: Effect of hormones on blood phosphate level

■ PHYSIOLOGY OF BONE

Bone or **osseous tissue** is a specialized rigid connective tissue that forms the skeleton. It consists of special type of cells and tough **intercellular matrix** of ground substance. The matrix is formed by organic substances like **collagen** and it is strengthened by the deposition of mineral salts like calcium phosphate and calcium carbonate. Throughout the life, bone is renewed by the process of bone formation and bone resorption.

■ FUNCTIONS OF BONE

1. *Protective function:* Protects soft tissues and vital organs of the body
2. *Mechanical function:* Supports the body and brings out various movements of the body by their attachment to the muscles and tendons
3. *Metabolic function:* Plays an important role in the metabolism homeostasis of calcium and phosphate in the body.
4. *Hemopoietic function:* Red bone marrow in the bones is the site of production of blood cells.

■ CLASSIFICATION OF BONE

Depending upon the size and shape, the bones are classified into five types:
1. Long bones: Bones of the limbs
2. Short bones: Bones in the wrist and ankle
3. Flat bones: Skull bones, mandible, scapula, etc.
4. Irregular bones: Vertebra
5. Sesamoid bones: Patella.

■ PARTS OF BONE

Long bones are formed by a cylindrical tube of bone tissue, which has three portions:
1. Diaphysis: Midportion or midshaft
2. Epiphysis: Wider extremity or the head on either end
3. Metaphysis: Portion between the diaphysis and the epiphysis (Fig. 68.8).

   In growing age, a layer of cartilage called **epiphyseal cartilage** or **epiphyseal plate** or **growth plate** is present in between epiphysis and metaphysis. Epiphyseal plate is responsible for the longitudinal growth of the bones.

■ COMPOSITION OF BONE

Bone consists of the tough organic matrix to which the bone salts are deposited.

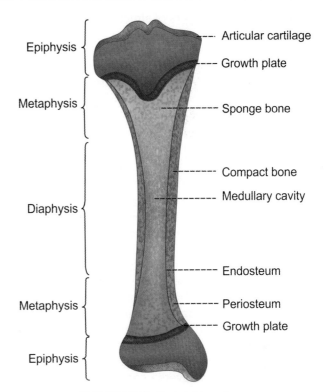

FIGURE 68.8: Parts of long bone

Matrix

Bone matrix is composed of protein fibers called **collagen fibers,** which are embedded in the gelatinous ground substance. These collagen fibers form about 90% of the bone. The ground substance is formed by ECF and **proteoglycans.** Proteoglycans are **chondroitin sulfate** and **hyaluronic acid,** which are concerned with the regulation and deposition of bone salts.

Bone Salts

The crystalline salts present in bones are called **hydroxyapatites,** which contain calcium and phosphate. Apart from these substances, some other salts like sodium, potassium, magnesium and carbonate are also present in the bone. The salts of the bone strengthen the bone matrix.

■ STRUCTURE OF BONE

Bone is covered by an outer white fibrous connective layer called **periosteum** and an inner dense fibrous membrane called endosteum. The tendons from the muscles are attached to periosteum. The heads (epiphysis) of bone are covered by a **hyaline cartilage.** It forms the synovial joint with adjoining bones.

Bones have two layers of structures:
1. Outer compact bone
2. Inner spongy bone.

In most of the bones, both compact and spongy forms are present. However, the thickness of each type varies in different regions. The epiphysis contains large amount of spongy bone and outer thin compact bone. In diaphysis, the amount of compact bone is more and the spongy bone is very thin.

Compact Bone

Compact or cortical bone is the hard and dense material forming about 80% of bone in the body. Its main functions are mechanical function and the protection of bone marrow.

Compact bone consists of minute cylindrical structures called **osteones** or **Haversian systems** (Fig. 68.9), which are formed by concentric layers of collagen. Collagen lamellae are called **Haversian lamellae.** In the center of each osteon, there is a canal called **Haversian canal** that contains the blood vessels, lymph vessels and nerve fibers. The Haversian systems communicate with each other by transverse canals called **Volkmann canal.**

Within the Haversian systems, there are small cavities called **lacunae,** inside which the **osteocytes** are trapped. Osteocytes send long processes called **canaliculi.** The canaliculi from neighboring osteocytes unite to form tight junctions.

Marrow cavity

Compact bone has a large narrow cavity called **marrow cavity** or medullary cavity, which contains yellow bone marrow.

Spongy Bone

Spongy or **trabecular** or **cancellous bone** forms 20% of bone in the body and it contains red bone marrow. It is made of **bone spicules,** which are separated by spaces.

■ TYPES OF CELLS IN BONE

Bone has three major types of cells:
1. Osteoblasts
2. Osteocytes
3. Osteoclasts.

1. Osteoblasts

Osteoblasts are the bone cells concerned with bone formation **(osteoblastic activity).** These cells are situated in the outer surface of bone, the marrow cavity and

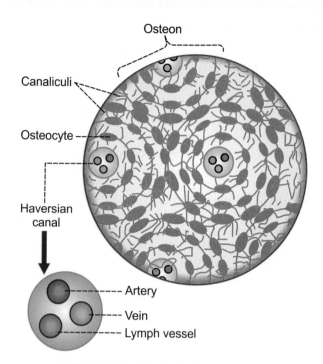

FIGURE 68.9: Structure of compact bone

epiphyseal plate. The osteoblasts arise from the giant multinucleated primitive cells called the **osteoprogenitor** cells. Differentiation of osteoprogenitor cells into osteoblasts (Table 68.1) is accelerated by some hormones and some bone proteins called **skeletal growth factors.** These growth factors stimulate the growth of osteoblasts also.

Functions of osteoblasts

i. Role in the formation of bone matrix

Osteoblasts are responsible for the synthesis of bone matrix by secreting type I collagen and a protein called **matrix gla protein** (MGP) or **osteocalcin.** Other proteins involved in the matrix synthesis are also produced by the osteoblasts. Such proteins are transforming growth factor (TGF), insulin-like growth factor (IGF), fibroblast growth factor (FGF) and platelet-derived growth factor (PDGF).

ii. Role in calcification

Osteoblasts are rich in enzyme alkaline phosphatase, which is necessary for deposition of calcium in the bone matrix **(calcification).**

iii. Synthesis of proteins

Osteoblasts synthesize the proteins called matrix gla protein and osteopontin, which are involved in the calcification.

Fate of osteoblasts

After taking part in bone formation, the osteoblasts differentiate into osteocytes, which are trapped inside the lacunae of calcified bone.

2. Osteocytes

Osteocytes are the bone cells concerned with maintenance of bone. Osteocytes are small flattened and rounded cells, embedded in the bone lacunae. These cells are the major cells in developed bone and are derived from the matured osteoblasts. The cytoplasmic processes from osteocytes run into canaliculi and ramify throughout the bone matrix. The processes from neighboring osteocytes have contact with each other forming tight junctions.

Functions of osteocytes

i. Help to maintain the bone as living tissue because of their metabolic activity
ii. Maintain the exchange of calcium between the bone and ECF.

3. Osteoclasts

Osteoclasts are the bone cells that are concerned with bone resorption **(osteoclastic activity)**. Osteoclasts are the **giant phagocytic multinucleated cells** found in the lacunae of bone matrix. These bone cells are derived from hemopoietic stem cells via monocytes colony forming units-M (CFU-M).

Functions of osteoclasts

i. Responsible for bone resorption during bone remodeling
ii. Synthesis and release of lysosomal enzymes necessary for bone resorption into the bone resorbing compartment.

■ BONE GROWTH

Embryo has a cartilaginous skeleton. The **cartilage** is composed of large amount of solid but flexible matrix. The matrix is derived from a protein called **chondrin,** that is secreted by the **cartilage cells** or **chondriocytes.** Some of the cartilage is converted into bones.

Ossification and Calcification

Ossification is the conversion of cartilage into bone. At the time of birth, the skeleton consists of 50% cartilage and 50% bone. At the age of 2 years and thereafter, the skeleton consists 35% cartilage and 65% bone.

Ossification is carried out by the osteoblasts, which enter the cartilage and lay down the matrix around them. Osteoblasts synthesize collagen fibers, which produce the matrix called osteoid. Then, calcium is deposited on the matrix. The deposition of calcium is called calcification.

Growth in Length

During growth, the epiphysis at the end of each long bone is separated from diaphysis by a plate of proliferative cartilage termed as **epiphyseal plate.**

Increase in the length of the bone occurs due to the formation of new bone from epiphyseal plate. The thickness of the epiphyseal plate reduces as the length of bone increases. Increase in length of the bone occurs as long as the epiphyseal plates remain separated from diaphysis (shaft). The growth of the bone stops when the epiphysis fuses with the shaft. The process by which epiphysis fuses with shaft is called the **epiphyseal fusion** or closure. It occurs usually at the time of puberty. Width of the bone increases due to increase in thickness of periosteum or the outer layers of compact bone.

■ BONE REMODELING

Bone remodeling is a dynamic lifelong process in which old bone is resorbed and new bone is formed. Usually, it takes place in groups of bone cells called the **basic multicellular units** (BMU). The entire process of remodeling extends for about 100 days in compact bone and about 200 days in spongy bone.

Processes of bone remodeling

1. Bone resorption: Destruction of bone matrix and removal of calcium (osteoclastic activity).
2. Bone formation: Development and mineralization of new matrix (osteoblastic activity).

Bone Resorption – Osteoclastic Activity

Osteoclastic activity is the process that involves destruction of bone matrix, followed by removal of calcium. Osteoclasts are responsible for bone resorption by their osteoclastic activity.

Part of the bone to be resorbed is known as bone resorbing compartment. The osteoclast present in this compartment attaches itself to the periosteal or endosteal surface of bone through villi-like membranous extensions. This process is mediated by the surface receptors called **integrins.** At the point of attachment, a ruffled border is formed by folding of the cell membrane.

Resorption of that particular compartment occurs by some substances released from membranous extensions of osteoclasts such as:
1. Collagenase
2. Phosphatase

3. Lysosomal enzymes
4. Acids like citric acid and lactic acid.

Sequence of events during bone resorption

1. Citric acid and lactic acid cause acidification of the area and decrease pH to 4
2. Lysosomal enzymes are activated at this pH
3. Activated enzymes digest or dissolve the collagen
4. Enzymes also dissolve the hydroxyapatite and form solution of bone salts
5. All the dissolved materials are now released into ECF
6. Some elements enter the blood
7. Remaining elements are cleaned up by the macrophages
8. A shallow cavity is formed in the bone resorbing compartment.

Bone Formation – Osteoblastic Activity

Osteoblastic activity is the process which involves the synthesis of collagen and formation of bone matrix that is mineralized. Osteoblasts are concerned with bone formation. Osteoblasts synthesize and release collagen into the shallow cavity formed after resorption in the bone resorbing compartment. The collagen fibers arrange themselves in regular units and form the organic matrix called osteoid.

Mineralization

Mineralization is the process by which the minerals are deposited on bone matrix. Mineralization starts about 10 to 12 days after the formation of osteoid. First, a large quantity of calcium phosphate is deposited. Afterwards, the hydroxide and bicarbonate ions are gradually added causing the formation of **hydroxyapatite crystals.** The process of mineralization is accelerated by the enzyme alkaline phosphatase, secreted by osteoblast. The process also requires the availability of adequate amount of calcium and phosphate in the ECF.

The completely mineralized bone surrounds the osteoblast. Now, the synthetic activity of osteoblast is reduced slowly and the cell is converted into osteocytes. Later, the bone is arranged in concentric lamellae on the inner surface of the cavity. At the end of the formation of new bone, the cavity is reduced to form Haversian canal.

Significance of Bone Remodeling

In children

1. Thickness of bone increases
2. Bone obtains strength in proportion to the growth

3. Shape of the bone is realtered in relation to growth of the body.

In adults

1. Toughness of bone is maintained
2. Mechanical integrity of skeleton is ensured throughout life
3. Blood calcium level is maintained.

Regulation of Bone Remodeling

Bone remodeling occurs continuously throughout the life. So a balance is maintained always between the bone resorption and bone formation.

However, in persons like athletes, soldiers and others, in whom the bone stress is more, the bone becomes heavy and strong. It is because of the stimulation of osteoblastic activity and mineralization of bone by repeated physical stress.

Apart from the physical stress, a variety of hormonal substances and growth factors are involved in regulation of bone resorption and bone formation (Table 68.1).

■ REPAIR OF BONE AFTER FRACTURE

The process of healing after bone fracture involves joining of broken ends by the deposition of new bone.

Stages of Bone Repair after Fracture

1. Formation of **hematoma** between the broken ends of bone and surrounding soft tissues. Hematoma means swelling or mass of blood clot confined to a tissue or space due to rupture of blood vessel
2. Development of acute inflammation
3. Phagocytosis of hematoma, debris and fragments of bone by macrophages
4. Formation of granular tissue and development of new blood vessels
5. Development of new osteoblasts and formation of new bone called callus
6. Spreading of new bone to fill the gap between the broken ends of bones
7. Reshaping of new bone by osteoclasts, which remove excess callus and formation of canal in the new bone.

■ APPLIED PHYSIOLOGY – DISEASES OF BONE

1. Osteoporosis

Osteoporosis is the bone disease characterized by the loss of bone matrix and minerals. Osteoporosis means **'porous bones'**.

TABLE 68.1: Factors regulating bone remodeling

Event	Stimulating factors	Inhibiting Factors
Bone formation	1. Growth hormone 2. Calcitonin 3. Insulin 4. Testosterone 5. Estrogen 6. Insulin-like growth factor 7. Transforming growth factor-β 8. Skeletal growth factor 9. Bone-derived growth factor 10. Platelet-derived growth factor	Cortisol
Mineralization	1. Calcitonin 2. Insulin 3. Vitamin D	Cortisol
Bone resorption	1. Parathormone 2. Thyroxine 3. Cortisol 4. Prostaglandins 5. Interleukin-1 6. Estrogen 7. Calcitonin	Testosterone

Causes of osteoporosis

Osteoporosis occurs due to excessive bone resorption and decreased bone formation. Osteoporosis is common in women after 60 years. The various risk factors are given in Box 68.1.

Manifestations of osteoporosis

Loss of bone matrix and minerals leads to loss of bone strength, associated with architectural deterioration of bone tissue. Ultimately, the bones become fragile with high risk of fracture. Commonly affected bones are vertebrae and hip.

2. Rickets

Rickets is the bone disease in children, characterized by inadequate mineralization of bone matrix. It occurs due to vitamin D deficiency. Vitamin D deficiency develops due to insufficiency in diet or due to inadequate exposure to sunlight.

BOX 68.1: Risk factors for osteoporosis

1. Sedentary life
2. Genetic factor
3. Early menopause or ovariectomy
4. Excessive smoking
5. Excessive alcohol or caffeine intake
6. Prolonged high intake of protein
7. Prolonged medication with drugs like corticosteroids and cyclosporin
8. Endocrine disorders like hypothyroidism, Cushing syndrome, acromegaly and hypogonadism.

Deficiency of vitamin D affects the reabsorption of calcium and phosphorus from renal tubules, resulting in **calcium deficiency.** It causes inadequate mineralization of epiphyseal growth plate in growing bones. This defect produces various manifestations.

Causes of rickets

Causes of rickets are given in Table 68.2.

Features of rickets

i. Collapse of chest wall: Due to the flattening of sides of thorax with prominent sternum. This deformity of the chest with projecting sternum is called **pigeon chest** or **chicken chest** or **pectus carinatum.**
ii. Rachitic rosary: A visible swelling where the ribs join their cartilages. It is because of the development of nodules at sternal end of ribs, which forms the rachitic rosary
iii. Kyphosis: Extreme forward curvature of the upper back bone (thoracic spine) with convexity backward (forward bending). Severe kyphosis

TABLE 68.2: Common causes of rickets and osteomalacia

Deficiency of vitamin D	Low dietary intake Inadequate synthesis in skin Reduced absorption from intestine
Renal diseases	Chronic renal failure Dialysis-induced bone disease Renal tubular acidosis.

causes formation of a hump (protuberance) which is called **humpback, hunchback** or **Pott curvature**

  iv. Lordosis: Extreme forward curvature of back bone in lumbar region: also called **hollow back** or **saddle back**

  v. Scoliosis: Lateral curvature of spine

  vi. Harrison sulcus: A groove in rib cage due to pulling of diaphragm inwards

  vii. Bowing of hands and legs

  viii. Enlargement of liver and spleen

  ix. Tetany: In advanced stages, the patient may die because of tetany, involving the respiratory muscles.

3. *Osteomalacia*

Rickets in adults is called **osteomalacia** or **adult rickets.**

Causes of osteomalacia

Osteomalacia occurs because of deficiency of vitamin D. It also occurs due to prolonged damage of kidney (renal rickets).

Features of osteomalacia

  i. Vague pain

  ii. Tenderness in bones and muscles

  iii. **Myopathy** leading to **waddling gait** (gait means the manner of walking). In waddling gait, the feet are wide apart and walk resembles that of a duck

  iv. Occasional hypoglycemic tetany.

Endocrine Functions of Pancreas

Chapter 69

- ■ ISLETS OF LANGERHANS
- ■ INSULIN
- ■ GLUCAGON
- ■ SOMATOSTATIN
- ■ PANCREATIC POLYPEPTIDE
- ■ REGULATION OF BLOOD GLUCOSE LEVEL
- ■ APPLIED PHYSIOLOGY

■ ISLETS OF LANGERHANS

Endocrine function of pancreas is performed by the islets of Langerhans. Human pancreas contains about 1 to 2 million islets.

Islets of Langerhans consist of four types of cells:
1. A cells or α-cells, which secrete glucagon
2. B cells or β-cells, which secrete insulin
3. D cells or δ-cells, which secrete somatostatin
4. F cells or PP cells, which secrete pancreatic polypeptide.

■ INSULIN

■ SOURCE OF SECRETION

Insulin is secreted by B cells or the β-cells in the islets of Langerhans of pancreas.

■ CHEMISTRY AND HALF-LIFE

Insulin is a polypeptide with 51 amino acids and a molecular weight of 5,808. It has two amino acid chains called α and β chains, which are linked by disulfide bridges. The α-chain of insulin contains 21 amino acids and β-chain contains 30 amino acids. The biological half-life of insulin is 5 minutes.

■ PLASMA LEVEL

Basal level of insulin in plasma is 10 μU/mL.

■ SYNTHESIS

Synthesis of insulin occurs in the rough endoplasmic reticulum of β-cells in islets of Langerhans. It is synthesized as **preproinsulin,** that gives rise to **proinsulin.** Proinsulin is converted into insulin and C peptide through a series of peptic cleavages. C peptide is a connecting peptide that connects α and β chains. At the time of secretion, C peptide is detached.

Preproinsulin → Proinsulin
Peptic cleavage ↓
Insulin

■ METABOLISM

Binding of insulin to insulin receptor is essential for its removal from circulation and degradation. Insulin is degraded in liver and kidney by a cellular enzyme called **insulin protease** or **insulin-degrading enzyme.**

■ ACTIONS OF INSULIN

Insulin is the important hormone that is concerned with the regulation of carbohydrate metabolism and blood glucose level. It is also concerned with the metabolism of proteins and fats.

1. *On Carbohydrate Metabolism*

Insulin is the only antidiabetic hormone secreted in the body, i.e. it is the only hormone in the body that reduces blood glucose level. Insulin reduces the blood glucose level by its following actions on carbohydrate metabolism:

i. *Increases transport and uptake of glucose by the cells*

Insulin facilitates the transport of glucose from blood into the cells by increasing the permeability of cell membrane to glucose. Insulin stimulates the rapid uptake of glucose by all the tissues, particularly liver, muscle and adipose tissues. But, it is not required for glucose uptake in some tissues such as brain (except hypothalamus), renal tubules, mucous membrane of intestine and RBCs. Insulin also increases the number of glucose transporters, especially GLUT 4 in the cell membrane. *Glucose transporters:* Usually, glucose is transported into the cells by **sodium-glucose symport pump.** In addition to symport pump, most of the cells have another type of transport proteins called **glucose transporters (GLUT).** So far, seven types of GLUT are identified (GLUT 1–7). Among these, **GLUT4** is insulin sensitive and it is located in cytoplasmic vesicles. It is present in large numbers in muscle fibers and adipose cells.

When insulin-receptor complex is formed in the membrane of such cells, the vesicles containing GLUT4 are attracted towards the membrane and GLUT4 is released into the membrane. Now, GLUT4 starts transporting the glucose molecules from extracellular fluid (ECF) into the cell. The advantage of GLUT4 is that it transports glucose at a faster rate.

ii. *Promotes peripheral utilization of glucose*

Insulin promotes the peripheral utilization of glucose. In presence of insulin, glucose which enters the cell is oxidized immediately. The rate of utilization depends upon the intake of glucose.

iii. *Promotes storage of glucose – glycogenesis*

Insulin promotes the rapid conversion of glucose into glycogen (glycogenesis), which is stored in the muscle and liver. Thus, glucose is stored in these two organs in the form of glycogen. Insulin activates the enzymes which are necessary for glycogenesis. In liver, when glycogen content increases beyond its storing capacity, insulin causes conversion of glucose into fatty acids.

iv. *Inhibits glycogenolysis*

Insulin prevents glycogenolysis, i.e. the breakdown of glycogen into glucose in muscle and liver.

v. *Inhibits gluconeogenesis*

Insulin prevents gluconeogenesis, i.e. the formation of glucose from proteins by inhibiting the release of amino acids from muscle and by inhibiting the activities of enzymes involved in gluconeogenesis.

Thus, insulin decreases the blood glucose level by:
  i. Facilitating transport and uptake of glucose by the cells
  ii. Increasing the peripheral utilization of glucose
  iii. Increasing the storage of glucose by converting it into glycogen in liver and muscle
  iv. Inhibiting glycogenolysis
  v. Inhibiting gluconeogenesis.

2. *On Protein Metabolism*

Insulin facilitates the synthesis and storage of proteins and inhibits the cellular utilization of proteins by the following actions:
  i. Facilitating the transport of amino acids into the cell from blood, by increasing the permeability of cell membrane for amino acids
  ii. Accelerating protein synthesis by influencing the transcription of DNA and by increasing the translation of mRNA
  iii. Preventing protein catabolism by decreasing the activity of cellular enzymes which act on proteins
  iv. Preventing conversion of proteins into glucose.

Thus, insulin is responsible for the conservation and storage of proteins in the body.

3. *On Fat Metabolism*

Insulin stimulates the synthesis of fat. It also increases the storage of fat in the adipose tissue.

Actions of insulin on fat metabolism are:

i. *Synthesis of fatty acids and triglycerides*

Insulin promotes the transport of excess glucose into cells, particularly the liver cells. This glucose is utilized for the synthesis of fatty acids and triglycerides. Insulin promotes the synthesis of lipids by activating the enzymes which convert:
  a. Glucose into fatty acids
  b. Fatty acids into triglycerides.

ii. *Transport of fatty acids into adipose tissue*

Insulin facilitates the transport of fatty acids into the adipose tissue.

iii. *Storage of fat*

Insulin promotes the storage of fat in adipose tissue by inhibiting the enzymes which degrade the triglycerides.

4. *On Growth*

Along with growth hormone, insulin promotes growth of body by its anabolic action on proteins. It enhances the transport of amino acids into the cell and synthesis of proteins in the cells. It also has the **protein-sparing effect,** i.e. it causes conservation of proteins by increasing the glucose utilization by the tissues.

Houssay Animal

The importance of insulin and growth hormone in the growth of the body is demonstrated by Houssay animal. Houssay animal is one in which both anterior pituitary and pancreas are removed. Administration of either insulin or growth hormone alone does not induce growth in this animal. However, the administration of both the hormones stimulates the growth. This proves the synergistic actions of these two hormones on growth.

■ MODE OF ACTION OF INSULIN

On the target cells, insulin binds with the receptor protein and forms the insulin-receptor complex. This complex executes the action by activating the intracellular enzyme system.

Insulin Receptor

Insulin receptor is a glycoprotein with a molecular weight of 340,000. It is present in almost all the cells of the body.

Subunits of insulin receptor

Insulin receptor is a **tetramer,** formed by four glycoprotein subunits (two α-subunits and two β-subunits). The α-subunits protrude out of the cell and the β-subunits protrude inside the cell (Fig. 69.1). The α and β subunits are linked to each other by disulfide bonds. Intracellular surfaces of α-subunits have the enzyme activity – **protein kinase (tyrosine kinase)** activity.

When insulin binds with α-subunits of the receptor protein, the tyrosine kinase at the β-subunit (that protrudes into the cell) is activated by means of autophosphorylation.

Activated tyrosine kinase acts on many intracellular enzymes by phosphorylating or dephosphorylating them so that some of the enzymes are activated while others are inactivated.

Thus, insulin action is exerted on the target cells by the activation of some intracellular enzymes and by the inactivation of other enzymes.

■ REGULATION OF INSULIN SECRETION

Insulin secretion is mainly regulated by blood glucose level.

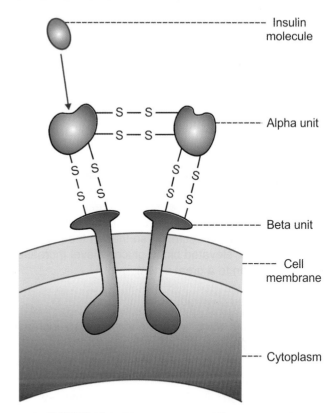

FIGURE 69.1: Diagram showing the structure of insulin receptor. S–S = Disulfide bond.

In addition, other factors like amino acids, lipid derivatives, gastrointestinal and endocrine hormones and autonomic nerve fibers also stimulate insulin secretion.

1. Role of Blood Glucose Level

When blood glucose level is normal (80 to 100 mg/dL), the rate of insulin secretion is low (up to 10 µU/minute). When blood glucose level increases between 100 and 120 mg/dL, the rate of insulin secretion rises rapidly to 100 µU/minute. When blood glucose level rises above 200 mg/dL, the rate of insulin secretion also rises very rapidly up to 400 µU/minute.

Biphasic effect of glucose

Action of blood glucose on insulin secretion is biphasic.
   i. Initially, when blood glucose level increases after a meal, the release of insulin into blood increases rapidly. Within few minutes, concentration of insulin in plasma increases up to 100 µU/mL from the basal level of 10 µU/mL. It is because of release of insulin that is stored in pancreas. Later, within 10 to 15 minutes, the insulin concentration in the blood reduces to half the value, i.e. up to 40 to 50 µU/mL of plasma.

ii. After 15 to 20 minutes, the insulin secretion rises once again. This time it rises slowly but steadily. It reaches the maximum between 2 and 2½ hours. The prolonged increase in insulin release is due to the formation of new insulin molecules continuously from pancreas (Fig. 69.2).

2. *Role of Proteins*

Excess amino acids in blood also stimulate insulin secretion. Potent amino acids are **arginine** and **lysin.** Without any increase in blood glucose level, the amino acids alone can cause a slight increase in insulin secretion. However, amino acids potentiate the action of glucose on insulin secretion so that, in the presence of amino acids, elevated blood glucose level increases insulin secretion to a great extent.

3. *Role of Lipid Derivatives*

The β-ketoacids such as acetoacetate also increase insulin secretion.

4. *Role of Gastrointestinal Hormones*

Insulin secretion is increased by some of the gastrointestinal hormones such as gastrin, secretin, CCK and GIP.

5. *Role of Endocrine Hormones*

Diabetogenic hormones like glucagon, growth hormone and cortisol also stimulate insulin secretion, indirectly.

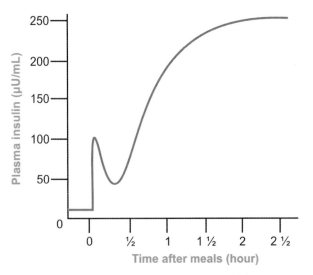

FIGURE 69.2: Changes in plasma level of insulin after meals. Increase in blood glucose level after meals produces biphasic effect on plasma level of insulin.

All these diabetogenic hormones increase the blood glucose level, which stimulates β-cells of islets of Langerhans. So insulin secretion is increased.

Prolonged hypersecretion of these hormones causes exhaustion of β-cells, resulting in diabetes mellitus.

6. *Role of Autonomic Nerves*

Stimulation of parasympathetic nerve to the pancreas (right vagus) increases insulin secretion. Chemical neurotransmitter involved is acetylcholine. Stimulation of sympathetic nerves inhibits the secretion of insulin and the neurotransmitter is noradrenaline.

However, the role of these nerves on the regulation of insulin secretion under physiological conditions is not clear.

■ GLUCAGON

■ SOURCE OF SECRETION

Glucagon is secreted from **A cells** or **α-cells** in the islets of Langerhans of pancreas. It is also secreted from **A cells** of stomach and **L cells** of intestine.

■ CHEMISTRY AND HALF-LIFE

Glucagon is a polypeptide with a molecular weight of 3,485. It contains 29 amino acids. Half-life of glucagon is 3 to 6 minutes.

■ SYNTHESIS

Glucagon is synthesized from the preprohormone precursor called **preproglucagon** in the α-cells of islets. Preproglucagon is converted into **proglucagon,** which gives rise to glucagon.

■ METABOLISM

About 30% of glucagon is degraded in liver and 20% in kidney. The cleaved glucagon fragments are excreted through urine. 50% of the circulating glucagon is degraded in blood itself by enzymes such as **serine** and **cysteine proteases.**

■ ACTIONS OF GLUCAGON

Actions of glucagon are antagonistic to those of insulin (Table 69.1). It increases the blood glucose level, peripheral utilization of lipids and the conversion of proteins into glucose.

1. *On Carbohydrate Metabolism*

Glucagon increases the blood glucose level by:
  i. Increasing glycogenolysis in liver and releasing glucose from the liver cells into the blood.

TABLE 69.1: Differences between insulin and glucagon

Features	Insulin	Glucagon
Source of secretion	β-cells of islets of langerhans	α-cells of islets of langerhans
Action on carbohydrate metabolism	*Decreases blood glucose level by:* 1. Facilitating transport and uptake of glucose by all cells except liver cells 2. Increasing peripheral utilization of glucose 3. Increasing glycogenesis in liver and muscle 4. Preventing glycogenolysis 5. Preventing gluconeogenesis	*Increases blood glucose level by:* 1. Facilitating glucose transport into liver cells 2. Increasing glycogenolysis 3. Increasing gluconeogenesis
Action on protein metabolism	1. Facilitates amino acid transport 2. Accelerates protein synthesis 3. Prevents protein catabolism 4. Prevents conversion of proteins into glucose	1. Increases transport of amino acids into liver cells 2. Increases utilization of amino acids for gluconeogenesis
Action on fat metabolism	1. Increases synthesis and storage of fat 2. No ketogenic effect	1. Increases lipolysis 2. Promotes ketogenesis
Blood fatty acids	Decreases	Increases
Hypersecretion leads to	Hypoglycemia	Hyperglycemia
Hyposecretion leads to	Diabetes mellitus	Hypoglycemia

Glucagon does not induce glycogenolysis in muscle

ii. Increasing gluconeogenesis in liver by:
 a. Activating the enzymes, which convert pyruvate into phosphoenol pyruvate
 b. Increasing the transport of amino acids into the liver cells. The amino acids are utilized for glucose formation.

2. On Protein Metabolism

Glucagon increases the transport of amino acids into liver cells. The amino acids are utilized for gluconeogenesis.

3. On Fat Metabolism

Glucagon shows lipolytic and ketogenic actions. It increases lipolysis by increasing the release of free fatty acids from adipose tissue and making them available for peripheral utilization. The lipolytic activity of glucagon, in turn promotes ketogenesis (formation of ketone bodies) in liver.

4. Other Actions

Glucagon:
 i. Inhibits the secretion of gastric juice
 ii. Increases the secretion of bile from liver.

■ MODE OF ACTION OF GLUCAGON

On the target cells (mostly liver cells), glucagon combines with receptor and activates adenyl cyclase via G protein. Adenyl cyclase causes the formation of cyclic adenosine monophosphate (AMP) which brings out the actions of glucagon. Glucagon receptor is a peptide with a molecular weight of 62,000.

■ REGULATION OF GLUCAGON SECRETION

Secretion of glucagon is controlled mainly by glucose and amino acid levels in the blood.

1. Role of Blood Glucose Level

Important factor that regulates the secretion of glucagon is the decrease in blood glucose level. When blood glucose level decreases below 80 mg/dL of blood, α-cells of islets of Langerhans are stimulated and more glucagon is released. Glucagon, in turn increases the blood glucose level. On the other hand, when blood glucose level increases, α-cells are inhibited and the secretion of glucagon decreases.

2. Role of Amino Acid Level in Blood

Increase in amino acid level in blood stimulates the secretion of glucagon. Glucagon, in turn converts the amino acids into glucose.

3. Role of Other Factors

Factors which increase glucagon secretion:
 i. Exercise
 ii. Stress
 iii. Gastrin

   iv. Cholecystokinin (CCK)
   v. Cortisol.

Factors which inhibit glucagon secretion:

   i. Somatostatin
   ii. Insulin
   iii. Free fatty acids
   iv. Ketones.

■ SOMATOSTATIN

■ SOURCE OF SECRETION

Somatostatin is secreted from:
1. Hypothalamus
2. D cells (δ-cells) in islets of Langerhans of pancreas
3. D cells in stomach and upper part of small intestine.

■ CHEMISTRY AND HALF-LIFE

Somatostatin is a polypeptide. It is synthesized in two forms, namely somatostatin-14 (with 14 amino acids) and somatostatin-28 (with 28 amino acids). Both the forms have similar actions. Half-life of somatostatin is 2 to 4 minutes.

■ SYNTHESIS

Somatostatin is synthesized from the precursor prosomatostatin. Prosomatostatin is converted mostly into somatostatin-14 in the D cells of islets in pancreas. However, in the intestine, large amount of somatostatin-28 is produced from prosomatostatin.

■ METABOLISM

Somatostatin is degraded in liver and kidney.

■ ACTIONS OF SOMATOSTATIN

1. Somatostatin acts within islets of Langerhans and, inhibits β and α cells, i.e. it inhibits the secretion of both glucagon and insulin
2. It decreases the motility of stomach, duodenum and gallbladder
3. It reduces the secretion of gastrointestinal hormones gastrin, CCK, GIP and VIP
4. Hypothalamic somatostatin inhibits the secretion of GH and TSH from anterior pituitary. That is why, it is also called **growth hormone-inhibitory hormone** (GHIH).

■ MODE OF ACTION OF SOMATOSTATIN

Somatostatin brings out its actions through cAMP.

■ REGULATION OF SECRETION OF SOMATOSTATIN

Pancreatic Somatostatin

Secretion of pancreatic somatostatin is stimulated by glucose, amino acids and CCK. The tumor of D cells of islets of Langerhans causes hypersecretion of somatostatin. It leads to hyperglycemia and other symptoms of diabetes mellitus.

Gastrointestinal Tract Somatostatin

Secretion of somatostatin in GI tract is increased by the presence of chyme-containing glucose and proteins in stomach and small intestine.

■ PANCREATIC POLYPEPTIDE

■ SOURCE OF SECRETION

Pancreatic polypeptide is secreted by F cells or PP cells in the islets of Langerhans of pancreas. It is also found in small intestine.

■ CHEMISTRY AND HALF-LIFE

Pancreatic polypeptide is a polypeptide with 36 amino acids. Its half-life is 5 minutes.

■ SYNTHESIS

Pancreatic polypeptide is synthesized from pre-prohormone precursor called **prepropancreatic** polypeptide in the PP cells of islets.

■ METABOLISM

Pancreatic polypeptide is degraded and removed from circulation mainly in kidney.

■ ACTIONS OF PANCREATIC POLYPEPTIDE

Exact physiological action of pancreatic polypeptide is not known. It is believed to increase the secretion of glucagon from α-cells in islets of Langerhans.

■ MODE OF ACTION OF PANCREATIC POLYPEPTIDE

Pancreatic polypeptide brings out its actions through cAMP.

■ REGULATION OF SECRETION

Secretion of pancreatic polypeptide is stimulated by the presence of chyme containing more proteins in the small intestine.

■ REGULATION OF BLOOD GLUCOSE LEVEL (BLOOD GLUCOSE LEVEL)

■ NORMAL BLOOD GLUCOSE LEVEL

In normal persons, blood glucose level is controlled within a narrow range. In the early morning after overnight **fasting,** the blood glucose level is low ranging between 70 and 110 mg/dL of blood. Between first and second hour after meals **(postprandial),** the blood glucose level rises to 100 to 140 mg/dL. Glucose level in blood is brought back to normal at the end of second hour after the meals.

Blood glucose regulating mechanism is operated through liver and muscle by the influence of the pancreatic hormones – insulin and glucagon. Many other hormones are also involved in the regulation of blood glucose level. Among all the hormones, insulin is the only hormone that reduces the blood glucose level and it is called the **antidiabetogenic hormone.** The hormones which increase blood glucose level are called **diabetogenic hormones** or **anti-insulin hormones.**

Necessity of Regulation of Blood Glucose Level

Regulation of blood glucose (sugar) level is very essential because, glucose is the only nutrient that is utilized for energy by many tissues such as brain tissues, retina and germinal epithelium of the gonads.

■ ROLE OF LIVER IN THE MAINTENANCE OF BLOOD GLUCOSE LEVEL

Liver serves as an important **glucose buffer system.** When blood glucose level increases after a meal, the excess glucose is converted into glycogen and stored in liver. Afterwards, when blood glucose level falls, the glycogen in liver is converted into glucose and released into the blood. The storage of glycogen and release of glucose from liver are mainly regulated by insulin and glucagon.

■ ROLE OF INSULIN IN THE MAINTENANCE OF BLOOD GLUCOSE LEVEL

Insulin decreases the blood glucose level and it is the only antidiabetic hormone available in the body (Refer the actions of insulin on carbohydrate metabolism in this Chapter).

■ ROLE OF GLUCAGON IN THE MAINTENANCE OF BLOOD GLUCOSE LEVEL

Glucagon increases the blood glucose level (Refer actions of glucagon on carbohydrate metabolism in this Chapter).

■ ROLE OF OTHER HORMONES IN THE MAINTENANCE OF BLOOD GLUCOSE LEVEL

Other hormones which increase the blood glucose level are:
1. Growth hormone (Chapter 66)
2. Thyroxine (Chapter 67)
3. Cortisol (Chapter 70)
4. Adrenaline (Chapter 71).

Thus, liver helps to maintain the blood glucose level by storing glycogen when blood glucose level is high after meals; and by releasing glucose, when blood glucose level is low after 2 to 3 hours of food intake. Insulin helps to control the blood glucose level, especially after meals, when it increases. Glucagon and other hormones help to maintain the blood glucose level by raising it in between the meals.

■ APPLIED PHYSIOLOGY

■ HYPOACTIVITY – DIABETES MELLITUS

Diabetes mellitus is a metabolic disorder characterized by high blood glucose level, associated with other manifestations. **'Diabetes'** means **'polyuria'** and **'mellitus'** means **'honey'.** The name 'diabetes mellitus' was coined by Thomas Willis, who discovered sweetness of urine from diabetics in 1675.

In most of the cases, diabetes mellitus develops due to deficiency of insulin.

Classification of Diabetes Mellitus

There are several forms of diabetes mellitus, which occur due to different causes. Diabetes may be primary or secondary. Primary diabetes is unrelated to another disease. Secondary diabetes occurs due to damage or disease of pancreas by another disease or factor.

Recent classification divides primary diabetes mellitus into two types, Type I and Type II. Differences between the two types are given in Table 69.2.

Type I Diabetes Mellitus

Type I diabetes mellitus is due to deficiency of insulin because of destruction of β-cells in islets of Langerhans. This type of diabetes mellitus may occur at any age of life. But, it usually occurs before 40 years of age and the persons affected by this require insulin injection. So it is also called **insulin-dependent diabetes mellitus (IDDM).** When it develops at infancy or childhood, it is called juvenile diabetes.

Type I diabetes mellitus develops rapidly and progresses at a rapid phase. It is not associated with **obesity,** but may be associated with **acidosis** or ketosis.

Causes of type I diabetes mellitus

1. Degeneration of β-cells in the islets of Langerhans of pancreas
2. Destruction of β-cells by viral infection
3. Congenital disorder of β-cells
4. Destruction of β-cells during autoimmune diseases. It is due to the development of antibodies against β-cells (Refer Chapter 17 for details).

Other forms of type 1 diabetes mellitus

1. **Latent autoimmune diabetes in adults (LADA):** LADA or slow onset diabetes has slow onset and slow progress than IDDM and it occurs in later life after 35 years. It may be difficult to distinguish LADA from type II diabetes mellitus, since pancreas takes longer period to stop secreting insulin.
2. **Maturity onset diabetes** in young individuals **(MODY):** It is a rare inherited form of diabetes mellitus that occurs before 25 years. It is due to hereditary defects in insulin secretion.

Type II Diabetes Mellitus

Type II diabetes mellitus is due to insulin resistance (failure of insulin receptors to give response to insulin). So, the body is unable to use insulin. About 90% of diabetic patients have type II diabetes mellitus. It usually occurs after 40 years. Only some forms of Type II diabetes require insulin. In most cases, it can be controlled by oral hypoglycemic drugs. So it is also called **noninsulin-dependent diabetes mellitus (NIDDM).**

Type II diabetes mellitus may or may not be associated with ketosis, but often it is associated with obesity.

Causes for type II diabetes mellitus

In this type of diabetes, the structure and function of β-cells and blood level of insulin are normal. But insulin receptors may be less, absent or abnormal, resulting in insulin resistance.

Common causes of insulin resistance are:

1. Genetic disorders (significant factors causing type II diabetes mellitus)
2. Lifestyle changes such as bad eating habits and physical inactivity, leading to obesity
3. Stress.

Other forms of type II diabetes mellitus

1. Gestational diabetes: It occurs during pregnancy. It is due to many factors such as hormones secreted during pregnancy, obesity and lifestyle before and during pregnancy. Usually, diabetes disappears after delivery of the child. However, the woman has high risk of development of type II diabetes later.
2. **Pre-diabetes:** It is also called **chemical, subclinical, latent** or **borderline diabetes.** It is the stage between normal condition and diabetes. The person does not show overt (observable) symptoms of diabetes but there is an increase in blood glucose level. Though pre-diabetes is reversible, the affected persons are at a high risk of developing type II diabetes mellitus.

TABLE 69.2: Differences between type I and type II diabetes mellitus

Features	Type I (IDDM)	Type II (NIDDM)
Age of onset	Usually before 40 year	Usually after 40 year
Major cause	Lack of insulin	Lack of insulin receptor
Insulin deficiency	Yes	Partial deficiency
Immune destruction of β-cells	Yes	No
Involvement of other endocrine disorders	No	Yes
Hereditary cause	Yes	May or may not be
Need for insulin	Always	Not in initial stage May require in later stage
Insulin resistance	No	Yes
Control by oral hypoglycemic agents	No	Yes
Symptoms appear	Rapidly	Slowly
Body weight	Usually thin	Usually overweight
Stress-induced obesity	No	Yes
Ketosis	Yes	May or may not be

Secondary Diabetes Mellitus

Secondary diabetes mellitus is rare and only about 2% of diabetic patients have secondary diabetes. It may be temporary or may become permanent due to the underlying cause.

Causes of secondary diabetes mellitus

1. Endocrine disorders such as gigantism, acromegaly and Cushing's syndrome.
   Hyperglycemia in these conditions causes excess stimulation of β-cells. Constant and excess stimulation, in turn causes burning out and degeneration of β-cells. The β-cell exhaustion leads to permanent diabetes mellitus.
2. Damage of pancreas due to disorders such as chronic pancreatitis, cystic fibrosis and hemochromatosis (high iron content in body causing damage of organs)
3. Pancreatectomy (surgical removal)
4. Liver diseases such as hepatitis C and fatty liver
5. Autoimmune diseases such as celiac disease
6. Excessive use of drugs like antihypertensive drugs (beta blockers and diuretics), steroids, oral contraceptives, chemotherapy drugs, etc.
7. Excessive intake of alcohol and opiates.

Signs and Symptoms of Diabetes Mellitus

Various manifestations of diabetes mellitus develop because of three major setbacks of insulin deficiency.
1. Increased blood glucose level (300 to 400 mg/dL) due to reduced utilization by tissue
2. Mobilization of fats from adipose tissue for energy purpose, leading to elevated fatty acid content in blood. This causes deposition of fat on the wall of arteries and development of atherosclerosis
3. Depletion of proteins from the tissues.
   Following are the signs and symptoms of diabetes mellitus:

1. Glucosuria

Glucosuria is the loss of glucose in urine. Normally, glucose does not appear in urine. When glucose level rises above 180 mg/dL in blood, glucose appears in urine. It is the renal threshold level for glucose.

2. Osmotic diuresis

Osmotic diuresis is the diuresis caused by osmotic effects. Excess glucose in the renal tubules develops osmotic effect. Osmotic effect decreases the reabsorption of water from renal tubules, resulting in diuresis. It leads to polyuria and polydipsia.

3. Polyuria

Excess urine formation with increase in the frequency of voiding urine is called polyuria. It is due to the osmotic diuresis caused by increase in blood glucose level.

4. Polydipsia

Increase in water intake is called polydipsia. Excess loss of water decreases the water content and increases the salt content in the body. This stimulates the thirst center in hypothalamus. Thirst center, in turn increases the intake of water.

5. Polyphagia

Polyphagia means the intake of excess food. It is very common in diabetes mellitus.

6. Asthenia

Loss of strength is called asthenia. Body becomes very weak because of this. Asthenia occurs due to protein depletion, which is caused by lack of insulin. Lack of insulin causes decrease in protein synthesis and increase in protein breakdown, resulting in protein depletion. Protein depletion also occurs due to the utilization of proteins for energy in the absence of glucose utilization.

7. Acidosis

During insulin deficiency, glucose cannot be utilized by the peripheral tissues for energy. So, a large amount of fat is broken down to release energy. It causes the formation of excess **ketoacids,** leading to acidosis.

One more reason for acidosis is that the ketoacids are excreted in combination with sodium ions through urine **(ketonuria).** Sodium is exchanged for hydrogen ions, which diffuse from the renal tubules into ECF adding to acidosis.

8. Acetone breathing

In cases of severe ketoacidosis, acetone is expired in the expiratory air, giving the characteristic acetone or fruity breath odor. It is a **life-threatening** condition of severe diabetes.

9. Kussmaul breathing

Kussmaul breathing is the increase in rate and depth of respiration caused by severe acidosis.

10. Circulatory shock

Osmotic diuresis leads to dehydration, which causes circulatory shock. It occurs only in severe diabetes.

11. Coma

Due to Kussmaul breathing, large amount of carbon dioxide is lost during expiration. It leads to drastic reduction in the concentration of bicarbonate ions causing severe acidosis and coma. It occurs in severe cases of diabetes mellitus.

Increase in the blood glucose level develops hyperosmolarity of plasma which also leads to coma. It is called **hyperosmolar coma.**

Complications of Diabetes Mellitus

Prolonged hyperglycemia in diabetes mellitus causes dysfunction and injury of many tissues, resulting in some complications. Development of these complications is directly proportional to the degree and duration of hyperglycemia. However, the patients with well-controlled diabetes can postpone the onset or reduce the rate of progression of these complications.

Initially, the untreated chronic hyperglycemia affects the blood vessels, resulting in vascular complications like atherosclerosis. Vascular complications are responsible for the development of most of the complications of diabetes such as:
1. Cardiovascular complications like:
   i.   Hypertension
   ii. Myocardial infarction
2. Degenerative changes in retina called diabetic retinopathy
3. Degenerative changes in kidney known as diabetic nephropathy
4. Degeneration of autonomic and peripheral nerves called diabetic neuropathy.

Diagnostic Tests for Diabetes Mellitus

Diagnosis of diabetes mellitus includes the determination of:
1. Fasting blood glucose
2. Postprandial blood glucose
3. Glucose tolerance test (GTT)
4. Glycosylated (glycated) hemoglobin.

Determination of glycosylated hemoglobin is commonly done to monitor the glycemic control of the persons already diagnosed with diabetes mellitus.

Abnormal response in diagnostic tests

Abnormal response in diagnostic tests occurs in conditions like **pre-diabetes** (see above). There is an increased fasting blood glucose level or impaired (decreased) glucose tolerance.

Treatment for Diabetes Mellitus

Type I diabetes mellitus

Type I diabetes mellitus is treated by exogenous insulin. Since insulin is a polypeptide, it is degraded in GI tract if taken orally. So, it is generally administered by subcutaneous injection.

Type II diabetes mellitus

Type II diabetes mellitus is treated by oral hypoglycemic drugs. Patients with longstanding severe diabetes mellitus may require a combination of oral hypoglycemic drugs with insulin to control the hyperglycemia.

Oral hypoglycemic drugs are classified into three types.
1. *Insulin secretagogues:* These drugs decrease the blood glucose level by stimulating insulin secretion from β-cells. Sulfonylureas (tolbutamide, gluburide, glipizide, etc.) are the commonly available insulin secretagogues
2. *Insulin sensitizers:* These drugs decrease the blood glucose level by facilitating the insulin action in the target tissues. Examples are biguanides (metformin) and thiazolidinediones (pioglitazone and rosiglitazone)
3. *Alpha glucosidase inhibitors:* These drugs control blood glucose level by inhibiting α-glucosidase. This intestinal enzyme is responsible for the conversion of dietary and other complex carbohydrates into glucose and other monosaccharides, which can be absorbed from intestine. Examples of α-glucosidase inhibitors are acarbose and meglitol.

■ HYPERACTIVITY – HYPERINSULINISM

Hyperinsulinism is the hypersecretion of insulin.

Cause of Hyperinsulinism

Hyperinsulinism occurs due to the tumor of β-cells in the islets of Langerhans.

Signs and Symptoms of Hyperinsulinism

1. *Hypoglycemia*

Blood glucose level falls below 50 mg/dL.

2. *Manifestations of central nervous system*

Manifestations of central nervous system occur when the blood glucose level decreases. All the manifestations are together called **neuroglycopenic symptoms.**

Initially, the activity of neurons increases, resulting in nervousness, tremor all over the body and sweating. If not treated immediately, it leads to **clonic convulsions** and **unconsciousness.** Slowly, the convulsions cease and **coma** occurs due to the damage of neurons.

Adrenal Cortex

- ■ IMPORTANCE OF ADRENAL GLANDS
- ■ FUNCTIONAL ANATOMY
- ■ HISTOLOGY OF ADRENAL CORTEX
- ■ HORMONES
- ■ SYNTHESIS, TRANSPORT AND FATE OF ADRENOCORTICAL HORMONES
- ■ MINERALOCORTICOIDS
- ■ GLUCOCORTICOIDS
- ■ ADRENAL SEX HORMONES
- ■ EXOGENOUS STEROIDS
- ■ APPLIED PHYSIOLOGY

■ IMPORTANCE OF ADRENAL GLANDS

Adrenal glands are called the **'life-saving glands'** or **'essential endocrine glands'.** It is because the absence of adrenocortical hormones causes death within 3 to 15 days and absence of adrenomedullary hormones, drastically decreases the resistance to mental and physical stress.

■ FUNCTIONAL ANATOMY OF ADRENAL GLANDS

There are two adrenal glands. Each gland is situated on the upper pole of each kidney. Because of the situation, adrenal glands are otherwise called **suprarenal glands.** Each gland weighs about 4 g.

■ PARTS OF ADRENAL GLAND

Adrenal gland (Fig. 70.1) is made of two distinct parts:
1. **Adrenal cortex:** Outer portion, constituting 80% of the gland
2. **Adrenal medulla:** Central portion, constituting 20% of the gland.
   These two parts are different from each other in development, structure and functions. Adrenal medulla develops from the neural crest, which gives origin to sympathetic nervous system. So, its secretions and

functions resemble that of sympathetic nervous system. Adrenal cortex develops from the **mesonephros,** which give rise to the renal tissues. It secretes entirely a different group of hormones known as **corticosteroids.**

■ HISTOLOGY OF ADRENAL CORTEX

Adrenal cortex is formed by three layers of structure. Each layer is distinct from one another.
1. Outer zona glomerulosa
2. Middle zona fasciculata
3. Inner zona reticularis.

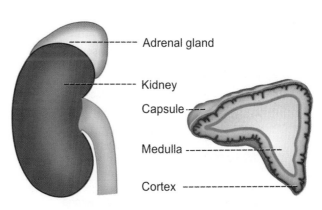

FIGURE 70.1: Adrenal gland

■ HORMONES OF ADRENAL CORTEX

Adrenocortical hormones are steroids in nature, hence the name **'corticosteroids'.** Based on their functions, corticosteroids are classified into three groups:
1. Mineralocorticoids
2. Glucocorticoids
3. Sex hormones.

■ SYNTHESIS, TRANSPORT AND FATE OF ADRENOCORTICAL HORMONES

■ SYNTHESIS

All adrenocortical hormones are steroid in nature and are synthesized mainly from cholesterol that is absorbed directly from the circulating blood. Small quantity of cholesterol is also synthesized within the cortical cells from acetylcoenzyme A (acetyl-CoA). Synthesis of aldosterone is given in Fig. 70.2.

■ TRANSPORT

Mineralocorticoids

Mineralocorticoids are transported in blood by binding with plasma proteins, especially globulins. The binding is loose and 50% of these hormones are present in free form.

Glucocorticoids

Glucocorticoids are transported by a special plasma protein known as **glucocorticoids-binding globulin** or **transcortin.** Ninety four percent of glucocorticoids are transported by this protein, whereas about 6% of them

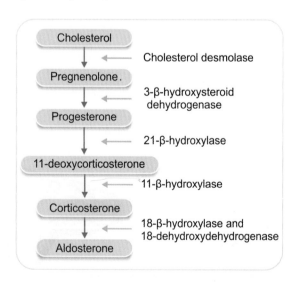

FIGURE 70.2: Synthesis of aldosterone

are found free in plasma. Albumin plays a very little role in glucocorticoid transport.

Sex Hormones

Adrenal sex hormones are transported by another special plasma protein known as **sex hormone-binding globulin.**

■ FATE OF CORTICOSTEROIDS

Corticosteroids are degraded mainly in the liver and conjugated to form glucuronides and to a lesser extent, form sulfates. About 25% of corticosteroids are excreted in bile and feces and remaining 75%, in the urine.

■ MINERALOCORTICOIDS

Mineralocorticoids are the corticosteroids that act on the minerals (electrolytes), particularly sodium and potassium.
  Mineralocorticoids are:
1. Aldosterone
2. 11-deoxycorticosterone.

■ SOURCE OF SECRETION

Mineralocorticoids are secreted by zona glomerulosa of adrenal cortex.

■ CHEMISTRY AND HALF-LIFE

Mineralocorticoids are C_{21} steroids having 21 carbon atoms. Half-life of mineralocorticoids is 20 minutes.

■ DAILY OUTPUT AND PLASMA LEVEL

Daily output and plasma level of mineralocorticoids are given in Table 70.1.

■ FUNCTIONS OF MINERALOCORTICOIDS

Ninety percent of mineralocorticoid activity is provided by aldosterone.

Life-saving Hormone

Aldosterone is very essential for life and it maintains the osmolarity and volume of ECF. It is usually called

TABLE 70.1: Daily output and plasma level of mineralocorticoids

Hormone	Daily output (µg)	Plasma level (µg/dL)
Aldosterone	0.15	0.006
11-Deoxycorticosterone	0.2	0.006

life-saving hormone because, its absence causes death within 3 days to 2 weeks. Aldosterone has three important functions.

It increases:
1. Reabsorption of sodium from renal tubules
2. Excretion of potassium through renal tubules
3. Secretion of hydrogen into renal tubules.
Actions of aldosterone are:

1. On Sodium Ions

Aldosterone acts on the distal convoluted tubule and the collecting duct and increases the reabsorption of sodium. During hypersecretion of aldosterone, the loss of sodium through urine is only few milligram per day. But during hyposecretion of aldosterone, the loss of sodium through urine increases **(hypernatriuria)** up to about 20 g/day. It proves the importance of aldosterone in regulation of sodium ion concentration and osmolality in the body.

2. On Extracellular Fluid Volume

When sodium ions are reabsorbed from the renal tubules, simultaneously water is also reabsorbed. Water reabsorption is almost equal to sodium reabsorption; so the net result is the increase in ECF volume.

Even though aldosterone increases the sodium reabsorption from renal tubules, the concentration of sodium in the body does not increase very much because water is also reabsorbed simultaneously.

But still, there is a possibility for mild increase in concentration of sodium in blood (mild hypernatremia). It induces thirst, leading to intake of water which again increases the ECF volume and blood volume.

3. On Blood Pressure

Increase in ECF volume and the blood volume finally leads to increase in blood pressure.

Aldosterone escape or escape phenomenon

Aldosterone escape refers to escape of the kidney from **salt-retaining effects** of excess administration or secretion of aldosterone, as in the case of primary hyperaldosteronism.

Mechanism of aldosterone escape

When aldosterone level increases, there is excess retention of sodium and water. This increases the volume of ECF and blood pressure. **Aldosterone-induced** high blood pressure decreases the ECF volume through two types of reactions:
  i. It stimulates secretion of **atrial natriuretic peptide** (ANP) from atrial muscles of the heart:

ANP causes excretion of sodium in spite of increase in aldosterone secretion
  ii. It causes **pressure diuresis** (excretion of excess salt and water by high blood pressure) through urine. This decreases the salt and water content in ECF, in spite of hypersecretion of aldosterone (Fig. 70.3).

Besides ANP, two more natriuretic peptides called **brain natriuretic peptide** (BNP) and **C-type natriuretic peptide** (CNP) are also secreted by cardiac muscle (Chapter 72). BNP and CNP also have similar actions of ANP on sodium excretion.

Significance of aldosterone escape

Because of aldosterone escape, edema does not occur.

4. On Potassium Ions

Aldosterone increases the potassium excretion through the renal tubules. When aldosterone is deficient, the potassium ion concentration in ECF increases leading to hyperkalemia. Hyperkalemia results in serious cardiac toxicity, with weak contractions of heart and development of arrhythmia. In very severe conditions, it may cause cardiac death. When aldosterone secretion increases, it leads to **hypokalemia** and **muscular weakness.**

5. On Hydrogen Ion Concentration

While increasing the sodium reabsorption from renal tubules, aldosterone causes tubular secretion of hydro-

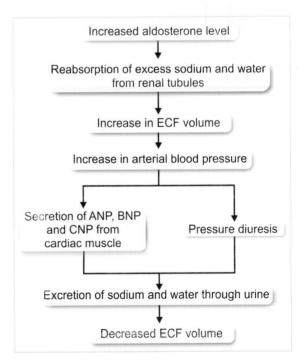

FIGURE 70.3: Aldosterone escape

gen ions. To some extent, secretion of hydrogen ions is in exchange for sodium ions. It obviously reduces the hydrogen ion concentration in the ECF. In normal conditions, aldosterone is essential to maintain acid-base balance in the body. In hypersecretion, it causes **alkalosis** and in hyposecretion, it causes **acidosis.**

6. *On Sweat Glands and Salivary Glands*

Aldosterone has almost the similar effect on sweat glands and salivary glands as it shows on renal tubules. Sodium is reabsorbed from sweat glands under the influence of aldosterone, thus the loss of sodium from the body is prevented. Same effect is shown on saliva also. Thus, aldosterone helps in the conservation of sodium in the body.

7. *On Intestine*

Aldosterone increases sodium absorption from the intestine, especially from colon and prevents loss of sodium through feces. Aldosterone deficiency leads to **diarrhea,** with loss of sodium and water.

■ MODE OF ACTION

Aldosterone acts through the messenger RNA (mRNA) mechanism.

Sequence of Events

1. Since aldosterone is lipid soluble, it diffuses readily into the cytoplasm of the tubular epithelial cells through the lipid layer of the cell membrane
2. In the cytoplasm, aldosterone binds with the specific receptor protein
3. Aldosterone-receptor complex diffuses into the nucleus where it binds to deoxyribonucleic acid (DNA) and causes formation of mRNA
4. The mRNA diffuses back into the cytoplasm and causes protein synthesis along with ribosomes. Most of the synthesized proteins are in the form of enzymes. One of such enzymes is sodium-potassium ATPase, which helps in the transport of sodium and potassium.

■ REGULATION OF SECRETION

Aldosterone secretion is regulated by four important factors (Fig. 70.4) which are given below in the order of their potency:

1. Increase in potassium ion (K^+) concentration in ECF
2. Decrease in sodium ion (Na^+) concentration in ECF
3. Decrease in ECF volume
4. Adrenocorticotropic hormone (ACTH).

Increase in the concentration of potassium ions is the most effective stimulant for aldosterone secretion.

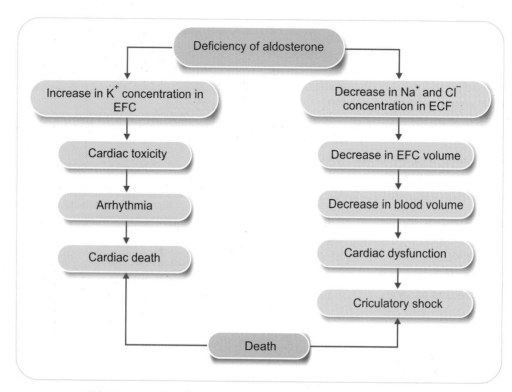

FIGURE 70.4: Importance of aldosterone. ECF = Extracellular fluid.

It acts directly on the zona glomerulosa and increases the secretion of aldosterone. Decrease in sodium ion concentration and ECF volume stimulates aldosterone secretion through **renin-angiotensin mechanism.** Renin secreted from juxtaglomerular apparatus of kidney acts on angiotensinogen in the plasma and converts it into angiotensin I, which is converted into angiotensin II by converting enzyme (ACE) secreted by lungs. Angiotensin II acts on the zona glomerulosa to secrete more aldosterone. Aldosterone in turn, increases the retention of sodium and water and excretion of potassium. This leads to increase in the sodium ion concentration and ECF volume.

Now, the increased sodium ion concentration and the ECF volume inhibit the juxtaglomerular apparatus and stop the release of renin. So, angiotensin II is not formed and release of aldosterone from adrenal cortex is stopped (Fig. 70.5).

Adrenocorticotropic hormone mainly stimulates the secretion of glucocorticoids. It has only a mild stimulating effect on aldosterone secretion.

■ GLUCOCORTICOIDS

Glucocorticoids act mainly on glucose metabolism.
Glucocorticoids are:
1. Cortisol
2. Corticosterone
3. Cortisone.

■ SOURCE OF SECRETION

Glucocorticoids are secreted mainly by zona fasciculata of adrenal cortex. A small quantity of glucocorticoids is also secreted by zona reticularis. Synthesis of cortisol is given in Fig. 70.6.

■ CHEMISTRY AND HALF-LIFE

Glucocorticoids are C_{21} steroids having 21 carbon atoms. Half-life of cortisol is 70 to 90 minutes and that of corticosterone is 50 minutes. Half-life of cortisone is not known.

■ DAILY OUTPUT AND PLASMA LEVEL

Daily output and plasma level of glucocorticoids are given in Table 70.2.

■ FUNCTIONS OF GLUCOCORTICOIDS

Cortisol or hydrocortisone is more potent and it has 95% of glucocorticoid activity. Corticosterone is less potent,

TABLE 70.2: Daily output and plasma level of glucocorticoids

Hormone	Daily output (µg)	Plasma level (µg/dL)
Cortisol	10.0	13.9
Corticosterone	3.0	0.4

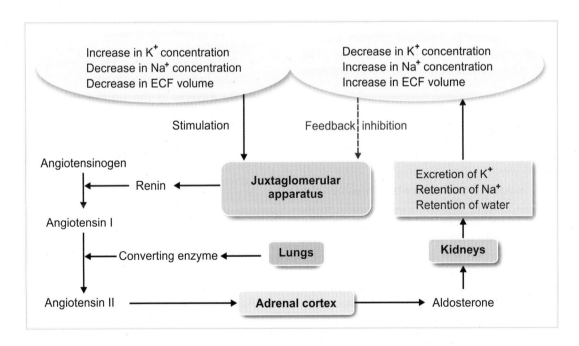

FIGURE 70.5: Regulation of aldosterone secretion

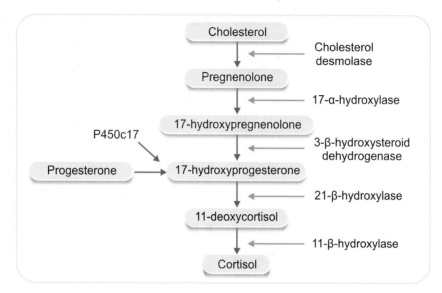

FIGURE 70.6: Synthesis of cortisol

showing only 4% of glucocorticoid activity. Cortisone with 1% activity is secreted in minute quantity.

Life-protecting Hormone

Like aldosterone, cortisol is also essential for life but in a different way. Aldosterone is a life-saving hormone, whereas cortisol is a life-protecting hormone because, it helps to withstand the stress and trauma in life.

Glucocorticoids have metabolic effects on carbohydrates, proteins, fats and water. These hormones also show mild mineralocorticoid effect. Removal of adrenal glands in human beings and animals causes disturbances of metabolism. Exposure to even mild harmful stress after **adrenalectomy,** leads to **collapse** and **death.**

1. On Carbohydrate Metabolism

Glucocorticoids increase the blood glucose level by two ways:

i. By promoting gluconeogenesis in liver from amino acids: Glucocorticoids enhance the breakdown of proteins in extrahepatic cells, particularly the muscle. It is followed by release of amino acids into circulation. From blood, amino acids enter the liver and get converted into glucose (gluconeogenesis)

ii. By inhibiting the uptake and utilization of glucose by peripheral cells: This action is called **anti-insulin action** of glucocorticoids.

Hypersecretion of glucocorticoids increases the blood glucose level, resulting in hyperglycemia, glucosuria and adrenal diabetes. Hyposecretion of

these hormones causes hypoglycemia and fasting during adrenal insufficiency will be fatal. It decreases blood glucose level to a great extent, resulting in death.

2. On Protein Metabolism

Glucocorticoids promote the catabolism of proteins, leading to:

i. Decrease in cellular proteins
ii. Increase in plasma level of amino acids
iii. Increase in protein content in liver.

Glucocorticoids cause catabolism of proteins by the following methods:

i. By releasing amino acids from body cells (except liver cells), into the blood
ii. By increasing the uptake of amino acids by hepatic cells from blood. In hepatic cells, the amino acids are used for the synthesis of proteins and carbohydrates (gluconeogenesis).

Thus, glucocorticoids cause mobilization of proteins from tissues other than liver. In hypersecretion of glucocorticoids, there is excess catabolism of proteins, resulting in muscular wasting and **negative nitrogen balance.**

3. On Fat Metabolism

Glucocorticoids cause mobilization and redistribution of fats. Actions on fats are:

i. Mobilization of fatty acids from adipose tissue
ii. Increasing the concentration of fatty acids in blood
iii. Increasing the utilization of fat for energy.

Glucocorticoids decrease the utilization of glucose. At the same time, these hormones mobilize fats and make the fatty acids available for utilization, by which energy is liberated. It leads to the formation of a large amount of ketone bodies. It is called **ketogenic effect** of glucocorticoids.

Hypersecretion of glucocorticoids causes an abnormal type of **obesity** by increasing the deposition of fat in certain areas such as abdomen, chest, face and buttocks.

4. On Water Metabolism

Glucocorticoids play an important role in the maintenance of water balance, by accelerating excretion of water. The adrenal insufficiency causes water retention and **water intoxication** after intake of large quantity of water.

5. On Mineral Metabolism

Glucocorticoids enhance the retention of sodium and to lesser extent, increase the excretion of potassium. Thus, hypersecretion of glucocorticoids causes edema, hypertension, hypokalemia and muscular weakness. Glucocorticoids decrease the blood calcium by inhibiting its absorption from intestine and increasing the excretion through urine.

6. On Bone

Glucocorticoids stimulate the bone resorption **(osteoclastic activity)** and inhibit bone formation and mineralization **(osteoblastic activity).** So, in hypersecretion of glucocorticoids, **osteoporosis** occurs.

7. On Muscles

Glucocorticoids increase the catabolism of proteins in muscle. So, hypersecretion causes muscular weakness due to loss of protein.

8. On Blood Cells

Glucocorticoids decrease the number of circulating eosinophils by increasing the destruction of eosinophils in reticuloendothelial cells. These hormones also decrease the number of basophils and lymphocytes and increase the number of circulating neutrophils, RBCs and platelets.

9. On Vascular Response

Presence of glucocorticoids is essential for the constrictor action of adrenaline and noradrenaline. In adrenal insufficiency, the blood vessels fail to respond to adrenaline and noradrenaline, leading to vascular collapse.

10. On Central Nervous System

Glucocorticoids are essential for normal functioning of nervous system. Insufficiency of these hormones causes personality changes like irritability and lack of concentration. Sensitivity to olfactory and taste stimuli increases in adrenal insufficiency.

11. Permissive Action of Glucocorticoids

Permissive action of glucocorticoids refers to execution of actions of some hormones only in the presence of glucocorticoids.
Examples:
  i. Calorigenic effect of glucagon
  ii. Lipolytic effect of catecholamines
  iii. Vascular effects of catecholamines
  iv. Bronchodilator effect of catecholamines.

12. On Resistance to Stress

Exposure to any type of stress, either physical or mental, increases the secretion of adrenocorticotropic hormone (ACTH), which in turn increases glucocorticoid secretion. The increase in glucocorticoid level is very essential for survival during stress conditions, as it offers high resistance to the body against stress.

Glucocorticoids enhance the resistance by the following ways:
  i. Immediate release and transport of amino acids from tissues to liver cells for the synthesis of new proteins and other substances, which are essential to withstand the stress
  ii. Release of fatty acids from cells for the production of more energy during stress
  iii. Enhancement of vascular response to catecholamines and fatty **acid-mobilizing action** of catecholamines, which are necessary to withstand the stress
  iv. Prevention of severity of other changes in the body caused by stress.

13. Anti-inflammatory Effects

Inflammation is defined as a localized protective response induced by injury or destruction of tissues. When the tissue is injured by mechanical or chemical factors, some substances are released from the affected area. These substances produce series of reactions in the affected area:

i. Chemical substances such as histamine, serotonin, leukotrienes, prostaglandins and bradykinin, which are released from damaged tissue cause vasodilatation and **erythema** (rushing of blood) in the affected area

ii. From blood, many leukocytes, particularly neutrophils and monocytes infiltrate the affected area. Leukocytes play an important role in the **defensive mechanism** (Chapter 16)

iii. Vasodilator substances released in the affected area increase the permeability of capillary membrane, resulting in oozing out of fluid from blood into interstitial space

iv. Coagulation occurs in the interstitial fluid because of fibrinogen and other proteins, which are leaked out from blood

v. Finally, **edema** occurs in that area which may be non-pitting type because of hard clot formation.

Glucocorticoids prevent the inflammatory reactions. Even if inflammation has already started, the glucocorticoids cause an early resolution of inflammation and rapid healing.

Glucocorticoids prevent the inflammatory changes by:

i. Inhibiting the release of chemical substances from damaged tissues and thereby preventing vasodilatation and erythema in the affected area

ii. Causing vasoconstriction through the permissive action on catecholamines. This also prevents rushing of blood to the injured area

iii. Decreasing the permeability of capillaries and preventing loss of fluid from plasma into the affected tissue

iv. Inhibiting the migration of leukocytes into the affected area

v. Suppressing T cells and other leukocytes, so that there is reduction in the reactions of tissues which enhance the inflammatory process.

14. Anti-allergic Actions

Corticosteroids prevent various reactions in allergic conditions as in the case of inflammation.

15. Immunosuppressive Effects

Glucocorticoids suppress the immune system of the body by decreasing the number of circulating T lymphocytes. It is done by suppressing proliferation of T cells and the lymphoid tissues (lymph nodes and thymus). Glucocorticoids also prevent the release of interleukin-2 by T cells.

Thus, hypersecretion or excess use of glucocorticoids decreases the immune reactions against all foreign bodies entering the body. It leads to severe infection causing death.

Immunological reactions, which are common during **organ transplantation,** may cause **rejection** of the transplanted tissues. Glucocorticoids are used to suppress the immunological reactions because of their immunosuppressive action.

■ MODE OF ACTION

Glucocorticoids bind with receptors to form hormone-receptor complex, which activates DNA to form mRNA. mRNA causes synthesis of enzymes, which alter the cell function.

■ REGULATION OF SECRETION

Anterior pituitary regulates glucocorticoid secretion by secreting adrenocorticotropic hormone (ACTH). ACTH secretion is regulated by hypothalamus through corticotropin-releasing factor (CRF).

Role of Anterior Pituitary – ACTH

Anterior pituitary controls the activities of adrenal cortex by secreting ACTH. ACTH is mainly concerned with the regulation of cortisol secretion and it plays only a minor role in the regulation of mineralocorticoid secretion.

Source of secretion

ACTH is secreted by the basophilic chromophilic cells of anterior pituitary.

Chemistry, plasma level and half-life

ACTH is a single chained polypeptide with 39 amino acids. The daily output of this hormone is 10 ng and the concentration in plasma is 3 ng/dL. Half-life of ACTH is 10 minutes.

Synthesis

ACTH is synthesized from a protein called prepro-opiomelanocortin (POMC). Along with ACTH, the POMC gives rise to some more byproducts called β-lipotropin, γ-lipotropin and β-endorphin. Two more byproducts, namely **α-melanocyte-stimulating hormone** (α-MSH) and **β-melanocyte-stimulating hormone** (β-MSH) are also secreted in animals. However, MSH activity is shown by ACTH and other byproducts from POMC in human beings.

Actions

ACTH is necessary for the structural integrity and secretory activity of adrenal cortex. It has other functions also.

Actions of ACTH on adrenal cortex (Adrenal actions)

1. Maintenance of structural integrity and vascularization of zona fasciculata and zona reticularis of adrenal cortex. In hypophysectomy, these two layers in the adrenal cortex are atrophied
2. Conversion of cholesterol into pregnenolone, which is the precursor of glucocorticoids. Thus, adrenocorticotropic hormone is responsible for the synthesis of glucocorticoids
3. Release of glucocorticoids
4. Prolongation of glucocorticoid action on various cells.

Other (Nonadrenal) actions of ACTH

1. Mobilization of fats from tissues
2. Melanocyte-stimulating effect. Because of structural similarity with melanocyte-stimulating hormone (MSH), ACTH shows melanocyte-stimulating effect. It causes darkening of skin by acting on melanophores, which are the cutaneous pigment cells containing melanin.

Mode of action of ACTH

ACTH acts by the formation of cyclic AMP.

Role of Hypothalamus

Hypothalamus also plays an important role in the regulation of cortisol secretion by controlling the ACTH secretion through **corticotropin-releasing factor** (CRF). It is also called **corticotropin-releasing hormone.** CRF reaches the anterior pituitary through the hypothalamo-hypophyseal portal vessels.

CRF stimulates the corticotropes of anterior pituitary and causes the synthesis and release of ACTH.

CRF secretion is induced by several factors such as emotion, stress, trauma and **circadian rhythm.** CRF in turn, causes release of ACTH, which induces glucocorticoid secretion.

Feedback Control

Cortisol regulates its own secretion through **negative feedback** control by inhibiting the release of CRF from hypothalamus and ACTH from anterior pituitary (Fig. 70.7).

Circadian rhythm of ACTH

ACTH secretion follows circadian rhythm (Chapter 149), i.e. it varies in different periods of the day. The rate of secretion of both ACTH and CRF is high in the morning and low in the evening. Hypothalamus plays an important role in the **circadian fluctuations of ACTH** secretion.

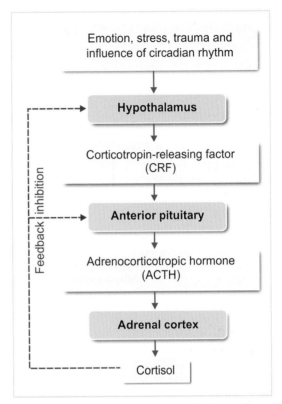

FIGURE 70.7: Regulation of cortisol secretion

■ ADRENAL SEX HORMONES

Adrenal sex hormones are secreted mainly by zona reticularis. Zona fasciculata secretes small quantities of sex hormones. Adrenal cortex secretes mainly the male sex hormones, which are called **androgens.** But small quantity of **estrogen** and **progesterone** are also secreted by adrenal cortex. Synthesis of sex hormones is given in Fig. 70.8.

Androgens secreted by adrenal cortex:
1. Dehydroepiandrosterone
2. Androstenedione
3. Testosterone.

Dehydroepiandrosterone is the most active adrenal androgen. Androgens, in general, are responsible for masculine features of the body (Chapter 74). But in normal conditions, the adrenal androgens have insignificant physiological effects, because of the low amount of secretion both in males and females.

In **congenital hyperplasia** of adrenal cortex or tumor of zona reticularis, an excess quantity of androgens is secreted. In males, it does not produce any special effect because, large quantity of androgens are produced by testes also. But in females, the androgens produce **masculine features.** Some of the androgens are converted into testosterone. Testosterone is responsible

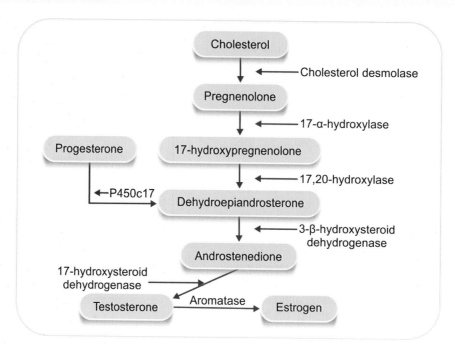

FIGURE 70.8: Synthesis of adrenal sex hormones

for the androgenic activity in adrenogenital syndrome or congenital adrenal hyperplasia.

■ EXOGENOUS STEROIDS

Corticosteroids are used as drugs since long. Exogenous steroids are extracted from adrenal cortex of animals or prepared artificially.

Commercially available synthetic drugs with corticosteroid effects are widely used. These drugs are either used as replacement of natural hormones (replacement therapy) in patients with deficiency disorders such as Addison disease or to treat a variety of other conditions such as arthritis, allergic conditions, asthma, skin disorders, etc.

■ SYNTHETIC STEROIDS

Synthetic steroids that are commonly used are:
1. **Cortisone** and **hydrocortisone,** which are used for replacement therapy have both glucocorticoid and mineralocorticoid effects
2. **Prednisolone** has more glucocorticoid activity than mineralocorticoid activity
3. **Fludrocortisone** (9-fluorocortisol) has more mineralocorticoid activity than glucocorticoid activity. It has most potent mineralocorticoid effect.
4. **Dexamethasone** has only glucocorticoid effect.

■ APPLIED PHYSIOLOGY

■ HYPERACTIVITY OF ADRENAL CORTEX

Hypersecretion of adrenocortical hormones leads to the following conditions:
1. Cushing syndrome
2. Hyperaldosteronism
3. Adrenogenital syndrome.

■ CUSHING SYNDROME

Cushing syndrome is a disorder characterized by obesity.

Causes

Cushing syndrome is due to the hypersecretion of glucocorticoids, particularly cortisol. It may be either due to pituitary origin or adrenal origin.

If it is due to pituitary origin, it is known as **Cushing disease.** If it is due to adrenal origin it is called **Cushing syndrome.** Generally, these two terms are used interchangeably.

Pituitary Origin

Increased secretion of ACTH causes hyperplasia of adrenal cortex, leading to hypersecretion of glucocorticoid. ACTH secretion is increased by:
   i. Tumor in pituitary cells, particularly in basophilic cells which secrete ACTH

ii. Malignant tumor of non-endocrine origin like cancer of lungs or abdominal viscera

iii. Hypothalamic disorder causing hypersecretion of corticotropin-releasing hormone.

Adrenal Origin

Cortisol secretion is increased by:
i. Tumor in zona fasciculata of adrenal cortex
ii. Carcinoma of adrenal cortex
iii. Prolonged treatment of chronic inflammatory diseases like rheumatoid arthritis, with high dose of exogenous glucocorticoids
iv. Prolonged treatment with high dose of ACTH, which stimulates adrenal cortex to secrete excess glucocorticoids.

Recently, Cushing syndrome is classified into two types:
i. **ACTH-dependent Cushing syndrome** which is due to hypersecretion of ACTH
ii. **ACTH-independent Cushing syndrome** in which the secretion of ACTH is normal. The syndrome develops due to abnormal membrane receptors for some peptides like interleukin-1, gonadotropin-releasing hormone and gastric inhibitory polypeptide in the cells of zona fasciculata. The binding of these peptides to the abnormal receptors increases secretion of glucocorticoids, resulting in Cushing syndrome. Cushing syndrome that is developed by treatment with exogenous glucocorticoids also belongs to this type.

Signs and Symptoms

i. Characteristic feature of this disease is the disproportionate distribution of body fat, resulting in some abnormal features:
  a. *Moon face:* The edematous facial appearance due to fat accumulation and retention of water and salt
  b. *Torso:* Fat accumulation in the chest and abdomen. Arms and legs are very slim in proportion to **torso** (torso means trunk of the body)
  c. *Buffalo hump:* Due to fat deposit on the back of neck and shoulder
  d. *Pot belly:* Due to fat accumulation in upper abdomen (Fig. 70.9).
ii. *Purple striae:* Reddish purple stripes on abdomen due to three reasons:
  a. Stretching of abdominal wall by excess subcutaneous fat

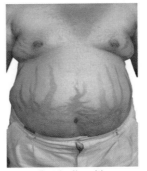 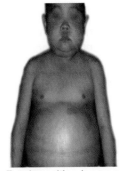

Pot belly with purple striae

Fat deposition in upper abdomen, thorax and face (moon face) with thin hands

FIGURE 70.9: Cushing syndrome
(*Courtesy:* Prof Mafauzy Mohamad)

  b. Rupture of subdermal tissues due to stretching
  c. Deficiency of collagen fibers due to protein depletion.
iii. Thinning of extremities
iv. Thinning of skin and subcutaneous tissues due to protein depletion caused by increased catabolism of proteins
v. Aconthosis: Skin disease characterized by darkened skin patches in certain areas such as axilla, neck and groin
vi. Pigmentation of skin, especially in ACTH-dependent type due to hypersecretion of ACTH which has got melanocyte-stimulating effect
vii. Facial plethora: Facial redness
viii. Hirsutism: Heavy growth of body and facial hair
ix. Weakening of muscles because of protein depletion
x. Bone resorption and osteoporosis due to protein depletion. Bone becomes susceptible to easy fracture
xi. Hyperglycemia due to gluconeogenesis (from proteins) and inhibition of peripheral utilization of glucose. Hyperglycemia leads to glucosuria and adrenal diabetes
xii. Hypertension by the mineralocorticoid effects of glucocorticoids – retention of sodium and water results in increase in ECF volume and blood volume, leading to hypertension
xiii. Immunosuppression resulting in susceptibility for infection
xiv. Poor wound healing.

Tests for Cushing Syndrome

i. Observation of external features
ii. Determination of blood sugar and cortisol levels
iii. Analysis of urine for 17-hydroxysteroids.

Treatment for Cushing Syndrome

Treatment depends upon the cause of the disease. Treatment may include cortisol-inhibiting drugs, surgical removal of pituitary or adrenal tumor, radiation or chemotherapy.

Nelson syndrome

Nelson syndrome is a disorder that develops after surgical removal of both adrenal glands. It is because of the growth of pituitary tumor that secretes excess ACTH. The features include headache and visual problems. Nelson syndrome can be treated with radiation or surgical removal of the pituitary gland.

■ HYPERALDOSTERONISM

Increased secretion of aldosterone is called hyperaldosteronism.

Causes and Types

Depending upon the causes, hyperaldosteronism is classified into two types:
  i. Primary hyperaldosteronism
  ii. Secondary hyperaldosteronism.

Primary Hyperaldosteronism

Primary hyperaldosteronism is otherwise known as **Conn syndrome.** It develops due to tumor in zona glomerulosa of adrenal cortex. In primary hyper-aldosteronism, edema does not occur because of escape phenomenon.

Secondary Hyperaldosteronism

Secondary hyperaldosteronism occurs due to extra adrenal causes such as:
  i.   Congestive cardiac failure
  ii. Nephrosis
  iii. Toxemia of pregnancy
  iv. Cirrhosis of liver.

Signs and Symptoms

  i.   Increase in ECF volume and blood volume
  ii. Hypertension due to increase in ECF volume and blood volume
  iii. Severe depletion of potassium, which causes renal damage. The kidneys fail to produce concentrated urine. It leads to polyuria and polydipsia

  iv. Muscular weakness due to potassium depletion
  v. Metabolic alkalosis due to secretion of large amount of hydrogen ions into the renal tubules. Metabolic alkalosis reduces blood calcium level causing tetany.

■ ADRENOGENITAL SYNDROME

Under normal conditions, adrenal cortex secretes small quantities of androgens which do not have any significant effect on sex organs or sexual function. However, secretion of abnormal quantities of adrenal androgens develops adrenogenital syndrome. Testosterone is responsible for the **androgenic activity** in adrenogenital syndrome.

Causes

Adrenogenital syndrome is due to the tumor of zona reticularis in adrenal cortex.

Symptoms

Adrenogenital syndrome is characterized by the tendency for the development of secondary sexual character of opposite sex.

Symptoms in females

Increased secretion of androgens causes development of male secondary sexual characters. The condition is called **adrenal virilism.** Symptoms are:
  i.   Masculinization due to increased muscular growth
  ii. Deepening of voice
  iii. Amenorrhea
  iv. Enlargement of clitoris
  v.   Male type of hair growth.

Symptoms in males

Sometimes, the tumor of estrogen secreting cells produces more than normal quantity of estrogens in males. It produces some symptoms such as:
  i.   Feminization
  ii. Gynecomastia (enlargement of breast)
  iii. Atrophy of testis
  iv. Loss of interest in women.

■ HYPOACTIVITY OF ADRENAL CORTEX

Hyposecretion of adrenocortical hormones leads to the following conditions:
  1. Addison disease or chronic adrenal insufficiency
  2. Congenital adrenal hyperplasia.

■ ADDISON DISEASE OR CHRONIC ADRENAL INSUFFICIENCY

Addison disease is the failure of adrenal cortex to secrete corticosteroids.

Types of Addison Disease

i. Primary Addison disease due to adrenal cause
ii. Secondary Addison disease due to failure of anterior pituitary to secrete ACTH
iii. Tertiary Addison disease due failure of hypothalamus to secrete corticotropin-releasing factor (CRF).

Causes for Primary Addison Disease

i. Atrophy of adrenal cortex due to autoimmune diseases
ii. Destruction of the gland because of tuberculosis
iii. Destruction of hormone-secreting cells in adrenal cortex by malignant tissues
iv. Congenital failure to secrete cortisol
v. Adrenalectomy and failure to take hormone therapy.

Signs and Symptoms

Signs and symptoms develop in Addison disease because of deficiency of both cortisol and aldosterone. Common signs and symptom are:

i. Pigmentation of skin and mucous membrane due to excess ACTH secretion, induced by cortisol deficiency. ACTH causes pigmentation by its melanocyte-stimulating action
ii. Muscular weakness
iii. Dehydration with loss of sodium
iv. Hypotension
v. Decreased cardiac output and decreased workload of the heart, leading to decrease in size of the heart
vi. Hypoglycemia
vii. Nausea, vomiting and diarrhea. Prolonged vomiting and diarrhea cause dehydration and loss of body weight
viii. Susceptibility to any type of infection
ix. Inability to withstand any stress, resulting in Addisonian crisis (see below).

Tests for Addison Disease

i. Measurement of blood level of cortisol and aldosterone
ii. Measurement of amount of steroids excreted in urine.

Addisonian Crisis or Adrenal Crisis or Acute Adrenal Insufficiency

Adrenal crisis is a common symptom of Addison disease, characterized by sudden collapse associated with an increase in need for large quantities of glucocorticoids. The condition becomes fatal if not treated in time.

Causes

i. Exposure to even mild stress
ii. Hypoglycemia due to fasting
iii. Trauma
iv. Surgical operation
v. Sudden withdrawal of glucocorticoid treatment.

■ CONGENITAL ADRENAL HYPERPLASIA

Congenital adrenal hyperplasia is a congenital disorder, characterized by increase in size of adrenal cortex. Size increases due to abnormal increase in the number of steroid-secreting cortical cells.

Causes

Even though the size of the gland increases, cortisol secretion decreases. It is because of the congenital deficiency of the enzymes necessary for the synthesis of cortisol, particularly, 21-hydroxylase.

Lack of this enzyme reduces the synthesis of cortisol, resulting in ACTH secretion from pituitary by feedback mechanism. ACTH stimulates the adrenal cortex causing hyperplasia, with accumulation of lipid droplets. Hence, it is also called **congenital lipid adrenal**

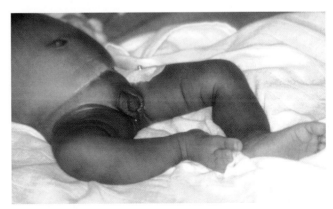

FIGURE 70.10: Congenital adrenal hyperplasia (Macro-genitosomia praecox) (*Courtesy:* Prof Mafauzy Mohamad)

hyperplasia. Cortisol cannot be synthesized because of lack of 21-hydroxylase. Therefore, due to the constant simulation of adrenal cortex by ACTH, the secretion of androgens increases. It results in sexual abnormalities such as virilism.

Symptoms

In boys

Adrenal hyperplasia produces a condition known as **macrogenitosomia praecox** (Fig. 70.10).

Features of macrogenitosomia praecox:
  i. Precocious body growth, causing stocky appearance called **infant Hercules**
  ii. Precocious sexual development with enlarged penis even at the age of 4 years.

In girls

In girls, adrenal hyperplasia produces masculinization. It is otherwise called **virilism.** In some cases of genetic disorders, the female child is born with external genitalia of male type. This condition is called **pseudohermaphroditism.**

Adrenal Medulla

■ INTRODUCTION

Medulla is the inner part of adrenal gland and it forms 20% of the mass of adrenal gland. It is made up of interlacing cords of cells known as **chromaffin cells.** Chromaffin cells are also called **pheochrome cells** or **chromophil cells.** These cells contain fine granules which are stained brown by potassium dichromate.

Types of chromaffin cells

Adrenal medulla is formed by two types of chromaffin cells:

1. Adrenaline-secreting cells (90%)
2. Noradrenaline-secreting cells (10%).

■ HORMONES OF ADRENAL MEDULLA

Adrenal medullary hormones are the amines derived from **catechol** and so these hormones are called **catecholamines.**

Catecholamines secreted by adrenal medulla

1. Adrenaline or epinephrine
2. Noradrenaline or norepinephrine
3. Dopamine.

■ PLASMA LEVEL OF CATECHOLAMINES

1. Adrenaline   :   3 µg/dL
2. Noradrenaline :   30 µg/dL
3. Dopamine   :   3.5 µg/dL

■ HALF-LIFE OF CATECHOLAMINES

Half-life of catecholamines is about 2 minutes.

■ SYNTHESIS OF CATECHOLAMINES

Catecholamines are synthesized from the amino acid **tyrosine** in the chromaffin cells of adrenal medulla (Fig. 71.1). These hormones are formed from **phenylalanine** also. But phenylalanine has to be converted into tyrosine.

Stages of Synthesis of Catecholamines

1. Formation of tyrosine from phenylalanine in the presence of enzyme **phenylalanine hydroxylase**
2. Uptake of tyrosine from blood into the chromaffin cells of adrenal medulla by active transport
3. Conversion of tyrosine into dihydroxyphenylalanine **(DOPA)** by **hydroxylation** in the presence of **tyrosine** hydroxylase

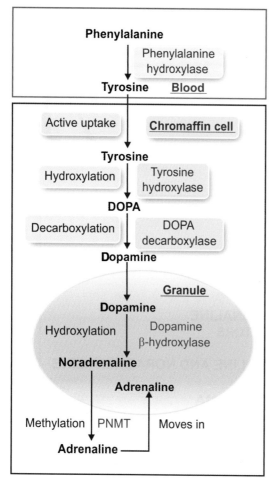

FIGURE 71.1: Synthesis of catecholamines. DOPA = Di-hydroxyphenylalanine, PNMT = Phenylethanolamine-N-methyltransferase.

4. **Decarboxylation** of DOPA into dopamine by **DOPA decarboxylase**
5. Entry of dopamine into granules of chromaffin cells
6. **Hydroxylation** of dopamine into noradrenaline by the enzyme dopamine **beta-hydroxylase**
7. Release of noradrenaline from granules into the cytoplasm
8. **Methylation** of noradrenaline into adrenaline by the most important enzyme called **phenylethanolamine-N-methyltransferase (PNMT)**. PNMT is present in chromaffin cells.

■ METABOLISM OF CATECHOLAMINES

Eighty five percent of noradrenaline is taken up by the sympathetic adrenergic neurons. Remaining 15% of noradrenaline and adrenaline are degraded (Fig. 71.2).

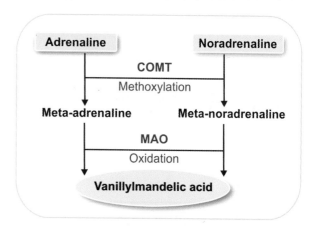

FIGURE 71.2: Metabolism of catecholamines. COMT = Catechol-O-methyltransferase, MAO = Monoamine oxidase.

Stages of Metabolism of Catecholamines

1. **Methoxylation** of adrenaline into **meta-adrenaline** and noradrenaline into **metanoradrenaline** in the presence of 'catechol-O-methyltransferase' (COMT). **Meta-adrenaline** and meta-noradrenaline are together called metanephrines
2. **Oxidation** of metanephrines into **vanillylmandelic acid (VMA)** by **monoamine oxidase (MAO)**

Removal of Catecholamines

Catecholamines are removed from body through urine in three forms:
   i. 15% as free adrenaline and free noradrenaline
   ii. 50% as free or conjugated meta-adrenaline and meta-noradrenaline
   iii. 35% as vanillylmandelic acid (VMA).

■ ACTIONS OF ADRENALINE AND NORADRENALINE

Adrenaline and noradrenaline stimulate the nervous system. Adrenaline has significant effects on metabolic functions and both adrenaline and noradrenaline have significant effects on cardiovascular system.

■ MODE OF ACTION OF ADRENALINE AND NORADRENALINE – ADRENERGIC RECEPTORS

Actions of adrenaline and noradrenaline are executed by binding with receptors called adrenergic receptors, which are present in the target organs.

Adrenergic receptors are of two types:
1. **Alpha-adrenergic receptors,** which are subdivided into alpha-1 and alpha-2 receptors
2. **Beta-adrenergic receptors,** which are subdivided into beta-1 and beta-2 receptors.

Refer Table 71.1 for the mode of action of these receptors.

■ ACTIONS

Circulating adrenaline and noradrenaline have similar effect of sympathetic stimulation. But, the effect of adrenal hormones is prolonged 10 times more than that of sympathetic stimulation. It is because of the slow inactivation, slow degradation and slow removal of these hormones.

Effects of adrenaline and noradrenaline on various target organs depend upon the type of receptors present in the cells of the organs. Adrenaline acts through both alpha and beta receptors equally. Noradrenaline acts mainly through alpha receptors and occasionally through beta receptors.

1. On Metabolism (via Alpha and Beta Receptors)

Adrenaline influences the metabolic functions more than noradrenaline.
  i. General metabolism: Adrenaline increases oxygen consumption and carbon dioxide removal. It increases basal metabolic rate. So, it is said to be a calorigenic hormone
 ii. Carbohydrate metabolism: Adrenaline increases the blood glucose level by increasing the glycogenolysis in liver and muscle. So, a large quantity of glucose enters the circulation
iii. Fat metabolism: Adrenaline causes mobilization of free fatty acids from adipose tissues. Catecholamines need the presence of glucocorticoids for this action.

2. On Blood (via Beta Receptors)

Adrenaline decreases blood coagulation time. It increases RBC count in blood by contracting smooth muscles of splenic capsule and releasing RBCs from spleen into circulation.

3. On Heart (via Beta Receptors)

Adrenaline has stronger effects on heart than noradrenaline. It increases overall activity of the heart, i.e.
  i. Heart rate (**chronotropic effect**)
 ii. Force of contraction (**inotropic effect**)
iii. Excitability of heart muscle (**bathmotropic effect**)
 iv. Conductivity in heart muscle (**dromotropic effect**).

4. On Blood Vessels (via Alpha and Beta-2 Receptors)

Noradrenaline has strong effects on blood vessels. It causes constriction of blood vessels throughout the body via alpha receptors. So it is called '**general vasoconstrictor**'. Vasoconstrictor effect of noradrenaline increases total peripheral resistance.

Adrenaline also causes constriction of blood vessels. However, it causes dilatation of blood vessels in skeletal muscle, liver and heart through beta-2 receptors. So, the total peripheral resistance is decreased by adrenaline.

Catecholamines need the presence of glucocorticoids, for these vascular effects.

5. On Blood Pressure (via Alpha and Beta Receptors)

Adrenaline increases **systolic blood pressure** by increasing the force of contraction of the heart and cardiac output. But, it decreases **diastolic blood pressure** by reducing the total peripheral resistance. Noradrenaline increases **diastolic pressure** due to general vasoconstrictor effect by increasing the total peripheral resistance. It also increases the **systolic blood pressure** to a slight extent by its actions on heart. The action of catecholamines on blood pressure needs the presence of glucocorticoids.

TABLE 71.1: Adrenergic receptors

Receptor	Mode of action	Response
Alpha-1 receptor	Activates IP$_3$ through phospholipase C	Mediates more of noradrenaline actions than adrenaline actions
Alpha-2 receptor	Inhibits adenyl cyclase and cAMP	
Beta-1 receptor	Activates adenyl cyclase and cAMP	Mediates actions of adrenaline and noradrenaline equally
Beta-2 receptor	Activates adenyl cyclase and cAMP	Mediates more of adrenaline actions than noradrenaline actions

IP$_3$ = Inositol triphosphate

Thus, hypersecretion of catecholamines leads to hypertension.

6. *On Respiration (via Beta-2 Receptors)*

Adrenaline increases rate and force of respiration. Adrenaline injection produces apnea, which is known as **adrenaline apnea.** It also causes **bronchodilation.**

7. *On Skin (via Alpha and Beta-2 Receptors)*

Adrenaline causes contraction of **arrector pili.** It also increases the secretion of sweat.

8. *On Skeletal Muscle (via Alpha and Beta-2 Receptors)*

Adrenaline causes severe contraction and quick fatigue of skeletal muscle. It increases glycogenolysis and release of glucose from muscle into blood. It also causes **vasodilatation** in skeletal muscles.

9. *On Smooth Muscle (via Alpha and Beta Receptors)*

Catecholamines cause contraction of smooth muscles in the following organs:
  i. Splenic capsule
  ii. Sphincters of gastrointestinal (GI) tract
  iii. Arrector pili of skin
  iv. Gallbladder
  v. Uterus
  vi. Dilator pupillae of iris
  vii. Nictitating membrane of cat.

Catecholamines cause relaxation of smooth muscles in the following organs:
  i. Non-sphincteric part of GI tract (esophagus, stomach and intestine)
  ii. Bronchioles
  iii. Urinary bladder.

10. *On Central Nervous System (via Beta Receptors)*

Adrenaline increases the activity of brain. Adrenaline secretion increases during **'fight or flight reactions'** after exposure to stress. It enhances the cortical arousal and other facilitatory functions of central nervous system.

11. *Other Effects of Catecholamines*

  i. On salivary glands (via alpha and beta-2 receptors): Cause vasoconstriction in salivary gland, leading to mild increase in salivary secretion
  ii. On sweat glands (via beta-2 receptors): Increase the secretion of apocrine sweat glands
  iii. On lacrimal glands (via alpha receptors): Increase the secretion of tears
  iv. On ACTH secretion (via alpha receptors): Adrenaline increases ACTH secretion
  v. On nerve fibers (via alpha receptors): Adrenaline decreases the latency of action potential in the nerve fibers, i.e. electrical activity is accelerated
  vi. On renin secretion (via beta receptors): Increase the rennin secretion from juxtaglomerular apparatus of the kidney.

■ REGULATION OF SECRETION OF ADRENALINE AND NORADRENALINE

Adrenaline and noradrenaline are secreted from adrenal medulla in small quantities even during rest. During stress conditions, due to **sympathoadrenal discharge,** a large quantity of catecholamines is secreted. These hormones prepare the body for fight or flight reactions.

Catecholamine secretion increases during exposure to cold and hypoglycemia also.

■ DOPAMINE

Dopamine is secreted by adrenal medulla. Type of cells secreting this hormone is not known. Dopamine is also secreted by dopaminergic neurons in some areas of brain, particularly basal ganglia. In brain, this hormone acts as a neurotransmitter.

Injected dopamine produces the following effects:
1. Vasoconstriction by releasing norepinephrine
2. Vasodilatation in mesentery
3. Increase in heart rate via beta receptors
4. Increase in systolic blood pressure. Dopamine does not affect diastolic blood pressure.

Deficiency of dopamine in basal ganglia produces nervous disorder called parkinsonism (Chapter 151).

■ APPLIED PHYSIOLOGY – PHEOCHROMOCYTOMA

Pheochromocytoma is a condition characterized by hypersecretion of catecholamines.

Cause

Pheochromocytoma is caused by tumor of chromophil cells in adrenal medulla. It is also caused rarely by tumor of sympathetic ganglia **(extra-adrenal pheochromocytoma).**

Signs and Symptoms

Characteristic feature of pheochromocytoma is hypertension. This type of hypertension is known as **endocrine** or **secondary hypertension.**

Other features:
1. Anxiety
2. Chest pain
3. Fever
4. Headache
5. Hyperglycemia
6. Metabolic disorders
7. Nausea and vomiting
8. Palpitation
9. Polyuria and glucosuria
10. Sweating and flushing
11. Tachycardia
12. Weight loss.

Tests for Pheochromocytoma

Pheochromocytoma is detected by measuring metanephrines and vanillylmandelic acid in urine and catecholamines in plasma.

Endocrine Functions of Other Organs

Chapter 72

```
■ PINEAL GLAND
    ■ SITUATION AND STRUCTURE
    ■ FUNCTIONS
■ THYMUS
    ■ SITUATION
    ■ FUNCTIONS
■ KIDNEYS
    ■ ERYTHROPOIETIN
    ■ THROMBOPOIETIN
    ■ RENIN
    ■ 1,25-DIHYDROXYCHOLECALCIFEROL
    ■ PROSTAGLANDINS
■ HEART
    ■ ATRIAL NATRIURETIC PEPTIDE
    ■ BRAIN NATRIURETIC PEPTIDE
    ■ C-TYPE NATRIURETIC PEPTIDE
```

■ PINEAL GLAND

■ SITUATION AND STRUCTURE

Pineal gland or **epiphysis** is located in the diencephalic area of brain above the hypothalamus. It is a small cone-shaped structure with a length of about 10 mm.

Pineal gland has two types of cells:
1. Large epithelial cells called parenchymal cells
2. Neuroglial cells.

In adults, the pineal gland is **calcified.** But, the epithelial cells exist and secrete the hormonal substance.

■ FUNCTIONS

Pineal gland has two functions:
1. It controls the sexual activities in animals by regulating the seasonal fertility. However, the pineal gland plays little role in regulating the sexual functions in human being
2. It secretes the hormonal substance called melatonin.

Melatonin

Source of secretion

Melatonin is secreted by the parenchymal cells of pineal gland.

Chemistry

Melatonin is an **indole** (N-acetyl-5-methoxytryptamine).

Actions of melatonin

Melatonin acts mainly on gonads. Its action differs from species to species. In some animals, it stimulates the gonads while in other animals, it inhibits the gonads.

In humans, it inhibits the onset of puberty by inhibiting the gonads.

Diurnal variation in melatonin secretion

Melatonin secretion is more in darkness than in daylight. In animals, the secretion of melatonin varies according to activities in different periods of the day, i.e. **circadian** rhythm (Chapter 149). Hypothalamus is responsible for the circadian fluctuations of melatonin secretion.

■ THYMUS

■ SITUATION

Thymus is situated in front of trachea, below the thyroid gland. Thymus is small in newborn infants and gradually enlarges till puberty and then decreases in size.

■ FUNCTIONS

Thymus has lymphoid function and endocrine function. It plays an important role in development of immunity in the body.

Thymus has two functions:
1. Processing the T lymphocytes
2. Endocrine function.

1. *Processing the T Lymphocytes*

Thymus plays an essential role in the development of immunity by processing the T lymphocytes (Chapter 17). The lymphocytes which are produced in bone marrow are processed in thymus into T lymphocytes. It occurs during the period between 3 months before birth and 3 months after birth. So, the removal of thymus 3 months after birth, will not affect the cell-mediated immunity.

2. *Endocrine Function of Thymus*

Thymus secretes two hormones:
  i. Thymosin
  ii. Thymin.

Thymosin

Thymosin is a peptide. It accelerates lymphopoiesis and proliferation of T lymphocytes.

Thymin

Thymin is also called **thymopoietin.** It suppresses the neuromuscular activity by inhibiting acetylcholine release. Hyperactivity of thymus causes myasthenia gravis.

■ KIDNEYS

Kidneys secrete five hormonal substances:
1. Erythropoietin
2. Thrombopoietin
3. Renin
4. 1,25-dihydroxycholecalciferol (calcitriol)
5. Prostaglandins.

Recently, it is discovered that kidney secretes small quantity of C-type natriuretic peptide (see below).

■ ERYTHROPOIETIN

Source of Secretion

Endothelial cells of peritubular capillaries in the kidney secrete erythropoietin. The stimulant for its secretion is hypoxia. Erythropoietin is a glycoprotein with 165 amino acids.

Action of Erythropoietin

Erythropoietin stimulates the bone marrow and causes erythropoiesis. More details are given in Chapter 10.

■ THROMBOPOIETIN

Source of Secretion

Thrombopoietin is a glycoprotein. It is secreted by kidneys and liver.

Action of Thrombopoietin

Thrombopoietin stimulates the production of platelets.

■ RENIN

Source of Secretion

The granular cells of juxtaglomerular apparatus of the kidney secrete renin.

Actions of Renin

When renin is released into the blood, it acts on a specific plasma protein called **alpha-2 globulin.** It is also called angiotensinogen or **renin substrate.**

Renin converts angiotensinogen into angiotensin I, which is converted into angiotensin II by a converting enzyme. The other details of renin and angiotensin II are given in Chapter 50.

■ 1,25-DIHYDROXYCHOLECALCIFEROL – CALCITRIOL

Formation of 1,25-dihydroxycholecalciferol

1,25-dihydroxycholecalciferol is otherwise known as **calcitriol** or **activated vitamin D.** It is formed from cholecalciferol, which is present in skin and intestine. The cholecalciferol (vitamin D3) from skin or intestine is converted into 25-hydroxycholecalciferol in liver. This in turn, is activated into 1,25-dihydroxycholecalciferol by parathormone in kidney (refer Chapter 68).

Actions of 1,25-Dihydroxycholecalciferol

The activated vitamin D plays an important role in the maintenance of blood calcium level. It acts on the intestinal epithelium and enhances absorption of calcium from intestine into the blood. Details are given in Chapter 68.

■ PROSTAGLANDINS

Source of Secretion

Prostaglandins secreted from kidney are PGA_2 and PGE_2. These hormones are secreted by juxtaglomerular cells and type I interstitial cells present in medulla of kidney.

Action of Prostaglandins

Prostaglandins decrease the blood pressure by systemic vasodilatation, diuresis and natriuresis. Details of prostaglandins are given in Chapter 73.

■ HEART

Heart secretes the hormones atrial natriuretic peptide and brain natriuretic peptide. Recently, another peptide called C-type natriuretic peptide is found in heart.

■ ATRIAL NATRIURETIC PEPTIDE

Atrial natriuretic peptide (ANP) is a polypeptide with 28 amino acids. It is secreted by **atrial musculature** of the heart. Recently, it is found in hypothalamus of brain also. However, its action in brain is not known.

ANP is secreted during overstretching of atrial muscles in conditions like increase in blood volume. ANP, in turn increases excretion of sodium (followed by water excretion) through urine and helps in the maintenance of extracellular fluid (ECF) volume and blood volume. It also lowers blood pressure.

Effect of ANP on Sodium Excretion

Atrial natriuretic peptide increases excretion of sodium ions through urine by:
1. Increasing glomerular filtration rate by relaxing **mesangeal cells** and dilating afferent arterioles

2. Inhibiting sodium reabsorption from distal convoluted tubules and collecting ducts in kidneys
3. Increasing the secretion of sodium into the renal tubules.

Escape phenomenon

Thus, ANP is responsible for escape phenomenon and prevention of edema in **primary hyperaldosteronism,** in spite of increased ECF volume (Refer Chapter 70 for details).

Effect of ANP on Blood Pressure

ANP decreases the blood pressure by:
1. Vasodilatation by relaxing the smooth muscle fibers, mainly in arterioles and venules
2. Inhibiting renin secretion from juxtaglomerular apparatus of kidney
3. Inhibiting vasoconstrictor effect of angiotensin II
4. Inhibiting vasoconstrictor effects of catecholamines.

■ BRAIN NATRIURETIC PEPTIDE

Brain natriuretic peptide (BNP) is also called B-type natriuretic peptide. It is a polypeptide with 32 amino acids. It is secreted by the cardiac muscle. It is also secreted in some parts of the brain. The stimulant for its secretion is not known.

BNP has same actions of ANP (see above). On brain, its actions are not known.

Clinical Importance of BNP

Measurement of plasma level of BNP (BNP test) is becoming an important diagnostic tool for heart diseases. Normally, blood contains very small amount of BNP. However, in conditions like heart failure, BNP level is increased in blood.

■ C-TYPE NATRIURETIC PEPTIDE

C-type natriuretic peptide (CNP) is the newly discovered peptide hormone. It is a 22 amino acid peptide. Initially, it was identified in brain. Now, it is known to be secreted by several tissues which include myocardium, endothelium of blood vessels, gastrointestinal tract and kidneys. The functions of this hormone are not fully studied. It is believed that it has similar action of atrial natriuretic peptide.

Local Hormones

- ■ INTRODUCTION
- ■ LOCAL HORMONES SYNTHESIZED IN TISSUES
  - ■ PROSTAGLANDINS AND ITS RELATED HORMONES
  - ■ OTHER LOCAL HORMONES SYNTHESIZED IN TISSUES
- ■ LOCAL HORMONES PRODUCED IN BLOOD
  - ■ KININS

■ INTRODUCTION

Local hormones are the substances which act on the same area of their secretion or in immediate neighborhood. The endocrine hormones are secreted in one place but execute their actions on some other remote place.

Local hormones are usually released in an inactive form and are activated by some conditions or substances.

Classification of Local Hormones

Local hormones are classified into two types:
- I. Hormones synthesized in tissues
- II. Hormones synthesized in blood.

■ LOCAL HORMONES SYNTHESIZED IN TISSUES

Local hormones synthesized in the tissues are:
1. Prostaglandins and related substances
2. Other local hormones synthesized in tissues.

■ PROSTAGLANDINS AND ITS RELATED HORMONES

Prostaglandins and other hormones which are derived from **arachidonic acid** are collectively called **eicosanoids**. The eicosanoids are:
1. Prostaglandins
2. Thromboxanes
3. Prostacyclin
4. Leukotrienes
5. Lipoxins

Synthesis of eicosanoids

Phospholipids of the cell membrane are released by the action of phospholipase A_2. Phospholipids are converted into arachidonic acid. Arachidonic acid is converted into an **endoperoxide** called **prostaglandin G_2** (PGG_2), which is converted into **prostaglandin H_2** (PGH_2). PGH_2 gives rise to **prostaglandins, prostacyclin** and **thromboxanes** (Fig. 73.1).

1. Prostaglandins

Prostaglandins were first discovered and isolated from human semen by Ulf von Euler of Sweden, in 1930. He thought that these hormones were secreted by prostate gland hence the name prostaglandins. However, now it is believed that almost all the tissues of the body including renal tissues (Chapter 72) synthesize prostaglandins.

Chemistry

Prostaglandins are unsaturated fatty acids with a cyclopentane ring and 20 carbon atoms.

Synthesis

Prostaglandins are synthesized from arachidonic acid.

Types

A variety of prostaglandins are identified. Active forms of prostaglandins are PGA_2, PGD_2, PGE_2 and PGF_2.

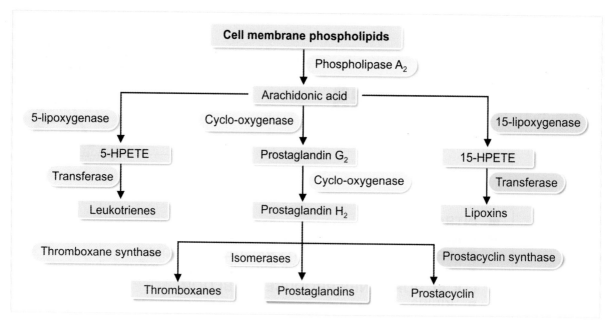

FIGURE 73.1: Synthesis of prostaglandins and related hormones.
HPETE = Hydroperoxyeicosatetraenoic acid

Actions

Prostaglandins show variety of physiological actions in the body. Various actions of prostaglandins are:

   i. *On blood:* Prostaglandins accelerate the capacity of RBCs to pass through minute blood vessels.
  ii. *On blood vessels:* PGE_2 causes vasodilatation.
 iii. *On GI tract:* The prostaglandins reduce gastric secretion. In experimental animals, prostaglandins inhibit the formation of peptic ulcer.
  iv. *On respiratory system:* PGE_2 causes bronchodilatation.
   v. *On lipids:* Some of the prostaglandins are antilipolytic agents. These hormones inhibit the release of free fatty acids from adipose tissue.
  vi. *On nervous system:* In brain, prostaglandins control or alter the actions of neurotransmitters.
 vii. *On reproduction:* Prostaglandins play an important role in regulating the reproductive cycle. These hormones also cause degeneration of corpus luteum **(luteolysis).** Prostaglandins increase the receptive capacity of cervical mucosa for sperms and cause **reverse peristaltic movement** of uterus and fallopian tubes during coitus. This in turn, increases the velocity of sperm transport in female genital tract.

Prostaglandins (PGE_2) play an important role during parturition and facilitate labor by increasing the force of uterine contractions. Prostaglandins are secreted from uterine tissues, fetal membranes and placenta. Their concentration increases in maternal blood and amniotic fluid at the time of **labor.** Prostaglandins increase the force of uterine contractions by elevating the concentration of calcium ions in the smooth muscle fibers of uterus.

When injected **intra-amniotically** during pregnancy, prostaglandins induce **abortion.** When injected during last stages of pregnancy, prostaglandins induce labor.

viii. *On kidney:* The prostaglandins stimulate juxtaglomerular apparatus and enhance the secretion of renin, diuresis and natriuresis.

Mode of action of prostaglandins

Prostaglandins mainly act by the formation of second messenger cyclic AMP.

2. *Thromboxanes*

Thromboxanes are derived from arachidonic acid.
Thromboxanes are of two types:

   i. Thromboxane A_2, which is secreted in platelets
  ii. Thromboxane B_2, the metabolite of thromboxane A_2.

Actions

Thromboxane A_2:

   i. Causes vasoconstriction
  ii. Plays an important role in hemostasis by accelerating aggregation of platelets
 iii. Accelerates clot formation.

3. *Prostacyclin*

Prostacyclin is also a derivative of arachidonic acid. It is produced in the endothelial cells and smooth muscle cells of blood vessels.

Actions

It causes vasodilatation and inhibits platelet aggregation.

4. *Leukotrienes*

Leukotrienes are derived from arachidonic acid via 5-hydroperoxyeicosatetraeonic acid (5-HPETE). Leukotrienes are the mediators of **allergic responses**. These hormones also promote inflammatory reactions.

The release of leukotrienes increases when some allergic agents combine with antibodies like IgE.

Actions

Leukotrienes cause:
 i. Bronchiolar constriction
 ii. Arteriolar constriction
 iii. Vascular permeability
 iv. Attraction of neutrophils and eosinophils towards the site of inflammation.

5. *Lipoxins*

Lipoxins are also derived from arachidonic acid via 15-hydroperoxyeicosatetraeonic acid (15-HPETE). Lipoxins are of two types namely, lipoxin A and lipoxin B.

Actions

Lipoxin A causes dilation of minute blood vessels. Both the types inhibit the cytotoxic effects of killer T cells.

■ OTHER LOCAL HORMONES SYNTHESIZED IN TISSUES

In addition to prostaglandins and related hormonal substances, tissues secrete some more hormones which are listed below:
 1. Acetylcholine
 2. Serotonin
 3. Histamine
 4. Substance P
 5. Heparin
 6. Leptin
 7. Gastrointestinal hormones.

1. *Acetylcholine*

Acetylcholine is the cholinergic neurotransmitter (Chapter 164). It is the transmitter substance at neuromuscular junction. It is also secreted by other nerve endings and other cells.

Source of secretion

 i. Presynaptic terminals
 ii. Preganglionic parasympathetic nerve
 iii. Postganglionic parasympathetic nerve
 iv. Preganglionic sympathetic nerve
 v. Postganglionic sympathetic cholinergic nerves such as:
  a. Nerves supplying eccrine sweat glands
  b. Sympathetic vasodilator nerves in skeletal muscle
 vi. Nerves in amacrine cells of retina
 vii. Mast cell
 viii. Gastric mucosa
 ix. Lungs
 x. Many regions of brain.

Actions

Acetylcholine:
 i. Produces excitatory function of synapse by opening the sodium channels
 ii. Activates smooth muscles in GI tract, urinary tract and skeletal muscles
 iii. Inhibits cardiac function
 iv. Causes vasodilatation.

Destruction

Acetylcholine is very quick in action. Immediately after executing the action, it is destroyed by **acetylcholinesterase**. This enzyme is present in **basal lamina** of the **synaptic cleft.**

2. *Serotonin*

Serotonin is otherwise known as 5-hydroxytryptamine.

Source of secretion

Serotonin is secreted in the following structures:
 i. Hypothalamus
 ii. Limbic system
 iii. Cerebellum
 iv. Spinal cord

v. Retina
vi. Gastrointestinal tract
vii. Lungs
viii. Platelets.

Actions

Serotonin:
i. Is an inhibitory substance (Chapter 141)
ii. Inhibits impulses of pain sensation in posterior gray horn of spinal cord
iii. Causes mood depression and induces sleep (Chapter160)
iv. Causes vasoconstriction.

3. Histamine

Source of secretion

Histamine is secreted in nerve endings of hypothalamus, limbic cortex and other parts of cerebral cortex and spinal cord. Histamine is also released from tissues during allergic condition, inflammation or damage.

Actions

i. It is an excitatory neurotransmitter substance
ii. Histamine released from tissues causes vasodilatation and enhances the capillary permeability for fluid and plasma proteins from blood into the affected tissues. So, the accumulation of fluid with proteins develops local edema
iii. In GI tract, histamine increases the motility.

4. Substance P

Source of secretion

i. Nerve endings (first order neurons of pain pathway) in spinal cord and retina (Chapters 141 and 145)
ii. GI tract (by the presence of chyme).

Actions

i. Substance P is the neurotransmitter for pain
ii. It is also the neurotransmitter substance in GI tract. In GI tract, it increases the mixing and propulsive movements of small intestine.

5. Heparin

Source of secretion

i. Mast cells
ii. Basophils.

Actions

Heparin is a naturally produced anticoagulant (Refer Chapter 20 for other details).

6. Leptin

Leptin (in Greek, it means thin) is a protein hormone with 167 amino acids.

Source of secretion

Leptin is secreted by adipocytes in adipose tissues.

Actions

Leptin plays an important role in controlling the adipose tissue and food intake. Leptin acts on hypothalamus and inhibits the feeding center, resulting in stoppage of food intake (Chapter 149). At the same time, it also stimulates the metabolic reactions involved in utilization of fat stored in adipose tissue for energy. Thus, the circulating leptin level informs the brain about the energy storage and the necessity to regulate metabolic reactions, food intake and body weight.

Mode of action of leptin

Refer Chapter 149 for mode of leptin and leptin receptors.

7. Gastrointestinal Hormones

Gastrointestinal hormones are explained in Chapter 44.

■ LOCAL HORMONES PRODUCED IN BLOOD

Local hormones produced in the blood are:
1. Serotonin
2. Angiotensinogen
3. Kinins.

Serotonin is described above. Angiotensinogen is explained in Chapter 50.

■ KININS

Kinins are biologically active protein hormones which are circulating in blood. Kinins are of two types:
1. Bradykinin
2. Kallidin.

Along with other proteins of their family, kinins form the **kinin system** or **kinin-kallikrein system.**

Formation of Kinins

Kinins are cleaved from their precursors which are of two types:

1. **High-molecular-weight kinogen (HMW kinogen)** – precursor of bradykinin
2. **Low-molecular-weight kinogen (LMW kinogen)** – precursor of kallidin.

The cleavage of kinins from their precursors occurs by proteases called kallikreins, which are of two types, plasma kallikrein and tissue kallikrein.

Formation of bradykinin from HMW kinogen

HMW kinogen is α-2-globulin secreted in liver. It is hydrolyzed by plasma kallikrein to form bradykinin. Plasma kallikrein is circulating in blood in its inactive form called **prekallikrein.** Prekallikrein is converted into active **kallikrein** by activated factor XII, which initiates the intrinsic pathway of blood coagulation. Kallikrein also activates factor XII (see below).

Formation of kallidin LMW kinogen

LMW kinogen is secreted in many tissues. It is hydrolyzed by tissue kallikrein to form kallidin, which is also known as **lysylbradykinin.** Tissue kallikrein is present in many tissues like salivary glands, pancreas, intestine, sweat glands, kidneys and prostate.

Actions of Kinins

Bradykinin:

1. Dilates the blood vessels and decreases the blood pressure. It is considered as a potent vasodilator
2. Increases the blood flow throughout the body by its vasodilator action
3. Increases permeability of capillaries during inflammatory conditions, resulting in edema in the affected area
4. Stimulates pain receptors
5. Causes contraction of extravascular smooth muscles, especially smooth muscles of intestine.

Kallidin:

Kallidin is also a vasodilator hormone.

Actions of Kallikreins

1. Kallikreins hydrolyze the kinogens to form kinins (see above)
2. Along with HMW kinogen, the plasma kallikrein activates factor XII during blood coagulation (Chapter 20)
3. Kallikreins are potent **vasodilators.**

QUESTIONS IN ENDOCRINOLOGY

■ LONG QUESTIONS

1. Enumerate the hormones secreted by pituitary gland. Describe the actions and regulation of secretion of growth hormone. Write in brief about effects of hypersecretion of anterior pituitary gland.
2. Give an account of hypothalamo-hypophyseal relations.
3. Describe the synthesis, storage, release, transport, functions and regulation of secretion of thyroid hormones.
4. Explain the functions and regulation of secretion of parathormone. Add a note on the disorders of parathormone.
5. What is the importance of calcium in the body? Explain the regulation of blood calcium level. Add a note on tetany.
6. Enlist the hormones secreted by pancreas. Explain the functions and regulation of secretion of insulin.
7. Describe in detail the regulation of blood sugar level.
8. Classify the hormones secreted by adrenal cortex. Explain the actions and regulation of secretion of cortisol.
9. Enumerate the corticosteroids. Describe the actions and regulation of secretion of aldosterone.
10. What are catecholamines? Explain the synthesis, metabolism, actions and regulation of secretion of catecholamines.

■ SHORT QUESTIONS

1. Mechanism of hormonal action.
2. Mechanism of action of protein hormones.
3. Mechanism of action of steroid hormones.
4. Second messenger.
5. Growth hormone.
6. Thyroid-stimulating hormone.
7. Adrenocorticotropic hormone.
8. Gonadotropins.
9. Somatomedin.
10. Oxytocin.
11. Antidiuretic hormone.
12. Neuroendocrine reflex.
13. Milk ejection reflex.
14. Disorders of anterior pituitary gland.
15. Gigantism.
16. Acromegaly.
17. Dwarfism.
18. Acromicria.
19. Simmond disease.
20. Fröhlich syndrome.
21. Disorders of posterior pituitary gland.
22. Hypothalamo-hypophyseal relations.
23. Diabetes insipidus.
24. Synthesis of thyroid hormones.
25. Thyroglobulin.
26. Thyroxine.
27. Hyperthyroidism/thyrotoxicosis/Graves disease.
28. Hypothyroidism.
29. Goiter.
30. Cretinism.
31. Myxedema.
32. Antithyroid substances.
33. Parathormone.
34. Tetany.
35. Hypercalcemia/hypocalcemia.
36. Insulin.
37. Glucagon.
38. Somatostatin.
39. Diabetes mellitus.
40. Hyperinsulinism.
41. Cortisol.
42. Non-metabolic actions of cortisol.
43. Aldosterone.
44. Aldosterone escape.
45. Adrenal androgens.
46. Cushing syndrome or disease.
47. Hyperaldosteronism.
48. Atrial natriuretic peptide or endocrine function of heart.
49. Adrenogenital syndrome.
50. Virilism.
51. Addison disease.
52. Addisonian crisis.
53. Synthesis of catecholamines.
54. Actions of catecholamines.
55. Adrenergic receptors.
56. Dopamine.
57. Pheochromocytoma.
58. Functions of pineal gland.
59. Melatonin.
60. Functions of thymus.
61. Endocrine functions of kidney.
62. Local hormones.
63. Prostaglandins.
64. Acetylcholine.
65. Leptin.
66. Kinins.

Section
7

Reproductive System

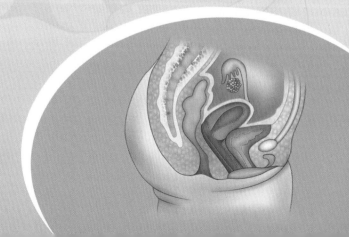

Male Reproductive System

Chapter
74

■ INTRODUCTION

Reproductive system ensures the continuation of species. **Gonads** are the primary reproductive organs which produce the gametes (egg or ovum); a pair of testes (singular = testis) produces sperms in males and a pair of ovaries produces ovum in females.

Normally, most of the animals including humans are either definite males or definite females. However, in some organisms like earthworms and snails, both sexes may be present in the same organism and this condition is known as **hermaphroditism.**

In humans and most of the higher animals, reproduction occurs sexually, i.e. by mating. However, there are some species like insects which can produce offsprings without mating.

Reproductive organs include:
1. Primary sex organs
2. Accessory sex organs.

Primary Sex Organs

Testes are the primary sex organs or gonads in males.

Accessory Sex Organs

Accessory sex organs in males are:
1. Seminal vesicles
2. Prostate gland

3. Urethra
4. Penis.

External and Internal Genitalia

Reproductive organs are generally classified into two groups, namely external genitalia (genital organs) and internal genitalia. External genital organs in males are scrotum, penis and urethra. Remaining sex organs constitute the internal genitalia.

■ FUNCTIONAL ANATOMY OF TESTES

Testes are the **primary sex organs** or gonads in males. There are two testes in almost all the species. In human beings, both the testes are ovoid or walnut-shaped bodies that are located and suspended in a sac-like structure called **scrotum.**

Each testis weighs about 15 to 19 g and measures about 5 × 3 cm. Testis is made up of about 900 coiled tubules known as **seminiferous tubules,** which produce sperms. Seminiferous tubules continue as the vas efferens, which form the **epididymis.** It is continued as **vas deferens.**

Vas deferens is also called **ductus deferens, spermatic deferens** or **sperm duct.** From epididymis in scrotum, the vas deferens extends on its one side upwards into abdominal cavity via inguinal canal. Terminal portion of vas deferens is called **ampulla** (Fig. 74.1). Ampulla of vas deferens joins ducts of seminal vesicle of same side, to form **ejaculatory duct.**

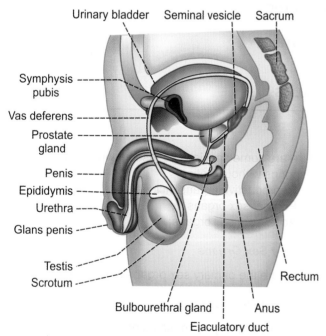

Urinary bladder   Seminal vesicle   Sacrum

Symphysis pubis

Vas deferens

Prostate gland

Penis

Epididymis

Urethra

Glans penis

Testis

Scrotum

Rectum

Bulbourethral gland   Anus

Ejaculatory duct

FIGURE 74.1: Male reproductive system and other organs of pelvis

Thus, there are two ejaculatory ducts each of which receives sperm from vas deferens and secretions of seminal vesicle on its own side. Both the ejaculatory ducts empty into a single **urethra.** Actually, ejaculatory ducts open into prostatic part of urethra.

■ COVERINGS OF TESTIS

Each testis is enclosed by three coverings.

1. Tunica Vasculosa

Tunica vasculosa is the innermost covering. It is made up of connective tissue and it is rich in blood vessels

2. Tunica Albuginea

Tunica albuginea is the middle covering. It is a dense fibrous capsule

3. Tunica Vaginalis

Tunica vaginalis is the outermost closed cleft like covering, formed by **mesothelial cells.** It is formed by visceral and parietal layers, which glide on one another and allow free movement of testes. Visceral layer of tunica vaginalis adheres to tunica albuginea and the parietal layer lines the inner surface of the scrotum.

Anterior and lateral surfaces of testis are covered by all the three layers. Posterior surface is covered by tunica albuginea only.

■ PARENCHYMA OF TESTIS

Lobules of Testis

Tunica albuginea on the posterior surface of testis is thickened to form the **mediastinum testis.** From this, the connective tissue septa called **septula testis** radiate into testis and bind with tunica albuginea at various points. Because of this, testis is divided into a number of **pyramidal lobules,** with bases directed towards the periphery and the apices towards the mediastinum (Fig. 74.2).

The septula do not form complete partition so the lobules of testis anastomose with one another at many places. Each testis has about 200 to 300 lobules.

Seminiferous Tubules

Each lobule contains 1 to 4 coiled tubules known as the seminiferous tubules, which are surrounded and supported by interlobular connective tissue. Seminiferous tubules do not end bluntly, but form single, double or triple arches. Limbs of an arch are not in the same lobule (fig. 74.2). Other details of seminiferous tubules are given below.

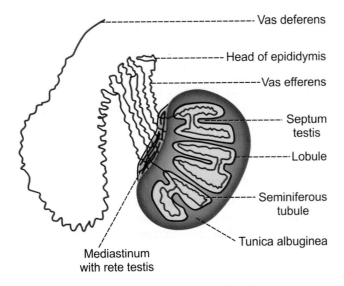

FIGURE 74.2: Structure of testis

Rete Testis

Rete testis is a network of thin-walled channels present in mediastinum. All the seminiferous tubules open into the rete testis.

Vas Efferens

From rete testis, 8 to 15 tubules called vas efferens arise. Vas efferens join together and form the head of epididymis and then converge to form the duct of epididymis (Fig. 74.3).

Epididymis

Duct of epididymis is an enormously convoluted tubule, with a length of about 4 meter. It begins at head, where it receives vas efferens.

Vas Deferens

At the caudal pole of testis, epididymis turns sharply upon itself and continues as vas deferens, without any definite demarcation.

Interstitial Cells of Leydig

Interstitial cells of Leydig are the hormone secreting cells of testis, lying in between the seminiferous tubules.

■ SEMINIFEROUS TUBULES

Seminiferous tubules are thread-like convoluted tubular structures which produce the spermatozoa or sperms. There are about 400 to 600 seminiferous tubules in each testis. Each tubule is 30 to 70 cm long with a diameter of 150 to 300 μ.

Wall of the seminiferous tubule is formed by three layers:

1. Outer capsule or tunica propria, formed by fibro-elastic connective tissue
2. Thin homogeneous basement membrane
3. Complex stratified epithelium, which consists of two types of cells:
   i. Spermatogenic cells or germ cells
   ii. Sertoli cells or supporting cells.

Spermatogenic Cells

Spermatogenic cells or germ cells present in seminiferous tubules are **precursor cells** of spermatozoa. These cells lie in between **Sertoli cells** and are arranged in an orderly manner in 4 to 8 layers.

In children, the testis is not fully developed. Therefore, the **spermatogenic cells** are in primitive stage called **spermatogonia.** With the onset of puberty, spermatogonia develop into sperms through different stages.

Stages of spermatogenic cells

Different stages of spermatogenic cells seen from periphery to the lumen of seminiferous tubules are:

1. Spermatogonium
2. Primary spermatocyte
3. Secondary spermatocyte
4. Spermatid.

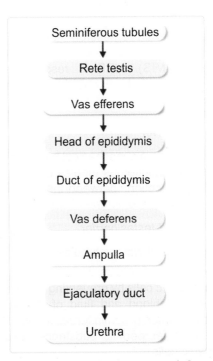

FIGURE 74.3: Pathway for the passage of sperms

Sertoli Cells

Sertoli cells are the **supporting cells** for spermatogenic cells in seminiferous tubules. These cells are also called **sustentacular cells** or **nurse cells.**

Sertoli cells are the large and tall irregular columnar cells, extending from basement membrane to lumen of the seminiferous tubule. Germ cells present in seminiferous tubule are attached to Sertoli cells by means of cytoplasmic connection. This attachment between germ cells and Sertoli cells exists till the matured spermatozoa are released into the lumen of seminiferous tubules.

Functions of Sertoli cells

Sertoli cells provide support, protection and nourishment for the spermatogenic cells present in seminiferous tubules.

Sertoli cells:

1. Support and **nourish** the spermatogenic cells till the spermatozoa are released from them
2. Secrete the enzyme **aromatase,** which converts androgens into estrogen
3. Secrete **androgen-binding protein** (ABP), which is essential for testosterone activity, especially during spermatogenesis
4. Secrete **estrogen-binding protein** (EBP)
5. Secrete **inhibin,** which inhibits FSH release from anterior pituitary
6. Secrete **activin,** which has opposite action of inhibin (increases FSH release)
7. Secrete **müllerian regression factor** (MRF) in fetal testes. MRF is also called **müllerian inhibiting substance** (MIS). MRF is responsible for the regression of müllerian duct during sex differentiation in fetus.

Blood-testes Barrier

Blood-testes barrier is a mechanical barrier that separates blood from seminiferous tubules of the testes. It is formed by tight junctions between the adjacent Sertoli cells, near the basal membrane of seminiferous tubule.

Functions of blood-testes barrier

1. Protection of seminiferous tubules

Blood-testes barrier protects the seminiferous tubules and spermatogenic cells by preventing the entry of toxic substances from blood and fluid of the surrounding tissues into the lumen of seminiferous tubules. However, blood-testes barrier permits substances essential for spermatogenic cells.

Substances prevented by blood-testes barrier:
 i. Large molecules including proteins, polysaccharides and cytotoxic substances
 ii. Medium-sized molecules like galactose.

Substances permitted by blood-testes barrier:
 i. Nutritive substances essential for spermatogenic cells
 ii. Hormones necessary for spermatogenesis
 iii. Water.

2. Prevention of autoimmune disorders

Blood-testes barrier also prevents the development of autoimmune disorders by inhibiting the movement of antigenic products of spermatogenesis, from testis into blood.

Damage of blood-testes barrier

Blood-testes barrier is commonly damaged by trauma or viral infection like **mumps.** Whenever, the blood-testes barrier is damaged the sperms enter the blood. The immune system of the body is activated, resulting in the production of **autoantibodies** against sperms. The antibodies destroy the germ cells, leading to consequent **sterility.**

■ FUNCTIONS OF TESTES

Testes performs two functions:
1. Gametogenic function: Spermatogenesis
2. Endocrine function: Secretion of hormones.

■ GAMETOGENIC FUNCTIONS OF TESTES – SPERMATOGENESIS

Spermatogenesis is the process by which the male gametes called **spermatozoa** (sperms) are formed from the primitive **spermatogenic cells** (spermatogonia) in the testis (Fig. 74.4). It takes 74 days for the formation of sperm from a **primitive germ cell.** Throughout the process of spermatogenesis, the spermatogenic cells have cytoplasmic attachment with Sertoli cells. **Sertoli cells** supply all the necessary materials for spermatogenesis through the cytoplasmic attachment.

■ STAGES OF SPERMATOGENESIS

Spermatogenesis occurs in four stages:
1. Stage of proliferation
2. Stage of growth
3. Stage of maturation
4. Stage of transformation.

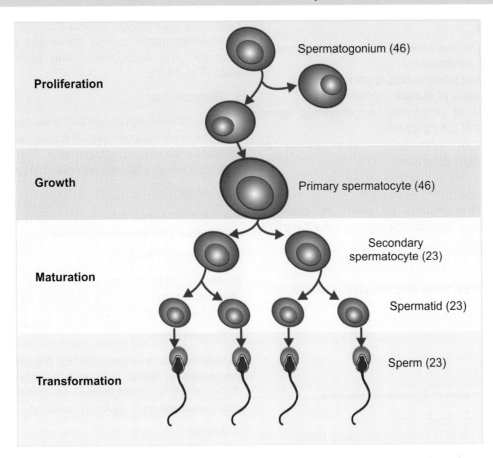

FIGURE 74.4: Spermatogenesis. Number in parenthesis indicate chromosomal number

1. *Stage of Proliferation*

Each **spermatogonium** contains **diploid number** (23 pairs) of chromosomes. One member of each pair is from maternal origin and the other one from paternal origin. The 23 pairs include 22 pairs of **autosomal chromosomes** and one pair of **sex chromosomes.** Sex chromosomes are one X chromosome and one Y chromosome.

During the proliferative stage, spermatogonia divide by mitosis, without any change in chromosomal number. In man, there are usually seven generations of spermatogonia. The last generation enters the stage of growth as **primary spermatocyte.**

During this stage, the spermatogonia migrate along with Sertoli cells towards the lumen of seminiferous tubule.

2. *Stage of Growth*

In this stage, the primary spermatocyte grows into a large cell. Apart from growth, there is no other change in spermatocyte during this stage.

3. *Stage of Maturation*

After reaching the full size, each primary spermatocyte quickly undergoes meiotic or maturation division, which occurs in two phases:

First phase

In the first phase, each **primary spermatocyte** divides into two **secondary spermatocytes.** The significance of the first meiotic division is that each secondary spermatocyte receives only the **haploid** or **half the number of chromosomes.** 23 chromosomes include 22 autosomes and a X or a Y chromosome.

Second phase

During this phase, each secondary spermatocyte undergoes second meiotic division, resulting in two smaller cells called **spermatids.** Each spermatid has **haploid** number of chromosomes.

4. *Stage of Transformation*

There is no further division. Spermatids are transformed into matured **spermatozoa** (sperms), by means of **spermeogenesis** and released by **spermination.**

Spermeogenesis

Spermeogenesis is the process by which spermatids become matured spermatozoa.

Changes taking place during spermeogenesis:
  i. Condensation of nuclear material
  ii. Formation of acrosome, mitochondrial spiral filament and tail structures
  iii. Removal of extraneous (extra volume of nonessential) cytoplasm.

Spermination

Spermination is the process by which the matured sperms are released from Sertoli cells into the lumen of seminiferous tubules.

Refer Chapter 77 for structure of sperm.

■ **FACTORS AFFECTING SPERMATOGENESIS**

Spermatogenesis is influenced by:
  1. Sertoli cells
  2. Hormones
  3. Other factors.

1. *Role of Sertoli Cell in Spermatogenesis*

Sertoli cells influence spermatogenesis by:
  i. Supporting and nourishing the germ cells
  ii. Providing hormonal substances necessary for spermatogenesis
  iii. Secreting androgen-binding protein (ABP), which is essential for testosterone activity, particularly on spermatogenesis
  iv. Releasing sperms into the lumen of seminiferous tubules (spermination).

2. *Role of Hormones in Spermatogenesis*

Spermatogenesis is influenced by many hormones, which act either directly or indirectly: Table 74.1 gives the hormones essential for each stage of spermatogenesis.

Hormones necessary for spermatogenesis are:
  i. Follicle-stimulating hormone (FSH)
  ii. Testosterone
  iii. Estrogen
  iv. Luteinizing hormone (LH)
  v. Growth hormone (GH)
  vi. Inhibin
  vii. Activin.

i. *Follicule-stimulating hormone*

Follicule-stimulating hormone is responsible for the **initiation of spermatogenesis.** It binds with Sertoli cells and spermatogonia and induces the proliferation of spermatogonia. It also stimulates the formation of estrogen and androgen-binding protein from Sertoli cells (Fig. 74.5).

ii. *Testosterone*

Testosterone is responsible for the sequence of remaining stages in spermatogenesis. It is also responsible for the **maintenance of spermatogenesis.** Testosterone activity is largely influenced by androgen-binding protein.

iii. *Estrogen*

Estrogen is formed from testosterone in Sertoli cells. It is necessary for **spermeogenesis.**

iv. *Luteinizing Hormone*

In males, this hormone is called **interstitial cell-stimulating** hormone. It is essential for the **secretion of testosterone** from Leydig cells.

v. *Growth Hormone*

Growth hormone is essential for the **general metabolic processes** in testis. It is also necessary for the proliferation of spermatogonia. In pituitary dwarfs, the spermatogenesis is severely affected.

vi. *Inhibin*

Inhibin is a peptide hormone and serves as a transforming growth factor. It is secreted by Sertoli cells. In females, it is secreted by granulosa cells of ovarian follicles. Its secretion is stimulated by FSH.

Inhibin plays an important role in the **regulation of spermatogenesis** by inhibiting FSH secretion through feedback mechanism. FSH secreted from anterior pituitary induces spermatogenesis by stimulating Sertoli cells. It also stimulates the secretion of inhibin from Sertoli cells. So, when the rate of spermatogenesis increases, there is a simultaneous increase in inhibin secretion also. Inhibin in turn, acts on anterior pituitary and inhibits the secretion of FSH, leading to decrease in the pace of spermatogenesis.

TABLE 74.1: Hormones necessary for spermatogenesis

Stage of spermatogenesis	Hormones necessary
Stage of proliferation	Follicle-stimulating hormone Growth hormone
Stage of growth	Testosterone Growth hormone
Stage of maturation	Testosterone Growth hormone
Stage of transformation	Testosterone Estrogen

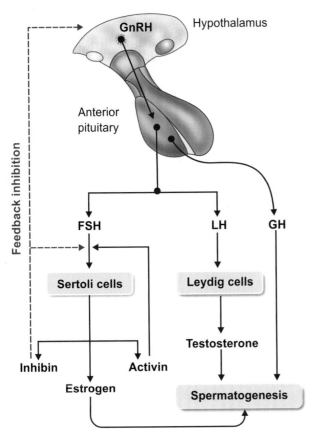

FIGURE 74.5: Role of hormones in spermatogenesis. Blue arrow = Stimulation, Red dotted arrow = inhibition, GnRH = Gonadotropin-releasing hormone, FSH = Follicle-stimulating hormone, LH = Lutinizing hormone, GH = Growth hormone.

It is believed that inhibin also inhibits FSH secretion indirectly by inhibiting GnRH secretion from hypothalamus.

vii. *Activin*

Activin is also a peptide hormone secreted in gonads along with inhibin. The exact location of its secretion in testis is not known. It is suggested that activin is secreted by Sertoli cells and Leydig cells.

Activin has opposite actions of inhibin. It increases the secretion of FSH and accelerates spermatogenesis.

3. *Role of Other Factors in Spermatogenesis*

i. *Increase in body temperature*

Increase in body temperature prevents spermato-genesis. Normally, the temperature in scrotum is about 2°C less than the body temperature. This low temperature is essential for spermatogenesis. When the temperature increases, the spermatogenesis stops. It is very common in **cryptorchidism** (undescended testes).

In cryptorchidism, the testes are in the abdomen, where the temperature is always higher than that of scrotum. High temperature in the abdomen causes degeneration of seminiferous tubules and stoppage of spermatogenesis.

ii. *Diseases*

Infectious diseases such as mumps cause degeneration of seminiferous tubules and stoppage of spermatogenesis.

■ ENDOCRINE FUNCTIONS OF TESTES

■ HORMONES SECRETED BY TESTES

Testes secrete male sex hormones, which are collectively called the **androgens.**

Androgens secreted by testes are:
1. Testosterone
2. Dihydrotestosterone
3. Androstenedione.

Among these three androgens, testosterone is secreted in large quantities. However, dihydro-testosterone is more active.

Female sex hormones, namely estrogen and progesterone are also found in testes. Two more hormones activin and inhibin are also secreted in testes. However, these two hormones do not have **androgenic actions.**

Source of Secretion of Androgens

Androgens are secreted in large quantities by testes and in small quantity by adrenal cortex.

Testes

In testes, androgens are secreted by the interstitial cells of Leydig, which form 20% of mass of adult testis. Leydig cells are numerous in newborn male baby and in adult male. But in childhood, these cells are scanty or nonexisting. So, the secretion of androgens occurs in newborn babies and after puberty.

Adrenal cortex

Androgens secreted by zona reticularis of adrenal cortex are testosterone, androstenedione and dehydroepiandrosterone. Adrenal androgens do not have any significant physiological actions because of their small quantity. In abnormal conditions, the hypersecretion of adrenal androgens results in sexual disorders (Chapter 70).

Chemistry

Testosterone is a C_{19} steroid.

Synthesis

Androgens are steroid hormones synthesized from cholesterol. Androgens are also synthesized directly from acetate. Synthesis of male sex hormones is given in Fig. 70.2, Chapter 70.

Plasma Level and Transport

Plasma level of testosterone in an adult male varies between 300 and 700 ng/dL. In adult female, the testosterone level is 30 to 60 mg/dL.

Two thirds of testosterone is transported in plasma by **gonadal steroid-binding globulin.** It is β-globulin in nature and it is also called **sex steroid-binding globulin.** The remaining one third of testosterone is transported by **albumin.**

Metabolism

In many target tissues, testosterone is converted into **dehydrotestosterone,** which is the most active androgen. In some of the tissues such as adipose tissue, hypothalamus and liver, testosterone is converted into **estradiol.** Major portion of testosterone is degraded in liver. It is converted into inactive forms of **androsterone** and **dehydroepiandrosterone.** These two substances are later conjugated and excreted through urine.

■ TESTOSTERONE SECRETION IN DIFFERENT PERIODS OF LIFE

Testosterone secretion starts at 7th week of fetal life by fetal genital ridge. Fetal testes begin to secrete testosterone at about 2nd to 4th month of fetal life. In fetal life, testosterone secretion from testes is stimulated by human chorionic gonadotropins, secreted by placenta.

But in childhood, practically no testosterone is secreted approximately until 10 to 12 years of age. Afterwards, the testosterone secretion starts and it increases rapidly at the onset of puberty and lasts through most of the remaining part of life. The secretion starts decreasing after 40 years and becomes almost zero by the age of 90 years (Fig. 74.6).

■ FUNCTIONS OF TESTOSTERONE

In general, testosterone is responsible for the distinguishing characters of masculine body. It also plays an important role in fetal life.

Functions of Testosterone in Fetal Life

Testosterone performs three functions in fetus:
1. Sex differentiation in fetus

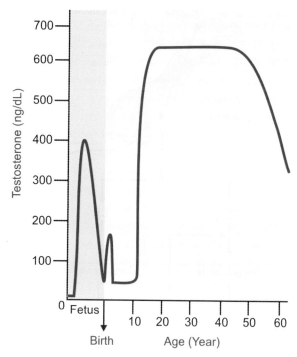

FIGURE 74.6: Plasma testosterone in different ages of male humans

2. Development of accessory sex organs
3. Descent of the testes.

1. Sex differentiation in fetus

Sex chromosomes are responsible for the determination of sex of the fetus (Chapter 84), whereas testosterone is responsible for the sex differentiation of fetus.

Fetus has two genital ducts:
  i. **Müllerian duct,** which gives rise to female accessory sex organs such as vagina, uterus and fallopian tube
  ii. **Wolffian duct,** which gives rise to male accessory sex organs such as epididymis, vas deferens and seminal vesicles.

If testosterone is secreted from the genital ridge of the fetus at about 7th week of intrauterine life, the müllerian duct system disappears and male sex organs develop from Wolffian duct.

In addition to testosterone, **müllerian regression factor** (MRF) secreted by Sertoli cells is also responsible for regression of müllerian duct.

In the absence of testosterone, Wolffian duct regresses and female sex organs develop from müllerian duct.

2. Development of accessory sex organs and external genitalia

Testosterone is also essential for the growth of the external genitalia, viz. penis and scrotum and other accessory sex organs, namely genital ducts, seminal vesicles and prostate.

3. Descent of testes

Descent of testes is the process by which testes enter scrotum from abdominal cavity. Initially, testes are developed in the abdominal cavity and are later pushed down into the scrotum through inguinal canal, just before birth. The process by which testes enter the scrotum is called the descent of testes. Testosterone is necessary for descent of testes.

Cryptorchidism

Cryptorchidism is a congenital disorder characterized by the failure of one or both the testes to descent from abdomen into scrotum. In such case, the testes are called **undescended testes.** Males with untreated testes are prone for **testicular cancer.**

Treatment

Administration of testosterone or gonadotropic hormones (which stimulate Leydig cells) causes descent of testes, provided the **inguinal canal** is large enough to allow the passage of testes. Surgery is required if the inguinal canal is narrow.

Functions of Testosterone in Adult Life

Testosterone has two important functions in adult:
1. Effect on sex organs
2. Effect on secondary sexual characters.

1. Effect on sex organs

Testosterone increases the size of penis, scrotum and the testes after puberty. All these organs are enlarged at least 8 folds between the onset of puberty and the age of 20 years, under the influence of testosterone. Testosterone is also necessary for spermatogenesis.

2. Effect on secondary sexual characters

Secondary sexual characters are the physical and behavioral characteristics that distinguish the male from female. These characters appear at the time of puberty in humans. Testosterone is responsible for the development of secondary sexual characters in males.

Secondary sexual characters in males:

i. Effect on muscular growth

One of the most important male sexual characters is the development of musculature after puberty. Muscle mass increases by about 50%, due to the anabolic effect of testosterone on proteins. Testosterone accelerates the transport of amino acids into the muscle cells, synthesis of proteins and storage of proteins. Testosterone also decreases the breakdown of proteins.

ii. Effect on bone growth

After puberty, testosterone increases the thickness of bones by increasing the bone matrix and deposition of calcium. It is because of the **protein anabolic activity** of testosterone. Deposition of calcium is secondary to the increase in bone matrix.

In addition to increase in the size and strength of bones, testosterone also causes early fusion of epiphyses of long bones with shaft. So, if testes are removed before puberty, the fusion of epiphyses is delayed and the height of the person increases.

iii. Effect on shoulder and pelvic bones

Testosterone causes broadening of shoulders and it has a specific effect on pelvis, which results in:
  a. Lengthening of pelvis
  b. Funnel-like shape of pelvis.
  c. Narrowing of pelvic outlet.
   Thus, pelvis in males is different from that of females, which is broad and round or oval in shape.

iv. Effect on skin

Testosterone increases the thickness of skin and ruggedness of subcutaneous tissue. These changes in skin are due to the deposition of proteins in skin. It also increases the quantity of melanin pigment, which is responsible for the deepening of the skin color.

Testosterone enhances the secretory activity of sebaceous glands. So, at the time of puberty, when the body is exposed to sudden increase in testosterone secretion, the excess secretion of sebum leads to development of **acne** on the face. After few years, the skin gets adapted to testosterone secretion and the acne disappears.

v. Effect on hair distribution

Testosterone causes male type of hair distribution on the body, i.e. hair growth over the pubis, along linea alba up to umbilicus, on face, chest and other parts of the body such as back and limbs. In males, the pubic hair has the base of the triangle downwards where as in females it is upwards. Testosterone decreases the hair growth on the head and may cause baldness, if there is genetic background.

vi. *Effect on voice*

At the time of adolescence, the boys have a **cracking voice.** It is because of the testosterone effect, which causes:

a. Hypertrophy of laryngeal muscles
b. Enlargement of larynx and lengthening
c. Thickening of vocal cords.

Later, the cracking voice changes gradually into a typical adult male voice with a bossing sound.

vii. *Effect on basal metabolic rate*

At the time of puberty and earlier part of adult life, the testosterone increases the basal metabolic rate to about 5% to 10% by its anabolic effects on protein metabolism.

viii. *Effect on electrolyte and water balance*

Testosterone increases the sodium reabsorption from renal tubules, along with water reabsorption. It leads to increase in ECF volume.

ix. *Effect on blood*

Testosterone has got **erythropoietic action.** So, after puberty, testosterone causes mild increase in RBC count. It also increases the blood volume by increasing the water retention and ECF volume.

■ MODE OF ACTION OF TESTOSTERONE

Testosterone combines with receptor proteins. The testosterone-receptor complex migrates to nucleus, binds with a nuclear protein and induces the DNA-RNA transcription process. In 30 minutes, the RNA polymer is activated and the concentration of RNA increases. The quantity of DNA also increases.

So, the testosterone primarily stimulates the protein synthesis in the target cells, which are responsible for the development of secondary sexual characters.

Testosterone is converted into dihydrotestosterone (DHT) in the target cells of some accessory sex organs such as epididymis and penis. DHT combines with receptor proteins and the DHT-receptor complex induces the DNA-RNA transcription process. DHT-receptor complex is more stable than testosterone-receptor complex.

In brain, testosterone is converted into estrogen (estradiol).

■ REGULATION OF TESTOSTERONE SECRETION

In Fetus

During fetal life, the testosterone secretion from testes is stimulated by **human chorionic gonadotropin,** which has the properties similar to those of luteinizing hormone. Human chorionic gonadotropin stimulates the development of Leydig cells in the fetal testes and promotes testosterone secretion.

In Adults

Luteinizing hormone (LH) or **interstitial cell stimulating** hormone (ICSH) stimulates the Leydig cells and the quantity of testosterone secreted is directly proportional to the amount of LH available.

Secretion of LH from anterior pituitary gland is stimulated by luteinizing hormone releasing hormone (LHRH) from hypothalamus.

Feedback Control

Testosterone regulates its own secretion by **negative feedback** mechanism. It acts on hypothalamus and inhibits the secretion of LHRH. When LHRH secretion is inhibited, LH is not released from anterior pituitary, resulting in stoppage of testosterone secretion from testes. On the other hand, when testosterone production is low, lack of inhibition of hypothalamus leads to secretion of testosterone through LHRH and LH (Fig. 74.7).

■ ANABOLIC STEROIDS

Anabolic steroids are the synthetic forms of testosterone, which are used to increase the growth of muscles and bones. Like androgens, these steroids also increase the growth of muscles and bones by accelerating protein synthesis (anabolic effect). These drugs are also called **anabolic-androgenic steroids** (AAS).

Therapeutic Uses of Anabolic Steroids

1. Growth stimulation
2. Bone marrow stimulation
3. Hormone replacement therapy
4. Induction of puberty in males.

Abuse of Anabolic Steroids

Anabolic steroids are commonly used by athletes to improve their performances during competitions, particularly in professional sports. Organizations of many sports have banned the use of anabolic steroids by their athletes.

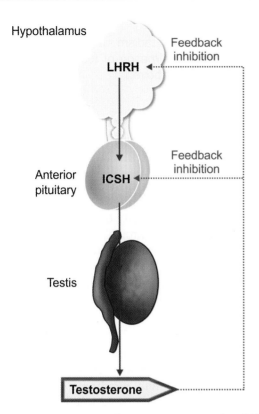

FIGURE 74.7: Regulation of testosterone secretion. LHRH = Luteinizing hormone-releasing hormone, ICSH = Interstitial cell-stimulating hormone.

■ PRODUCTION OF FEMALE SEX HORMONES IN MALES

In addition to androgens, female sex hormones are also produced in testes.

Estrogen

Small amount of estrogen is produced in males. Estrogen level in plasma of normal adult male is 12 to 34 pg/mL. Estrogens have three sources of production in males.

1. Adrenal Cortex

Adrenal cortex secretes small quantity of estrogen. Refer Chapter 70 for details.

2. Testes

Up to 20% of estrogen in males is produced in testes. Estrogen is formed from androgens in Sertoli cells of testes, by the influence of the enzyme aromatase.

3. Other Organs

About 80% of estrogen is formed from androgens in other organs, particularly liver.

Progesterone

Progesterone is also produced from androgens in males though the quantity is very less. Plasma progesterone level in normal adult male is 0.3 ng/mL.

■ MALE ANDROPAUSE OR CLIMACTERIC

Male andropause or climacteric is the condition in men, characterized by emotional and physical changes in the body, due to low androgen level with aging. It is also called **viropause.**

After the age of 50, testosterone secretion starts declining. It is accompanied by decrease in number and secretory activity of Leydig cells. Low level of testosterone increases the secretion of FSH and LH, which leads to some changes in the body. It does not affect most of the men. But some men develop symptoms similar to those of **female menopausal syndrome** (Chapter 82). Common symptoms are hot flashes, illusions of suffocation and mood changes.

■ APPLIED PHYSIOLOGY

■ EFFECTS OF EXTIRPATION OF TESTES

Extirpation (removal) of testes is called castration. Effects of castration depend upon the age when testes are removed.

1. Effects of Extirpation of Testes before Puberty – Eunuchism

If a boy looses the testes before puberty, he continues to have infantile sexual characters throughout his life and this condition is called eunuchism. Height of the person is slightly more but the bones are weak and thin. Muscles become weak and shoulder remains narrow.

Sex organs do not increase in size and the male secondary sexual characters do not develop. The voice remains like that of a child.

There is abnormal deposition of fat on buttocks, hip, pubis and breast, resembling the feminine distribution.

2. Effects of Extirpation of Testes Immediately after Puberty

If testes are removed after puberty, some of the male secondary sexual characters revert to those of a child and other masculine characters are retained.

Sex organs are depressed. Seminal vesicles and prostate undergo atrophy. Penis remains smaller. Voice remains mostly masculine but other secondary sexual characters like masculine hair distribution, musculature and thickness of bones are lost. There may be loss of sexual desire and sexual activities.

3. *Effect of Extirpation of Testes in Adults*

Removal of testes in adults does not cause loss of secondary sexual characters. But, accessory sex organs start degenerating. The sexual desire is not totally lost. Erection occurs but ejaculation is rare because of degeneration of accessory sex organs and lack of sperms.

■ HYPERGONADISM IN MALES

Hypergonadism is the condition characterized by hypersecretion of sex hormones from gonads.

Cause

Hypergonadism in males is mainly due to the tumor of Leydig cells. It is common in **prepubertal boys** who develop **precocious pseudopuberty.**

Symptoms

There is a rapid growth of musculature and bones. But, the height of the person is less because of early closure of epiphysis. There is excess development of sex organs and secondary sexual characters.

The tumors also secrete estrogenic hormones, which cause **gynecomastia** (the enlargement of breasts).

■ HYPOGONADISM IN MALES

Hypogonadism is a condition characterized by reduction in the functional activity of gonads.

Causes

Hypogonadism in males is due to various abnormalities of testes:
1. Congenital nonfunctioning of testes
2. Under-developed testes due to absence of human chorionic gonadotropins in fetal life
3. Cryptorchidism, associated with partial or total degeneration of testes
4. Castration
5. Absence of androgen receptors in testes
6. Disorder of the gonadotropes (cells secreting gona-dotropins) in anterior pituitary
7. Hypothalamic disorder.

Signs and Symptoms

Clinical picture of male hypogonadism depends upon whether the testicular deficiency develops before or after puberty.

Before puberty

Features of hypogonadism are similar to those developed due to extirpation of testes before puberty, which are described above.

After puberty

Symptoms are similar to those developed due to the removal of testes after puberty (see above).

In adults

Same symptoms, which develop after extirpation of testes, occur in this condition.

Hypogonadism caused by testicular disorders increases the gonadotropin secretion and the condition is called **hypergonadotropic hypogonadism.** Hypogonadism that occurs due to deficiency of gonadotropins (pituitary or hypothalamic disorder) is called **hypogonadotropic hypogonadism.**

Fröhlich Syndrome

Fröhlich syndrome is the disorder characterized by obesity and hypogonadism in adolescent boys. It is also called **adiposogenital syndrome** or **hypothalamic eunuchism.** Refer Chapter 66 for details.

■ ACCESSORY SEX ORGANS IN MALES

Seminal Vesicles

Seminal vesicles are explained in Chapter 75.

Prostate gland

Prostate gland is explained in Chapter 76.

Urethra

Urethra in male has both reproductive and urinary functions. Refer Chapter 57 for details of urethra. Urethra contains mucus glands throughout its length, which are called **glands of Littre.** The bilateral **bulbourethral glands** or **Cowper** glands also open into the urethra.

Penis

Penis is the male genital organ. Urethra passes through penis and opens to the exterior. Penis is formed by three erectile tissue masses, i.e. a paired **corpora cavernosa** and an unpaired **corpus spongiosum.** Corpus spongiosum surrounds the urethra and terminates distally to form **glans penis.**

Seminal Vesicles

- ■ STRUCTURE OF SEMINAL VESICLES
- ■ PROPERTIES AND COMPOSITION OF SEMINAL FLUID
  - ■ PROPERTIES
  - ■ COMPOSITION
- ■ FUNCTIONS OF SEMINAL FLUID
  - ■ NUTRITION TO SPERMS
  - ■ CLOTTING OF SEMEN
  - ■ FERTILIZATION

■ STRUCTURE OF SEMINAL VESICLES

Seminal vesicles are the paired glands situated in lower abdomen on either side of prostate gland behind urinary bladder. Each seminal vesicle is a hollow sac of irregular shape and is lined by complexly folded mucous membrane.

Epithelial cells of the mucous membrane are secretory in nature and secrete seminal fluid. Duct of seminal vesicle from each side joins with **ampulla of vas deferens** to form **ejaculatory duct.** Thus seminal fluid is emptied into ejaculatory ducts, which open into urethra. Refer Chapter 57 for details.

■ PROPERTIES AND COMPOSITION OF SEMINAL FLUID

■ PROPERTIES

Seminal fluid is mucoid and viscous in nature. It is neutral or slightly alkaline in reaction. It adds to the bulk of semen as it forms 60% of the total semen.

■ COMPOSITION

Seminal vesicles secrete several important substances. Refer Figure 77.1 for the products of seminal fluid.

■ FUNCTIONS OF SEMINAL FLUID

■ NUTRITION TO SPERMS

Fructose and other nutritive substances in seminal fluid are utilized by sperms after being ejaculated into the female genital tract.

■ CLOTTING OF SEMEN

Immediately after ejaculation, semen **clots** because of the conversion of fibrinogen from seminal fluid into fibrin.

■ FERTILIZATION

Prostaglandin of seminal fluid enhances fertilization of ovum by:

1. Increasing the receptive capacity of cervical mucosa for sperms
2. Initiating **reverse peristaltic movement** of uterus and fallopian tubes. This in turn, increases the rate of transport of sperms in female genital tract during coitus (oxytocin is also responsible for this process).

Prostate Gland

> - ■ STRUCTURE OF PROSTATE GLAND
> - ■ PROPERTIES AND COMPOSITION OF PROSTATIC FLUID
>   - ■ PROPERTIES
>   - ■ COMPOSITION
> - ■ FUNCTIONS OF PROSTATIC FLUID
>   - ■ MAINTENANCE OF SPERM MOTILITY
>   - ■ CLOTTING OF SEMEN
>   - ■ LYSIS OF COAGULUM
> - ■ APPLIED PHYSIOLOGY – ENLARGEMENT OF PROSTATE GLAND

■ STRUCTURE OF PROSTATE GLAND

Human prostate gland weighs about 40 g. It consists of 20 to 30 separate glands, which open separately into the urethra. These glands are **tubuloalveolar** in nature. Epithelial lining of these glands is made up of columnar cells. Prostate secretes **prostatic fluid,** which is emptied into **prostatic urethra** through **prostatic sinuses** (Chapter 57).

■ PROPERTIES AND COMPOSITION OF PROSTATIC FLUID

■ PROPERTIES

Prostate fluid is a thin, milky and alkaline fluid. It forms 30% of total semen.

■ COMPOSITION

Refer Figure 77.1 for the products secreted by prostate gland.

■ FUNCTIONS OF PROSTATIC FLUID

■ MAINTENANCE OF SPERM MOTILITY

Prostatic fluid provides optimum pH for the motility of sperms. Generally, sperms are nonmotile at a pH of less than 6.0. There are some factors, which decrease the pH and motility of sperm both in vas deferens and female genital tract.

In vas deferens

End products of metabolic activities in the sperm make the fluid in vas deferens acidic, so that the sperms are nonmotile.

In female genital tract

Vaginal secretions in females are highly acidic with a pH of 3.5 to 4.0. So, when semen is ejaculated into female genital tract at coitus, sperms are nonmotile initially.

However, the alkaline prostatic secretion, which is also present in semen neutralizes the acidity in vagina and maintains a pH of 6.0 to 6.5. At this pH, the sperms become motile and chances of fertilization are enhanced.

■ CLOTTING OF SEMEN

The clotting enzymes present in prostatic fluid convert fibrinogen (from seminal vesicles) into **coagulum.** It is essential for holding the sperms in uterine cervix.

■ LYSIS OF COAGULUM

The coagulum is dissolved by fibrinolysin of prostatic fluid, so that the sperms become motile.

■ **APPLIED PHYSIOLOGY –**
  ENLARGEMENT OF PROSTATE GLAND

Enlargement of prostate gland is of two types:
  1. Benign enlargement
  2. Malignant enlargement.

1. *Benign enlargement*

Hyperplasia of glandular structures and connective tissues causes benign **(nonmalignant)** enlargement of prostate gland. It occurs in some men after 60 years of age, due to unknown causes.

Enlarged prostate gland stretches the urethra and obstructs urine outflow from bladder.

Common symptoms are increase in the frequency of urination, difficulty in urination, dribbling of urine after urination and occasional renal failure.

2. *Malignant enlargement*

Malignant enlargement **(cancer)** of prostate gland also causes obstruction of urinary passage. In addition, the **metastasis** (spread of cancer from primary site to other places) affects the other tissues, particularly bones.

Semen

- ■ INTRODUCTION
- ■ NATURE OF SEMEN
- ■ PROPERTIES OF SEMEN
- ■ COMPOSITION OF SEMEN
  - ■ SPERM
  - ■ PRODUCTS FROM SEMINAL VESICLES
  - ■ PRODUCTS FROM PROSTATE GLAND
- ■ SEMEN ANALYSIS
- ■ QUALITIES OF SEMEN REQUIRED FOR FERTILITY
- ■ APPLIED PHYSIOLOGY

■ INTRODUCTION

Semen is a white or grey fluid that contains sperms. It is the collection of fluids from testes, seminal vesicles, prostate gland and bulbourethral glands. Semen is discharged during sexual act and the process of discharge of semen is called **ejaculation.**

Testes contribute sperms. Prostate secretion gives milky appearance to the semen. Secretions from seminal vesicles and bulbourethral glands provide mucoid consistency to semen.

■ NATURE OF SEMEN

At the time of ejaculation, human semen is liquid in nature. Immediately, it coagulates and after some time it becomes liquid once again **(secondary liquefaction).**

Fibrinogen secreted from the seminal vesicle is converted into a weak **coagulum** by the clotting enzymes secreted from prostate gland. Coagulum is liquefied after about 30 minutes, as it is lysed by fibrinolysin produced in prostate gland.

When semen is ejaculated, the sperms are non-motile due to the viscosity of coagulum. When the coagulum dissolves, the sperms become motile.

■ PROPERTIES OF SEMEN

1. Specific gravity : 1.028
2. Volume : 2 mL to 6 mL per ejaculation
3. Reaction : It is alkaline with a pH of 7.5. Alkalinity is due to the prostate fluid.

■ COMPOSITION OF SEMEN

Semen contains 10% sperms and 90% of fluid part, which is called **seminal plasma.** Seminal plasma contains the products from seminal vesicle and prostate gland (Fig. 77.1). It also has small amount of secretions from the mucus glands, particularly the bulbourethral glands.

■ SPERM

Sperm is the **male gamete (reproductive cell),** developed in the testis. It is also called **spermatozoon** (plural = spermatozoa). Matured sperm is 60 µ long.

Sperm Count

Total count of sperm is about 100 to 50 million/mL of semen. **Sterility** occurs when the sperm count falls below 20 million/mL.

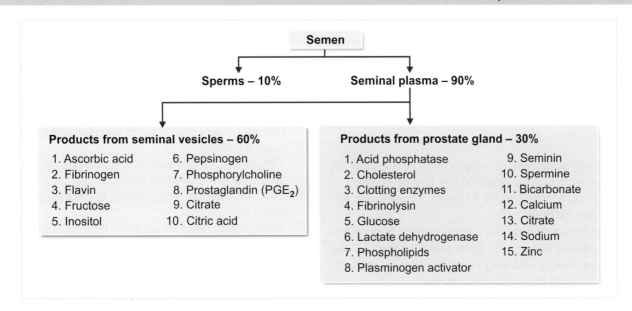

FIGURE 77.1: Composition of semen

Though the sperms can be stored in male genital tract for longer periods, after ejaculation the survival time is only about 24 to 48 hours at a temperature equivalent to body temperature.

Rate of motility of sperm in female genital tract is about 3 mm/minute. Sperms reach the fallopian tube in about 30 to 60 minutes after sexual intercourse. Uterine contractions during sexual act facilitate the movement of sperms.

Structure of Sperm

Sperm consists of four parts (Fig. 77.2):
1. Head
2. Neck
3. Body
4. Tail.

1. Head

Head of sperm is oval in shape (in front view), with a length of 3 to 5 μ and width of up to 3 μ. Anterior portion of head is thin.

Head is covered by a thin cell membrane and it is formed by a condensed nucleus with a thin cytoplasm. Anterior two thirds of the head is called **acrosome** or **galea capitis.**

Acrosome

Acrosome is the thick cap like anterior part of sperm head. It develops from Golgi apparatus and it is made up of mucopolysaccharide and acid phosphatase. Acrosome also contains hyaluronidase and proteolytic

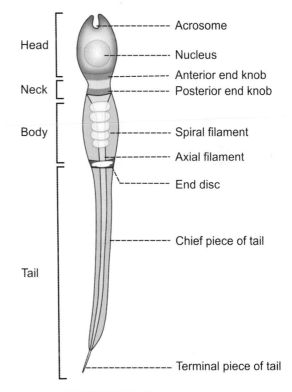

FIGURE 77.2: Human sperm

enzymes, which are essential for the sperm to fertilize the ovum.

2. Neck

Head is connected to the body by a short neck. Its anterior end is formed by thick disk-shaped anterior end knob, which is also called **proximal centriole.** Posterior end is formed by another similar structure known as **posterior end knob.** It gives rise to the **axial filament** of body.

Often, the neck and body of sperm are together called **midpiece.**

3. Body

Body is cylindrical with a length of 5 to 9 μ and the thickness of 1 μ. The body of the sperm consists of a central core called **axial filament,** covered by thin cytoplasmic capsule.

Axial filament starts from posterior end knob of the neck. It passes through the body and a perforated disc called **end disk** or **end ring centriole.** Finally, the axial filament reaches the tail as **axial thread.**

In the body, the axial filament is surrounded by a closely wound spiral filament consisting of mitochondria.

4. Tail

Tail of the sperm consists of two segments:
  i. *Chief or main piece:* It is enclosed by cytoplasmic capsule and has an axial thread. It is 40 to 50 μ long
  ii. *Terminal or end piece:* It has only the axial filament.

■ PRODUCTS FROM SEMINAL VESICLES

Products of seminal vesicles are given in Figure 77.1.

■ PRODUCTS FROM PROSTATE GLAND

Products of prostate gland are given in Figure 77.1.

■ SEMEN ANALYSIS

Analysis of semen evaluates the qualities of semen, which is useful to investigate the infertility.

Parameters of semen analysis:
1. Volume
2. Reaction and pH
3. Liquefaction
4. Sperm count
5. Morphology of sperm
6. Motility of sperms
7. Pus cells and RBCs
8. Fructose level.

■ QUALITIES OF SEMEN REQUIRED FOR FERTILITY

Minimum required qualities of semen for fertility are:
1. Volume of semen per ejaculation must be at least 2 mL
2. Sperm count must be at least 20 million/mL
3. Number of sperms in each ejaculation must be at least 40 million
4. 75% of sperms per ejaculation must be alive
5. 50% of sperms must be motile
6. 30% of sperms must have normal shape and structure
7. Sperms with head defect must be less than 35%
8. Sperms with midpiece defect must be less than 20%
9. Sperms with tail defect must be less than 20%.

■ APPLIED PHYSIOLOGY

Azoospermia

Azoospermia is the condition characterized by lack of sperm in semen. It is a **congenital** disease. It is also caused by excess use of corticosteroids and androgens.

Oligozoospermia

Oligozoospermia is the low sperm count with less than 20 million of sperms/mL of semen. Oligozoospermia causes **infertility.**

Teratozoospermia

Teratozoospermia is the condition characterized by presence of sperms with abnormal morphology. It is also called **teratospermia.** It occurs in **Crohn's disease, Hodgkin disease** and **celiac disease.** The abnormal morphology of sperm results in **infertility.**

Aspermia

Aspermia is the lack of semen. It occurs due to retrograde ejaculation. **Retrograde ejaculation** is the entrance of semen into urinary bladder instead of entering urethra. It is due to dysfunction of sphincter of the bladder, which is caused by prostatic surgery or excess use of drugs. Aspermia leads to **infertility.**

Oligospermia

Oligospermia is a genetic disorder characterized by low volume of semen.

Hematospermia

Hematospermia is the appearance of blood in sperm. It occurs due to infection of urethra or prostate. It is also common in **congenital bleeding disorder.**

Female Reproductive System

- ■ **FEMALE REPRODUCTIVE ORGANS**
  - ■ **PRIMARY SEX ORGANS**
  - ■ **ACCESSORY SEX ORGANS**
  - ■ **FUNCTIONAL ANATOMY OF ACCESSORY SEX ORGANS**
- ■ **SEXUAL LIFE IN FEMALES**
  - ■ **FIRST PERIOD**
  - ■ **SECOND PERIOD**
  - ■ **THIRD PERIOD**

■ FEMALE REPRODUCTIVE ORGANS

Female reproductive system comprises of primary sex organs and accessory sex organs (Fig. 78.1).

■ PRIMARY SEX ORGANS

Primary sex organs are a pair of ovaries, which produce eggs or ova and secrete female sex hormones, the

estrogen and progesterone. Details of structure and functions of ovary are given in Chapter 79.

■ ACCESSORY SEX ORGANS

Accessory sex organs in females are:

1. *A system of genital ducts:* Fallopian tubes, uterus, cervix and vagina (Figs. 78.2 and 78.3)

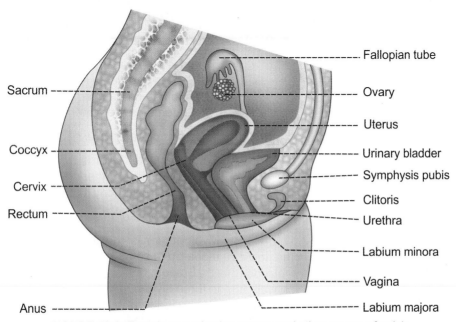

FIGURE 78.1: Female reproductive organs and other organs of pelvis

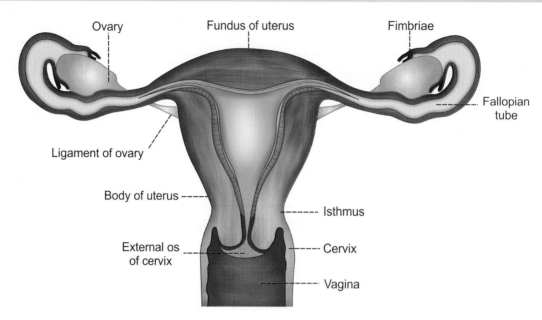

FIGURE 78.2: Female reproductive system

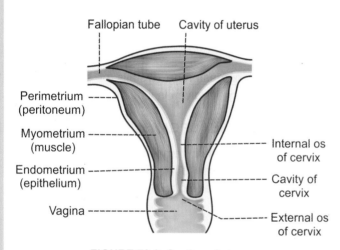

FIGURE 78.3: Section of uterus

2. *External genitalia:* Labia majora, labia minora and clitoris.

Mammary glands are not the female genital organs but are the important glands of female reproductive system.

■ FUNCTIONAL ANATOMY OF ACCESSORY SEX ORGANS

Uterus

Uterus is otherwise known as **womb.** It lies in the pelvic cavity, in between the rectum and urinary bladder. Uterus is a hollow muscular organ with a thick wall. It has a central cavity, which opens into vagina through cervix. On either side at its upper part, the fallopian tubes open. Uterus communicates with peritoneal cavity through fallopian tubes.

Virgin uterus is pyriform in shape and is flattened anteroposteriorly. It measures about 7.5 cm in length, 5 cm in breadth at its upper part and about 2.5 cm in thickness. There is a constriction almost at the middle of uterus called **isthmus.**

Divisions of uterus

Uterus is divided into three portions:
1. Fundus (above the entrance points of fallopian tubes)
2. Body (between fundus and isthmus)
3. Cervix (below isthmus).

Structure of uterus

Uterus is made up of three layers:
1. Serous or outer layer
2. Myometrium or middle muscular layer
3. Endometrium or inner mucus layer.

1. *Serous or outer layer*

Serous or outer layer is the covering of uterus derived from peritoneum. Anteriorly, it covers the uterus completely, but posteriorly it covers only up to the isthmus.

2. *Myometrium or middle muscular layer*

Myometrium is the thickest layer of uterus and it is made up of smooth muscle fibers.

Smooth muscle fibers of myometrium are arranged in three layers:
   i. External myometrium with transversely arranged muscle fibers

ii. Middle myometrium with muscle fibers arranged longitudinally, obliquely and transversely

iii. Internal myometrium with circular muscle fibers.

Muscular layer is interdisposed with blood vessels, nerve fibers, lymphatic vessels and areolar tissues.

3. *Endometrium or inner mucus layer*

Endometrium is smooth and soft with pale red color. It is made up of ciliated columnar epithelial cells.

Surface of the endometrium has minute orifices, through which tubular follicles of endometrium open. Endometrium also contains connective tissue in which the uterine glands are present. Uterine glands are lined by ciliated columnar epithelial cells.

Changes in uterus

Uterus changes its size, structure and function in different phases of sexual life.

Just before menstruation, uterus is enlarged, becomes more vascular. The endometrium thickens with more blood supply. This layer is desquamated during menstruation and reformed after menstrual period.

During pregnancy, uterus is enlarged very much with increase in weight. After parturition (delivery), it comes back to its original size but the cavity remains larger. In old age, uterus is atrophied.

Cervix

Cervix is the lower constricted part of uterus. It is divided into two portions:

1. Upper supravaginal portion, which communicates with body of uterus through **internal os** (orifice) of cervix. Mucus membrane of this portion has glandular follicles, which secrete mucus.

2. Lower vaginal portion, which projects into the anterior wall of the vagina and it communicates with vagina through **external os** (orifice) of cervix. Mucus membrane of this portion is formed by stratified epithelial cells.

Vagina

Vagina is a short tubular organ. It is lined by mucus membrane, which is formed by stratified epithelial cells.

■ SEXUAL LIFE IN FEMALES

Lifespan of a female is divided into three periods.

■ FIRST PERIOD

First period extends from birth to puberty. During this period, primary and accessory sex organs do not function. These organs remain quiescent. Puberty occurs at the age of 12 to 15 years.

■ SECOND PERIOD

Second period extends from onset of puberty to the onset of menopause. First menstrual cycle is known as **menarche.** Permanent stoppage of the menstrual cycle in old age is called **menopause,** which occurs at the age of about 45 to 50 years. During the period between menarche and menopause, women menstruate and reproduce.

■ THIRD PERIOD

Third period extends after menopause to the rest of the life.

Ovary

Chapter 79

- ■ INTRODUCTION
- ■ FUNCTIONAL ANATOMY OF OVARY
  - ■ MEDULLA
  - ■ CORTEX
- ■ OVARIAN HORMONES
  - ■ ESTROGEN
  - ■ FUNCTIONS OF ESTROGEN
  - ■ PROGESTERONE
  - ■ FUNCTIONS OF PROGESTERONE

■ INTRODUCTION

Ovary is the gonad or **primary sex organs** in females. A woman has two ovaries. Ovaries have two functions, gametogenic and endocrine functions. Gametogenic function is the production and release of **ovum** or egg, which is the **female gamete** (reproductive cell). Endocrine function of ovaries is the secretion of female sex hormones.

■ FUNCTIONAL ANATOMY OF OVARY

Ovaries are flattened ovoid bodies, with dimensions of 4 cm in length, 2 cm in width and 1 cm in thickness. Each ovary is attached at hilum to the broad ligament, by means of mesovarium and ovarian ligament.

Each ovary has two portions:
1. Medulla
2. Cortex.

■ MEDULLA

Medulla or zona vasculosa is the central deeper portion of the ovary. It has the stroma of loose connective tissues. It contains blood vessels, lymphatics, nerve fibers and bundles of smooth muscle fibers near the hilum.

■ CORTEX

Cortex is the outer broader portion and has compact cellular layers. It is interrupted at the hilum, where the medulla is continuous with **mesovarium.** Cortex is lined by the germinal epithelium underneath a fibrous layer known as **'tunica albuginea'.**

Cortex consists of the following structures:
i. Glandular structures, which represent ovarian follicles at different stages
ii. Connective tissue cells
iii. Interstitial cells, which are clusters of epithelial cells with fine lipid granules formed mainly from theca interna.

Ovarian Follicles

In the intrauterine life, outer part of cortex contains the **germinal epithelium,** which is derived from the **germinal ridges.** When fetus develops, the germinal epithelium gives rise to a number of primordial ova. The primordial ova move towards the inner substance of cortex. A layer of spindle cells called **granulose cells** from the ovarian stroma surround the ova. Primordial ovum along with granulosa cells is called the **primordial follicle** (Fig. 79.1).

At 7th or 8th month of intrauterine life, about 6 million primordial follicles are found in the ovary. But at the time of birth, only 1 million primordial follicles are seen in both the ovaries and the rest of the follicles degenerate. At the time of puberty, the number decreases further to about 300,000 to 400,000. After menarche, during every menstrual cycle, one of the follicles matures

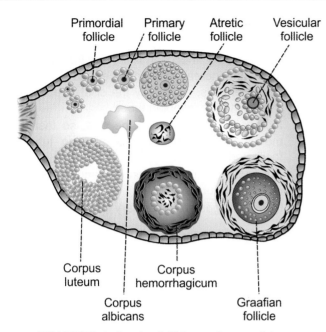

Primordial follicle   Primary follicle   Atretic follicle   Vesicular follicle

Corpus luteum   Corpus hemorrhagicum

Corpus albicans   Graafian follicle

FIGURE 79.1: Ovarian follicles and corpus luteum

and releases its ovum. During every menstrual cycle, only one ovum is released from any one of the ovaries.

During every cycle, many of the follicles degenerate. The degeneration of the follicles is called **atresia** and the degenerated follicles are known as **atretic follicles.** The atretic follicles become fibrous and the fibrotic follicles are called the **corpus fibrosa.** Atresia occurs at all levels of follicles. Usually, the degenerated follicles disappear without leaving any scar.

Functions of Ovaries

Ovaries are the primary sex organs in females. Functions of ovaries are:
1. Secretion of female sex hormones
2. Oogenesis
3. Menstrual cycle.

Sex hormones are discussed in this Chapter. Oogenesis and menstrual cycle are explained in the next Chapter.

■ OVARIAN HORMONES

Ovary secretes the female sex hormones estrogen and progesterone. Ovary also secretes few more hormones, namely inhibin (Chapter 80), relaxin (Chapter 84) and small quantities of androgens.

■ ESTROGEN

Source of Secretion

In a normal non-pregnant woman, estrogen is secreted in large quantity by theca interna cells of ovarian follicles

and in small quantity by corpus luteum of the ovaries. Estrogen secretion is predominant at the later stage of follicular phase before ovulation (Chapter 80).

Estrogen is derived from androgens, particularly androstenedione, which is secreted in theca interna cells. Androstenedione migrates from theca cells to granulosa cells, where it is converted into estrogen by the activity of the enzyme aromatase.

A small quantity of estrogen is also secreted by adrenal cortex. In pregnant woman, a large amount of estrogen is secreted by the placenta.

Chemistry

Estrogen is a C_{18} steroid.

Different Forms

Estrogen is present in three forms in plasma:
1. β-estradiol
2. Estrone
3. Estriol.

All the three forms of estrogen are present in significant quantities in plasma. The quantity and potency of β-estradiol are more than those of estrone and estriol.

Plasma Level

Plasma level of estrogen in females at normal reproductive age varies during different phases of menstrual cycle. In follicular phase, it is 30 to 200 pg/mL (Fig. 80.4). In normal adult male, estrogen level is 12 to 34 pg/mL.

Half-life

Half-life of estrogen is 30 to 60 minutes.

Synthesis

The different forms of estrogen are synthesized from the cholesterol or acetate. If estrogen is formed from acetate, first acetate is converted into cholesterol.

Pathway for synthesis of estrogen

Acetate → Cholesterol → Pregnenolone
↓
Estrogen ← Testosterone ← Progesterone

During synthesis of estrogen, progesterone and testosterone are synthesized first (Fig. 70.2). Then, before leaving the ovaries, almost all the testosterone and much of the progesterone are converted into estrogen. About 1/15 of testosterone is secreted into the plasma of the female by the ovaries.

Transport in Plasma

Estrogen is transported mainly by the plasma protein, **albumin.** A small quantity of estrogen is also transported by **globulin.** The binding of estrogen with the plasma protein is loose, so that the hormones are released into the tissues easily.

Metabolism

Estrogen is degraded mainly in the liver. Here, it is conjugated with glucuronides and sulfates. About one fifth of the conjugated products are excreted in the bile. Most of the remaining part is excreted in the urine. Liver also converts the potent active beta estradiol into the almost inactive estrogen, the estriol.

■ FUNCTIONS OF ESTROGEN

Major function of estrogen is to promote cellular proliferation and tissue growth in the sexual organs and in other tissues, related to reproduction. In childhood, the estrogen is secreted in small quantity. During puberty, the secretion increases sharply, resulting in changes in the sexual organs. Effects of estrogen are:

1. Effect on Ovarian Follicles

Estrogen promotes the growth of ovarian follicles by increasing the proliferation of the follicular cells. It also increases the secretory activity of theca cells (Refer Chapter 80 for details).

2. Effect on Uterus

Estrogen produces the following changes in uterus:
  i. Enlargement of uterus to about double of its childhood size due to the proliferation of endometrial cells
  ii. Increase in the blood supply to endometrium
  iii. Deposition of glycogen and fats in endometrium
  iv. Proliferation and dilatation of blood vessels of endometrium
  v. Proliferation and dilatation of the endometrial glands, which become more tortuous with increased blood flow
  vi. Increase in the spontaneous activity of the uterine muscles and their sensitivity to oxytocin
  vii. Increase in the contractility of the uterine muscles.

All these changes prepare uterus for pregnancy.

3. Effect on Fallopian Tubes

Estrogen:
  i. Acts on the mucosal lining of the fallopian tubes and increases the number and size of the epithelial cells, especially the ciliated epithelial cells lining the fallopian tubes
  ii. Increases the activity of the cilia, so that the movement of ovum in the fallopian tube is facilitated
  iii. Enhances the proliferation of glandular tissues in fallopian tubes.

All these changes are necessary for the fertilization of ovum.

4. Effect on Vagina

Estrogen:
  i. Changes the vaginal epithelium from cuboidal into stratified type; the stratified epithelium is more resistant to trauma and infection
  ii. Increases the layers of the vaginal epithelium by proliferation
  iii. Reduces the pH of vagina, making it more acidic.

All these changes are necessary for the prevention of certain common vaginal infections such as **gonorrheal vaginitis.** Such infections can be cured by the administration of estrogen.

5. Effect on Secondary Sexual Characters

Estrogen is responsible for the development of secondary sexual characters (Chapter 74) in females.

Secondary sexual characters in female

  i. *Hair distribution:* Hair develops in the pubic region and axilla. In females, pubic hair has the base of the triangle upwards. Body hair growth is less. Scalp hair grows profusely
  ii. *Skin:* Skin becomes soft and smooth. Vascularity of skin also increases
  iii. *Body shape:* Shoulders become narrow, hip broadens, thighs converge and the arms diverge. Fat deposition increases in breasts and buttocks
  iv. *Pelvis:*
    a. Broadening of pelvis with increased transverse diameter
    b. Round or oval shape of pelvis
    c. Round or oval=shaped pelvic outlet.

Thus, pelvis in females is different from that of males, which is funnel shaped.

iv. *Voice:* Larynx remains in prepubertal stage, which produces high-pitch voice.

6. Effect on Breast

Estrogen causes:

i. Development of stromal tissues of breasts
ii. Growth of an extensive ductile system
iii. Deposition of fat in the ductile system.

All these effects prepare the breasts for lactation. Estrogen causes development of lobules and alveoli of the breasts, to some extent. However, progesterone is necessary for the full growth of breast and prolactin is necessary for its function.

7. Effect on Bones

Estrogen increases **osteoblastic activity.** So, at the time of puberty, the growth rate increases enormously. But, at the same time, estrogen causes early fusion of the epiphysis with the shaft. This effect is much stronger in females than the similar effect of testosterone in males. As a result, the growth of the females usually ceases few years earlier than in the males.

In old age, the estrogen is not secreted or it becomes scanty. It leads to **osteoporosis,** in which the bones become extremely weak and **fragile.** Because of this, the bones are highly susceptible for **fractures** (Chapter 68).

8. Effect on Metabolism

i. On protein metabolism

Estrogen induces anabolism of proteins, by which it increases the total body protein.

ii. On fat metabolism

Estrogen causes deposition of fat in the subcutaneous tissues, breasts, buttocks and thighs. The overall specific gravity of the female body is considerably lesser than that of males because of fat deposition.

9. Effect on Electrolyte Balance

Estrogen causes sodium and water retention from the renal tubules. This effect is normally insignificant but in pregnancy, it becomes more significant.

Mode of Action of Estrogen

Estrogen receptors situated on nuclear membrane of target cells are of two types namely **α and β estrogen receptors.** The α-estrogen receptors are present in uterus, liver, heart and kidneys. The β estrogen receptors are present in ovaries and other tissues.

Estrogen acts through genes.

Regulation of Estrogen Secretion

Estrogen secretion is regulated by follicle-stimulating hormone (FSH) released from anterior pituitary. Release of FSH is stimulated by the gonadotropin-releasing hormone (GnRH) secreted from hypothalamus.

Theca cells and granulosa cells have many FSH receptors. After binding with the receptors, FSH acts via cAMP and stimulates the secretory activities of theca and granulosa cells. Estrogen inhibits secretion of FSH and GnRH by **negative feedback.** Inhibin secreted by granulosa cells (Chapter 80) also decreases estrogen secretion, by inhibiting the secretion of FSH and GnRH (Fig. 79.2).

■ PROGESTERONE

Source of Secretion

In non-pregnant woman, a small quantity of progesterone is secreted by theca interna cells of ovaries during the first half of menstrual cycle, i.e. during follicular stage. But, a large quantity of progesterone is secreted during the latter half of each menstrual cycle, i.e. during secretory phase by the corpus luteum. Small amount of progesterone is secreted from adrenal cortex also.

In pregnant woman, large amount of progesterone is secreted by the corpus luteum in the first trimester. In the second trimester, corpus luteum degenerates. Placenta

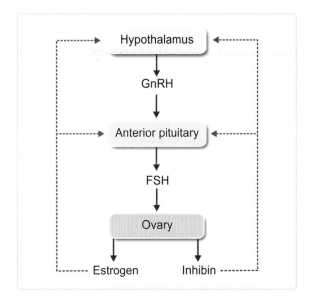

FIGURE 79.2: Regulation of estrogen secretion. Red dotted lines indicate inhibition.

secretes large quantity of progesterone in second and third trimesters.

Chemistry

Progesterone is a C_{21} steroid.

Half-life

Half-life of progesterone is 4 to 5 minutes.

Synthesis

Progesterone is synthesized from acetate or cholesterol in the ovaries, along with estrogen (Fig. 70.2, Chapter 70).

Plasma Level

Plasma level of progesterone in females at normal reproductive age varies during different phases of menstrual cycle. In follicular phase, it is about 0.9 ng/mL (Fig. 80.4). In normal adult male, progesterone level is 0.3 ng/mL.

Transport in Blood

Like estrogen, progesterone is also transported in the blood by the plasma proteins – **albumin** and **globulin.**

Metabolism

Within few minutes after secretion, almost all the progesterone is degraded into other steroids, which do not have progesterone effect. The degradation occurs in liver. The main end product of progesterone degradation is pregnanediol, which is conjugated with glucuronic acid and excreted in the urine.

■ FUNCTIONS OF PROGESTERONE

Progesterone is concerned mainly with the final preparation of the uterus for pregnancy and the breasts for lactation. The effects of progesterone are:

1. Effect on Fallopian Tubes

Progesterone promotes the secretory activities of mucosal lining of the fallopian tubes. Secretions of fallopian tubes are necessary for nutrition of the fertilized ovum, while it is in fallopian tube before implantation.

2. Effect on the Uterus

Progesterone promotes the secretory activities of uterine **endometrium** during the secretory phase of the menstrual cycle. Thus, the uterus is prepared for implantation of the fertilized ovum.

Progesterone:
  i. Increases the thickness of the endometrium by increasing the number and size of the cells
     Thickness of endometrium increases from 1 mm thickness at the beginning of secretory phase to about 5 to 6 mm at the end of secretory phase.
 ii. Increases the size of uterine glands and these glands become more tortuous
iii. Increases the secretory activities of epithelial cells of uterine glands
 iv. Increases the deposition of lipid and glycogen in the stromal cells of endometrium
  v. Increases the blood supply to endometrium. It is due to increase in size of the vessels and vasodilatation
 vi. Decreases the frequency of uterine contractions during pregnancy. Because of this, the expulsion of the implanted ovum is prevented.

3. Effect on Cervix

Progesterone increases the thickness of cervical mucosa and thereby inhibits the transport of sperm into uterus. This effect is utilized in the contraceptive actions of minipills.

4. Effect on the Mammary Glands

Progesterone promotes the development of lobules and alveoli of mammary glands by proliferating and enlarging the alveolar cells. It also makes the breasts secretory in nature. It makes the breasts to swell by increasing the secretory activity and fluid accumulation in the subcutaneous tissue.

5. Effect on Hypothalamus

Progesterone inhibits the release of LH from hypothalamus through feedback effect. This effect is utilized for its contraceptive action.

6. Thermogenic Effect

Progesterone increases the body temperature after ovulation. The mechanism of thermogenic action is not known. It is suggested that progesterone increases the body temperature by acting on hypothalamic centers for temperature regulation.

7. Effect on Respiration

During luteal phase of menstrual cycle and during pregnancy, progesterone increases the ventilation via respiratory center. This decreases the partial pressure of carbon dioxide in the alveoli.

8. *Effect on Electrolyte Balance*

Progesterone increases the reabsorption of sodium and water from the renal tubules. However, in large doses, it is believed to cause excretion of sodium and water. This may be due to an indirect effect, i.e. progesterone combines with the same receptors, which bind with aldosterone. So, the action of aldosterone is blocked, leading to the excretion of sodium and water.

Mode of Action of Progesterone

The progesterone receptors situated on the nuclear membrane of target cells are of two types, namely A-progesterone receptors and B-progesterone receptors. Exact location of each type of progesterone receptor is not clear.

Like estrogen, progesterone also acts through genes.

Regulation of Progesterone Secretion

LH from anterior pituitary activates the corpus luteum to secrete progesterone. Secretion of LH is influenced by the gonadotropin-releasing hormone secreted in hypothalamus. Progesterone inhibits the release of LH from anterior pituitary by **negative feedback.**

Menstrual Cycle

■ INTRODUCTION

■ DEFINITION

Menstrual cycle is defined as cyclic events that take place in a rhythmic fashion during the reproductive period of a woman's life. Menstrual cycle starts at the age of 12 to 15 years, which marks the onset of puberty. The commencement of menstrual cycle is called **menarche.** Menstrual cycle ceases at the age of 45 to 50 years. Permanent cessation of menstrual cycle in old age is called **menopause.**

■ DURATION OF MENSTRUAL CYCLE

Duration of menstrual cycle is usually 28 days. But, under physiological conditions, it may vary between 20 and 40 days.

■ CHANGES DURING MENSTRUAL CYCLE

During each menstrual cycle, series of changes occur in ovary and accessory sex organs.

These changes are divided into 4 groups:
1. Ovarian changes
2. Uterine changes

3. Vaginal changes
4. Changes in cervix.
   All these changes take place simultaneously.

OVARIAN CHANGES DURING MENSTRUAL CYCLE

Changes in the ovary during each menstrual cycle occur in two phases:
A. Follicular phase
B. Luteal phase.
   Ovulation occurs in between these two phases.

FOLLICULAR PHASE

Follicular phase extends from the 5th day of the cycle until the time of ovulation, which takes place on 14th day. Maturation of ovum with development of ovarian follicles takes place during this phase.

Ovarian Follicles

Ovarian follicles are glandular structures present in the cortex of ovary. Each follicle consists of the ovum surrounded by epithelial cells, namely **granulosa cells.** The follicles gradually grow into a matured follicle through various stages.

Different follicles:

1. Primordial follicle
2. Primary follicle
3. Vesicular follicle
4. Matured follicle or graafian follicle.

1. *Primordial Follicle*

At the time of puberty, both the ovaries contain about 400,000 primordial follicles. Diameter of the primordial follicle is about 15 to 20 μ and that of ovum is about 10 μ.

Each primordial follicle has an ovum, which is incompletely surrounded by the granulosa cells (Chapter 79, Fig. 79.1). These cells provide nutrition to the ovum during childhood.

Granulosa cells also secrete the **oocyte maturation inhibiting factor,** which keeps ovum in the immature stage. All the ova present in the ovaries are formed before birth. No new ovum is developed after birth.

At the onset of puberty, under the influence of FSH and LH the primordial follicles start growing through various stages.

2. *Primary Follicle*

Primordial follicle becomes the primary follicle, when ovum is completely surrounded by the granulosa cells.

During this stage, the follicle and the ovum increase in size. Diameter of the follicle increases to 30 to 40 μ and that of ovum increases to about 20 μ. The follicle is not covered by a definite connective tissue capsule.

Changes taking place during development of primary follicle

i. Proliferation of granulosa cells and increase in size of the follicle
ii. Increase in size of the ovum
iii. Onset of formation of connective tissue capsule around the follicle.
   Primary follicles develop into vesicular follicles.

3. *Vesicular Follicle*

Under the influence of FSH, about 6 to 12 primary follicles start growing and develop into vesicular follicles.

Changes taking place during the development of vesicular follicle
i. Changes in granulosa cells
ii. Changes in ovum
iii. Formation of capsule.

i. *Changes in granulosa cells*

a. First, the proliferation of granulosa cells occurs
b. A cavity called **follicular cavity** or **antrum** is formed in between the granulosa cells
c. Antrum is filled with a serous fluid called the **liquor folliculi**
d. With continuous proliferation of granulosa cells, the follicle increases in size
e. Antrum with its fluid also increases in size
f. Ovum is pushed to one side and it is surrounded by granulosa cells, which forms the **germ hill** or **cumulus oophorus**
g. Granulosa cells, which line the antrum form **membrana granulosa**
h. Cells of germ hill become columnar and form **corona radiata.**

ii. *Changes in ovum*

a. First, the ovum increases in size and its diameter increases to 100 to 150 μ
b. Nucleus becomes larger and vesicular
c. Cytoplasm becomes granular
d. Thick membrane is formed around the ovum, which is called zona pellucida
e. A narrow cleft appears between ovum and zona pellucida. This cleft is called **perivitelline space.**

iii. Formation of capsule

Spindle cells from the stroma of ovarian cortex are modified and form a covering sheath around the follicle. The covering sheath is known as **follicular sheath** or **theca folliculi.**

Theca folliculi divides into two layers:
a. Theca interna
b. Theca externa.

a. Theca interna

Theca interna is the inner vascular layer with loose connective tissue. This layer also contains special type of epithelial cells with lipid granules and some delicate collagen fibers.

Epithelial cells become secretory in nature and start secreting the female sex hormones, especially estrogen. Hormones are released into the fluid of antrum.

b. Theca externa

Theca externa is the outer layer of follicular capsule and consists of thickly packed fibers and spindle-shaped cells.

After about 7th day of menstrual cycle, one of the vesicular follicles outgrows others and becomes the dominant follicle. It develops further to form graafian follicle. Other vesicular follicles degenerate and become **atretic** by means of **apoptosis.**

4. Graafian Follicle

Graafian follicle is the matured ovarian follicle with maturing ovum (Fig. 80.1). It is named after the Dutch physician and anatomist, **Regnier De Graaf.**

Changes taking place during the development of graafian follicle

   i. Size of the follicle increases to about 10 to 12 mm. It extends through the whole thickness of ovarian cortex
  ii. At one point, the follicle encroaches upon tunica albuginea and protrudes upon surface of the ovary. This protrusion is called **stigma.** At the stigma, the tunica albuginea becomes thin
 iii. Follicular cavity becomes larger and distended with fluid
 iv. Ovum attains maximum size
  v. Zona pellucida becomes thick
 vi. Corona radiata becomes prominent
vii. Small spaces filled with fluid appear between the cells of germ hill, outside the corona radiata. These spaces weaken the attachment of the ovum to the follicular wall
viii. Theca interna becomes prominent. Its thickness becomes double with the formation of rich capillary network

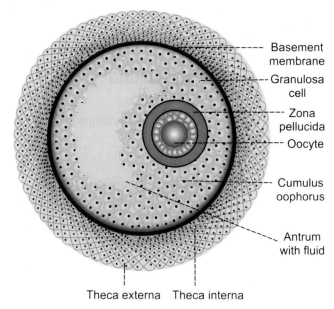

FIGURE 80.1: Graafian follicle

Basement membrane
Granulosa cell
Zona pellucida
Oocyte
Cumulus oophorus
Antrum with fluid
Theca externa   Theca interna

 ix. On the 14th day of menstrual cycle, graafian follicle is ready for the process of ovulation.

■ OVULATION

Ovulation is the process by which the graafian follicle ruptures with consequent **discharge of ovum** into the abdominal cavity. It is influenced by LH. Ovulation occurs on 14th day of menstrual cycle in a normal cycle of 28 days. The ovum enters the fallopian tube.

Process of Ovulation

Mechanism of ovulation is not known clearly. Process of ovulation is explained in the next Chapter.

Stages of ovulation
1. Rupture of graafian follicles takes place at the stigma
2. Follicular fluid oozes out
3. Germ hillock is freed from wall
4. Ovum is expelled out into the abdominal cavity along with some amount of fluid and granulosa cells
5. From abdominal cavity, the ovum enters the fallopian tube through the fimbriated end.

Other details are given in the next Chapter.

Ovum becomes **haploid** before or during ovulation by the formation of polar bodies. After ovulation, the ovum is viable only for 24 to 48 hours. So it must be fertilized within that time.

Fertilized ovum is called **zygote.** Zygote moves from fallopian tube and reaches the uterus on 3rd day after ovulation. It is **implanted** in the uterine wall on 6th or 7th day.

If fertilization does not occur, ovum degenerates. Generally, only one ovum is released from one of the ovaries.

■ LUTEAL PHASE

Luteal phase extends between 15th and 28th day of menstrual cycle. During this phase, corpus luteum is developed and hence this phase is called luteal phase (Fig. 80.2).

Corpus Luteum

Corpus luteum is a glandular yellow body, developed from the ruptured graafian follicle after the release of ovum. It is also called **yellow body.**

Development of Corpus Luteum

Soon after the rupture of graafian follicle and release of ovum, the follicle is filled with **blood.** Now the follicle is called **corpus hemorrhagicum.** The blood clots slowly. Corpus hemorrhagicum does not degenerate immediately. It is transformed into corpus luteum.

Follicular cavity closes gradually by the healing of the wound. Blood clot is gradually replaced by a **serous**

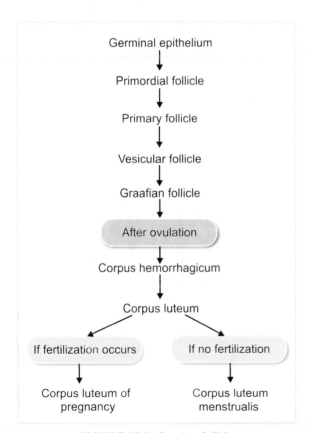

FIGURE 80.2: Ovarian follicle

fluid containing fibrin. Corpus luteum obtains a diameter of 15 mm and remains in the ovary till the end of the cycle.

Structure of Corpus Luteum

In the corpus luteum, **granulosa cells** and **theca interna cells** are transformed into **lutein cells** called granulosa lutein cells and theca lutein cells. The process which transforms the granulosa and theca cells into lutein cells is called **luteinization.**

Granulosa lutein cells contain fine lipid granules and the yellowish pigment granules. The **yellowish pigment** granules give the characteristic yellow color to corpus luteum.

Theca lutein cells contain only lipid granules and not the yellow pigment.

Follicular cavity is greatly reduced with irregular outline. It is filled with the serous fluid and remnants of blood clots.

Functions of Corpus Luteum

1. *Secretion of hormones*

Corpus luteum acts as a **temporary endocrine gland.** It secretes large quantity of progesterone and small amount of estrogen. Granulosa lutein cells secrete **progesterone** and theca lutein cells secrete **estrogen.** LH influences the secretion of these two hormones.

2. *Maintenance of pregnancy*

If pregnancy occurs, corpus luteum remains active for about 3 months, i.e. until placenta develops. Hormones secreted by corpus luteum during this period maintain the pregnancy.

Abortion occurs if corpus luteum becomes inactive or removed before third month of pregnancy, i.e. before placenta starts secreting the hormones.

Fate of Corpus Luteum

Fate of corpus luteum depends upon whether ovum is fertilized or not.

1. *If the ovum is not fertilized*

If fertilization does not take place, the corpus luteum reaches the maximum size about one week after ovulation. During this period, it secretes large quantity of progesterone with small quantity of estrogen. Then, it degenerates into the **corpus luteum menstrualis** or **spurium.** The cells decrease in size and the corpus luteum becomes smaller and involuted. Afterwards, the corpus luteum menstrualis is transformed into a whitish scar called **corpus albicans.** The process by which corpus luteum undergoes regression is called **luteolysis.**

2. *If ovum is fertilized*

If ovum is fertilized and pregnancy occurs, the corpus luteum persists and increases in size. It attains a diameter of 20 to 30 mm and it is transformed into **corpus luteum graviditatis (verum)** or **corpus luteum of pregnancy.** It remains in the ovary for 3 to 4 months. During this period, it secretes large amount of progesterone with small quantity of estrogen, which are essential for the maintenance of pregnancy. After 3 to 4 months, placenta starts secreting these hormones and corpus luteum degenerates.

■ UTERINE CHANGES DURING MENSTRUAL CYCLE

During each menstrual cycle, along with ovarian changes, uterine changes also occur simultaneously (Fig. 80.3).

Uterine changes occur in three phases:
1. Menstrual phase
2. Proliferative phase
3. Secretory phase.

■ MENSTRUAL PHASE

After ovulation, if pregnancy does not occur, the thickened **endometrium** is shed or **desquamated.** This desquamated endometrium is expelled out through vagina along with blood and tissue fluid. The process of shedding and exit of uterine lining along with blood and fluid is called **menstruation** or **menstrual bleeding.** It lasts for about 4 to 5 days. This period is called menstrual phase or **menstrual period.** It is also called **menses, emmenia** or **catamenia.**

The day when bleeding starts is considered as the first day of the menstrual cycle.

Two days before the onset of bleeding, that is on 26th or 27th day of the previous cycle, there is a sudden reduction in the release of estrogen and progesterone from ovary. Decreased level of these two hormones is responsible for menstruation.

Changes in Endometrium during Menstrual Phase

i. Lack of estrogen and progesterone causes sudden involution of endometrium
ii. It leads to reduction in the thickness of endometrium, up to 65% of original thickness
iii. During the next 24 hours, the tortuous blood vessels in the endometrium undergo severe constriction. Endometrial vasoconstriction is because of three reasons:
   a. Involution of endometrium
   b. Actions of vasoconstrictor substances like prostaglandin, released from tissues of involuted endometrium
   c. Sudden lack of estrogen and progesterone (which are vasodilators)
iv. Vasoconstriction leads to **hypoxia,** which results in **necrosis** of the endometrium
v. Necrosis causes rupture of blood vessels and oozing of blood
vi. Outer layer of the **necrotic endometrium** is separated and passes out along with blood
vii. This process is continued for about 24 to 36 hours

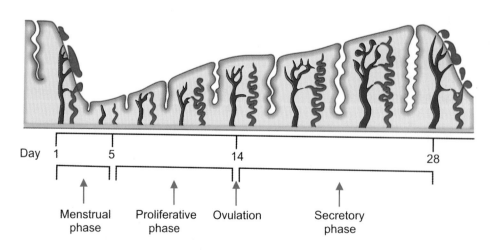

FIGURE 80.3: Uterine changes during menstrual cycle

viii. Within 48 hours after the reduction in the secretion of estrogen and progesterone, the superficial layers of endometrium are completely desquamated

ix. Desquamated tissues and the blood in the endometrial cavity initiate the contraction of uterus

x. Uterine contractions expel the blood along with desquamated uterine tissues to the exterior through vagina.

During normal menstruation, about 35 mL of **blood** along with 35 mL of **serous fluid** is expelled. The blood clots as soon as it oozes into the uterine cavity. **Fibrinolysin** causes **lysis of clot** in uterine cavity itself, so that the expelled menstrual fluid does not clot. However, in the pathological conditions involving uterus, the lysis of blood clot does not occur. So the menstrual fluid comes out with blood clot.

Menstruation stops between 3rd and 7th day of menstrual cycle. At the end of menstrual phase, the thickness of endometrium is only about 1 mm. This is followed by proliferative phase.

■ PROLIFERATIVE PHASE

Proliferative phase extends usually from 5th to 14th day of menstruation, i.e. between the day when menstruation stops and the day of ovulation. It corresponds to the follicular phase of ovarian cycle.

At the end of menstrual phase, only a thin layer (1 mm) of endometrium remains, as most of the endometrial stroma is desquamated.

Changes in Endometrium during Proliferative Phase

i. Endometrial cells proliferate rapidly

ii. Epithelium reappears on the surface of endometrium within the first 4 to 7 days

iii. Uterine glands start developing within the endometrial stroma

iv. Blood vessels appear in the stroma

v. Proliferation of endometrial cells occurs continuously, so that the endometrium reaches the thickness of 3 to 4 mm at the end of proliferative phase.

All these uterine changes during proliferative phase occur because of the influence of estrogen released from ovary. On 14th day, ovulation occurs under the influence of LH. This is followed by secretory phase.

■ SECRETORY PHASE

Secretory phase extends between 15th and 28th day of the menstrual cycle, i.e. between the day of ovulation and the day when menstruation of next cycle commences.

After ovulation, corpus luteum is developed in the ovary. It secretes a large quantity of progesterone along with a small amount of estrogen. Estrogen causes further proliferation of cells in uterus, so that the endometrium becomes more thick. Progesterone causes further enlargement of endometrial stroma and further growth of glands.

Under the influence of progesterone, the endometrial glands commence their secretory function. Many changes occur in the endometrium before commencing the secretory function.

Changes in Endometrium during Secretory Phase

i. Endometrial glands become more tortuous. Because of increase in size, the glands become tortuous to get accommodated within the endometrium

ii. Cytoplasm of stromal cells increases because of the deposition of glycogen and lipids

iii. Many new blood vessels appear within endometrial stroma. Blood vessels also become tortuous

iv. Blood supply to endometrium increases

v. Thickness of endometrium increases up to 6 mm.

Actually, secretory phase is the preparatory period, during which the uterus is prepared for implantation of ovum. All these uterine changes during secretory phase occur due to the influence of estrogen and progesterone. Estrogen is responsible for repair of damaged endometrium and growth of the glands. Progesterone is responsible for further growth of these structures and secretory activities in the endometrium.

If a fertilized ovum is implanted during this phase and if the implanted ovum starts developing into a fetus, then further changes occur in the uterus for the survival of the developing fetus. If the implanted ovum is unfertilized or if pregnancy does not occur, menstruation occurs after this phase and a new cycle begins.

■ CHANGES IN CERVIX AND VAGINA DURING MENSTRUAL CYCLE

■ CHANGES IN CERVIX DURING MENSTRUAL CYCLE

Mucus membrane of the cervix also shows cyclic changes during different phases of menstrual cycle.

Proliferative Phase

During proliferative phase, the mucus membrane of cervix becomes thinner and more alkaline due to the influence of estrogen. It helps in the survival and motility of spermatozoa.

Secretory Phase

During secretory phase, the mucus membrane of cervix becomes more thick and adhesive because of actions of progesterone.

■ VAGINAL CHANGES DURING MENSTRUAL CYCLE

Proliferative Phase

Epithelial cells of vagina are cornified. Estrogen is responsible for this.

Secretory Phase

Vaginal epithelium proliferates due to the actions of progesterone. It is also infiltrated with leukocytes. These two changes increase the resistance of vagina for infection.

■ REGULATION OF MENSTRUAL CYCLE

Regulation of menstrual cycle is a complex process that is carried out by a well organized regulatory system. The regulatory system is a highly integrated system, which includes hypothalamus, anterior pituitary and ovary with its growing follicle. In the whole scenario, the growing follicle has a vital role to play.

■ HORMONES INVOLVED IN REGULATION

The regulatory system functions through the hormones of **hypothalamo-pituitary-ovarian axis.**

Hormones involved in the regulation of menstrual cycle are:
1. Hypothalamic hormone: GnRH
2. Anterior pituitary hormones: FSH and LH
3. Ovarian hormones: Estrogen and progesterone.
   Hormonal level during menstrual cycle is shown in Fig. 80.4.

Hypothalamic Hormone – GnRH

GnRH triggers the cyclic changes during menstrual cycle by stimulating secretion of FSH and LH from anterior pituitary. GnRH secretion depends upon two factors:
  i. External factors like psychosocial events, which act on hypothalamus via cortex and many other brain centers
 ii. Feedback effects of ovarian changes via ovarian hormones.

Anterior Pituitary Hormones – FSH and LH

FSH and LH modulate the ovarian and uterine changes by acting directly and/or indirectly via ovarian hormones. FSH stimulates the recruitment and growth of immature ovarian follicles. LH triggers ovulation and sustains corpus luteum.

Secretion of FSH and LH is under the influence of GnRH.

Ovarian Hormones – Estrogen and Progesterone

Estrogen and progesterone which are secreted by follicle and corpus luteum, show many activities during menstrual cycle. Ovarian follicle secretes large quantity of estrogen and corpus luteum secretes large quantity of progesterone.

Estrogen secretion reaches the peak twice in each cycle; once during follicular phase just before ovulation and another one during luteal phase (Fig. 80.4). On the other hand, progesterone is virtually absent during follicular phase till prior to ovulation. But it plays a critical role during luteal phase.

Estrogen is responsible for the growth of follicles. Both the steroids act together to produce the changes in uterus, cervix and vagina.

Both the ovarian hormones are under the influence of GnRH, which acts via FSH and LH. In addition, the secretion of GnRH, FSH and LH is regulated by ovarian hormones.

■ REGULATION OF OVARIAN CHANGES

Follicular Phase

1. The **biological clock** responsible to trigger the cyclic events is the **pulsatile secretion of GnRH,** at about every 2 hours (due to some mechanism that is not understood clearly)
2. Pulsatile release of GnRH stimulates the secretion of FSH and LH from anterior pituitary
3. LH induces the synthesis of androgens from theca cells of growing follicle
4. FSH promotes **aromatase activity** in granulosa cells of the follicle (Chapter 79), resulting in the conversion of androgens into estrogen. It also promotes follicular development
5. Estrogen is responsible for development and growth of graafian follicle. It also stimulates the secretory activities of theca cells
6. Estrogen also exerts a **double feedback control** on GnRH
   i. Initially, when estrogen secretion is moderate, it exerts a **negative feedback control** on GnRH so that GnRH secretion is inhibited. This leads to decrease in secretion of FSH and LH (negative feedback)
   ii. During later period of follicular phase, when a large amount of estrogen is secreted by the

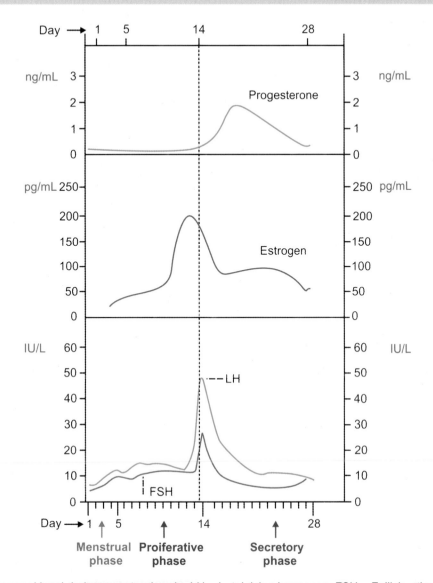

FIGURE 80.4: Hormonal level during menstrual cycle. LH = Luteinizing hormones, FSH = Follicle-stimulating hormone.

maturing follicle, it exerts a **positive feedback effect** on GnRH secretion. Now, GnRH secretion is increased, resulting in secretion of large quantity of FSH and LH. This in turn, facilitates the growth of graafian follicle

7. In addition, estrogen shows the following actions:
   i. Increases the number of FSH and LH receptors on the granulosa cells of follicles and increases the sensitivity of these cells for FSH and LH
   ii. Facilitates the faster growth of graafian follicle
8. LH is necessary to provide the final touches for the growth of graafian follicle. It stimulates the secretion of estrogen. At the same time, it stimulates the theca cells to secrete progesterone.

Ovulation

LH is important for ovulation. Without LH, ovulation does not occur even with a large quantity of FSH. The need for excessive secretion of LH for ovulation is known as **ovulatory surge for LH** or **luteal surge.**

Prior to ovulation, a large quantity of LH is secreted due to **positive feedback effect** of estrogen on GnRH, as mentioned above.

Luteal Phase

Role of LH

Ovarian changes during luteal phase depend mainly on LH.

Luteinizing hormone:

1. Induces development of corpus luteum from the follicle (devoid of ovum) by converting the granulosa cells into lutein cells
2. Stimulates corpus luteum to secrete progesterone and estrogen
3. Necessary for the maintenance of corpus luteum.

Role of FSH

FSH also plays a role during luteal phase.
Follicle-stimulating hormone:

1. Maintains the secretory activity of corpus luteum
2. Stimulates lutein cells to secrete inhibin, which in turn inhibits FSH secretion.

If the ovum is not fertilized or if implantation of ovum does not take place, the changes in the level of the hormones produce some effects on corpus luteum which are:

1. Progesterone and estrogen secreted from corpus luteum, inhibit the secretion of FSH and LH from anterior pituitary by **negative feedback**
2. Granulosa lutein cells secrete another hormone called inhibin (which is also secreted by Sertoli cells of testes in males: Chapter 74). Inhibin also inhibits the secretion of FSH and LH by **negative feedback**
3. In the absence of FSH and LH, the corpus luteum becomes inactive
4. Finally, the corpus luteum regresses by means of luteolysis; so progesterone and estrogen are not available
5. Absence of progesterone and estrogen induces the secretion of GnRH from hypothalamus
6. GnRH stimulates the secretion of FSH and LH from anterior pituitary
7. FSH and LH stimulate the new immature follicles, resulting in the commencement of next cycle.

■ REGULATION OF UTERINE CHANGES

Uterine changes during menstrual cycle are influenced by estrogen and progesterone.

Proliferative Phase

During proliferative stage, the repair of the damaged endometrium occurs mainly by estrogen.
Estrogen stimulates:

1. Proliferation of cells in endometrial stroma
2. Development of uterine glands and appearance of blood vessels in the endometrial stroma.

Secretory Phase

Secretory phase of uterine changes, coincides with luteal phase of ovarian cycle. Under the influence of FSH and LH from anterior pituitary, the corpus luteum secretes large amount of progesterone and small amount of estrogen. Progesterone is responsible for endometrial changes along with estrogen during this phase.
Progesterone stimulates:

1. Growth of endometrial glands and makes them more tortuous
2. Growth of blood vessels and makes them also tortuous, leading to increase in blood flow to endometrium
3. Secretory activities of endometrial glands.

Thus, during the secretory phase, the structure, blood flow and secretory functions of uterus are influenced by estrogen and progesterone secreted by corpus luteum.

Menstrual Phase

If pregnancy does not occur, menstrual phase occurs:

1. During the last two days of secretory phase, i.e. two days prior to onset of menstruation, the secretion of large quantity of progesterone and estrogen from corpus luteum inhibits the secretion of FSH and LH from anterior pituitary, by negative feedback
2. In the absence of LH and FSH, the corpus luteum becomes inactive and starts regressing
3. **Sudden withdrawal** (absence) of ovarian hormones progesterone and estrogen occurs
4. It leads to **menstrual bleeding.**

Lack of ovarian hormones causes the release of gonadotropins once again from anterior pituitary. It results in the onset of development of new follicles in ovary and the cycle repeats.

■ APPLIED PHYSIOLOGY – ABNORMAL MENSTRUATION

■ MENSTRUAL SYMPTOMS

Menstrual symptoms are the unpleasant symptoms with discomfort, which appear in many women during menstruation. These symptoms are due to hormonal withdrawal, leading to cramps in uterine muscle before or during menstruation.

Common Menstrual Symptoms

1. Abdominal pain
2. Dysmenorrhea (menstrual pain)
3. Headache

4. Occasional nausea and vomiting
5. Irritability
6. Depression
7. **Migraine** (neurological disorder, characterized by intense headache causing disability).

■ PREMENSTRUAL SYNDROME

Premenstrual syndrome (PMS) is the symptom of stress that appears before the onset of menstruation. It is also called **premenstrual stress syndrome, premenstrual stress** or **premenstrual tension.** It lasts for about 4 to 5 days prior to menstruation. Symptoms appear due to salt and water retention caused by estrogen.

Common Features

1. Mood swings
2. Anxiety
3. Irritability
4. Emotional instability
5. Headache
6. Depression
7. Constipation
8. Abdominal cramping
9. Bloating (abdominal swelling).

■ ABNORMAL MENSTRUATION

1. **Amenorrhea:** Absence of menstruation
2. **Hypomenorrhea:** Decreased menstrual bleeding
3. **Menorrhagia:** Excess menstrual bleeding
4. **Oligomenorrhea:** Decreased frequency of menstrual bleeding
5. **Polymenorrhea:** Increased frequency of menstruation
6. **Dysmenorrhea:** Menstruation with pain
7. **Metrorrhagia:** Uterine bleeding in between menstruations.

■ ANOVULATORY CYCLE

Anovulatory cycle is the menstrual cycle in which ovulation does not occur. The menstrual bleeding occurs but the release of ovum does not occur. It is common during puberty and few years before menopause. When it occurs before menopause, it is called **perimenopause.** If it occurs very often during childbearing years, it leads to infertility.

Common Causes

1. Hormonal imbalance
2. Prolonged strenuous exercise program
3. Eating disorders
4. Hypothalamic dysfunctions
5. Tumors in pituitary gland, ovary or adrenal gland
6. Long-term use of drugs like steroidal oral contraceptives.

Ovulation

- ■ INTRODUCTION
- ■ PROCESS OF OVULATION
- ■ HORMONAL REGULATION OF OVULATION
- ■ DETERMINATION OF OVULATION TIME
  - ■ DETERMINATION OF BASAL BODY TEMPERATURE
  - ■ DETERMINATION OF HORMONAL EXCRETION IN URINE
  - ■ DETERMINATION OF HORMONAL LEVEL IN PLASMA
  - ■ ULTRASOUND SCANNING
  - ■ CERVICAL MUCUS PATTERN
- ■ SIGNIFICANCE OF DETERMINING OVULATION TIME

■ INTRODUCTION

Ovulation is the process by which the **graafian follicle** in the ovary ruptures and the **ovum** is released into the abdominal cavity. Ovulation occurs on the 14th day of menstrual cycle in a normal cycle of 28 days.

The ovum, which is released into the abdominal cavity, enters the fallopian tube through the fimbriated end of the tube. Usually, only one ovum is released from any one of the ovaries. LH is responsible for ovulation.

■ PROCESS OF OVULATION

Prior to ovulation, large amount of LH is secreted (luteal surge). This causes changes in the graafian follicle leading to ovulation.

Stages of Ovulation

1. Graafian follicle moves towards the periphery of ovary
2. New blood vessels are formed in the ovary by actions of LH and progesterone
3. These blood vessels protrude into the wall of the follicle
4. This increases the blood flow to the follicle
5. Now, prostaglandin is released from granulosa cells of the follicle
6. It causes leakage of plasma into the follicle
7. Just before ovulation the follicle swells and protrudes against the capsule of the ovary. This protrusion is called **stigma**
8. Then, progesterone activates the proteolytic enzymes present in the cells of theca interna
9. These enzymes weaken the follicular capsule and cause degeneration of the stigma
10. After about 30 minutes, fluid begins to ooze from the follicle through the stigma
11. It decreases the size of the follicle causing rupture of stigma
12. Now, ovum is released from the follicle along with fluid and plenty of small granulosa cells into the abdominal cavity (Fig. 81.1).

■ HORMONAL REGULATION OF OVULATION

Hormonal regulation of ovulation is discussed in the previous chapter.

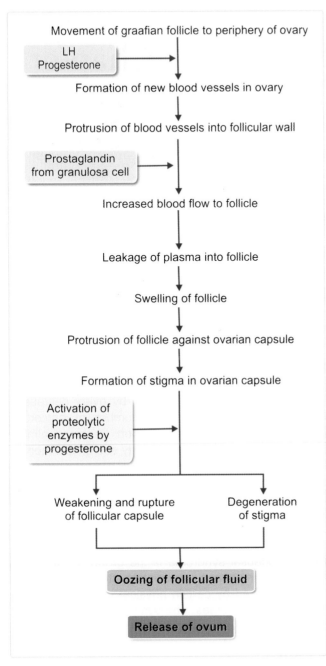

FIGURE 81.1: Process of ovulation

■ DETERMINATION OF OVULATION TIME

Various methods are available to determine the ovulation time. In human beings, usually indirect methods are adopted such as:
1. Determination of basal body temperature
2. Determination of hormonal excretion in urine
3. Determination of hormonal level in plasma
4. Ultrasound scanning
5. Cervical mucus pattern.

■ DETERMINATION OF BASAL BODY TEMPERATURE

Body temperature is measured for few days during the mid period of menstrual cycle. Temperature is measured in the morning by placing the thermometer in rectum or vagina. There is a slight fall in the basal temperature just prior to ovulation. And the temperature increases after ovulation. The alteration in the temperature is very mild and it is about ± 0.3°C to 0.5°C. The increase in temperature is due to the **thermogenic effect** of **progesterone** (Chapter 79).

■ DETERMINATION OF HORMONAL EXCRETION IN URINE

At the time of ovulation, there is an increase in the urinary excretion of metabolic end products of estrogen and progesterone. The end products of estrogen metabolism are estrone, estriol and 17-β-estradiol. The end product of progesterone metabolism is **pregnanediol.**

■ DETERMINATION OF HORMONAL LEVEL IN PLASMA

Plasma level of FSH, LH, estrogen and progesterone is measured. Hormone level is altered at the time of ovulation and after ovulation.

At the time of ovulation:

   i. FSH level decreases
  ii. LH level increases
 iii. Estrogen level increases.

After ovulation:

Progesterone level increases.

■ ULTRASOUND SCANNING

Process of ovulation can be observed in ultrasound scanning.

■ CERVICAL MUCUS PATTERN

When the cervical mucus spread on a slide is examined under microscope, it shows a **fern pattern.** This pattern disappears after ovulation.

■ SIGNIFICANCE OF DETERMINING OVULATION TIME

Determination of ovulation time is helpful for family planning by **rhythm method** (Chapter 88).

Menopause

■ CLIMACTERIC AND MENOPAUSE
■ CAUSE FOR MENOPAUSE
■ CHANGES DURING MENOPAUSE
    ■ CAUSE
    ■ SYMPTOMS
    ■ TREATMENT – HORMONE REPLACEMENT THERAPY (HRT)

■ CLIMACTERIC AND MENOPAUSE

Climacteric is the period in old age when reproductive system undergoes changes due to the decreased secretion of sex hormones, estrogen and progesterone. It occurs at the age of 45 to 55. In females, climacteric is accompanied by menopause.

Menopause is defined as the period when permanent cessation of menstruation takes place. Normally, it occurs at the age of 45 to 55 years.

In some women, the menstruation stops suddenly. In others, the menstrual flow decreases gradually during every cycle and finally it stops. Sometimes irregular menstruation occurs with lengthening or shortening of the period with less or more flow.

Early menopause may occur because of surgical removal of ovaries (**ovariectomy**) or uterus (**hysterectomy**) as a part of treatment for abnormal menstruation. Usually, females with short menstrual cycle attain menopause earlier than the females with longer cycle. Cigarette smoking causes earlier onset of menopause.

■ CAUSE FOR MENOPAUSE

Due to advancement of age, the atrophy of ovaries occurs. It leads to the cessation of menstrual cycle causing menopause. Throughout a woman's sexual life, about 450 of the primordial follicles grow into graafian follicles and ovulate, while thousands of the follicles degenerate.

At the age of 45 years, only few primordial follicles remain in the ovary to be stimulated by FSH and LH. Now, the production of estrogen by ovary decreases due to the decrease in the number of primordial follicles. When estrogen secretion becomes almost zero, FSH and LH are continuously secreted. When all the primordial follicles are atrophied, estrogen secretion stops completely.

■ CHANGES DURING MENOPAUSE – POSTMENOPAUSAL SYNDROME

Postmenopausal syndrome is the group of symptoms that appear in women immediately after menopause. It is characterized by certain physical, physiological and psychological changes. The symptoms start appearing soon after the ovaries stop functioning.

■ CAUSE

Major cause for the symptoms is the lack of estrogen and progesterone. Symptoms may persist till the body gets acclimatized to the absence of estrogen and progesterone.

■ SYMPTOMS

Symptoms do not appear in all women. Some women develop mild symptoms and some women develop severe symptoms, which last for few months to few years.

Symptoms of postmenopausal syndrome:

1. *Hot flashes characterized by extreme flushing of the skin:* Hot flashes start with **discomfort** in the abdomen and **chill** followed by the feeling of heat spreading towards the head. Then the face becomes red followed by sweating and exhaustion.
2. *Vasomotor instability:* Wide fluctuation in blood pressure may be present. Blood pressure increases suddenly and it comes back to normal automatically.
3. Fatigue
4. Nervousness
5. Emotional outburst like crying and anger
6. Mental depression
7. Insomnia
8. Palpitation
9. Vertigo
10. Headache
11. Numbness or tingling sensation
12. Urinary disturbances such as increased frequency of micturition
13. *Long-term effects of estrogen lack such as osteoporosis and atherosclerosis:* **Osteoporosis** is the bone disease resulting in reduction in bone mass. And the bones become susceptible for fracture. **Atherosclerosis** is the condition characterized by deposition of cholesterol on the wall of the blood vessels.

■ TREATMENT – HORMONE REPLACEMENT THERAPY

Most of the women manage it very well. But, about 15% of the women need treatment. In many cases, psychotherapy works very well. If it fails, hormone replacement therapy (HRT) is given. Daily administration of estrogen in small quantities will reverse the symptoms. The combination of estrogen and progesterone is considered to be more advantageous because progesterone prevents the **estrogen-induced cancer** and **hyperplasia of myometrium.** Dose of the hormones should be gradually reduced to prevent the reoccurrence of **postmenopausal symptoms.**

Infertility

- ■ **DEFINITION**
- ■ **INFERTILITY IN MALES**
  - ■ **CAUSES**
- ■ **INFERTILITY IN FEMALES**
  - ■ **CAUSES**

■ DEFINITION

Infertility is the inability to produce the offspring. In females, it is the inability to conceive a child by natural process or inability to carry pregnancy till the completion of term. Infertility occurs due to various factors such as immature reproductive system, defective reproductive system, endocrine disorders, etc.

■ INFERTILITY IN MALES

■ CAUSES

1. Decreased Sperm Count – Oligozoospermia

Normal sperm count in a male is about 100 to 150 millions/mL of semen. Infertility occurs when the sperm count decreases below 20 millions/mL of semen. Sperm count decreases because of disruption of seminiferous tubules or acute infection in testis. In some males, there is possibility of sterility (permanent inability to produce offspring) because of absence of spermatogenesis as in the case of cryptorchidism or underdeveloped testis (Chapter 74).

2. Abnormal Sperms

Sometimes, the sperm count may be normal, but the structure of the sperm may be abnormal. The sperms may be without tail and nonmotile or with two heads or with abnormal head. When a large number of abnormal sperms are produced infertility occurs (Chapter 77).

3. Obstruction of Reproductive Ducts

Obstruction of reproductive ducts like vas deferens leads to infertility.

4. Other Disorders

  i. Cryptorchidism
  ii. Trauma
  iii. Mumps
  iv. Long-term use of drugs
  v. Alcoholism
  vi. Genetic disorders
  vii. Hypothalamic disorders
  viii. Disorders of pituitary, thyroid and pancreas.

■ INFERTILITY IN FEMALES

■ CAUSES

1. Abnormalities of Ovary

Sometimes, a thick capsule develops around the ovaries and prevents ovulation. In some women, ovaries develop cysts (membranous sac containing fluid) or become fibrotic (hardened tissues resulting from lymphedema).

In these conditions, maturation and release of ovum does not occur.

2. Abnormalities of Uterus

A type of endometrial tissue similar to uterine endometrium grows in the pelvic cavity surrounding the uterus, fallopian tubes and ovaries. It is called endometriosis. And, pregnancy does not occur in this condition.

In some cases, there is low grade infection or inflammation or abnormal hormonal stimulation in the cervix. It leads to the abnormal secretion of thick mucus in cervix, which prevents entry of sperm and fertilization of ovum.

3. Absence of Ovulation

Ovulation does not occur in some females, because of hyposecretion of gonadotropic hormones. Quantities of these hormones are not sufficient enough to cause maturation of ovum or release of ovum. The cycle without ovulation is known as anovulatory cycle.

4. Other Disorders

   i.   Diabetes mellitus
   ii.   Renal diseases
   iii.   Liver diseases
   iv.   Hypothalamic disorders
   v.   Disorders of pituitary gland, thyroid and adrenal glands.

Pregnancy and Parturition

■ **INTRODUCTION**
■ **FERTILIZATION OF THE OVUM**
■ **SEX CHROMOSOMES AND SEX DETERMINATION**
  ■ SEX CHROMOSOMES
  ■ SEX DETERMINATION
■ **IMPLANTATION**
■ **DEVELOPMENT OF PLACENTA AND EMBRYO**
■ **MATERNAL CHANGES DURING PREGNANCY**
  ■ STRUCTURAL CHANGES
  ■ INCREASE IN BODY WEIGHT
  ■ METABOLIC CHANGES
  ■ CHANGES IN PHYSIOLOGICAL SYSTEMS
■ **GESTATION PERIOD**
■ **PARTURITION**
  ■ BRAXTON HICKS CONTRACTIONS
  ■ FALSE LABOR CONTRACTIONS
  ■ STAGES OF PARTURITION
  ■ MECHANISM OF LABOR
  ■ ROLE OF UTERUS
  ■ ROLE OF CERVIX
  ■ ROLE OF HORMONES

■ INTRODUCTION

Ovum is released from graafian follicle of ovary into the abdominal cavity at the time of ovulation.

From abdominal cavity, ovum enters fallopian tube through the **fimbriated end.** Entry of ovum is facilitated by movement of cilia present in the inner surface of fimbriated end.

Ovum of matured follicle in the ovary is in **primary oocyte** stage with **diploid number** (23 pairs) of chromosomes. Just before ovulation, meiotic division takes place in the ovum. Primary oocyte divides into a **secondary oocyte** and a **first polar body.** First polar body is expelled out. **Secondary oocyte** contains only 23 chromosomes **(haploid).** Remaining 23 chromosomes are lost in the expelled first polar body.

Thus, when the ovum is released into abdominal cavity during ovulation, it is in the secondary oocyte stage with haploid number of chromosomes.

■ FERTILIZATION OF THE OVUM

Fertilization refers to **fusion** (union) of male and female gametes (sperm and ovum) to form a new offspring.

If sexual intercourse occurs at ovulation time and semen is ejaculated in the vagina, the sperms travel through the vagina and uterus to reach the fallopian tube. Sperms reach the ovarian end of fallopian tube within 30 to 60 minutes.

Movement of the sperm through uterus is facilitated by the **antiperistaltic contractions** of uterine muscles. Uterine contractions are induced by oxytocin, which is secreted from posterior pituitary by neuroendocrine reflex during sexual intercourse (Chapter 66). Uterine contractions are also facilitated by **prostaglandin** (PGE_2) present in male seminal fluid.

Among 200 to 300 millions of sperms entering female genital tract, only a few thousand sperms reach the spot near the ovum. Among these few thousand sperms, only one succeeds in fertilizing the ovum.

During fertilization, the sperm enters the ovum by penetrating the multiple layers of granulosa cells known as **corona radiata** present around the ovum. It is facilitated by **hyaluronidase** and **proteolytic enzymes** present in acrosome of sperm. Proteolytic enzymes from acrosome of the successful sperm diffuse through the structures of zona pellucida and inactivate the other sperms entering the ovum.

Penetrating movement of sperm is enabled by a protein called **CatSper** present in the tail portion of the sperm. It is a tunnel-shaped protein and forms the ion channel for entry of calcium into sperm cell.

Immediately after fertilization, ovum, which is in secondary oocyte stage, divides into a matured ovum and a **second polar body.** Second polar body is expelled. Nucleus of matured ovum becomes female pronucleus with 23 chromosomes, which include **22 autosomes** and one sex chromosome called **X chromosome.**

Simultaneously, head of sperm swells and becomes male pronucleus. Then 23 chromosomes of the sperm and 23 chromosomes of ovum arrange themselves to reform the 23 pairs of chromosomes in the fertilized ovum.

■ SEX CHROMOSOMES AND SEX DETERMINATION

■ SEX CHROMOSOMES

All the dividing cells in the body have 23 pairs of chromosomes. Among the 23 pairs, 22 pairs are called **somatic chromosomes** or **autosomes.** Remaining one pair of chromosomes is called **sex chromosomes.** Sex chromosomes are X and Y chromosomes.

■ SEX DETERMINATION

Sex chromosomes are responsible for sex determination. During fertilization of ovum, 23 chromosomes from ovum and 23 chromosomes from the sperm unite together to form the 23 pairs (46) of chromosomes in the fertilized ovum. Now, sex determination occurs. Ovum contains the X chromosome. Sperm has either X chromosome or Y chromosome. When the ovum is fertilized by a sperm with X chromosome, the child will be female with XX chromosome. And, if the ovum is fertilized by a sperm

with Y chromosome, the sex of the child will be male with XY chromosome. So, the sex of the child depends upon the male partner.

Role of testosterone in **sex differentiation** is explained in Chapter 74.

■ IMPLANTATION

Implantation is the process by which the fertilized ovum called **zygote** implants (fixes itself or gets attached) in the endometrial lining of uterus.

After the fertilization, the ovum is known as zygote. Zygote takes 3 to 5 days to reach the uterine cavity from fallopian tube. While travelling through the fallopian tube, the zygote receives its nutrition from the secretions of fallopian tube.

After reaching the uterus, the developing zygote remains freely in the uterine cavity for 2 to 4 days before it is implanted. Thus, it takes about 1 week for implantation after the day of fertilization. During the stay in uterine cavity before implantation, the zygote receives its nutrition from the secretions of endometrium, which is known as **uterine milk.**

Just before implantation, the zygote develops into **morula** and then the implantation starts. A layer of spherical cells called trophoblast cells is formed around morula. Trophoblast cells release proteolytic enzymes over the surface of endometrium. These enzymes digest the cells of the endometrium. Now, morula moves through the digested part of endometrium and implants itself.

■ DEVELOPMENT OF PLACENTA AND EMBRYO

Already uterus is prepared by progesterone secreted from the corpus luteum during secretory phase of menstrual cycle. After implantation, placenta develops between morula and endometrium.

When implantation occurs, there is further increase in the thickness of endometrium because of continuous secretion of progesterone from corpus luteum. At this stage, the endometrial stromal cells are called **decidual cells** and the endometrium at the implanted area is called **decidua.**

Now the **trophoblastic cells** of morula develop into cords, which are attached with decidual portion of endometrium. Blood capillaries grow into these cords from the blood vessels of the newly formed embryo. At about 16th day after fertilization, heart of embryo starts pumping the blood into the **trophoblastic cords.**

At the same time, blood sinusoids develop around the trophoblastic cords. These sinusoids receive blood from the mother.

Trophoblastic cells form some vascular projections into which fetal capillaries grow. These vascular projections become **placental villi.**

Thus, the final form of **placenta** has got the fetal part and the maternal part.

Fetal part of placenta contains the two umbilical arteries, which carry fetal blood to the placental villi through the capillaries. The blood returns back to fetus through umbilical vein. Maternal part of placenta is formed by uterine arteries through which blood flows into sinusoids that surround the villi. The blood returns back to mother's body through uterine vein.

Functions of placenta are described in detail in Chapter 85.

■ MATERNAL CHANGES DURING PREGNANCY

During pregnancy, the changes are noticed in various organs, body weight, the metabolic activities and functional status of different physiological systems in the mother.

■ STRUCTURAL CHANGES

Various structural changes are noticed in the primary sex organs, accessory sex organs and in the mammary glands during pregnancy.

1. Ovaries

Follicular changes do not appear in ovary and ovulation does not occur because the secretion of FSH and LH from anterior pituitary is inhibited. Corpus luteum enlarges and secretes a large quantity of progesterone and little estrogen, which are essential for maintaining the pregnancy. It continues for 3 months and then, corpus luteum degenerates. By this time placenta develops fully and takes over the function of secreting estrogen and progesterone. It continues throughout the period of pregnancy thus inhibiting the secretion of FSH and LH.

2. Uterus

When the fetus grows, uterus undergoes changes in volume, size, shape and weight.

i. Volume

Volume of uterus increases gradually due to fetal growth. From almost zero volume, uterus reaches about 5 to 7 liters at the end of pregnancy. Out of this, 50% of the volume is due to the fetus and rest is due to the placenta, amniotic fluid, etc.

ii. Size

Size of the uterus also increases due to:
a. **Hyperplasia** (increase in number of cells) of myometrium
b. **Hypertrophy** (increase in size of the cells) of myometrium
c. Growth of fetus.

iii. Shape

The shape of non-pregnant uterus is **pyriform.** As the fetus grows, at the 12th week of pregnancy, it becomes **globular.** Then, once again it becomes pyriform gradually.

iv. Weight

Non-pregnant uterus weighs about 30 to 50 g. The weight increases as the pregnancy advances. At the end of pregnancy, the uterine weight increases to about 1,000 to 1,200 g.

v. Histological changes

Endometrium shows formation of decidua, which is the bed for the fertilized ovum during the initial stages of pregnancy. Later, by the end of 3 months, three layers of decidua are formed:
a. Decidua basalis, which is the maternal part
b. Decidua capsularis that surrounds fetal sac
c. Decidua parietalis, which lines rest of uterine wall.

After the 3rd month, the decidua capsularis and parietalis fuse together.

3. Vagina

Vagina increases in size and its color changes to violet due to increased blood supply. There is deposition of **glycogen** in the epithelial cells.

4. Cervix

In cervix, the number of glands, blood supply and mucus secretion increase. The tough cervix becomes soft and it is closed by **mucus plug.**

5. Fallopian Tube

The number of epithelial cells and blood supply increase in fallopian tubes.

6. Mammary Glands

Size of the mammary glands increases because of development of new ducts and alveoli, deposition of fat and increased vascularization. Pigmentation of nipple and areola occurs.

■ INCREASE IN BODY WEIGHT

Average weight gained by the body during pregnancy is about 12 kg. Approximate weight of various structures, which adds to the weight gain:

1. Fetus   : 3.5 kg
2. Amniotic fluid   : 2.0 kg
3. Placenta   : 1.5 kg
4. Increase in maternal : 5.0 kg
   body weight

If proper **prenatal care** is not taken, the body weight increases greatly by about 20 to 30 kg.

■ METABOLIC CHANGES

The metabolic activities are accelerated in the body due to increased secretion of various hormones like thyroxine, cortisol and sex hormones.

1. *Basal Metabolic Rate*

Increase in the secretion of various hormones especially thyroxine increases the basal metabolic rate by about 15% in the later stages of pregnancy.

2. *Protein Metabolism*

The anabolism of proteins increases during pregnancy. Positive nitrogen balance occurs. The deposition of proteins increases in the uterus.

3. *Carbohydrate Metabolism*

Blood glucose level increases leading to **glucosuria**. **Ketosis** develops either due to less food or more vomiting. Because of all these reasons, there is **hyperplasia** of beta cells of islets of Langerhans in pancreas leading to increase in secretion of insulin. Inspite of this, there is possibility of developing **diabetes in pregnancy** or **latent diabetes** after delivery.

4. *Lipid Metabolism*

During pregnancy, there is deposition of about 3 to 4 kg of fat in the maternal body. It also increases the blood cholesterol level and ketosis.

5. *Water and Mineral Metabolism*

Estrogen and progesterone are secreted by corpus luteum in the first trimester and by placenta later. These hormones increase the retention of sodium and water. Secretion of aldosterone increases during pregnancy. Aldosterone in turn increases the reabsorption of sodium from renal tubules. Apart from water and sodium retention, there is retention of calcium and phosphorus as well. Calcium and phosphorus are necessary for the growing fetus.

■ CHANGES IN PHYSIOLOGICAL SYSTEMS

1. *Blood*

The blood volume increases by about 20% or about 1 L. This increase is mainly because of increase in plasma volume. It causes hemodilution. Because of great demand for iron by the fetus, the mother usually develops anemia. It can be rectified by proper prenatal care and iron replacement.

2. *Cardiovascular System*

Cardiac output

Generally, cardiac output increases by about 30% in the first trimester. After the 3rd month, cardiac output starts decreasing and reaches almost the normal level in the later stages of pregnancy.

Blood pressure

Arterial blood pressure remains unchanged during the first trimester. During the second trimester, there is a slight decrease in blood pressure. It is due to the diversion of blood to uterine sinuses. And, hypertension develops if proper prenatal care is not taken.

Pre-eclampsia

Pre-eclampsia is the **hypertensive** disorder of pregnancy. It is otherwise known as **toxemia of pregnancy**. About 3% to 4% of the pregnant women suffer from this. It usually occurs during last trimester of pregnancy.

Cause for hypertension

1. Release of vasoconstrictor substances from placenta
2. Hypersecretion of adrenal hormones and other hormones, which cause vasoconstriction
3. Development of autoimmune processes induced by the presence of placenta or fetus.

Other symptoms associated with hypertension

1. Decreased blood flow to kidney and thickening of glomerular capillary membrane, leading to reduction in GFR and urinary output
2. Retention of sodium and water
3. Decreased urinary output along with retention of sodium and water results in increased extracellular fluid volume and edema
4. Excretion of proteins through urine.

Eclampsia

Eclampsia is the serious condition of pre-ecclampsia characterized by severe **vascular spasm,** dangerous **hypertension** and **convulsive muscular contractions** almost like **seizures.** It occurs just before, during or immediately after delivery. It leads to **death,** if timely treatment is not given.

Features of eclampsia

1. Spasm of blood vessels
2. Very severe hypertension
3. Renal failure
4. Liver failure
5. Heart failure
6. Convulsions
7. Coma.

Treatment for eclampsia

Treatment should be immediate. It includes administration of quick acting vasodilator drugs or termination of pregnancy.

3. Respiratory System

Overall activity of respiratory system increases slightly. Tidal volume, pulmonary ventilation and oxygen utilization are increased.

4. Excretory System

Renal blood flow and GFR increase resulting in increase in urine formation. It is because of increase in fluid intake and the increased excretory products from fetus. The urine becomes diluted with the specific gravity of 1,025. In the first trimester, the frequency of micturition increases because of the pressure exerted by the uterus on bladder.

5. Digestive System

During the initial stages of pregnancy, the **morning sickness** occurs in mother. It involves **nausea, vomiting** and **giddiness.** This is because of the hormonal imbalance. The motility of GI tract decreases by progesterone and constipation is common. **Indigestion** and **hypochlorhydria** (decrease in the amount of hydrochloric acid in gastric juice) also occur.

6. Endocrine System

i. *Anterior pituitary*

During pregnancy, the size of anterior pituitary increases by about 50%. And secretion of corticotropin, thyrotropin and prolactin increases. However, the secretion of FSH and LH decreases very much. It is because of negative feedback control by estrogen and progesterone, which are continuously secreted from corpus luteum initially and placenta later on.

ii. *Adrenal cortex*

There is moderate increase in secretion of cortisol, which helps in the mobilization of amino acids from the mother's tissues to the fetus. Aldosterone secretion also increases. It reaches the maximum at the end of pregnancy. Along with estrogen and progesterone, aldosterone is responsible for the retention of water and sodium.

iii. *Thyroid gland*

The size and the secretory activity of thyroid gland increase during pregnancy. The increased secretion of thyroxine helps in the preparation of mammary glands for lactation. It is also responsible for increase in basal metabolic rate.

iv. *Parathyroid glands*

Parathyroid glands also show an increase in the size and secretory activity. Parathormone is responsible for maintenance of calcium level in mother's blood in spite of loss of large amount of calcium to fetus.

7. Nervous System

There is general excitement of nervous system during pregnancy. It leads to the **psychological imbalance** such as change in the moods, excitement or depression in the early stages of pregnancy. During the later months of pregnancy, the woman becomes very much excited because of anticipation of delivery of the baby, labor pain, etc.

■ GESTATION PERIOD

Gestation period refers to the pregnancy period. The average gestation period is about 280 days or 40 weeks from the date of last menstrual period (LMP). Traditionally, it is calculated as 10 lunar months. However, in terms of modern calendar it is calculated as 9 months and 7 days. If the menstrual cycle is normal 28 day cycle, the fertilization of ovum by the sperm occurs on 14th day after LMP. Thus the actual duration of human pregnancy is 280 – 14 = 266 days. If the pregnancy ends before 28th week, it is referred as miscarriage. If the pregnancy ends before 37th week, then it is considered as premature labor.

■ PARTURITION

Parturition is the expulsion or delivery of the fetus from the mother's body. It occurs at the end of pregnancy. The process by which the delivery of fetus occurs is called **labor.** It involves various activities such as contraction of uterus, dilatation of cervix and opening of vaginal canal.

■ BRAXTON HICKS CONTRACTIONS

Braxton Hicks contractions are the weak, irregular, short and usually painless uterine contractions, which start after 6th week of pregnancy. These contractions are named after the British doctor, **John Braxton Hicks** who discovered them in 1872. It is suggested that these contractions do not induce cervical dilatation but may cause softening of cervix. Often called the **practice contractions,** Braxton Hicks contractions help the uterus practice for upcoming labor. Sometimes these contractions cause discomfort.

Braxton Hicks contractions are triggered by several factors such as:
1. Touching the abdomen
2. Movement of fetus in uterus
3. Physical activity
4. Sexual intercourse
5. Dehydration.

■ FALSE LABOR CONTRACTIONS

While nearing the time of delivery, the Braxton Hicks contractions become intense and are called **false labor contractions.** The false labor contractions are believed to help cervical dilatation.

■ STAGES OF PARTURITION

Parturition occurs in three stages:

First Stage

First, the strong uterine contractions called **labor contractions** commence. Labor contractions arise from fundus of uterus and move downwards so that the head of fetus is pushed against cervix. It results in dilatation of cervix and opening of vaginal canal. Exact cause for the onset of labor is not known. This stage extends for a variable period of time.

Second Stage

In this stage, the fetus is delivered out from uterus through cervix and vaginal canal. This stage lasts for about 1 hour.

Third Stage

During this stage, the placenta is detached from the decidua and is expelled out from uterus. It occurs within 10 to 15 minutes after the delivery of the child.

■ MECHANISM OF LABOR

The slow and weak contractions of uterus commence at about a month before parturition. Later, the contractions gradually obtain strength and finally are converted into labor contractions at the time of labor. Exact cause for the onset of labor contractions is not known. It is strongly believed that the labor contractions are induced by the signal from fetus. And during labor, reflexes from uterus and cervix produce the powerful uterine contractions. Thus, uterus and cervix play an important role in labor. Many hormones are also involved during parturition.

■ ROLE OF UTERUS

Once started, the uterine contractions cause the development of more and more strong contractions. That is, the irritation of uterine muscle during initial contraction leads to further reflex contractions. It is called **positive feedback** mechanism. It plays an important role, not only in producing more number of uterine contractions but also the contractions to become more and more powerful.

■ ROLE OF CERVIX

Cervix also plays an important role in increasing the strength of uterine contractions. When the head of fetus is forced against the cervix during the first stage of labor, the cervix stretches. It causes stimulation of muscles of cervix, which in turn results in reflex contractions of uterus.

■ ROLE OF HORMONES

Hormones involved in the process of parturition:

Maternal Hormones

1. Oxytocin
2. Prostaglandins
3. Cortisol
4. Catecholamines
5. Relaxin.

Fetal Hormones

1. Oxytocin
2. Cortisol
3. Prostaglandins.

Placental Hormones

1. Estrogen
2. Progesterone
3. Prostaglandins.

Estrogen

Estrogen is continuously secreted along with progesterone throughout the gestation period. However, in the later period, the quantity of estrogen released is much greater than that of progesterone.

Estrogen:

i. Increases the force of uterine contractions
ii. Increases the number of oxytocin receptors in uterine wall
iii. Accelerates the synthesis of prostaglandin from uterus.

Progesterone

Progesterone plays an important role in labor indirectly by its sudden withdrawal at the end of pregnancy.

Throughout the period of gestation, progesterone suppresses uterine contractions. It also inhibits the synthesis of prostaglandin (PGE_2), which is necessary for uterine contraction. Progesterone inhibits prostaglandin synthesis by inhibiting the release of the enzyme phospholipase A, which is essential for prostaglandin synthesis.

Sudden decrease in progesterone secretion at the end of gestation period increases the uterine contractions and PGE_2 synthesis.

Oxytocin

Oxytocin:

i. Causes contraction of smooth muscle of uterus and enhances labor. During the later stages of pregnancy, the number of receptors for oxytocin increases in the wall of uterus by the influence of estrogen. Because of this, the uterus becomes more sensitive to oxytocin.
ii. Stimulates the release of prostaglandins in the decidua.

Oxytocin is released in large quantity during labor. It is due to **neuroendocrine reflex.** During the movement of fetus through cervix, the receptors on the cervix are stimulated and start discharging a large number of impulses. Impulses are carried to hypothalamus by the somatic nerve fibers and result in the release of a large quantity of oxytocin, which enhances labor. The release of more amount of oxytocin occurs due to **positive feedback** (Chapter 66).

Relaxin

Relaxin is secreted from maternal ovary (corpus luteum) during the initial period of pregnancy. It is secreted in large quantity at the time of labor by placenta and mammary glands (Chapter 87).

Relaxin:

i. Helps labor by softening the cervix and loosening the ligaments of symphysis pubis, so that the dilatation of cervix occurs
ii. Increases the number of receptors for oxytocin in the myometrium
iii. Simultaneously suppresses the inhibitory action of progesterone on uterine contraction so that the uterus starts contracting
iv. Facilitates the development of mammary glands.

Prostaglandins

In recent times, prostaglandins are considered to play a vital role in labor. Prostaglandins particularly PGE_2 facilitate labor by increasing the force of uterine contractions. The prostaglandins are secreted from uterine tissues, fetal membranes and placenta. Their concentration is increased in maternal blood and amniotic fluid at the time of labor.

Prostaglandins increase the force of uterine contractions by elevating the intracellular concentration of calcium ions in the uterine muscles.

Catecholamines

It is believed that the circulating adrenaline and noradrenaline also might increase the uterine contraction through alpha adrenergic receptors.

Cortisol

At the time of labor, hypothalamus releases large quantity of corticotropin-releasing hormone, which increases the release of cortisol from the adrenal cortex. Cortisol enhances the uterine contraction and plays an important role in helping the mother to withstand the stress during labor.

Placenta

■ INTRODUCTION

Placenta is a temporary membranous vascular organ that develops in females during pregnancy. It is expelled after childbirth. Placenta forms a link between the fetus and mother. It is considered as an anchor for the growing fetus. It is not only the physical attachment between the fetus and mother, but also forms the physiological connection between the two.

Placenta is implanted in the wall of the uterus. It is formed from both embryonic and maternal tissues. So, it consists of two parts namely the fetal part and the mother's part. It is connected to the fetus by umbilical cord, which contains blood vessels and connective tissue. Development of placenta is explained in Chapter 84.

The delivery of fetus is followed by the expulsion of placenta. After expulsion of the placenta, the umbilical cord is cut. The site of attachment of placenta in the center of anterior abdomen of fetus is called navel or umbilicus.

■ FUNCTIONS OF PLACENTA

■ NUTRITIVE FUNCTION

Nutritive substances, electrolytes and hormones necessary for the development of fetus diffuse from mother's blood into fetal blood through placenta.

■ EXCRETORY FUNCTION

Metabolic end products and other waste products from the fetal body are excreted into the mother's blood through placenta.

■ RESPIRATORY FUNCTION

Fetal lungs are non-functioning and placenta forms the respiratory organ for fetus. Oxygen necessary for fetus is received by diffusion from the maternal blood and carbon dioxide from fetal blood diffuses into the mother's blood through placenta.

Exchange of Respiratory Gases between Fetal Blood and Maternal Blood

Exchange of respiratory gases between fetal blood and maternal blood occurs mainly because of pressure gradient. Partial pressure of oxygen in the maternal blood is 50 mm Hg. In fetal blood, the partial pressure of oxygen is 30 mm Hg. This pressure gradient of 20 mm Hg causes the diffusion of oxygen into the fetal blood.

This pressure gradient is very low, compared to the gradient existing between partial pressure of oxygen in arterial blood and alveoli in adults. Still, an adequate quantity of oxygen is available for fetus.

It is because of two reasons:

1. The hemoglobin in fetal blood has 20 times more affinity for oxygen than the adult hemoglobin

2. The concentration of hemoglobin is about 50% more in fetal blood than in adult blood.

Bohr effect and Double Bohr effect

Bohr effect is the decrease in the affinity of hemoglobin for oxygen due to increased carbon dioxide tension. When carbon dioxide tension decreases, the affinity of hemoglobin for oxygen is increased. All the metabolic end products including carbon dioxide are completely excreted from fetus into the maternal blood. This develops low partial pressure of carbon dioxide in fetal blood. So, the affinity of fetal hemoglobin for oxygen increases resulting in diffusion of more amount of oxygen from mother's blood into fetal blood.

At the same time, because of entrance of fetal carbon dioxide into maternal blood, partial pressure of carbon dioxide is very high in mother's blood. It decreases the affinity of mother's hemoglobin for oxygen resulting in diffusion of more amount of oxygen into the fetal blood.

Double Bohr effect is the operation of Bohr effect in both fetal blood and maternal blood.

■ ENDOCRINE FUNCTION

Hormones secreted by placenta are:
1. Human chorionic gonadotropin
2. Estrogen
3. Progesterone
4. Human chorionic somatomammotropin
5. Relaxin.

1. Human Chorionic Gonadotropin

Human chorionic gonadotropin (hCG) is a glycoprotein. Its chemical structure is similar to that of LH.

Actions of hCG

i. *On corpus luteum:* hCG is responsible for the preservation and the secretory activity of corpus luteum. Progesterone and estrogen secreted by corpus luteum are essential for the maintenance of pregnancy. Deficiency or absence of hCG during the first 2 months of pregnancy leads to termination of pregnancy (abortion), because of involution of corpus luteum.

ii. *On fetal testes:* Action of hCG on fetal testes is similar to that of LH in adults. It stimulates the interstitial cells of Leydig and causes secretion of testosterone. The testosterone is necessary for the development of sex organs in male fetus.

2. Estrogen

Placental estrogen is similar to ovarian estrogen in structure and function.

Actions of placental estrogen

i. *On uterus:* Causes enlargement of the uterus so that, the growing fetus can be accommodated.

ii. *On breasts:* Responsible for the enlargement of the breasts and growth of the duct system in the breasts.

iii. *On external genitalia:* Causes enlargement of the female external genitalia.

iv. *On pelvis:* Relaxes pelvic ligaments. It facilitates the passage of the fetus through the birth canal at the time of labor.

3. Progesterone

Placental progesterone is similar to ovarian progesterone in structure and function.

Actions of placental progesterone

i. *On endometrium of uterus:* Accelerates the proliferation and development of decidual cells in the endometrium of uterus. The decidual cells are responsible for the supply of nutrition to the embryo in the early stage.

ii. *On the movements of uterus:* Inhibits the contraction of muscles in the pregnant uterus. It is an important function of progesterone as it prevents expulsion of fetus during pregnancy.

iii. *On breasts:* Causes enlargement of breasts and growth of duct system of the breasts.

Progesterone is responsible for further development and preparation of mammary glands for lactation.

4. Human Chorionic Somatomammotropin

Human chorionic somatomammotropin (HCS) is a protein hormone secreted from placenta. It is often called placental lactogen. It acts like prolactin and growth hormone secreted from pituitary. So, it is believed to act on mammary glands and to enhance the growth of fetus by influencing the metabolic activities. It increases the amount of glucose and lipids in the maternal blood, which are transferred to fetus.

Actions of HCS

i. *On breasts:* In experimental animals, adminis-tration of HCS causes enlargement of mammary glands and induces lactation. That is why, it is

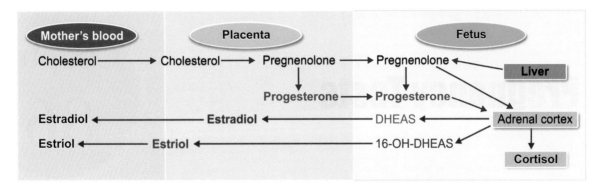

FIGURE 85.1: Fetoplacental unit. DHEAS = Dehydroepiandrosterone sulfate, 16-OH-DHEAS = 16-hydoxy-dehydroepiandrosterone sulfate.

named as mammotropin. However, the action of this hormone on the breasts of pregnant women is not known.

ii. *On protein metabolism:* HCS acts like GH on protein metabolism. It causes anabolism of proteins and accumulation of proteins in the fetal tissues. Thus, the growth of fetus is enhanced.

iii. *On carbohydrate metabolism:* It reduces the peripheral utilization of glucose in the mother leading to availability of large quantity of glucose to the growing fetus.

iv. *On lipid metabolism:* It mobilizes fat from the adipose tissue of the mother. A large amount of free fatty acid is made available as the source of energy in the mother's body. It compensates the loss of glucose from the mother's blood to fetus.

5. *Relaxin*

Relaxin is a polypeptide, which is secreted by corpus luteum. It is also secreted in large quantity by placenta and mammary glands at the time of labor (Refer Chapter 84).

■ FETOPLACENTAL UNIT

Fetoplacental unit refers to the interaction between fetus and placenta in the formation of steroid hormones. The interaction between fetus and placenta occurs because some of the enzymes involved in steroid synthesis present in fetus are absent in placenta and those enzymes, which are absent in fetus are present in placenta.

Due to this interaction during synthesis of steroid hormones, fetus and placenta are together called fetoplacental unit (Fig. 85.1).

■ FUNCTIONS OF FETOPLACENTAL UNIT

Placenta and fetus interact with each other in the synthesis of steroid hormones in the following manner:

1. Cholesterol, which is the precursor for steroid hormones, is obtained by placenta from mother's blood
2. Placenta synthesizes pregnenolone from cholesterol
3. From pregnenolone, progesterone is formed
4. Some amount of the pregnenolone from placenta enters fetus. Fetal liver also produces a small quantity of pregnenolone
5. Pregnenolone from placenta and fetal liver forms the substrate for the formation of two substances in the adrenal gland of the fetus:
   i. Dehydroepiandrosterone sulfate (DHEAS)
   ii. 16-hydroxy-dehydroepiandrosterone sulfate (16-OH-DHEAS).

   Some of the DHEAS is also hydroxylated into 16-OH-DHEAS in fetal liver
6. DHEAS and 16-OH-DHEAS are transported back into the placenta to form estrogen
7. Estradiol is synthesized from DHEAS and estriol from 16-OH-DHEAS. These two forms of estrogen enter mother's blood
8. Some amount of the progesterone enters the fetus from placenta
9. From this progesterone, cortisol and corticosterone are synthesized in fetal adrenal glands.

Pregnancy Tests

```
■ INTRODUCTION
■ BIOLOGICAL TEST
■ IMMUNOLOGICAL TESTS
```

■ INTRODUCTION

Pregnancy test is the test used to detect or confirm pregnancy. The basis of pregnancy tests is to determine the presence of the **human chorionic gonadotropin (hCG)** in the urine of woman suspected for pregnancy. Both biological and immunological tests are available to determine the presence of hCG in the urine of the pregnant woman.

■ BIOLOGICAL TESTS

These tests are performed by using experimental animals. The biological tests for pregnancy can be performed only after 2 or 3 weeks of conception so that, the concentration of hCG in urine is sufficient to show the result.

■ ASCHHEIM-ZONDEK TEST

Aschheim-Zondek test was the first test invented for confirming the pregnancy. It depends upon the ovarian changes in immature mice caused by hCG. The immature mice do not ovulate naturally.

Ovulation occurs only if hCG is injected. 2 mL of urine from the woman suspected for pregnancy is injected daily for 2 days into the immature mice. 5 days after injection of urine, the mice are killed. The ovaries are examined for the presence of corpora lutea (plural for corpus luteum) and hemorrhages, which indicates ovulation. Ovulation is due to the presence of hCG in urine.

■ KUPPERMAN TEST

Kupperaman test is the modification of Aschheim-Zondek test, in order to save time. In this, an immature rat is used instead of immature mice. About 2 mL of urine is injected subcutaneously into immature rat and ovarian changes are observed after 6 hours. If the urine is injected intraperitoneally, the ovarian changes can be observed within 2 hours.

■ FRIEDMAN TEST

In this test, 10 to 15 mL of urine is injected intravenously into rabbit and ovulation is observed by examining the ovaries after 48 hours.

■ HOGBEN TEST

In this test, about 20 to 30 ml of urine is concentrated and injected into the dorsal lymph sac of South African toad, *Xenopus levis*. If hCG is present in the urine, it causes ovulation after 12 hours.

■ GALLI-MAININI TEST

In this test, 2 mL of urine is injected into the male amphibian (toad or frog). hCG in urine causes expulsion of spermatozoa within 2 hours.

Biological tests are outdated after the development of immunological tests.

Disadvantages of Biological Tests

Biological tests for pregnancy are replaced by immunological tests because of several disadvantages:
1. The biological test require animals
2. Tests can be performed only after 2 to 3 weeks of pregnancy so that sufficient quantity of hCG is excreted in urine
3. Results are not obtained quickly; one has to wait for 2 to 48 hours
4. Tests involve tedious procedures such as sacrificing the animals.

■ IMMUNOLOGICAL TESTS

Presence of hCG is also determined by using immunological techniques. Immunological tests are based on **double antigen-antibody reactions.** Commonly performed immunological test is known as **Gravindex test.**

■ PRINCIPLE

Principle is to determine the agglutination of sheep RBCs coated with hCG. Latex particles could also be used instead of sheep RBCs.

■ REQUISITES

1. *Antiserum from Rabbit*

Urine from a pregnant woman is collected and hCG is isolated. This hCG is injected into a rabbit.

The rabbit develops **antibodies against hCG.** The antibodies are called **hCG antibody or anti-hCG.** The rabbit's blood is obtained and serum is separated. The serum containing hCG antibody is called **rabbit antiserum** or **hCG antiserum.** It is readily available in the market.

2. *Red Blood Cells from Sheep*

RBCs are obtained from sheep blood and are coated with pure hCG obtained from urine of the pregnant women. Nowadays, instead of sheep RBCs, the rubberized synthetic particles called the **latex particles** are used.

3. *Urine*

Fresh urine sample of the woman, who needs to confirm pregnancy is used for Gravindex test.

■ PROCEDURE

1. One drop of hCG antiserum is taken on a glass slide. One drop of urine from the woman who wants to confirm pregnancy is added to this and both are mixed well.
2. Now, one drop of latex particles is added to this and mixed.

■ OBSERVATION AND RESULT

Result is determined by observing the agglutination of latex particles added to mixer of hCG antiserum and woman's urine.

Absence of Agglutination of Latex Particles

If hCG is present in urine, it is agglutinated by antibodies of antiserum and all the antibodies are fully used up. No

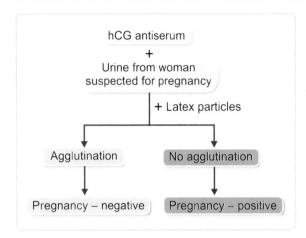

FIGURE 86.1: Immunological test for pregnancy

free antibody is available. Agglutination of hCG molecules by antibodies is not visible because it is colorless.

Later when latex particles are added, these particles are not agglutinated because, free antibody is not available. Thus, absence of agglutination of latex particles indicates that the woman is pregnant.

Presence of Agglutination of Latex Particles

If urine without hCG is mixed with antiserum, the antibodies are freely available. When latex particles are added, the antibodies cause agglutination of these latex particles. Agglutination of latex particles can be seen clearly even with naked eye. Thus, presence of agglutination of latex particles indicates that, the woman is not pregnant (Fig. 86.1).

■ ADVANTAGES OF IMMUNOLOGICAL TESTS FOR PREGNANCY

1. Immunological tests are more accurate
2. Result is obtained quickly within few minutes
3. These tests can be carried out very easily. The procedure is not cumbersome, as in the case of biological tests
4. Immunological tests can be performed on 5th day of conception. By biological methods, the tests can be performed only after 2 or 3 weeks of conception. It is because, the concentration of hCG required for producing changes in the animals is excreted in urine only after 2 or 3 weeks of pregnancy
5. Recently available immunological tests are more sensitive and involve single step method. Test kit is available in the form of cards. These **pregnancy test** cards can be used even in the first few days of conception. Most sensitive test can detect hCG level as low as 20 mIU/mL.

Mammary Glands and Lactation

> ■ DEVELOPMENT OF MAMMARY GLANDS
> ■ ROLE OF HORMONES IN GROWTH OF MAMMARY GLANDS
> ■ LACTATION
> ■ BREAST MILK

■ DEVELOPMENT OF MAMMARY GLANDS

■ AT BIRTH

At the time of birth, mammary gland is **rudimentary** and consists of only a tiny nipple and few radiating ducts from it.

■ AT CHILDHOOD

Till puberty, there is no difference in the structure of mammary gland between male and female.

■ AT PUBERTY

At the time of puberty and afterwards there is a vast change in the structure of female mammary gland due to hormonal influence. The beginning of changes in mammary gland is called **thelarche.** It occurs at the time of puberty, just before **menarche** (Chapter 80). At puberty, there is growth of duct system and formation of glandular tissue. During every sexual cycle, at the time of menstruation there is slight regression and in between the phases of menstruation, proliferative changes occur. On the whole, progressive enlargement occurs, which is also due to the deposition of fat.

■ DURING PREGNANCY

During pregnancy, the mammary glands enlarge to a great extent accompanied by marked changes in structure. During first half of pregnancy, the duct system develops further with appearance of many new alveoli. No milk is secreted by the gland now.

During the second half, there is enormous growth of glandular tissues and the development is completed for the production of milk just before the end of gestation period.

■ ROLE OF HORMONES IN GROWTH OF MAMMARY GLANDS

Various hormones are involved in the development and growth of breasts at different stages:
1. Estrogen
2. Progesterone
3. Prolactin
4. Placental hormones
5. Other hormones.

■ 1. ESTROGEN

Growth of Ductile System

Estrogen causes growth and branching of **duct system;** so the normal development of duct system in breasts at puberty depends upon estrogen. Estrogen is also responsible for the accumulation of fat in breasts.

■ 2. PROGESTERONE

Growth of Glandular Tissue

The development of stroma of the mammary glands depends upon progesterone activity. Progesterone also stimulates the development of **glandular tissues.**

■ 3. PROLACTIN

Prolactin is necessary for **milk secretion.** However, it also plays an important role in growth of mammary glands during pregnancy.

Normally, prolactin is inhibited by prolactin-inhibiting hormone secreted from hypothalamus. However, prolactin secretion starts increasing from 5th month of pregnancy. At that time, it acts directly on the mammary glands and causes proliferation of epithelial cells of alveoli.

■ 4. PLACENTAL HORMONES

Estrogen and progesterone secreted from placenta are essential for further development of mammary glands during pregnancy. Both the hormones stimulate the proliferation of ducts and glandular cells during pregnancy.

■ 5. OTHER HORMONES

Growth hormone, thyroxine and cortisol enhance the overall growth and development of mammary glands in all stages. Relaxin also facilitates the development of mammary glands. It is secreted by corpus luteum, mammary glands and placenta. Its major function is to facilitate dilatation of cervix during labor (Chapter 84).

■ LACTATION

Lactation means synthesis, secretion and ejection of milk.
Lactation involves two processes:
A. Milk secretion
B. Milk ejection.

■ MILK SECRETION

Synthesis of milk by alveolar epithelium and its passage through the duct system is called milk secretion.
Milk secretion occurs in two phases:
1. Initiation of milk secretion or lactogenesis
2. Maintenance of milk secretion or galactopoiesis.

1. *Initiation of Milk Secretion or Lactogenesis*

Although small amount of milk secretion occurs at later months of pregnancy, a free flow of milk occurs only after the delivery of the child. The milk, which is secreted initially before parturition is called **colostrum.**

Colostrum is lemon yellow in color and it is rich in protein (particularly globulins) and salts. But its sugar content is low. It contains almost all the components of milk except fat.

Role of hormones in lactogenesis

Prolactin is responsible for lactogenesis. During pregnancy, particularly in later months, large quantity of prolactin is secreted. But the activity of this hormone is suppressed by estrogen and progesterone secreted by placenta. Because of this, lactation is prevented during pregnancy.

Immediately after the delivery of the baby and expulsion of placenta, there is sudden loss of estrogen and progesterone. Now, the prolactin is free to exert its action on breasts and to promote lactogenesis.

2. *Maintenance of Milk Secretion or Galactopoiesis*

Galactopoiesis depends upon the hormones like growth hormone, thyroxine and cortisol, which are essential for continuous supply of glucose, amino acids, fatty acids, calcium and other substances necessary for the milk production (Fig. 87.1).

Role of hypothalamus in galactopoiesis

Galactopoiesis occurs till 7 to 9 months after delivery of child provided feeding the baby with mother's milk is continued till then. In fact, the milk production is continued only if feeding the baby is continued. Suckling of nipple by the baby is responsible for continuous milk production.

When the baby suckles, the impulses from touch receptors around the nipple stimulate hypothalamus. It is suggested that hypothalamus releases some prolactin-releasing factors, which cause the prolactin secretion from anterior pituitary. Prolactin acts on glandular tissues and maintains the functional activity of breast for subsequent nursing.

■ MILK EJECTION

Milk ejection is the discharge of milk from mammary gland. It depends upon suckling exerted by the baby and on contractile mechanism in breast, which expels milk from alveoli into the ducts.

Milk ejection is a reflex phenomenon. It is called **milk ejection reflex** or **milk let-down reflex.** It is a **neuroendocrine reflex.**

Milk Ejection Reflex

Milk ejection reflex is explained in Chapter 66.

■ EFFECT OF LACTATION ON MENSTRUAL CYCLE

Woman who nurses her child regularly does not have menstrual cycle for about 24 to 30 weeks after delivery.

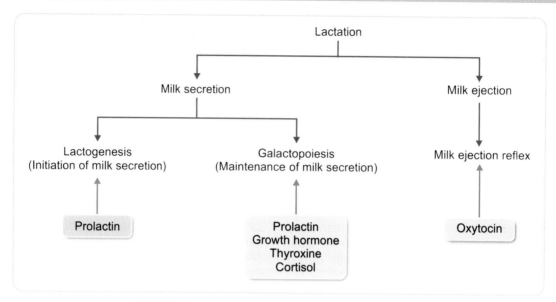

FIGURE 87.1: Process of lactation and role of hormones

It is because, regular nursing the baby stimulates prolactin secretion continuously. Prolactin inhibits GnRH secretion resulting in suppression of gonadotropin secretion. In the absence of gonadotropin, the ovaries become inactive and ovulation does not occur.

When the frequency of nursing the baby decreases (after about 24 weeks) the secretion of GnRH and gonadotropins starts slowly. When sufficient quantity of gonadotropins is secreted, the menstrual cycle starts.

■ BREAST MILK

Breast or human milk forms the primary source of nutrition for infants.

■ COMPOSITION

Breast milk contains about 88.5% of water and 11.5% of solids. Important solids are lactose, lactalbumin, iron, vitamins A and D and minerals.

■ ADVANTAGES OF BREAST MILK

Breast milk is always considered superior to animal milk (cow milk or goat milk) because it consists of sufficient quantity of all the substances necessary for infants like iron, vitamins and minerals.

Besides nourishment of infant, the breast milk also provides several antibodies, which help the infant resist the infection by lethal bacteria. Even some neutrophils and macrophages are secreted in milk. These phagocytic cells protect the infant by destroying microbes in the infant's body.

■ DISADVANTAGES OF ANIMAL MILK

1. It causes irritation of GI tract and anemia
2. Excess proteins and fats in animal milk are difficult to digest and absorb by the infants
3. High content of casein is harder to digest resulting in GI bleeding and anemia
4. High concentrations of sodium and potassium in animal milk causes overstraining of immature kidneys in infants
5. Low iron content in animal milk develops iron deficiency anemia
6. It has low content of vitamins and essential fatty acids.

Fertility Control

- ■ INTRODUCTION
- ■ RHYTHM METHOD (SAFE PERIOD)
- ■ MECHANICAL BARRIERS – PREVENTION OF ENTRY OF SPERM INTO UTERUS
- ■ CHEMICAL METHODS
- ■ ORAL CONTRACEPTIVES (PILL METHOD)
  - ■ CLASSICAL OR COMBINED PILLS
  - ■ SEQUENTIAL PILLS
  - ■ MINIPILLS OR MICROPILLS
  - ■ DISADVANTAGES AND ADVERSE EFFECTS OF ORAL CONTRACEPTIVES
  - ■ LONG-TERM CONTRACEPTIVES
- ■ INTRAUTERINE CONTRACEPTIVE DEVICE (IUCD)
  - ■ MECHANISM OF ACTION OF IUCD
  - ■ DISADVANTAGES OF IUCD
- ■ MEDICAL TERMINATION OF PREGNANCY (MTP) – ABORTION
  - ■ DILATATION AND CURETTAGE (D AND C)
  - ■ VACUUM ASPIRATION
  - ■ ADMINISTRATION OF PROSTAGLANDIN
- ■ SURGICAL METHOD (STERILIZATION) – PERMANENT METHOD
  - ■ TUBECTOMY
  - ■ VASECTOMY

■ INTRODUCTION

Fertility control is the use of any method or device to prevent pregnancy. It is also called **birth control, family planning** or **contraception.** Fertility control techniques may be temporary or permanent. Several methods are available for fertility control.

■ RHYTHM METHOD (SAFE PERIOD)

Rhythm method of fertility control is based on the time of ovulation. After ovulation, i.e. on the 14th day of menstrual cycle, the ovum is fertilized during its passage through fallopian tubes. Its viability is only for 2 days after ovulation and should be fertilized within this period.

Sperms survive only for about 24 to 48 hours after ejaculation in the female genital tract. If sexual intercourse occurs during this period, i.e. between few days before and few days after ovulation, there is chance of pregnancy. This period is called the **dangerous period.** Pregnancy can be avoided if there is no sexual intercourse during this period. The prevention of pregnancy by avoiding sexual mating during this period is called rhythm method.

The periods, when pregnancy does not occur are 4 to 5 days after menstrual bleeding and 5 to 6 days before the onset of next cycle. These periods are together called **safe period.**

Advantages and Disadvantages

It is one of the most successful methods of fertility control provided the woman knows the exact day of ovulation. However, it is not a successful method because of various reasons. Basic knowledge about the menstrual cycle is necessary to determine the day of ovulation. Self-restraint is essential to avoid sexual intercourse. Because of the practical difficulties, this method is not popular.

■ MECHANICAL BARRIERS – PREVENTION OF ENTRY OF SPERM INTO UTERUS

Mechanical barriers are used to prevent the entry of sperm into uterine cavity. These barriers are called **condoms.** The **male condom** is a leak proof sheath, made of latex. It covers the penis and does not allow entrance of semen into the female genital tract during coitus.

In females, the commonly used condom is **cervical cap** or **diaphragm.** It covers the cervix and prevents entry of sperm into uterus.

■ CHEMICAL METHODS

Chemical substances, which destroy the sperms, are applied in female genital tract before coitus. Destruction of sperms is called **spermicidal action.** The spermicidal substances are available in the form of foam tablet, jelly, cream and paste.

■ ORAL CONTRACEPTIVES (PILL METHOD)

Oral contraceptives are the drugs taken by mouth (pills) to prevent pregnancy. These pills prevent pregnancy by inhibiting maturation of follicles and ovulation. This leads to alteration of normal menstrual cycle. The menstrual cycle becomes the anovulatory cycle.

This method of fertility control is called **pill method** and pills are called **contraceptive pills** or **birth control pills.** These pills contain synthetic estrogen and progesterone.

Contraceptive pills are of three types:
1. Classical or combined pills
2. Sequential pills
3. Minipills or micropills.

■ 1. CLASSICAL OR COMBINED PILLS

Classical or combined pills contain a moderate dose of synthetic estrogen like ethinyl estradiol or mestranol and a mild dose of synthetic progesterone like norethindrone or norgestrol.

Pills are taken daily from 5th to 25th day of menstrual cycle. The withdrawal of the pills after 25th day causes menstrual bleeding. The intake of pills is resumed again after 5th day of the next cycle.

Mechanism of Action

During the continuous intake of the pills, there is relatively large amount of estrogen and progesterone in the blood.

It suppresses the release of gonadotropins, FSH and LH from pituitary by means of feedback mechanism. Lack of FSH and LH prevents the maturation of follicle, and ovulation. In addition, progesterone increases the thickness of mucosa in cervix, which is not favorable for transport of sperm. When the pills are withdrawn after 21 days the menstrual flow starts.

■ 2. SEQUENTIAL PILLS

Sequential pills contain a high dose of estrogen along with moderate dose of progesterone. These pills also prevent ovulation.

Sequential pills are taken in two courses:
i. Daily for 15 days from 5th to 20th day of the menstrual cycle and then
ii. During the last 5 days, i.e. 23rd to 28th day.

■ 3. MINIPILLS OR MICROPILLS

Minipills contain a low dose of only progesterone and are taken throughout the menstrual cycle. It prevents pregnancy without affecting ovulation. The progesterone increases the thickness of cervical mucosa, so that the transport of sperms is inhibited. It also prevents implantation of ovum.

■ DISADVANTAGES AND ADVERSE EFFECTS OF ORAL CONTRACEPTIVES

About 40% of women who use contraceptive pills may have minor transient side effects. However, long term use of oral contraceptives causes some serious side effects. Some of the side effects are rare, but may be dangerous.

Following are the disadvantages and adverse effects of oral contraceptives:
1. Major practical difficulty is the regular intake of the pills
2. May not be suitable for women having disorders such as diabetes, cardiovascular diseases or liver diseases
3. Clotting tendency of blood due to suppressed production of anticoagulants in liver
4. Hypertension and heart attack
5. Increases the risk of stroke
6. Tenderness of breast and risk of breast cancer (but may decrease the risk of ovarian and uterine cancer).

■ LONG-TERM CONTRACEPTIVES

To avoid taking pills daily, the long-term contraceptives are used. These contraceptives are in the form of implants containing mainly progesterone. The implants, which are inserted beneath the skin release the drug slowly and prevent fertility for 4 to 5 years. Though it seems to be effective, it may produce amenorrhea.

■ INTRAUTERINE CONTRACEPTIVE DEVICE (IUCD) – PREVENTION OF FERTILIZATION AND IMPLANTATION OF OVUM

Fertilization and the implantation of ovum are prevented by inserting some object made from metal or plastic into uterine cavity. Such object is called intrauterine contraceptive device (IUCD).

■ MECHANISM OF ACTION OF IUCD

Intrauterine contraceptive device prevents fertilization and **implantation of the ovum.** The IUCD with copper content has **spermicidal action** also. The IUCD which is loaded with synthetic progesterone slowly releases progesterone. Progesterone causes thickening of cervical mucus and prevents entry of sperm into uterus.

The common IUCDs are **Lippes loop,** which is 'S' shaped and made of plastic and copper T, which is made up of copper. It is inserted into the uterine cavity by using some special applicator.

■ DISADVANTAGES OF IUCD

IUCD has some disadvantages. It has the tendency to:
1. Cause heavy bleeding in some women
2. Promote infection
3. Come out of uterus accidentally.

■ MEDICAL TERMINATION OF PREGNANCY (MTP) – ABORTION

Abortion is done during first few months of pregnancy. This method is called medical termination of pregnancy (MTP). There are three ways of doing MTP (Table 88.1).

■ DILATATION AND CURETTAGE (D AND C)

In this method, the cervix is dilated and the implanted ovum or zygote is removed.

■ VACUUM ASPIRATION

The implanted ovum is removed by vacuum aspiration method. This is done up to 12 weeks of pregnancy.

■ ADMINISTRATION OF PROSTAGLANDIN

Administration of prostaglandin like PGE_2 and PGF_2 intravaginally increases uterine contractions resulting in abortion.

TABLE 88.1: Contraceptive methods in males and females

	Males	Females
Rhythm method		Safe period
Condom	Male condom	Cervical cap Diaphragm
Chemical methods		Chemical substances applied in genital tract
Oral contraceptives		Classical pills Sequential pills Mini pills
Implants		Intrauterine contraceptive device: Lippe loop Copper T
Medical termination of pregnancy (MTP)		Dilation and curettage Vacuum aspiration Prostaglandin administration
Surgical method (sterilization)	Vasectomy	Tubectomy

■ SURGICAL METHOD (STERILIZATION) – PERMANENT METHOD

Permanent sterility is obtained by surgical methods. It is also called sterilization.

■ TUBECTOMY

In tubectomy, the fallopian tubes are cut and both the cut ends are ligated. It prevents entry of ovum into uterus. The operation is done through vaginal orifice in the postpartum period. During other periods, it is done by abdominal incision. Tubectomy is done quickly (in few minutes) by using a **laparoscope.**

Though tubectomy causes permanent sterility, if necessary **recanalization** of fallopian tube can be done using plastic tube by another surgical procedure.

■ VASECTOMY

In vasectomy, the vas deferens is cut and the cut ends are ligated. So the sperms cannot enter the ejaculatory duct and the semen is devoid of sperms. It is done by surgical procedure with **local anesthesia.** If necessary, the **recanalization** of vas deferens can be done with plastic tube.

QUESTIONS IN REPRODUCTIVE SYSTEM

■ LONG QUESTIONS

1. Describe the functions of testis and regulation of testicular functions.
2. Describe the actions and regulation of secretion of testosterone.
3. What are the female sex hormones? Explain their actions.
4. What is menstrual cycle? Explain the ovarian changes taking place during menstrual cycle.
5. Describe the uterine changes during menstrual cycle.
6. Give an account of menstrual cycle and explain the hormonal regulation of menstrual cycle.
7. Give an account of lactation. And, add a note on the role of various hormones in the development of mammary glands and lactation.

■ SHORT QUESTIONS

1. Gametogenic function of testis or spermatogenesis.
2. Endocrine functions of testis.
3. Sertoli cells.
4. Testosterone.
5. Cryptorchidism.
6. Secondary sexual characters in males.
7. Puberty in males.
8. Seminal vesicles.
9. Prostate gland.
10. Semen.
11. Spermatozoa.
12. Effects of removal of testes.
13. Hyper and hypogonadism in males.
14. Estrogen.
15. Progesterone.
16. Follicle-stimulating hormone.
17. Luteinizing hormone.
18. Gonadotropins.
19. Secondary sexual characters in females.
20. Puberty in females.
21. Ovarian follicles.
22. Graafian follicle.
23. Ovulation.
24. Corpus luteum.
25. Hormonal regulation of menstrual cycle.
26. Menopause.
27. Infertility in females.
28. Infertility in males.
29. Maternal changes during pregnancy.
30. Functions of placenta.
31. Placental hormones.
32. Fetoplacental unit.
33. Parturition.
34. Pregnancy tests.
35. Role of hormones in lactation.
36. Prolactin.
37. Lactation.
38. Milk ejection reflex.
39. Oxytocin.
40. Safe period/Rhythm method.
41. Condoms.
42. Oral contraceptives.
43. IUCD.
44. MTP.
45. Vasectomy.
46. Tubectomy.
47. Contraceptive methods in females.
48. Contraceptive methods in males.

Section 8

Cardiovascular System

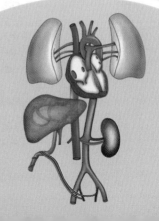

Introduction to Cardiovascular System

■ CARDIOVASCULAR SYSTEM

Cardiovascular system includes **heart** and **blood vessels.** Heart pumps blood into the blood vessels. Blood vessels circulate the blood throughout the body. Blood transports nutrients and oxygen to the tissues and removes carbon dioxide and waste products from the tissues.

■ HEART

Heart is a muscular organ that pumps blood throughout the circulatory system. It is situated in between two lungs in the mediastinum. It is made up of four chambers, two atria and two ventricles. The musculature of ventricles is thicker than that of atria. Force of contraction of heart depends upon the muscles.

■ RIGHT SIDE OF THE HEART

Right side of the heart has two chambers, **right atrium** and **right ventricle.** Right atrium is a thin walled and low pressure chamber. It has got the pacemaker known as sinoatrial node that produces cardiac impulses and atrioventricular node that conducts the impulses to the ventricles.

Right atrium receives venous (deoxygenated) blood via two large veins:

1. **Superior vena cava** that returns venous blood from the head, neck and upper limbs

2. **Inferior vena cava** that returns venous blood from lower parts of the body (Fig. 89.1).

Right atrium communicates with right ventricle through tricuspid valve. Wall of right ventricle is thick. Venous blood from the right atrium enters the right ventricle through this valve.

From the right ventricle, pulmonary artery arises. It carries the venous blood from right ventricle to lungs. In the lungs, the deoxygenated blood is oxygenated.

■ **LEFT SIDE OF THE HEART**

Left side of the heart has two chambers, **left atrium** and **left ventricle.** Left atrium is a thin walled and low pressure chamber. It receives oxygenated blood from the lungs through pulmonary veins. This is the only exception in the body, where an artery carries venous blood and vein carries the arterial blood.

Blood from left atrium enters the left ventricle through mitral valve (bicuspid valve). Wall of the left ventricle is very thick. Left ventricle pumps the arterial blood to different parts of the body through **systemic aorta.**

■ **SEPTA OF THE HEART**

Right and left atria are separated from one another by a fibrous septum called **interatrial septum.** Right

and left ventricles are separated from one another by **interventricular septum.** The upper part of this septum is a membranous structure, whereas the lower part of it is muscular in nature.

■ **LAYERS OF WALL OF THE HEART**

Heart is made up of three layers of tissues:
1. Outer pericardium
2. Middle myocardium
3. Inner endocardium.

■ **PERICARDIUM**

Pericardium is the outer covering of the heart. It is made up of two layers:
  i. Outer parietal pericardium
  ii. Inner visceral pericardium.

The space between the two layers is called **pericardial cavity** or **pericardial space** and it contains a thin film of fluid.

i. *Outer Parietal Pericardium*

Parietal pericardium forms a strong protective sac for the heart. It helps also to anchor the heart within the mediastinum.

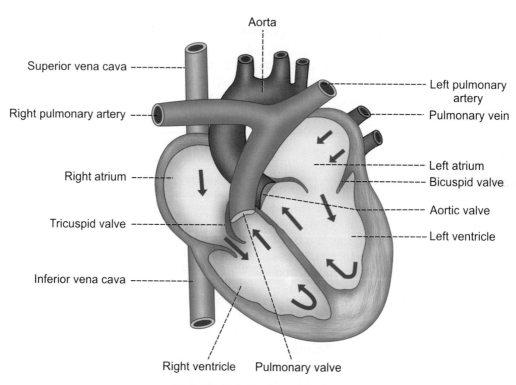

FIGURE 89.1: Section of the heart

Parietal pericardium is made up two layers:
a. Outer fibrous layer
b. Inner serous layer.

Fibrous layer

Fibrous layer of the parietal pericardium is formed by thick fibrous connective tissue. It is attached to the diaphragm and it is continuous with tunica adventitia (outer wall) of the blood vessels, entering and leaving the heart. It is attached with diaphragm below. Because of the fibrous nature, it protects the heart from over stretching.

Serous layer

Serous layer is formed by mesothelium, together with a small amount of connective tissue. Mesothelium contains squamous epithelial cells which secrete a small amount of fluid, which lines the pericardial space. This fluid prevents friction and allows free movement of heart within pericardium, when it contracts and relaxes. The total volume of this fluid is only about 25 to 35 mL.

ii. Inner Visceral Pericardium

Inner visceral pericardium lines the surface of myocardium. It is made up of flattened epithelial cells. This layer is also known as **epicardium.**

■ MYOCARDIUM

Myocardium is the middle layer of wall of the heart and it is formed by cardiac muscle fibers or cardiac myocytes. Myocardium forms the bulk of the heart and it is responsible for pumping action of the heart. Unlike skeletal muscle fibers, the cardiac muscle fibers are involuntary in nature.

Refer Chapter 28 for features of cardiac muscles.
Myocardium has three types of muscle fibers:
i. Muscle fibers which form contractile unit of heart
ii. Muscle fibers which form pacemaker
iii. Muscle fibers which form conductive system.

i. Muscle Fibers which Form Contractile Unit of Heart

These cardiac muscle fibers are striated and resemble the skeletal muscle fibers in structure. Cardiac muscle fiber is bound by **sarcolemma.** It has a centrally placed nucleus. **Myofibrils** are embedded in the sarcoplasm. **Sarcomere** of the cardiac muscle has all the contractile proteins, namely actin, myosin, troponin and tropomyosin. **Sarcotubular system** in cardiac muscle is similar to that of skeletal muscle.

Important difference between skeletal muscle and cardiac muscle is that the cardiac muscle fiber is branched and the skeletal muscle is not branched.

Intercalated disk

Intercalated disk is a tough double membranous structure, situated at the junction between the branches of neighboring cardiac muscle fibers. It is formed by the fusion of the membrane of the cardiac muscle branches (Fig. 89.2).

Intercalated disks form **adherens junctions,** which play an important role in the contraction of cardiac muscle as a single unit (Chapter 2).

Syncytium

Syncytium means tissue with cytoplasmic continuity between adjacent cells. However, cardiac muscle is like a **physiological syncytium,** since there is no continuity of the cytoplasm and the muscle fibers are separated from each other by cell membrane. At the sides, the membranes of the adjacent muscle fibers fuse together to form **gap junctions.** Gap junction is permeable to ions and it facilitates the rapid conduction of action potential from one fiber to another. Because of this, all the cardiac muscle fibers act like a single unit, which is referred as syncytium.

Syncytium in human heart has two portions, syncytium of atria and the syncytium of ventricles. Both the portions of syncytium are connected by a thick non-conducting fibrous ring called the **atrioventricular ring.**

ii. Muscle Fibers which Form the Pacemaker

Some of the muscle fibers of heart are modified into a specialized structure known as pacemaker. These muscle fibers forming the pacemaker have less striation.

Pacemaker

Pacemaker is structure in the heart that generates the impulses for heart beat. It is formed by **pacemaker cells**

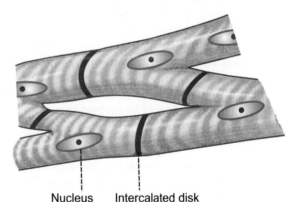

Nucleus   Intercalated disk

FIGURE 89.2: Cardiac muscle fibers

called **P cells.** Sinoatrial (SA) node forms the pacemaker in human heart. Details of pacemaker are given in next chapter.

iii. *Muscle Fibers which Form Conductive System*

Conductive system of the heart is formed by modified cardiac muscle fibers. Impulses from SA node are transmitted to the atria directly. However, the impulses are transmitted to ventricles through various components of conducting system, which are explained in the next chapter.

■ ENDOCARDIUM

Endocardium is the inner most layer of heart wall. It is a thin, smooth and glistening membrane. It is formed by a single layer of endothelial cells, lining the inner surface of the heart. Endocardium continues as endothelium of the blood vessels.

■ VALVES OF THE HEART

There are four valves in human heart. Two valves are in between atria and the ventricles called atrioventricular valves. Other two are the semilunar valves, placed at the opening of blood vessels arising from ventricles, namely systemic aorta and pulmonary artery. Valves of the heart permit the flow of blood through heart in only one direction.

Atrioventricular Valves

Left atrioventricular valve is otherwise known as **mitral valve** or **bicuspid valve.** It is formed by two valvular **cusps** or flaps (Fig. 89.3). Right atrioventricular valve is known as **tricuspid valve** and it is formed by three cusps.

Brim of the atrioventricular valves is attached to atrioventricular ring, which is the fibrous connection between the atria and ventricles. Cusps of the valves are attached to **papillary muscles** by means of **chordae tendineae.** Papillary muscles arise from inner surface of the ventricles. Papillary muscles play an important role in closure of the cusps and in preventing the back flow of blood from ventricle to atria during ventricular contraction.

Atrioventricular valves open only towards ventricles and prevent the backflow of blood into atria.

Semilunar Valves

Semilunar valves are present at the openings of systemic aorta and pulmonary artery and are known as **aortic valve** and **pulmonary valve** respectively. Because of the

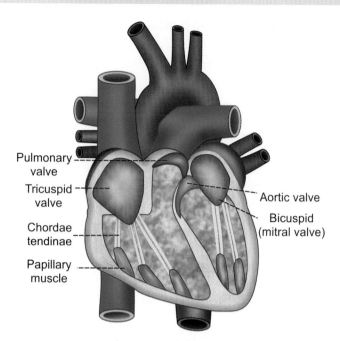

FIGURE 89.3: Valves of the heart

half moon shape, these two valves are called semilunar valves. Semilunar valves are made up of three flaps.

Semilular valves open only towards the aorta and pulmonary artery and prevent the backflow of blood into the ventricles.

■ ACTIONS OF THE HEART

Actions of the heart are classified into four types:
1. Chronotropic action
2. Inotropic action
3. Dromotropic action
4. Bathmotropic action.

■ CHRONOTROPIC ACTION

Chronotropic action is the frequency of heartbeat or heart rate. It is of two types:
  i. **Tachycardia** or increase in heart rate
  ii. **Bradycardia** or decrease in heart rate.

■ INOTROPIC ACTION

Force of contraction of heart is called inotropic action. It is of two types:
  i. Positive inotropic action or increase in the force of contraction
  ii. Negative inotropic action or decrease in the force of contraction.

■ DROMOTROPIC ACTION

Dromotropic action is the conduction of impulse through heart. It is of two types:

i. Positive dromotropic action or increase in the velocity of conduction

ii. Negative dromotropic action or decrease in the velocity of conduction.

■ BATHMOTROPIC ACTION

Bathmotropic action is the excitability of cardiac muscle. It is also of two types:

i. Positive bathmotropic action or increase in the excitability of cardiac muscle

ii. Negative bathmotropic action or decrease in the excitability of cardiac muscle.

Regulation of Actions of Heart

All the actions of heart are continuously regulated. It is essential for the heart to cope up with the needs of the body. All the actions are altered by stimulation of nerves supplying the heart or some hormones or hormonal substances secreted in the body.

■ BLOOD VESSELS

Vessels of circulatory system are the aorta, arteries, arterioles, capillaries, venules, veins and venae cavae. Structural differences between different blood vessels are given in Table 89.1.

■ ARTERIAL SYSTEM

Arterial system comprises the aorta, arteries and arterioles. Walls of the aorta and arteries are formed by three layers:

1. Outer **tunica adventitia,** which is made up of connective tissue layer. It is the continuation of fibrous layer of parietal pericardium.

2. Middle **tunica media,** which is formed by smooth muscles

3. Inner **tunica intima,** which is made up of endothelium. It is the continuation of endocardium.

Aorta, arteries and arterioles have two laminae of elastic tissues:

i. **External elastic lamina** between tunica adventitia and tunica media

ii. **Internal elastic lamina** between tunica media and tunica intima.

Aorta and arteries have more elastic tissues and the arterioles have more smooth muscles.

Arterial branches become narrower and their walls become thinner while reaching the periphery. Aorta has got the maximum diameter of about 25 mm. Diameter of the arteries is gradually decreased and at the end arteries, it is about 4 mm. It further decreases to 30 μ in the arterioles and ends up with 10 μ in the terminal arterioles. **Resistance** (peripheral resistance) is offered to blood flow in the arterioles and so these vessels are called **resistant vessels.**

Arterioles are continued as capillaries, which are small, thin walled vessels having a diameter of about 5 to 8 μ. Capillaries are functionally very important because, the exchange of materials between the blood and the tissues occurs through these vessels.

■ VENOUS SYSTEM

From the capillaries, venous system starts and it includes venules, veins and venae cavae. Capillaries end in venules, which are the smaller vessels with thin muscular wall than the arterioles. Diameter of the venules is about 20 μ. At a time, a large quantity of blood is held in venules and hence the venules are called **capacitance vessels.** Venules are continued as veins, which have the diameter of 5 mm. Veins form superior and inferior venae cavae, which have a diameter of about 30 mm.

TABLE 89.1: Structural and dimensional differences between different blood vessel walls

Blood vessel	Diameter	Thickness of the wall	Elastic tissue	Smooth muscle fibers	Fibrous tissue
Aorta	25 mm	2 mm	More	Less	More
Artery	4 mm	1 mm	More	More	Moderate
Arteriole	30 μ	6 μ	Moderate	More	Moderate
Terminal arteriole	10 μ	2 μ	Less	More	Moderate
Capillary	8 μ	0.5 μ	Absent	Absent	Moderate
Venule	20 μ	1 μ	Absent	Absent	Less
Vein	5 mm	0.5 mm	Less	More	Moderate
Vena cava	30 mm	1.5 mm	Less	More	More

Walls of the veins and venae cavae are made up of inner endothelium, elastic tissues, smooth muscles and outer connective tissue layer. In the veins and venae cavae, the elastic tissue is less but the smooth muscle fibers are more.

■ COMPLICATIONS IN BLOOD VESSELS

Aorta and Arteries

Arterial blood vessels are highly susceptible for arteriosclerosis and atherosclerosis. **Arteriosclerosis** is the disease of the arteries, associated with hardening, thickening and loss of elasticity in the wall of the vessels. **Atherosclerosis** is the disease marked by the narrowing of lumen of arterial vessel due to deposition of cholesterol.

Arterioles

When the tone of the smooth muscles in the arterioles increases, hypertension occurs.

Capillaries

Permeability of the capillary membrane may increase resulting in shock or edema due to leakage of fluid, proteins and other substances from blood.

Veins

Inflammation of the wall of veins leads to the formation of intravascular clot called **thrombosis**. The clot gets dislodged, as **thrombus**. The thrombus travels through blood and causes **embolism**. Embolism obstructs the blood flow to vital organs such as brain, heart and lungs, leading to many complications.

■ DIVISIONS OF CIRCULATION

Blood flows through two divisions of circulatory system:
1. Systemic circulation
2. Pulmonary circulation.

■ SYSTEMIC CIRCULATION

Systemic circulation is otherwise known as **greater circulation** (Fig. 89.4). Blood pumped from left ventricle passes through a series of blood vessels, arterial system

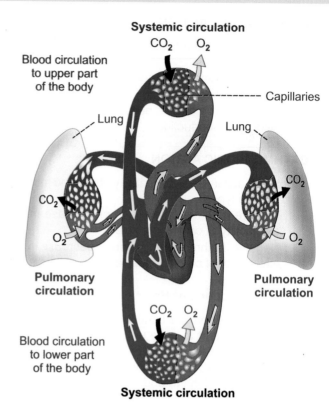

FIGURE 89.4: Systemic and pulmonary circulation

and reaches the tissues. Exchange of various substances between blood and the tissues occurs at the capillaries.

After exchange of materials, blood enters the venous system and returns to right atrium of the heart. From right atrium, blood enters the right ventricle.

Thus, through systemic circulation, oxygenated blood is supplied from heart to the tissues and venous blood returns to the heart from tissues.

■ PULMONARY CIRCULATION

Pulmonary circulation is otherwise called **lesser circulation.** Blood is pumped from right ventricle to lungs through pulmonary artery. Exchange of gases occurs between blood and alveoli of the lungs at pulmonary capillaries. Oxygenated blood returns to left atrium through the pulmonary veins.

Thus, left side of the heart contains oxygenated or arterial blood and the right side of the heart contains deoxygenated or venous blood.

Properties of Cardiac Muscle

■ EXCITABILITY

■ DEFINITION

Excitability is defined as the ability of a living tissue to give response to a stimulus. In all the tissues, initial response to a stimulus is electrical activity in the form of action potential. It is followed by mechanical activity in the form of contraction, secretion, etc.

■ ELECTRICAL POTENTIALS IN CARDIAC MUSCLE

Refer Chapter 31 for basics of electrical potentials in the muscle.

Resting Membrane Potential

Resting membrane potential in:

Single cardiac muscle fiber	:	-85 to -95 mV
Sinoatrial (SA) node	:	-55 to -60 mV
Purkinje fibers	:	-90 to -100 mV.

Action Potential

Action potential in cardiac muscle is different from that of other tissues such as skeletal muscle, smooth muscle and nervous tissue. Duration of the action potential in cardiac muscle is 250 to 350 msec (0.25 to 0.35 sec).

Phases of action potential

Action potential in a single cardiac muscle fiber occurs in four phases:

1. Initial depolarization
2. Initial repolarization
3. A plateau or final depolarization
4. Final repolarization.

1. Initial Depolarization

Initial depolarization is very rapid and it lasts for about 2 msec (0.002 sec). Amplitude of depolarization is about + 20 mV (Fig. 90.1).

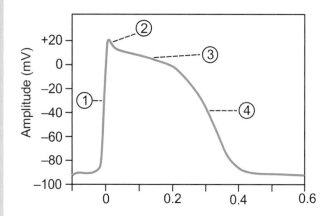

FIGURE 90.1: Action potential in ventricular muscle. 1 = Depolarization, 2 = Initial rapid repolarization, 3 = Plateau, 4 = Final repolarization.

2. *Initial Repolarization*

Immediately after depolarization, there is an initial rapid repolarization for a short period of about 2 msec. The end of rapid repolarization is represented by a notch.

3. *Plateau or Final Depolarization*

Afterwards, the muscle fiber remains in depolarized state for sometime before further repolarization. It forms the plateau (stable period) in action potential curve. The plateau lasts for about 200 msec in atrial muscle fibers and for about 300 msec in ventricular muscle fibers. Due to long plateau in action potential, the contraction time is also longer in cardiac muscle by 5 to 15 times than in skeletal muscle.

4. *Final Repolarization*

Final repolarization occurs after the plateau. It is a slow process and it lasts for about 50 to 80 msec before the re-establishment of resting membrane potential.

■ IONIC BASIS OF ACTION POTENTIAL

1. *Initial Depolarization*

Initial depolarization (first phase) is because of rapid opening of fast **sodium channels** and the **rapid influx of sodium ions,** as in the case of skeletal muscle fiber.

2. *Initial Repolarization*

Initial repolarization is due to the transient (short duration) opening of **potassium channels** and **efflux of a small quantity of potassium ions** from the muscle fiber. Simultaneously, the fast sodium channels close

suddenly and slow sodium channels open, resulting in **slow influx** of low quantity of **sodium ions.**

3. *Plateau or Final Depolarization*

Plateau is due to the slow opening of **calcium channels.** These channels are kept open for a longer period and cause influx of large number of **calcium ions.** Already the slow sodium channels are opened, through which slow influx of sodium ions continues. Because of the entry of calcium and sodium ions into the muscle fiber, positivity is maintained inside the muscle fiber, producing prolonged depolarization, i.e. plateau. Calcium ions entering the muscle fiber play an important role in the contractile process.

4. *Final Repolarization*

Final repolarization is due to **efflux of potassium ions.** Number of potassium ions moving out of the muscle fiber exceeds the number of calcium ions moving in. It makes negativity inside, resulting in final repolarization. Potassium efflux continues until the end of repolarization.

Restoration of Resting Membrane Potential

At the end of final repolarization, all sodium ions, which had entered the cell throughout the process of action potential move out of the cell and potassium ions move into the cell, by activation of **sodium-potassium pump.** Simultaneously, excess of calcium ions, which had entered the muscle fiber also move out through sodium-calcium pump. Thus, the resting membrane potential is restored.

■ SPREAD OF ACTION POTENTIAL THROUGH CARDIAC MUSCLE

Action potential spreads through cardiac muscle very rapidly because of the presence of gap junctions between the cardiac muscle fibers. Gap junctions are permeable junctions and allow free movement of ions and so the action potential spreads rapidly from one muscle fiber to another fiber.

Action potential is transmitted from atria to ventricles through the fibers of specialized conductive system, which is explained later in this chapter.

■ RHYTHMICITY

■ DEFINITION

Rhythmicity is the ability of a tissue to produce its own impulses regularly. It is also called **autorhythmicity** or

self-excitation. Property of rhythmicity is present in all the tissues of heart. However, heart has a specialized excitatory structure, from which the discharge of impulses is rapid. This specialized structure is called pacemaker. From here, the impulses spread to other parts through the specialized conductive system.

■ PACEMAKER

Pacemaker is the structure of heart from which the impulses for heartbeat are produced. It is formed by the **pacemaker cells** called **P cells.** In mammalian heart, the pacemaker is sinoatrial node (SA node). It was Lewis Sir Thomas, who named SA node as pacemaker of heart, in 1918.

Sinoatrial Node

Sinoatrial (SA) node is a small strip of modified cardiac muscle, situated in the superior part of lateral wall of right atrium, just below the opening of superior vena cava. The fibers of this node do not have contractile elements. These fibers are continuous with fibers of atrial muscle, so that the impulses from the SA node spread rapidly through atria.

Other parts of heart such as atrioventricular (AV) node, atria and ventricle also can produce the impulses and function as pacemakers. Still, SA node is called the pacemaker because the rate of production of impulse (rhythmicity) is more in SA node than in other parts. It is about 70 to 80/minute.

Experimental Evidences

Experimental evidences to prove that SA node is the pacemaker in **mammalian heart:**
1. Stimulation of SA node accelerates the heart rate
2. Destruction of SA node causes immediate stoppage of the heartbeat. After sometime, atrioventricular node becomes the pacemaker and starts generating the impulses. So the heart starts beating, but the rate is slow.
3. Local cooling of SA node decreases the heart rate
4. Local warming of SA node increases the heart rate
5. Electrical activity starts first in SA node.

Spread of Impulses from SA Node

Mammalian heart has got a specialized conductive system, by which the impulses from SA node spreads to other parts of the heart (see below).

Rhythmicity of Different Parts of Human Heart

1. SA node : 70 to 80/minute
2. AV node : 40 to 60/minute
3. Atrial muscle : 40 to 60/minute
4. Purkinje fibers : 35 to 40/minute
5. Ventricular muscle : 20 to 40/minute.

Pacemaker in Amphibian Heart

Sinus venosus is the pacemaker in amphibian heart. It is experimentally proved by:
1. Applying Stannius ligatures
2. When sinus venosus is warmed by warm Ringer solution, heart rate increases
3. When sinus venosus is cooled by cold Ringer solution, heart rate decreases
4. Electrical activity starts first in sinus venosus.

Stannius ligature experiment

Stannius ligature experiment was demonstrated by German biologist **Stannius** in a **pithed frog.** Ligature means tying. **Pithing** is a process by which the brain and spinal cord are severed by using a needle, to abolish all the reflex activities during the experiment. Pithed frog is technically dead but some of its organs such as heart, continue to function for some time.

Chest wall of a pithed frog is opened and heart is exposed. A bent pin is fixed at the tip of ventricle and attached to a recording device by means of a thread. After recording the normal heartbeats (**normal cardiogram** or **sinus rhythm**), a ligature is applied between the sinus venosus and right auricle. It is called first Stannius ligature.

When this ligature is applied, the heart stops beating immediately. It is because the impulses produced by sinus venosus cannot be conducted to the other chambers of the heart. However, the sinus contractions are continued. After sometime, auricular muscle becomes the pacemaker and starts producing the impulses for heartbeat, but at a slower rate. Auricular contraction occurs first, followed by ventricular contraction. This rhythm of the heart is called **auriculoventricular rhythm** (Fig. 90.2).

When a second ligature is applied between auricles and ventricle, the heart stops beating again, because impulses from auricles cannot reach the ventricle. After few minutes, the ventricle produces its **own impulses** and starts beating but at a much slower rate. The slow independent ventricular rhythm is called **idioventricular rhythm.** Thus, all the three parts of the heart, sinus venosus, auricular musculature and ventricular musculature have the property of rhythmicity. However, sinus venosus is the pacemaker because it produces the impulses at a faster rate.

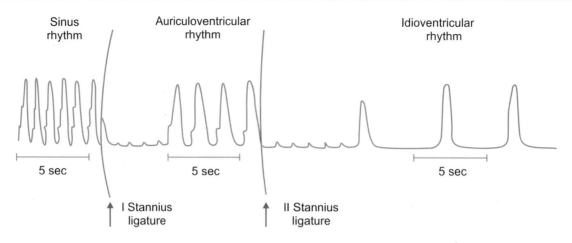

FIGURE 90.2: Effect of Stannius ligatures on frog's heart

Spread of Impulses from Sinus Venosus

Amphibian heart does not have any specialized conductive system. Pacemaker in amphibian heart is the sinus venosus and impulses from **sinus venosus** spreads through the muscles of auricles and ventricle.

Rhythmicity of Different Parts of Amphibian Heart

1. Sinus venosus   : 40 to 60/minute
2. Auricular muscle   : 20 to 40/minute
3. Ventricular muscle : 15 to 20/minute.

■ ELECTRICAL POTENTIAL IN SA NODE

Resting Membrane Potential – Pacemaker Potential

Pacemaker potential is the unstable resting membrane potential in SA node. It is also called prepotential.

Electrical potential in SA node is different from that of other cardiac muscle fibers. In SA node, each impulse triggers the next impulse. It is mainly due to the unstable resting membrane potential.

Resting membrane potential in SA node has a negativity of –55 to –60 mV. It is different from the negativity of –85 to –95 mV in other cardiac muscle fibers.

Action Potential

Depolarization starts very slowly and the threshold level of –40 mV is reached very slowly. After the threshold level, rapid depolarization occurs up to +5 mV. It is followed by rapid repolarization. Once again, the resting membrane potential becomes unstable and reaches the threshold level slowly (Fig. 90.3).

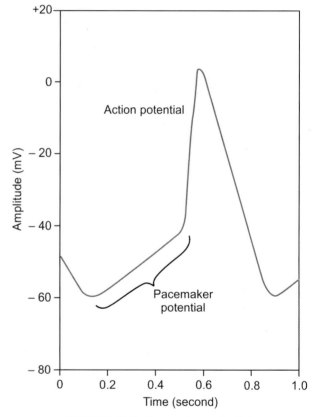

FIGURE 90.3: Pacemaker potential

Ionic Basis of Electrical Activity in Pacemaker

Pacemaker potential or resting membrane potential

Resting membrane potential is not stable in the SA node. To start with, the sodium ions leak into the pacemaker fibers and cause slow depolarization. This slow depolarization forms the initial part of pacemaker potential. Then, the **calcium channels** start opening. At the beginning, there is a slow **influx of calcium ions** causing further depolarization in the same slower rate. It forms the later part of the pacemaker potential.

Thus, the initial part of pacemaker potential is due to slow **influx of sodium ions** and the later part is due to the slow influx of calcium ions.

Depolarization

When the negativity is decreased to –40 mV, which is the **threshold level,** the action potential starts with rapid depolarization. The depolarization occurs because of influx of more calcium ions. Unlike in other tissues, the depolarization in SA node is mainly due to the influx of calcium ions, rather than sodium ions.

Repolarization

After rapid depolarization, repolarization starts. It is due to the efflux of potassium ions from pacemaker fibers. Potassium channels remain open for a longer time, causing efflux of **more potassium ions.** It leads to the development of more negativity, beyond the level of resting membrane potential. It exists only for a short period. Then, the slow depolarization starts once again, leading to the development of **pacemaker potential,** which triggers the next action potential.

■ CONDUCTIVITY

Human heart has a specialized conductive system, through which impulses from SA node are transmitted to all other parts of the heart (Fig. 90.4).

■ CONDUCTIVE SYSTEM IN HUMAN HEART

Conductive system of the heart is formed by the modified cardiac muscle fibers. These fibers are the specialized cells, which conduct the impulses rapidly from SA node to the ventricles. Conductive tissues of the heart are also called the junctional tissues.

Components of Conductive System in Human Heart

1. AV node
2. Bundle of His
3. Right and left bundle branches
4. Purkinje fibers.

SA node is situated in right atrium, just below the opening of superior vena cava. AV node is situated in right posterior portion of intra-atrial septum. Impulses from SA node are conducted throughout right and left atria. Impulses also reach the AV node via some specialized fibers called internodal fibers.

There are three types of internodal fibers:
1. Anterior internodal fibers of Bachman
2. Middle internodal fibers of Wenckebach
3. Posterior internodal fibers of Thorel.

All these fibers from SA node converge on AV node and interdigitate with fibers of AV node. From AV node, the **bundle of His** arises. It divides into right and left branches, which run on either side of the interventricular septum. From each branch of bundle of His, many **Purkinje fibers** arise and spread all over the ventricular myocardium.

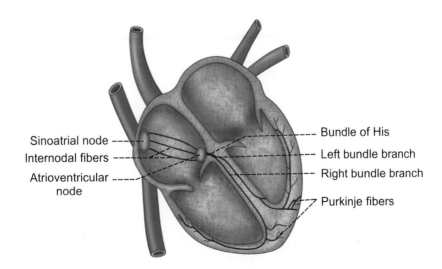

Sinoatrial node
Internodal fibers
Atrioventricular node

Bundle of His
Left bundle branch
Right bundle branch
Purkinje fibers

FIGURE 90.4: Sinoatrial node and conductive system of the heart

■ VELOCITY OF IMPULSES AT DIFFERENT PARTS OF CONDUCTIVE SYSTEM

1. Atrial muscle fibers   :   0.3 meter/second
2. Internodal fibers   :   1.0 meter/second
3. AV node   :   0.05 meter/second
4. Bundle of His   :   0.12 meter/second
5. Purkinje fibers   :   4.0 meter/second
6. Ventricular muscle fibers :   0.5 meter/second.

Thus, the velocity of impulses is maximum in Purkinje fibers and minimum at AV node.

■ CONTRACTILITY

Contractility is ability of the tissue to shorten in length (contraction) after receiving a stimulus. Various factors affect the contractile properties of the cardiac muscle. Following are the contractile properties:

■ ALL-OR-NONE LAW

According to all-or-none law, when a stimulus is applied, whatever may be the strength, the whole cardiac muscle gives maximum response or it does not give any response at all. Below the threshold level, i.e. if the strength of stimulus is not adequate, the muscle does not give response.

All-or-none law is demonstrated in the **quiescent (quiet) heart** of frog. Heart is made quiescent by applying the first Stannius ligature in between the sinus venosus and right auricle.

Ventricle is stimulated by placing the electrode at the base of ventricle.

First, one stimulus is applied with a minimum strength of 1 volt at the base of ventricle and the contraction is recorded. Then, after 20 seconds, the strength of stimulus is increased to 2 volt and the stimulus is applied.

The curve is recorded. The procedure is repeated by increasing the strength every time and applying the stimulus with an interval of 20 seconds (Fig. 90.5).

Amplitude of all contractions remains the same, irrespective of increasing the strength of stimulus. This shows that cardiac muscle obeys all-or-none law.

Cause for All-or-none law

All-or-none law is applicable to whole cardiac muscle. It is because of **syncytial** arrangement of cardiac muscle. In the case of skeletal muscle, all-or-none law is applicable only to a single muscle fiber.

■ STAIRCASE PHENOMENON

When the ventricle of a quiescent heart of frog is stimulated at a short interval of 2 seconds, without changing the strength, the force of contraction increases gradually for the first few contractions and then it remains same. Gradual increase in the force of contraction is called staircase phenomenon.

Cause for Staircase Phenomenon

Staircase phenomenon occurs because of **beneficial effect** (Chapter 30), which facilitates the force of successive contraction. So, there is a gradual increase in force of contraction (Fig. 90.5).

■ SUMMATION OF SUBLIMINAL STIMULI

When a stimulus with a subliminal strength is applied, the quiescent heart does not show any response. When few stimuli with same subliminal strength are applied in succession, the heart shows response by contraction, due to the summation of stimuli.

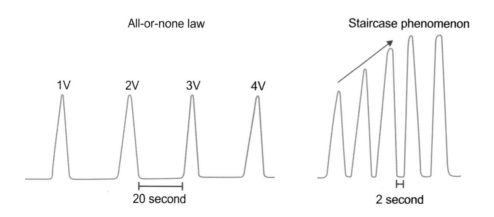

FIGURE 90.5: All-or-none law and staircase phenomenon in cardiac muscle

■ REFRACTORY PERIOD

Refractory period is the period in which the muscle does not show any response to a stimulus. It is of two types:
1. Absolute refractory period
2. Relative refractory period.

Absolute Refractory Period

Absolute refractory period is the period during which the muscle does not show any response at all, whatever may be the strength of the stimulus. It is because, the depolarization occurs during this period. So, a second depolarization is not possible.

Relative Refractory Period

Relative refractory period is the period during which the muscle shows response if the strength of stimulus is increased to maximum. It is the stage at which the muscle is in repolarizing state.

Refractory Period in Skeletal Muscle

In skeletal muscle, the refractory period is short. Absolute refractory period extends during the first half of latent period, measuring about 0.005 sec. Relative refractory period extends during the second half of latent period measuring 0.005 sec. So, the total refractory period is 0.01 sec.

Refractory Period in Cardiac Muscle

Cardiac muscle has a **long refractory period** compared to skeletal muscle. Absolute refractory period extends throughout the contraction period of cardiac muscle and its duration is 0.27 sec. Relative refractory period extends during first half of relaxation period, which is about 0.26 sec. So, the total refractory period is 0.53 sec.

Significance of Long Refractory Period in Cardiac Muscle

Long refractory period in cardiac muscle has three advantages:
1. Summation of contractions does not occur
2. Fatigue does not occur
3. Tetanus does not occur.

Demonstration of Refractory Period in Heart

Refractory period is demonstrated in the heart of a pithed frog. Refractory period can be recorded in beating heart as well as the quiescent heart.

Refractory period in beating heart

First, normal cardiogram is recorded with the heart of a pithed frog. The impulses for heartbeat arise from the sinus venosus. An electrical (external) stimulus is applied by keeping the electrode at the base of the ventricle. When the stimulus is applied during systole, the heart does not show any response. It is because the absolute refractory period extends throughout systole (Fig. 90.6).

When a stimulus is applied during diastole, the heart contracts because, diastole is the relative refractory period. This contraction of the heart is called **extrasystole** or **premature contraction.** Etrasystole is followed by the stoppage of heart in diastole for a while. This diastole is longer than the diastole after regular

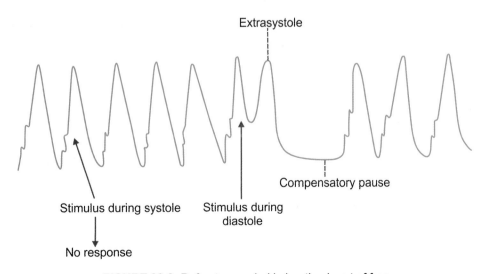

FIGURE 90.6: Refractory period in beating heart of frog

contraction. Temporary stoppage of the heart before it starts contracting is called **compensatory pause**. Duration of extrasystole and compensatory pause is equivalent to the duration of two cardiac cycles.

Cause for compensatory pause

A natural impulse from sinus venosus arrives at the time of contraction period of extrasystole. As this period is absolute refractory period, the natural impulse cannot cause contraction of heart. And the heart has to wait for the arrival of next natural impulse from sinus venosus. Till the arrival of next impulse, the heart stops in diastole.

Refractory period in quiescent heart

Frog's heart is made quiescent by applying the first Stannius ligature. Electrode is placed over the base of ventricle. When two stimuli are applied successively in such a way that the second stimulus falls during contraction period, the heart contracts only once. It is because of the first stimulus. There is no response to second stimulus because systole is the absolute

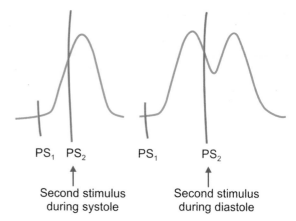

FIGURE 90.7: Refractory period in quiescent heart of a frog. PS$_1$ = Point of first stimulus, PS$_2$ = Point of second stimulus.

refractory period. However, when a second stimulus is applied during diastole, the heart contracts again and second contraction superimposes over the first one. This shows that the relative refractory period extends during diastole (Fig. 90.7).

Cardiac Cycle

Chapter
91

■ DEFINITION

Cardiac cycle is defined as the succession of (sequence of) **coordinated events** taking place in the heart during each beat. Each heartbeat consists of two major periods called systole and diastole. During systole, heart contracts and pumps the blood through arteries. During diastole, heart relaxes and blood is filled in the heart. All these changes are repeated during every heartbeat, in a cyclic manner.

■ EVENTS OF CARDIAC CYCLE

Events of cardiac cycle are classified into two:
1. Atrial events
2. Ventricular events.

■ DIVISIONS AND DURATION OF CARDIAC CYCLE

When the heart beats at a normal rate of 72/minute, duration of each cardiac cycle is about 0.8 second.

■ ATRIAL EVENTS

Atrial events are divided into two divisions:

1. Atrial systole	= 0.11 (0.1) sec
2. Atrial diastole	= 0.69 (0.7) sec.

■ VENTRICULAR EVENTS

Ventricular events are divided into two divisions:

1. Ventricular systole	= 0.27 (0.3) sec
2. Ventricular diastole	= 0.53 (0.5) sec.

In clinical practice, the term 'systole' refers to ventricular systole and 'diastole' refers to ventricular diastole. Ventricular systole is divided into two subdivisions and ventricular diastole is divided into five subdivisions.

Ventricular Systole

	Time (second)
1. Isometric contraction	= 0.05
2. Ejection period	= 0.22
	0.27

Ventricular Diastole

1. Protodiastole	= 0.04
2. Isometric relaxation	= 0.08
3. Rapid filling	= 0.11
4. Slow filling	= 0.19
5. Last rapid filling	= 0.11
	0.53

Among the atrial events, atrial systole occurs during the last phase of ventricular diastole. Atrial diastole is not considered as a separate phase, since it coincides with the whole of ventricular systole and earlier part of ventricular diastole.

■ DESCRIPTION OF ATRIAL EVENTS

■ ATRIAL SYSTOLE

Atrial systole is also known as **last rapid filling phase** or **presystole.** It is usually considered as the last phase of ventricular diastole. Its duration is 0.11 second.

During this period, only a small amount, i.e. 10% of blood is forced from atria into ventricles. Atrial systole is not essential for the maintenance of circulation. Many persons with atrial fibrillation survive for years, without suffering from circulatory insufficiency. However, such persons feel difficult to cope up with physical stress like exercise.

Pressure and Volume Changes

During atrial systole, the intra-atrial pressure increases. Intraventricular pressure and ventricular volume also increase but slightly.

Fourth Heart Sound

Contraction of atrial musculature causes the production of fourth heart sound.

■ ATRIAL DIASTOLE

After atrial systole, the atrial diastole starts. Simultaneously, ventricular systole also starts. Atrial diastole lasts for about 0.7 sec (accurate duration is 0.69 sec). This long atrial diastole is necessary because, this is the period during which atrial filling takes place. Right atrium receives deoxygenated blood from all over the body through superior and inferior venae cavae. Left atrium receives oxygenated blood from lungs through pulmonary veins.

Atrial Events Vs Ventricular Events

Out of 0.7 sec of atrial diastole, first 0.3 sec (0.27 sec accurately) coincides with ventricular systole. Then, ventricular diastole starts and it lasts for about 0.5 sec (0.53 sec accurately). Later part of atrial diastole coincides with ventricular diastole for about 0.4 sec. So, the heart relaxes as a whole for 0.4 sec. Figure 91.1 shows the correlation between atrial and ventricular events of cardiac cycle.

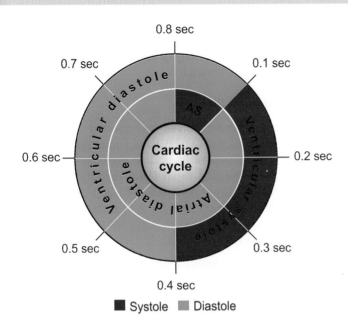

0.8 sec
0.7 sec
0.1 sec
0.6 sec — Cardiac cycle — 0.2 sec
0.5 sec
0.3 sec
0.4 sec

■ Systole   ■ Diastole

FIGURE 91.1: Atrial and ventricular events of cardiac cycle

■ DESCRIPTION OF VENTRICULAR EVENTS

■ ISOMETRIC CONTRACTION PERIOD

Isometric contraction period in cardiac cycle is the first phase of ventricular systole. It lasts for 0.05 second. Isometric contraction is the type of muscular contraction characterized by increase in tension, without any change in the length of muscle fibers. Isometric contraction of ventricular muscle is also called **isovolumetric contraction.**

Immediately after atrial systole, the atrioventricular valves are closed due to increase in ventricular pressure. Semilunar valves are already closed. Now, ventricles contract as closed cavities, in such a way that there is no change in the volume of ventricular chambers or in the length of muscle fibers. Only the tension increases in ventricular musculature.

Because of increased tension in ventricular musculature during isometric contraction, the pressure increases sharply inside the ventricles.

First Heart Sound

Closure of atrioventricular valves at the beginning of this phase produces first heart sound.

Significance of Isometric Contraction

During isometric contraction period, the ventricular pressure increases greatly. When this pressure

increases above the pressure in the aorta and pulmonary artery, the semilunar valves open. Thus, the pressure rise in ventricle, caused by isometric contraction is responsible for the **opening of semilunar valves,** leading to ejection of blood from the ventricles into aorta and pulmonary artery.

■ EJECTION PERIOD

Due to the opening of semilunar valves and isotonic contraction of ventricles, blood is ejected out of both the ventricles. Hence, this period is called ejection period. Duration of this period is 0.22 second. Ejection period is of two stages:

1. First Stage or Rapid Ejection Period

First stage starts immediately after the opening of semilunar valves. During this stage, a large amount of blood is rapidly ejected from both the ventricles. It lasts for 0.13 second.

2. Second Stage or Slow Ejection Period

During this stage, the blood is ejected slowly with much less force. Duration of this period is 0.09 second.

End-systolic Volume

Ventricles are not emptied at the end of ejection period and some amount of blood remains in each ventricle. Amount of blood remaining in ventricles at the end of ejection period (i.e. at the end of systole) is called end-systolic volume. It is 60 to 80 mL per ventricle.

Measurement of end-diastolic volume

End-systolic volume is measured by **radionuclide angiocardiography** (multigated acquisition – **MUGA scan**) and **echocardiography.** It is also measured by cardiac **catheterization,** computed tomography **(CT) scan** and magnetic resonance imaging **(MRI)** (Chapter 109).

Ejection Fraction

Ejection fraction refers to the fraction (or portion) of end-diastolic volume (see below) that is ejected out by each ventricle per beat. From 130 to 150 mL of end-diastolic volume, 70 mL is ejected out by each ventricle (stroke volume). Normal ejection fraction is 60% to 65%.

Determination of ejection fraction

Ejection fraction (E_f) is the stroke volume divided by end-diastolic volume expressed in percentage. Stroke volume (SV) is, end-diastolic volume (EDV) minus end-systolic volume (ESV).

Ejection fraction is calculated as:

$$E_f = \frac{SV}{EDV} = \frac{EDV - ESV}{EDV}$$

Where,

E_f = Ejection fraction
SV = Stroke volume
EDV = End-diastolic volume
ESV = End-systolic volume.

Significance of determining ejection fraction

Ejection fraction is the measure of left ventricular function. Clinically, it is considered as an important index for assessing the ventricular contractility. Ejection fraction decreases in **myocardial infarction** and **cardiomyopathy.**

■ PROTODIASTOLE

Protodiastole is the first stage of ventricular diastole, hence the name protodiastole. Duration of this period is 0.04 second. Due to the ejection of blood, the pressure in aorta and pulmonary artery increases and pressure in ventricles drops.

When intraventricular pressure becomes less than the pressure in aorta and pulmonary artery, the semilunar valves close. Atrioventricular valves are already closed (see above). No other change occurs in the heart during this period. Thus, protodiastole indicates only the end of systole and beginning of diastole.

Second Heart Sound

Closure of semilunar valves during this phase produces second heart sound.

■ ISOMETRIC RELAXATION PERIOD

Isometric relaxation is the type of muscular relaxation, characterized by decrease in tension without any change in the length of muscle fibers. Isometric relaxation of ventricular muscle is also called **isovolumetric relaxation.**

During isometric relaxation period, once again all the valves of the heart are closed (Fig. 91.2). Now, both the ventricles relax as closed cavities without any change in volume or length of the muscle fiber. Intraventricular pressure decreases during this period. Duration of isometric relaxation period is 0.08 second.

Significance of Isometric Relaxation

During isometric relaxation period, the ventricular pressure decreases greatly. When the ventricular pressure becomes less than the pressure in the atria, the

atrioventricular valves open. Thus, the fall in pressure in the ventricles, caused by isometric relaxation is responsible for the **opening of atrioventricular valves,** resulting in filling of ventricles.

■ RAPID FILLING PHASE

When atrionventricular valves are opened, there is a sudden rush of blood (which is accumulated in atria during atrial diastole) from atria into ventricles. So, this period is called the first rapid filling period. Ventricles also relax isotonically. About 70% of filling takes place during this phase, which lasts for 0.11 second.

Third Heart Sound

Rushing of blood into ventricles during this phase causes production of third heart sound.

■ SLOW FILLING PHASE

After the sudden rush of blood, the ventricular filling becomes slow. Now, it is called the slow filling. It is also called **diastasis.** About 20% of filling occurs in this phase. Duration of slow filling phase is 0.19 second.

■ LAST RAPID FILLING PHASE

Last rapid filling phase occurs because of atrial systole. After slow filling period, the atria contract and push a small amount of blood into ventricles. About 10% of ventricular filling takes place during this period. Flow of additional amount of blood into ventricle due to atrial systole is called **atrial kick.**

End-diastolic Volume

End-diastolic volume is the amount of blood remaining in each ventricle at the end of diastole. It is about 130 to 150 mL per ventricle.

Measurement of end-diastolic volume

End-diastolic volume is measured by the same methods, which are used to measure end-systolic volume (see above).

■ INTRA-ATRIAL PRESSURE CHANGES DURING CARDIAC CYCLE

■ SIGNIFICANCE

Pressure in the atria is called the intra-atrial pressure. Intra-atrial pressure is responsible for opening of the atrioventricular valves and ventricular filling. It is also the main factor for the development of venous pulse.

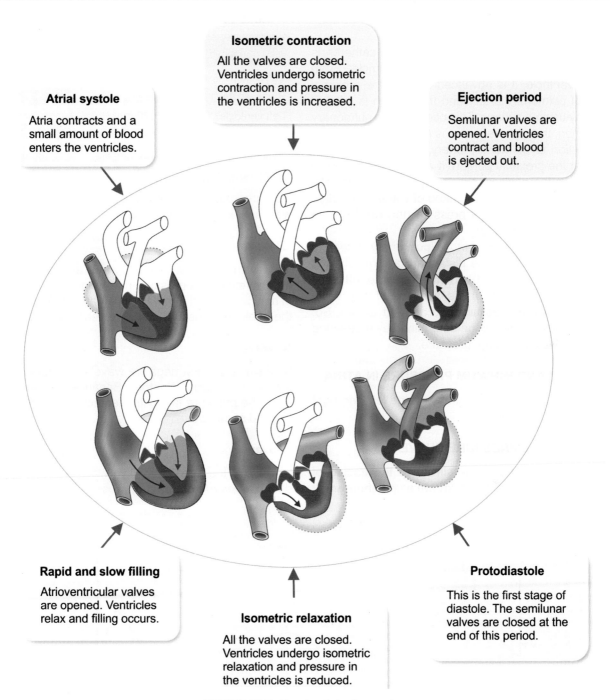

Atrial systole

Atria contracts and a small amount of blood enters the ventricles.

Isometric contraction

All the valves are closed. Ventricles undergo isometric contraction and pressure in the ventricles is increased.

Ejection period

Semilunar valves are opened. Ventricles contract and blood is ejected out.

Rapid and slow filling

Atrioventricular valves are opened. Ventricles relax and filling occurs.

Isometric relaxation

All the valves are closed. Ventricles undergo isometric relaxation and pressure in the ventricles is reduced.

Protodiastole

This is the first stage of diastole. The semilunar valves are closed at the end of this period.

FIGURE 91.2: Events of cardiac cycle

■ METHODS OF STUDY

Right atrial pressure is recorded directly by cardiac **catheterization** (Chapter 98). Left atrial pressure is determined indirectly by measuring pulmonary capillary wedge pressure, which reflects the left atrial pressure accurately.

Pulmonary Capillary Wedge Pressure

Pulmonary capillary wedge pressure is the pressure exerted in the pulmonary capillary bed after obstructing the proximal part of pulmonary artery.

Pulmonary capillary wedge pressure is measured by using a **balloon-tipped multilumen cardiac catheter**

(Swan-Ganz catheter). Tip of the catheter is not open but a pressure transducer is attached to it.

By means of venous puncture, the catheter is guided through right atrium into right ventricle. From the right ventricle, it is advanced towards the proximal portion of pulmonary artery and the balloon is inflated with air by using a syringe. This occludes the pulmonary artery. Then, the catheter alone is advanced further into distal portion of pulmonary artery, leaving the inflated balloon at the proximal portion. It allows the catheter to float in a wedge position. Now the pressure existing in the pulmonary capillary bed ahead of catheter is called pulmonary capillary wedge pressure (the word wedge refers to being obstructed).

When the proximal part of pulmonary artery is obstructed, pressure in the distal part falls rapidly and after about 10 seconds, it becomes equal to left atrial pressure. It is because of the absence of any valve between pulmonary capillary bed and left atrium. So, the left atrial pressure can be determined by measuring pulmonary capillary wedge pressure.

■ MAXIMUM AND MINIMUM PRESSURE IN ATRIA

Maximum and minimum pressures in the left and right atria are given in Table 91.1.

■ INTRA-ATRIAL PRESSURE CURVE

Intra-atrial pressure curve is similar to the tracing of jugular venous pulse, which is known as **phlebogram**. It

TABLE 91.1: Pressure changes during cardiac cycle

Area	Maximum pressure	Minimum pressure
Left atrium	7 to 8 mm Hg	0 to 2 mm Hg
Right atrium	5 to 6 mm Hg	0 to 2 mm Hg
Left ventricle	120 mm Hg	5 mm Hg
Right ventricle	25 mm Hg	2 to 3 mm Hg
Systemic aorta	120 mm Hg	80 mm Hg
Pulmonary artery	25 mm Hg	7 to 8 mm Hg

has three positive waves, a, c and v and three negative waves, x, x_1 and y (Fig. 91.3).

'a' Wave

'a' wave is the first positive wave and occurs during **atrial systole.** The pressure rises sharply up to 5 mm Hg in right atrium and 7 mm Hg in left atrium. After reaching the peak, the pressure starts decreasing.

'x' Wave

'x' wave is the first negative wave and appears during the onset of **atrial diastole.** Because of relaxation of atria, the pressure falls. Atrioventricular valves close at the end of this wave.

'c' Wave

'c' wave is the second positive wave and this appears during **isometric contraction.** Rise in pressure is due to

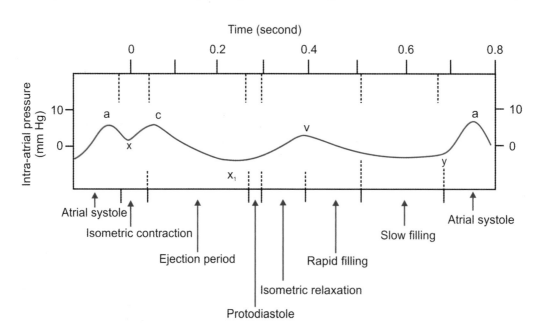

FIGURE 91.3: Intra-arterial pressure changes during cardiac cycle.
a, c, v = Positive waves. x, x_1, y = Negative waves.

the **closure of atrioventricular valves** and the increased intraventricular pressure.

When atrioventricular valves close, there is a little back flow of blood towards atria. When the intraventricular pressure increases, there is bulging of AV valves into the atria. Because of these two factors, the atrial pressure rises.

'x₁' Wave

'x_1' wave is the second negative wave and appears during **ejection period.** During ejection period, the contraction of ventricular musculature pulls the atrioventricular ring towards the ventricles. This causes fall in atrial pressure.

'v' Wave

'v' wave is the third positive wave, which is obtained during **atrial diastole.** It shows a gradual increase in atrial pressure due to filling of blood in atria (venous return).

'y' Wave

'y' wave is the third negative wave and appears after the **opening of AV valves** when the blood rushes from atria into ventricles. So, the pressure in the atria falls.

■ INTRAVENTRICULAR PRESSURE CHANGES DURING CARDIAC CYCLE

■ SIGNIFICANCE

Intraventricular pressure is the pressure developed inside the ventricles of the heart. It is essential for the circulation of blood, because the flow of blood through systemic and pulmonary circulation depends upon the pressure at which the blood is pumped out of ventricles. Thus, intraventricular pressure is essential for the circulation of blood.

■ METHODS OF STUDY

Intraventricular pressure is measured by cardiac catheterization.

■ MAXIMUM AND MINIMUM PRESSURE IN VENTRICLES

There is some difference in the pressure in right ventricle and left ventricle. The pressure is always more in left ventricle than in the right ventricle. Maximum and minimum pressures in the ventricles are given in Table 91.1.

■ INTRAVENTRICULAR PRESSURE CURVE

Intraventricular pressure curve has seven segments (Fig. 91.4).

'A-B' Segment

'A-B' segment is a positive wave and appears during **atrial systole.** Rise in pressure during this period is due to the entry of a small amount of blood into the ventricles because of atrial systole. The pressure rises to about 6 to 7 mm Hg in the right ventricle and to about 7 to 8 mm Hg in the left ventricle.

'B' indicates the **closure of atrioventricular valves.**

'B-C' Segment

'B-C' segment appears during **isometric contraction.** During isometric contraction period, there is a sharp rise in the intraventricular pressure.

'C' denotes the **opening of semilunar valves.**

'C-D' Segment

'C-D' segment appears during **ejection period.** During ejection period, the pressure in the ventricles rises to the peak and then falls down. First part of the curve indicates the maximum ejection and the pressure increases to the maximum. Second part of the curve represents the slow ejection phase when the pressure decreases.

Maximum pressure rise in right ventricle is about 25 mm Hg and the maximum pressure rise in left ventricle is about 120 mm Hg, during the peak of this wave. Maximum pressure in the left ventricle is 4 to 5 times more than that in the right ventricle, because of the thick wall of the left ventricle.

'D-E' Segment

'D-E' segment appears during **protodiastole.** Pressure decreases slightly due to the starting of ventricular relaxation.

'E' indicates the **closure of semilunar valves.**

'E-F' Segment

'E-F' segment is obtained during **isometric relaxation.** There is a sharp fall in the intraventricular pressure during this phase. Pressure in the ventricle falls below the pressure in the atria and this causes the opening of atrioventricular valves.

'F' represents the **opening of atrioventricular valves.**

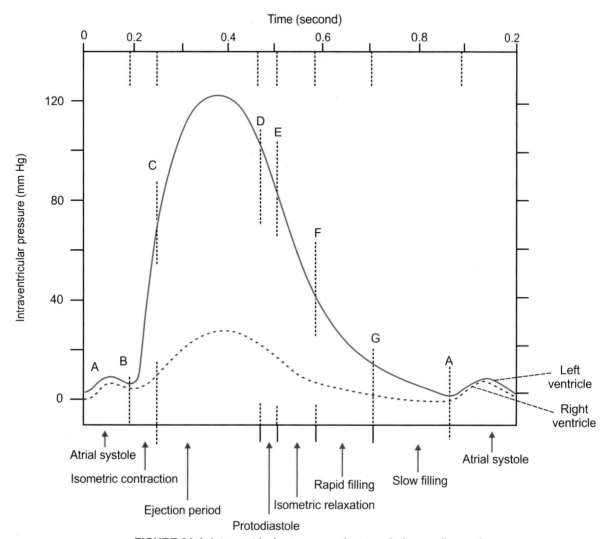

FIGURE 91.4: Intraventricular pressure changes during cardiac cycle

'F-G' Segment

'F-G' segment appears during **rapid filling phase.** In spite of filling of blood, pressure decreases in the ventricles. It is because of the relaxation of the ventricles.

'G-A' Segment

'G-A' segment is the last part of intraventricular pressure curve. It is obtained during **slow filling phase.** Because of continuous relaxation of ventricles during slow filling period, the ventricular pressure decreases further.

■ AORTIC PRESSURE CHANGES DURING CARDIAC CYCLE

■ SIGNIFICANCE

Aortic pressure is the pressure developed in the aorta. It is necessary to maintain the blood flow through the circulatory system.

■ METHOD OF STUDY

Changes in aortic pressure during the cardiac cycle are recorded by using **catheter.**

■ MAXIMUM AND MINIMUM PRESSURE IN AORTA

Pressure in systemic aorta is always higher than that of pulmonary artery. It is because of the higher pressure in left ventricle than in the right ventricle. Maximum and minimum pressures in aorta are given in Table 91.1. Minimum pressure in systemic aorta is much greater than the minimum pressure in the left ventricle. It is due to the presence of elastic tissues in the aorta, which enable the aorta to recoil and maintain the minimum pressure at a higher level.

■ AORTIC PRESSURE CURVE

During the ejection period of the cardiac cycle, the pressure in the aorta increases and reaches the peak.

During diastole, it reduces gradually and reaches the minimum level. At the time of closure of semilunar valves, an incisura occurs due to back flow of some blood towards the ventricles (Fig. 91.5).

■ VENTRICULAR VOLUME CHANGES DURING CARDIAC CYCLE

■ SIGNIFICANCE

Volume of blood in the ventricles is an important factor to maintain cardiac output and blood circulation.

■ METHODS OF STUDY

1. *By using Henderson Cardiometer*

This study is done only in animals. Cardiometer is a cup-shaped device with an outlet. At the top, it is closed by means of a rubber diaphragm. A small hole is made in the diaphragm, through which the ventricles of the animal are pushed. Cardiometer is connected to a recording device like **Marey tambour** (a small stainless steel capsule covered by rubber membrane) or **polygraph**, to record the volume changes (Fig. 99.1).

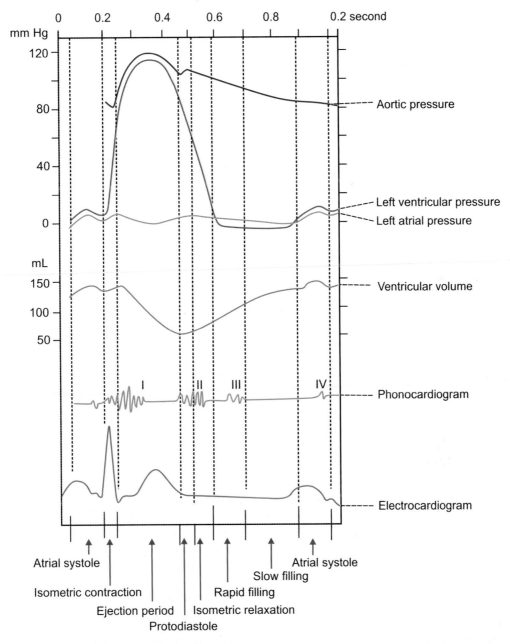

FIGURE 91.5: Comprehensive diagram showing ECG, phonocardiogram, pressure changes and volume changes during cardiac cycle

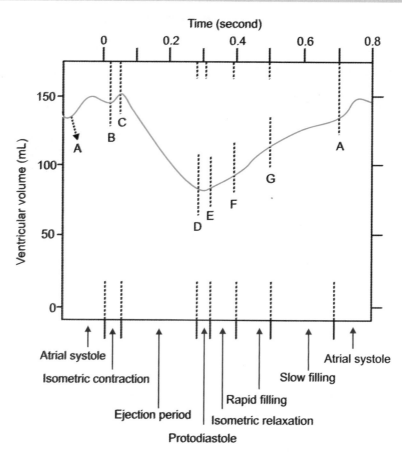

FIGURE 91.6: Ventricular volume changes during cardiac cycle

2. By Angiography

Angiography is the **radiographic study** of heart and blood vessels using a **radiopaque contrast** medium. During angiography, it is possible to measure the ventricular dimensional area and thickness of ventricular wall. From the values obtained, the ventricular volume is calculated.

■ VOLUME OF BLOOD IN RIGHT AND LEFT VENTRICLES

End-diastolic Volume and End-systolic Volume

Amount of blood is the same in both right and left ventricles. Maximum volume of blood in each ventricle after filling (end-diastolic volume) is 130 to 150 mL. Minimum volume of blood left in the ventricles at the end of ejection period (end of systolic volume) is 60 to 80 mL.

See above for measurement of end-diastolic volume and end-systolic volume.

Ejection Fraction

Ejection fraction (E_f) is the stroke volume divided by end-diastolic volume, expressed in percentage. See above for determination and significance of determining ejection period.

■ VENTRICULAR VOLUME CURVE

Ventricular volume curve recorded by using **Henderson cardiometer** has seven segments (Fig. 91.6).

'A-B' Segment

'A-B' segment wave is because of **atrial systole** or last filling phase of ventricles, during which a small amount of blood enters the ventricles from the atria. It increases the ventricular volume slightly.

'B' indicates the **closure of atrioventricular valves.**

'B-C' Segment

'B-C' segment is a positive wave, which is obtained during **isometric contraction.** Actually, the ventricular volume is not altered during isometric contraction. However, the slight upward deflection of this wave is an artifact. It is because the heart thrusts itself into the cardiometer during isometric contraction.

'C' represents the **opening of semilunar valves.**

'C-D' Segment

'C-D' segment occurs during **ejection period.** Initially, there is a sharp fall in the ventricular volume. This occurs during rapid ejection. Later, during slow ejection period, the blood leaves the ventricles slowly. So the ventricular volume decreases slowly.

'D-E' Segment

'D-E' segment part of the ventricular volume curve is recorded during **protodiastole.** There is no change in the ventricular volume during protodiastole.

'E' denotes the closure of semilunar valves.

'E-F' Segment

'E-F' segment appears during **isometric relaxation period** of the cardiac cycle. Actually, the ventricular volume is not altered during isometric relaxation. However, there is a slight upward deflection in the curve due to artifact. It is because of the entrance of blood into coronary artery from aorta during this period. It increases the pressure within the cardiometer.

'F' indicates the **opening of atrioventricular valves.**

'F-G' Segment

'F-G' segment appears during **rapid filling phase.** Rapid rise in ventricular volume is due to sudden rush of blood after the opening of atrioventricular valves.

'G-A' Segment

'G-A' segment is recorded during **slow filling phase.** Ventricular volume increases slowly because of slow filling.

Heart Sounds

■ INTRODUCTION

Heart sounds are the sounds produced by mechanical activities of heart during each cardiac cycle.

Heart sounds are produced by:
1. Flow of blood through cardiac chambers
2. Contraction of cardiac muscle
3. Closure of valves of the heart.

Heart sounds are heard by placing the ear over the chest or by using a stethoscope or microphone. These sounds are also recorded graphically.

■ DIFFERENT HEART SOUNDS

Four heart sounds are produced during each cardiac cycle:
1. First heart sound
2. Second heart sound
3. Third heart sound
4. Fourth heart sound.

First and second heart sounds are called **classical heart sounds** and are heard by using the stethoscope.

These two sounds are more prominent and resemble the spoken words 'LUB, (or LUBB) and 'DUBB' (or DUP), respectively.

Third heart sound is a mild sound and it is not heard by using stethoscope in normal conditions. But it can be heard by using a microphone. Fourth heart sound is an inaudible sound. It becomes audible in pathological conditions only. This sound is studied only by graphic registration, i.e. the phonocardiogram.

■ IMPORTANCE OF HEART SOUNDS

Study of heart sounds has important diagnostic value in clinical practice because alteration in the heart sounds indicates cardiac diseases involving valves of the heart.

■ DESCRIPTION OF HEART SOUNDS

■ FIRST HEART SOUND

First heart sound is produced during **isometric contraction** period and earlier part of **ejection period** (Table 92.1).

TABLE 92.1: Heart sounds

Features	First heart sound	Second heart sound	Third heart sound	Fourth heart sound
Occurs during	Isometric contraction period and part of ejection period	Protodiastole and part of isometric relaxation	Rapid filling phase	Atrial systole
Characteristics	Long, soft and low pitched Resembles the word 'LUBB'	Short, sharp and high pitched Resembles the word 'DUP'	Low pitched	Inaudible sound
Cause	Closure of atrioventricular valves	Closure of semilunar valves	Rushing of blood into ventricle	Contraction of atrial musculature
Duration (sec)	0.10 to 0.17	0.10 to 0.14	0.07 to 0.10	0.02 to 0.04
Frequency (cycles per sec)	25 to 45	50	1 to 6	1 to 4
Relation with ECG	Coincides with peak of 'R' wave	Precedes or appears 0.09 second after peak of 'T' wave	Between 'T' wave and 'P' wave	Between 'P' wave and 'Q' wave
Number of vibrations in phonocardiogram	9 to 13	4 to 6	1 to 4	1 to 2

Causes

Major cause for first heart sound is the sudden and synchronous (simultaneous) closure of **atrioventricular valves.** However, some other factors are also involved. Four types of factors are responsible for the production of the first heart sound.

1. Valvular factor

Synchronous closure of atrioventricular valves set up the vibrations in the **valvular leaflets** and **chordae tendineae.** These vibrations are mainly responsible for the production of the first heart sound.

2. Vascular factor

Rush of blood from the ventricles into aorta and pulmonary artery during ejection period is also responsible for the production of the first heart sound.

3. Muscular factor

Myocardial tension and the contraction of ventricular muscle during isometric contraction and the ejection periods also add to the production of the first heart sound.

4. Atrial factor

Vibrations produced by the atrial systole also play a role in the production of the first heart sound.

Characteristics

First heart sound is a long, soft and low-pitched sound. It resembles the spoken word **'LUBB'.** The duration of this sound is 0.10 to 0.17 second. Its frequency is 25 to 45 cycles/second.

Applied Physiology

1. Reduplication of first heart sound

Reduplication means splitting of the heart sound. First heart sound is split when the atrioventricular valves do not close simultaneously **(asynchronous closure).** Splitting of first heart sound in normal conditions **(physiological splitting)** is rare. **Pathological splitting** of first heart sound occurs in stenosis of atrioventricular valves and atrial septal defect.

2. Soft first heart sound

Heart sound becomes soft when the intensity of sound decreases. A soft first heart sound is heard in low blood pressure, severe heart failure, myocardial infarction and myxedema.

3. Loud or accentuated first heart sound

First heart sound becomes louder or accentuated (becoming prominent) in conditions like mitral stenosis, **Wolff-Parkinson-White syndrome** and acute rheumatic fever. It is loud in patients with thin chest wall also.

4. Cannon sound

Cannon sound refers to the loud first heart sound that is heard intermittently. It is heard in ventricular tachycardia and complete atrioventricular block.

First Heart Sound and ECG

First heart sound coincides with peak of 'R' wave in ECG.

■ SECOND HEART SOUND

Second heart sound is produced at the end of **protodiastolic period.**

Cause

Second heart sound is produced due to the sudden and synchronous closure of the **semilunar valves.**

Characteristics

Second heart sound is a short, sharp and high-pitched sound. It resembles the spoken word **'DUBB'** (or DUP). Duration of second heart sound is 0.10 to 0.14 second. Its frequency is 50 cycles/second.

Applied Physiology

1. Reduplication of second heart sound

Splitting of second heart sound occurs due to asynchronous closure of semilunar valves. It may occur both in physiological and pathological conditions.

Physiological splitting: It occurs during deep inspiration. Normally, aortic valve closes prior to the closure of pulmonary valve. Interval between the two valves widens during inspiration and narrows during expiration.

Increased negative intrathoracic pressure during deep inspiration increases lung expansion and venous return into right atrium. However, the venous return from lungs to left atrium is reduced during this condition. Because of increased venous return in right atrium and subsequent increase in blood volume in right ventricle, pulmonary valve is kept open for slightly longer time than the aortic valve. So, the pulmonary valve closes little later than the aortic valve causing splitting of second heart sound.

Pathological splitting: The splitting of second heart sound occurs during pulmonary stenosis, right bundle branch block and right ventricular hypertrophy.

Reverse splitting: It is the splitting of second heart sound, in which aortic valve closes after the closure of pulmonary valve. It is due to the delay in emptying of left ventricle. It is also called **paradoxical splitting** (paradoxical = contradictory or opposite). Reverse splitting is common in left bundle-branch block, aortic stenosis and left ventricular hypertrophy.

2. Loud or accentuated second heart sound

Loud or accentuated second heart sound is produced by the closure of either aortic valve or pulmonary valve. Aortic valve produces loud sound during systemic hypertension and **coarctation** (narrowing) of aorta.

Pulmonary valve produces loud sound during pulmonary hypertension.

3. Soft second heart sound

Second heart sound becomes soft in heart failure.

Second Heart Sound and ECG

Second heart sound coincides with the 'T' wave in ECG. Sometimes, it may precede the 'T' wave or it may commence after the peak of 'T' wave.

■ THIRD HEART SOUND

Third heart sound is a low-pitched sound that is produced during **rapid filling period** of the cardiac cycle. It is also called ventricular gallop or protodiastolic gallop, as it is produced during earlier part of diastole.

Usually, the third heart sound is **inaudible** by stethoscope and it can be heard only by using microphone.

Causes

Third heart sound is produced by the **rushing of blood** into ventricles and vibrations set up in the ventricular wall during rapid filling phase. It may also be due to vibrations set up in chordae tendineae.

Characteristics

Third heart sound is a short and low-pitched sound. Duration of this sound is 0.07 to 0.10 second. Its frequency is 1 to 6 cycles/second.

Conditions when Third Heart Sound becomes Audible by Stethoscope

Third heart sound can be heard by stethoscope in children and athletes. Pathological conditions when third heart sound becomes loud and audible by stethoscope are aortic regurgitation, cardiac failure and cardiomyopathy with dilated ventricles.

When third heart sound is heard by stethoscope, the condition is called **triple heart sound** (see below). Third heart sound is usually heard best with the bell of stethoscope placed at the apex beat area, when the patient is in left **lateral decubitus** (lying on left side) position.

Third Heart Sound and ECG

Third heart sound appears between 'T' and 'P' waves of ECG.

■ FOURTH HEART SOUND

Normally, the fourth heart sound is an **inaudible** sound. It becomes audible only in pathological conditions. It is studied only by graphical recording, i.e. by phonocardiography. This sound is produced during **atrial systole** (late diastole) and it is considered as the physiologic atrial sound. It is also called **atrial gallop** or **presystolic gallop.**

Causes

Fourth heart sound is produced by contraction of **atrial musculature** and vibrations are set up in atrial musculature, flaps of the atrioventricular valves during systole. It is also due to the vibrations set up in the ventricular myocardium because of ventricular distention during atrial systole.

Characteristics

Fourth heart sound is a short and low-pitched sound. Duration of this sound is 0.02 to 0.04 second. Its frequency is 1 to 4 cycles/second.

Conditions when Fourth Heart Sound becomes Audible

Fourth heart sound becomes audible by stethoscope when the ventricles become stiff. Ventricular stiffness occurs in conditions like ventricular hypertrophy, long standing hypertension and aortic stenosis. To overcome the ventricular stiffness, the atria contract forcefully, producing audible fourth heart sound.

When fourth heart sound is heard by stethoscope, the condition is called **triple heart sound** (see below). It is usually heard best with the bell of stethoscope placed at the apex beat area, when the patient is in supine or left semilateral position.

Fourth Heart Sound and ECG

Fourth heart sound coincides with the interval between the end of 'P' wave and the onset of 'Q' wave.

■ TRIPLE AND QUADRUPLE HEART SOUNDS

■ TRIPLE HEART SOUND OR GALLOP RHYTHM

Triple heart sound or **triple rhythm** is an **abnormal rhythm** of heart, characterized by three clear heart sounds during each heart beat. It is due to an abnormal third or fourth heart sound that is heard besides first and second heart sounds. It is also called **gallop rhythm,** since it resembles the sound of a horse's gallop. Usually, it is indicative of serious cardiovascular disease.

Conditions when Triple Heart Sound is Produced

Triple heart sound is produced in conditions like myocardial infarction and severe hypertension.

■ QUADRUPLE HEART SOUND

Quadruple heart sound is an abnormal rhythm of heart, characterized by four clear heart sounds during each heart beat. It is also called **quadruple rhythm.** It is due to third and fourth heart sounds that are heard besides first and second heart sounds. It is also called **quadruple gallop.**

Quadruple heart sound is also indicative of serious cardiovascular disease.

Conditions when Quadruple Heart Sound is Produced

Quadruple heart sound is produced in patients with congestive heart failure.

Summation Gallop

Whenever there is tachycardia in patients with quadruple heart sound, the third and fourth heart sounds merge together and give rise to a single sound. This sound is called **summation gallop** and it resembles gallop rhythm.

■ METHODS OF STUDY OF HEART SOUNDS

Heart sounds are studied by three methods:
1. By using stethoscope
2. By using microphone
3. By using phonocardiogram.

■ BY STETHOSCOPE

First and second heart sounds are heard on the auscultation areas, by using the stethoscope. The chest piece of the stethoscope is placed over four areas on the chest, which are called auscultation areas.

Auscultation Areas

i. Mitral area (Bicuspid area)

Mitral area is in the left 5th intercostal space, about 10 cm away from the midline (midclavicular line). Sound produced by the closure of mitral valve (first heart

sound) is transmitted well into this area. It is also called **apex beat area** because apex beat is felt in this area.
Apex beat

Apex beat is the thrust of the apex of ventricles, against the chest wall during systole.

ii. Tricuspid area

Tricuspid area is on the xiphoid process. Sound produced by the closure of tricuspid valve (first heart sound) is transmitted well into this area.

iii. Pulmonary area

Pulmonary area is on the left 2nd intercostal space, close to sternum. Sound produced by the closure of pulmonary valve (second heart sound) is heard well on this area.

iv. Aortic area

Aortic area is over the right 2nd intercostal space, close to the sternum. On this area, the sound produced by the closure of aortic valve (second heart sound) is heard well.

First heart sound is best heard in mitral and tricuspid areas. However, it is heard in other areas also but the intensity is less. Similarly, the second heart sound is best heard in pulmonary and aortic areas. It is also heard in other areas with less intensity.

■ BY MICROPHONE

A highly sensitive microphone is placed over the chest. The heart sounds are amplified by means of an **amplifier** and heard by using a **loudspeaker.** First, second and third heart sounds are heard by this method.

■ BY PHONOCARDIOGRAM

Phonocardiography is the technique used to record the heart sounds. Phonocardiogram is the graphical record of heart sounds. It is done by placing an electronic **sound transducer** over the chest. This transducer is connected to a recording device like polygraph. All the four heart sounds can be recorded in phonocardiogram. It helps to analyze the frequency of the sound waves.

Appearance of Heart Sounds in Phonocardiogram

In phonocardiogram, the heart sounds are recorded in the following manner (Fig. 91.6).

First heart sound

First heart sound is recorded as single group of waves. The waves are of small amplitude to start with. Later, the amplitude rapidly rises and falls to form **crescendo** and **diminuendo** series of waves. About 9 to 13 waves appear.

Second heart sound

Second heart sound appears as single group of waves, which have same amplitude. About 4 to 6 waves are recorded.

Third heart sound

Third heart sound is found in phonocardiogram with only 1 to 4 waves grouped together.

Fourth heart sound

Mostly, the fourth heart sound merges with first heart sound. If it appears as separate form, it has 1 to 2 waves with very low amplitude.

Cardiac Murmur

- ■ INTRODUCTION
  - ■ CAUSES OF MURMUR
- ■ CLASSIFICATION OF MURMUR
  - ■ SYSTOLIC MURMUR
  - ■ DIASTOLIC MURMUR
  - ■ CONTINUOUS MURMUR

■ INTRODUCTION

Cardiac murmur is the abnormal or unusual heart sound. It is also called **abnormal heart sound** or **cardiac bruit.** Cardiac murmur is heard by stethoscope, along with normal heart sounds.

Cardiac murmur is heard by placing chest piece of stethoscope over the auscultatory areas. Murmur due to disease of a particular valve is heard well over the auscultatory area of that valve. Sometimes, the murmur is felt by palpation as **'thrills'.** In some patients, murmur is heard without any aid, even at a distance of few feet away from the patient.

■ CAUSES OF MURMUR

Cardiac murmur is produced because of change in the pattern of blood flow. Normally, blood flows in **streamline** through the heart and blood vessels. However, during abnormal conditions like valvular diseases, the blood flow becomes **turbulent.** It produces the cardiac murmur.

Murmur is produced because of valvular diseases, septal defects and vascular defects (Table 93.1).

Valvular Diseases

Valvular diseases are of two types:
1. Stenosis
2. Incompetence.

1. Stenosis

Stenosis means narrowing of heart valve. Blood flows rapidly with turbulence through the narrow orifice of the valve, resulting in murmur.

TABLE 93.1: Causes for cardiac murmur

Type of murmur	Causes
Systolic murmur	1. Incompetence of atrioventricular valves 2. Stenosis of semilunar valves 3. Anemia 4. Septal defect 5. Coarctation of aorta
Diastolic murmur	1. Stenosis of atrioventricular valves 2. Incompetence of semilunar valves
Continuous murmur	1. Patent ductus arteriosus

2. Incompetence

Incompetence refers to weakening of the heart valve. When the valve becomes weak, it cannot close properly. It causes back flow of blood, resulting in **turbulence.** This disease is also called **regurgitation** or **valvular insufficiency.**

■ CLASSIFICATION OF MURMUR

Cardiac murmur is classified into three types:
A. Systolic murmur
B. Diastolic murmur
C. Continuous murmur.

■ SYSTOLIC MURMUR

Systolic murmur is the murmur which is produced during systole. It is produced in the following conditions:

1. Incompetence of Atrioventricular Valves

When the atrioventricular valves become weak, these valves cannot close completely. It causes **regurgitation** of blood from ventricles to the atria during ventricular systole, producing the murmur. It is a **harsh blowing sound** with high frequency.

2. Stenosis of Semilunar Valves

During stenosis of aortic valve, the left ventricular pressure raises up to 300 mm Hg during systole. It causes a greater turbulence in the blood flow. The vibrations of this sound can be felt as **'thrills'** by palpation over lower neck region and upper chest. In severe conditions, the sound is heard even a few feet away from the affected person. It is a **harsh** and a **loud sound.**

3. Murmur due to Anemia

A systolic murmur is heard in severe anemia because of reduced viscosity and accelerated flow of blood.

4. Septal Defect

During interventricular septal defect, blood flows from left ventricle to right ventricle during systole. It produces a systolic murmur. Septal defect is a rare disorder.

5. Coarctation of Aorta

Coarctation of aorta is a congenital disorder, characterized by the narrowing of a part of systemic aorta. A loud murmur is produced during systole and it is heard in the earlier part of diastole also.

■ DIASTOLIC MURMUR

Diastolic murmur is the murmur that is produced during diastole. It is produced in the following conditions:

1. Stenosis of Atrioventricular Valves

When the atrioventricular valves become narrow, the turbulence of blood flow occurs during diastole, i.e. when blood enters the ventricles from atria. Murmur due to stenosis of mitral valve is heard better at mitral area. Murmur due to stenosis of tricuspid valve is heard best at tricuspid area. It is a **weak sound** with low frequency.

Sometimes, murmur due to mitral stenosis cannot be heard by stethoscope, due to low frequency. But it can be felt as a mild thrill over mitral area of the chest.

2. Incompetence of Semilunar Valves

Murmur is produced during the regurgitation of blood from aorta into the ventricle, through incompetent semilunar valve during diastole. It is like a **blowing sound** with low frequency.

■ CONTINUOUS MURMUR

Continuous murmur is the murmur that is heard in conditions such as patent ductus arteriosus.

Patent Ductus Arteriosus

Intact ductus arteriosus is called patent ductus arteriosus (Chapter 114). A continuous murmur is heard in this condition. However, intensity of the sound is more during systole and less during diastole. Because of this, it is also called **machinery murmur.**

It is a **harsh blowing sound** and is heard best in the pulmonary area. The murmur is heard 1 year after birth.

Electrocardiogram (ECG)

■ DEFINITIONS

Electrocardiography

Electrocardiography is the **technique** by which electrical activities of the heart are studied. The spread of excitation through myocardium produces local electrical potential. This low-intensity current flows through the body, which acts as a **volume conductor.** This current can be picked up from surface of the body by using suitable electrodes and recorded in the form of electrocardiogram. This technique was discovered by Dutch physiologist, **Einthoven Willem,** who is considered the father of electrocardiogram (ECG).

Electrocardiograph

Electrocardiograph is the **instrument** (machine) by which electrical activities of the heart are recorded.

Electrocardiogram

Electrocardiogram (ECG or EKG from electrokardiogram in Dutch) is the record or **graphical registration** of electrical activities of the heart, which occur prior to the onset of mechanical activities. It is the **summed electrical activity** of all cardiac muscle fibers recorded from surface of the body.

■ USES OF ECG

Electrocardiogram is useful in determining and diagnosing the following:
1. Heart rate
2. Heart rhythm
3. Abnormal electrical conduction
4. Poor blood flow to heart muscle (ischemia)
5. Heart attack

6. Coronary artery disease
7. Hypertrophy of heart chambers.

■ ELECTROCARDIOGRAPHIC GRID

The paper that is used for recording ECG is called ECG paper. ECG machine amplifies the electrical signals produced from the heart and records these signals on a moving ECG paper.

Electrocardiographic grid refers to the markings (lines) on ECG paper. ECG paper has horizontal and vertical lines at regular intervals of 1 mm. Every 5th line (5 mm) is thickened.

■ DURATION

Time duration of different ECG waves is plotted horizontally on X-axis.

On X-axis

1 mm = 0.04 second
5 mm = 0.20 second

■ AMPLITUDE

Amplitude of ECG waves is plotted vertically on Y-axis.

On Y-axis

1 mm = 0.1 mV
5 mm = 0.5 mV

■ SPEED OF THE PAPER

Movement of paper through the machine can be adjusted by two speeds, 25 mm/second and 50 mm/second. Usually, speed of the paper during recording is fixed at 25 mm/second. If heart rate is very high, speed of the paper is changed to 50 mm/second.

■ ECG LEADS

ECG is recorded by placing series of electrodes on the surface of the body. These electrodes are called ECG leads and are connected to the ECG machine.

Electrodes are fixed on the limbs. Usually, right arm, left arm and left leg are chosen. Heart is said to be in the center of an **imaginary equilateral triangle** drawn by connecting the roots of these three limbs. This triangle is called Einthoven triangle.

Einthoven Triangle and Einthoven Law

Einthoven triangle is defined as an equilateral triangle that is used as a model of standard limb leads used to record electrocardiogram. Heart is presumed to lie in the center of Einthoven triangle.

Electrical potential generated from the heart appears simultaneously on the roots of the three limbs, namely the left arm, right arm and the left leg.

Refer next Chapter for Einthoven law.

ECG is recorded in 12 leads, which are generally classified into two categories.
  I. Bipolar leads
  II. Unipolar leads.

■ BIPOLAR LIMB LEADS

Bipolar limb leads are otherwise known as **standard limb leads.** Two limbs are connected to obtain these leads and both the electrodes are **active recording electrodes,** i.e. one electrode is positive and the other one is negative (Fig. 94.1).

Standard limb leads are of three types:
  a. Limb lead I
  b. Limb lead II
  c. Limb lead III.

Lead I

Lead I is obtained by connecting right arm and left arm. Right arm is connected to the negative terminal of the instrument and the left arm is connected to the positive terminal.

Lead II

Lead II is obtained by connecting right arm and left leg. Right arm is connected to the negative terminal of the instrument and the left leg is connected to the positive terminal.

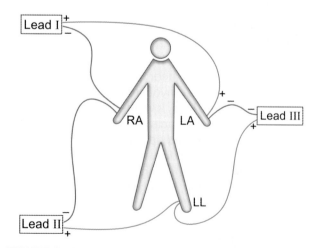

FIGURE 94.1: Position of electrodes for standard limb leads
RA = Right arm, LA = Left arm, LL=Left leg.

Lead III

Lead III is obtained by connecting left arm and left leg. Left arm is connected to the negative terminal of the instrument and the left leg is connected to the positive terminal.

■ UNIPOLAR LEADS

Here, one electrode is **active electrode** and the other one is an **indifferent electrode.** Active electrode is positive and the indifferent electrode is serving as a **composite negative electrode.**

Unipolar leads are of two types:
1. Unipolar limb leads
2. Unipolar chest leads.

1. Unipolar Limb Leads

Unipolar limb leads are also called **augmented limb leads** or **augmented voltage leads.** Active electrode is connected to one of the limbs. Indifferent electrode is obtained by connecting the other two limbs through a resistance.

Unipolar limb leads are of three types:
   i. aVR lead
   ii. aVL lead
   iii. aVF lead.

i. aVR lead

Active electrode is from right arm. Indifferent electrode is obtained by connecting left arm and left leg.

ii. aVL lead

Active electrode is from left arm. Indifferent electrode is obtained by connecting right arm and left leg.

iii. aVF lead

Active electrode is from left leg (foot). Indifferent electrode is obtained by connecting the two upper limbs.

2. Unipolar Chest Leads

Chest leads are also called **'V' leads** or **precardial chest leads.** Indifferent electrode is obtained by connecting the three limbs, viz. left arm, left leg and right arm, through a **resistance** of 5000 ohms. Active electrode is placed on six points over the chest (Fig. 94.2). This electrode is known as the chest electrode and the six points over the chest are called V_1, V_2, V_3, V_4, V_5 and V_6. V indicates vector, which shows the direction of current flow.

Position of chest leads:
   V_1 : Over 4th intercostal space near right sternal margin
   V_2 : Over 4th intercostal space near left sternal margin

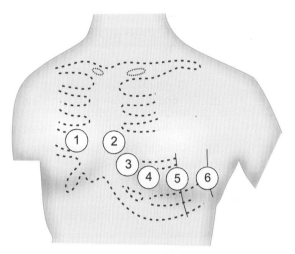

FIGURE 94.2: Position of electrodes for chest leads (V_1 to V_6)

   V_3 : In between V_2 and V_4
   V_4 : Over left 5th intercostal space on the mid clavicular line
   V_5 : Over left 5th intercostal space on the anterior axillary line
   V_6 : Over left 5th intercostal space on the mid axillary line.

■ WAVES OF NORMAL ECG

Normal ECG consists of waves, complexes, intervals and segments. Waves of ECG recorded by limb lead II are considered as the typical waves. Normal electrocardiogram has the following waves, namely P, Q, R, S and T (Table 94.1 and Fig. 94.3). Einthoven had named the waves of ECG starting from the middle of the English alphabets (P) instead of starting from the beginning (A).

Major Complexes in ECG

1. 'P' wave, the atrial complex
2. 'QRS' complex, the initial ventricular complex
3. 'T' wave, the final ventricular complex
4. 'QRST', the ventricular complex.

■ 'P' WAVE

'P' wave is a positive wave and the first wave in ECG. It is also called **atrial complex.**

Cause

'P' wave is produced due to the **depolarization** of **atrial musculature.** Depolarization spreads from SA node to all parts of atrial musculature. **Atrial repolarization** is not

TABLE 94.1: Waves of normal ECG

Wave/Segment	From – To	Cause	Duration (second)	Amplitude (mV)
P wave	–	Atrial depolarization	0.1	0.1 to 0.12
QRS complex	Onset of Q wave to the end of S wave	Ventricular depolarization and atrial repolarization	0.08 to 0.10	Q = 0.1 to 0.2 R = I S = 0.4
T wave	–	Ventricular repolarization	0.2	0.3
P-R interval	Onset of P wave to onset of Q wave	Atrial depolarization and conduction through AV node	0.18 (0.12 to 0.2)	–
Q-T interval	Onset of Q wave and end of T wave	Ventricular depolarization and ventricular repolarization	0.4 to 0.42	–
S-T segment	End of S wave and onset of T wave	Isoelectric	0.08	–

recorded as a separate wave in ECG because it merges with ventricular repolarization (QRS complex).

Duration

Normal duration of 'P' wave is 0.1 second.

Amplitude

Normal amplitude of 'P' wave is 0.1 to 0.12 mV.

Morphology

'P' wave is normally positive (upright) in leads I, II, aVF, V_4, V_5 and V_6. It is normally negative (inverted) in aVR. It is variable in the remaining leads, i.e. it may be positive, negative, biphasic or flat (Fig. 94.4).

Clinical Significance

Variation in the duration, amplitude and morphology of 'P' wave helps in the diagnosis of several cardiac problems such as:

1. *Right atrial hypertrophy:* 'P' wave is tall (more than 2.5 mm) in lead II. It is usually pointed
2. *Left atrial dilatation or hypertrophy:* It is tall and broad based or M shaped
3. *Atrial extrasystole:* Small and shapeless 'P' wave, followed by a small compensatory pause
4. *Hyperkalemia:* 'P' wave is absent or small
5. *Atrial fibrillation:* 'P' wave is absent
6. *Middle AV nodal rhythm:* 'P' wave is absent
7. *Sinoatrial block:* 'P' wave is inverted or absent
8. *Atrial paroxysmal tachycardia:* 'P' wave is inverted
9. *Lower AV nodal rhythm:* 'P' wave appears after QRS complex.

■ 'QRS' COMPLEX

'QRS' complex is also called the **initial ventricular complex.** 'Q' wave is a small negative wave. It is continued as the tall 'R' wave, which is a positive wave. 'R' wave is followed by a small negative wave, the 'S' wave.

Cause

'QRS' complex is due to **depolarization** of **ventricular musculature.** 'Q' wave is due to the depolarization of basal portion of interventricular septum. 'R' wave is due to the depolarization of apical portion of interventricular septum and apical portion of ventricular muscle. 'S' wave is due to the depolarization of basal portion of ventricular muscle near the atrioventricular ring.

Duration

Normal duration of 'QRS' complex is between 0.08 and 0.10 second.

Amplitude

Amplitude of 'Q' wave = 0.1 to 0.2 mV.
Amplitude of 'R' wave = 1 mV.
Amplitude of 'S' wave = 0.4 mV.

Morphology

'Q' wave is normally small with amplitude of 4 mm or less. It is less than 25% of amplitude of 'R' wave in leads I, II, aVL, V_5 and V_6. In the remaining leads, its amplitude is < 0.2 mm.

From chest leads V_1 to V_6, 'R' wave becomes gradually larger. It is smaller in V_6 than V_5. 'S' wave is large in V_1 and larger in V_2. It gradually becomes smaller from V_3 to V_6.

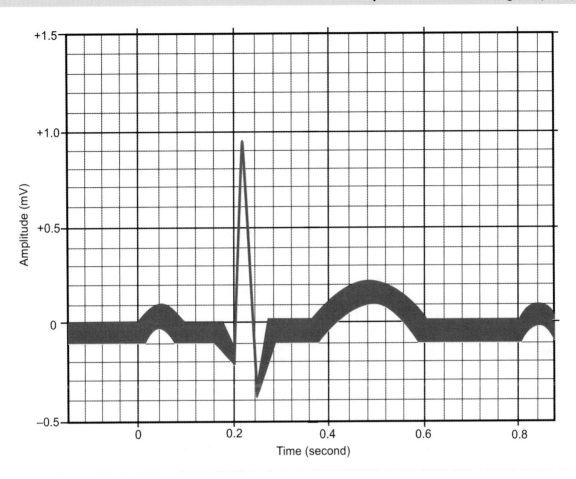

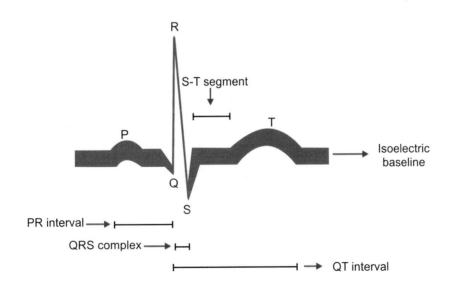

FIGURE 94.3: Waves of normal ECG

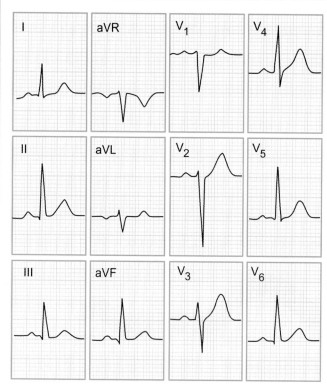

FIGURE 94.4: 12-lead ECG
(*Courtesy:* Dr Atul Ruthra)

Clinical Significance

Variation in the duration, amplitude and morphology of 'QRS' complex helps in the diagnosis of several cardiac problems such as:

1. *Bundle branch block:* QRS is prolonged or deformed
2. *Hyperkalemia:* QRS is prolonged.

■ 'T' WAVE

'T' wave is the **final ventricular complex** and is a positive wave.

Cause

'T' wave is due to the **repolarization** of **ventricular musculature.**

Duration

Normal duration of 'T' wave is 0.2 second.

Amplitude

Normal amplitude of 'T' wave is 0.3 mV.

Morphology

'T' wave is normally positive in leads I, II and V_5 and V_6. It is normally inverted in lead aVR. It is variable in the other leads, i.e. it is positive, negative or flat.

Clinical Significance

Variation in duration, amplitude and morphology of 'T' wave helps in the diagnosis of several cardiac problems such as:

1. *Acute myocardial ischemia:* Hyperacute 'T' wave develops. Hyperacute 'T' wave refers to a tall and broad-based 'T' wave, with slight asymmetry.
2. *Old age, hyperventilation, anxiety, myocardial infarction, left ventricular hypertrophy and pericarditis:* 'T' wave is small, flat or inverted
3. *Hypokalemia:* 'T' wave is small, flat or inverted
4. *Hyperkalemia:* 'T' wave is tall and tented.

■ 'U' WAVE

'U' wave is not always seen. It is also an insignificant wave in ECG. It is supposed to be due to **repolarization** of **papillary muscle.**

Clinical Significance

Appearance of 'U' wave in ECG indicates some clinical conditions such as:

1. *Hypercalcemia, thyrotoxicosis and hypokalemia:* 'U' wave appears. It is very prominent in hypokalemia.
2. *Myocardial ischemia:* Inverted 'U' wave appears.

■ INTERVALS AND SEGMENTS OF ECG

■ 'P-R' INTERVAL

'P-R' interval is the interval between the onset of 'P' wave and onset of 'Q' wave.

'P-R' interval signifies the atrial depolarization and conduction of impulses through AV node. It shows the duration of conduction of the impulses from the SA node to ventricles through atrial muscle and AV node.

'P' wave represents the atrial depolarization. Short **isoelectric** (zero voltage) period after the end of 'P' wave represents the time taken for the passage of depolarization within AV node.

Duration

Normal duration of 'P-R interval' is 0.18 second and varies between 0.12 and 0.2 second. If it is more than 0.2 second, it signifies the delay in the conduction of impulse from SA node to the ventricles. Usually, the delay occurs in the AV node. So it is called the **AV nodal delay.**

Clinical Significance

Variation in the duration of 'P-R' intervals helps in the diagnosis of several cardiac problems such as:

1. It is prolonged in bradycardia and first degree heart block

2. It is shortened in tachycardia, Wolf-Parkinson-White syndrome, Lown-Ganong-Levine syndrome, Duchenne muscular dystrophy and type II glycogen storage disease.

■ 'Q-T' INTERVAL

'Q-T' interval is the interval between the onset of 'Q' wave and the end of 'T' wave.

'Q-T' interval indicates the ventricular depolarization and ventricular repolarization, i.e. it signifies the electrical activity in ventricles.

Duration

Normal duration of Q-T interval is between 0.4 and 0.42 second.

Clinical Significance

1. 'Q-T' interval is prolonged in long 'Q-T' syndrome, myocardial infarction, myocarditis, hypocalcemia and hypothyroidism
2. 'Q-T' interval is shortened in short 'Q-T' syndrome and hypercalcemia.

■ 'S-T' SEGMENT

'S-T' segment is the time interval between the end of 'S' wave and the onset of 'T' wave. It is an isoelectric period.

J Point

The point where 'S-T' segment starts is called 'J' point. It is the junction between the QRS complex and 'S-T' segment.

Duration of 'S-T' Segment

Normal duration of 'S-T' segment is 0.08 second.

Clinical Significance

Variation in the duration of 'S-T' segment and its deviation from isoelectric base indicates the pathological conditions such as:
1. Elevation of 'S-T' segment occurs in anterior or inferior myocardial infarction, left bundle branch block and acute pericarditis. In athletes, 'S-T' segment is usually elevated
2. Depression of 'S-T' segment occurs in acute myocardial ischemia, posterior myocardial infarction, ventricular hypertrophy and hypokalemia

3. 'S-T' segment is prolonged in hypocalcemia
4. 'S-T' segment is shortened in hypercalcemia.

■ 'R-R' INTERVAL

'R-R' interval is the time interval between two consecutive 'R' waves.

Significance

'R-R' interval signifies the duration of one cardiac cycle.

Duration

Normal duration of 'R-R' interval is 0.8 second.

Significance of Measuring 'R-R' Interval

Measurement of 'R-R' interval helps to calculate:
1. Heart rate
2. Heart rate variability.

1. Heart Rate

Heart rate is calculated by measuring the number of 'R' waves per unit time.

Calculation of heart rate

Time is plotted horizontally (X-axis). On X-axis, interval between two thick lines is 0.2 sec (see above). Time duration for 30 thick lines is 6 seconds. Number of 'R' waves (QRS complexes) in 6 seconds (30 thick lines) is counted and multiplied by 10 to obtain heart rate. For the sake of convenience, the ECG paper has special time marking at every 3 seconds. So it is easy to find the time duration of 6 seconds.

2. Heart Rate Variability

Heart rate variability (HRV) refers to the beat-to-beat variations. Under resting conditions, the ECG of healthy individuals exhibits some periodic variation in 'R-R' intervals. This rhythmic phenomenon is known as **respiratory sinus arrhythmia** (RSA), since it fluctuates with the phases of respiration. 'R-R' interval decreases during inspiration and increases during expiration (Chapter 96).

Significance of Heart Rate Variability

HRV decreases in many clinical conditions like:
1. Cardiovascular dysfunctions such as hypertension
2. Diabetes mellitus
3. Psychiatric problems such as panic and anxiety.

Vector

■ INTRODUCTION

Cardiac vector is the direction at which electrical potential generated in the heart travels at an instant. It is also called **cardiac axis.**

Vector is represented by an arrow. Arrowhead shows the **direction** of electrical potential. Length of the arrow represents the **amplitude** (magnitude or voltage) of the potential.

■ INSTANTANEOUS MEAN VECTOR

Current flows in all directions. Mean direction of flow of electrical potential at one instance is known as instantaneous mean vector or instantaneous summated vector (Fig. 95.1).

For example, when current flows through interventricular septum from the base of ventricles towards apex, the electrical potential generated by flow of current travels in different directions as follows:

1. Electrical potential travels downwards through the interventricular septum, towards the apical part, i.e. from depolarized part of septum towards non-depolarized (polarized) part of septum. This potential is strong.
2. Through the inner surface of ventricles, the potential travels upwards from apical part towards the base. Magnitude of this potential is very weak.

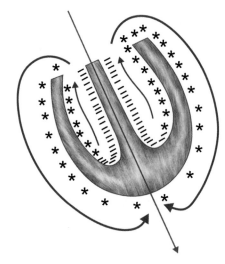

FIGURE 95.1: Instantaneous mean vector when current flows through interventricular septum of the heart

3. Through the outer surface of heart, the electrical potential travels downwards. It has a higher magnitude.

Though the potential travels in all directions in this instance, the potential flowing downwards (from base to apex of the heart) is much greater in magnitude than the potential flowing in other directions. Thus, the mean direction of flow of electrical potential in this instance is downwards. This downward vector is called instantaneous mean vector or instantaneous summated vector at this instance.

■ DEGREE OF INSTANTANEOUS MEAN VECTOR

While recording electrocardiogram (ECG) in different limb leads, the degree of vector is altered. Direction of current flow is always from negative point towards the positive point. When the electrical potential flows in a horizontal plane from right side towards left side of the heart, the degree of vector is zero (Fig. 95.2).

■ DEGREE OF INSTANTANEOUS MEAN VECTOR AT DIFFERENT LIMB LEADS

Standard Limb Lead I (Right Arm and Left Arm)

In this instance, the electrical potential travels from right side (negative point) of the heart towards the left side (positive point) in the horizontal plane. So, the degree of vector is considered as zero.

Standard Limb Lead II (Right Arm and Left Leg)

Vector is from above downwards and slightly towards left, i.e. at 60°.

Standard Limb Lead III (Left Arm and Left Leg)

Here, vector is from above downwards and slightly towards right at 120°.

Lead Augmented Vector Right (aVR)

Vector is from below towards upper part of the heart and slightly towards right at 210°.

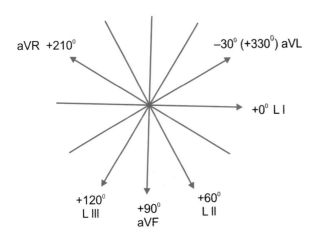

FIGURE 95.2: Degree of instantaneous vector at different leads

Lead Augmented Vector Front (aVF)

Vector is from above downwards at 90°.

Lead Augmented Vector Left (aVL)

In this, the vector is from below, towards upper part of the heart and slightly towards left, at –30° or at +330°.

■ CALCULATED VECTOR OR MEAN QRS VECTOR

Instantaneous mean vector cannot be determined by the recording of ECG. But, another vector can be calculated by measuring the amplitude of QRS complex from the ECG, recorded in standard limb leads. It is called the calculated vector or mean QRS vector.

It is also called the electrical axis of the heart or cardiac vector.

Calculated cardiac vector is useful in the diagnosis of heart diseases.

■ CALCULATION OF MEAN QRS VECTOR

Calculation of mean QRS vector depends upon the fact that if the amplitude of QRS complex is determined from ECG recorded at any two standard limb leads, the amplitude of QRS complex in the remaining lead can be known from the calculation.

Amplitude is measured in mm. For determining the amplitude of QRS complex, first the height of R wave is measured. From this value, height of negative wave Q or S (whichever is more) is deducted. The calculation is based on Einthoven triangle.

Einthoven Triangle

Refer previous Chapter for Einthoven triangle.

Steps for Calculation of Mean QRS Vector

1. An equilateral triangle is drawn on a plain paper. This triangle represents Einthoven triangle. Each side of this triangle represents one standard limb lead.
2. From the midpoint of each side, a perpendicular line is drawn towards the center. Meeting point of the perpendicular lines represents center of electrical activity in the heart (Fig. 95.3).
3. On each side of triangle, the amplitude of QRS complex is plotted from midpoint towards the positive point of the lead. For example, the amplitude of QRS complex in lead I is 10 mm and in lead II, it is 16 mm (Fig. 95.4).
4. In the triangle, upper side represents lead I and in this lead, the left is positive. So, a 10 mm line is drawn

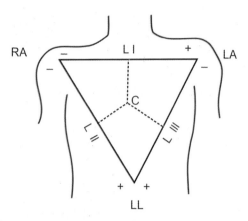

FIGURE 95.3: Einthoven triangle. C = Center of electrical activity, RA = Right arm, LA = Left arm, LL = Left leg, LI, LII and LIII = Standard limb leads.

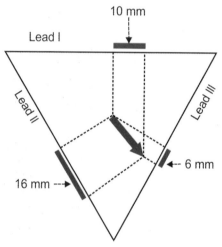

FIGURE 95.4: Calculation of cardiac vector. Arrow in the center indicates the cardiac vector.

on upper side from the midpoint, towards left (positive). This 10 mm distance along the axis of lead I is called **projected vector** for lead I.

5. In the same way, the projected vector for Lead II is drawn on the right side of the triangle
6. From the positive end of each projected vector another perpendicular line is drawn towards interior of the triangle
7. Now an arrow is drawn between center of electrical activity and the meeting point of perpendicular lines from positive end of projected vectors (Fig. 95.5).

    This arrow shows the vector. Arrowhead is drawn towards positive end, i.e. downwards.
8. Degree and the length of the arrow are measured. Degree denotes the direction of vector and length denotes the magnitude.

Amplitude of QRS Complex in Lead III

Amplitude (electrical potential) of QRS complex in lead III can be calculated by applying Einthoven law.

Einthoven law

Einthoven law states that potential differences between the bipolar leads measured simultaneously will, at any given moment, have the values II = I + III. That is, the potential of any wave or complex in lead II of ECG is equal to the sum of potentials in lead I and lead III. Einthoven law is the modification of Kirchhoff's law of voltage.

Kirchhoff's law of voltage

According to Kirchhoff law, the algebraic sum of voltage rise in a closed circuit is equal to the algebraic sum of voltage drops.

Application of Einthoven law in calculating QRS complex

By applying Einthoven law, amplitude (electrical potential) of QRS complex in one lead can be mathematically calculated, by summing up or subtracting the amplitude in other two leads, depending upon the potentials of these leads.

For example, amplitude of QRS in lead II = I + III and the amplitude of QRS in lead III = II − I. Thus, in this case of Einthoven triangle mentioned above, amplitude of QRS in lead I is 1 mV and lead II is 1.6 mV. Thus, the amplitude of QRS in lead III is 0.6 mV. It can also be measured from the triangle drawn to calculate the vector (Fig. 95.5).

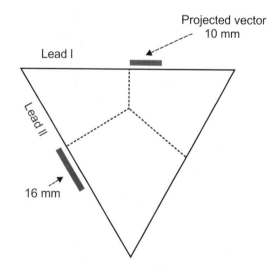

FIGURE 95.5: Determination of vector in Lead I and Lead II

■ VECTORAL ANALYSIS

Mean QRS vector (cardiac axis) in normal conditions is at about +59°. It varies between −30° and +110°.

When the axis deviates towards the left, i.e. in anti-clockwise direction, away from −30°, it is called left axis deviation. When the axis deviates towards the right (clockwise direction), away from +110°, it is known as right axis deviation.

Left axis deviation

Left axis deviation occurs in left ventricular hypertrophy, left bundle-branch block and posterior wall infarction.

Right axis deviation

Right axis deviation occurs due to right ventricular hypertrophy, right bundle-branch block and anterior wall infarction.

■ VECTOR CARDIOGRAM

From the recording of the electrocardiogram, only the calculated vector, i.e. cardiac axis is determined. Instantaneous mean vector cannot be determined by the electrocardiogram, but it can be determined by means of vector cardiogram.

Vector cardiogram is the simultaneous recording of electrical potential in different axis across the heart above, downward and sideward. It is obtained by using a cathode-ray oscilloscope. The technique is equal to connecting the tops of all instantaneous mean vectors in the series of 3 loops. It is done by means of a sophisticated electronic device along with oscilloscope.

Each loop of electronic connection is used to record different vector cardiogram called P vector cardiogram, QRS vector cardiogram and T vector cardiogram.

Arrhythmia

- ■ **DEFINITION**
- ■ **CLASSIFICATION**
- ■ **NORMOTOPIC ARRHYTHMIA**
  - ■ SINUS ARRHYTHMIA
  - ■ SINUS TACHYCARDIA
  - ■ SINUS BRADYCARDIA
- ■ **ECTOPIC ARRHYTHMIA**
  - ■ HEART BLOCK
  - ■ EXTRASYSTOLE
  - ■ PAROXYSMAL TACHYCARDIA
  - ■ ATRIAL FLUTTER
  - ■ ATRIAL FIBRILLATION
  - ■ VENTRICULAR FIBRILLATION
- ■ **ABNORMAL PACEMAKER**
- ■ **ARTIFICIAL PACEMAKER**
- ■ **CURRENT OF INJURY**

■ DEFINITION

Arrhythmia refers to **irregular heartbeat** or disturbance in the rhythm of heart. In arrhythmia, heartbeat may be fast or slow or there may be an extra beat or a missed beat. It occurs in physiological and pathological conditions.

■ CLASSIFICATION

In arrhythmia, SA node may or may not be the pacemaker. If SA node is not the pacemaker, any other part of the heart such as atrial muscle, AV node and ventricular muscle becomes the pacemaker.

Accordingly, arrhythmia is classified into two types:
A. Normotopic arrhythmia
B. Ectopic arrhythmia.

■ NORMOTOPIC ARRHYTHMIA

Normotopic arrhythmia is the irregular heartbeat, in which SA node is the pacemaker.

Normotopic arrhythmia is of three types:
1. Sinus arrhythmia
2. Sinus tachycardia
3. Sinus bradycardia.

■ SINUS ARRHYTHMIA

Sinus arrhythmia is a normal rhythmical increase and decrease in heart rate, in relation to respiration. It is also called **respiratory sinus arrhythmia** (RSA). Normal sinus rhythm means the normal heartbeat with SA node as the pacemaker.

Normal heart rate is 72 per minute. However, under physiological conditions, in a normal healthy person, heart rate varies according to the phases of respiratory cycle. Heart rate increases during inspiration and decreases during expiration.

ECG Changes

ECG is normal during sinus arrhythmia. Only the duration of R-R interval varies rhythmically according to phases

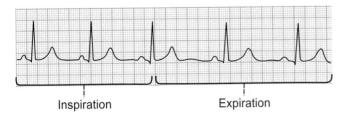

Inspiration   Expiration

FIGURE 96.1: ECG in sinus arrhythmia. Normal P-QRS-T. R-R interval is shortened during inspiration and prolonged during expiration (*Courtesy:* Dr Atul Ruthra).

of respiration (Fig. 96.1). It is shortened during inspiration and prolonged during expiration (Chapter 94).

Cause

Sinus arrhythmia is due to fluctuation in the discharge of impulses from SA node (Fig. 96.2). During inspiration, the lungs are inflated and the intrathoracic pressure decreases. This increases the venous return. Inflation of lungs stimulates the stretch receptors of lungs, which send impulses to vasodilator area (cardioinhibitory center) through afferent fibers of vagus. It leads to reflex inhibition of vasodilator area and reduction in

vagal tone. Because of these two factors, heart rate increases. Simultaneously, increased venous return initiates **Bainbridge reflex** that causes increase in heart rate (Chapter 101).

During expiration, the lungs are deflated and intrathoracic pressure increases. This decreases the venous return. During deflation of lungs, the stretch receptors are not stimulated and vasodilator area is not inhibited. So, vagal tone increases, resulting in decreased heart rate. Simultaneously, decreased venous return abolishes Bainbridge reflex. It also decreases the heart rate.

■ SINUS TACHYCARDIA

Sinus tachycardia is the increase in discharge of impulses from SA node, resulting in increase in heart rate. Discharge of impulses from SA node is very rapid and the heart rate increases up to 100/minute and sometimes up to 150/minute.

ECG Changes

ECG is normal in sinus tachycardia, except for short R-R intervals because of increased heart rate (Fig. 96.3).

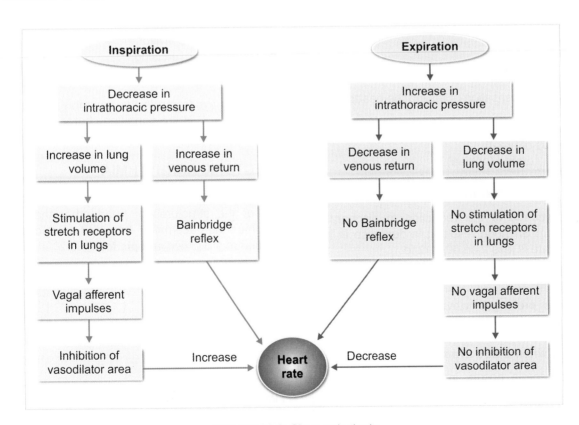

FIGURE 96.2: Sinus arrhythmia

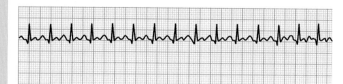

FIGURE 96.3: ECG in sinus tachycardia. Normal P-QRS-T. R-R interval is shortened. Heart rate is more than 100/min (*Courtesy:* Dr Atul Ruthra).

Conditions when Sinus Tachycardia Occurs

Sinus tachycardia occurs in physiological as well as pathological conditions.

Physiological conditions when tachycardia occurs

1. Exercise
2. Emotion
3. High altitude
4. Pregnancy.

Pathological conditions when tachycardia occurs

1. Fever
2. Anemia
3. Hyperthyroidism
4. Hypersecretion of catecholamines
5. Cardiomyopathy
6. Valvular heart disease
7. Hemorrhagic shock.

Features of Sinus Tachycardia

1. Palpitations (sensation of feeling the heartbeat)
2. Dizziness
3. Fainting
4. Shortness of breath
5. Chest discomfort (angina).

■ SINUS BRADYCARDIA

Sinus bradycardia is the reduction in discharge of impulses from SA node resulting in decrease in heart rate. Heart rate is less than 60/minute.

ECG Changes

ECG shows prolonged waves and prolonged R-R interval (Fig. 96.4).

Conditions when Sinus Bradycardia Occurs

Sinus bradycardia occurs in both physiological and pathological conditions. It occurs during sleep. It is common in athletes due to the cardiovascular reflexes, in response to increased force of contraction of heart.

Physiological conditions when sinus bradycardia occurs

1. Sleep
2. Athletic heart.

Pathological conditions when sinus bradycardia occurs

1. Disease of SA node
2. Hypothermia
3. Hypothyroidism
4. Heart attack
5. Congenital heart disease
6. Degenerative process of aging
7. Obstructive jaundice
8. Increased intracranial pressure
9. Use of certain drugs like beta blockers, channel blockers, digitalis and other **antiarrhythmic drugs**
10. Atherosclerosis. Bradycardia due to **atherosclerosis** of carotid artery, at the region of carotid sinus is called **carotid sinus syndrome.**

Features of Sinus Bradycardia

1. Sick sinus syndrome
2. Fatigue
3. Weakness
4. Shortness of breath
5. Lack of concentration
6. Difficulty in exercising.

Sick sinus syndrome

Sick sinus syndrome is the common feature of sinus bradycardia. It is the condition characterized by dizziness and unconsciousness.

■ ECTOPIC ARRHYTHMIA

Ectopic arrhythmia is the abnormal heartbeat, in which one of the structures of heart other than SA node becomes the pacemaker. Impulses produced by these structures are called **ectopic foci.**

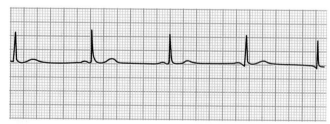

FIGURE 96.4: ECG in sinus bradycardia. Normal P-QRS-T. R-R interval is prolonged. Heart rate is less than 60/min. (*Courtesy:* Dr Atul Ruthra).

Subtypes of Ectopic Arrhythmia

Ectopic arrhythmia is further divided into two subtypes:

1. Homotopic arrhythmia, in which the impulses for heartbeat arise from any part of conductive system
2. Heterotopic arrhythmia, in which the impulses arise from the musculature of heart other than conductive system.

Different Ectopic Arrhythmia

1. Heart block
2. Extrasystole
3. Paroxysmal tachycardia
4. Atrial flutter
5. Atrial fibrillation
6. Ventricular fibrillation.

■ HEART BLOCK

Heart block is the blockage of impulses generated by SA node in the conductive system. Because of the blockage, the impulses cannot reach the cardiac musculature, resulting in ectopic arrhythmia. Based on the area affected, the heart block is classified into two types (Fig. 96.5):

1. Sinoatrial block
2. Atrioventricular block.

Sinoatrial Block – AV Nodal Rhythm

Sinoatrial block is the failure of impulse transmission from SA node to AV node. It is also called **sinus block.** During sinoatrial block, heart stops beating. Immediately, AV node takes over the pacemaker function and produces the impulses. This leads to AV nodal (atrioventricular) rhythm.

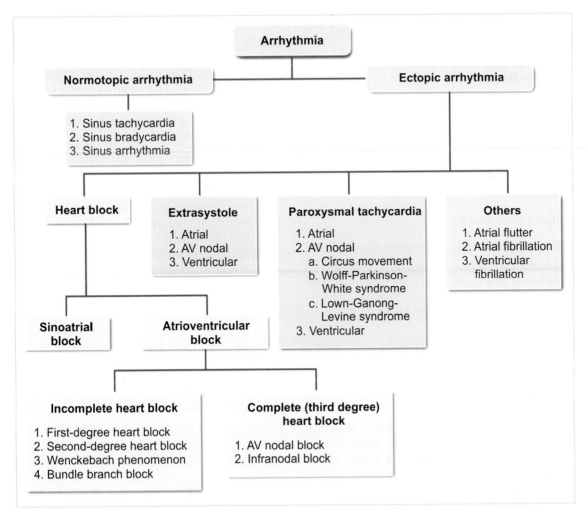

FIGURE 96.5: Classification of arrhythmia. AV = Atrioventricular.

Sinoatrial block is due to the defect in internodal fibers and it occurs suddenly. Initially, the heart stops for a while. Then after few seconds, the AV node becomes the pacemaker and the heart starts beating with decreased rate of 40 to 60/minute.

Impulses may be discharged from any part of AV node, viz.

1. In upper nodal rhythm, the impulses are discharged from the upper part of AV node. In this rhythm, the P wave of ECG is inverted. QRS complex and T wave are normal

2. In middle nodal rhythm, the impulses are by the middle part of AV node. Here, all the chambers of the heart contract simultaneously. P wave of ECG is absent as it merges with QRS complex

3. In lower nodal rhythm, the impulses are produced by the lower part of AV node. In this condition, ventricular contraction occurs prior to atrial contraction as the impulses reach the ventricles prior to the atria. In ECG, QRS complex appears prior to P wave and R-P interval is obtained instead of P-R interval. It is called **reversed heart block.**

Atrioventricular Block

Atrioventricular block is the heart block in which the impulses are not transmitted from atria (from AV node) to ventricles because of defective conductive system.

Atrioventricular block is of two categories:

1. Incomplete heart block
2. Complete heart block.

1. Incomplete Heart Block

Incomplete heart block is the condition in which the transmission of impulses from atria to ventricles is slowed down and not blocked completely. Impulses reach ventricles late.

Incomplete heart block is of four types:

i. First degree heart block
ii. Second degree heart block
iii. Wenckebach phenomenon
iv. Bundle branch block.

i. First degree heart block

First degree heart block is the heart block in which the conduction of impulses through AV node is very slow, i.e. the AV nodal delay is longer. It is also called **delayed conduction.** In ECG, the P-R interval is very much prolonged and is more than 0.2 second.

First degree heart block is common in young adults and trained athletes. It is also caused by rheumatic fever and some drugs. It does not produce any symptom.

ii. Second degree heart block

Second degree heart block is the type of heart block in which some of the impulses produced by SA node fail to reach the ventricles. It is also called the **partial heart block.** When some of the impulses from SA node fail to reach the ventricles, one ventricular contraction occurs for every 2, 3 or 4 atrial contractions, i.e. 2 : 1, 3 : 1 or 4 : 1. In ECG, the ventricular complex (QRST) is missing accordingly.

During frequent development of second degree heart block, bradycardia occurs.

iii. Wenckebach phenomenon or syndrome

Wenckebach phenomenon is a type of heart block characterized by progressive increase in AV nodal delay, resulting in missing of one beat. Afterwards, the conduction of impulse is normal or slightly delayed. In ECG, the progressive lengthening of P-R interval is noticed till QRST complex disappears.

iv. Bundle branch block

Bundle branch block (BBB) is the heart block that occurs during dysfunction of right or left branch of bundle of His. During this type of block, the impulse from atria reaches unaffected ventricle first. Then, from here, the impulse travels to the affected side. So, ECG shows normal ventricular rate, but the QRS complex is prolonged or deformed.

2. Complete Heart Block (Third degree heart block)

Complete heart block is the condition in which the impulses produced by SA node cannot reach the ventricles. It is also called **complete atrioventricular block** or third degree heart block. Because of this, the ventricles beat in their own rhythm, independent of atrial beat. It is called **idioventricular rhythm.**

Complete heart block occurs due to any one of the following causes:

i. Disease of AV node, which leads to AV nodal block
ii. Defective conductive system below the level of AV node, causing infranodal block.

i. AV nodal block

In this type of block, a part of AV node is defective and the unaffected part becomes the pacemaker. Rhythmicity of AV node is about 45 to 60/minute.

ii. Infranodal block

Infranodal block is the heart block in which the impulses from SA node are blocked in the branches of bundle of His (below the level of AV node). In this condition, the distal part of the conductive system (i.e. the Purkinje fibers) becomes the pacemaker. The rhythmicity of Purkinje fibers is about 35/minute. Sometimes, a part of ventricular musculature becomes the pacemaker and the ventricular rate in such conditions is about 20/minute.

Third degree heart block is the serious one since it decreases the pumping action of the heart. Very often, it results in Stokes-Adams syndrome. It may also cause heart failure.

Stokes-Adams syndrome

Stokes-Adams syndrome is the sudden attack of dizziness and unconsciousness caused by heart block. It may be accompanied by convulsions also. In many patients suffering from heart block, the complete heart block occurs intermittently. When the block occurs, the ventricles stop beating immediately. **Ectopic pacemaker** (AV node, Purkinje fiber or ventricular muscle) starts functioning only after 5 to 30 seconds.

During this time, the blood circulation is affected because of lack of ventricular output. Brain cannot withstand the stoppage of blood supply and oxygen supply even for 5 seconds. Before the onset of discharge from ectopic pacemaker, dizziness and fainting occurs. If the discharge of impulses from ectopic pacemaker is delayed beyond 30 seconds, death occurs.

■ EXTRASYSTOLE

Extrasystole and Compensatory Pause

Extrasystole is the premature contraction of the heart before its normal contraction. It is caused by an ectopic focus (discharge of an impulse from any part of the heart other than the SA node). The ectopic focus produces an extra beat of the heart that is always followed by a compensatory pause. Compensatory pause is the period during which the heart stops in relaxed state.

Cause for the compensatory pause

In the cardiac muscle, absolute refractory period extends throughout contraction period. When the heart is in extrasystole (because of ectopic focus), an impulse is discharged from natural pacemaker, SA node. As this natural impulse reaches the myocardium during the contraction period of extrasystole, the myocardium does not give response, because it is refractory now. For the next beat, the heart has to wait till the discharge of next natural impulse from SA node. During this time, the heart stops in diastole. It is the cause for compensatory pause (Chapter 90).

Parts of the heart which give origin for ectopic foci are AV node, bundle of His, atrial musculature and ventricular musculature.

Accordingly, extrasystole is divided into three types:
1. Atrial extrasystole
2. Nodal extrasystole
3. Ventricular extrasystole.

1. *Atrial Extrasystole*

Atrial extrasystole is the premature contraction produced by a stimulus arising from atrial muscle. In this condition, an extra P wave appears immediately after the regular T wave. P wave is small and shapeless. The P-R interval of this beat is short.

2. *Nodal Extrasystole*

Nodal extrasystole is caused by stimulus arising from AV node. P wave is merged with QRS complex and all the chambers of the heart contract together.

3. *Ventricular Extrasystole*

Ventricular extrasystole is the extrasystole that is caused by stimulus from ventricular muscle. In this condition, an extra QRS complex follows the regular T wave. This QRS complex is prolonged as the impulse is conducted through ventricular muscle and not through the conductive system. This QRS complex also has a high voltage. T wave of this beat is inverted.

Conditions when Extrasystole Occurs

Extrasystole is associated with organic diseases of the heart. Particularly, any ischemic area of ventricular musculature can produce an ectopic focus.

Other conditions which produce extrasystole:
  i. Emotions
  ii. Severe exhaustion
  iii. Excessive ingestion of coffee or alcohol
  iv. Excessive smoking
  v. Hyperthyroidism
  vi. Reflexes elicited from abnormal viscera.

■ PAROXYSMAL TACHYCARDIA

Paroxysmal tachycardia is the sudden attack of increased heart rate due to ectopic foci arising from atria, AV node or ventricle. It is also called **Bouveret-Hoffmann syndrome.**

Increase in heart rate due to ectopic foci arising from either atria or AV node is called **supraventricular** tachycardia (SVT). It differs from ventricular tachycardia, which does not depend upon atria or AV node. The attack lasts for a period of few seconds to few hours. It also stops suddenly. After the attack, heart functions normally. Symptoms include palpitations, chest pain, rapid breathing and dizziness.

Paroxysmal tachycardia is of three types:

1. Atrial paroxysmal tachycardia
2. AV nodal paroxysmal tachycardia
3. Ventricular paroxysmal tachycardia.

1. *Atrial Paroxysmal Tachycardia*

Atrial paroxysmal tachycardia is the sudden increase in heart rate caused by ectopic impulses discharged from atrial musculature. Heart rate is 150 to 220/minute. P wave in ECG is inverted, with normal QRST.

2. *AV Nodal Paroxysmal Tachycardia – Bundle of Kent*

AV nodal paroxysmal tachycardia is the sudden increase in heart rate caused by ectopic foci arising from AV node due to a temporary block in the conductive system. It also involves circus movement. This type of tachycardia is very common in some healthy persons who have got an additional conductive system. This system is formed by some abnormal junctional tissues constituting a structure called bundle of Kent. Bundle of Kent connects the atria and ventricles directly, so the conduction is very rapid than through the regular conductive system.

Circus movement – Re-entry and atrial echo beat

Circus movement is defined as circuitous propagation of impulses around a structural or functional obstruction, resulting in re-entry of the impulse and **re-excitation** of heart. When there is a sudden and temporary block in normal conductive system, the impulses from SA node reach the ventricle through bundle of Kent. By this time, the blockage in normal conductive system disappears. Now, the impulse, which passes through bundle of Kent, after exciting the ventricular muscle, travels in the opposite direction through the normal conductive system and finally, it re-enters the AV node. Re-entered impulse activates the AV node and depolarizes the atria, resulting in atrial contraction. It is called **atrial echo beat.**

Re-entered nodal impulse simultaneously spreads to ventricle through normal conductive system, completing the circus movement. This circus movement is repeated producing tachycardia called AV nodal paroxysmal tachycardia. ECG shows normal QRST complex. But P wave is mostly absent.

Wolff-Parkinson-White syndrome

Wolff-Parkinson-White syndrome is the condition characterized by repeated attacks of AV nodal paroxysmal tachycardia in persons with bundle of Kent. ECG shows short P-R interval with normal QRS complex and T wave.

Lown-Ganong-Levin syndrome

Lown-Ganong-Levin syndrome is another condition characterized by AV nodal paroxysmal tachycardia. This occurs in persons who have got another type of abnormal conductive fibers like bundle of Kent. These fibers also connect atria and distal part of conductive system directly bypassing the AV node. So the impulse from SA node reaches ventricle through the abnormal conductive fibers. After exciting the ventricular muscle, the impulse travels in opposite direction through normal conductive system and finally, it re-enters the AV node. The re-entered impulse activates the AV node causing atrial contraction. ECG shows short P-R interval with normal QRS complex and T wave.

3. *Ventricular Paroxysmal Tachycardia*

Ventricular paroxysmal tachycardia is the sudden increase in heart rate caused by ectopic foci arising from ventricular musculature. Sometimes, a part of ventricular muscle, particularly an ischemic area is excited abnormally, followed by a series of extrasystole. This condition is dangerous as the circus movement is developed within ventricular muscle. This circus movement leads to ventricular fibrillation, which is fatal.

■ ATRIAL FLUTTER

Atrial flutter is an arrhythmia characterized by rapid ineffective atrial contractions, caused by ectopic foci originating from atrial musculature. It is often associated with atrial paroxysmal tachycardia. Both the atria beat rapidly like the wings of a bird, hence the name atrial flutter.

Atrial rate is about 250 to 350/minute. Maximum number of impulses conducted by AV node is about 230 to 240 /minute. So, during atrial flutter, the second degree of heart block occurs. The ratio between atrial beats and ventricular beats is 2 : 1 or sometimes 3 : 1.

Atrial flutter is common in patients suffering from cardiovascular diseases such as hypertension and coronary artery disease. Initially, it is marked by palpitations that are unnoticed. However, prolonged atrial flutter may lead to atrial fibrillation or heart failure.

■ ATRIAL FIBRILLATION

Atrial fibrillation is the type of arrhythmia characterized by rapid and irregular atrial contractions at the rate of 300 to 400 beats/minute. It is mostly due to circus movement of impulses within atrial musculature. P wave is absent in ECG.

Atrial fibrillation is common in old people and patients with heart diseases. Though it is not life-threatening, it may cause complications. If it continues for long time, it may cause blood clot and blockage of blood flow to vital organs.

■ VENTRICULAR FIBRILLATION

Ventricular fibrillation is the dangerous cardiac arrhythmia, characterized by rapid and irregular twitching of ventricles. Ventricles beat very rapidly and irregularly due to the circus movement of impulses within ventricular muscle. The rate reaches 400 to 500/minute. This is triggered by ventricular extrasystole. This type of arrhythmia is serious as it leads to death, since the ventricles cannot pump blood.

Ventricular fibrillation is very common during electric shock and during ischemia of conductive system. It also occurs in other conditions like coronary occlusion, chloroform anesthesia, cyclopropane anesthesia, trauma of heart and disturbances of heart (due to improper handling) during cardiac surgery.

■ ABNORMAL PACEMAKER

Abnormal pacemaker is the part of the heart other than SA node that becomes the pacemaker and discharges ectopic foci. Various types of arrhythmia develop when an abnormal pacemaker is activated. These arrhythmias are already described in this Chapter.

Common abnormal pacemakers:
1. Atrioventricular node
2. Atrial musculature
3. Ventricular musculature.

1. AV Node as Pacemaker

When AV node becomes the pacemaker, the following arrhythmias occur:
  i. AV nodal rhythm
  ii. AV nodal extrasystole
  iii. AV nodal paroxysmal tachycardia.

2. Atrial Musculature as Pacemaker

Following arrhythmias occur if atrial musculature becomes the pacemaker:
  i. Atrial extrasystole
  ii. Atrial paroxysmal tachycardia

  iii. Wolff-Parkinson-White syndrome
  iv. Lown-Ganong-Levine syndrome
  v. Atrial flutter
  vi. Atrial fibrillation.

3. Ventricular Musculature as Pacemaker

If ventricular muscle becomes the pacemaker, following arrhythmias are developed:
  i. Ventricular extrasystole
  ii. Ventricular paroxysmal tachycardia
  iii. Ventricular fibrillation.

■ ARTIFICIAL PACEMAKER

Artificial pacemaker is a small **electronic device** that is surgically implanted to regulate abnormal heartbeat. It contains a battery powered **pulse generator,** that produces electrical impulses capable of stimulating the heart. This pacemaker is implanted under the skin over the chest of the patient. Pulses generated by this device are transmitted to the heart through electrodes. Electrodes connected to the device are inserted and passed through a vein and positioned in the heart chambers. The device has a **lithium battery** that may last for 10 to 15 years. The outer casing of the pacemaker is usually made of titanium, which is rarely rejected by body's immune system.

Pulse generator of the pacemaker has multiple functions. It is programmed to cope up with the needs of the individual patient.

■ CURRENT OF INJURY

Current of injury means flow of current from an injured region of heart to the unaffected part. When ischemia occurs in any part of the ventricular musculature due to coronary occlusion, that part of ventricle becomes depolarized either partially or completely and the repolarization does not occur. It causes flow of current from affected (depolarized) part to unaffected part of the ventricular muscle.

Current of injury in myocardial infarction affects the ECG pattern and cardiac vector. In ECG, the J point and ST segments are displaced (Chapter 94). Deviation of cardiac axis is also common during the current of injury.

Cardiac Axis

In the infarction of anterior wall of the ventricle, the cardiac axis (vector) is deviated to right up to +150° due to current of injury and in the posterior wall infarction, there is left axis deviation up to −95°.

Effect of Changes in Electrolyte Concentration on Heart

■ INTRODUCTION

Distribution of electrolytes in extracellular fluid and intracellular fluid is responsible for the electrical activity of the tissues including myocardium. Thus, any change in the concentration of any electrolyte will definitely alter the electrical activity of cardiac muscle.

■ EFFECT OF CHANGES IN SODIUM ION CONCENTRATION

Normal sodium ion concentration in blood is 135 to 145 mEq/L. Change in concentration of sodium ion does not alter the electrical activity of heart severely. Only the low level of sodium ion in body fluids reduces the electrical activity of cardiac muscle and electrocardiogram (ECG) shows low-voltage waves.

Changes in the concentration of potassium and calcium ions have significant effects on heart.

■ EFFECT OF CHANGES IN POTASSIUM ION CONCENTRATION

Normal potassium ion concentration in blood is about 3.5 to 5 mEq/L. Changes in ECG appear when the potassium level increases to 6 mEq/L (hyperkalemia) or when it decreases to 2 mEq/L (hypokalemia).

■ EFFECT OF HYPERKALEMIA

Hyperkalemia decreases:
1. Resting membrane potential, leading to hyper-polarization
2. Excitability of the muscle.

Effects of hyperkalemia on the excitability of cardiac muscle, depend upon the severity of hyperkalemia.

Changes in ECG When Potassium Level Increases to 6 or 7 mEq/L

T wave is tall and tented. P-R interval and QRS complex are normal.

Changes in ECG When Potassium Level Increases to 8 mEq/L

P-R interval and the duration of QRS complex are prolonged because, hyperkalemia decreases the rate of conduction. P wave may be small.

Changes in ECG When Potassium Level Increases beyond 9 mEq/L

Severe hyperkalemia makes the atrial muscle unexcitable. So, P wave is absent in ECG. QRS complex merges with T wave. This condition is fatal because, it leads to ventricular fibrillation or stoppage of heart in diastole, due to the lack of excitability.

■ EFFECT OF HYPOKALEMIA

Hypokalemia decreases the sensitivity of heart muscle.

Changes in ECG When Potassium Level Falls to 2 mEq/L

1. S-T segment is depressed
2. T wave is small, flat or inverted
3. U wave appears. Sometimes, the U wave merges with T wave. Because of this, the Q-T interval is mistaken for being prolonged.

Changes in ECG When Potassium Level Falls below 2 mEq/L

1. Depression of S-T segment below the isoelectric baseline
2. Inversion of T wave
3. Appearance of prominent U wave
4. Prolongation of P-R interval.

■ EFFECT OF CHANGES IN CALCIUM ION CONCENTRATION

Normal concentration of calcium ion in blood is 9 to 11 mg/dL (4.5 to 5.5 mEq/L). Mostly, hypocalcemia affects the heart, rather than hypercalcemia.

■ EFFECT OF HYPERCALCEMIA

Hypercalcemia is the elevation in blood calcium level. It increases the excitability and contractility of the heart muscle. In clinical conditions, the effect of hypercalcemia is very rare.

Changes in ECG

1. Shortening of duration of S-T segment
2. Shortening of QT interval
3. Appearance of U wave.

Calcium Rigor

Stoppage of the heart in systole, due to hypercalcemia is called the calcium rigor. It can be demonstrated in experimental animals by infusing large quantity of calcium. Calcium rigor is a reversible phenomenon and the heart starts functioning normally, when the calcium ions are washed.

■ EFFECT OF HYPOCALCEMIA

Hypocalcemia is the reduction in blood calcium level. It reduces the excitability of the cardiac muscle.

Changes in ECG

1. Prolongation of S-T segment
2. Prolongation of Q-T interval
3. Appearance of a prominent U wave.

■ EXPERIMENTAL EVIDENCES

Effects of ions on heart are demonstrated experimentally by perfusion of heart from animals such as frog and rabbit.

Cardiac Output

Chapter 98

■ INTRODUCTION

Cardiac output is the amount of blood pumped from each ventricle. Usually, it refers to left ventricular output through aorta. Cardiac output is the most important factor in cardiovascular system, because rate of blood flow through different parts of the body depends upon cardiac output.

■ DEFINITIONS AND NORMAL VALUES

Usually, cardiac output is expressed in three ways:

1. Stroke volume
2. Minute volume
3. Cardiac index.

However, in routine clinical practice, cardiac output refers to minute volume.

■ STROKE VOLUME

Stroke volume is the amount of blood pumped out by each ventricle during each beat.

Normal value: 70 mL (60 to 80 mL) when the heart rate is normal (72/minute).

■ MINUTE VOLUME

Minute volume is the amount of blood pumped out by each ventricle in one minute. It is the product of stroke volume and heart rate:

Minute volume = Stroke volume × Heart rate

Normal value: 5 L/ventricle/minute.

■ CARDIAC INDEX

Cardiac index is the minute volume expressed in relation to square meter of body surface area. It is defined as the amount of blood pumped out per ventricle/minute/ square meter of the body surface area.

Normal value: 2.8 ± 0.3 L/square meter of body surface area/minute (in an adult with average body surface area of 1.734 square meter and normal minute volume of 5 L/minute).

■ EJECTION FRACTION

Ejection fraction is the fraction of end diastolic volume that is ejected out by each ventricle. Normal ejection fraction is 60% to 65%. Refer Chapter 91 for details.

■ CARDIAC RESERVE

Cardiac reserve is the maximum amount of blood that can be pumped out by heart above the normal value. Cardiac reserve plays an important role in increasing the cardiac output during the conditions like exercise. It is essential to withstand the stress of exercise.

Cardiac reserve is usually expressed in percentage. In a normal young healthy adult, the cardiac reserve is 300% to 400%. In old age, it is about 200% to 250%. It increases to 500% to 600% in athletes. In cardiac diseases, the cardiac reserve is minimum or nil.

■ VARIATIONS IN CARDIAC OUTPUT

■ PHYSIOLOGICAL VARIATIONS

1. *Age:* In children, cardiac output is less because of less blood volume. Cardiac index is more than that in adults because of less body surface area.
2. *Sex:* In females, cardiac output is less than in males because of less blood volume. Cardiac index is more than in males, because of less body surface area.
3. *Body build:* Greater the body build, more is the cardiac output.
4. *Diurnal variation:* Cardiac output is low in early morning and increases in day time. It depends upon the basal conditions of the individuals.
5. *Environmental temperature:* Moderate change in temperature does not affect cardiac output. Increase in temperature above 30°C raises cardiac output.
6. *Emotional conditions:* Anxiety, apprehension and excitement increases cardiac output about 50% to 100% through the release of catecholamines, which increase the heart rate and force of contraction.
7. *After meals:* During the first one hour after taking meals, cardiac output increases.
8. *Exercise:* Cardiac output increases during exercise because of increase in heart rate and force of contraction.
9. *High altitude:* In high altitude, the cardiac output increases because of increase in secretion of adrenaline. Adrenaline secretion is stimulated by hypoxia (lack of oxygen).
10. *Posture:* While changing from recumbent to upright position, the cardiac output decreases.
11. *Pregnancy:* During the later months of pregnancy, cardiac output increases by 40%.
12. *Sleep:* Cardiac output is slightly decreased or it is unaltered during sleep.

■ PATHOLOGICAL VARIATIONS

Increase in Cardiac Output

Cardiac output increases in the following conditions:
1. *Fever:* Due to increased oxidative processes
2. *Anemia:* Due to hypoxia
3. *Hyperthyroidism:* Due to increased basal metabolic rate.

Decrease in Cardiac Output

Cardiac output decreases in the following conditions:
1. *Hypothyroidism:* Due to decreased basal metabolic rate
2. *Atrial fibrillation:* Because of incomplete filling of ventricles
3. *Incomplete heart block with coronary sclerosis or myocardial degeneration:* Due to defective pumping action of the heart
4. *Congestive cardiac failure:* Because of weak contractions of heart
5. *Shock:* Due to poor pumping and circulation
6. *Hemorrhage:* Because of decreased blood volume.

■ DISTRIBUTION OF CARDIAC OUTPUT

The whole amount of blood pumped out by the right ventricle goes to lungs. But, the blood pumped by the left ventricle is distributed to different parts of the body.

Fraction of cardiac output distributed to a particular region or organ depends upon the metabolic activities of that region or organ.

Distribution of Blood Pumped out of Left Ventricle

Distribution of blood pumped out of left ventricle to different organs and the percentage of cardiac output are given in Table. 98.1. Heart, which pumps the blood to all other organs, receives the least amount of blood. Liver receives maximum amount of blood.

■ FACTORS MAINTAINING CARDIAC OUTPUT

Cardiac output is maintained (determined) by four factors:
1. Venous return
2. Force of contraction
3. Heart rate
4. Peripheral resistance.

■ 1. VENOUS RETURN

Venous return is the amount of blood which is returned to heart from different parts of the body. When it increases, the ventricular filling and cardiac output are increased. Thus, cardiac output is **directly proportional** to venous return, provided the other factors (force of contraction, heart rate and peripheral resistance) remain constant.

Venous return in turn, depends upon five factors:
- i. Respiratory pump
- ii. Muscle pump
- iii. Gravity
- iv. Venous pressure
- v. Sympathetic tone.

i. Respiratory Pump

Respiratory pump is the respiratory activity that helps the return of blood, to heart during inspiration. It is also called **abdominothoracic pump.** During inspiration,

TABLE 98.1: Distribution of blood pumped out of left ventricle

Organ	Amount of blood (mL/ minute)	Percentage
Liver	1,500	30
Kidney	1,300	26
Skeletal muscles	900	18
Brain	800	16
Skin, bone and GI tract	300	6
Heart	200	4
Total	5,000	100

thoracic cavity expands and makes the intrathoracic pressure more negative. It increases the diameter of inferior vena cava, resulting in increased venous return. At the same time, descent of diaphragm increases the intra-abdominal pressure, which compresses abdominal veins and pushes the blood upward towards the heart and thereby the venous return is increased (Fig. 98.1).

Respiratory pump is much stronger in forced respiration and in severe muscular exercise.

ii. Muscle Pump

Muscle pump is the muscular activity that helps in return of the blood to heart. During muscular activities, the veins are compressed or squeezed. Due to the presence of valves in veins, during compression the blood is moved towards the heart (Fig. 98.2). When muscular activity increases, the venous return is more.

When the skeletal muscles contract, the vein located in between the muscles is compressed. Valve of the vein

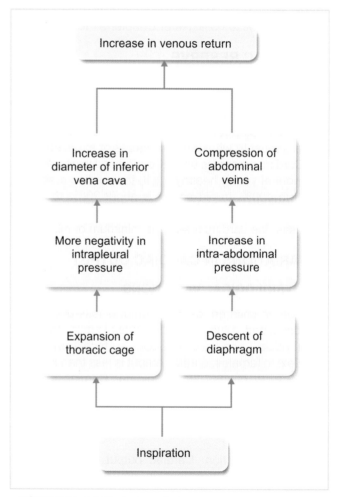

FIGURE 98.1: Effect of respiratory pump on venous return

proximal to the contracting muscles (Fig. 98.2 A) is opened and the blood is propelled towards the heart. Valve of the vein distal to the muscles is closed by the back flow of blood.

During relaxation of the muscles (Fig. 98.2 B), the valve proximal to muscles closes and prevents the back flow of blood. The valve distal to the muscles opens and allows the blood to flow upwards.

iii. Gravity

Gravitational force reduces the venous return. When a person stands for a long period, gravity causes pooling of blood in the legs, which is called **venous pooling.** Because of venous pooling, the amount of blood returning to heart decreases.

iv. Venous Pressure

Venous pressure also affects the venous return. Pressure in the venules is 12 to 18 mm Hg. In the smaller and larger veins, the pressure gradually decreases. In the great veins, i.e. inferior vena cava and superior vena cava, the pressure falls to about 5.5 mm Hg. At the junction of venae cavae and right atrium, it is about 4.6 mm Hg. Pressure in the right atrium is still low and it alters during cardiac action. It falls to zero during atrial diastole. This pressure gradient at every part of venous tree helps as a driving force for venous return.

v. Sympathetic Tone

Venous return is aided by sympathetic or vasomotor tone (Chapter 103), which causes constriction of venules. Venoconstriction pushes the blood towards heart.

■ 2. FORCE OF CONTRACTION

Cardiac output is **directly proportional** to the force of contraction, provided the other three factors remain constant. According to **Frank-Starling law,** force of contraction of heart is directly proportional to the initial length of muscle fibers, before the onset of contraction.

Force of contraction depends upon preload and afterload.

Preload

Preload is the stretching of the cardiac muscle fibers at the end of diastole, just before contraction. It is due to increase in ventricular pressure caused by filling of blood during diastole. Stretching of muscle fibers increases their length, which increases the force of contraction and cardiac output.

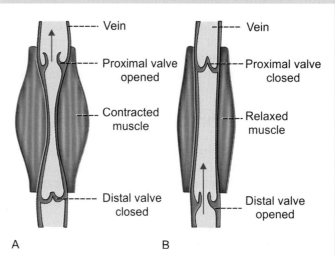

FIGURE 98.2: Mechanism of muscle pump. A. During contraction of the muscle; B. During relaxation of the muscle.

Thus, force of contraction of heart and cardiac output are **directly proportional** to preload.

Afterload

Afterload is the force against which ventricles must contract and eject the blood. Force is determined by the arterial pressure. At the end of isometric contraction period, semilunar valves are opened and blood is ejected into the aorta and pulmonary artery. So, the pressure increases in these two vessels. Now, the ventricles have to work against this pressure for further ejection. Thus, the afterload for left ventricle is determined by aortic pressure and afterload for right ventricular pressure is determined by pressure in pulmonary artery.

Force of contraction of heart and cardiac output are **inversely proportional** to afterload.

■ 3. HEART RATE

Cardiac output is **directly proportional** to heart rate provided, the other three factors remain constant. Moderate change in heart rate does not alter the cardiac output. If there is a marked increase in heart rate, cardiac output is increased.

If there is marked decrease in heart rate, cardiac output is decreased.

■ 4. PERIPHERAL RESISTANCE

Peripheral resistance is the resistance offered to blood flow at the peripheral blood vessels. Peripheral resistance is the resistance or load against which the heart has to pump the blood. So, the cardiac output is **inversely proportional** to peripheral resistance.

Resistance is offered at **arterioles** so, the arterioles are called **resistant vessels.** In the body, maximum peripheral resistance is offered at the **splanchnic region.** Other details of peripheral resistance are given in Chapter 102.

■ MEASUREMENT OF CARDIAC OUTPUT

Cardiac output is measured by direct methods and indirect methods. Direct methods are used only in animals. Indirect methods are used both in animals and human beings.

■ MEASUREMENT OF CARDIAC OUTPUT BY DIRECT METHODS

Direct methods used to measure cardiac output in animals:

1. By using cardiometer
2. By using flowmeter.

1. By Using Cardiometer

This is described in Chapter 91.

2. By Using Flowmeter

Mechanical flowmeter

Mechanical flowmeter is used to measure cardiac output or the amount of blood flow to any organ. It is used only in animals. It has an inlet, a measuring device in the middle and an outlet. Aorta or the artery entering any organ is cut. Inlet and outlet of the flowmeter are inserted into cut ends of the blood vessel. When the blood passes through the flowmeter, the measuring device determines the amount of blood flow (Fig. 99.1).

Electromagnetic flowmeter

Principle: Principle of this flowmeter is to develop an electromagnetic field by means of two coils of wire. If the coils are placed on either side of a blood vessel, the electromagnetic field is produced around the vessel. When blood flows through the vessel, there is an alteration in the electromagnetic field. By using appropriate electrodes, the changes in the magnetic field can be detected. By connecting electrodes to an electronic device, velocity of blood flow is determined on the basis of changes in the magnetic field. From the velocity of blood flow, the volume of blood flow is calculated.

Instrument: An **electromagnetic probe** is devised with the electromagnetic coils and the electrodes. The probe has a cleft and it is fixed in such a way that the intact blood vessel passes through the cleft. The probe almost encircles the blood vessel. The probe is connected to the electronic device to measure the volume of blood flow.

Advantage of this flowmeter is that the blood vessel need not be cut open.

Ultrasonic Doppler flowmeter

Principle: Ultrasound is the sound with very high frequency. It is very much beyond the audible range of human ears. The waves of the **ultrasound** are transmitted through a blood vessel. These sound waves are called **transmitted waves.** While passing through the blood vessels, the sound waves hit against the blood cells, particularly the red blood cells and are reflected back. Frequency of the **reflected waves** is different from that of the transmitted waves. This effect is called the **Doppler effect** (named after the discoverer **Johann Christian Doppler**). Alteration in the frequency of reflected waves depends upon the velocity of blood flowing through the blood vessel. By detecting the differences between frequencies of transmitted and reflected sound waves, the velocity of blood flow and then the volume of blood flow are determined.

Instrument: Ultrasonic device has piezoelectric crystals, which produce the **ultrasonic waves** and act as sensors to receive the reflected waves. This device is connected to an electronic equipment, which detects the difference between the frequencies of transmitted and reflected waves and thereby, determines the velocity of blood flow and the volume of blood flow.

Disadvantages of Direct Methods

i. Direct methods to measure cardiac output can be used only in animals
ii. Blood vessel has to be cut open at the risk of animal's life
iii. While using cardiometer, the size of the cardiometer must be suitable for the size of the heart
iv. While using mechanical flowmeter, diameter of inlet and the outlet of the flowmeter must be equivalent to the diameter of the blood vessel.

■ MEASUREMENT OF CARDIAC OUTPUT BY INDIRECT METHODS

Several methods are available to measure cardiac output. Each method has got its own advantages and disadvantages. Generally, the safe and accurate method is preferred. In view of safety, always non-invasive methods are preferred. The invasive method is also accepted provided, it gives accurate results. In addition to providing measurement of cardiac output, nowadays the methods are expected to provide other hemodynamic data and some useful information about the structure and movements of valves and chambers of the heart.

Invasive and Non-invasive Methods

Invasive method refers to a procedure which involves invasion or penetration of healthy tissues, organs or parts of the body, by means of perforation, puncture, incision, injection or catheterization. Non-invasive method means the procedure that does not involve invasion or penetration of tissues, organs or parts of the body.

Different Indirect Methods

Indirect methods used to measure cardiac output:
1. By using Fick principle
2. Indicator (dye) dilution technique
3. Thermodilution technique
4. Ultrasonic Doppler transducer technique
5. Doppler echocardiography
6. Ballistocardiography.

1. By Using Fick Principle

Adolph Fick described Fick principle in 1870. According to this principle, the amount of a substance taken up by an organ (or by the whole body) or given out in a unit of time is the product of amount of blood flowing through the organ and the arteriovenous difference of the substance across the organ.

$$\text{Amount of substance taken or given} = \text{Amount of blood flow/minute} \times \text{Arteriovenous difference}$$

For example,

Amount of blood flowing through lungs is 5,000 mL/minute
O_2 content in arterial blood = 20 mL/100 mL of blood
O_2 content in venous blood = 15 mL/100 mL of blood

$$\text{Amount of oxygen moved from lungs to blood} = \text{Amount of blood flow/minute} \times \text{Arteriovenous difference of } O_2$$

$$= 5,000 \times \frac{20-15}{100}$$

$$= 5,000 \times \frac{5}{100} = 250$$

Amount of oxygen moved from lungs to blood
= 250 mL/minute

Modification of Fick principle to measure cardiac output

Fick principle is modified to measure the cardiac output or a part of cardiac output (amount of blood to an organ). Thus, cardiac output or the amount of blood flowing through an organ in a given unit of time is determined by the formula:

$$\text{Cardiac output} = \frac{\text{Amount of substance taken or given by the organ/minute}}{\text{Arteriovenous difference of the substance across the organ}}$$

By modifying Fick principle, cardiac output is measured in two ways:
i. By using oxygen consumption
ii. By using carbon dioxide given out.

Measurement of Cardiac Output by Using Oxygen Consumption

Fick principle is used to measure the cardiac output by determining the amount of oxygen consumed in the body in a given period of time and dividing this value by the arteriovenous difference across the lungs.

$$\text{Cardiac output} = \frac{O_2 \text{ consumed (in mL/minute)}}{\text{Arteriovenous } O_2 \text{ difference}}$$

Oxygen consumption: Amount of oxygen consumed is measured by using a **respirometer** or **BMR apparatus (Benedict Roth apparatus).**

Oxygen content in arterial blood: Blood is collected from any artery to determine the oxygen content in arterial blood. Oxygen content is determined by blood gas analysis.

Oxygen content in venous blood: Only mixed venous blood is used to determine the oxygen content of venous blood, since oxygen content is different in different veins. Mixed venous blood is collected from right atrium or pulmonary artery. It is done by introducing a **catheter** through basilar vein of forearm. Oxygen is determined from this blood by **blood gas analysis** (Fig. 98.3).

Calculation

For example, in a subject, the following data are obtained:

O_2 consumed (by lungs) = 250 mL/minute
O_2 content in arterial blood = 20 mL/100 mL of blood
O_2 content in venous blood = 15 mL/100 mL of blood

$$\text{Cardiac output} = \frac{O_2 \text{ consumed (in mL/minute)}}{\text{Arteriovenous } O_2 \text{ difference}}$$

$$= \frac{250}{5/100} = \frac{250 \times 100}{5}$$

$$= 5,000 \text{ mL/minute}$$

5 mL of oxygen is taken by 100 mL of blood while passing through the lungs. Thus, 250 mL of oxygen is taken by 5,000 mL of blood. Since cardiac output is equivalent to the amount of blood passing through pulmonary circulation, the cardiac output = 5 L/minute.

Measurement of Cardiac Output by Using Carbon Dioxide

Cardiac output is also measured by knowing the arteriovenous difference of carbon dioxide and amount of carbon dioxide given out (removed) by lungs (Fig. 98.4). Thus:

$$\text{Cardiac output} = \frac{CO_2 \text{ evolved (in mL/minute)}}{\text{Arteriovenous } CO_2 \text{ difference}}$$

Calculation

For example, in a subject
CO$_2$ removed by lungs   = 200 mL/minute
CO$_2$ content in arterial blood = 56 mL/100 mL of blood
CO$_2$ content in venous blood   = 60 mL/100 mL of blood

$$\text{Cardiac output} = \frac{200}{60 - 56 \text{ mL/100 mL}}$$

$$= \frac{200 \times 100}{4}$$

$$= 5,000 \text{ mL} = 5 \text{ L/minute}$$

Since cardiac output is equal to the amount of blood passing through lungs (pulmonary circulation), the cardiac output = 5 L/minute

Nitrous oxide is also used to measure cardiac output by applying Fick principle.

Advantage of measurement of cardiac output by Fick principle

The results are accurate.

Disadvantage

Fick principle is an invasive method and involves the insertion of catheter through subject vein.

2. Indicator (Dye) Dilution Method

Indicator dilution technique is described in detail in Chapter 6. Marker substance used to measure cardiac output is lithium chloride.

Advantage

The results are accurate.

Disadvantage

Indicator dilution method is an invasive method and involves injection of marker substance.

3. Thermodilution Technique

Cardiac output can also be measured by thermodilution technique or **thermal indicator method.** This method is the modified indicator dilution method. It is the popular method to measure cardiac output.

In this method, a known volume of cold sterile solution is injected into the right atrium via inferior vena

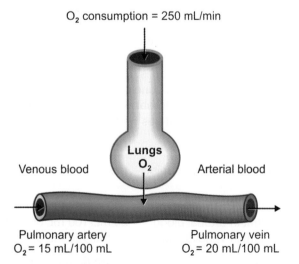

O$_2$ consumption = 250 mL/min

Venous blood   **Lungs O$_2$**   Arterial blood

Pulmonary artery
O$_2$ = 15 mL/100 mL

Pulmonary vein
O$_2$ = 20 mL/100 mL

FIGURE 98.3: Oxygen consumption

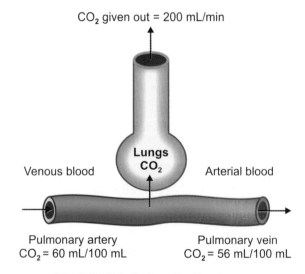

CO$_2$ given out = 200 mL/min

Venous blood   **Lungs CO$_2$**   Arterial blood

Pulmonary artery
CO$_2$ = 60 mL/100 mL

Pulmonary vein
CO$_2$ = 56 mL/100 mL

FIGURE 98.4: Carbon dioxide given out

cava by using a catheter. Cardiac output is measured by determining the resultant change in the blood temperature in pulmonary artery. For this purpose, two **thermistors (temperature transducers)** are used. One of them is placed in the inferior vena cava and the second one is placed in pulmonary artery. A pulmonary artery catheter is used to place the thermistors in their positions.

A known quantity of cold saline or cold dextrose solution is injected into inferior vena cava. Thermistors determine the temperature of blood entering the heart via inferior vena cava and temperature of blood leaving the heart via pulmonary artery. From the values of temperature, cardiac output is measured by applying indicator dilution technique.

Advantages

Results are accurate in this method. Even low cardiac output can be measured. Saline is also harmless. Catheter is also used to determine hemodynamic pressures and to collect mixed venous blood.

Disadvantage

Thermodilution technique is an invasive method and it requires catheterization.

Continuous cardiac output measurement catheter

Cardiac output can be measured continuously by using a modified pulmonary artery catheter called **continuous cardiac output measurement catheter** (CCO catheter). CCO catheter works on thermodilution principle. Instead of injecting cold saline, a heating filament which delivers heat directly to blood is used. The heating filament is fitted to the ventricular portion of the catheter. Cardiac output is measured as done in thermodilution technique. This method is commonly used in intensive care unit (ICU).

4. Esophageal Ultrasonic Doppler Transducer Technique

Esophageal ultrasonic doppler transducer technique involves insertion of a flexible probe into midthoracic part of esophagus. A pulse wave ultrasonic **Doppler transducer** is fixed at the tip of the probe. This transducer calculates the velocity of blood flow in descending aorta (refer ultrasonic Doppler flow meter for details). The diameter of aorta is determined by echocardiography (see below). Cardiac output is calculated by using the values of velocity of blood flow and diameter of aorta.

Advantages

The cardiac output can be measured continuously. This can be used during cardiac surgery.

Disadvantages

Esophageal ultrasonic doppler transducer is an invasive method and results are less accurate.

5. Doppler Echocardiography

Doppler echocardiography is a method for detecting the direction and velocity of moving blood within the heart. This is also a popular method to measure cardiac output.

Echocardiography is a **diagnostic procedure,** which uses the ultrasound waves (more than 20,000 Hz) to produce the image of the heart muscle. Ultrasound waves which reflect or echo off the heart can determine the size, shape, movement of the valves and chambers and the flow of blood through the heart.

During echocardiographic examination, the patient lies bare-chested on the examination table. A special gel is spread over the chest to help the transducer make good contact and slide smoothly over the skin. The transducer is a small hand operated device, which is attached to machine by a flexible cable. The transducer is placed against the chest. The transducer produces and directs ultrasound waves into the chest. Some of the waves get reflected (or echoed) back to the transducer. The reflection of sound waves depends upon the type of tissues and blood. The reflected sound waves are received by the transducer and translated into an image of the heart and displayed on a monitor or recorded on paper or tape.

Echocardiography may also show the abnormalities in functioning of heart valves or damage to the myocardium from an earlier heart attack.

When **Doppler principle** is applied in echocardio-graphy, it enables the determination of direction, rate and other characteristics of blood flow. Doppler echocardiography is based upon the changes in frequency of the reflected sound waves from red blood cells (refer ultrasonic Doppler flow meter for details).

By Doppler echocardiography, the velocity of blood flow through aortic valve is determined. The diameter of the aorta is determined by simple echocardiography. From these values, cardiac output is calculated.

Advantage

Doppler echocardiography is a non-invasive technique. It also provides other useful information about the structures and movements of valves and chambers of heart.

Disadvantage

Doppler echocardiography method provides less accurate results. It requires well trained operator.

6. *Ballistocardiographic Method*

Ballistocardiography is the technique to record the movements of the body caused by **ballistic recoil,** associated with contraction of heart and ejection of blood. It is based on **Newton's third law of motion** (for every action there is an equal and opposite reaction). When heart pumps blood into aorta and pulmonary artery, a recoiling force is exerted against heart and the body. It is similar to that of ballistic recoil when a bullet is fired from a riffle.

Pulsations due to this ballistic recoil can be recorded graphically by making the subject to lie on a suspended bed, movable in the long axis of the body. The cardiac output is determined by analyzing the graph obtained.

Advantage

The only advantage of ballistocardiography is that it is a non-invasive method.

Disadvantage

Ballistocardiography is not a commonly used technique because it involves cumbersome procedures for calibrating the equipment and analyzing the graph. It also does not provide accurate results.

■ CARDIAC CATHETERIZATION

■ DEFINITION

Catheter is a thin radiopaque tube, made up of elastic web, rubber, plastic, glass or metal. Cardiac catheterization is an invasive procedure in which a catheter is inserted **intravascularly** into any chamber of the heart or a blood vessel.

Cardiac catheterization is helpful to study the different variables of hemodynamics, both in normal and diseased states. Cardiac catheterization was discovered by a German medical student Werner Forsmann, who practiced this technique first on himself.

■ CONDITIONS WHEN CARDIAC CATHETERIZATION IS PERFORMED

Cardiac catheterization is generally performed:
1. When clinical assessments indicate rapid deterioration of patient's health and immediate treatment. This is the most common condition when cardiac catheterization is needed.
2. Whenever there is a need to confirm the suspected cardiac disease of a patient
3. Whenever there is need to determine anatomical and physiological status of heart and blood vessels.

■ PROCEDURE

Cardiac catheterization is performed by insertion of catheter into the peripheral blood vessel through skin, by needle puncture. This procedure is called **percutaneous insertion** of catheter.

Left Heart Catheterization

Left heart catheterization is done by passing a catheter through femoral artery, brachial artery or axillary artery. Catheter is guided into left ventricle under fluoroscopic observation via aorta. From left ventricle, the catheter is advanced into left atrium.

In patients with aortic stenosis or **prosthetic** (artificial) **valve,** the direct left ventricular puncture is performed. Under local anesthesia, a needle with a catheter is inserted through the thoracic wall at the level of apex beat. When the needle enters left ventricle, the catheter is advanced through the needle into left ventricle and later the needle is removed.

Latest technology includes catheterization through radial artery, which is called **transradial catheterization.**

Right Heart Catheterization

Right heart catheterization is usually performed by venous puncture via femoral vein. Catheter can also be introduced via internal jugular vein, subclavian vein or medial vein. Under **fluoroscopic observation,** the catheter is advanced into right atrium. From right atrium, it can be guided into right ventricle and also into pulmonary artery.

■ USES OF CARDIAC CATHETERIZATION

Cardiac catheterization is useful for both diagnostic and therapeutic purposes. It gives crucial information about the need for cardiac surgery, coronary angioplasty and other **therapeutic procedures.** It also gives information about anticipated risks and reversibility in the patient's condition during **cardiac surgery** or other **therapeutic interventions.**

Diagnostic Uses of Cardiac Catheterization

1. Blood samples are collected during cardiac catheterization to measure oxygen saturation and the concentration of ischemic metabolites like lactate
2. Cardiac output is measured by using Fick principle, indicator dilution technique or thermodilution technique during cardiac catheterization

3. Angiography is done with the help of catheterization. Angiography or **arteriography** is the diagnostic or **therapeutic radiography (imaging technique),** in which the fluoroscopic picture is used to visualize the blood filled structures like cardiac chambers, arteries and veins of heart and other blood vessels, by using a **radiopaque contrast** medium. It is used to determine the obstruction or occlusion of coronary blood vessels or other blood vessels. It is also used to determine the anomalies of coronary blood vessels.

4. Various pressures are determined by attaching a pressure transducer to the cardiac catheter.

Right heart catheterization is used to measure:
   i. Right atrial pressure
   ii. Right ventricular pressure
   iii. Pulmonary arterial pressure
   iv. Pulmonary capillary wedge pressure.

Left heart catheterization is used to measure:
   i. Aortic pressure
   ii. Left ventricular pressure
   iii. Left atrial pressure.

Therapeutic Uses of Cardiac Catheterization – Interventional Cardiology

Cardiac catheterization is performed for various therapeutic procedures. Interventional cardiology is a branch of cardiology that deals with performance of traditional surgical procedures by cardiac catheterization. It helps in:
1. Thrombolysis
2. Percutaneous transluminal coronary angioplasty
3. Laser coronary angioplasty
4. Catheter ablation.

1. Thrombolysis

Thrombolysis **(reperfusion therapy)** is the procedure used to break up and dissolve a **thrombus** (clot) in the coronary artery of patient affected by acute myocardial infarction due to coronary thrombus. Cardiac catheterization is used for intracoronary administration of **thrombolytic agents** which cause thrombolysis.

Thrombolytic agents:
   i. Tissue plasminogen activator
   ii. Streptokinase
   iii. Urokinase.

All these thrombolytic agents convert plaminogen into plasmin, which degrades fibrin in clot and restore normal blood flow.

2. Percutaneous transluminal coronary angioplasty

Coronary angioplasty means the correction of narrowed or totally obstructed lumen of blood vessels by mechanical methods. In percutaneous transluminal coronary angioplasty (PTCA), a narrowed coronary artery is dilated by inflating a balloon attached to the tip of catheter that is introduced into the blood vessel. Sometimes, a **stent** (expandable wire mesh) is introduced into the corrected blood vessel by the catheter to keep the vessel in dilated state.

3. Laser coronary angioplasty

Catheter is also used to emit laser (Light amplification by stimulated emission of radiation) energy. Laser energy which is emitted into the occluded coronary artery vaporizes the atherosclerotic plaque in the diseased vessel. This technique is called laser coronary angioplasty.

4. Catheter ablation

Catheter ablation is the procedure to destroy (ablate) an area of cardiac tissue that blocks the electrical pathway or produces abnormal electrical impulses, resulting in cardiac arrhythmia such as supraventricular tachycardia (SVT) or Wolff-Parkinson-White syndrome (Chapter 96).

It involves advancing a catheter (with electrodes attached to its tip) towards the heart via either femoral vein or subclavian vein. When the catheter enters right atrium, arrhythmia is induced. Then the electrodes at the tip of catheter record the electrical potentials. By using these recordings, the area of faulty electrical site is pinpointed. This procedure is called **electrical mapping.**

Once the damaged site is confirmed, **radiofrequency energy** is used to destroy the small amount of tissue that disturbs the electrical flow through the heart. Thus, the healthy heart rhythm is restored. Tissue is also destroyed by freezing with intense cold **(cryoablation).**

Heart-lung Preparation

■ INTRODUCTION
■ PROCEDURE
■ USES OF HEART-LUNG PREPARATION

■ INTRODUCTION

Heart-lung preparation is an experimental set up, devised by **Starling.** It is used to demonstrate the effects of various factors on the activities of heart, particularly heart rate and cardiac output. This preparation is also used to record the cardiac function curves.

■ PROCEDURE

Heart-lung preparation is usually done in dogs. After giving **anesthesia,** neck of the dog is opened and a **tracheal cannula** is inserted into the trachea. Tracheal cannula is connected to a **respiratory pump,** so that respiration in the animal is controlled artificially, to avoid any disturbance during the experimental procedure (Fig. 99.1).

Then, chest is opened and an **arterial cannula** is inserted into one of the branches of aorta. All the other branches from arch of aorta and descending aorta are ligated. Arterial cannula is connected to two instruments:

1. **Mercury manometer** to measure the arterial blood pressure
2. **Air bottle,** which provides elasticity artificially (as in the case of arterial wall).

Thus, the blood ejected from left ventricle passes into air bottle through the arterial cannula and rubber tubes. From the air bottle, the blood is diverted through a tube which provides **artificial resistance.** Air bottle is also connected to a **pressure bottle.** Pressure bottle is attached to a pressure pump. This pump is used to maintain the pressure within the set up.

Artificial resistance is offered by applying pressure surrounding the **resistance tube.** Resistance tube is also connected to a manometer.

After passing through the resistance tube, blood is allowed to flow through a **warming glass coil,** which is kept inside a water bath with a heater. Temperature of water bath is controlled, so that the temperature of blood could be maintained.

Warming coil is connected to a **venous reservoir** through a flowmeter, which determines the amount of blood flow (cardiac output). Venous reservoir is connected to superior vena cava by a rubber tube. A screw type clamp is fitted to the rubber tube. This clamp is used to adjust the amount of blood returning to heart (venous return). A **thermometer** is also fitted to the tube to note the temperature of blood.

A third mercury manometer is connected to the inferior vena cava. It is used to determine the venous pressure. A cardiometer is fitted to the ventricle. This cardiometer is connected to a recording device like **Marey tambour** or **polygraph,** to record the ventricular volume changes.

Pulmonary circulation is kept intact for continuous oxygenation of blood.

■ USES OF HEART-LUNG PREPARATION

Thus, in this set up, the heart works as an isolated organ. So, the effects of various factors can be demonstrated on the activities of heart, like heart rate, ventricular volume and cardiac output.

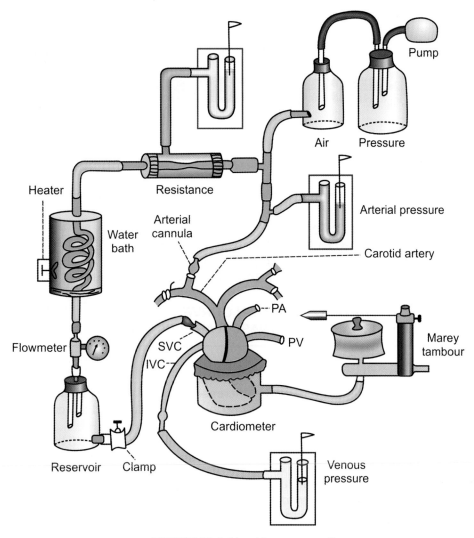

FIGURE 99.1: Heart-lung preparation.
SVC = Superior vena cava, IVC = Inferior vena cava, PA = Pulmonary artery, PV = Pulmonary vein.

Examples

1. When venous return decreases, stroke volume decreases
2. When venous return increases, stroke volume increases
3. When resistance increases, cardiac output decreases
4. When resistance decreases, cardiac output increases
5. Heart-lung preparation is also used to record two types of cardiac function curves:
   i. Cardiac output curves
   ii. Venous return curves.

   Though the cardiac function curves are obtained in experiments using the animals, these curves represent the functions of the ventricles in human heart also (Chapter 100).

Cardiac Function Curves

■ INTRODUCTION

Cardiac function curves are **Frank-Starling curves,** which demonstrate the capacity of ventricles to pump blood and to maintain blood circulation throughout the body. Most of the cardiac function curves are obtained from animal experiments, by using heart-lung preparation. However, these curves are considered to represent the functions of ventricles in human heart.

Cardiac function curves are of two types:
1. Cardiac output curves
2. Venous return curves.

■ CARDIAC OUTPUT CURVES

Cardiac output curves are the curves that show the relationship between cardiac output and right atrial pressure. Right atrial pressure, in turn, depends upon venous return.

■ NORMAL CARDIAC OUTPUT CURVES

Normally, left ventricular output is 5 L/minute, when the pressure in right atrium is 2 mm Hg. When the atrial pressure rises between 4 and 8 mm Hg, the left ventricular output also increases. It increases to about two and a half times of normal (basal) output, i.e. the output increases to about 13 to 14 L/minute. This is the maximum limit for increase in cardiac output. Further

increase in right atrial pressure does not increase the ventricular output and the curve shows a **plateau** (Fig. 100.1).

Right ventricular output is 5 L/minute, when the right atrial pressure is zero. This reaches the maximum, i.e. 13 to 14 L/minute when the atrial pressure increases between 2 and 4 mm Hg (Fig. 100.1).

Thus, the cardiac output curves demonstrate that cardiac output is directly proportional to atrial pressure up to a certain extent (as explained above).

Plateau of the curve shows that the heart can control the output by itself if the atrial pressure rises beyond +8 mm Hg. It is due to the fact that in normal conditions, venous return is decreased when atrial pressure raises above +8 mm Hg.

■ FACTORS AFFECTING CARDIAC OUTPUT CURVES

Shifting of cardiac output curve to left indicates increase in cardiac output and shifting to right indicates decrease in cardiac output. The conditions which shift the cardiac output curve to left or right are discussed below:

Shift to Left

When there is an abnormal increase in the functioning of the heart **(hypereffective heart),** the cardiac output curve is shifted to left, indicating **increase in cardiac output.**

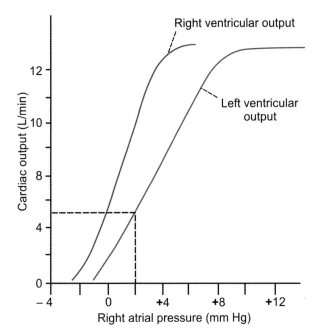

FIGURE 100.1: Normal cardiac output curves

Conditions when shift to left occurs

1. Combined stimulation of sympathetic and the parasympathetic nerves supplying the heart: It causes hyperexcitation of the heart, resulting in increased rate and force of contraction. The cardiac output increases up to 25 L/minute (i.e. the plateau is shifted to left). Increase in output is about twice the maximum output in normal conditions (13 to 14 L/minute).
2. Hypertrophy of heart: It increases cardiac output up to 10 to 19 L/minute. It is because of increase in force of contraction.
3. Excitation (by cardiac nerves) of the heart along with hypertrophy of the ventricles: In this condition, the cardiac output is elevated above 35 L/minute. It occurs in Marathon runners. Increase in cardiac output is an important factor for prolonged running time of Marathon runners.

Shift to Right

When the functioning of heart decreases **(hypoeffective heart),** cardiac output curve is shifted to right, indicating **decrease in cardiac output.**

Conditions when shift to right occurs

1. Stimulation of parasympathetic nerve fibers of the heart
2. Inhibition of sympathetic nerves to heart
3. Myocardial infarction
4. Diseases of the valves in the heart
5. Congenital heart diseases.

■ EFFECT OF EXTRACARDIAC PRESSURE ON CARDIAC OUTPUT CURVE

Extracardiac pressure is the pressure outside the heart. Intrapleural pressure is the major extracardiac pressure. When it increases above the normal level, i.e. from –6 to –2 mm Hg or becomes positive, the venous return decreases, resulting in decrease in cardiac output. Cardiac output curve is shifted to right. It happens in opening of thoracic cage and in positive pressure breathing.

When the intrapleural pressure decreases, i.e. when it becomes more negative, the venous return increases and the cardiac output also increases. The curve is shifted towards left. It is common in **negative pressure breathing.**

Cardiac Tamponade

Cardiac tamponade is the mechanical compression of heart due to accumulation of fluid in **pericardial space.** In addition to intrapleural pressure, accumulation of fluid in pericardial space also increases the extracardiac pressure and compresses the heart. In cardiac tamponade, the cardiac output decreases and output curve is shifted to right.

■ VENOUS RETURN CURVES

Venous return curves are the curves which demonstrate the relationship between venous return (blood flow in vascular system) and right atrial pressure. Venous return curves are also called **systemic vascular function curves.**

Normally, 5 L of blood returns to heart every minute. When right atrial pressure increases, venous return decreases due to **backpressure.** When venous return decreases, the cardiac output also decreases (Fig. 100.2).

■ ANALYSIS OF CARDIAC FUNCTION CURVES

Relation of cardiac output and venous return with right atrial pressure is determined when cardiac output curves and venous return curves are merged together (Fig. 100.3).

■ COUPLING OF CARDIAC AND VASCULAR FUNCTIONS

Cardiac output represents cardiac function and venous return represents vascular function. Coupling or merging of cardiac output (cardiac function) curves and venous return (vascular function) curves shows that when venous return is normal (5 L/minute), the cardiac output as well as the right atrial pressure are normal.

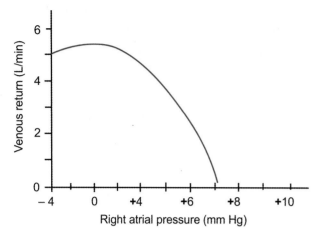

FIGURE 100.2: Venous return curve

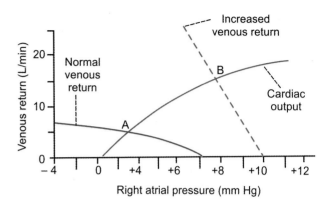

FIGURE 100.3: Analysis of cardiac function curves

Relation between cardiac output and venous return under normal conditions is represented by (A). When the venous return increases (B), the cardiac output also increases along with increase in right atrial pressure. Thus, any factor that alters venous return alters the cardiac output also.

Heart Rate

- ■ **HEART RATE**
  - ■ NORMAL HEART RATE
  - ■ TACHYCARDIA
  - ■ BRADYCARDIA
- ■ **REGULATION OF HEART RATE**
- ■ **VASOMOTOR CENTER – CARDIAC CENTER**
  - ■ VASOCONSTRICTOR AREA
  - ■ VASODILATOR AREA
  - ■ SENSORY AREA
- ■ **MOTOR (EFFERENT) NERVE FIBERS TO HEART**
  - ■ PARASYMPATHETIC NERVE FIBERS
  - ■ SYMPATHETIC NERVE FIBERS
- ■ **SENSORY (AFFERENT) NERVE FIBERS FROM HEART**
- ■ **FACTORS AFFECTING VASOMOTOR CENTER – REGULATION OF VAGAL TONE**
  - ■ IMPULSES FROM HIGHER CENTERS
  - ■ IMPULSES FROM RESPIRATORY CENTERS
  - ■ IMPULSES FROM BARORECEPTORS
  - ■ IMPULSES FROM CHEMORECEPTORS
  - ■ IMPULSES FROM RIGHT ATRIUM
  - ■ IMPULSES FROM OTHER AFFERENT NERVES
  - ■ BEZOLD-JARISCH REFLEX

■ HEART RATE

■ NORMAL HEART RATE

Normal heart rate is 72/minute. It ranges between 60 and 80 per minute.

■ TACHYCARDIA

Tachycardia is the increase in heart rate above 100/minute.

Physiological Conditions when Tachycardia Occurs

1. Childhood
2. Exercise
3. Pregnancy
4. Emotional conditions such as anxiety.

Pathological Conditions when Tachycardia Occurs

1. Fever
2. Anemia
3. Hypoxia
4. Hyperthyroidism
5. Hypersecretion of catecholamines
6. Cardiomyopathy
7. Diseases of heart valves.

■ BRADYCARDIA

Bradycardia is the decrease in heart rate below 60/minute.

Physiological Conditions when Bradycardia Occurs

1. Sleep
2. Athletes.

Pathological Conditions when Bradycardia Occurs

1. Hypothermia
2. Hypothyroidism
3. Heart attack
4. Congenital heart disease
5. Degenerative process of aging
6. Obstructive jaundice
7. Increased intracranial pressure.

Drugs which Induce Bradycardia

1. Beta blockers
2. Channel blockers
3. Digitalis and other antiarrhythmic drugs.

■ REGULATION OF HEART RATE

Heart rate is maintained within normal range constantly. It is subjected for variation during normal physiological conditions such as exercise, emotion, etc. However, under physiological conditions, the altered heart rate is quickly brought back to normal. It is because of the perfectly tuned regulatory mechanism in the body.

Heart rate is regulated by the nervous mechanism, which consists of three components:

A. Vasomotor center
B. Motor (efferent) nerve fibers to the heart
C. Sensory (afferent) nerve fibers from the heart.

■ VASOMOTOR CENTER – CARDIAC CENTER

Vasomotor center is the nervous center that regulates the heart rate. It is the same center in brain, which regulates the blood pressure. It is also called the cardiac center.

Vasomotor center is bilaterally situated in the **reticular formation** of medulla oblongata and lower part of pons.

Areas of Vasomotor Center

Vasomotor center is formed by three areas:
1. Vasoconstrictor area
2. Vasodilator area
3. Sensory area.

■ VASOCONSTRICTOR AREA – CARDIOACCELERATOR CENTER

Situation

Vasoconstrictor area is situated in the reticular formation of medulla in floor of IV ventricle and it forms the lateral portion of vasomotor center. It is otherwise known as **pressor area** or cardioaccelerator center.

Function

Vasoconstrictor area increases the heart rate by sending accelerator impulses to heart, through **sympathetic nerves.** It also causes constriction of blood vessels. Stimulation of this center in animals increases the heart rate and its removal or destruction decreases the heart rate.

Control

Vasoconstrictor area is under the control of **hypothalamus** and **cerebral cortex.**

■ VASODILATOR AREA – CARDIOINHIBITORY CENTER

Situation

Vasodilator area is also situated in the reticular formation of medulla oblongata in the floor of IV ventricle. It forms the medial portion of vasomotor center. It is also called **depressor area** or cardioinhibitory center.

Function

Vasodilator area decreases the heart rate by sending inhibitory impulses to heart through vagus nerve. It also causes dilatation of blood vessels. Stimulation of this area in animals with weak electric stimulus decreases the heart rate and stimulation with a strong stimulus stops the heartbeat. When this area is removed or destroyed, heart rate increases.

Control

Vasodilator area is under the control of **cerebral cortex** and **hypothalamus.** It is also controlled by the impulses from baroreceptors, chemoreceptors and other sensory impulses via afferent nerves.

■ SENSORY AREA

Situation

Sensory area is in the posterior part of vasomotor center, which lies in **nucleus of tractus solitarius** in medulla and pons.

Function

Sensory area receives sensory impulse via glosso-pharyngeal nerve and vagus nerve from periphery, particularly, from the baroreceptors. In turn, this area controls the vasoconstrictor and vasodilator areas.

■ MOTOR (EFFERENT) NERVE FIBERS TO HEART

Heart receives efferent nerves from both the divisions of autonomic nervous system. Parasympathetic fibers arise from the medulla oblongata and pass through vagus nerve. Sympathetic fibers arise from upper thoracic (T1 to T4) segments of spinal cord (Fig. 101.1).

■ PARASYMPATHETIC NERVE FIBERS

Parasympathetic nerve fibers are the cardioinhibitory nerve fibers. These nerve fibers reach the heart through the cardiac branch of vagus nerve.

Origin

Parasympathetic nerve fibers supplying heart arise from the **dorsal nucleus of vagus.** This nucleus is situated in the floor of fourth ventricle in medulla oblongata and is in close contact with vasodilator area.

Distribution

Preganglionic parasympathetic nerve fibers from dorsal nucleus of vagus reach the heart by passing through the main trunk of vagus and **cardiac branch of vagus.** After reaching the heart, preganglionic fibers terminate on postganglionic neurons. Postganglionic fibers from these neurons innervate heart muscle.

Most of the fibers from right vagus terminate in sinoatrial (SA) node. Remaining fibers supply the atrial muscles and atrioventricular (AV) node. Most of the fibers from left vagus supply AV node and some fibers supply the atrial muscle and SA node.

Ventricles do not receive the vagus nerve supply. Few fibers are located in the bases of ventricles, but the functions of these nerve fibers are not known.

Function

Vagus nerve is cardioinhibitory in function and carries inhibitory impulses from vasodilator area to the heart.

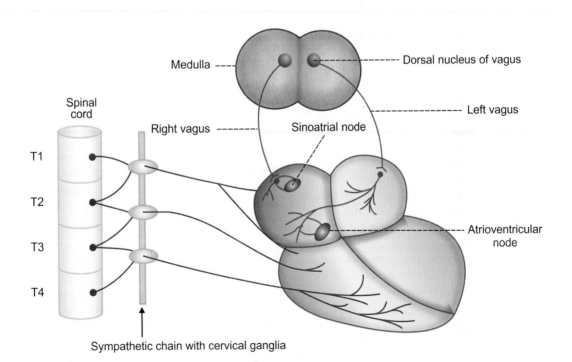

FIGURE 101.1: Nerve supply to heart

Vagal Tone

Vagal tone is the continuous stream of inhibitory impulses from vasodilator area to heart via vagus nerve. Heart rate is kept under control because of vagal tone.

These impulses reach the heart and exert inhibitory effect on heart. Heart rate is inversely proportional to vagal tone. In experimental animals (dog), removal of vagal input (by sectioning vagus) increases the heart rate. This proves the existence of vagal tone. Under resting conditions, vagal tone dominates sympathetic tone (see below).

Impulses from different parts of the body regulate the heart rate through vasomotor center, by altering the vagal tone. Vagal tone is also called **cardioinhibitory tone** or **parasympathetic tone.**

Effect of Stimulation of Vagus Nerve

Effect of stimulation of right vagus nerve – Vagal escape

Right vagus supplies mainly SA node. Stimulation of right vagus in experimental animals such as dog, with a weak stimulus causes reduction in heart rate and force of contraction. Stimulation with strong stimulus causes stoppage of heart due to inhibition of SA node. If the stimulus is continued for some time, the ventricle starts beating; but the rate of contraction is slower than before. This is because of vagal escape.

Vagal escape refers to escape of ventricle from inhibitory effect of vagal stimulation. If stimulation of vagus nerve is stopped, heart starts beating normally (Fig. 101.2).

Cause for vagal escape

Stimulation of right vagus stops the heartbeat due to inhibition of SA node and atria. However, ventricles are not supplied by vagus. So, the ventricles are not inhibited by vagal stimulation. Because of this, when stoppage of heart beat is continued for some time (by vagal stimulation), a part of ventricular musculature becomes pacemaker and starts producing impulses. It results in contraction of ventricles, which is called vagal escape.

Thus, vagal escape includes only ventricular contractions. However, the rhythmicity of ventricular muscle is less and it is about 20/minute.

Effect of stimulation of left vagus nerve – heart block

Left vagus supplies mainly the AV node. Stimulation of left vagus in dog with a weak stimulus causes a slight

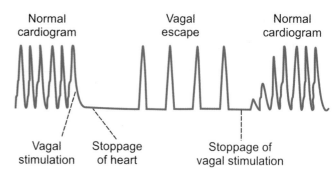

FIGURE 101.2: Effect of vagal stimulation on frog heart

reduction in rate of ventricular contraction. Stimulation of left vagus causes inhibition of AV node. Because of inhibition of AV node, some of the impulses from SA node are not conducted to ventricles. This is called the **partial heart block.** The ratio between atrial contraction and ventricular contraction is 2 : 1, 3 : 1 or 4 : 1, depending upon the strength of stimulus.

Stimulation of left vagus with strong stimulus causes stoppage of ventricular contraction, which is called **complete heart block.** This is because of the complete inhibition of AV node. The prolongation of stimulation causes **idioventricular rhythm,** which is different from the rhythm of atrial contraction.

Mode of Action of Vagus Nerve

Vagus nerve inhibits the heart by secreting the neurotransmitter substance known as **acetylcholine.**

■ SYMPATHETIC NERVE FIBERS

Sympathetic nerve fibers supplying the heart have cardioacceleratory function.

Origin

Preganglionic fibers of the sympathetic nerves to heart arise from lateral gray horns of the first 4 thoracic (T1 to T4) segments of the spinal cord. These segments of the spinal cord receive fibers from vasoconstrictor area of vasomotor center.

Course and Distribution

Preganglionic fibers reach the superior, middle and inferior **cervical sympathetic ganglia** situated in the sympathetic chain. Inferior cervical sympathetic ganglion fuses with first thoracic sympathetic ganglion, forming **stellate ganglion.** From these ganglia, the postganglionic fibers arise.

Postganglionic fibers form three nerves:
1. Superior cervical sympathetic nerve, which innervates larger arteries and base of the heart
2. Middle cervical sympathetic nerve, which supplies the rest of the heart
3. Inferior cervical sympathetic nerve, which serves as **sensory (afferent) nerve** from the heart.

Function

Sympathetic nerves are cardioaccelerators in function and carry cardioaccelerator impulses from vasoconstrictor area to the heart.

Sympathetic Tone

Sympathetic tone or **cardioaccelerator tone** is the continuous stream of impulses produced by the vasoconstrictor area. Impulses pass through sympathetic nerves and accelerate the heart rate.

Under normal conditions, the vagal tone is dominant over sympathetic tone. Whenever vagal tone is reduced or abolished, the sympathetic tone becomes powerful. It is generally believed that the sympathetic tone does not play an important role in the regulation of cardiac function under resting physiological conditions. However, it plays a definite role in increasing the heart rate during emergency conditions.

Rate of contraction of a completely denervated heart of dog is higher than the rate of an innervated heart in resting conditions. This shows that under resting conditions, the vagal tone is **dominant** over sympathetic tone.

Effect of Stimulation of Sympathetic Nerves

Stimulation of sympathetic nerves increases the rate and force of contraction of heart. The effect depends upon the strength of stimulus.

Mode of Action of Sympathetic Nerves

Cardioacceleration by sympathetic stimulation is due to the release of neurotransmitter substance, **noradrenaline.**

■ SENSORY (AFFERENT) NERVE FIBERS FROM HEART

Afferent (sensory) nerve fibers from the heart pass through **inferior cervical sympathetic nerve.** These nerve fibers carry sensations of stretch and pain from the heart to brain via spinal cord.

■ FACTORS AFFECTING VASOMOTOR CENTER – REGULATION OF VAGAL TONE

Vasomotor center regulates the cardiac activity by receiving impulses from different sources in the body. After receiving the impulses from different sources, the vasodilator area alters the vagal tone and modulates the activities of the heart.

Various sources from which the impulses reach the vasomotor center:

■ 1. IMPULSES FROM HIGHER CENTERS

Vasomotor center is mainly controlled by the impulses from higher centers in cerebral cortex and hypothalamus.

Cerebral Cortex

Area 13 in cerebral cortex is concerned with emotional reactions of the body. During emotional conditions, this area sends inhibitory impulses to the vasodilator area. This causes reduction in vagal tone, leading to increase in heart rate.

Hypothalamus

Hypothalamus influences the heart rate via vasomotor center. Stimulation of posterior and lateral hypothalamic nuclei causes **tachycardia.** Stimulation of preoptic and anterior nuclei causes **bradycardia.**

■ 2. IMPULSES FROM RESPIRATORY CENTERS

In forced breathing, heart rate increases during inspiration and decreases during expiration. This variation is called **respiratory sinus arrhythmia.** This is common in some children and in some adults even during quiet breathing.

Sinus arrhythmia is due to the alteration of vagal tone because of impulses arising from respiratory centers during inspiration. These impulses inhibit the vasodilator area, resulting in decreased vagal tone and increased heart rate. During expiration, the respiratory center stops sending impulses to vasodilator center. Now, vagal tone increases, leading to decrease in heart rate.

■ 3. IMPULSES FROM BARORECEPTORS – MAREY REFLEX

Baroreceptors

Baroreceptors are the receptors which give response to change in blood pressure. These receptors are also called **pressoreceptors.**

Situation

Depending upon the situation, baroreceptors are divided into two types:

1. Carotid baroreceptors, situated in carotid sinus, which is present in the wall of internal carotid artery near the bifurcation of common carotid artery.
2. Aortic baroreceptors, situated in the wall of arch of aorta.

Nerve Supply

Carotid baroreceptors are supplied by **Hering nerve,** which is the branch of glossopharyngeal (IX cranial) nerve. Aortic baroreceptors are supplied by **aortic nerve,** which is a branch of vagus (X cranial) nerve (Fig. 101.3).

Nerve fibers from the baroreceptors reach the nucleus of tractus solitarius, which is situated adjacent to vasomotor center in medulla oblongata.

Function – Marey Reflex

Baroreceptors regulate the heart rate through Marey reflex. Stimulus for this reflex is increase in blood pressure.

Marey reflex is a **cardioinhibitory reflex** that decreases heart rate when blood pressure increases. Whenever blood pressure increases, the aortic and carotid baroreceptors are stimulated and stimulatory impulses are sent to nucleus of tractus solitarius via Hering nerve and aortic nerve (afferent nerves). Now, the nucleus of tractus solitarius stimulates vasodilator area, which in turn increases the vagal tone, leading to decrease in heart rate (Fig. 101.4). Marey reflex includes **aortic reflex** and **carotid sinus reflex.**

When pressure is less, the baroreceptors are not stimulated. So, no impulses go to nucleus of tractus solitarius. There are no inhibitory impulses to the heart and heart rate is not decreased. Thus, the heart rate is inversely proportional to blood pressure.

Marey law

According to Marey law, the pulse rate (which represents heart rate) is inversely proportional to blood pressure.

Baroreceptors induce the Marey reflex only during resting conditions. So, in many conditions such as exercise, there is an increase in both blood pressure and heart rate.

■ 4. IMPULSES FROM CHEMORECEPTORS

Chemoreceptors

Chemoreceptors are receptors giving response to change in chemical constituents of blood, particularly oxygen, carbon dioxide and hydrogen ion concentration.

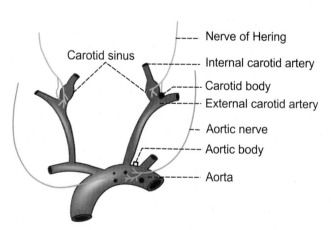

FIGURE 101.3: Nerve supply to baroreceptors and chemoreceptors

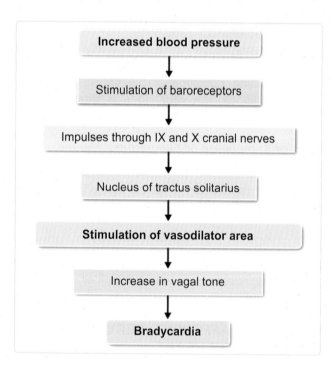

FIGURE 101.4: Marey (cardioinhibitory) reflex

Situation

Peripheral chemoreceptors are situated in the carotid body and aortic body, adjacent to baroreceptors.

Structure

Chemoreceptors are made up of two types of cells, type I or **glomus cells** and type II or **sustentacular cells.** Glomus cells have afferent nerve endings, which are stimulated by hypoxia. Type II cells are **glial cells** and provide support for type I cells.

Nerve Supply

Chemoreceptors in the carotid body are supplied by **Hering nerve,** which is the branch of glossopharyngeal nerve. Chemoreceptors in the aortic body are supplied by **aortic nerve** which is the branch of vagus nerve (Fig. 101.3).

Function

Whenever there is hypoxia, hypercapnea and increased hydrogen ions concentration in the blood, the chemoreceptors are stimulated and inhibitory impulses are sent to vasodilator area. Vagal tone decreases and heart rate increases. Chemoreceptors play a major role in maintaining respiration than the heart rate.

Sinoaortic Mechanism and Buffer Nerves

Sinoaortic mechanism is the mechanism of baroreceptors and chemoreceptors in carotid and aortic regions, that regulates heart rate, blood pressure and respiration. The nerves supplying these receptors are called **buffer nerves.**

■ 5. IMPULSES FROM RIGHT ATRIUM – BAINBRIDGE REFLEX

Bainbridge reflex is a **cardioaccelerator reflex** that increases the heart rate when venous return is increased. Since this reflex arises from right atrium, it is also called **right atrial reflex.**

Increase in venous return causes distention of right atrium and stimulation of **stretch receptors,** situated in the wall of right atrium. Stretch receptors, in turn, send inhibitory impulses through **inferior cervical sympathetic**

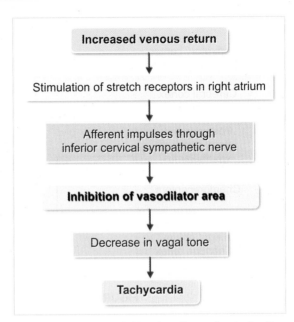

FIGURE 101.5: Bainbridge (cardioaccelerator) reflex

nerve to vasodilator area of vasomotor center. Vasodilator area is inhibited, resulting in decrease in vagal tone and increase in heart rate (Fig. 101.5).

■ 6. IMPULSES FROM OTHER AFFERENT NERVES

Stimulation of sensory nerves produces varying effects.

Examples:

i. Stimulation of receptors in nasal mucous membrane causes **bradycardia.** Impulses from nasal mucous membrane pass via the branches of V cranial nerve and decrease the heart rate.

ii. Most of the painful stimuli cause tachycardia and some cause **bradycardia.** Impulses are transmitted via pain nerve fibers (Fig. 101.6).

■ 7. BEZOLD-JARISCH REFLEX

Bezold-Jarisch reflex is the reflex characterized by bradycardia and hypotension, caused by stimulation of **chemoreceptors** present in the wall of left ventricles by substances such as alkaloids. It is also called **coronary**

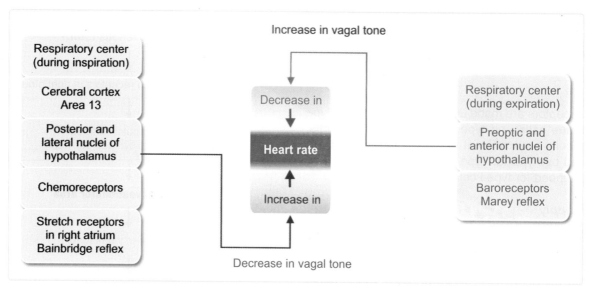

FIGURE 101.6: Factors regulating vagal tone and heart rate

chemoreflex. Vagal fibers form the afferent and efferent pathways of this reflex.

Conditions when Bezold-Jarisch Reflex Occurs

Bezold-Jarisch reflex is a pathological reflex and it does not occur in physiological conditions.

Conditions when this reflex occurs:
1. Myocardial infarction
2. Administration of thrombolytic agents
3. Hemorrhage
4. Aortic stenosis
5. Syncope.

Hemodynamics

■ INTRODUCTION

Dynamics means study of motion. **Hemodynamics** refers to the study of movement of blood through circulatory system.

Major function of cardiovascular system is to pump the blood and to circulate it through different parts of the body. It is essential for the maintenance of pressure and other physical factors within the blood vessels, so that the volume of blood supplied to different parts of the body is adequate. Circulatory system is designed for carrying out all these actions.

■ MEAN VOLUME OF BLOOD FLOW

■ DEFINITION AND FORMULA

Mean volume of blood flow is the volume of blood which flows into the region of circulatory system in a given unit of time. It is the product of mean velocity and the cross-sectional area of the vascular bed.

Q = V × A

Where,

Q = Quantity of blood
V = Velocity of blood flow
A = Cross-sectional area of the blood vessel.

■ IMPORTANCE

In terms of transport of foodstuffs and oxygen to the tissues and waste products away from the tissues, mean volume of blood flow is of greater physiological importance than linear velocity.

■ METHODS OF STUDY

1. By Using Flowmeters

Different types of flowmeters are described in Chapter 98.

2. By Using Plethysmograph

Plethysmograph is an instrument used for measuring the volume of an enclosed organ.

3. By Venous Occlusion Plethysmography

In this, the venous outflow from an organ is stopped by clamping the vein, without disturbing the artery. Blood flow into the organ causes a corresponding increase in its volume for the first few seconds. This increase in volume is recorded graphically. Amount of blood flow is determined by proper calibration of the graph.

4. By Fick Principle

Fick principle is explained in the measurement of cardiac output in Chapter 98.

■ TYPES OF BLOOD FLOW

Blood flow through a blood vessel is of two types:
1. Streamline or laminar flow
2. Turbulent flow.

1. Streamline Flow

Streamline flow is a **silent flow.** Within the blood vessel, a very thin layer of blood is in contact with the vessel wall. It does not move or moves very slowly. Next layer within the vessel has a low momentum. Next layer of blood has a slightly higher momentum. Gradually, the momentum increases in the inner layers, so that the momentum is greatest in the center of the stream. This type of flow is known as streamline flow and it

does not produce any sound within the vessel (Fig. 102.1). Streamline flow occurs only at velocities up to a critical level.

2. Turbulent Flow

Turbulent flow is the **noisy flow.** When the velocity of blood flow increases above critical level, the flow becomes turbulent. Turbulent flow creates sounds.

Reynolds number

Critical velocity at which the flow becomes turbulent is known as Reynolds number.

Formula to determine Reynolds number:

$$N_R = \frac{PDV}{\eta}$$

N_R = Reynolds number
P = Density of the blood
D = Diameter of the vessel
V = Velocity of the flow
η = Viscosity of the blood

■ FACTORS DETERMINING VOLUME OF BLOOD FLOW

Volume of blood flow is determined by five factors:
1. Pressure gradient
2. Resistance to blood flow
3. Viscosity of blood
4. Diameter of blood vessels
5. Velocity of blood flow.

1. Pressure Gradient

Volume of blood flowing through any blood vessel is **directly proportional** to the pressure gradient. Pressure gradient is the pressure difference between the two ends of the blood vessel.

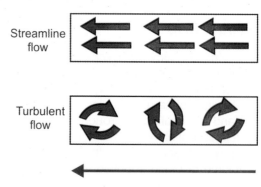

FIGURE 102.1: Streamline flow and turbulent flow

Formula to determine pressure gradient

Pressure gradient = $P_1 - P_2$

Where,

P_1 = Pressure at proximal end of the vessel

P_2 = Pressure at distal end of the vessel.

Maximum pressure gradient exists between the aorta and the inferior vena cava. The pressure in aorta is 120 mm Hg and the pressure in inferior vena cava is 0 mm Hg. So, the pressure gradient is 120 – 0 = 120 mm Hg. Pressure gradient in different areas of vascular bed is given in Table 102.1.

2. Resistance to Blood Flow (Peripheral Resistance)

Volume of blood flow is **inversely proportional** to the resistance. Resistance is the friction, tension or hindrance, against which the blood has to flow. Peripheral resistance means the resistance offered to blood flow in peripheral blood vessels. Though resistance exists in all the blood vessels to some extent, it is remarkable in the peripheral vessels, particularly the arterioles.

Determinants of peripheral resistance

i. Radius of blood vessels
ii. Pressure gradient
iii. Viscosity of blood.

Peripheral resistance is inversely related to radius of the blood vessel, i.e. lesser the radius, more will be the resistance. Radius of the arterioles is very less. It is because the arterioles remain partially constricted all the time due to sympathetic tone. So, the resistance is more. Hence, the **arterioles** are called **resistant vessels.**

Formula to determine resistance

$$\text{Resistance} = \frac{\text{Pressure gradient}}{\text{Volume of blood flow}}$$

$$= \frac{P_1 - P_2}{Q}$$

3. Viscosity of Blood

Volume of blood flow is inversely proportional to the viscosity of blood. Viscosity is the friction of blood against the wall of the blood vessel. Isaac Newton described viscosity as the internal friction or lack of slipperiness. Viscosity influences the blood flow through resistance.

Factors determining viscosity

RBC count is the main factor which determines the viscosity of the blood. Another factor determining viscosity is plasma protein, mainly albumin.

When hemoconcentration occurs as in case of burns or in polycythemia, the viscosity increases and the velocity of blood flow decreases, so the volume of blood reaching the organ is decreased.

4. Diameter of Blood Vessels

Volume of blood flow is directly proportional to the diameter of the blood vessels. When the diameter of a segment of blood vessel is considered, the aorta has the maximum diameter and capillary has got the minimum diameter. But, in circulation, the diameter of the vessel is considered in relation to the cross-sectional area through which the blood flows.

TABLE 102.1: Pressure gradient in different areas of vascular bed

Blood vessels	P_1 (mm Hg)	P_2 (mm Hg)	Pressure gradient (mm Hg)
Between aorta and vena cava	120	0	120
Between two ends of aorta	120	100	20
Between beginning of arteries and end of arterioles	100	30	70
Between arterial and venous ends of capillaries	30	15	15
Between two ends of venules	15	10	5
Between two ends of veins	10	0	10
Between two ends of vena cava	0	– 2	– 2

P_1 = Pressure at proximal end of the blood vessel, P_2 = Pressure at distal end of the blood vessel, Pressure gradient = $P_1 - P_2$.

Cross-sectional area is progressively increased as the arteries ramify and as the distance from the heart is increased. Cross-sectional area of each branch is smaller, but the sum of the cross-sectional areas of all the branches is always greater than that of the parent vessel. In this way, the aorta has got less cross-sectional area of 4 cm², compared to that of capillaries, which is 2,500 cm².

But, the cross-sectional area is subjected to variations under physiological and pathological conditions. Diameter of the aorta depends upon the elasticity of the wall and its recoiling tendency helps in maintaining the flow and pressure. Diameter of the arterioles depends upon the **sympathetic tone.**

5. *Velocity of Blood Flow*

Volume of blood flow is **directly proportional** to the velocity of blood flow. Velocity of blood flow is the rate at which blood flows through a particular region. It is described later in this chapter.

■ HAGEN-POISEUILLE EQUATION

Hagen and Poiseuille have worked on dynamics extensively. Equation which explains the relationship between different variables of dynamics, is named after them. Variables of dynamics are applied to hemodynamics also.

According to Hagen-Poiseuille equation, volume (Q) of any fluid flowing through a rigid tube is:
1. Directly proportional to pressure gradient $(P_1 - P_2)$
2. Directly proportional to the fourth power of radius (r^4)
3. Inversely proportional to the length of the tube (L).

$$\text{Thus, } Q = K\,\frac{(P_1 - P_2) \times r^4}{L}$$

K is the constant for fluid flowing at a temperature. It is directly proportional to temperature of the fluid. Viscosity of the fluid is also affected by the temperature. Viscosity is inversely proportional to temperature of the fluid. Therefore in the equation, the constant 'K' is expressed as the reciprocal of viscosity (η).

$$\text{So, } Q = \frac{(P_1 - P_2) \times r^4}{L \times \eta}$$

Volume of flow of fluid is always expressed in a given unit of time. π/8 is the arithmetic value derived while determining volume of fluid flowing in a given unit of time. So, the equation has to be rewritten as:

$$Q = \frac{(P_1 - P_2) \times r^4}{L \times \eta \times \pi/8}$$

$$= \frac{(P_1 - P_2) \times \pi r^4}{8\,(L \times \eta)}$$

$$\text{Thus, } Q = \frac{(P_1 - P_2)\,\pi r^4}{8\,(L \times \eta)}$$

■ WINDKESSEL EFFECT

Windkessel effect is the recoiling effect of blood vessels that converts the **pulsatile flow** of blood into a **continuous flow.** Blood vessels showing the windkessel effect are known as **windkessel vessels.**

Mean velocity of the blood that flows through the aorta is more than 50 cm/second, but it is not constant. During systole, it increases up to 120 cm/second and during diastole, it becomes almost negative. This variation is noticed even in the larger arteries.

During systole, velocity of blood flow reaches maximum, because of the force created by contraction of the heart. Therefore, the maximum volume of blood is pumped into the aorta. During diastole, this force is absent and the volume of blood entering the aorta is zero. Thus, the flow of blood into the aorta is not continuous. This type of flow is called pulsatile flow.

However, the flow of blood through other blood vessels is continuous. It is because of the behavioral pattern of aorta and to a little extent, the behavioral pattern of larger arteries. During systole, the aorta is completely dilated and during diastole, it recoils. The elastic recoiling of this vessel creates the continuous momentum of blood. So, the pulsatile flow of blood is converted into a continuous flow.

This effect was named as windkessel effect by **Otto Frank,** in 1899. Windkessel is a German word used for an **'elastic reservoir'.**

Thus, the windkessel vessels play an important role in maintaining the continuous flow of blood through the circulatory tree by acting as a **second pump,** the **first pump** being the heart.

■ VELOCITY OF BLOOD FLOW

■ DEFINITION

Velocity of blood flow is the rate at which blood flows through a particular region of the body. It mainly depends upon the diameter or cross-sectional area of blood vessel.

■ MEAN VELOCITY OF BLOOD FLOW IN DIFFERENT VESSELS

Mean velocity (cm/second) of blood flow in different blood vessels:

Large arteries	:	50.00
Small arteries	:	5.00
Arterioles	:	0.50
Capillaries	:	0.05
Venules	:	0.10
Small veins	:	1.00
Large veins	:	2.00

■ METHODS OF STUDY

1. By Using Flowmeters

Flowmeters are described in Chapter 98.

2. By Hemodromography

Hemodromography is a technique by which the velocity of blood is continuously recorded.

■ FACTORS MAINTAINING VELOCITY

Three factors are responsible for the maintenance of the velocity of blood flow:
1. Cardiac output
2. Cross-sectional area of the blood vessel
3. Viscosity of the blood.

1. Cardiac Output

Velocity of blood flow is **directly proportional** to cardiac output. Increase in cardiac output leads to increase in the velocity of blood flow in all parts of the circulation.

2. Cross-sectional Area of Blood Vessels

Velocity of blood flow is **inversely proportional** to the total cross-sectional area of the vascular bed, through which the blood circulates. Cross-sectional area increases progressively as the arteries ramify. Cross-sectional area of each branch is smaller, but the sum of the cross-sectional areas of all the branches is always greater than that of the parent vessel. So, velocity of blood flow is decreased as the distance from the heart is increased.

3. Viscosity of Blood

Velocity of blood flow is **inversely proportional** to the viscosity of blood. If viscosity is more, the velocity of blood flow is reduced (See in Factors maintaining volume of blood flow). It is because of the friction of blood against arterial wall, which is more when viscosity of blood is increased.

■ PHASIC CHANGES IN THE VELOCITY OF BLOOD FLOW

Velocity of blood flow is altered according to the phases of cardiac cycle. Blood flows in the large arteries at a greater speed during systole than during diastole. In common carotid artery, the velocity reaches 50 cm/sec during systole and it is only 30 cm/sec during diastole.

■ CIRCULATION TIME

■ DEFINITION

Circulation time is the time taken by blood to travel through a part or whole of the circulatory system.

If a substance is injected into a vein, the time taken by it to appear in the blood of the same vein or in the corresponding vein on the opposite side shows the total circulation time.

Similarly, if the transit is from vein to the lungs, it shows the circulation time through pulmonary circuit and if it is from vein to capillaries, it shows the time for flow through pulmonary circuit, left heart and arteries to capillaries, i.e. the total circulation time minus the time for venous return.

■ MEASUREMENT OF CIRCULATION TIME

Circulation time is measured by introducing some easily recognized substance into bloodstream and determining the time when the substance appears at a given point **(end point)** in the circulation.

The injected substance must produce some characteristic response at its end point, so that its appearance could be easily recognized. Introduction of the substance into circulation is done by injecting through median cubital vein or directly into the heart.

Substances used for Measuring Circulation Time

1. Histamine: Causes flushing of face due to vasodilatation
2. Dehydrocholine (20%): Gives a bitter taste when it reaches the tongue
3. Ether or acetone: Detectable in breath by smell
4. Sodium cyanide (small dose): Causes hyperpnea when it reaches the carotid artery (by acting on baroreceptors)
5. Dye fluorescein: Identified at the end point by yellow color; it is used for total circulation time
6. Radioactive substances: Detected at various points of the body by using an ionization chamber.

■ TYPICAL CIRCULATION TIMES

1. Arm vein to arm vein (total circulation time): 25 seconds (22 to 28), determined by using dye fluorescein
2. Arm vein to face: 24 seconds, determined by using histamine
3. Arm vein to tongue: 11 seconds (8 to 16), determined by using dehydrocholine
4. Arm vein to lung (pulmonary circulatory time): 6 seconds (4 to 6), determined by using ether or acetone
5. Arm vein to heart (shortest circulation time): 4 seconds, determined by using radioactive substances
6. Arm vein to carotid artery: 14 seconds (12 to 15), determined by using sodium cyanide.

■ TOTAL CIRCULATION TIME AND HEARTBEAT

Number of heartbeat/total circulation time, however, remains the same for human beings and all the animals, i.e. about 30/total circulation time.

■ CONDITIONS ALTERING CIRCULATION TIME

Circulation time is decreased when the velocity of blood flow is increased and the circulation time is more when the velocity is less.

Conditions when Circulation Time is Prolonged (Sluggish Blood Flow)

1. Myxedema: Due to decreased metabolic activity
2. Polycythemia: Due to increased viscosity of blood
3. Cardiac failure: Due to inability of the heart to pump blood.

Conditions when Circulation Time is Shortened (Rapid Blood Flow)

1. Exercise: Due to increased cardiac activity and vasodilatation
2. Adrenaline administration: Due to increased cardiac activity
3. Hyperthyroidism: Due to increased metabolic activity
4. Anemia: Due to decreased blood volume and less viscosity
5. Decrease in peripheral resistance: Due to vasodilatation.

■ LOCAL REGULATION OF BLOOD FLOW – AUTOREGULATION

■ INTRODUCTION

Autoregulation means the regulation of blood flow to an organ by the organ itself. It is defined as the **intrinsic ability** of an organ to regulate a constant blood flow, in spite of changes in the perfusion pressure (arterial pressure – venous pressure).

Normally, a sudden increase or decrease in arterial blood pressure momentarily increases or decreases the blood flow. Local mechanisms start functioning and the blood flow is brought to relatively normal level within few minutes.

Autoregulatory response is independent of neural and hormonal influences. So, it is the **intrinsic capacity** of the organ.

■ ROLE OF PRESSURES IN AUTOREGULATION

Perfusion Pressure and Effective Perfusion Pressure

Generally, the term perfusion pressure refers to balance between the pressure in blood vessels on either side of the organ, i.e. arterial pressure minus venous pressure ($P_A - P_V$) across the organ.

However, the blood flow to any organ or region of the body depends up on the effective perfusion pressure. Effective perfusion pressure is the perfusion pressure divided by resistance in the blood vessels.

Formula to determine effective perfusion pressure

$$EFP = \frac{P_A - P_V}{R}$$

EFP = Effective perfusion pressure
P_A = Arterial pressure
P_V = Venous pressure
R = Resistance

But basically, the major factor that determines the perfusion pressure and effective perfusion pressure is the **mean arterial pressure.** The normal mean arterial blood pressure is about 93 mm Hg. Usually, blood flow through an organ is kept constant when the mean arterial pressure increases up to 170 mm Hg or when it falls till 60 mm Hg (the range varies slightly in different organs). However, beyond this range, the autoregulation fails and the blood flow is altered in relation to rise or fall in pressure.

■ THEORIES OF AUTOREGULATION

Autoregulation is explained by two theories:
1. Myogenic theory
2. Metabolic theory.

1. *Myogenic Theory*

According to this theory, the intrinsic contractile property of the smooth muscle fibers present in the blood vessels is responsible for autoregulation. It is known that the sudden stretching of blood vessels causes contraction of smooth muscle fibers present in the wall of the vessels, particularly small arteries and arterioles. So, when the arterial blood pressure increases suddenly, the stretching of the blood vessels immediately causes vasoconstriction and thereby, the blood flow is controlled.

Stretching of blood vessels due to increased blood pressure increases the flow of calcium ions into the cells from ECF. Calcium influx causes contraction of smooth muscles in the blood vessels, leading to vasoconstriction.

On the other hand, when the blood pressure is less, the stretching of blood vessels is less causing vasodilatation and increase in blood flow.

2. *Metabolic Theory*

According to metabolic theory the normal blood flow is maintained by the metabolic end products. Normally, the flow of blood washes away the metabolic end products. When the blood flow is reduced, there is accumulation of metabolites. These metabolites dilate the blood vessels and bring the blood flow back to normal. Conversely, when blood flow increases, the vasodilator metabolites are washed out of the tissues quickly. It leads to vasoconstriction and the volume of blood flow becomes normal.

Common vasodilators of metabolic origin:
 i. Adenosine
 ii. Carbon dioxide
 iii. Lactate
 iv. Hydrogen.

■ AUTOREGULATION IN SOME VITAL ORGANS

Volume of blood flow is regulated by local mechanisms in almost all the tissues of the body. However, auto-regulation is more effective in some of the **vital organs** like **kidney** (Chapter 51), **heart** (Chapter 108) and **brain** (Chapter 109). Mechanism of autoregulation also varies slightly in these organs.

Arterial Blood Pressure

Chapter 103

- **DEFINITIONS AND NORMAL VALUES**
  - SYSTOLIC BLOOD PRESSURE
  - DIASTOLIC BLOOD PRESSURE
  - PULSE PRESSURE
  - MEAN ARTERIAL PRESSURE
- **VARIATIONS**
  - PHYSIOLOGICAL VARIATIONS
  - PATHOLOGICAL VARIATIONS
- **DETERMINANTS OF ARTERIAL BLOOD PRESSURE**
  - CENTRAL FACTORS
  - PERIPHERAL FACTORS
- **REGULATION OF ARTERIAL BLOOD PRESSURE**
- **NERVOUS MECHANISM**
  - VASOMOTOR CENTER
  - VASOCONSTRICTOR FIBERS
  - VASODILATOR FIBERS
  - MECHANISM OF ACTION OF VASOMOTOR CENTER
- **RENAL MECHANISM**
  - BY REGULATION OF EXTRACELLULAR FLUID VOLUME
  - THROUGH RENIN-ANGIOTENSIN MECHANISM
- **HORMONAL MECHANISM**
  - HORMONES WHICH INCREASE BLOOD PRESSURE
  - HORMONES WHICH DECREASE BLOOD PRESSURE
- **LOCAL MECHANISM**
  - LOCAL VASOCONSTRICTORS
  - LOCAL VASODILATORS
- **MEASUREMENT OF ARTERIAL BLOOD PRESSURE**
  - DIRECT METHOD
  - INDIRECT METHOD
- **APPLIED PHYSIOLOGY**
  - HYPERTENSION
  - HYPOTENSION

■ DEFINITIONS AND NORMAL VALUES

Arterial blood pressure is defined as the lateral pressure exerted by the column of blood on wall of arteries. The pressure is exerted when blood flows through the arteries. Generally, the term 'blood pressure' refers to arterial blood pressure.

Arterial blood pressure is expressed in four different terms:
1. Systolic blood pressure
2. Diastolic blood pressure
3. Pulse pressure
4. Mean arterial blood pressure.

■ SYSTOLIC BLOOD PRESSURE

Systolic blood pressure (systolic pressure) is defined as the **maximum pressure** exerted in the arteries **during systole** of heart.

Normal systolic pressure: 120 mm Hg (110 mm Hg to 140 mm Hg).

■ DIASTOLIC BLOOD PRESSURE

Diastolic blood pressure (diastolic pressure) is defined as the **minimum pressure** exerted in the arteries **during diastole** of heart.

Normal diastolic pressure: 80 mm Hg (60 mm Hg to 80 mm Hg).

■ PULSE PRESSURE

Pulse pressure is the difference between the systolic pressure and diastolic pressure.

Normal pulse pressure: 40 mm Hg (120 – 80 = 40).

■ MEAN ARTERIAL BLOOD PRESSURE

Mean arterial blood pressure is the average pressure existing in the arteries. It is not the arithmetic mean of systolic and diastolic pressures. It is the diastolic pressure plus one third of pulse pressure. To determine the mean pressure, diastolic pressure is considered than the systolic pressure. It is because, the diastolic period of cardiac cycle is longer (0.53 second) than the systolic period (0.27 second).

Normal mean arterial pressure: 93 mm Hg (80 + 13 = 93).

Formula to calculate mean arterial blood pressure:

Mean arterial blood pressure
= Diastolic pressure + 1/3 of pulse pressure

$$= 80 + \frac{40}{3} = 93.3 \text{ mm Hg}$$

■ VARIATIONS

Blood pressure is altered in physiological and pathological conditions. Systolic pressure is subjected for variations easily and quickly and its variation occurs in a wider range. Diastolic pressure is not subjected for easy and quick variations and its variation occurs in a narrow range.

■ PHYSIOLOGICAL VARIATIONS

1. Age

Arterial blood pressure increases as age advances.

Systolic pressure in different age

Newborn	:	70 mm Hg
After 1 month	:	85 mm Hg
After 6 month	:	90 mm Hg
After 1 year	:	95 mm Hg
At puberty	:	120 mm Hg
At 50 years	:	140 mm Hg
At 70 years	:	160 mm Hg
At 80 years	:	180 mm Hg

Diastolic pressure in different age

Newborn	:	40 mm Hg
After 1 month	:	45 mm Hg
After 6 month	:	50 mm Hg
After 1 year	:	55 mm Hg
At puberty	:	80 mm Hg
At 50 years	:	85 mm Hg
At 70 years	:	90 mm Hg
At 80 years	:	95 mm Hg

2. Sex

In females, up to the period of menopause, arterial pressure is 5 mm Hg, less than in males of same age. After menopause, the pressure in females becomes equal to that in males of same age.

3. Body Built

Pressure is more in obese persons than in lean persons.

4. Diurnal Variation

In early morning, the pressure is slightly low. It gradually increases and reaches the maximum at noon. It becomes low in evening.

5. After Meals

Arterial blood pressure is increased for few hours after meals due to increase in cardiac output.

6. During Sleep

Usually, the pressure is reduced up to 15 to 20 mm Hg during deep sleep. However, it increases slightly during sleep associated with dreams.

7. Emotional Conditions

During excitement or anxiety, the blood pressure is increased due to release of adrenaline.

8. After Exercise

After moderate exercise, systolic pressure increases by 20 to 30 mm Hg above the basal level due to increase in rate and force of contraction and stroke volume. Normally, diastolic pressure is not affected by moderate exercise. It is because, the diastolic pressure depends upon peripheral resistance, which is not altered by moderate exercise.

After severe muscular exercise, systolic pressure rises by 40 to 50 mm Hg above the basal level. But, the diastolic pressure reduces because the peripheral resistance decreases in severe muscular exercise. More details are given in Chapter 117.

■ PATHOLOGICAL VARIATIONS

Pathological variations of arterial blood pressure are hypertension and hypotension. Refer applied physiology of this chapter for details.

■ DETERMINANTS OF ARTERIAL BLOOD PRESSURE – FACTORS MAINTAINING ARTERIAL BLOOD PRESSURE

Some factors are necessary to maintain normal blood pressure. These factors are called **local factors**, **mechanical factors** or determinants of blood pressure (Table 103.1).

Types of Local Factors

Local factors are divided into two types:
A. Central factors, which are pertaining to the heart:
  1. Cardiac output
  2. Heart rate
B. Peripheral factors, which are pertaining to blood and blood vessels:
  3. Peripheral resistance

4. Blood volume
5. Venous return
6. Elasticity of blood vessels
7. Velocity of blood flow
8. Diameter of blood vessels
9. Viscosity of blood.

■ CENTRAL FACTORS

1. Cardiac Output

Systolic pressure is **directly proportional** to cardiac output. Whenever the cardiac output increases, the systolic pressure is increased and when cardiac output is less, the systolic pressure is reduced. Cardiac output increases in muscular exercise, emotional conditions, etc. So in these conditions, the systolic pressure is increased. In conditions like myocardial infarction, the cardiac output decreases, resulting in fall in systolic pressure.

2. Heart Rate

Moderate changes in heart rate do not affect arterial blood pressure much. However, marked alteration in the heart rate affects the blood pressure by altering cardiac output (Chapter 98).

■ PERIPHERAL FACTORS

3. Peripheral Resistance

Peripheral resistance is the important factor, which maintains diastolic pressure. Diastolic pressure is **directly proportional** to peripheral resistance. Peripheral resistance is the resistance offered to the blood flow at the periphery. Resistance is offered at arterioles, which are called the resistant vessels. When peripheral resistance increases, diastolic pressure is increased and when peripheral resistance decreases, the diastolic pressure is decreased.

TABLE 103.1: Local factors determining arterial blood pressure

Arterial blood pressure	Factors
Arterial blood pressure is directly proportional to	1. Cardiac output 2. Heart rate 3. Peripheral resistance 4. Blood volume 5. Venous return 6. Velocity of blood flow 7. Viscosity of blood
Arterial blood pressure is inversely proportional to	1. Elasticity of blood vessel 2. Diameter of blood vessel

4. *Blood Volume*

Blood pressure is **directly proportional** to blood volume. Blood volume maintains the blood pressure through the venous return and cardiac output. If the blood volume increases, there is an increase in venous return and cardiac output, resulting in elevation of blood pressure (Fig. 103.1).

5. *Venous Return*

Blood pressure is **directly proportional** to venous return. When venous return increases, there is an increase in ventricular filling and cardiac output, resulting in elevation of arterial blood pressure.

6. *Elasticity of Blood Vessels*

Blood pressure is **inversely proportional** to the elasticity of blood vessels. Due to elastic property, the blood vessels are distensible and are able to maintain the pressure. When the elastic property is lost, the blood vessels become rigid **(arteriosclerosis)** and pressure increases as in old age. Deposition of cholesterol, fatty acids and calcium ions produce rigidity of blood vessels and **atherosclerosis,** leading to increased blood pressure.

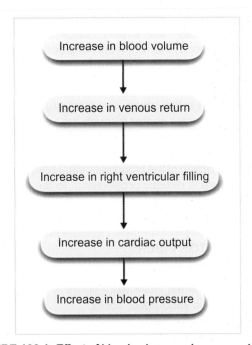

FIGURE 103.1: Effect of blood volume and venous return on arterial blood pressure

7. *Velocity of Blood Flow*

Pressure in a blood vessel is **directly proportional** to the velocity of blood flow. If the velocity of blood flow increases, the resistance is increased. So, the pressure is increased.

8. *Diameter of Blood Vessels*

Arterial blood pressure is **inversely proportional** to the diameter of blood vessel. If the diameter decreases, the peripheral resistance increases, leading to increase in the pressure.

9. *Viscosity of Blood*

Arterial blood pressure is **directly proportional** to the viscosity of blood. When viscosity of blood increases, the frictional resistance is increased and this increases the pressure.

■ REGULATION OF ARTERIAL BLOOD PRESSURE

Arterial blood pressure varies even under physiological conditions. However, immediately it is brought back to normal level because of the presence of well organized regulatory mechanisms in the body. Body has four such regulatory mechanisms to maintain the blood pressure within normal limits (Fig. 103.2):

A. Nervous mechanism or short-term regulatory mechanism
B. Renal mechanism or long-term regulatory mechanism
C. Hormonal mechanism
D. Local mechanism.

■ NERVOUS MECHANISM FOR REGULATION OF BLOOD PRESSURE – SHORT-TERM REGULATION

Nervous regulation is rapid among all the mechanisms involved in the regulation of arterial blood pressure. When the pressure is altered, nervous system brings the pressure back to normal within few minutes. Although nervous mechanism is **quick in action,** it operates only for a short period and then it adapts to the new pressure. Hence, it is called short-term regulation. The nervous mechanism regulating the arterial blood pressure operates through the vasomotor system.

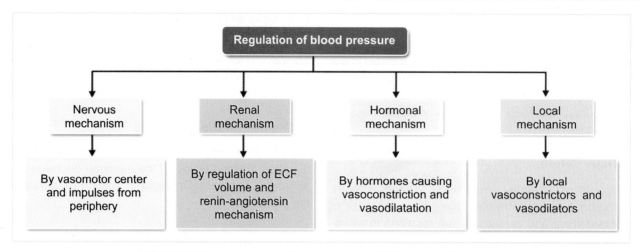

FIGURE 103.2: Regulation of blood pressure. ECF = Extracellular fluid.

Vasomotor System

Vasomotor system includes three components:
1. Vasomotor center
2. Vasoconstrictor fibers
3. Vasodilator fibers.

■ VASOMOTOR CENTER

Vasomotor center is bilaterally situated in the reticular formation of medulla oblongata and the lower part of the pons.
Vasomotor center consists of three areas:
  i. Vasoconstrictor area
  ii. Vasodilator area
  iii. Sensory area.

i. *Vasoconstrictor Area*

Vasoconstrictor area is also called the **pressor area.** It forms the lateral portion of vasomotor center. Vasoconstrictor area sends impulses to blood vessels through sympathetic vasoconstrictor fibers. So, the stimulation of this area causes vasoconstriction and rise in arterial blood pressure. This area is also concerned with acceleration of heart rate (Chapter 101).

ii. *Vasodilator Area*

Vasodilator area is otherwise called **depressor area.** It forms the medial portion of vasomotor center. This area suppresses the vasoconstrictor area and causes vasodilatation. It is also concerned with cardioinhibition (Chapter 101).

iii. *Sensory Area*

Sensory area is in the nucleus of tractus solitarius, which is situated in posterolateral part of medulla and pons. This area receives sensory impulses via glossopharyngeal and vagal nerves from the periphery, particularly from the baroreceptors. Sensory area in turn, controls the vasoconstrictor and vasodilator areas.

■ VASOCONSTRICTOR FIBERS

Vasoconstrictor fibers belong to the sympathetic division of autonomic nervous system. These fibers cause vasoconstriction by the release of neurotransmitter substance, **noradrenaline.** Noradrenaline acts through alpha receptors of smooth muscle fibers in blood vessels.
Vasoconstrictor fibers play major role than the vasodilator fibers in the regulation of blood pressure.

Vasomotor Tone

Vasomotor tone is the continuous discharge of impulses from vasoconstrictor center through the vasoconstrictor fibers. Vasomotor tone plays an important role in regulating the pressure by producing a constant partial state of constriction of the blood vessels. Thus, the arterial blood pressure is directly proportional to the vasomotor tone. Vasomotor tone is also called **sympathetic vasoconstrictor tone** or **sympathetic tone.**

■ VASODILATOR FIBERS

Vasodilator fibers are of three types:
  i. Parasympathetic vasodilator fibers
  ii. Sympathetic vasodilator fibers
  iii. Antidromic vasodilator fibers.

i. *Parasympathetic Vasodilator Fibers*

Parasympathetic vasodilator fibers cause dilatation of blood vessels by releasing **acetylcholine.**

ii. Sympathetic Vasodilator Fibers

Some of the sympathetic fibers cause vasodilatation in certain areas, by secreting **acetylcholine.** Such fibers are called **sympathetic vasodilator** or **sympathetic cholinergic fibers.** Sympathetic cholinergic fibers, which supply the blood vessels of skeletal muscles, are important in increasing the blood flow to muscles by vasodilatation, during conditions like exercise.

Sympathetic cholinergic vasodilator fibers form the important part of vasomotor system. Signals for the vasodilator fibers are generated in cerebral cortex. Signals are relayed through the fibers from cerebral cortex to lateral gray horn of the spinal cord via hypothalamus, midbrain and medulla. In the spinal cord, these impulses activate the preganglionic sympathetic fibers. These fibers in turn, activate the postganglionic fibers. Postganglionic fibers cause dilatation of blood vessels by secreting acetylcholine.

iii. Antidromic Vasodilator Fibers

Normally, the impulses produced by a cutaneous receptor (like pain receptor) pass through sensory nerve fibers. But, some of these impulses pass through the other branches of the axon in the opposite direction and reach the blood vessels supplied by these branches. These impulses now dilate the blood vessels. It is called the **antidromic** or **axon reflex** and the nerve fibers are called antidromic vasodilator fibers (see Fig. 113.1, Chapter 113).

■ MECHANISM OF ACTION OF VASOMOTOR CENTER IN THE REGULATION OF BLOOD PRESSURE

Vasomotor center regulates the arterial blood pressure by causing vasoconstriction or vasodilatation. However, its actions depend upon the impulses it receives from other structures such as baroreceptors, chemoreceptors, higher centers and respiratory centers. Among these structures, baroreceptors and chemoreceptors play a major role in the short-term regulation of blood pressure.

1. Baroreceptor Mechanism

Baroreceptors are the receptors, which give response to change in blood pressure. Baroreceptors are also called **pressoreceptors.**

Situation

Baroreceptors are situated in the **carotid sinus** and wall of the **aorta** (Refer Chapter 101).

Nerve supply

Refer Chapter 101 and Figure 101.3.

Functions

Role of baroreceptors when blood pressure increases

When arterial blood pressure rises rapidly, baroreceptors are activated and send stimulatory impulses to **nucleus of tractus solitarius** through glossopharyngeal and vagus nerves. Now, the nucleus of tractus solitarius acts on both vasoconstrictor area and vasodilator areas of vasomotor center. It inhibits the vasoconstrictor area and excites the vasodilator area.

Inhibition of vasoconstrictor area reduces vasomotor tone. Reduction in vasomotor tone causes vasodilatation, resulting in decreased peripheral resistance. Simultaneous excitation of vasodilator center increases vagal tone (Chapter 101). This decreases the rate and force of contraction of heart, leading to reduction in cardiac output. These two factors, i.e. decreased peripheral resistance and reduced cardiac output bring the arterial blood pressure back to normal level (Fig. 103.3).

Role of baroreceptors when blood pressure decreases

The fall in arterial blood pressure or the occlusion of common carotid arteries decreases the pressure in carotid sinus. This causes inactivation of baroreceptors. Now, there is no inhibition of vasoconstrictor center or excitation of vasodilator center. Therefore, the blood pressure rises.

Information regarding blood pressure within the range of 50 to 200 mm Hg (mean arterial pressure) reaches the vasomotor center through the carotid baroreceptors. Information about the blood pressure range of 100 to 200 mm Hg goes through aortic baroreceptors.

Both carotid and aortic baroreceptors are stimulated by the rising pressure than the steady pressure and their response depends upon the rate of increase in the blood pressure.

Since the baroreceptor mechanism acts against the rise in arterial blood pressure, it is called **pressure buffer mechanism** or system and the nerves from baroreceptors are called the **buffer nerves.**

2. Chemoreceptor Mechanism

Chemoreceptors are the receptors giving response to change in chemical constituents of blood. Peripheral chemoreceptors influence the vasomotor center.

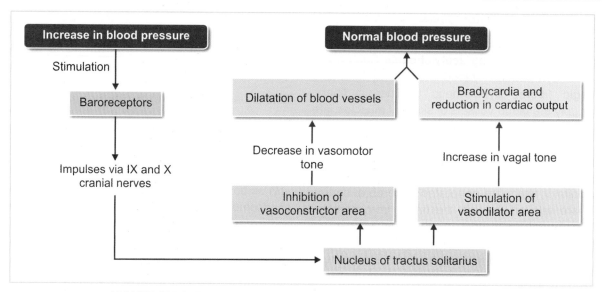

FIGURE 103.3: Regulation of blood pressure by baroreceptor mechanism

Situation

Peripheral chemoreceptors are situated in the carotid body and aortic body (Chapter 101).

Nerve supply

Refer Chapter 101 and Figure 101.3.

Function

Peripheral chemoreceptors are sensitive to lack of oxygen, excess of carbon dioxide and hydrogen ion concentration in blood. Whenever blood pressure decreases, blood flow to chemoreceptors decreases, resulting in decreased oxygen content and excess of carbon dioxide and hydrogen ion. These factors excite the chemoreceptors, which send impulses to stimulate vasoconstrictor center. Blood pressure rises and blood flow increases. Chemoreceptors play a major role in maintaining respiration rather than blood pressure (Chapter 126).

Sinoaortic mechanism

Mechanism of action of baroreceptors and chemoreceptors in carotid and aortic region constitute sinoaortic mechanism. Nerves supplying the baroreceptors and chemoreceptors are called **buffer nerves** because these nerves regulate the heart rate (Chapter 101), blood pressure and respiration (Chapter 126).

3. *Higher Centers*

Vasomotor center is also controlled by the impulses from the two higher centers in the brain.

i. Cerebral cortex

Area 13 in cerebral cortex is concerned with emotional reactions. During emotional conditions, this area sends impulses to vasomotor center. Vasomotor center is activated, the vasomotor tone is increased and the pressure rises.

ii. Hypothalamus

Stimulation of posterior and lateral nuclei of hypo-thalamus causes vasoconstriction and increase in blood pressure. Stimulation of preoptic area causes vasodilatation and decrease in blood pressure. Impulses from hypothalamus are mediated via vasomotor center.

4. *Respiratory Centers*

During the beginning of expiration, arterial blood pressure increases slightly, i.e. by 4 to 6 mm Hg. It decreases during later part of expiration and during inspiration because of two factors:

i. Radiation of impulses from respiratory centers towards vasomotor center at different phases of respiratory cycle

ii. Pressure changes in thoracic cavity, leading to alteration of venous return and cardiac output.

■ RENAL MECHANISM FOR REGULATION OF BLOOD PRESSURE – LONG-TERM REGULATION

Kidneys play an important role in the long-term regulation of arterial blood pressure. When blood pressure alters slowly in several days/months/years, the nervous mechanism adapts to the altered pressure and looses the sensitivity for the changes. It cannot regulate the pressure any more. In such conditions, the renal mechanism operates efficiently to regulate the blood pressure. Therefore, it is called long-term regulation.

Kidneys regulate arterial blood pressure by two ways:

1. By regulation of ECF volume
2. Through renin-angiotensin mechanism.

■ BY REGULATION OF EXTRACELLULAR FLUID VOLUME

When the blood pressure increases, kidneys excrete large amounts of water and salt, particularly sodium, by means of **pressure diuresis** and pressure natriuresis. Pressure diuresis is the excretion of large quantity of water in urine because of increased blood pressure. Even a slight increase in blood pressure doubles the water excretion. Pressure natriuresis is the excretion of large quantity of sodium in urine.

Because of **diuresis** and **natriuresis,** there is a decrease in ECF volume and blood volume, which in turn brings the arterial blood pressure back to normal level.

When blood pressure decreases, the reabsorption of water from renal tubules is increased. This in turn, increases ECF volume, blood volume and cardiac output, resulting in restoration of blood pressure.

■ THROUGH RENIN-ANGIOTENSIN MECHANISM

Source of renin secretion, formation of angiotensin and conditions when renin is secreted are described in Chapter 50.

Actions of Angiotensin II

When blood pressure and ECF volume decrease, renin secretion from kidneys is increased. It converts angiotensinogen into angiotensin I. This is converted into angiotensin II by ACE (angiotensin-converting enzyme).

Angiotensin II acts in two ways to restore the blood pressure:

i. It causes constriction of arterioles in the body so that the peripheral resistance is increased and blood pressure rises. In addition, angiotensin II causes constriction of afferent arterioles in kidneys, so that glomerular filtration reduces. This results in retention of water and salts, increases ECF volume to normal level. This in turn increases the blood pressure to normal level.

ii. Simultaneously, angiotensin II stimulates the adrenal cortex to secrete aldosterone. This hormone increases reabsorption of sodium from renal tubules. Sodium reabsorption is followed by water reabsorption, resulting in increased

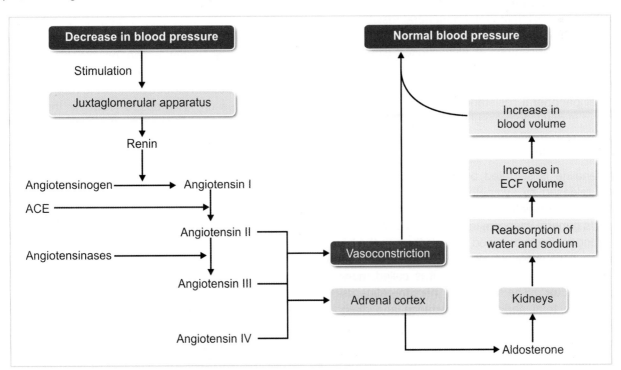

FIGURE 103.4: Regulation of blood pressure by renin-angiotensin mechanism. ACE = Angiotensin-converting enzyme.

ECF volume and blood volume. It increases the blood pressure to normal level (Fig. 103.4).

Actions of Angiotensin III and Angiotensin IV

Like angiotensin II, the angiotensins III and IV also increase the blood pressure and stimulate adrenal cortex to secrete aldosterone (Chapter 50).

■ HORMONAL MECHANISM FOR REGULATION OF BLOOD PRESSURE

Many hormones are involved in the regulation of blood pressure. Hormones, which increase or decrease the arterial blood pressure are listed in Table 103.2.

■ HORMONES WHICH INCREASE BLOOD PRESSURE

Hormones, which increase the arterial blood pressure have different mechanism of action.

1. Adrenaline

Adrenaline is secreted by the adrenal medulla. It is also released by sympathetic postganglionic nerve endings. Adrenaline regulates the blood pressure by acting through heart and blood vessels. It increases systolic pressure by increasing the force of contraction of the heart and cardiac output. It decreases diastolic pressure by reducing the total peripheral resistance.

Adrenaline causes constriction of blood vessels through alpha receptors. It also causes dilatation of blood vessels through β_2-receptors in some areas of the body like skeletal muscle, liver and heart. So, the total peripheral resistance is reduced leading to decrease in diastolic pressure (Chapter 71).

2. Noradrenaline

Noradrenaline is secreted by the adrenal medulla. It is also released by sympathetic postganglionic nerve endings. Noradrenaline increases diastolic pressure due to its general vasoconstrictor effect (Chapter 71). It has stronger effects on blood vessels than on the heart. It causes constriction of all blood vessels throughout the body via alpha receptors. So it is called 'general vasoconstrictor'. The action of noradrenaline is to increase the total peripheral resistance and diastolic pressure.

It also increases the systolic pressure slightly, by increasing the force of contraction of heart.

3. Thyroxine

Thyroxine secreted form thyroid gland increases systolic pressure but decreases the diastolic pressure. It increases the systolic pressure by increasing cardiac output. The cardiac output is increased because of increase in the blood volume and force of contraction of the heart (Chapter 67).

Thyroxine has indirect action on diastolic pressure. Large quantities of metabolites are produced during increased metabolic activity induced by thyroxine. These metabolites cause vasodilatation, leading to decrease in peripheral resistance. It causes decrease in diastolic pressure.

Generally, mean arterial pressure is not altered by the activity of thyroxine. Systolic pressure is increased and the diastolic pressure is decreased. So, only the pulse pressure increases.

4. Aldosterone

Aldosterone is secreted from adrenal cortex. It causes retention of sodium and water and thereby, increases the ECF fluid volume and blood volume, leading to increase in blood pressure. Thus, an increase in the secretion of aldosterone increases the blood pressure by increasing the blood volume (Chapter 70).

5. Vasopressin

Vasopressin or ADH, which is secreted by posterior pituitary has a potent action on the blood vessels, particularly the arteries. It causes constriction of the arteries in all parts of the body. Due to the vasoconstriction, the blood pressure is increased. However, the amount of this hormone required to cause the **vasopressor effect** is very much high than the amount required to cause the **antidiuretic effect** (Chapter 66).

6. Angiotensins

Angiotensin II, III and IV, which are obtained from angiotensinogen cause constriction of systemic arterioles and elevate blood pressure (Chapter 50).

7. Serotonin

Serotonin is otherwise known as **5-hydroxytryptamine.** Serotonin is secreted from many sources (refer Chapter 73 for details). It increases the blood pressure by vasoconstriction.

TABLE 103.2: Hormones involved in regulation of arterial blood pressure

Hormones which increase arterial blood pressure	Hormones which decrease arterial blood pressure
1. Adrenaline*	1. Vasoactive intestinal polypeptide (VIP)
2. Noradrenaline	2. Bradykinin
3. Thyroxine*	3. Prostaglandin
4. Aldosterone	4. Histamine
5. Vasopressin	5. Acetylcholine
6. Angiotensin	6. Atrial natriuretic peptide
7. Serotonin	7. Brain natriuretic peptide
	8. C-type natriuretic peptide

*Adrenaline and thyroxine increase systolic pressure but decrease diastolic pressure.

■ HORMONES WHICH DECREASE BLOOD PRESSURE

Following hormones decrease the arterial blood pressure by causing vasodilatation:

1. *Vasoactive Intestinal Polypeptide*

Vasoactive intestinal polypeptide (VIP) is secreted in the stomach and small intestine. A small amount of this hormone is also secreted in large intestine. VIP is a vasodilator and causes dilatation of peripheral blood vessels and decrease in blood pressure.

2. *Bradykinin*

Bradykinin is produced in blood during the conditions like inflammation. During such conditions, the enzyme in the blood called kallikrein is activated. It acts on α_2-globulin to form kallidin, which is converted into bradykinin (Chapter 73).

Bradykinin is a vasodilator substance and causes reduction in blood pressure.

3. *Prostaglandins*

Prostaglandin PGE_2 is a vasodilator substance. It is secreted from almost all tissues of the body (Chapter 73). It decreases blood pressure.

4. *Histamine*

Histamine is secreted in nerve endings of hypothalamus, limbic cortex and other parts of cerebral cortex. Histamine is also released from tissues during allergic conditions, inflammation or damage (Chapter 73).

Histamine causes vasodilatation and decreases the blood pressure.

5. *Acetylcholine*

Acetylcholine is the cholinergic neurotransmitter released from many sources (Chapter 73). Acetylcholine causes vasodilatation and decreases the blood pressure.

6. *Atrial Natriuretic Peptide*

Atrial natriuretic peptide (ANP) is a hormone secreted by the atrial musculature of heart. It causes dilatation of blood vessels and decreases the blood pressure (Chapter 72).

7. *Brain Natriuretic Peptide*

Brain natriuretic peptide (BNP) is a hormone secreted by the atrial musculature of heart. Like ANP, this hormone also causes dilatation of blood vessels and decreases the blood pressure (Chapter 72).

8. *C-type Natriuretic Peptide*

C-type natriuretic peptide (CNP) is secreted by several tissues including myocardium and vascular endothelium (Chapter 71). CNP decreases blood pressure by vasodilatation.

■ LOCAL MECHANISM FOR REGULATION OF BLOOD PRESSURE

In addition to nervous, renal and hormonal mechanisms, some local substances also regulate the blood pressure. The local substances regulate the blood pressure by vasoconstriction or vasodilatation.

■ LOCAL VASOCONSTRICTORS

Local vasoconstrictor substances are derived from vascular endothelium. These substances are called **endothelium-derived constricting factors** (EDCF). Common EDCF are endothelins (ET), which are peptides with 21 amino acids. Three types of endothelins ET1, ET2 and ET3 are identified so far.

Endothelins are produced by stretching of blood vessels. These peptides act by activating phospholipase, which in turn activates prostacyclin and thromboxane A_2. These two substances cause constriction of blood vessels and increase the blood pressure.

■ LOCAL VASODILATORS

Local vasodilators are of two types:
1. Vasodilators of metabolic origin
2. Vasodilators of endothelial origin.

Vasodilators of Metabolic Origin

Vasodilators of metabolic origin are carbon dioxide, lactate, hydrogen ions and adenosine (Table 103.3).

Vasodilators of Endothelial Origin

Nitric oxide (NO) is an endothelium-derived relaxing factor (EDRF). It is synthesized from arginine. Nitric oxide synthesis is stimulated by acetylcholine, bradykinin, VIP, substance P and platelet breakdown products. As nitric oxide is a vasodilator, deficiency of this leads to constant vasoconstriction and hypertension.

Other functions of nitric oxide are penile erection with vasodilatation and engorgement of corpora cavernosa, activation of macrophages in brain, destruction of cancer cells and relaxation of smooth muscles of gastrointestinal tract.

Types of nitric oxide

   i. NO_3 (nitrate)
  ii. NO^+ (nitrosonium cation)
 iii. NO^- (nitroxyl anion).

■ MEASUREMENT OF ARTERIAL BLOOD PRESSURE

Blood pressure was first measured in horse in 1733, by **Stephen Hales,** with a long tube of about 9 feet length. Later, **Poiseuille** reduced the length of the tube to one foot and used mercury to balance the column of blood.

In 1847, **Ludwig** placed a float on the top of **mercury column** and made continuous recording possible. Introduction of rubber tubing, anesthesia and **manometer** enabled the accurate measurement of blood pressure.

Blood pressure is measured by two methods:

A. Direct method
B. Indirect method.

■ DIRECT METHOD

Direct method to measure arterial blood pressure is employed only in animals. Animal is given suitable anesthesia, then the neck is opened and a tracheal cannula is inserted into the trachea. This tracheal cannula is connected to a respiratory pump, so that the respiration in the animal is controlled artificially to avoid any disturbance during the experimental procedure. A venous cannula is inserted through the femoral vein. It is used to infuse saline to compensate blood loss during experimental procedure.

Carotid artery is cannulated and connected to a **mercury manometer.** By using a **kymograph,** the blood pressure can be recorded continuously in the form of graph. The **cannula** inserted into carotid artery can also be connected to an electronic pressure transducer, which in turn is connected to a recording device like **polygraph** to obtain the recordings.

■ INDIRECT METHOD

Indirect method is used to measure arterial blood pressure in man as well as in animals.

Apparatus

Apparatus used to measure blood pressure in human beings is called **sphygmomanometer.** Along with sphygmomanometer, **stethoscope** is also necessary to measure blood pressure.

Principle

When an external pressure is applied over the artery, the blood flow through it is obstructed. And the pressure required to cause occlusion of blood flow indicates the pressure inside the vessel.

Procedure

Brachial artery is usually chosen because of convenience. The arm cuff of sphygmomanometer is tied around upper arm, above the cubital fossa. Cuff should not be too tight or too loose. It is connected to sphygmomanometer. Now, blood pressure can be measured by three methods.

  1. Palpatory method
  2. Auscultatory method
  3. Oscillatory method.

1. Palpatory method

First, the **radial pulse** is felt. While feeling the pulse, pressure is increased in the cuff by inflating air into it, with the help of a hand pump. While doing this, mercury column in the sphygmomanometer shows the pressure in the cuff.

When pressure is increased in the arm cuff, brachial artery is compressed and blood flow is obstructed. So,

TABLE 103.3: Local substances involved in the regulation of arterial blood pressure

Local vasoconstrictors (Endothelins)	Local vasodilators	
	Metabolic products	Endothelins (ET)
EDCF:		EDRF:
1. ET1	1. Carbon dioxide	1. Nitric oxide
2. ET2	2. Lactate	
3. ET3	3. Hydrogen	
	4. Adenosine	

radial pulse disappears. When radial pulse disappears, the pressure is further increased by about 20 mm Hg. Then, the pressure in the cuff is slowly reduced by releasing the valve of the hand pump, i.e. the cuff is deflated slowly. This is done by feeling the pulse and simultaneously watching the mercury column in the apparatus. Pressure is noted when the pulse reappears. This pressure indicates the systolic pressure.

Disadvantage of palpatory method is that the diastolic pressure cannot be measured.

2. Auscultatory method

Auscultatory method is the most accurate method to determine arterial blood pressure. After determining the systolic pressure in palpatory method, the pressure in the cuff is raised by about 20 mm Hg above that level, so that the brachial artery is occluded due to compression. Now, the chest piece of the stethoscope is placed over the antecubital fossa and the arm cuff is slowly deflated. While doing so, series of sounds are heard through the stethoscope. These sounds are known as **Korotkoff sounds,** named after the discoverer Korotkoff (1905). While reducing the pressure, Korotkoff sounds have five phases:

First phase – appearance of tapping sound

While decreasing the pressure from arm cuff, the occlusion of the artery is relieved and when blood starts flowing through the artery, first sound appears suddenly. In a normal person, it appears, when the pressure is reduced to 120 mm Hg. It is a clear **tapping sound.**

Appearance of tapping sound indicates **systolic pressure.** When the pressure is reduced further by 10 mm Hg from the initial level, this sound slowly becomes louder.

Second phase – appearance of murmuring sound

Following the clear taping sound, a murmuring sound is heard when the pressure is reduced further by about 15 mm Hg.

Third phase – appearance of gong sound

After the murmuring sound, a very clear and louder sound is heard. It is of **gong type.** It is heard while reducing the pressure by another 15 mm Hg.

Fourth phase – appearance of muffled sound

Next to the gong type sound, a mild and muffled sound is heard when the pressure is decreased further by 5 mm Hg.

Fifth phase – disappearance of muffled sound

Muffling sound disappears. **Disappearance** of this sound indicates **diastolic pressure.**

Thus, in auscultatory method, the appearance of clear tapping sound during first phase indicates the systolic pressure and disappearance of the muffling sound in fifth phase shows diastolic pressure.

3. Oscillatory method

When pressure in the arm cuff is increased above the level of systolic pressure, the artery is occluded due to compression. At this stage, the mercury column in the manometer remains static. When the pressure is gradually reduced, some oscillations occur at the top of the mercury column. While deflating the cuff further, the amplitude and duration of oscillations increase suddenly. It denotes systolic pressure. When the cuff pressure is reduced further, the amplitude and duration of oscillations is reduced. It reflects the diastolic pressure.

Because of its inaccuracy, this method is not followed in routine clinical practice. By connecting the manometer to an appropriate recording device, the oscillations of mercury column can be recorded graphically.

Automatic Blood Pressure Instrument

Nowadays automatic blood pressure instrument is widely used. The instrument has a **microprocessor-driven air pump,** which automatically inflates the arm cuff at a fixed pressure value. Then, it records the pressure oscillation pattern during a stepwise deflation. The principle of measuring pressure depends up on the non-linear properties of brachial arterial wall, which induce non-constant oscillations of the cuff pressure during deflation. The sensors in the instrument detect the oscillometric waves and determine the systolic pressure, diastolic pressure, pulse pressure and mean arterial pressure. The instrument determines the pulse rate also.

Automatic instrument does not need expert personnel to measure the blood pressure since it has the self-measuring facilities. However, the accuracy of oscillometric method is still controversial.

Microprocessor controlled blood pressure **monitors** that are fixed around wrist or finger are also available.

■ APPLIED PHYSIOLOGY

Pathological variations of arterial blood pressure:
  A. Hypertension
  B. Hypotension.

■ HYPERTENSION

Definition

Hypertension is defined as the persistent high blood pressure. Clinically, when the systolic pressure remains elevated above 150 mm Hg and diastolic pressure remains elevated above 90 mm Hg, it is considered as hypertension. If there is increase only in systolic pressure, it is called **systolic hypertension.**

Types of Hypertension

Hypertension is divided into two types:
1. Primary hypertension or essential hypertension
2. Secondary hypertension.

1. Primary Hypertension or Essential Hypertension

Primary hypertension is the elevated blood pressure in the absence of any underlying disease. It is also called essential hypertension. Arterial blood pressure is increased because of increased peripheral resistance, which occurs due to some unknown cause.

 Primary hypertension is of two types:
  i. Benign hypertension
  ii. Malignant hypertension.

i. Benign hypertension

Benign hypertension is the high blood pressure that does not cause any problem. It is defined as the essential hypertension that runs a relatively long and symptomless course. In early stages of this condition, there is moderate increase in blood pressure, with systolic pressure of 200 mm Hg and the diastolic pressure of about 100 mm Hg. However, in resting conditions and sleep, the blood pressure returns to normal level. Later, there is a further increase in blood pressure and it does not come back to normal level in resting conditions. Persistent increase in pressure over the years causes development of vascular, cardiac or renal diseases.

ii. Malignant hypertension

Malignant hypertension is a severe form of hypertension with a rapid course leading to progressive cardiac and renal diseases. It is also called **accelerated hypertension.** In this case, the blood pressure is elevated to a great extent. Systolic pressure rises to about 250 mm Hg and diastolic pressure rises to 150 mm Hg. It is always developed due to the combined effects of primary and secondary hypertension. Malignant hypertension cause severe damage of tunica intima of small blood vessels and organs like eye (retina), heart, brain and kidneys. It is a **fatal disease,** since it causes death within few years.

2. Secondary Hypertension

Secondary hypertension is the high blood pressure due to some underlying disorders. The different forms of secondary hypertension are:

i. Cardiovascular hypertension

Cardiovascular hypertension is produced due to the cardiovascular disorders such as:
  a. Atherosclerosis: Hardening of blood vessels due to fat deposition
  b. Coarctation of aorta: Narrowing of aorta.

ii. Endocrine hypertension

Endocrine hypertension is developed because of hyper-activity of some endocrine glands:
  a. Pheochromocytoma: Tumor in adrenal medulla, resulting in excess secretion of catecholamines
  b. Hyperaldosteronism: Excess secretion of aldosterone from adrenal cortex
  c. Cushing syndrome: Excess secretion of glucocorticoids from adrenal cortex.

iii. Renal hypertension

Renal diseases causing hypertension:
  a. Stenosis of renal arteries
  b. Tumor of juxtaglomerular cells, leading to excess production of angiotensin II
  c. Glomerulonephritis.

iv. Neurogenic hypertension

Nervous disorders producing hypertension:
  a. Increased intracranial pressure
  b. Lesion in tractus solitarius
  c. Sectioning of nerve fibers from carotid sinus.

v. Hypertension during pregnancy

Some pregnant women develop hypertension because of **toxemia of pregnancy.** Arterial blood pressure is elevated by the low glomerular filtration rate and retention of sodium and water. It may be because of some autoimmune processes during pregnancy or release of some vasoconstrictor agents from placenta or due to the excessive secretion of hormones causing rise in blood pressure. Hypertension is associated with **convulsions** in **eclampsia** (Chapter 84).

Experimental Hypertension

Hypertension can be produced in experimental animals by various methods. These methods correlate with the causes of hypertension in human beings.

 Experimental hypertension is produced by the following methods:
1. Clamping the renal artery
2. Denervation of baroreceptors in carotid sinus and aortic arch

3. Injections of corticosteroids
4. Infusion of salt with aldosterone.

Goldblatt hypertension

Goldblatt hypertension is one of the experimental hypertension produced in dogs by Goldblatt and it is named after him. He removed one kidney of the dog and clamped the artery of other kidney. It produced slow and steady increase in arterial pressure. The elevation of blood pressure was due to excessive secretion of renin from intact kidney, leading to the formation of a large quantity of angiotensin II. It is known as 'one kidney Goldblatt hypertension'. Hypertension is also developed when the artery of one kidney is clamped without doing anything with the kidney of the other side. It is called 'two kidney Goldblatt hypertension'. It is due to the renin-angiotensin mechanism and retention of salts.

Manifestations of Hypertension

Severe manifestations of primary hypertension:
1. Renal failure
2. Left ventricular failure
3. Myocardial infarction
4. Cerebral hemorrhage
5. Retinal hemorrhage.

Treatment of Hypertension

Secondary hypertension is cured by treating the disease causing hypertension. Primary hypertension can be controlled but cannot be cured.

Following are the **antihypertensive drugs** to control primary hypertension:

1. Beta adrenoceptor blockers

Beta adrenoceptor blockers or **beta antagonists (adrenergic beta blockers** or beta blockers) block the effect of sympathetic nerves on heart and blood vessels by binding with beta adrenoceptors, so that there is reduction in cardiac output and inhibition of vasoconstriction, leading to fall in blood pressure.

2. Alpha adrenoceptor blockers

Alpha adrenoceptor blockers or alpha **antagonists (adrenergic alpha blockers** or alpha blockers) block the effect of sympathetic nerves on blood vessels by binding with alpha adrenoceptors, leading to vasodilatation and fall in blood pressure.

3. Calcium channel blockers

Calcium channel blockers are drugs, which block the calcium channels in myocardium and thereby, reduce

the contractility of myocardium. It causes decrease in cardiac output and fall in blood pressure.

4. Vasodilators

Vasodilator agents reduce blood pressure by vasodilatation.

5. Diuretics

Diuretics cause diuresis and reduce the ECF volume and blood volume. So, blood pressure is decreased.

6. Inhibitors of angiotensin-converting enzyme (ACE inhibitors)

ACE inhibitors reduce the blood pressure by blocking the formation of angiotensin.

7. Depressors of vasomotor center

Depressor drugs act on vasomotor center and reduce the vasomotor tone. So, vasoconstriction is prevented.

8. Angiotensin II receptor blockers

Angiotensin II receptor blockers or antagonists are the antihypertensive drugs that decrease the blood pressure by blocking the effect of angiotensin II (vasoconstriction and secretion of aldosterone).

■ HYPOTENSION

Definition

Hypotension is the low blood pressure. When the systolic pressure is less than 90 mm Hg, it is considered as hypotension.

Types

1. Primary hypotension
2. Secondary hypotension.

1. Primary hypotension

Primary hypotension is the low blood pressure that develops in the absence of any underlying disease and develops due to some unknown cause. It is also called **essential hypotension.** Frequent fatigue and weakness are the common symptoms of this condition. However, the persons with primary hypotension are not easily susceptible to heart or renal disorders.

2. Secondary hypotension

Secondary hypotension is the hypotension that occurs due to some underlying diseases. Diseases, which cause hypotension are:
   i. Myocardial infarction
   ii. Hypoactivity of pituitary gland
   iii. Hypoactivity of adrenal glands

iv. Tuberculosis
v. Nervous disorders.

Orthostatic hypotension

Orthostatic hypotension is the sudden fall in blood pressure while standing for some time. It is due to the effect of gravity. It develops in persons affected by myasthenia gravis or some nervous disorders like tabes dorsalis, syringomyelia and diabetic neuropathy. Common symptom of this condition is **orthostatic syncope.** Syncope is described in detail in Chapter 116.

Venous Pressure

- ■ **DEFINITION AND NORMAL VALUES**
  - ■ **VENOUS PRESSURE IN EXTREMITIES OF THE BODY**
  - ■ **VENOUS PRESSURE IN CENTRAL AND PERIPHERAL VEINS**
- ■ **VARIATIONS OF VENOUS PRESSURE**
  - ■ **PHYSIOLOGICAL VARIATIONS**
  - ■ **PATHOLOGICAL VARIATIONS**
- ■ **MEASUREMENT**
  - ■ **DIRECT METHOD**
  - ■ **INDIRECT METHOD**
- ■ **FACTORS REGULATING VENOUS PRESSURE**
  - ■ **LEFT VENTRICULAR CONTRACTION OR *VIS A TERGO***
  - ■ **RIGHT ATRIAL PRESSURE OR *VIS A FRONTE***
  - ■ **RESISTANCE OR *VIS A LATRE***
  - ■ **VOLUME OF VENOUS BLOOD**
  - ■ **PERIPHERAL RESISTANCE**
  - ■ **GRAVITY AND POSTURE**
- ■ **EFFECT OF RESPIRATION ON VENOUS PRESSURE**
  - ■ **VALSALVA MANEUVER**
  - ■ **MÜELLER MANEUVER**

■ DEFINITION AND NORMAL VALUES

Venous pressure is the pressure exerted by the contained blood in the veins. The pressure in vena cava and right atrium is called **central venous pressure.** The pressure in peripheral veins is called **peripheral venous pressure.**

Pressure is not same in all the veins. It varies in different veins in the extremities of the body and also varies from central veins to peripheral veins.

■ VENOUS PRESSURE IN EXTREMITIES OF THE BODY

Venous pressure is less in the parts of the body above the level of the heart and it is more in parts below the level of the heart. Pressure in:

Jugular vein: 5.1 mm Hg (6.9 cm H_2O)
Dorsal venous arch of foot: 13.2 mm Hg (17.9 cm H_2O).
(1 mm Hg pressure = 1.359 cm H_2O pressure)

■ VENOUS PRESSURE IN CENTRAL AND PERIPHERAL VEINS

Pressure is greater in peripheral veins than in central veins. Pressure in:
Antecubital vein: 7.1 mm Hg (9.6 cm H_2O)
Superior vena cava: 4.6 mm Hg (6.2 cm H_2O).

■ VARIATIONS OF VENOUS PRESSURE

Venous pressure is altered both in physiological and pathological conditions.

■ PHYSIOLOGICAL VARIATIONS

Venous pressure increases in:
1. Changing from standing to supine position
2. Tilting the body
3. Forced expiration (Valsalva maneuver)
4. Contraction of abdominal and limb muscles
5. Effect of gravity during prolonged travelling or standing
6. Excitement.

■ PATHOLOGICAL VARIATIONS

Venous pressure increases in:
1. Low cardiac output
2. Congestive heart failure
3. Venous obstruction
4. Failure of valves in veins
5. Paralysis of muscles
6. Immobilization of parts of body
7. Renal failure.

Venous pressure decreases in:
1. Severe hemorrhage
2. Surgical shock.

■ MEASUREMENT OF VENOUS PRESSURE

■ DIRECT METHOD

Central venous pressure is measured by a catheter introduced through median cubital vein of forearm. Position of tip of the catheter is checked by fluoroscopy. Other end of catheter is connected to a manometer, which measures the pressure. Peripheral venous pressure is measured by using a needle connected to a manometer.

■ INDIRECT METHOD

Measurement of venous pressure is done by using an apparatus designed by Ranger. By this apparatus, collapse of the vein is noticed by the reflection of light through a transparent device. Pressure required to cause the collapse of peripheral vein denotes the pressure in the particular vein.

■ FACTORS REGULATING VENOUS PRESSURE

■ 1. LEFT VENTRICULAR CONTRACTION OR *VIS A TERGO*

Left ventricular contraction is also called *vis a tergo* or force from behind. It forces the blood through the arteries, arterioles, capillaries and veins to the right atrium. Venous pressure is **directly proportional** to left ventricular pressure. By the time blood passes through capillaries and reaches the venules, the pressure becomes less than 8 mm Hg and when it reaches right atrium, the pressure may be less than 1 mm Hg.

■ 2. RIGHT ATRIAL PRESSURE OR *VIS A FRONTE*

Right atrial pressure is also called *vis a fronte* or force from front. It determines the venous return. It is also called central venous pressure, which in turn regulates the peripheral venous pressure. Normal right atrial pressure is 0 mm Hg.

■ 3. RESISTANCE OR *VIS A LATRE*

Resistance offered to blood flow through the veins is also called *vis a latre* or force from side. Venous pressure is **directly proportional** to the resistance, which is due to venous tone and extravascular factors. Because of the thin-walled nature, veins and venules are compressed by the extravascular factors such as:
   i. Compression of arm vein while passing over first rib
   ii. Compression of neck veins in erect posture due to fall in pressure and by atmospheric pressure
   iii. Compression of abdominal veins by increased intra-abdominal pressure
   iv. Compression of veins while passing in between the muscles.

■ 4. VOLUME OF VENOUS BLOOD

Venous pressure is **directly proportional** to the volume of blood in the venous system.

■ 5. PERIPHERAL RESISTANCE

Venous pressure is **inversely proportional** to peripheral resistance. When peripheral resistance is more, arterioles constrict and the veins are filled with less blood. Hence, the pressure decreases. When peripheral resistance is less, the veins are filled with more blood and venous pressure increases.

■ 6. GRAVITY AND POSTURE

Pressure is more in the veins below the level of heart and the pressure is less in veins above the level of heart.

Weight of the column of blood in veins influences the venous pressure. During prolonged standing, the pressure in lower extremities is more (90 cm H_2O). It is

TABLE 104.1: Valsalva maneuver Vs Müeller maneuver

Features	Valsalva maneuver	Müeller maneuver
1. Intrathoracic pressure	Increases up to +50 mm Hg	Decreases up to –70 mm Hg
2. Central vein in thorax	Compressed	Dilated and blood rushes
3. Venous return to right atrium	Decreases	Increases
4. Peripheral venous pressure	Increases to 30 cm H_2O	Decreases to 3 cm H_2O
5. Central venous pressure	Decreases	Increases

because of pooling of blood in the legs due to gravity. It increases the weight of the column of blood, leading to increase in pressure. During the movement, the venous pressure in foot decreases.

In head region, the venous pressure is –10 cm H_2O because of the hydrostatic suction below the skull. So, there is always a negative venous pressure in the head.

■ EFFECT OF RESPIRATION ON VENOUS PRESSURE

During normal quiet breathing, the central venous pressure is altered in accordance with intrathoracic pressure. Thus, during inspiration, the central venous pressure decreases because of decreased intrathoracic pressure. During expiration, it increases because of increased intrathoracic pressure.

The effect of respiration on venous pressure is demonstrated by some procedures which exaggerate these effects on venous pressure. Such procedures are Valsalva maneuver and Mueller maneuver.

■ VALSALVA MANEUVER OR VALSALVA EXPERIMENT

Valsalva maneuver is the forced expiratory effort with closed glottis. It is performed by attempting to exhale forcibly, while keeping the mouth and nose closed.

Effects of Valsalva Maneuver

During this maneuver, the intrathoracic pressure becomes positive and increases greatly. It may reach +50 mm Hg. High intrathoracic pressure produces the following effects (Table 104.1):
1. Compression of central vein in thorax
2. Decrease in venous return to right atrium
3. Increase in peripheral venous pressure to about 30 cm H_2O, due to accumulation of blood in peripheral veins such as veins of neck, face and limbs
4. Decrease in central venous pressure.

Uses of Valsalva Maneuver

1. Valsalva maneuver is used as a diagnostic tool to evaluate the cardiovascular disorders. Best example is the 30 minutes endurance test.
2. Valsalva maneuver is practiced to relieve chest pain
3. It is used to correct the abnormal heart rhythms.

30 seconds endurance test

The subject is asked to blow against sphygmomanometer, in which the pressure is maintained at 40 mm Hg for 30 seconds. Then the changes in heart rate, blood pressure or murmurs are observed to evaluate the cardiovascular disorders.

■ MÜELLER MANEUVER OR MÜELLER EXPERIMENT

Müeller maneuver or experiment is the forced inspiratory effort with closed glottis. It is performed by attempting to inhale forcibly, while keeping the mouth and nose closed. It is also called reverse Valsalva maneuver.

Effects of Müeller Maneuver

During this maneuver, the intrathoracic pressure decreases greatly (becomes more negative). It is about –70 mm Hg. This pressure produces the following effects (Table 104.1):
1. Dilatation of right atrium and central vein because of increase in negative intrathoracic pressure
2. Rapid emptying of blood from peripheral veins into the central veins and increase in venous return to right atrium
3. Decrease in peripheral venous pressure to less than 3 to 4 cm H_2O
4. Increase in central venous pressure.

Uses of Müeller Maneuver

Müeller maneuver is used to evaluate:
1. Upper respiratory tract problems
2. Sleep apnea syndrome.

Capillary Pressure

```
■ INTRODUCTION
■ REGIONAL VARIATIONS
■ MEASUREMENT
■ REGULATION
■ CAPILLARY ONCOTIC PRESSURE
```

■ INTRODUCTION

Definition

Capillary pressure is the pressure exerted by the blood contained in capillary. It is also called **capillary hydrostatic pressure.**

Significance

Capillary pressure is responsible for the exchange of various substances between blood and interstitial fluid through capillary wall.

Normal Values

Generally, the pressure in the arterial end of the capillary is about 30 to 32 mm Hg and in venous end it is 15 mm Hg. However, capillary pressure varies depending upon the function of the organ or region of the body.

■ REGIONAL VARIATIONS

Regional variation in capillary pressure is in relation to the physiological activities of the particular region. So, it has some functional significance. Capillary pressure remarkably varies in kidneys and lungs.

Capillary Pressure in Kidneys

In kidneys, the glomerular capillary pressure is high. It is about 60 mm Hg. This high capillary pressure is responsible for glomerular filtration.

Capillary Pressure in Lungs

In lungs, the pulmonary capillary pressure is low and it is about 7 mm Hg. It favors exchange of gases between blood and alveoli.

■ MEASUREMENT

Direct Method

Capillary pressure was first measured by **EM Landis,** when he was a medical student. Minute vessels in the web of foot in a frog were cannulated by using micropipette, with a diameter of 5 μ at the tip with the aid of microscope. The cannula was connected to a manometer.

This method was later followed to measure capillary pressure in other organs.

Indirect Method

Indirect method is based upon the principle of exerting an external pressure necessary to obstruct the flow of blood in capillaries. The capillaries are observed under microscope.

■ REGULATION

Arterioles play an important role in regulating the capillary pressure and the pressure in capillaries is considered as a function of arteriolar resistance.

When the arterioles constrict, resistance increases in arterioles, which raises the arterial blood pressure. At

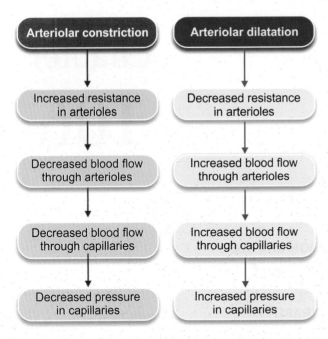

FIGURE 105.1: Regulation of capillary pressure

the same time, the volume of blood flowing into capillaries decreases, leading to fall in capillary pressure.

On the other hand, during dilatation of arterioles, the resistance decreases and arterial blood pressure decreases. But the capillary pressure increases because of increase in volume of blood flowing into capillaries (Fig. 105.1).

■ CAPILLARY ONCOTIC PRESSURE

Capillary membrane is permeable to all substances except plasma proteins. So, the plasma proteins stay within the capillaries and exert some pressure which is called oncotic pressure or colloidal osmotic pressure. Normal oncotic pressure is about 25 mm Hg. Among the plasma proteins, albumin exerts 70% of oncotic pressure.

Oncotic pressure plays an important role in filtration across capillary membrane, particularly in renal glomerular capillaries.

Arterial Pulse

■ INTRODUCTION

Arterial pulse is defined as the pressure changes transmitted in the form of waves through arterial wall and blood column from heart to periphery.

When heart contracts, the blood is ejected into aorta with great force. It causes distension of this blood vessel and a rise in pressure. A pressure wave is produced on the elastic wall of the aorta. It travels rapidly from the heart and can be felt after a brief interval, at any superficial peripheral artery like radial artery at wrist.

Pulse rate is the accurate measure of heart rate, except in conditions like pulses deficit (see below).

■ TRANSMISSION OF PULSE

Central arterial pulse is transmitted to the peripheral arteries as **peripheral arterial pulse.** Formation and transmission of pulse wave depends upon the elasticity of blood vessels. Thus, when the walls of the arteries are more distensible, the pressure rise is less and so the transmission of pulse is less. When the arterial wall loses its elastic property and becomes rigid as in old age, the pressure rise is more and the transmission of pulse is also more.

Pulse is not transmitted to capillaries because capillaries are devoid of elastic tissues.

■ VELOCITY OF TRANSMISSION OF PULSE

Average velocity at which the pulse wave is transmitted varies between 7 and 9 meter/second. Pulse travels faster than the blood. Maximum velocity of blood flow in the body (in larger arteries) is only 50 cm/second.

■ DELAY IN TRANSMISSION OF PULSE

At the arteries, pulse is felt after a short interval from the beginning of ventricular systole. This delay is very small and it can be measured only by accurate recording. The delay is directly proportional to the distance from heart.

Delay of pulse at:
1. Common carotid artery: 0.01 to 0.02 second
2. Radial artery: About 0.08 second.

■ METHODS OF RECORDING ARTERIAL PULSE

■ BY MANOMETER

In animals, pulse is recorded by inserting a cannula into the dissected artery. This cannula is connected to a manometer or any recording device.

■ BY DUDGEON SPHYGMOGRAPH

Dudgeon sphygmograph is tied to the wrist in such a way that, a small plate rests on the skin over radial artery. Movements of arterial wall are magnified by a series of levers and are recorded on a moving strip of smoked paper. This instrument is outdated and it is replaced by electronic pulse transducers.

■ BY ELECTRONIC PULSE TRANSDUCER

Pulse transducer is placed over the finger and tied. This device throws light on the blood vessel through skin. Sensor of the transducer detects the light rays reflected from the flowing blood. Alteration in frequency of the reflected light rays is amplified and recorded by connecting the transducer to a recording device like polygraph. The record shows finger pulse volume, which represents the arterial pulse tracing.

■ INTERPRETATION OF ARTERIAL PULSE TRACING

Pulse recorded in **radial artery** or **femoral artery** is the **typical peripheral pulse** (Fig. 106.1). Peripheral pulse tracing has three main features:

1. *Anacrotic Limb*

Anacrotic limb or primary wave is the ascending limb or upstroke. It is due to the rise in pressure during systole.

2. *Catacrotic Limb*

Catacrotic limb is the descending limb or downstroke. It is due to the fall in pressure during diastole.

3. *Catacrotic Notch*

In the upper part of the catacrotic limb of pulse tracing, a small notch appears. It is known as catacrotic notch or incisura. This notch is produced by the backflow of blood during the closure of semilunar valves at the beginning of diastolic period, which produces slight increase in the pressure.

4. *Precatacrotic and Postcatacrotic Waves*

The wave appearing before the catacrotic notch is called precatacrotic wave. The wave appearing after the notch is called postcatacrotic wave.

■ PULSE POINTS

Usually, pulse is palpated on the radial artery because it is easily approachable and placed superficially. However, arterial pulse can be felt in different areas on the body. These areas are called pulse points. Pulse points and the area of palpation are given in Table 106.1.

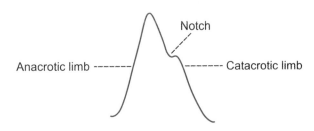

FIGURE 106.1: Radial pulse tracing

TABLE 106.1: Pulse points

Pulse point	Area of palpation
1. Temporal pulse	Over the temple, in front of ear on superficial temporal artery
2. Facial pulse	On facial artery at the angle of jaw
3. Carotid pulse	In the neck along anterior border of sternocleidomastoid muscle on common carotid artery
4. Axillary pulse	In axilla on axillary artery
5. Brachial pulse	In cubital fossa along medial border of biceps muscle on brachial artery
6. Radial pulse	Over the thumbside of wrist between tendons of brachioradialis and flexor carpi radialis muscles on radial artery
7. Ulnar pulse	Over the little fingerside of wrist on ulnar artery
8. Femoral pulse	In the groin on femoral artery
9. Popliteal pulse	Behind knee, in the popliteal fossa on popliteal artery
10. Dorsalis pedis pulse	Over the dorsum of foot on dorsalis pedis artery
11. Tibial pulse	Over the back of the ankle, behind medial malleolus on posterior tibial artery

■ EXAMINATION OF RADIAL PULSE

Examination of pulse is a valuable clinical procedure. Pulse represents the heartbeat. By examining pulse, important information regarding cardiac function such as rate of contraction, rhythmicity, etc. can be obtained. In addition, an experienced physician can determine the mean arterial pressure by hardness of pulse and its amplitude.

Method of Examining Radial Pulse

Subject is made to sit comfortably with forearm placed in mid or semi prone position, with wrist slightly flexed. The observer must stand by the right side of the subject. Tips of the middle three fingers (index finger, middle finger and ring finger) are placed over the radial artery below the wrist at the base of thumb. Light pressure is applied by the fingers until the pulse is felt. If necessary, the fingers are moved around till the pulse is felt.

Index finger is used to occlude blood flow from radial artery. **Ring finger** is used to occlude retrograde flow of blood from ulnar artery through palmar arch. **Middle finger** is used to assess the pulse.

Observations during Examination of Pulse

1. Rate
2. Rhythm
3. Character
4. Volume
5. Condition of blood vessel wall
6. Delayed pulse.

■ 1. RATE

Pulse rate is the number of pulse per minute. It has to be counted at least for 30 seconds. Pulse rate in adults is 72/minute.

Pulse Rate at Different Age

In fetus	: 150 to 180/minute
At birth	: 130 to 140/minute
At 10 years of age	: 90/minute
After puberty	: 72/minute.

Variations

Conditions that alter the heart rate alter pulse rate also.

Pulse rate increases during:

  i. Exercise
  ii. Pregnancy
  iii. Emotional conditions
  iv. Fever
  v. Anemia
  vi. Hypersecretion of catecholamines
  vii. Hyperthyroidism.

Pulse rate decreases during:

  i. Sleep
  ii. Hypothermia
  iii. Hypothyroidism
  iv. Incomplete heart block.

■ 2. RHYTHM

Rhythm is the regularity of pulse. It refers to interval between beats. Under normal conditions, the pulse appears at regular intervals. Rhythm of the pulse becomes irregular in conditions like atrial fibrillation, extrasystole and other types of arrhythmia (Chapter 96).

Pulse with irregular rhythm is of two types:
  i. Regularly irregular pulse
  ii. Irregularly irregular pulse.

■ 3. CHARACTER

Character denotes the tension on the vessel wall produced by the waves of pulse. It is usually evaluated at right carotid artery. Normally, it is not possible to detect the different waves of the pulse or slight variations in the character or form of the pulse. However, it becomes more prominent in some abnormal conditions such as anacrotic pulse, water hammer pulse, pulsus paradoxus, etc. which are explained later in this chapter.

■ 4. VOLUME

Volume is the determination of movement of the vessel wall, produced by the transmission of pulse wave. It is also a measure of pulse pressure. It depends upon the condition of the blood vessel.

■ 5. CONDITION OF THE BLOOD VESSEL WALL

Condition of wall of the blood vessel is assessed by feeling the radial artery and rolling it against the underlying bones. Normally, the wall of the vessel is not palpable in children and young adults. However, in old age the wall of the vessel becomes rigid and palpable. In abnormal conditions like arteriosclerosis, it is felt as a hard rope.

■ 6. DELAYED PULSE

Sometimes, the arrival of pulse in certain peripheral arteries is delayed. It is an important feature to be noted because it is useful in diagnosis of certain diseases.

Types of delayed pulse:
  i. Femoral delay
  ii. Radial-radial delay.

i. *Femoral Delay*

While palpating radial pulse and femoral pulse simultaneously, there is a short delay in the arrival of femoral pulse wave. Normally, it is negligible and unnoticed. However, the prolonged or noticeable delay in the arrival of femoral pulse indicates coarctation (narrowing) of aorta. This delay is called femoral delay, **radial femoral delay** or **radiofemoral delay.**

ii. *Radial-radial Delay*

When both the radial pulses are examined simultaneously, sometimes the arrival of pulse is delayed on one side. It is called **radio-radial delay** or radial-radial delay or **radial-radial inequality.** This indicates the narrowing of large artery due to atherosclerosis.

■ APPLIED PHYSIOLOGY – ABNORMAL PULSE

■ 1. PULSUS DEFICIT

Pulsus deficit is the abnormal condition in which the pulse rate is less than the heart rate. It occurs in atrial fibrillation, when the stroke volume is reduced. Because of reduced stroke volume, some of the pulse waves become weak and disappear before reaching the peripheral arteries. Pulsus deficit is the only condition in which pulse rate is less than the heart rate.

■ 2. PULSUS ALTERNANS

Pulsus alternans is the abnormal condition in which the amplitude of every second wave in pulse tracing is relatively smaller. It is because of the alternate variation in the force of ventricular contraction. However, the rhythm of the pulse is not altered. It is common in severe myocardial diseases, paroxysmal tachycardia and atrial fibrillation.

■ 3. ANACROTIC PULSE

Anacrotic pulse is the abnormal pulse, characterized by a slow ascending limb which has a notch called anacrotic notch. It is produced in aortic stenosis, when ejection is slow.

■ 4. THREADY PULSE OR WEAK PULSE

Thready or weak pulse is the abnormal pulse in which the volume of pulse becomes very feeble and is hardly felt at the arteries. It usually occurs whenever the stroke volume decreases or when there is severe vasoconstriction, as in the case of severe hemorrhage or severe chills. In these conditions, the sympathetic activity increases enormously, leading to generalized vasoconstriction.

■ 5. PULSUS PARADOXUS

Pulsus paradoxus is the condition when the pulse becomes very strong and very weak alternately, in relation to respiratory cycle. Normally, there is a slight increase in volume of pulse during inspiration and slight decrease in volume during expiration. But, it is hardly noticed. However, when it becomes very prominent, it is pathological. This type of pulse is noticed in cardiac tamponade (Chapter 100). It is also noticed in physiological conditions such as deep breathing.

■ 6. WATER HAMMER PULSE

Water hammer pulse is the abnormal pulse, characterized by a rapid upstroke and an equally rapid downstroke. It is also called **collapsing** or **Corrigan pulse.** It is seen in conditions like aortic regurgitation, patent ductus arteriosus and arteriovenous fistula. It is best felt by raising the arm of the subject and holding it by grasping the wrist with palm of the observer.

■ 7. ABNORMAL PULSE IN PATENT DUCTUS ARTERIOSUS

Patent ductus arteriosus is the permanent existence of ductus arteriosus. In fetus, the lungs are nonfunctioning. So, the blood which is pumped by right ventricle into the pulmonary artery, is diverted to systemic aorta through ductus arteriosus. Ductus arteriosus closes after birth. However, in some cases, it exists without closing (Fig. 106.2).

Pulse pressure wave is very much altered in this condition. Since, the blood flows from systemic aorta

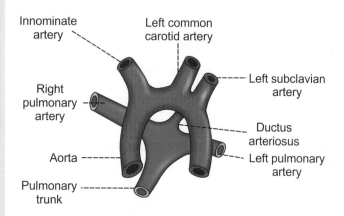

FIGURE 106.2: Diagram showing ductus arteriosus

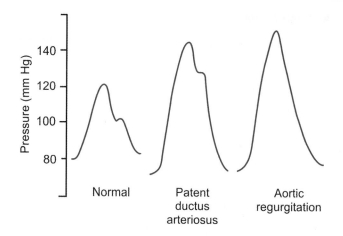

FIGURE 106.3: Radial pulse tracing in patent ductus arteriosus and aortic regurgitation

to pulmonary artery, after every ventricular systole, the blood flows out of aorta quickly. It decreases the diastolic pressure and the catacrotic limb of the pulse tracing falls below the level of 80 mm Hg.

Flow of blood from aorta to pulmonary artery increases the venous return to left side of the heart. So, left ventricular output increases, which in turn elevates the systolic pressure in arteries. Thus, in pulse tracing, the peak of the pulse wave is elevated above the level of 120 mm Hg. So, the pulse tracing in this condition reveals the increased pulse pressure (Fig. 106.3).

■ 8. ABNORMAL PULSE IN AORTIC REGURGITATION

Aortic regurgitation is the backflow of blood from aorta into left ventricle. It is common during incompetence of semilunar valve in aorta. It decreases the diastolic pressure. Because of backflow of blood, the left ventricular filling increases greatly, leading to increase in output and systolic pressure. Thus, the pulse tracing in aortic regurgitation is more or less similar to that in patent ductus arteriosus. Only difference is that in the tracing during aortic regurgitation, the incisura is very mild. And in severe conditions, when the aortic valve does not close, the incisura is absent (Fig. 106.3).

Venous Pulse

- ■ INTRODUCTION
- ■ SIGNIFICANCE
- ■ EXAMINATION OF VENOUS PULSE
- ■ METHODS TO RECORD VENOUS PULSE
- ■ RECORDING OF VENOUS PULSE – JUGULAR VENOUS PULSE TRACING
- ■ APPLIED PHYSIOLOGY – ABNORMAL VENOUS PULSE
  - ■ ELEVATED JUGULAR VENOUS PULSE
  - ■ KUSSMAUL SIGN
  - ■ ABNORMALITIES OF WAVES IN JUGULAR PULSE TRACING

■ INTRODUCTION

Venous pulse is defined as the pressure changes transmitted in the form of waves from right atrium to veins near heart. Venous pulse is observed only in larger veins near the heart such as jugular vein.

Observation of venous pulse is an integral part of the physical examination because it reflects right atrial pressure and the hemodynamic events in right atrium.

■ SIGNIFICANCE

1. Venous pulse recording is used to determine the rate of atrial contraction, just as the record of arterial pulse is used to determine the rate of ventricular contraction
2. Many phases of cardiac cycle can be recognized by means of venous pulse tracing
3. Venous pulse tracing is the simple and accurate method to measure the duration of different phases in diastole
4. Venous pulse also represents the atrial pressure changes taking place during cardiac cycle.

■ EXAMINATION OF VENOUS PULSE

Inspection of jugular vein pulsations is routinely done by bedside examination of neck veins. It provides valuable information about the cardiac function.

To observe the pulsation of internal jugular vein, head of the subject is tilted upwards at 45°. However, in patients with increased venous pressure, the head should be tilted as much as 90°. Pulsations of jugular vein can be noticed when light is passed across the skin overlying internal jugular vein with relaxed neck muscles. Simultaneous palpation of the left carotid artery helps the examiner confirm the venous pulsations.

■ METHODS TO RECORD VENOUS PULSE

A small **funnel** covered by thin **rubber membrane** is placed over the skin at the level of external jugular vein, in the **supraclavicular fossa.** Slight pressure is exerted to provide perfect contact between edge of the funnel and skin.

Pressure changes in the vein cause some oscillations in rubber membrane through the skin. The oscillations are transmitted through rubber tube to a recording device like **Marey tambour.** Nowadays, **electronic transducer** is used for this purpose.

The subject should be in such a position so as to avoid the effect of gravity, which tends to empty veins and reduce the amplitude of the venous pulse.

■ RECORDING OF VENOUS PULSE – JUGULAR VENOUS PULSE TRACING

Recording of jugular venous pulse is called **phlebogram.** It is similar to intra-atrial pressure curve (Fig. 107.1).

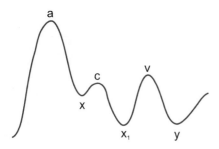

FIGURE 107.1: Phlebogram

Like intra-atrial pressure curve, phlebogram also has three positive waves, namely a, c, v and three negative waves namely x, x_1, y.

'a' Wave

'a' wave is the first positive wave. It is due to rise in atrial pressure during **atrial systole.** It precedes ventricular systole.

'x' Wave

'x' wave is a negative wave due to fall in atrial pressure. It coincides with **atrial diastole** and beginning of **ventricular systole.**

'c' Wave

'c' wave is a positive wave due to rise in atrial pressure during **isometric contraction period.** During this period, the atrioventricular valves bulge into the atria and increase the pressure in the atria slightly.

Earlier, it was thought that this wave was due to transmission of pulse from neighboring carotid artery. Hence, it was called 'c' wave.

'x_1' Wave

'x_1' wave is a negative wave due to fall in atrial pressure during **ejection period.** During ejection period, the atrioventricular ring is pulled towards ventricles causing distention of atria. So, the atrial pressure falls.

'v' Wave

'v' wave is a positive wave due to rise in atrial pressure. The pressure increases because of filling of atria (venous return). It is obtained during **isometric relaxation period** or during atrial diastole.

'y' Wave

'y' wave is a negative wave which denotes fall in atrial pressure. Pressure falls due to the opening of atrioventricular valve and emptying of blood into the ventricle. This wave appears during **rapid and slow filling periods.** 'y' wave is followed by 'a' wave and the cycle is repeated.

■ APPLIED PHYSIOLOGY – ABNORMAL VENOUS PULSE

■ ELEVATED JUGULAR VENOUS PULSE

Elevated jugular venous pulse indicates the rise in right ventricular pressure.
   It occurs in:
1. Bradycardia
2. Pericardial effusion
3. Constrictive pericarditis
4. Tricuspid stenosis
5. Pulmonary hypertension.

■ KUSSMAUL SIGN

Kussmaul sign is the increase in venous distention and venous pressure. Normally, it occurs during inspiration.

Pathological Conditions when Kussmaul Sign occurs

1. Cardiac tamponade
2. Constrictive pericarditis
3. Restrictive cardiomyopathy
4. Right ventricular infarction.

■ ABNORMALITIES OF WAVES IN JUGULAR PULSE TRACING

1. *Elevation of 'a' Wave*

Elevation of 'a' wave occurs in:
   i. Tricuspid stenosis
   ii. Pulmonary hypertension.

2. *Cannon 'a' Wave*

Giant 'a' wave with abrupt fall (downward deflection) is called Cannon 'a' wave. It appears in:
   i. Complete heart block
   ii. Paroxysmal atrioventricular nodal tachycardia
   iii. Ventricular tachycardia.

3. *Abnormal 'v' Wave*

'v' wave becomes abnormal in tricuspid incompetence.

4. *Abnormal 'x' Wave*

Abnormal 'x' wave appears in:
   i. Atrial fibrillation
   ii. Cardiac temponade
   iii. Constrictive pericarditis.

5. *Abnormal 'y' Wave*

'y' wave becomes abnormal in:
   i. Tricuspid regurgitation
   ii. Constrictive pericarditis.

Coronary Circulation

■ DISTRIBUTION OF CORONARY BLOOD VESSELS

■ CORONARY ARTERIES

Heart muscle is supplied by two coronary arteries, namely right and left coronary arteries, which are the first branches of aorta. Arteries encircle the heart in the manner of a **crown,** hence the name coronary arteries (Latin word corona = crown).

Right and Left Coronary Arteries

Right coronary artery supplies whole of the right ventricle and posterior portion of left ventricle. Left coronary artery supplies mainly the anterior and lateral parts of left ventricle. There are many variations in diameter of coronary arteries.

Variations in Coronary Arteries

1. In 50% to 60% of human beings, the right coronary artery is larger (right dominant) and supplies more blood to heart than left coronary artery
2. In 15% to 20% of human beings, the left coronary artery is larger (left dominant)
3. In 20% to 30% of human beings, both arteries supply almost equal amount of blood.

Branches of Coronary Arteries

Coronary arteries divide and subdivide into smaller branches, which run all along the surface of the heart. Smaller branches are called **epicardiac arteries** and give rise to further smaller branches known as **final arteries** or **intramural vessels.** Final arteries run at right angles through the heart muscle, near the inner aspect of wall of the heart.

■ VENOUS DRAINAGE

Venous drainage from heart muscle is by three types of vessels.

1. Coronary Sinus

Coronary sinus is the larger vein draining 75% of total coronary flow. It drains blood from left side of the heart and opens into right atrium near tricuspid valve.

2. Anterior Coronary Veins

Anterior coronary veins drain blood from right side of the heart and open directly into right atrium.

3. Thebesian Veins

Thebesian veins drain deoxygenated blood from myocardium, directly into the concerned chamber of the heart.

■ PHYSIOLOGICAL SHUNT

Physiological shunt is the diverted route (diversion), through which the venous (deoxygenated) blood is mixed with arterial blood. Deoxygenated blood flowing from thebesian veins into cardiac chambers makes up the part of normal physiological shunt.

Other component of physiological shunt is the drainage of deoxygenated blood from bronchial circulation into pulmonary vein, without being oxygenated. Refer Chapter 119 for more details about physiological shunt.

■ CORONARY BLOOD FLOW AND ITS MEASUREMENT

■ NORMAL CORONARY BLOOD FLOW

Normal blood flow through coronary circulation is about 200 mL/minute. It forms 4% of cardiac output. It is about 65 to 70 mL/minute/100 g of cardiac muscle.

■ MEASUREMENT OF CORONARY BLOOD FLOW

Direct Method

Coronary blood flow is measured by using an **electromagnetic flowmeter.** It is directly placed around any coronary artery (refer Chapter 98 for details of electromagnetic flowmeter).

Indirect Method

1. By Fick principle

Coronary blood flow is measured by applying Fick principle (Chapter 98) using **nitrous oxide** (N_2O). The subject is asked to inhale a known quantity of the gas with atmospheric air. Then, blood samples are collected from an artery and from coronary sinus, by using a catheter. The blood flow is determined by using the formula:

$$\text{Blood flow} = \frac{\text{Amount of } N_2O \text{ taken up/minute}}{\text{Arteriovenous difference of } N_2O \text{ content}}$$

2. By using Doppler flowmeter

Piezoelectric crystals are used in the Doppler flowmeter probe, to transmit and receive the pulses of high frequency sound waves (Chapter 98). The Doppler flowmeter probe is mounted to a catheter and positioned at the ostium of right or left coronary artery to measure the velocity of phasic flow of blood. The cross-sectional area of the artery is determined by angiography. From velocity of blood flow and cross-sectional area, the volume of blood flow is calculated.

3. By videodensitometry

Videodensitometry is the technique used to measure both velocity of blood flow and the cross-sectional area of coronary arteries, simultaneously. From these two values, the coronary blood flow can be calculated.

■ PHASIC CHANGES IN CORONARY BLOOD FLOW

Blood flow through coronary arteries is not constant. It decreases during systole and increases during diastole (Fig. 108.1).

Intramural vessels or final arteries supplying myocardium are perpendicular to the cardiac muscles. So, during systole, the intramural vessels are compressed and blood flow is reduced. During diastole, the compression is released and the blood vessels are distended. So, the blood flow increases.

■ PHASIC CHANGES IN LEFT VENTRICLE

In left ventricle, during the onset of isometric contraction, blood flow declines sharply due to two reasons, namely increase in myocardial tissue pressure and decrease in aortic pressure.

During ejection period, rise in aortic pressure causes a sharp rise in flow into left coronary artery. However,

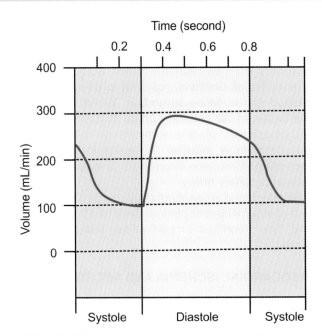

FIGURE 108.1: Phasic changes in coronary blood flow

the flow of blood through coronary capillaries is less. It is due to the high intramural myocardial pressure in the contracting ventricle. Decreased blood flow is maintained until the closure of aortic valve, i.e. till the end of systole.

During the onset of diastole, blood flow rises and it reaches the peak sharply. During the later part of diastole, the flow is reduced slightly along with decreasing aortic pressure. Once again, there is a sharp fall in flow during the onset of systole.

■ PHASIC CHANGES IN RIGHT VENTRICLE

A small amount of blood flows into right ventricle during systole. It is because the force of contraction is not as severe as in the case of left ventricle. Still, the amount of blood flowing is very much less than that during diastole.

■ FACTORS REGULATING CORONARY BLOOD FLOW

Autoregulation

Like any other organ, heart also has the capacity to regulate its own blood flow by autoregulation (Chapter 102). Coronary blood flow is not affected when mean arterial pressure varies between 60 and 150 mm Hg. Several factors are involved in the autoregulation mechanism.

Coronary blood flow is regulated mainly by local vascular response to the needs of cardiac muscle.

Factors regulating coronary blood flow:

1. Need for oxygen
2. Metabolic factors
3. Coronary perfusion pressure
4. Nervous factors.

■ 1. NEED FOR OXYGEN

Oxygen is the most important factor maintaining blood flow through the coronary blood vessels. Amount of blood passing through coronary circulation is directly proportional to the consumption of oxygen by cardiac muscle.

Even in resting condition, a large amount of oxygen, i.e. 70% to 80% is consumed from the blood by heart muscle than by any other tissues. In conditions associated with increased cardiac activity, the need for oxygen increases enormously.

Thus, the need for oxygen, i.e. hypoxia immediately causes coronary vasodilatation and increases the blood flow to heart.

■ 2. METABOLIC FACTORS

Coronary vasodilatation during hypoxic conditions occurs because of some metabolic products, which increase the coronary blood flow by vasodilatation.

Reactive Hyperemia

Reactive hyperemia is the increase in blood flow due to the vasodilator effects of metabolites.

Metabolic Products which Increase the Coronary Blood Flow

Adenosine

Adenosine is a potent vasodilator and it increases the blood flow to cardiac muscle. During hypoxia, ATP in the muscle is degraded in large amount, forming ADP. Some ADP molecules are further degraded into adenosine, which is released into tissue fluids of heart muscle.

Other substances

Other substances which increase the coronary blood flow by vasodilatation are:
  i. Potassium
  ii. Hydrogen
  iii. Carbon dioxide
  iv. Adenosine phosphate compounds.

■ 3. CORONARY PERFUSION PRESSURE

Perfusion pressure is the balance between mean arterial pressure and venous pressure (Chapter 102). Thus, coronary perfusion pressure is the balance between mean arterial pressure in aorta and the right atrial pressure. Since right aterial pressure is low, the mean arterial pressure becomes the major factor that maintains the coronary blood flow. Range of mean arterial pressure at which the coronary blood flow can be maintained is given above.

■ 4. NERVOUS FACTORS

Coronary blood vessels are innervated both by parasympathetic and sympathetic divisions of autonomic nervous system. It is not known whether the autonomic nerves have direct effect on blood flow in various conditions. However, these nerves influence the coronary blood flow indirectly by acting on the musculature of heart.

For example, stimulation of sympathetic nerves increases the rate and force of contraction of heart. This in turn, causes liberation of more metabolites which dilate the blood vessels and increase the coronary blood flow. Similarly, when parasympathetic nerves are stimulated, the cardiac functions are inhibited and the production of metabolites is less. Coronary blood flow decreases.

■ APPLIED PHYSIOLOGY – CORONARY ARTERY DISEASE

Coronary artery disease (CAD) is the heart disease that is caused by inadequate blood supply to cardiac muscle due to occlusion of coronary artery. It is also called coronary heart disease.

■ CORONARY OCCLUSION

Definition

Coronary occlusion is the partial or complete obstruction of the coronary artery.

Cause

Coronary occlusion is caused by atherosclerosis, a condition associated with deposition of cholesterol on the walls of the artery. In due course, this part of the arterial wall becomes fibrotic and it is called **atherosclerotic plaque.** The plaque is made up of cholesterol, calcium and other substances from blood. Because of the atherosclerotic plaque, the lumen of the coronary artery becomes narrow. In severe conditions, the artery is completely occluded.

Development of atherosclerotic plaque is common in coronary arteries near the origin from aorta. This plaque activates platelets, resulting in **thrombosis** and the blood clot is called **thrombus.** When three fourth of the lumen of the coronary artery is obstructed either by atherosclerotic plaque or thrombus, the blood flow to myocardium is reduced. It results in **ischemia** of myocardium. Coronary thrombosis is associated with **spasm** of coronary artery.

Smaller blood vessels are occluded by the thrombus or part of atherosclerotic plaque, detached from coronary artery. This thrombus or part of the plaque is called **embolus.**

■ MYOCARDIAL ISCHEMIA AND NECROSIS

Myocardial Ischemia

Myocardial ischemia is the reaction of a part of myocardium in response to hypoxia. Hypoxia develops when blood flow to a part of myocardium decreases severely due to occlusion of a coronary artery.

Blood flow is usually restored if a small quantum of myocardium is affected by ischemia due to obstruction of smaller blood vessels. It is due to rapid development of **coronary collateral arteries.**

Necrosis

Necrosis refers to death of cells or tissues by injury or disease in a localized area. Ischemia leads to necrosis of myocardium if a large part of myocardium is involved or the occlusion is severe involving larger blood vessels. Necrosis is irreversible.

■ MYOCARDIAL INFARCTION – HEART ATTACK

Myocardial infarction is the necrosis of myocardium caused by insufficient blood flow due to embolus, thrombus or vascular spasm. It is also called heart attack. In myocardial infarction, death occurs rapidly due to ventricular fibrillation.

Myocardial Stunning

Myocardial stunning is a type of transient mechanical dysfunction of heart, caused by a mild reduction in blood flow. A substantial reduction in coronary blood flow causes ischemia followed by necrosis. A mild reduction in blood flow causes only ischemia and it may not be sufficient to cause necrosis of myocardium. However, it produces some transient (short lived) mechanical disturbances or dysfunction of the heart. Since it is short lived, heart recovers completely from this.

Symptoms of Myocardial Infarction

Common symptoms of myocardial infarction:
1. Cardiac pain
2. Nausea
3. Vomiting
4. Palpitations
5. Difficulty in breathing
6. Extreme weakness
7. Sweating
8. Anxiety.

■ CARDIAC PAIN – ANGINA PECTORIS

Cardiac pain is the **chest pain** that is caused by myocardial ischemia. It is also called angina pectoris. It is the common manifestation of coronary artery disease. Pain starts beneath the sternum and radiates to the surface of left arm and left shoulder. Cardiac pain is a referred pain and it is felt over the body, away from heart. It is because, heart and left arm develop from the same dermatomal segment in embryo.

Cause for Cardiac Pain

Ischemia is mainly due to hypoxia. During myocardial ischemia, there is accumulation of anaerobic metabolic end products such as uric acid. Metabolites and other pain producing substances like substance P, histamine and kinin stimulate the sensory nerve endings, leading to pain.

Sensory Pathway

Sensory pathway from the heart is as follows:
1. Inferior cervical sympathetic nerve fibers (Chapter 101) carrying the sensations of pain (or stretch) from the heart reach the posterior gray horn of first 4 thoracic segments of spinal cord
2. Here, these fibers synapse with second order neurons (substantial gelatinosa of Rolando) of lateral spinothalamic tract
3. Fibers from substantial gelatinosa of Rolando form lateral spinothalamic tract and reach the sensory cortex via thalamus.

If hypoxia in myocardium is relieved by coronary collateral circulation or by treatment, the pain producing substances are washed away by blood flow.

Chronic Angina Pectoris

In chronic angina pectoris, the patient does not feel the pain normally. The pain is felt only when the workload of heart increases. The workload of the heart increases in conditions like exercise and emotional outburst.

When the frequency of angina attack increases, the patient is prone to develop acute myocardial infarction.

Treatment for Angina Pectoris

1. *By using drugs*

   i. *Vasodilator drugs:* Vasodilator drugs like glycerol trinitrate or sodium nitrite relieve the pain by dilating coronary arteries. However, the main therapeutic effect of such drugs is to dilate splanchnic blood vessels, which cause reduction in venous return, cardiac output, workload of the heart and oxygen consumption in myocardium so that, release of pain promoting substances is inhibited.

   ii. *Calcium **channel blockers:*** These drugs block the influx of calcium into the cells. When calcium influx is blocked, the myocardial contractility and workload of the heart are decreased.

   iii. *Sympathetic blocking agents:* Sympathetic blocking agents like propranolol **(beta blockers)** block the beta-adrenergic receptors and inhibit the cardiac activity. This decreases heart rate, stroke volume, workload on heart and oxygen consumption. It also stops the production of nociceptive substances in myocardium.

2. *By thrombolysis*

Refer Chapter 98.

3. *By surgical methods*

   i. *Aortic-coronary artery bypass graft:* Part of myocardium affected by coronary occlusion is detected by **angiography.** Then, the anastomosis is made between aorta and the coronary artery beyond occlusion, by a technique called aortic-coronary artery bypass graft. Mostly, a small vein from lower limb is used for anastomosis. Though this method can relieve the pain, it is not useful if the myocardium is damaged extensively.

   ii. *Percutaneous transluminal coronary angioplasty (PTCA):* Refer Chapter 98.

   iii. *Laser coronary angioplasty:* Refer Chapter 98.

Cerebral Circulation

Chapter

109

- ■ INTRODUCTION
- ■ CEREBRAL VESSELS AND NORMAL CEREBRAL BLOOD FLOW
- ■ MEASUREMENT OF CEREBRAL BLOOD FLOW
  - ■ KETY AND SCHMIDT NITROUS OXIDE METHOD
  - ■ BY USING RADIOACTIVE SUBSTANCES
  - ■ BY COMPUTERIZED AXIAL TOMOGRAPHY (CAT)
  - ■ BY POSITRON EMISSION TOMOGRAPHY (PET)
  - ■ BY MAGNETIC RESONANCE IMAGING (MRI)
- ■ REGULATION OF CEREBRAL BLOOD FLOW
  - ■ AUTOREGULATION
  - ■ CHEMICAL FACTORS
  - ■ NERVOUS FACTORS
- ■ APPLIED PHYSIOLOGY – STROKE

■ INTRODUCTION

Brain tissues need adequate blood supply continuously. Stoppage of blood flow to brain for 5 seconds leads to unconsciousness and for 5 minutes leads to irreparable damage to the brain cells.

■ CEREBRAL VESSELS AND NORMAL CEREBRAL BLOOD FLOW

Brain receives blood from the **basilar artery** and **internal carotid artery.** Branches of these arteries form **circle of Willis.** Venous drainage is by sinuses, which open into **internal jugular vein.**

Normally, brain receives 750 to 800 mL of blood per minute. It is about 15% to 16% of total cardiac output and about 50 to 55 mL/100 g of brain tissue per minute.

■ MEASUREMENT OF CEREBRAL BLOOD FLOW

■ 1. KETY AND SCHMIDT NITROUS OXIDE METHOD

Nitrous oxide method is an indirect method to measure the blood flow to the brain. It is based on **Fick principle** (Chapter 98). **Nitrous oxide** is used as an indicator substance in this method.

The subject is asked to inhale nitrous oxide at a low concentration, which is less than the amount required for anesthesia. After inhalation of the gas for about 10 minutes, the amount of nitrous oxide retained in the brain tissues becomes equal to the amount of nitrous oxide present in cerebral venous blood. Now, the concentration of nitrous oxide is determined in the arterial blood and cerebral venous blood and the cerebral blood flow is calculated by the formula:

$$\text{Cerebral blood flow} = \frac{\text{Amount of N}_2\text{O taken by brain}}{\text{Arteriovenous difference of N}_2\text{O}}$$

■ 2. BY USING RADIOACTIVE SUBSTANCES

Radioactive substances method is used to determine the amount of blood flow to different regions of the cerebral cortex. Radioactive substance is injected into the carotid artery. By measuring the radioactivity in the brain tissues using **radioactive detectors (scintillation counter),** the blood flowing through each area of brain is determined. Advantage of this method is that the blood flow to about 250 areas of cerebral cortex can be measured by using many radioactive detectors. Radioactive xenon and 2-deoxyglucose are the commonly used radioactive substances to measure the cerebral blood flow.

■ 3. BY COMPUTERIZED AXIAL TOMOGRAPHY

Computerized axial tomography (CT or CAT) scanning was introduced in 1970s. Tomography scanning is a process which combines many two dimensional X-ray images to generate cross sectional pictures of different organs or regions of the body. Advancement of technology resulted in combination of many three dimensional X-ray images of body structures and organs including brain. CT scan of brain is useful to determine brain damage and local changes in cerebral blood flow, while the subject performs a task.

■ 4. BY POSITRON EMISSION TOMOGRAPHY

Positron emission tomography (PET) scanner is a type of computerized tomography machine. A short-lived radioactive substance called radionuclide combined with sugar is injected into the patient. Radionuclide emits positrons (antiparticle or antimatter counterpart of electron). Positron emissions from radionuclide are detected by rotating the PET scanner around patient's head. PET is used to study blood volume, oxygen consumption, pH, glucose utilization, blood flow and the activity of receptors in brain cells.

■ 5. BY MAGNETIC RESONANCE IMAGING

Magnetic resonance imaging (MRI) is a different type of imaging technique. It involves polarization of hydrogen atoms in the soft tissues by using a large magnet and detecting the resonant signals (summation of the spinning energies within the living cells) from the tissues. Since the images are very clear, this technique is useful for scanning soft tissues, brain, spinal cord, abdomen, joints and malignant tissues. MRI is also used to measure blood flow to the organs such as brain. Measurement of blood flow to a part or area of the organ is called functional magnetic resonance imaging (fMRI).

■ REGULATION OF CEREBRAL BLOOD FLOW

Cerebral circulation is regulated by three factors:
1. Autoregulation
2. Chemical factors
3. Neural factors.

■ AUTOREGULATION

Like any other vital organ, brain also regulates its own blood flow by means of autoregulation (Chapter 102). However, the autoregulation in brain has got its own limitations. It depends upon:
  i. Effective perfusion pressure
  ii. Cerebral vascular resistance.
  Cerebral blood flow is directly proportional to the balance between effective perfusion pressure and the vascular resistance in brain.

i. *Effective Perfusion Pressure*

Effective perfusion pressure is the balance between the mean arterial blood pressure and venous pressure across the organ, divided by resistance (Chapter 102). Since venous pressure is zero in brain, mean arterial blood pressure plays an important role in regulating cerebral blood flow. Autoregulation is possible in brain if the mean arterial pressure is within the range of 60 mm Hg and 140 mm Hg. Autoregulation fails beyond this range on either side.

ii. *Cerebral Vascular Resistance*

When the vascular resistance is more, the blood flow to the brain is less. Resistance to blood flow in brain is offered by intracranial pressure, cerebrospinal fluid pressure and viscosity of blood.

Intracranial pressure and cerebrospinal fluid pressure

Increase in the intracranial pressure or the pressure exerted by the cerebrospinal fluid (CSF) compresses the cerebral blood vessels and decreases blood flow. These pressures are elevated in conditions like head injury. However, severe ischemic effects are avoided by some protective reflexes such as Cushing reflex.

Cushing reflex

Cushing reflex is a protective reflex that helps save the brain tissues from ischemic effects during the periods of reduced cerebral blood flow. It is also called **Cushing reaction,** response or phenomenon.

Increase in intracranial pressure or increase in CSF pressure compresses the cerebral blood vessels and decreases the blood flow. However, blood flow is decreased only for a short period. It is restored immediately by means of Cushing reflex. When cerebral blood flow decreases by the compression of cerebral arteries, the cerebral ischemia develops. Compression of blood vessels decreases the blood flow to vasomotor center also. Local hypoxia and hypercapnea activate vasomotor center, resulting in peripheral vasoconstriction and rise in the arterial pressure. The increased arterial pressure helps to restore the cerebral blood flow. Thus, Cushing reflex plays the most important role in maintaining the cerebral blood flow (Fig. 109.1).

Cushing reflex operates only when the rise in arterial blood pressure is proportional to increase in intracranial pressure. When the increase in intracranial pressure is very high and if it exceeds the arterial blood pressure, this

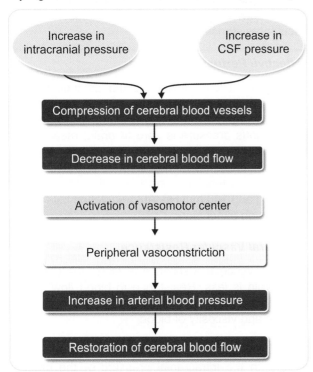

FIGURE 109.1: Schematic representation of Cushing reflex. CSF = Cerebrospinal fluid.

protective mechanism fails. And the cerebral ischemia becomes severe, leading to irreversible damage of the brain tissues.

Monro-Kellie doctrine

According to Monro-Kellie doctrine or principle, though the cerebral arteries are compressed by increased intracranial pressure or cerebrospinal fluid pressure, the volume of brain tissue is not affected. It is because the brain tissue is not compressible.

Viscosity

Increase in the viscosity of blood as in polycythemia, increases the cerebral vascular resistance and blood flow decreases. When viscosity decreases as in the case of anemia, the resistance is decreased and blood flow increases. Thus, the cerebral blood flow is inversely proportional to the viscosity of blood.

■ **CHEMICAL FACTORS**

Chemical factors which increase the cerebral blood flow:
  i.   Decreased oxygen tension
  ii. Increased carbon dioxide tension
  iii. Increased hydrogen ion concentration.

Carbon dioxide is the most important factor, as it causes dilatation of cerebral blood vessels, leading to increase in blood flow. A moderate increase in carbon dioxide tension does not alter the blood flow due to autoregulation. When arterial partial pressure of carbon dioxide rises above 45 mm Hg, the cerebral blood flow increases.

Carbon dioxide combines with water to form carbonic acid, which dissociates into bicarbonate ions and hydrogen ion. The hydrogen ion causes dilatation of blood vessels in brain.

Hypoxia increases cerebral blood flow by vasodilatation.

■ **NERVOUS FACTORS**

Cerebral blood vessels are supplied by sympathetic vasoconstrictor fibers. But, these fibers do not play any role in regulating cerebral blood flow under normal conditions. In pathological conditions like hypertension, the sympathetic nerves cause constriction of cerebral blood vessels, leading to reduction in blood flow. It prevents cerebral vascular hemorrhage and cerebral stroke.

■ APPLIED PHYSIOLOGY – STROKE

Definition

Stroke is the sudden death of neurons in localized area of brain due to inadequate blood supply. It is characterized by reversible or irreversible paralysis with other symptoms. Stroke is also called **cardiovascular accident** (CVA) or **brain attack.**

Types

Stroke is classified into two types:
1. **Ischemic stroke,** which occurs due to interruption of blood flow to a part of brain by thrombus or atherosclerotic embolus
2. **Hemorrhagic stroke,** which develops by the rupture of a blood vessel in the brain and spilling of blood into the surrounding areas.

Causes

Most common factors (risk factors) which causes stroke are:

1. Heart disease
2. Hypertension
3. High cholesterol in blood
4. High blood sugar (diabetes mellitus)
5. Heavy smoking
6. Heavy alcohol consumption.

Symptoms

Symptoms of stroke depend upon the area of brain that is damaged. Generally, stroke causes dizziness, loss of consciousness, coma or death.

Other features of stroke:
1. Weakness
2. Numbness or paralysis, particularly on one side of the body
3. Impairment of speech
4. Emotional disturbances
5. Loss of coordination
6. Loss of memory.

Splanchnic Circulation

- ■ INTRODUCTION
- ■ MESENTERIC CIRCULATION
  - ■ DISTRIBUTION OF BLOOD FLOW
  - ■ REGULATION OF MESENTERIC BLOOD FLOW
- ■ SPLENIC CIRCULATION
  - ■ IMPORTANCE OF SPLENIC CIRCULATION
  - ■ STORAGE OF BLOOD
  - ■ REGULATION OF BLOOD FLOW TO SPLEEN
- ■ HEPATIC CIRCULATION
  - ■ BLOOD VESSELS
  - ■ NORMAL BLOOD FLOW
  - ■ REGULATION OF BLOOD FLOW TO LIVER

■ INTRODUCTION

Splanchnic or visceral circulation constitutes three portions:

1. Mesenteric circulation supplying blood to GI tract
2. Splenic circulation supplying blood to spleen
3. Hepatic circulation supplying blood to liver.

Unique feature of splanchnic circulation is that the blood from mesenteric bed and spleen forms a major amount of blood flowing to liver. Blood flows to liver from GI tract and spleen through portal system.

■ MESENTERIC CIRCULATION

■ DISTRIBUTION OF BLOOD FLOW

Stomach : 35 mL/100 g/minute
Intestine : 50 mL/100 g/minute
Pancreas : 80 mL/100 g/minute.

■ REGULATION OF MESENTERIC BLOOD FLOW

Mesenteric blood flow is regulated by the following factors:

1. *Local Autoregulation*

Local autoregulation is the primary factor regulating blood flow through mesenteric bed (Chapter 102).

2. *Activity of Gastrointestinal Tract*

Contraction of the wall of the GI tract reduces blood flow due to compression of blood vessels. And relaxation of wall of GI tract increases the blood flow due to removal of compression on the vessel wall.

3. *Nervous Factor*

Mesenteric blood flow is regulated by sympathetic nerve fibers. Increase in sympathetic activity as in the case of emotional conditions or **'fight and flight reactions'** constrict the mesenteric blood vessels. So, more blood is diverted to organs like skeletal muscles, heart and brain, which need more blood during these conditions. Parasympathetic nerves do not have any direct action on the mesenteric blood vessels. But these nerves increase the contraction of GI tract which compresses the blood vessels, resulting in reduction in blood flow.

4. *Chemical Factors – Functional Hyperemia*

Functional hyperemia is the increase in mesenteric blood flow immediately after food intake. It is mainly because of **gastrin** and **cholecystokinin** secreted after food intake. In addition to these two GI hormones, digestive products of food substances such as glucose and fatty acids also cause vasodilatation and increase the mesenteric blood flow.

■ SPLENIC CIRCULATION

■ IMPORTANCE OF SPLENIC CIRCULATION

Spleen is the main reservoir for blood. Due to the dilatation of blood vessels, a large amount of blood is stored in spleen. And the constriction of blood vessels by sympathetic stimulation releases blood into circulation.

■ STORAGE OF BLOOD

In spleen, two structures are involved in storage of blood, namely **splenic venous sinuses** and **splenic pulp** (Chapter 25).

Small arteries and arterioles open directly into the venous sinuses. When spleen distends, sinuses swell and large quantity of blood is stored. Capillaries of splenic pulp are highly permeable. So, most of the blood cells pass through capillary membrane and are stored in the pulp.

Venous sinuses and the pulp are lined with **reticuloendothelial cells.**

■ REGULATION OF BLOOD FLOW TO SPLEEN

Blood flow to spleen is regulated by sympathetic nerve fibers.

■ HEPATIC CIRCULATION

■ BLOOD VESSELS

Liver receives blood from two sources:
1. Hepatic artery
2. Portal vein.
   More details are given in Chapter 40.

■ NORMAL BLOOD FLOW

Liver receives maximum amount of blood as compared to any other organ in the body since, most of the metabolic activities are carried out in the liver. Blood flow to liver is 1,500 mL/minute, which forms 30% of the cardiac output. It is about 100 mL/100 g of tissue/minute.

Normally, about 1,100 mL of blood flows through portal vein and remaining 400 mL of blood flows through hepatic artery. However, portal vein carries only about 25% of oxygen to liver. It is because it carries the blood, which has already passed through the blood vessels of GI tract, where oxygen might have been used. Hepatic artery transports 75% of oxygen to the liver.

■ REGULATION OF BLOOD FLOW TO LIVER

Blood flow to liver is regulated by the following factors:

1. *Systemic Blood Pressure*

Systemic blood pressure is the important factor responsible for blood flow to liver and hepatic blood flow is directly proportional to systemic blood pressure.

2. *Splenic Contraction*

During splenic contraction, blood flow to liver increases.

3. *Movements of Intestine*

Motility of intestine increases hepatic blood flow.

4. *Chemical Factors*

Chemical factors which increase the blood flow to liver by vasodilatation are:
   i. Excess carbon dioxide
   ii. Lack of oxygen
   iii. Increase in hydrogen ion concentration.

5. *Nervous Factors*

Sympathetic fibers to liver cause vasoconstriction in liver and decrease the blood flow.

Sympathetic fibers to liver and other portions of splanchnic circulation pass through splanchnic nerve. Role of parasympathetic fibers in hepatic circulation is not known.

Capillary Circulation

- ■ **INTRODUCTION**
  - ■ MICROCIRCULATION
  - ■ FEATURES OF CAPILLARIES
  - ■ DIMENSIONS OF CAPILLARIES
  - ■ VELOCITY AND VOLUME OF BLOOD FLOW
- ■ **STRUCTURE OF CAPILLARIES**
  - ■ ENDOTHELIAL CELLS
  - ■ PERICYTES
- ■ **PATTERN OF CAPILLARY SYSTEM**
  - ■ PREFERENTIAL CHANNELS
  - ■ TRUE CAPILLARIES
  - ■ ANATOMICAL AND PHYSIOLOGICAL SHUNTS
- ■ **PECULIARITIES OF CAPILLARY BLOOD FLOW**
- ■ **FUNCTIONS OF CAPILLARIES**
  - ■ DIFFUSION
  - ■ FILTRATION
  - ■ PINOCYTOSIS
- ■ **FACTORS CONTROLLING CAPILLARY CIRCULATION**
  - ■ NERVOUS FACTORS
  - ■ CHEMICAL FACTORS

■ INTRODUCTION

■ MICROCIRCULATION

Microcirculation refers to flow of blood through the minute blood vessels such as arterioles, capillaries and venules. Capillary circulation forms the major part of microcirculation. Human body contains about 10 billion capillaries.

Study of Capillary Circulation

Blood flow through capillaries is studied by focusing the capillaries under dissecting microscope. Frog's web, mesentery of mammals and fingernail bed of humans can be observed by using microscope.

■ FEATURES OF CAPILLARIES

1. Capillaries arise from arterioles and form the actual functional area of circulatory system, i.e. exchange of materials between blood and tissues
2. Structurally, capillaries are very narrow and short. However, quantitatively, these vessels outnumber the other blood vessels. About 10 billion capillaries are present in the body.
3. Each capillary lies in a very close proximity to the cells of the tissues at a distance of about 20 to 30 mm. This enables easy and rapid exchange of substances between blood and the tissues through interstitial fluid.

■ DIMENSIONS OF CAPILLARIES

Dimensions of capillaries are given in Table 111.1.

TABLE 111.1: Dimensions and details of capillaries

Dimensions/Details	Normal value
Total number of capillaries	10 billion
Surface area of all capillaries	500 to 700 sq m
Average length	0.5 to 1 mm
Average diameter	8 μ
Pressure at arterial end	30 to 32 mm Hg
Pressure at venous end	14 to 16 mm Hg
Velocity of blood flow	0.05 cm/second

■ VELOCITY AND VOLUME OF BLOOD FLOW

Average velocity of blood flow through capillaries is 0.05 cm/second. About 5% of total blood is present in capillaries.

■ STRUCTURE OF CAPILLARIES

Capillaries are formed by single layer of endothelial cells, which are wrapped around by pericytes.

■ ENDOTHELIAL CELLS

Endothelial cells of the capillaries are thin, flattened, nucleated polygonal cells joined together by a cement substance.

Capillaries do not have muscular coat. Yet, these blood vessels actively modify their own diameter in response to nervous, hormonal, chemical and physical stimuli. Endothelial cells themselves alter the diameter of capillaries by swelling or shrinking.

In most of the capillaries, adjacent endothelial cells leave a cleft called fenestra through which several substances may traverse the endothelium by means of transcytosis (Fig. 111.1). However, in cerebral capillaries the fenestra are absent because the endothelial cells fuse to each other by tight junctions (Chapter 163).

■ PERICYTES

Pericyte is a perivascular mesenchymal like cell associated with walls of small blood vessels such as capillaries and postcapillary vessels. It is similar to renal mesangial cell. It is also known as mural cell or Rouget cell (named after the discoverer Charles Rouget).

Pericytes extend long cytoplasmic processes, which wrap around the endothelial cells. Pericytes play important role in remodeling and maintenance of capillary system. These cells are contractile in nature and secrete several vasoactive agents, growth factors, extracellular matrix and components of basement membrane. Pericytes are also involved in regulation of blood flow through endothelial junctions particularly in conditions such as inflammation.

■ PATTERN OF CAPILLARY SYSTEM

Capillaries are disposed between arterioles and venules. From the arterioles, the meta-arterioles take origin (Fig. 111.2). From meta-arterioles, two types of capillaries arise:

1. Preferential channels
2. True capillaries.

■ 1. PREFERENTIAL CHANNELS

Preferential channels are also called continuous capillaries. After arising from meta-arterioles, these capillaries form a network and finally join the venules. Preferential channels or continuous capillaries have same diameter as meta-arterioles.

■ 2. TRUE CAPILLARIES

True capillaries also form a network and join the venules. Diameter of the true capillaries is less than that of the meta-arterioles.

Precapillary Sphincter

Beginning of true capillaries is encircled by smooth muscle fibers. It functions as a sphincter; so it is known as precapillary sphincter. It controls the blood flow through true capillaries.

■ ANATOMICAL AND PHYSIOLOGICAL SHUNTS

Anatomical Shunt

Anatomical shunt is the direct link between arterioles and venules. It is also called arteriovenous shunt. Flow

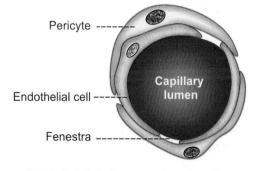

FIGURE 111.1: Cross section of capillary

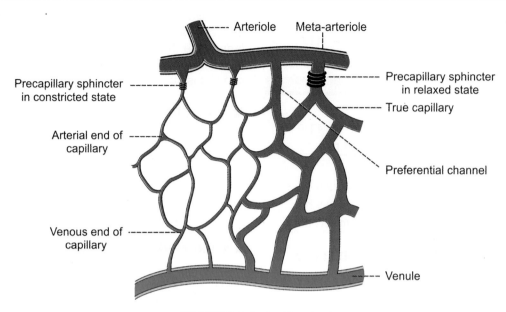

FIGURE 111.2: Capillary bed

of blood through the capillaries where exchange of nutrients, gases and other substances takes place is called nutritional flow. Blood flow through anatomical shunt is called non-nutritional flow. Non-nutritional blood flow occurs in many tissues of the body particularly during resting conditions when metabolic activities are low.

Physiological Shunt

Physiological shunt is the link between arterial and venous side of circulation provided by meta-arteriole. Many tissues of the body such as muscles do not have anatomical shunts. However, the meta-arteriole in these tissues acts as the physiological shunt between arterial and venous sides of the circulation. Non-nutritional blood flow occurs through physiological shunt under resting conditions.

Shunt in Capillaries Vs Shunt in Heart

Physiological shunt in capillaries is different from physiological shunt in heart. In capillaries, the oxygenated blood flows towards deoxygenated blood. But in heart, the deoxygenated blood flows towards the oxygenated blood (Chapter 108).

■ PECULIARITIES OF CAPILLARY BLOOD FLOW

1. Blood does not pass through capillary system continuously. It is because of the alternate cons-

triction and dilatation of meta-arterioles and the alternate opening and closure of precapillary sphincters.
2. Direction of blood flow through capillaries is not fixed as in the case of other blood vessels. Blood may flow in opposite direction in two adjacent capillaries.
3. In capillaries, blood flows as a single pile or single row of blood cells. In other blood vessels, the blood flows in either axial stream containing mainly blood cells or peripheral stream containing plasma.
4. Under resting conditions, most of the capillaries lie in collapsed state. Only during activity, all the capillaries open up and increase the vascularity.
5. Amount of blood flowing through the capillary system throughout the body is very low. It is only about 150 mL/minute.
6. Velocity of blood flow is least in capillaries. It is only about 0.05 cm/second. It facilitates exchange of substances between capillaries and tissues.

■ FUNCTIONS OF CAPILLARIES

Most important function of capillaries is the exchange of substances between blood and tissues. Oxygen, nutrients and other essential substances enter the tissues from capillary blood; carbon dioxide, metabolites and other unwanted substances are removed from the tissues by capillary blood.

Exchange of materials across the capillary endothelium occurs by the following processes:
1. Diffusion
2. Filtration
3. Pinocytosis.

■ DIFFUSION

Diffusion is the main process for exchange of gases, water, glucose, sodium, urea and many other substances. These substances diffuse through the intercellular clefts present in the endothelial wall of the capillaries. Diffusion occurs because of concentration gradient across the capillary wall.

■ FILTRATION

Site of filtration of substances through capillary membrane varies in different organs. In skeletal muscles, cardiac muscles, kidneys and intestine, filtration occurs through the slit pores present in capillary endothelium. Capillaries in other organs have discontinued endothelium through which filtration occurs.

Filtration of substances through capillary endothelium depends upon the net filtration pressure. Net filtration pressure is the balance between the driving pressures and the opposing pressures. It is well explained by Starling hypothesis (Chapter 52). Process of filtration is explained in Chapter 27.

■ PINOCYTOSIS

Larger molecules are transported across the capillary endothelium in the form of vesicles. Large molecules are packed as vesicles in the capillary endothelial cells. These vesicles are transported across the endothelial membrane by the process called pinocytosis (Chapter 3).

■ FACTORS CONTROLLING CAPILLARY CIRCULATION

Capillary blood flow is controlled by the nervous and chemical factors.

■ NERVOUS FACTORS

Capillaries are mainly supplied by the sympathetic vasoconstrictor fibers.

■ CHEMICAL FACTORS

Many chemical factors such as excess of carbon dioxide, increased hydrogen ion concentration, lack of oxygen, histamine and metabolites like lactic acid cause dilatation of capillaries. Serotonin causes constriction of capillaries.

Circulation through Skeletal Muscle

Chapter 112

> ■ INTRODUCTION
> ■ FACTORS REGULATING BLOOD FLOW TO SKELETAL MUSCLE
>   ■ MECHANICAL FACTORS
>   ■ CHEMICAL FACTORS
>   ■ NERVOUS FACTORS
> ■ APPLIED PHYSIOLOGY – VARICOSE VEINS

■ INTRODUCTION

During resting condition, blood flow to skeletal muscle is 4 to 7 mL/100 g/minute. During exercise, it increases to about 100 mL/100 g/minute.

■ FACTORS REGULATING BLOOD FLOW TO SKELETAL MUSCLE

Blood flow through skeletal muscle is regulated by three factors:
1. Mechanical factors
2. Chemical factors
3. Nervous factors.

■ MECHANICAL FACTORS

During contraction of the muscle, blood vessels are compressed and the blood flow decreases. And during relaxation of the muscle, compression of blood vessels is relieved and the blood flow increases.

In severe muscular exercise, blood flow increases in between the muscular contractions.

■ CHEMICAL FACTORS

Important chemical factors, which regulate the blood flow through skeletal muscles, are lack of oxygen, excess of carbon dioxide and increased hydrogen ion concentration. All these chemical factors increase the blood flow to muscle by causing vasodilatation.

■ NERVOUS FACTORS

Blood vessels of the skeletal muscles are mostly innervated by sympathetic nerve fibers and few parasympathetic nerve fibers are also seen. Special feature of sympathetic nerve fibers supplying the skeletal muscles is that these nerve fibers are **vasodilators** and not constrictors. Since the sympathetic nerve fibers cause dilatation of blood vessels in muscle by secreting acetylcholine, these nerve fibers are called **sympathetic vasodilator fibers** or **sympathetic cholinergic fibers.**

■ APPLIED PHYSIOLOGY – VARICOSE VEINS

Varicose vein is the vein that becomes irregularly swollen (twisted or tortuous) and enlarged. Superficial veins of the leg are mostly affected.

Causes for Varicose Vein

1. Permanent dilatation of veins due to **incompetence** of the valves of the veins or absence of muscular activity for long periods. So, varicose veins are common in the individuals with occupations, which require standing for long periods.
2. Thrombophlebitis (inflammation of vein associated with formation of thrombus).

Varicose veins may also develop in obese persons and pregnant women.

Varicose Vein in Obesity

Obesity is the major factor for varicose veins. Excess fat increases the pressure on veins of legs and aggravate the condition.

Varicose Vein in Pregnancy

During pregnancy, varicose veins develop because of two reasons:

1. Increased blood level of progesterone, which dilates the blood vessel
2. Enlarged uterus, which compresses the major veins in pelvic region leading to increase in venous pressure.

Cutaneous Circulation

Chapter 113

- ■ ARCHITECTURE OF CUTANEOUS BLOOD VESSELS
- ■ FUNCTIONS OF CUTANEOUS CIRCULATION
- ■ NORMAL BLOOD FLOW TO SKIN
- ■ REGULATION OF CUTANEOUS BLOOD FLOW
- ■ APPLIED PHYSIOLOGY – VASCULAR RESPONSES OF SKIN TO MECHANICAL STIMULI
  - ■ WHITE REACTION
  - ■ LEWIS TRIPLE RESPONSE

■ ARCHITECTURE OF CUTANEOUS BLOOD VESSELS

Architecture of cutaneous blood vessels is formed in the following manner:

1. **Arterioles** arising from the smaller arteries reach the base of **papillae of dermis** (Chapter 60)
2. Then, these arterioles turn horizontally and give rise to **meta-arterioles**
3. From meta-arterioles, hairpin-shaped **capillary loops** arise. Arterial limb of the loop ascends vertically in the papillae and turns to form a venous limb, which descends down.
4. After reaching the base of papillae, few venous limbs of neighboring papillae unite to form the **collecting venule**
5. Collecting venules anastomose with one another to form the **subpapillary venous plexus**
6. Subpapillary plexus runs horizontally beneath the bases of papillae and drain into **deeper veins.**

■ FUNCTIONS OF CUTANEOUS CIRCULATION

Cutaneous blood flow performs two functions:

1. Supply of nutrition to skin
2. Regulation of body temperature by heat loss.

■ NORMAL BLOOD FLOW TO SKIN

Under normal conditions, the blood flow to skin is about 250 mL/square meter/minute. When the body temperature increases, cutaneous blood flow increases up to 2,800 mL/square meter/minute because of cutaneous vasodilatation.

■ REGULATION OF CUTANEOUS BLOOD FLOW

Cutaneous blood flow is regulated mainly by body temperature. Hypothalamus plays an important role in regulating cutaneous blood flow.

When body temperature increases, the hypothalamus is activated. Hypothalamus in turn causes cutaneous vasodilatation by acting through medullary vasomotor center. Now, blood flow increases in skin. Increase in cutaneous blood flow causes the loss of heat from the body through sweat. When body temperature is low, vasoconstriction occurs in the skin. Therefore, the blood flow to skin decreases and prevents the heat loss from skin.

■ APPLIED PHYSIOLOGY – VASCULAR RESPONSES OF SKIN TO MECHANICAL STIMULI

Vascular responses of skin are the reactions developed in blood vessels of skin when some mechanical stimuli are applied over the surface of it.

Vascular responses of skin are of two types:

A. White reaction
B. Lewis triple response.

■ WHITE REACTION

White reaction is the response of the blood vessels in skin to a mechanical stimulus. When the surface of skin is stroked lightly with a pointed object, a pale line appears within 20 seconds. This line takes the path of the stroke. This response in skin is known as white reaction. Maximum intensity of the line is obtained in 1 minute and it fades away after 5 minutes.

White reaction is due to the **constriction of cutaneous capillaries.** Capillaries constrict because of the local stimulation of capillary wall and exertion of tension upon capillary wall. No nervous factor is involved in this process.

■ LEWIS TRIPLE RESPONSE

Lewis triple response is the vascular response of skin that includes three consecutive reactions of blood vessels of skin to a mechanical stimulus. It was discovered by **Lewis Sir Thomas** in 1927. He noticed that the vascular reactions of skin to various injuries occur in three stages and named these reactions as triple response.

Three reactions of this response:
1. Red reaction
2. Flare
3. Wheal.

1. *Red Reaction*

Red reaction is the appearance of a **red line** when a pointed instrument is drawn firmly over the surface of the skin. This reaction occurs over the line of the stroke. Red reaction appears within 15 seconds after the stroke. It obtains the maximum intensity at the end of 1 minute and disappears later gradually.

Red reaction is because of **dilatation of capillaries** due to mechanical stimulus. This reaction is purely a local response. It occurs due to the release of histamine-like substance from the tissues damaged by the stimulus. Lewis called it **'H' substance.**

Red reaction does not depend upon nervous factors. It occurs even after the sectioning or degeneration of nerves of skin.

2. *Flare*

If the stroke is applied with little more force or if the stroke is repeated on the same line, the red reaction spreads around the line of stroke. It spreads for about 10 cm from the line of stroke, depending upon the force applied. This is called flare or **spreading flush.** Flare appears within 30 seconds after appearance of red line. It also disappears later. Flare is due to **dilatation of arterioles.** It depends upon nervous mechanism and is due to **axon reflex.**

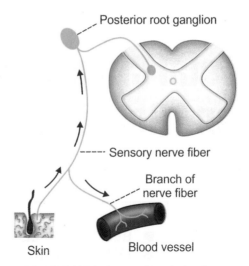

FIGURE 113.1: Axon reflex during flare

Axon Reflex

Axon reflex or antidromic reflex is the process by which the impulses are conducted in a direction opposite to the normal direction. Normally, the impulses produced by a cutaneous pain receptor pass through sensory nerve fiber towards the nerve cell body in posterior nerve root ganglion. Some of these impulses pass through the other branches of the same fiber in the opposite direction and reach the blood vessels supplied by these branches. Impulses now dilate the blood vessels. This is called the **antidromic** or axon reflex (Fig. 113.1). Nerve fibers transmitting the impulses in the opposite direction are called **antidromic vasodilator fibers.**

Flare occurs if the main trunk of nerves is cut. It does not occur when the nerves degenerate.

3. *Wheal*

When intensity of stimulus is severe, the surface of skin on the line of stroke is interrupted. A small elevation or swelling is seen in the surrounding area up to a height of 2 mm. It is called wheal or local edema.

Wheal appears within 3 minutes after the stimulus and it replaces the red line. Maximum height is obtained within 5 minutes and it disappears after several hours.

Wheal appears due to the leakage of fluid from capillaries. The permeability of capillary membrane is increased. Wheal does not depend upon nervous mechanism.

Dermographism

The process of embossing signs over skin is called dermographism. It is also called **writing on skin.** Some letters or designs can be embossed upon the skin over back or in the forearm in the same manner by which the wheal is produced.

Fetal Circulation and Respiration

Chapter 114

- ■ INTRODUCTION
- ■ BLOOD VESSELS IN FETUS
- ■ FETAL LUNGS
- ■ CHANGES IN CIRCULATION AND RESPIRATION AFTER BIRTH – NEONATAL CIRCULATION AND RESPIRATION
  - ■ FIRST BREATH OF THE CHILD
  - ■ FLOW OF BLOOD TO LUNGS
  - ■ CLOSURE OF FORAMEN OVALE
  - ■ REVERSAL OF BLOOD FLOW IN DUCTUS ARTERIOSUS
  - ■ CLOSURE OF DUCTUS VENOSUS
  - ■ CLOSURE OF DUCTUS ARTERIOSUS

■ INTRODUCTION

Fetal circulation is different from that of adults because of the presence of **placenta.** Since fetal lungs are non-functioning, placenta is responsible for exchange of gases between fetal blood and mother's blood. So, the blood from right ventricle is diverted to placenta.

Development of heart is completed at 4th week of intrauterine life and it starts beating at the rate of 65 per minute. Along with heart, the blood vessels also develop. Heart rate gradually increases and reaches the maximum rate of about 140 beats per minute just before birth.

Fetus is connected with the mother through placenta. Fetal blood passes to placenta through umbilical vessels and the maternal blood runs through uterine vessels. These two sets of blood vessels lie in close proximity in the placenta through which exchange of substances takes place between mother's blood and fetal blood. However, there is no direct admixture of maternal and fetal blood (Fig. 114.1).

■ BLOOD VESSELS IN FETUS

As **fetal lungs** are **non-functioning,** there is no necessity of large amount of blood to be pumped into lungs. Instead, the fetal heart pumps large quantity of blood into the placenta for exchange of substances. From

placenta, the **umbilical veins** collect the blood, which has more oxygen and nutrients. Umbilical vein passes through liver. Some amount of blood is supplied to liver from umbilical vein. However, a large quantity of blood is diverted from umbilical vein into the **inferior vena cava** through **ductus venosus.** Liver receives blood from portal vein also.

In liver, the oxygenated blood mixes slightly with deoxygenated blood and enters the right atrium via inferior vena cava. From right atrium, major portion of blood is diverted into left atrium via **foramen ovale.** Foramen ovale is an opening in intra-atrial septum.

Blood from upper part of the body enters the right atrium through superior vena cava. From right atrium, blood enters right ventricle. From here, blood is pumped into pulmonary artery. From pulmonary artery, blood enters the systemic aorta through **ductus arteriosus.** Only a small quantity of blood is supplied to fetal lungs. Blood from left ventricle is pumped into aorta. Fifty percent of blood from aorta reaches the placenta through **umbilical arteries.**

■ FETAL LUNGS

Pulmonary vascular resistance is the resistance offered to blood flow through pulmonary vascular bed. This resistance is very high in fetus because of the non-

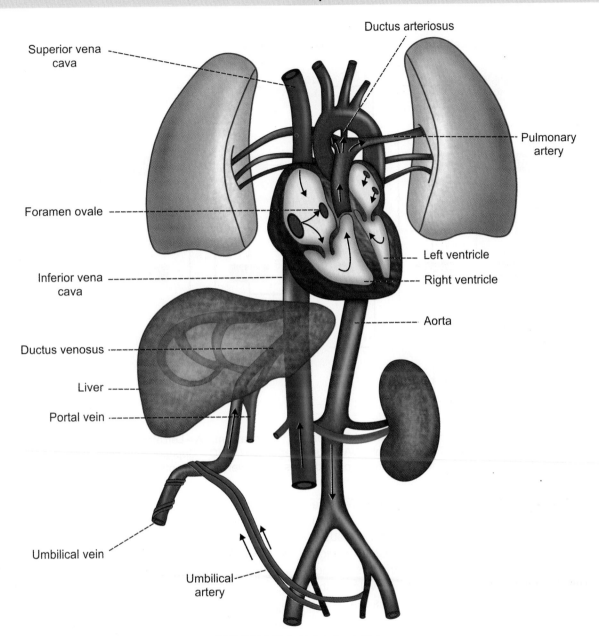

FIGURE 114.1: Fetal circulation

functioning of fetal lungs. The high resistance in fetal lungs increases the pressure in the blood vessels of lungs. Because of the high pressure, the blood is diverted from pulmonary artery into aorta via ductus arteriosus.

■ CHANGES IN CIRCULATION AND RESPIRATION AFTER BIRTH – NEONATAL CIRCULATION AND RESPIRATION

■ 1. FIRST BREATH OF THE CHILD

When fetus is delivered and umbilical cord is cut and tied, the lungs start functioning. When placental blood flow is cut off, there is sudden **hypoxia** and **hypercapnia.** Now,

the respiratory center is strongly stimulated by these two factors and the respiration starts. Initially, there is **gasping,** which is followed by normal respiration.

■ 2. FLOW OF BLOOD TO LUNGS

Lungs expand during the first breath of the infant. Expansion of lungs causes immediate reduction in the pulmonary vascular resistance and a sudden fall in pressure in the blood vessels of lungs. Therefore, the blood flow from pulmonary artery to lungs increases.

■ 3. CLOSURE OF FORAMEN OVALE

When blood starts flowing through the pulmonary circulation, the oxygenated blood from the lungs returns to

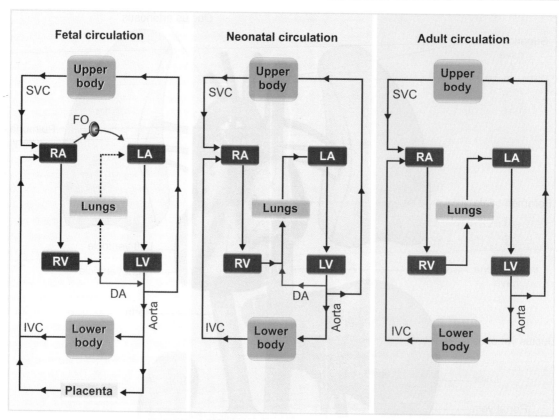

FIGURE 114.2: Fetal, neonatal and adult circulation. RA = Right atrium, LA = Left atrium, RV = Right ventricle, LV = Left ventricle, FO = Foramen ovale, DA = Ductus arteriosus, SVC = Superior vena cava, IVC = Inferior vena cava, Dashed blue line (Fetal circulation) indicates flow of very less quantity of blood.

left atrium. It causes increase in the left atrial pressure. Simultaneously, due to stoppage of blood from placenta, pressure in inferior vena cava is decreased. It leads to fall in right atrial pressure. Thus, the pressure in right atrium is less and the pressure in left atrium is already high. This causes the closure of foramen ovale. Within few days after birth, the foramen ovale closes completely and fuses with the atrial wall.

■ 4. REVERSAL OF BLOOD FLOW IN DUCTUS ARTERIOSUS

In fetus, since pulmonary arterial pressure is very high, the blood passes from pulmonary artery into aorta via ductus arteriosus. However, in neonatal life, since the systemic arterial pressure is more than pulmonary arterial pressure, the blood passes in **opposite direction** in ductus arteriosus, i.e. from systemic aorta into pulmo-

nary aorta (Fig. 114.2). The **reversed flow** in ductus arteriosus is heard as **continuous murmur** in infants.

■ 5. CLOSURE OF DUCTUS VENOSUS

Due to the contraction of smooth muscle near junction between umbilical vein and ductus venosus, the constriction and closure of ductus venosus occurs. Later, the ductus venosus becomes fibrous band.

■ 6. CLOSURE OF DUCTUS ARTERIOSUS

Ductus arteriosus starts closing due to narrowing. It closes completely after 2 days and the adult type of circulation starts. In some rare cases, the ductus arteriosus does not close. It remains intact producing a continuous murmur. This condition with intact ductus arteriosus is known as **patent ductus arteriosus** (Refer to Chapter 106).

Hemorrhage

Chapter 115

- ■ DEFINITION
- ■ TYPES AND CAUSES OF HEMORRHAGE
  - ■ ACCIDENTAL HEMORRHAGE
  - ■ CAPILLARY HEMORRHAGE
  - ■ INTERNAL HEMORRHAGE
  - ■ POSTPARTUM HEMORRHAGE
  - ■ HEMORRHAGE DUE TO PREMATURE DETACHMENT OF PLACENTA
- ■ COMPENSATORY EFFECTS OF HEMORRHAGE
  - ■ IMMEDIATE COMPENSATORY EFFECTS OF HEMORRHAGE
  - ■ DELAYED COMPENSATORY EFFECTS OF HEMORRHAGE

■ DEFINITION

Hemorrhage is defined as the excess loss of blood due to rupture of blood vessels.

■ TYPES AND CAUSES OF HEMORRHAGE

Hemorrhage occurs due to various reasons. Based on the cause, hemorrhage is classified into five categories:

■ 1. ACCIDENTAL HEMORRHAGE

Accidental hemorrhage occurs in road accidents and industrial accidents, which are very common in the developed and developing countries.

Accidental hemorrhage is of two types:
  i. Primary hemorrhage, which occurs immediately after the accident
  ii. Secondary hemorrhage, which takes place sometime (about few hours) after the accident.

■ 2. CAPILLARY HEMORRHAGE

Capillary hemorrhage is the bleeding due to the rupture of blood vessels, particularly capillaries. It is very common in brain (**cerebral hemorrhage**) and heart during cardiovascular diseases. The rupture of the capillary is followed by spilling of blood into the surrounding areas.

■ 3. INTERNAL HEMORRHAGE

Internal hemorrhage is the bleeding in viscera. It is caused by rupture of blood vessels in the viscera. The blood accumulates in viscera.

■ 4. POSTPARTUM HEMORRHAGE

Excess bleeding that occurs immediately after labor (delivery of the baby) is called postpartum hemorrhage. In some cases, it is very severe and leads to major complications.

■ 5. HEMORRHAGE DUE TO PREMATURE DETACHMENT OF PLACENTA

In some cases, the placenta is detached from the uterus of mother before the due date of delivery causing severe hemorrhage.

■ COMPENSATORY EFFECTS OF HEMORRHAGE

Many effects are observed during and after hemorrhage. Effects are different in acute hemorrhage and chronic hemorrhage.

Acute Hemorrhage

Acute hemorrhage is the sudden loss of large quantity of blood. It occurs in conditions like accidents. Decreased blood volume in acute hemorrhage causes **hypovolemic shock** (Chapter 116).

Chronic Hemorrhage

Chronic hemorrhage is the loss of blood either by internal or by external bleeding over a long period of time. Internal bleeding occurs in conditions like ulcer. External bleeding occurs in conditions like hemophilia and excess vaginal bleeding (menorrhagia). Chronic hemorrhage produces different types of effects such as anemia.

Compensatory Effects

After hemorrhage, series of compensatory reactions develop in the body to cope up with the blood loss.

Compensatory effects of hemorrhage are of two types.
A. Immediate compensatory effects
B. Delayed compensatory effects.

■ IMMEDIATE COMPENSATORY EFFECTS OF HEMORRHAGE

1. On Cardiovascular System

Reduced blood volume after hemorrhage decreases venous return, ventricular filling and cardiac output. In severe hemorrhage, there is fall in blood pressure also. However, when blood loss is slow or less, the arterial blood pressure is not affected much. If it is affected it is restored quickly.

During mild hemorrhage

During slow or mild hemorrhage when there is loss of a small amount of blood up to 350 to 500 mL the blood pressure decreases slightly and soon it returns back to normal.

Mechanism involved in maintenance of blood pressure:
  i. Usually when arterial blood pressure increases, the carotid and aortic baroreceptors are stimulated and send impulses to brain resulting in decrease in blood pressure (Chapter 103). During hemorrhage when the arterial blood pressure falls, baroreceptors become inactivated and stop discharging impulses.
  ii. This increases the vasomotor tone leading to vasoconstriction. This type of reflex vasoconstriction occurs in all regions of the body except brain and heart.
  iii. Vasoconstriction results in increase in the peripheral resistance
  iv. Loss of blood also causes reflex constriction of veins
  v. Venoconstriction enhances the venous return, ventricular filling and stroke volume
  vi. Thus, because of increased peripheral resistance and stroke volume the arterial blood pressure is restored
  vii. One more factor is involved in this mechanism. Vasoconstriction occurs in the organs having reservoir function such as skin, liver and spleen. Blood from these reservoir organs is directed into systemic circulation. This may compensate the volume of blood that is lost during hemorrhage.

During severe hemorrhage

When hemorrhage is severe with loss of about 1,500 to 2,000 mL of blood, the arterial blood pressure falls to a great extend. It is because of decreased venous return and stroke volume.

In the heart, the reflex tachycardia increases the quantity of metabolic products in myocardium. These metabolic products cause coronary vasodilatation.

2. On Skin

Vasoconstriction in skin, which occurs after hemorrhage decreases the cutaneous blood flow. It increases the deoxygenation of blood and large quantity of reduced hemoglobin is accumulated in cutaneous blood vessels. It results in greyish pallor color of skin.

Sometimes cyanosis develops in certain areas of the body. Skin also becomes cold due to less blood flow. Sweating is decreased.

3. On Tissue Fluid

Arteriolar constriction decreases the capillary pressure. Therefore, tissue fluid enters capillaries. It helps to compensate the blood loss. It also causes **hemodilution.**

4. On Kidneys

Constriction of afferent and efferent arterioles of kidneys after hemorrhage decreases the glomerular filtration rate (GFR) very much. Therefore, the urinary output decreases. The blood level of nitrogenous substances, particularly urea, increases resulting in uremia.

Severe hemorrhage leads to fall in arterial blood pressure and damage of renal tubules resulting in acute **renal failure.**

5. On Renin Secretion

Hypoxia produced after blood loss increases secretion of renin from kidney and the subsequent formation of angiotensin II. Angiotensin II helps in restoring blood pressure by producing generalized vasoconstriction. It also increases release of aldosterone from adrenal cortex. Aldosterone causes retention of sodium and this helps increasing the blood pressure. Angiotensins III and IV are also involved in restoring the blood pressure (Chapter 50).

6. On Secretion of Antidiuretic Hormone

Antidiuretic hormone (ADH) is released in large quantities immediately after the hemorrhage. It is probably due to increased osmolality of body fluid by aldosterone induced sodium retention. ADH promotes water retention and helps in restoring osmolality and volume of ECF.

7. On Secretion of Catecholamines

Sympathetic activity increases due to blood loss. It causes secretion of large quantities of catecholamines, which are also involved in restoring blood pressure by the vasoconstrictor effect.

8. On Respiration

Hemorrhage causes stagnant hypoxia because of decrease in venous return, cardiac output and velocity of blood flow. Hypoxia stimulates the chemoreceptors leading to increase in respiratory rate. The catecholamines, which are secreted in large quantities due to hemorrhage, increase the respiratory movements through **reticular activating system** (RAS).

9. On Nervous System

i. On brain

Though hemorrhage causes vasoconstriction in many organs of the body, it causes vasodilatation in brain. It is because of increased **sympathetic activity.** However, the blood flow to brain is not affected very much after hemorrhage because of **autoregulation.**

ii. On reticular formation

Catecholamines stimulate the RAS. It causes restlessness, anxiety and increased motor activity after hemorrhage. The respiratory movements are also accelerated due to stimulation of RAS.

iii. Fainting

When hemorrhage is severe, cardiac output decreases and blood pressure falls. The autoregulation in brain fails to cope up with the hypotension. So, the blood flow to brain decreases resulting in **fainting** (refer Chapter 116 for details).

iv. Cerebral ischemia

When the blood flow to brain is severely affected due to hypoxia, ischemia of the brain tissues develops within 5 minutes. It causes irreversible damage to brain tissues.

■ DELAYED COMPENSATORY EFFECTS OF HEMORRHAGE

If hemorrhage is not severe, some delayed compensatory reactions occur. These reactions help to restore blood volume, blood pressure and blood flow to different regions of the body.

Delayed reactions are:
1. Restoration of plasma volume
2. Restoration of plasma proteins
3. Restoration of red blood cell count and hemoglobin content.

1. Restoration of Plasma Volume

During the period of hemorrhage itself, tissue fluid starts entering the blood because of low capillary pressure. So, the plasma volume increases.

Because of increase in plasma volume, hemodilution occurs. So, the concentration of plasma proteins and hemoglobin is low. Transport of fluid from tissues is continued for long time after hemorrhage.

2. Restoration of Plasma Proteins

The reserve proteins stored in liver start mobilizing within few hours after hemorrhage. Liver also starts synthesizing the plasma proteins. Restoration of plasma proteins occurs within 3 to 4 days. Plasma proteins help to retain the fluid transported from tissues to blood.

3. Restoration of Red Blood Cell Count and Hemoglobin Content

Hypoxia that is developed after hemorrhage stimulates the secretion of erythropoietin from kidney. Erythropoietin in turn stimulates red bone marrow causing erythropoiesis. However, restoration of RBC count is a slow process. It takes about 4 to 6 weeks. Reticulocyte count increases in blood.

Hemoglobin content also comes back to normal level along with RBC count, if the diet contains adequate quantity of iron and proteins.

Circulatory Shock and Heart Failure

116

- ■ **DEFINITION**
- ■ **MANIFESTATIONS OF CIRCULATORY SHOCK**
- ■ **STAGES OF CIRCULATORY SHOCK**
  - ■ FIRST STAGE OR COMPENSATED STAGE
  - ■ SECOND STAGE OR PROGRESSIVE STAGE
  - ■ THIRD STAGE OR IRREVERSIBLE STAGE
- ■ **TYPES AND CAUSES OF CIRCULATORY SHOCK**
  - ■ SHOCK DUE TO DECREASED BLOOD VOLUME
  - ■ SHOCK DUE TO INCREASED VASCULAR CAPACITY
  - ■ SHOCK DUE TO CARDIAC DISEASES
  - ■ SHOCK DUE TO OBSTRUCTION OF BLOOD FLOW
- ■ **TREATMENT FOR CIRCULATORY SHOCK**
  - ■ BLOOD TRANSFUSION
  - ■ PLASMA TRANSFUSION
  - ■ ADMINISTRATION OF PLASMA SUBSTITUTES
  - ■ ADMINISTRATION OF SYMPATHOMIMETIC DRUGS
  - ■ ADMINISTRATION OF GLUCOCORTICOIDS
  - ■ OXYGEN THERAPY
  - ■ BY CHANGING THE POSTURE
- ■ **HEART FAILURE**
  - ■ INTRODUCTION
  - ■ CAUSES
  - ■ SIGNS AND SYMPTOMS
  - ■ TYPES
  - ■ COMPENSATED VERSUS DECOMPENSATED HEART FAILURE

■ DEFINITION

Shock is a general term that refers to the depression or suppression of body functions produced by any disorder. **Circulatory shock** refers to the shock developed by inadequate blood flow throughout the body. It is a **life-threatening** condition and it may result in death if the affected person is not treated immediately.

■ MANIFESTATIONS OF CIRCULATORY SHOCK

Characteristic feature of all types of circulatory shock is the insufficient blood flow to the tissues particularly

the brain. Major cause of decreased blood flow is the reduction in cardiac output.

Following are the manifestations of circulatory shock:

1. Whenever cardiac output is decreased, arterial blood pressure drops down
2. Low blood pressure produces reflex tachycardia and reflex vasoconstriction
3. Tachycardia decreases the diastolic period. So, filling of the heart reduces leading to decrease in stroke volume and systolic pressure. This decreases the pulse pressure below 20 mm Hg. Pulse also becomes feeble.

4. Stagnant hypoxia develops because of decreased velocity of blood flow
5. Skin becomes pale and cold due to the vaso-constriction
6. Along with hypoxia, cyanosis also develops in many parts of the body, particularly ear lobes and fingertips
7. Glomerular filtration rate (GFR) and urinary output are reduced due to fall in blood pressure and constriction of renal blood vessels
8. Metabolic activities of myocardium are accelerated because of reduced blood flow and increased heart rate. A large amount of lactic acid is produced, resulting in acidosis.
9. Acidosis decreases myocardial efficiency and pump-ing action of the heart leading to further reduction in cardiac output
10. So, the blood flow to vital organs is severely affected
11. Lack of blood flow to brain tissues produces ischemia resulting in fainting and irreparable damage of brain tissues
12. Finally the damage of brain tissues and cardiac arrest kill the victim.

■ STAGES OF CIRCULATORY SHOCK

Circulatory shock occurs in three stages:
1. First stage or compensated stage
2. Second stage or progressive stage
3. Third stage or irreversible stage.

■ FIRST STAGE OR COMPENSATED STAGE

First stage is also called **non-progressive stage.** When blood loss is less than 10% of total volume, the blood pressure decreases only moderately. And the regulatory mechanisms in the body operate successfully to re-establish normal blood pressure and normal blood flow throughout the body. Thus the shock becomes non-progressive and the person recovers. Regulatory mechanisms **involve negative feedback control.**

Regulatory mechanisms are:
i. Baroreceptor mechanism
ii. Renal mechanism
iii. ADH mechanism.

i. *Baroreceptor Mechanism*

Ischemic response by baroreceptors initiates strong sympathetic stimulation, which causes vasoconstriction and tachycardia (Fig. 116.1).

ii. *Renal Mechanism*

Kidneys release large amount of renin that increases the angiotensin II formation. Angiotensin II produces intense vasoconstriction and increases release of aldosterone from adrenal cortex. Aldosterone in turn promotes retention of water and salts by kidneys. This helps in restoration of blood volume.

iii. *ADH Mechanism*

Antidiuretic hormone (ADH) released from posterior pituitary increases retention of water by kidneys. ADH also enhances vasoconstriction.

Because of severe vasoconstriction caused by the regulatory mechanisms, normal blood pressure is re-established. Retention of water by kidneys and the consequent fluid shift mechanism that moves water from interstitial space and intestinal lumen restores the blood volume. And the person recovers if shock is not severe enough to progress further. With proper treatment, the progression can be arrested completely.

■ SECOND STAGE OR PROGRESSIVE STAGE

Second stage is also called **decompensated stage.** When the shock is severe, positive feedback system develops so that regulatory mechanisms become inadequate to compensate. And the shock enters progressive stage. With immediate and appropriate treatment, this stage of shock can be reversed.

During this stage, blood pressure falls to a low level, which is not adequate to maintain the blood flow to cardiac muscle. So the myocardium starts deteriorating because of lack of nutrition and oxygen. **Toxic substances** released from tissues also suppress the myocardium. Particularly, the bacterial toxin called **endotoxin affects** the myocardium severely (Fig. 116.2).

Loss of blood flow also causes suppression of vasomotor system and the sympathetic system. This causes further fall in blood pressure. Due to low pressure, **thrombosis** starts in small blood vessels like capillaries. Now the capillary permeability increases allowing passage of fluid from blood vessels into interstitial space. Finally because of tissue deterioration severe symptoms start appearing. And the shock progresses to irreversible stage.

■ THIRD STAGE OR IRREVERSIBLE STAGE

Third stage is the last stage prior to the collapse. It is also called **refractory stage.** Irreversible stage leads to death regardless of type of treatment offered to the patient. It is because the brain fails to function due to severe **cerebral ischemia.** The blood pressure falls drastically. Even the infusion of blood fails to restore blood pressure. Finally, cardiac failure occurs due to decrease in the myocardial activity and reduced arteriolar tone resulting in **death** of the affected person. Details of this stage are given in Figure 116.3.

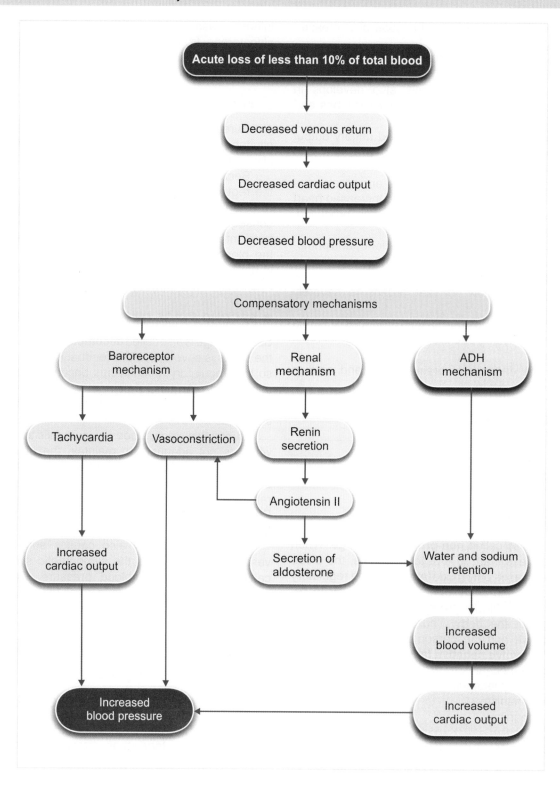

FIGURE 116.1: Compensated stage of circulatory shock. ADH = Antidiuretic hormone.

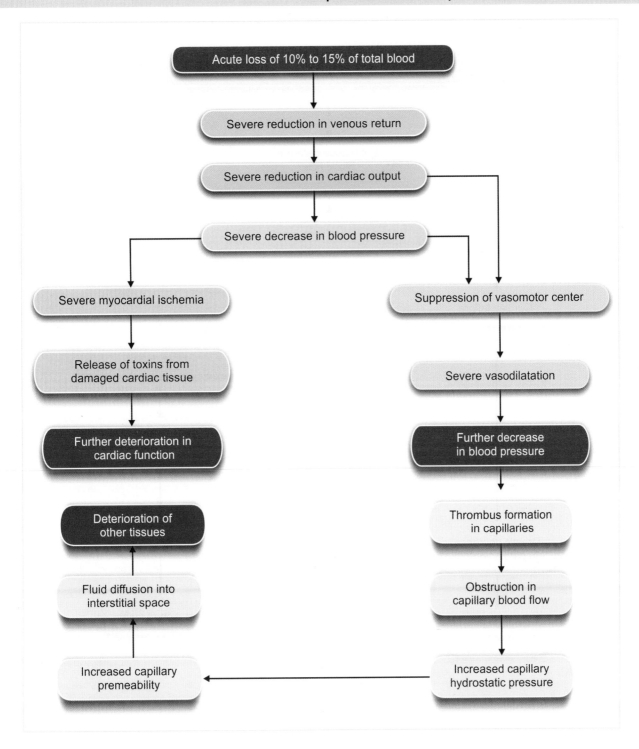

FIGURE 116.2: Progressive stage of circulatory shock

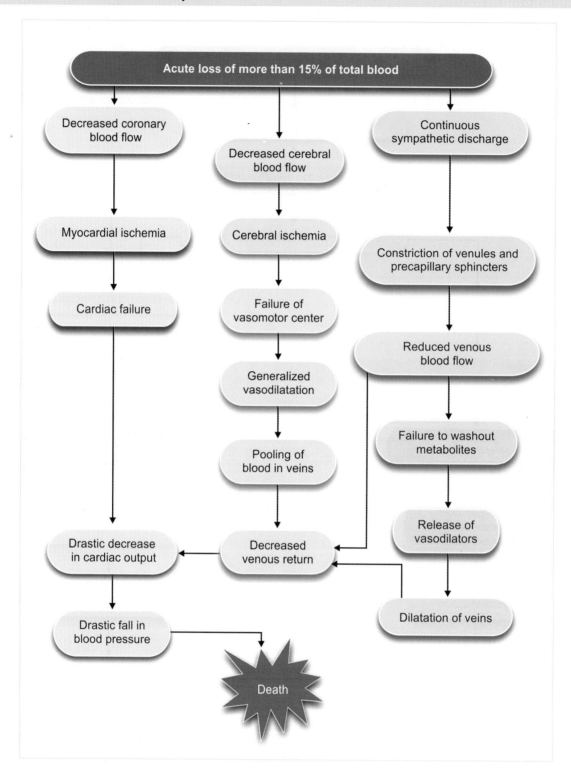

FIGURE 116.3: Irreversible stage of circulatory shock

■ TYPES AND CAUSES OF CIRCULATORY SHOCK

Circulatory shock is primarily classified into four types (Fig. 116.4).
A. Shock due to decreased blood volume
B. Shock due to increased vascular capacity
C. Shock due to cardiac disease
D. Shock due to obstruction of blood flow.

■ SHOCK DUE TO DECREASED BLOOD VOLUME – HYPOVOLEMIC SHOCK

Shock due to decreased blood volume is called hypovolemic shock or cold shock. It occurs when there is acute loss of at least 10% to 15% of blood. Loss of blood less than 10% may not produce any significant effect because of immediate compensatory mechanism.

Important Manifestations of Hypovolemic Shock

1. Decrease in cardiac output
2. Low blood pressure
3. Thin thready pulse
4. Pale and cold skin
5. Increase in respiratory rate
6. Restlessness or lethargy.

Pathological Conditions when Hypovolemic Shock Occurs

1. Hemorrhage: Hemorrhagic shock
2. Trauma: Traumatic shock
3. Surgery: Surgical shock
4. Burns: Burn shock
5. Dehydration: Dehydration shock.

1. *Hemorrhagic Shock*

Hemorrhagic shock is the shock due to hemorrhage. **Acute hemorrhage** as in the case of accident causes shock. **Chronic hemorrhage** as in ulcers does not produce shock. Details of effects of hemorrhage are given in the Chapter 115.

2. *Traumatic Shock*

Trauma means serious injury or wound caused by some external force. Shock caused by trauma is called traumatic shock. Shock occurs due to the damage of muscles and bones, which is common in battlefields and road accidents. Apart from loss of blood, the plasma escapes to the tissue spaces.

Following are the common symptoms of traumatic shock:

Crush syndrome

Crush syndrome is the condition characterized by renal failure when the limb of a person is crushed or compressed in traumatic condition. **Myoglobin** and some **toxic substances** released from affected muscles damage the renal tubular cells leading to **degeneration** of renal tubules. Stimulation of somatic afferents from the damaged muscles causes constriction of renal blood vessels. All these factors result in **renal failure.**

Reperfusion injury

Reperfusion injury refers to dysfunction of myocardium, blood vessels or any other tissue, which is induced by restoration of blood flow to previously ischemic tissue. It is also called **injury by reperfusion.**

Due to compression or damage during traumatic conditions, the ischemic tissues release some toxic substances. Later, when blood supply is restored to the

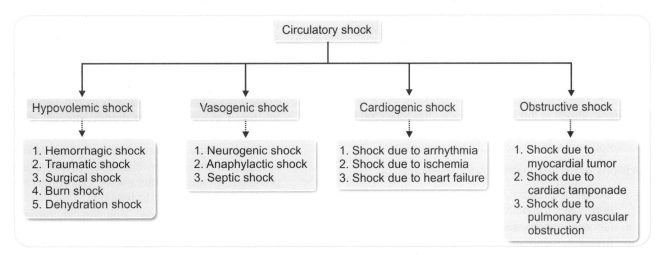

FIGURE 116.4: Different types of circulatory shock

tissues again, the **toxic substances** enter the tissues and cause further damage of the tissues. Common instance is myocardial reperfusion injury.

3. Surgical Shock

Surgical shock is the shock developed by surgical procedures. Surgical shock develops due to some reasons like internal hemorrhage, external hemorrhage and **dehydration** that occur during or after surgical procedures.

4. Burn Shock

Burn shock is the shock produced by the effects of burn. In burns, loss of plasma through the burnt surface is more than the loss of whole blood. It decreases the ECF volume and plasma volume, resulting in **hemoconcentration.** This leads to sluggish blood flow, which decreases the cerebral blood flow causing shock.

5. Dehydration Shock

Shock due to dehydration is called dehydration shock. Dehydration means decrease in water content of the body. It decreases the blood volume resulting in shock. Refer Chapter 6 for the causes of dehydration.

■ SHOCK DUE TO INCREASED VASCULAR CAPACITY – VASOGENIC SHOCK

In this case, the blood volume is normal. Shock occurs because of inadequate blood supply to the tissues due to increased vascular capacity. Capacity of the vascular system increases by the extensive dilatation of blood vessels. It is also known as vasogenic or **low resistance** or **distributive shock.**

Causes and Types of Vasogenic Shock

1. Sudden loss of vasomotor tone: Neurogenic shock
2. Anaphylaxis: Anaphylactic shock
3. Sepsis: Septic shock.

1. Neurogenic Shock

Neurogenic shock is the type of shock characterized by sudden depression of nervous system due to extensive vasodilatation caused by loss of vasomotor tone.

Conditions when neurogenic shock develops

i. Ischemia of brain: Severe ischemia in medulla depresses the activity of vasomotor center
ii. General anesthesia
iii. Spinal anesthesia
iv. Emotional conditions: Extreme emotions cause sudden and exaggerated activity of autonomic

nervous system, the subject faints because of neurogenic shock.

Syncope (Fainting)

Syncope or fainting is the sudden and transient (short-time) loss of consciousness and postural tone with spontaneous recovery. It occurs due to temporary inadequate cerebral blood flow.

Types of syncope:

i. *Vasovagal syncope or emotional fainting:* Fainting is caused by sudden stimulation of vagus nerve. It is also called **neurocardiogenic syncope.** It is due to extreme activation of parasympathetic division of autonomic nervous system. There is sudden decrease in heart rate (bradycardia) because of inhibition of myocardium by vagus. At the same time, the blood pressure also decreases (hypotension) due to severe vasodilatation by the parasympathetic nerve fibers (Fig. 116.5).

Simultaneously, sympathetic tone is decreased and it also causes vasodilatation leading to hypotension.

Because of bradycardia and hypotension, the cerebral blood flow decreases. This results in fainting. Vasovagal syncope is common in conditions like severe emotional distress and exertion.

ii. *Postural syncope:* Loss of consciousness because of **prolonged standing.** It is due to pooling of blood in lower limbs during prolonged standing resulting in decreased blood supply to the brain.

iii. *Micturition syncope:* Fainting during micturition. It is common in the patients who suffer from **orthostatic hypotension.** Fall in blood pressure while standing is called orthostatic hypotension (Chapter 103).

iv. *Effort syncope:* Fainting caused during exercise or any other strain. It is the common symptom in the patients with **stenosis of semilunar valves.** These patients faint during exercise or any other physical strain. It is due to the failure of the heart to increase the cardiac output, when the tissues need more blood flow.

v. *Cough syncope:* Fainting while coughing. Sometimes, severe cough increases intrathoracic pressure, which reduces the venous return and cardiac output leading to fainting.

vi. *Carotid sinus syncope:* Fainting in persons wearing dress with **tight collar.** Tight collar of the dress exerts pressure over the region of carotid sinus. This leads to reduction in heart rate, vasodilatation and fainting.

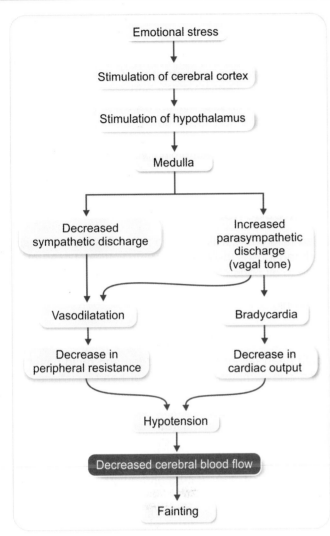

FIGURE 116.5: Schematic representation
of vasovagal syncope

2. Anaphylactic Shock

Anaphylaxis means **exaggerated allergic reaction** to a foreign protein or antigen or any other substance to which the person has been previously sensitized (Chapter 17). Shock that develops during **anaphylactic reactions** is called anaphylactic shock. Shock occurs because of vasodilatation and sudden fall in blood pressure. It is caused by the chemical mediators such as histamine that are secreted during anaphylactic reaction.

3. Septic Shock

Sepsis is the pathological condition characterized by the presence of pathogenic organisms or their toxins in blood or tissues. Shock developed during sepsis is known as septic shock or **blood poisoning.**

Conditions when septic shock occurs

   i. Infection of the uterus and fallopian tube, commonly occurring in abortion by instrumentation
   ii. Infection of peritoneum
   iii. Spreading of skin infection due to bacteria like streptococci or staphylococci
   iv. Spread of infection from any other part of the body.

Septic shock develops due to the depression of myocardium, dilatation of blood vessels and increased permeability of capillary membrane. All these effects occur due to the toxic substances released by bacteria. Septic shock is also called as **vasogenic, cardiogenic** or **hypovolemic shock.**

Endotoxin shock

Endotoxin shock is the shock developed by a bacterial toxin called endotoxin. Endotoxin is a lipopolysaccharide. It causes vasodilatation and depresses myocardial activity. It also activates the macrophages to release cytokines. Endotoxin shock is very common during the infection of alimentary tract by **gram-negative bacteria** like colon bacilli. It is actually released from dead bacteria. Endotoxin shock can also occur in urinary tract infection.

■ SHOCK DUE TO CARDIAC DISEASES – CARDIOGENIC SHOCK

Shock due to cardiac disease is also called cardiogenic shock.

Conditions when Cardiogenic Shock Occurs

1. Arrhythmia, particularly those which lead to reduced cardiac output
2. Depressed activity of myocardium due to ischemia
3. Congestive cardiac disease.

■ SHOCK DUE TO OBSTRUCTION OF BLOOD FLOW – OBSTRUCTIVE SHOCK

Shock developed due to the obstruction of blood flow through circulatory system is called obstructive shock.

Conditions when Obstructive Shock Occurs

1. Tumor in myocardium
2. Cardiac tamponade (Chapter 100)
3. Obstruction of blood vessels in lungs due to embolism.

■ TREATMENT FOR CIRCULATORY SHOCK

Treatment for shock is based on the cause of the shock. Following are the various measures taken during the treatment of shock.

■ BLOOD TRANSFUSION

Transfusion of whole blood is done in hypovolemic shock except burn shock.

■ PLASMA TRANSFUSION

Plasma transfusion is very useful in burns or other shocks in which there is loss of more plasma.

■ ADMINISTRATION OF PLASMA SUBSTITUTES

Plasma substitute is a solution of a substance that is used for transfusion instead of plasma. Plasma substitutes are used when plasma is not available.

Commonly used Plasma Substitutes

   i. Plasma expanders (solutions of sugar with high molecular weight such as dextran); such substances do not escape through capillary membrane
  ii. Concentrated human serum albumin
 iii. Hypertonic solutions, which cause drawing of fluid into blood from interstitial space.

■ ADMINISTRATION OF SYMPATHOMIMETIC DRUGS

Sympathomimetic drugs like epinephrine and norepine-phrine are useful in neurogenic and anaphylactic shocks, which occur due to vasodilatation. These two drugs restore the blood pressure by vasoconstriction. However, the sympathomimetic drugs should not be used for longer period since, these drugs induce severe myocardial activity. In traumatic and cardiogenic shocks, dopamine is used.

■ ADMINISTRATION OF GLUCOCORTICOIDS

Glucocorticoids are administered in serious conditions. Glucocorticoids increase the glucose metabolism in damaged tissues, prevent further damage of tissues and increase the myocardial activity.

■ OXYGEN THERAPY

Oxygen therapy is given only in severe conditions involving reduced oxygenation of tissues.

■ BY CHANGING THE POSTURE

This is the first measure to be taken in cases of hemorrhagic and neurogenic shock. The head down position (by raising the bed at the foot end) increases venous return, cardiac output and cerebral blood flow. However, this should not be used for longer periods because prolonged head down position might affect the ventilation. It is because of effect of the increased pressure exerted by abdominal viscera on diaphragm.

■ HEART FAILURE

■ INTRODUCTION

Heart failure or **cardiac failure** is the condition in which the heart looses the ability to pump sufficient amount of blood to all parts of the body. Heart failure may involve left ventricle or right ventricle or both. It may be acute or chronic.

Acute Heart Failure

Acute heart failure refers to sudden and rapid onset of signs and symptoms of abnormal heart functions. Its symptoms are severe initially. However, the symptoms last for a very short time and the condition improves rapidly. Usually it requires treatment.

Chronic Heart Failure

Chronic heart failure is the heart failure that is charac-terized by the symptoms that appear slowly over a period of time and become worst gradually.

Congestive Heart Failure

Congestive heart failure is a general term used to describe the heart failure resulting in accumulation of fluid in lungs and other tissues. When heart is not able to pump blood through aorta, the blood remains in heart. It results in dilatation of the chambers and accumulation of blood in veins **(vascular congestion). Fluid retention** and **pulmonary edema** also occur in this condition.

■ CAUSES OF HEART FAILURE

Common causes of heart failure are:
1. Coronary artery disease
2. Defective heart valves
3. Arrhythmia
4. Cardiac muscle disease such as cardiomyopathy
5. Hypertension
6. Congenital heart disease

7. Diabetes
8. Hyperthyroidism
9. Anemia
10. Lung disorders
11. Inflammation of cardiac muscle **(myocarditis)** due to viral infection, drugs, alcohol, etc.

■ SIGNS AND SYMPTOMS OF HEART FAILURE

Signs and Symptoms of Chronic Heart Failure

1. Fatigue and weakness
2. Rapid and irregular heartbeat
3. Shortness of breathing
4. Fluid retention and weight gain
5. Loss of appetite
6. Nausea and vomiting
7. Cough
8. Chest pain, if developed by myocardial infarction.

Signs and Symptoms of Acute Heart Failure

Signs and symptoms of acute heart failure may be same as chronic heart failure. But the signs and symptoms appear suddenly and severely. When heart starts to fail suddenly, the fluid accumulates in lungs causing pulmonary edema. It results in sudden and severe shortness of breath, cough with pink, foamy mucus and heart palpitations. It may lead to sudden death, if not attended immediately.

■ TYPES OF HEART FAILURE

1. Systolic Heart Failure

Systolic heart failure is the heart failure due to the decreased ability of heart to contract. It may involve right heart or left heart or both. It is caused either by muscular weakness or valvular defect. Ventricles may be filled with blood but cannot pump it out with sufficient force. Ejection fraction decreases to about 20%. So the amount of blood pumped to the body and to the lungs is decreased. As a result, more amount of blood remains in ventricle. Later the blood starts accumulating in lungs or systemic veins or both. Usually the ventricle enlarges in systolic heart failure.

2. Diastolic Heart Failure

Diastolic heart failure is the heart failure that occurs when the ventricles cannot relax properly due to the stiffening of cardiac muscle. So, there is reduction in ventricular filling and cardiac output.

3. Right Sided Heart Failure

Right sided heart failure occurs due to loss of pumping action of the right side of the heart. Because of loss of pumping action of right ventricle, blood accumulates in right atrium and blood vessels. It causes edema in the feet, ankles, legs and abdomen.

4. Left Sided Heart Failure

Left sided heart failure is due to the loss of pumping action of the left side of the heart. It causes congestion of lungs.

■ COMPENSATED VERSUS DECOMPENSATED HEART FAILURE

Chronic heart failure may be compensated or decompensated.

Compensated Heart Failure

Compensated heart failure is the heart failure with adequate cardiac output. Heart tries to maintain cardiac output by normal compensatory mechanisms such as increase in heart rate, increase in force of ventricular contraction and ventricular hypertrophy. In compensated heart failure, the symptoms are stable and features of fluid retention and pulmonary edema are absent. Eventually, in most of the patients the heart can no longer meet the demand even by compensatory mechanisms and this condition leads to decompensated heart failure.

Decompensated Heart Failure

Decompensated heart failure is the heart failure with inadequate cardiac output. It is characterized by deterioration and sudden and drastic worsening of cardiac function, resulting in death.

Cardiovascular Adjustments during Exercise

- ■ INTRODUCTION
- ■ TYPES OF EXERCISE
  - ■ DYNAMIC EXERCISE
  - ■ STATIC EXERCISE
- ■ AEROBIC AND ANAEROBIC EXERCISES
  - ■ AEROBIC EXERCISE
  - ■ ANAEROBIC EXERCISE
  - ■ METABOLISM IN AEROBIC AND ANAEROBIC EXERCISES
- ■ SEVERITY OF EXERCISE
  - ■ MILD EXERCISE
  - ■ MODERATE EXERCISE
  - ■ SEVERE EXERCISE
- ■ EFFECTS OF EXERCISE
  - ■ ON BLOOD
  - ■ ON BLOOD VOLUME
  - ■ ON HEART RATE
  - ■ ON CARDIAC OUTPUT
  - ■ ON VENOUS RETURN
  - ■ ON BLOOD FLOW TO SKELETAL MUSCLES
  - ■ ON BLOOD PRESSURE

■ INTRODUCTION

During exercise, there is an increase in metabolic needs of body tissues, particularly the muscles.

Various adjustments in the body during exercise are aimed at:

1. Supply of various metabolic requisites like nutrients and oxygen to muscles and other tissues involved in exercise
2. Prevention of increase in body temperature.

■ TYPES OF EXERCISE

Exercise is generally classified into two types depending upon the type of muscular contraction:

1. Dynamic exercise
2. Static exercise.

Cardiovascular changes are slightly different in these two types of exercise.

■ DYNAMIC EXERCISE

Dynamic exercise primarily involves the **isotonic muscular contraction.** It keeps the joints and muscles moving. Examples are swimming, bicycling, walking, etc. Dynamic exercise involves **external work,** which is the shortening of muscle fibers against load.

In this type of exercise, the heart rate, force of contraction, cardiac output and systolic blood pressure increase. However, the diastolic blood pressure is unaltered or decreased. It is because, during dynamic exercise, peripheral resistance is unaltered or decreased depending upon the severity of exercise.

■ STATIC EXERCISE

Static exercise involves **isometric muscular contraction** without movement of joints. Example is pushing heavy object. Static exercise does not involve **external work.**

During this exercise, apart from increase in heart rate, force of contraction, cardiac output and systolic blood pressure, the diastolic blood pressure also increases. It is because of increase in peripheral resistance during static exercise.

■ AEROBIC AND ANAEROBIC EXERCISES

Based on the type of metabolism involved, exercise is classified into two types:

1. Aerobic exercise
2. Anaerobic exercise.

The terms aerobic and anaerobic refer to the energy producing process during exercise. Aerobic means **'with air'** or **'with oxygen'**. Anaerobic means **'without air'** or **'without oxygen'**. Both aerobic and anaerobic exercises are required to maintain physical fitness.

■ AEROBIC EXERCISE

Aerobic exercise involves activities with lower intensity, which is performed for longer period. The energy is obtained by utilizing nutrients in the presence of oxygen and hence it is called aerobic exercise. At the beginning, the body obtains energy by burning glycogen stored in liver. After about 20 minutes, when stored glycogen is exhausted the body starts burning fat. Body fat is converted into glucose, which is utilized for energy.

Aerobic exercise requires large amount of oxygen to obtain the energy needed for prolonged exercise.

Examples of aerobic exercise:

1. Fast walking
2. Jogging
3. Running
4. Bicycling
5. Skiing
6. Skating
7. Hockey
8. Soccer
9. Tennis
10. Badminton
11. Swimming
12. Rowing.

■ ANAEROBIC EXERCISE

Anaerobic exercise involves exertion for short periods followed by periods of rest. It uses the muscles at high intensity and a high rate of work for a short period.

Body obtains energy by burning glycogen stored in the muscles without oxygen hence it is called anaerobic exercise.

Burning glycogen without oxygen liberates lactic acid. Accumulation of lactic acid leads to fatigue. Therefore, this type of exercise cannot be performed for longer period. And a recovery period is essential before going for another burst of anaerobic exercise. Anaerobic exercise helps to increase the muscle strength.

Examples of anaerobic exercise:

1. Pull-ups
2. Push-ups
3. Weightlifting
4. Sprinting
5. Any other rapid burst of strenuous exercise.

■ METABOLISM IN AEROBIC AND ANAEROBIC EXERCISES

When a person starts doing some exercise like jogging, bicycling or swimming, the muscles start utilizing energy. In order to have quick energy during the first few minutes, the muscles burn glycogen stored in them. During this period, fat is not burnt. Only glycogen is burnt and it is burnt without using oxygen. This is called **anaerobic metabolism.** Lactic acid is produced during this period. Presence of lactic acid causes some sort of burning sensation in the muscles particularly the muscles of arms, legs and back.

Muscles burn all the muscle glycogen within 3 to 5 minutes. If the person continues the exercise beyond this, glycogen stored in liver is converted into glucose, which is transported to muscles through blood. Now the body moves into **aerobic metabolism.** The glucose obtained from liver is burnt in the presence of oxygen. No more lactic acid is produced. So the burning sensation in the muscles disappears. Proper breathing is essential during this period so that adequate oxygen is supplied to the muscles to extract the energy from glucose. The supply of glucose from liver in combination with adequate availability of oxygen allows the person to continue the exercise.

Utilization of all the glycogen stored in liver is completed by about 20 minutes. If the exercise is continued beyond this, the body starts utilizing the fat. The stored fat called body fat is converted into carbohydrate, which is utilized by the muscles. This allows the person to do the exercise for a longer period.

■ SEVERITY OF EXERCISE

Cardiovascular and other changes in the body depend upon the severity of exercise also. Based on severity, the exercise is classified into three types.

■ 1. MILD EXERCISE

Mild exercise is the very simple form of exercise like slow walking. Little or no change occurs in cardiovascular system during mild exercise.

■ 2. MODERATE EXERCISE

Moderate exercise does not involve strenuous muscular activity. So, this type of exercise can be performed for a longer period. Exhaustion does not occur at the end of moderate exercise. The examples of this type of exercise are fast walking and slow running.

■ 3. SEVERE EXERCISE

Severe exercise involves strenuous muscular activity. The severity can be maintained only for short duration. Fast running for a distance of 100 or 400 meters is the best example of this type of exercise. Complete exhaustion occurs at the end of severe exercise.

■ EFFECTS OF EXERCISE ON CARDIOVASCULAR SYSTEM

■ 1. ON BLOOD

Mild hypoxia developed during exercise stimulates the juxtaglomerular apparatus to secrete erythropoietin. It stimulates the bone marrow and causes release of red blood cells. Increased carbon dioxide content in blood decreases the pH of blood.

■ 2. ON BLOOD VOLUME

More heat is produced during exercise and the thermo-regulatory system is activated. This in turn, causes secretion of large amount of sweat leading to:
  i. Fluid loss
  ii. Reduced blood volume
  iii. Hemoconcentration
  iv. Sometimes, severe exercise leads to even dehydration.

■ 3. ON HEART RATE

Heart rate increases during exercise. Even the thought of exercise or preparation for exercise increases the heart rate. It is because of impulses from cerebral cortex to medullary centers, which reduces vagal tone.

In moderate exercise, the heart rate increases to 180 beats/minute. In severe muscular exercise, it reaches 240 to 260 beats/minute. Increased heart rate during exercise is mainly because of **vagal withdrawal.** Increase in sympathetic tone also plays some role.

Increased heart rate during exercise is due to four factors:
  i. Impulses from proprioceptors, which are present in the exercising muscles; these impulses act through higher centers and increase the heart rate
  ii. Increased carbon dioxide tension, which acts through medullary centers
  iii. Rise in body temperature, which acts on cardiac centers via hypothalamus, increased temperature also stimulates SA node directly
  iv. Circulating catecholamines, which are secreted in large quantities during exercise.

■ 4. ON CARDIAC OUTPUT

Cardiac output increases up to 20 L/minute in moderate exercise and up to 35 L/minute during severe exercise. Increase in cardiac output is directly proportional to the increase in the amount of oxygen consumed during exercise.

During exercise, the cardiac output increases because of increase in heart rate and stroke volume. Heart rate increases because of **vagal withdrawal.** Stroke volume increases due to increased force of contraction. Because of vagal withdrawal, sympathetic activity increases leading to increase in rate and force of contraction.

■ 5. ON VENOUS RETURN

Venous return increases remarkably during exercise because of muscle pump, respiratory pump and splanchnic vasoconstriction (Chapter 98).

■ 6. ON BLOOD FLOW TO SKELETAL MUSCLES

There is a great increase in the amount of blood flowing to skeletal muscles during exercise. In resting condition, the blood supply to the skeletal muscles is 3 to 4 mL/100 g of the muscle/minute. It increases up to 60 to 80 mL in moderate exercise and up to 90 to 120 mL in severe exercise.

During the muscular activity, stoppage of blood flow occurs when the muscles contract. It is because of compression of blood vessels during contraction. And in between the contractions, the blood flow increases.

Sometimes the blood supply to muscles starts increasing even during the preparation for exercise. It is due to the sympathetic activity. Sympathetic nerves cause vasodilatation in muscles. The sympathetic nerve fibers causing vasodilatation in skeletal muscle are called **sympathetic cholinergic fibers** since these fibers secrete **acetylcholine** instead of noradrenaline.

Several other factors also are responsible for the increase in blood flow to muscles during exercise. All such factors increase the amount of blood flow to muscles by means of dilatation of blood vessels of the muscles. Such factors are:

  i. Hypercapnea
  ii. Hypoxia
  iii. Potassium ions
  iv. Metabolites like lactic acid
  v. Rise in temperature
  vi. Adrenaline secreted from adrenal medulla
  vii. Increased sympathetic cholinergic activity.

■ 7. ON BLOOD PRESSURE

During moderate isotonic exercise, the systolic pressure is increased. It is due to increase in heart rate and stroke volume. Diastolic pressure is not altered because peripheral resistance is not affected during moderate isotonic exercise.

In severe exercise involving isotonic muscular contraction, the systolic pressure enormously increases but the diastolic pressure decreases. Decrease in diastolic pressure is because of the decrease in peripheral resistance. Decrease in peripheral resistance is due to vasodilatation caused by metabolites.

During exercise involving isometric contraction, the peripheral resistance increases. So, the diastolic pressure also increases along with systolic pressure.

Blood Pressure after Exercise

Large quantities of metabolic end products are produced during exercise. These substances accumulate in the tissues, particularly the skeletal muscle. Metabolic end products cause vasodilatation. So, the blood pressure falls slightly below the resting level after the exercise. However, the pressure returns to resting level quickly as soon as the metabolic end products are removed from muscles.

QUESTIONS IN CARDIOVASCULAR SYSTEM

■ LONG QUESTIONS

1. Define cardiac cycle. Describe various events of cardiac cycle with pressure and volume changes.
2. Define electrocardiogram. Describe the waves, segments and intervals of normal ECG. Add a note on ECG leads.
3. Give the definitions, normal values and variations of cardiac output. Explain the factors regulating cardiac output.
4. What is cardiac output? Enumerate the various methods to measure cardiac output and explain the measurement of cardiac output by applying Fick principle.
5. Describe the innervation of heart and the regulation of heart rate.
6. Define arterial blood pressure. Describe the nervous regulation of arterial blood pressure.
7. Describe renal mechanism of (long term) regulation of arterial blood pressure.
8. What is the normal blood flow through coronary circulation? Explain the phasic changes, measurement and regulation of coronary blood blow.
9. Give an account of cerebral circulation.
10. Define hemorrhage. Explain various effects of hemorrhage.
11. Describe the cardiovascular and respiratory changes during exercise.

■ SHORT QUESTIONS

1. Action potential in cardiac muscle.
2. Pacemaker.
3. Pacemaker potential.
4. Conductive system in heart.
5. All-or-none law.
6. Refractory period in cardiac muscle.
7. Isometric contraction period.
8. Atrial pressure changes during cardiac cycle.
9. Ventricular pressure changes during cardiac cycle.
10. Ventricular volume changes during cardiac cycle.
11. Ejection fraction.
12. Heart sounds.
13. First and second heart sounds.
14. Phonocardiogram.
15. Cardiac murmurs.
16. Waves of normal ECG.
17. ECG leads.
18. Mean QRS vector.
19. Vectorcardiogram.
20. Sinus arrhythmia.
21. Heart block.
22. Extrasystole.
23. Stokes-Adams syndrome.
24. Abnormal pacemaker.
25. Current of injury.
26. Effect of electrolyte changes on heart.
27. Venous return.
28. Peripheral resistance.
29. Fick principle.
30. Cardiac catheterization.
31. Cardiac function curves.
32. Cardiac centers.
33. Nerve supply to heart.
34. Vagal tone.
35. Marey reflex.
36. Sinoaortic mechanism.
37. Buffer nerves.
38. Baroreceptors.
39. Chemoreceptors.
40. Bainbridge reflex.
41. Streamline and turbulent flow of blood.
42. Windkessel effect.
43. Mean volume of blood flow.
44. Velocity of blood flow.
45. Circulation time.
46. Autoregulation.
47. Determinants of arterial blood pressure.
48. Vasomotor center.
49. Vasomotor tone.
50. Nerve supply to blood vessels.
51. Renal regulation of blood pressure.
52. Vasoconstrictor substances.
53. Vasodilator substances.
54. Renin-angiotensin mechanism.
55. Hypertension.
56. Venous pressure.
57. Capillary pressure.
58. Arterial pulse.
59. Phlebogram.
60. Phasic changes in coronary blood flow.
61. Regulation of coronary circulation.
62. Coronary occlusion.
63. Myocardial infarction.
64. Angina pectoris.
65. Physiological shunt in heart.
66. Measurement of cerebral blood flow.

67. Regulation of cerebral blood flow.
68. Cushing reflex.
69. Stroke or cardiovascular accident.
70. Capillary circulation (microcirculation).
71. Shunt in capillaries.
72. Cutaneous circulation.
73. Vascular responses of skin.
74. Lewis triple response.

75. Fetal circulation.
76. Neonatal circulation.
77. Hemorrhage.
78. Manifestations of circulatory shock.
79. Syncope or fainting.
80. Vasovagal syncope.
81. Cardiovascular changes in moderate exercise.
82. Effect of exercise on blood pressure.

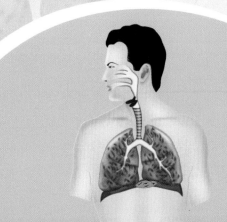

Section

9

Respiratory System and Environmental Physiology

Physiological Anatomy of Respiratory Tract

■ INTRODUCTION

Respiration is the process by which oxygen is taken in and carbon dioxide is given out. The first breath takes place only after birth. **Fetal lungs** are **non-functional.** So, during intrauterine life the exchange of gases between fetal blood and mother's blood occurs through placenta.

After the first breath, the respiratory process continues throughout the life. Permanent stoppage of respiration occurs only at death.

Normal Respiratory Rate at Different Age

Newborn	: 30 to 60/minute
Early childhood	: 20 to 40/minute
Late childhood	: 15 to 25/minute
Adult	: 12 to 16/minute.

■ TYPES OF RESPIRATION

Respiration is classified into two types:
1. **External respiration** that involves exchange of respiratory gases, i.e. oxygen and carbon dioxide between lungs and blood
2. **Internal respiration,** which involves exchange of gases between blood and tissues.

■ PHASES OF RESPIRATION

Respiration occurs in two phases:
1. **Inspiration** during which air enters the lungs from atmosphere

2. **Expiration** during which air leaves the lungs.

During normal breathing, inspiration is an active process and expiration is a passive process.

■ FUNCTIONAL ANATOMY OF RESPIRATORY TRACT

Respiratory tract is the anatomical structure through which air moves in and out. It includes nose, pharynx, larynx, trachea, bronchi and lungs (Fig. 118.1).

Pleura

Each lung is enclosed by a bilayered serous membrane called pleura or **pleural sac.** Pleura has two layers namely inner **visceral** and outer **parietal** layers. Visceral layer is attached firmly to the surface of the lungs. At hilum, it is continuous with parietal layer, which is attached to the wall of thoracic cavity.

Intrapleural Space or Pleural Cavity

Intrapleural space or pleural cavity is the narrow space in between the two layers of pleura.

Intrapleural Fluid

Intrapleural space contains a thin film of serous fluid called intrapleural fluid, which is secreted by the visceral layer of the pleura.

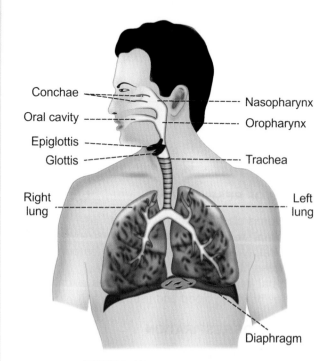

Conchae
Oral cavity
Epiglottis
Glottis
Right lung
Nasopharynx
Oropharynx
Trachea
Left lung
Diaphragm

FIGURE 118.1: Respiratory tract

Functions of intrapleural fluid

1. It functions as the lubricant to prevent friction between two layers of pleura
2. It is involved in creating the negative pressure called **intrapleural pressure** within intrapleural space.

Pleural Cavity in Abnormal Conditions

In some pathological conditions, the pleural cavity expands with accumulation of air **(pneumothorax),** water **(hydrothorax),** blood **(hemothorax)** or pus **(pyothorax).**

Tracheobronchial Tree

Trachea and bronchi are together called tracheobronchial tree. It forms a part of air passage.

Components of tracheobronchial tree

1. **Trachea** bifurcates into two main or **primary bronchi** called right and left bronchi
2. Each primary bronchus enters the lungs and divides into **secondary bronchi**
3. Secondary bronchi divide into **tertiary bronchi.** In right lung, there are 10 tertiary bronchi and in left lung, there are eight tertiary bronchi
4. Tertiary bronchi divide several times with reduction in length and diameter into many generations of **bronchioles**
5. When the diameter of bronchiole becomes 1 mm or less, it is called **terminal bronchiole**
6. Terminal bronchiole continues or divides into **respiratory bronchioles,** which have a diameter of 0.5 mm.

Upper and Lower Respiratory Tracts

Generally, respiratory tract is divided into two parts:
1. Upper respiratory tract that includes all the structures from nose up to vocal cords; vocal cords are the folds of mucous membrane within larynx that vibrates to produce the voice
2. Lower respiratory tract, which includes trachea, bronchi and lungs.

■ RESPIRATORY UNIT

Parenchyma of lungs is formed by respiratory unit that forms the **terminal portion** of respiratory tract. Respiratory unit is defined as the structural and functional unit of lung. Exchange of gases occurs only in this part of the respiratory tract.

■ STRUCTURE OF RESPIRATORY UNIT

Respiratory unit starts from the respiratory bronchioles (Fig. 118.2). Each respiratory bronchiole divides into

alveolar ducts. Each alveolar duct enters an enlarged structure called the **alveolar sac.** Space inside the alveolar sac is called **antrum.** Alveolar sac consists of a cluster of **alveoli.** Few alveoli are present in the wall of alveolar duct also.

Thus, respiratory unit includes:

1. Respiratory bronchioles
2. Alveolar ducts
3. Alveolar sacs
4. Antrum
5. Alveoli.

Each **alveolus** is like a pouch with the diameter of about 0.2 to 0.5 mm. It is lined by epithelial cells.

Alveolar Cells or Pneumocytes

Alveolar epithelium consists of alveolar cells or pneumocytes, which are of two types namely type I alveolar cells and type II alveolar cells.

Type I alveolar cells

Type I alveolar cells are the squamous epithelial cells forming about 95% of the total number of cells. These cells form the site of gaseous exchange between the alveolus and blood.

Type II alveolar cells

Type II alveolar cells are cuboidal in nature and form about 5% of alveolar cells. These cells are also called **granular pneumocytes.** Type II alveolar cells secrete **alveolar fluid** and **surfactant.**

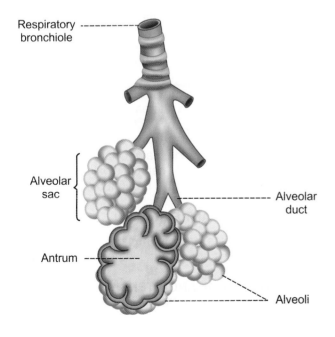

FIGURE 118.2: Respiratory unit

- Respiratory bronchiole
- Alveolar sac
- Antrum
- Alveolar duct
- Alveoli

■ RESPIRATORY MEMBRANE

Respiratory membrane is the membranous structure through which the exchange of gases occurs.

Respiratory membrane separates air in the alveoli from the blood in capillary. It is formed by the **alveolar membrane** and **capillary membrane.** Respiratory membrane has a surface area of 70 square meter and thickness of 0.5 micron. Structure of respiratory membrane is explained in Chapter 124 (See Fig. 124.1).

■ NON-RESPIRATORY FUNCTIONS OF RESPIRATORY TRACT

Besides primary function of gaseous exchange, the respiratory tract is involved in several non-respiratory functions of the body. Particularly, the lungs function as a defense barrier and metabolic organs, which synthesize some important compounds. Non-respiratory functions of the respiratory tract are:

■ 1. OLFACTION

Olfactory receptors present in the mucous membrane of nostril are responsible for **olfactory sensation.**

■ 2. VOCALIZATION

Along with other structures, larynx forms the **speech apparatus.** However, larynx alone plays major role in the process of vocalization. Therefore, it is called **sound box.**

■ 3. PREVENTION OF DUST PARTICLES

Dust particles, which enter the nostrils from air, are prevented from reaching the lungs by **filtration action** of the hairs in nasal mucous membrane. Small particles, which escape the hairs, are held by the **mucus** secreted by nasal mucous membrane. Those dust particles, which escape nasal hairs and nasal mucous membrane, are removed by the **phagocytic action** of **macrophages** in the alveoli.

Particles, which escape the protective mechanisms in nose and alveoli are thrown out by **cough** reflex and **sneezing** reflex (Chapter 126).

■ 4. DEFENSE MECHANISM

Lungs play important role in the **immunological** defense system of the body. Defense functions of the lungs are performed by their own defenses and by the presence of various types of cells in mucous membrane lining the alveoli of lungs. These cells are leukocytes, macrophages, mast cells, natural killer cells and dendritic cells.

i. *Lung's Own Defenses*

Epithelial cells lining the air passage secrete some innate immune factors called **defensins** and **cathelicidins.** These substances are the antimicrobial peptides, which play an important role in lung's natural defenses. Refer Chapter 17 for detail.

ii. *Defense through Leukocytes*

Leukocytes, particularly the neutrophils and lymphocytes present in the alveoli of lungs provide defense mechanism against bacteria and virus. **Neutrophils** kill the bacteria by phagocytosis. **Lymphocytes** develop immunity against bacteria.

iii. *Defense through Macrophages*

Macrophages engulf the dust particles and the pathogens, which enter the alveoli and thereby act as **scavengers** in lungs. Macrophages are also involved in the development of immunity by functioning as **antigen presenting cells.** When foreign organisms invade the body, the macrophages and other antigen presenting cells kill them. Later, the antigen from the organisms is digested into polypeptides. Polypeptide products are presented to T lymphocytes and B lymphocytes by the macrophages.

Macrophages secrete interleukins, tumor necrosis factors (TNF) and chemokines (Chapter 24). Interleukins and TNF activate the general immune system of the body (Chapter 17). Chemokines attract the white blood cells towards the site of any inflammation.

iv. *Defense through Mast Cell*

Mast cell is a large cell resembling the basophil. Mast cell produces the **hypersensitivity reactions** like allergy and anaphylaxis (Chapter 17). It secretes heparin, histamine, serotonin and hydrolytic enzymes.

v. *Defense through Natural Killer Cell*

Natural killer (NK) cell is a large granular cell, considered as the third type of lymphocyte. Usually NK cell is present in lungs and other lymphoid organs. Its granules contain hydrolytic enzymes, which destroy the microorganisms.

NK cell is said to be the first line of defense in specific immunity particularly **against viruses.**

It destroys the viruses and viral infected or damaged cells, which may form the tumors. It also destroys the malignant cells and prevents development of cancerous tumors. NK cells secrete interferons and the tumor necrosis factors (Chapter 17).

vi. *Defense through Dendritic Cells*

Dendritic cells in the lungs play important role in immunity. Along with macrophages, these cells function as antigen presenting cells.

■ 5. MAINTENANCE OF WATER BALANCE

Respiratory tract plays a role in water loss mechanism. During expiration, water evaporates through the expired air and some amount of body water is lost by this process.

■ 6. REGULATION OF BODY TEMPERATURE

During expiration, along with water, heat is also lost from the body. Thus, respiratory tract plays a role in heat loss mechanism.

■ 7. REGULATION OF ACID-BASE BALANCE

Lungs play a role in maintenance of acid-base balance of the body by regulating the carbon dioxide content in blood. Carbon dioxide is produced during various metabolic reactions in the tissues of the body. When it enters the blood, carbon dioxide combines with water to form carbonic acid. Since carbonic acid is unstable, it splits into hydrogen and bicarbonate ions.

$$CO_2 + H_2O \rightarrow H_2CO_3 \rightarrow H^+ + HCO_3^-$$

Entire reaction is reversed in lungs when carbon dioxide is removed from blood into the alveoli of lungs (Chapter 125).

$$H^+ + HCO_3^- \rightarrow H_2CO_3 \rightarrow CO_2 + H_2O$$

As carbon dioxide is a **volatile gas,** it is practically blown out by ventilation.

When metabolic activities are accelerated, more amount of carbon dioxide is produced in the tissues. Concentration of hydrogen ion is also increased. This leads to reduction in pH. Increased hydrogen ion concentration causes increased pulmonary ventilation (hyperventilation) by acting through various mechanisms like chemoreceptors in aortic and carotid bodies and in medulla of the brain (Chapter 126). Due to hyperventilation, excess of carbon dioxide is removed from body fluids and the pH is brought back to normal.

■ 8. ANTICOAGULANT FUNCTION

Mast cells in lungs secrete **heparin.** Heparin is an anticoagulant and it prevents the intravascular clotting.

■ 9. SECRETION OF ANGIOTENSIN-CONVERTING ENZYME

Endothelial cells of the pulmonary capillaries secrete the angiotensin-converting enzyme **(ACE).** It converts the angiotensin I into active angiotensin II, which plays an important role in the regulation of ECF volume and blood pressure (Chapter 50).

■ 10. SYNTHESIS OF HORMONAL SUBSTANCES

Lung tissues are also known to synthesize the hormonal substances, prostaglandins, acetylcholine and serotonin, which have many physiological actions in the body including regulation of blood pressure (Chapter 73).

■ RESPIRATORY PROTECTIVE REFLEXES

Respiratory protective reflexes are the reflexes that protect lungs and air passage from foreign particles. Respiratory process is modified by these reflexes in order to eliminate the foreign particles or to prevent the entry of these particles into the respiratory tract. Following are the respiratory protective reflexes:

■ COUGH REFLEX

Cough is a modified respiratory process characterized by forced expiration. It is a protective reflex and it is caused by **irritation of respiratory tract** and some other areas such as **external auditory canal** (see below).

Causes

Cough is produced mainly by irritant agents. It is also produced by several disorders such as cardiac disorders (congestive heart failure), pulmonary disorders (chronic obstructive pulmonary disease – COPD) and tumor in thorax, which may exert pressure on larynx, trachea, bronchi or lungs.

Mechanism

Cough begins with deep inspiration followed by forced expiration with closed glottis. This increases the intrapleural pressure above 100 mm Hg. Then, glottis opens suddenly with explosive outflow of air at a high velocity. Velocity of the airflow may reach 960 km/hour. It causes expulsion of irritant substances out of the respiratory tract.

Reflex Pathway

Receptors that initiate the cough are situated in several locations such as nose, paranasal sinuses, larynx, pharynx, trachea, bronchi, pleura, diaphragm, pericardium, stomach, external auditory canal and tympanic membrane.

Afferent nerve fibers pass via vagus, trigeminal, glossopharyngeal and phrenic nerves. The center for cough reflex is in the medulla oblongata.

Efferent nerve fibers arising from the medullary center pass through the vagus, phrenic and spinal motor nerves. These nerve fibers activate the primary and accessory respiratory muscles.

■ SNEEZING REFLEX

Sneezing is also a modified respiratory process characterized by forced expiration. It is a protective reflex caused by **irritation of nasal mucous** membrane.

Causes

Irritation of the nasal mucous membrane occurs because of dust particles, debris, mechanical obstruction of the airway and excess fluid accumulation in the nasal passages.

Mechanism

Sneezing starts with deep inspiration, followed by forceful expiratory effort with opened glottis resulting in expulsion of irritant agents out of respiratory tract.

Reflex Pathway

Sneezing is initiated by the irritation of nasal mucous membrane, the olfactory receptors and trigeminal nerve endings present in the nasal mucosa.

Afferent nerve fibers pass through the trigeminal and olfactory nerves. Sneezing center is in medulla oblongata. It is located diffusely in spinal nucleus of trigeminal nerve, nucleus solitarius and the reticular formation of medulla.

Efferent nerve fibers from the medullary center pass via trigeminal, facial, glossopharyngeal, vagus and intercostal nerves. These nerve fibers activate the pharyngeal, tracheal and respiratory muscles.

■ SWALLOWING (DEGLUTITION) REFLEX

Swallowing reflex is a respiratory protective reflex that prevents entrance of food particles into the air passage during swallowing.

While swallowing of the food, the respiration is arrested for a while. Temporary arrest of respiration is called apnea. Arrest of breathing during swallowing is called **swallowing apnea** or **deglutition apnea.** It takes place during pharyngeal stage, i.e. second stage of deglutition and prevents entry of food particles into the respiratory tract. Refer Chapter 43 for details.

Pulmonary Circulation

```
■ PULMONARY BLOOD VESSELS
    ■ PULMONARY ARTERY
    ■ BRONCHIAL ARTERY
    ■ PHYSIOLOGICAL SHUNT
■ CHARACTERISTIC FEATURES OF PULMONARY BLOOD VESSELS
■ PULMONARY BLOOD FLOW
■ PULMONARY BLOOD PRESSURE
■ MEASUREMENT OF PULMONARY BLOOD FLOW
■ REGULATION OF PULMONARY BLOOD FLOW
    ■ CARDIAC OUTPUT
    ■ VASCULAR RESISTANCE
    ■ NERVOUS FACTORS
    ■ CHEMICAL FACTORS
    ■ GRAVITY AND HYDROSTATIC PRESSURE
```

■ PULMONARY BLOOD VESSELS

Pulmonary blood vessels include **pulmonary artery,** which carries **deoxygenated blood** to alveoli of lungs and **bronchial artery,** which supply **oxygenated blood** to other structures of lungs (see below).

■ PULMONARY ARTERY

Pulmonary artery supplies deoxygenated blood pumped from right ventricle to alveoli of lungs (pulmonary circulation). After leaving the right ventricle, this artery divides into **right and left branches.** Each branch enters the corresponding lung along with primary bronchus. After entering the lung, branch of the pulmonary artery divides into small vessels and finally forms the **capillary plexus** that is in intimate relationship to alveoli. Capillary plexus is solely concerned with alveolar gas exchange. Oxygenated blood from the alveoli is carried to left atrium by one pulmonary vein from each side.

■ BRONCHIAL ARTERY

Bronchial artery arises from descending thoracic aorta. It supplies arterial blood to bronchi, connective tissue and other structures of lung stroma, visceral pleura and pulmonary lymph nodes. Venous blood from these structures is drained by two **bronchial veins** from each side. Bronchial veins from right side drain into **azygos vein** and the left bronchial veins drain into **superior hemiazygos** or **left superior intercostal veins.** However, the blood from distal portion of bronchial circulation is drained directly into the tributaries of **pulmonary veins.**

■ PHYSIOLOGICAL SHUNT

Definition

Physiological shunt is defined as a diversion through which the venous blood is mixed with arterial blood.

Components

Physiological shunt has two components:

1. Flow of deoxygenated blood from **bronchial circulation** into pulmonary veins without being oxygenated makes up part of normal physiological shunt
2. Flow of deoxygenated blood from **thebesian veins** into cardiac chambers directly (Chapter 108).

Venous Admixture and Wasted Blood

Physiological shunt results in venous admixture. Venous admixture refers to mixing of deoxygenated blood with oxygenated blood. Fraction of venous blood, which is not fully oxygenated is generally considered as wasted blood.

Normal Shunt Level and its Variations

Normal physiological shunt of venous blood to the left side of heart is 1% to 2% of cardiac output. In normal persons, it may increase up to 5% of cardiac output, which may be due to mismatching of ventilation-perfusion ratio within physiological limits.

Pathological increase in the shunt occurs in several conditions such as acute pulmonary infections and bronchiectasis (permanent dilatation of bronchi due to chronic pulmonary infections and inflammatory processes).

Physiological Shunt Vs Physiological Dead Space

Physiological shunt is analogous to physiological dead space (Chapter 122). Physiological shunt includes wasted blood and physiological dead space includes wasted air. Both wasted blood and wasted air exist on either side of alveolar membrane and both affect the ventilation-perfusion ratio (Chapter 122).

■ CHARACTERISTIC FEATURES OF PULMONARY BLOOD VESSELS

Following are the characteristic features of pulmonary blood vessels:
1. Pulmonary artery has a **thin wall.** Its thickness is only about one third of thickness of the systemic aortic wall. Wall of other pulmonary blood vessels is also thin.
2. Pulmonary blood vessels are **highly elastic** and more distensible
3. Smooth muscle coat is **not well developed** in the pulmonary blood vessels
4. True arterioles have less **smooth muscle** fibers
5. Pulmonary capillaries are **larger** than systemic capillaries. Pulmonary capillaries are also dense and have multiple anastomosis, so, each alveolus occupies a capillary basket.
6. Vascular resistance in pulmonary circulation is **very less;** it is only one tenth of systemic circulation
7. Pulmonary vascular system is a **low pressure system.** Pulmonary arterial pressure and pulmonary capillary pressure are very low (see below).

8. Pulmonary artery carries deoxygenated blood from heart to lungs and pulmonary veins carry oxygenated blood from lungs to heart
9. Physiological shunt is present.

■ PULMONARY BLOOD FLOW

Lungs receive the whole amount of blood that is pumped out from right ventricle. Output of blood per minute is same in both right and left ventricle. It is about 5 liter.

Thus, the lungs accommodate amount of blood, which is equal to amount of blood accommodated by all other parts of the body.

■ PULMONARY BLOOD PRESSURE

Pulmonary blood vessels are more distensible than systemic blood vessels. So the blood pressure is less in pulmonary blood vessels. Thus, the entire pulmonary vascular system is a **low pressure bed.**

Pulmonary Arterial Pressure

Systolic pressure : 25 mm Hg
Diastolic pressure : 10 mm Hg
Mean arterial pressure : 15 mm Hg.

Pulmonary Capillary Pressure

Pulmonary capillary pressure is about 7 mm Hg. This pressure is sufficient for exchange of gases between alveoli and blood.

■ MEASUREMENT OF PULMONARY BLOOD FLOW

Pulmonary blood flow is measured by applying Fick principle. Details are given in Chapter 98.

■ REGULATION OF PULMONARY BLOOD FLOW

Pulmonary blood flow is regulated by the following factors:
1. Cardiac output
2. Vascular resistance
3. Nervous factors
4. Chemical factors
5. Gravity and hydrostatic pressure.

■ 1. CARDIAC OUTPUT

Pulmonary blood flow is **directly proportional** to cardiac output. So, any factor that alters the cardiac output, also affects pulmonary blood flow.

Cardiac output is in turn regulated by four factors:
 i. Venous return
 ii. Force of contraction
 iii. Rate of contraction
 iv. Peripheral resistance.

Refer Chapter 98 for details of factors affecting cardiac output.

■ 2. VASCULAR RESISTANCE

Pulmonary blood flow is **inversely proportional** to the pulmonary vascular resistance. Pulmonary vascular resistance is low compared to systemic vascular resistance. Pulmonary vascular resistance is altered in different phases of respiration. During inspiration, pulmonary blood vessels are distended because of decreased intrathoracic pressure. This causes decrease in vascular resistance resulting in increased pulmonary blood flow (Fig. 119.1). During expiration, the pulmonary vascular resistance increases resulting in decreased blood flow.

During the conditions like exercise, the vascular resistance decreases and blood flow increases. It is influenced by the exercise-induced hypoxia and hypercapnea.

■ 3. NERVOUS FACTORS

Stimulation of sympathetic nerves under experimental conditions increases the pulmonary vascular resistance by vasoconstriction and the stimulation of parasympathetic, i.e. vagus nerve decreases the vascular resistance by vasodilatation.

However, under physiological conditions, it is doubtful whether autonomic nerves play any role in regulating the blood flow to lungs.

■ 4. CHEMICAL FACTORS

Excess of carbon dioxide or lack of oxygen causes vasoconstriction. The cause for pulmonary vasoconstriction by hypoxia is not known. But it has some significance. If some part of lungs is affected by hypoxia, there is constriction of capillaries in that area. Thus, blood is directed to the alveoli of neighboring area where gaseous exchange occurs.

■ 5. GRAVITY AND HYDROSTATIC PRESSURE

Normally in standing position, blood pressure in lower extremity of the body is very high and in upper parts above the level of heart, the pressure is low. This is because of the effect of gravitational force.

A similar condition is observed to some extent in lungs also. Pulmonary vascular pressure varies in different parts of the lungs:

i. *Apical Portion – Zone 1*

Normally, in the apical portion of lungs, pulmonary capillary pressure is almost same as alveolar pressure. So, the pulmonary arterial pressure is just sufficient for flow of blood into alveolar capillaries. However, if pulmonary arterial pressure decreases or if alveolar pressure increases, the capillaries are collapsed. This prevents flow of blood to alveoli. So, this zone of lung is called **area of zero blood flow** (Fig. 119.2).

Under these conditions, there is no gaseous exchange in this zone of lungs. So, it is considered as the part of physiological dead space, which is ventilated but not perfused. And, the ventilation-perfusion ratio increases. It may lead to growth of bacteria, particularly tubercle bacilli making this part of lungs susceptible for tuberculosis.

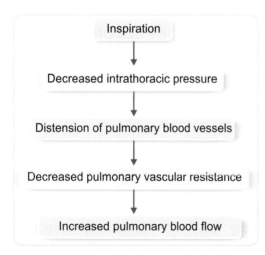

FIGURE 119.1: Schematic diagram showing increase in pulmonary blood flow during inspiration

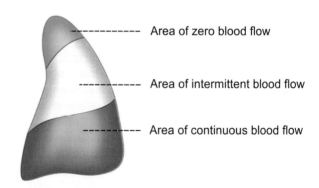

FIGURE 119.2: Pattern of blood flow in various areas of lungs

ii. *Midportion – Zone 2*

In the midportion of lungs, the pressure in alveoli is less than pulmonary systolic pressure and more than the pulmonary diastolic pressure. Because of this, the blood flow to the alveoli increases during systole and decreases during diastole. So, this zone of the lung is called **area of intermittent flow.** Ventilation-perfusion ratio is normal.

iii. *Lower Portion – Zone 3*

In the lower portion of lungs, the pulmonary arterial pressure is high and it is more than alveolar pressure both during systole and diastole. So the blood flows continuously. Hence, this part of lungs is called **area of continuous blood flow.** Ventilation-perfusion ratio decreases because of increased blood flow.

Mechanics of Respiration

- ■ **RESPIRATORY MOVEMENTS**
  - ■ INTRODUCTION
  - ■ MUSCLES OF RESPIRATION
  - ■ MOVEMENTS OF THORACIC CAGE
  - ■ MOVEMENTS OF LUNGS
- ■ **RESPIRATORY PRESSURES**
  - ■ INTRAPLEURAL PRESSURE
  - ■ INTRA-ALVEOLAR PRESSURE
- ■ **COMPLIANCE**
  - ■ DEFINITION
  - ■ NORMAL VALUES
  - ■ TYPES
  - ■ MEASUREMENT
  - ■ APPLIED PHYSIOLOGY
- ■ **WORK OF BREATHING**
  - ■ WORK DONE BY RESPIRATORY MUSCLES
  - ■ UTILIZATION OF ENERGY

■ RESPIRATORY MOVEMENTS

■ INTRODUCTION

Respiration occurs in two phases namely inspiration and expiration.

During inspiration, thoracic cage enlarges and lungs expand so that air enters the lungs easily. During expiration, the thoracic cage and lungs decrease in size and attain the preinspiratory position so that air leaves the lungs easily.

During normal quiet breathing, inspiration is the **active process** and expiration is the **passive process.**

■ MUSCLES OF RESPIRATION

Respiratory muscles are of two types:
1. Inspiratory muscles
2. Expiratory muscles.

However, respiratory muscles are generally classified into two types:
1. Primary or major respiratory muscles, which are responsible for change in size of thoracic cage during normal quiet breathing
2. Accessory respiratory muscles that help primary respiratory muscles during forced respiration.

Inspiratory Muscles

Muscles involved in inspiratory movements are known as inspiratory muscles.

Primary inspiratory muscles

Primary inspiratory muscles are the diaphragm, which is supplied by phrenic nerve (C3 to C5) and external intercostal muscles, supplied by intercostal nerves (T1 to T11).

Accessory inspiratory muscles

Sternocleidomastoid, scalene, anterior serrati, elevators of scapulae and pectorals are the accessory inspiratory muscles.

Expiratory Muscles

Primary expiratory muscles

Primary expiratory muscles are the internal intercostal muscles, which are innervated by intercostal nerves.

Accessory expiratory muscles

Accessory expiratory muscles are the abdominal muscles.

■ MOVEMENTS OF THORACIC CAGE

Inspiration causes enlargement of thoracic cage. Thoracic cage enlarges because of increase in **all diameters,** viz. anteroposterior, transverse and vertical diameters. Anteroposterior and transverse diameters of thoracic cage are increased by the elevation of ribs. Vertical diameter is increased by the descent of diaphragm.

In general, change in the size of thoracic cavity occurs because of the movements of four units of structures:
1. Thoracic lid
2. Upper costal series
3. Lower costal series
4. Diaphragm.

1. *Thoracic Lid*

Thoracic lid is formed by **manubrium sterni** and the first pair of ribs. It is also called **thoracic operculum.**

Movement of thoracic lid increases the **anteroposterior diameter** of thoracic cage. Due to the contraction of scalene muscles, the first ribs move upwards to a more horizontal position. This increases the anteroposterior diameter of upper thoracic cage.

2. *Upper Costal Series*

Upper costal series is constituted by second to sixth pair of ribs. Movement of upper costal series increases the **anteroposterior** and **transverse diameter** of the thoracic cage.

Movement of upper costal series is of two types:
i. Pump handle movement
ii. Bucket handle movement.

Pump handle movement

Contraction of external intercostal muscles causes elevation of these ribs and upward and forward movement of sternum. This movement is called pump handle movement. It increases **anteroposterior diameter** of the thoracic cage.

Bucket handle movement

Simultaneously, the central portions of these ribs (arches of ribs) move upwards and outwards to a more horizontal position. This movement is called bucket handle movement and it increases the **transverse diameter** of thoracic cage.

3. *Lower Costal Series*

Lower costal series includes seventh to tenth pair of ribs. Movement of lower costal series increases the **transverse diameter** of thoracic cage by bucket handle movement.

Bucket handle movement

Lower costal series of ribs also show bucket handle movement by swinging outward and upward. This movement increases the **transverse diameter** of the thoracic cage.

Eleventh and twelfth pairs of ribs are the floating ribs. These ribs are not involved in changing the size of thoracic cage.

4. *Diaphragm*

Movement of diaphragm increases the vertical diameter of thoracic cage. Normally, before inspiration the diaphragm is dome shaped with convexity facing upwards. During inspiration, due to the contraction, muscle fibers are shortened. But the central tendinous portion is drawn downwards so the diaphragm is flattened. Flattening of diaphragm increases the **vertical diameter** of the thoracic cage.

■ MOVEMENTS OF LUNGS

During inspiration, due to the enlargement of thoracic cage, the negative pressure is increased in the thoracic cavity. It causes expansion of the lungs. During expiration, the thoracic cavity decreases in size to the **pre-inspiratory position.** Pressure in the thoracic cage also comes back to the preinspiratory level. It compresses the lung tissues so that, the air is expelled out of lungs.

Collapsing Tendency of Lungs

Lungs are under constant threat to collapse even in resting conditions because of certain factors.

Factors Causing Collapsing Tendency of Lungs

Two factors are responsible for the collapsing tendency of lungs:

1. *Elastic property of lung tissues:* Elastic tissues of lungs show constant recoiling tendency and try to collapse the lungs
2. *Surface tension:* It is the tension exerted by the fluid secreted from alveolar epithelium on the surface of alveolar membrane.

   Fortunately, there are some factors, which save the lungs from collapsing.

Factors Preventing Collapsing Tendency of Lungs

In spite of elastic property of lungs and surface tension in the alveoli of lungs, the collapsing tendency of lungs is prevented by two factors:

1. *Intrapleural pressure:* It is the pressure in the pleural cavity, which is always negative (see below). Because of negativity, it keeps the lungs expanded and prevents the collapsing tendency of lungs produced by the elastic tissues.
2. *Surfactant:* It is a substance secreted in alveolar epithelium. It reduces surface tension and prevents the collapsing tendency produced by surface tension.

Surfactant

Surfactant is a **surface acting material** or agent that is responsible for lowering the surface tension of a fluid. Surfactant that lines the epithelium of the alveoli in lungs is known as **pulmonary surfactant** and it decreases the **surface tension** on the alveolar membrane.

Source of secretion of pulmonary surfactant

Pulmonary surfactant is secreted by two types of cells:

1. **Type II alveolar epithelial cells** in the lungs, which are called surfactant secreting alveolar cells or pneumocytes. Characteristic feature of these cells is the presence of microvilli on their alveolar surface.
2. **Clara cells,** which are situated in the bronchioles. These cells are also called bronchiolar exocrine cells.

Chemistry of surfactant

Surfactant is a **lipoprotein complex** formed by lipids especially phospholipids, proteins and ions.

1. *Phospholipids:* Phospholipids form about 75% of the surfactant. Major phospholipid present in the surfactant is **dipalmitoylphosphatidylcholine** (DPPC).
2. *Other lipids:* Other lipid substances of surfactant are triglycerides and phosphatidylglycerol (PG).
3. *Proteins:* Proteins of the surfactant are called specific surfactant proteins. There are four main surfactant proteins, called SP-A, SP-B, SP-C and SP-D. SP-A and SP-D are hydrophilic, while SP-B and SP-C are hydrophobic. Surfactant proteins are vital components of surfactant and the surfactant becomes inactive in the absence of proteins.
4. *Ions:* Ions present in the surfactant are mostly calcium ions.

Formation of surfactant

Type II alveolar epithelial cells and Clara cells have a special type of membrane bound organelles called **lamellar bodies,** which form the intracellular source of surfactant. Laminar bodies contain surfactant phospholipids and surfactant proteins. These materials are synthesized in endoplasmic reticulum and stored in laminar bodies.

By means of exocytosis, lipids and proteins of lamellar bodies are released into surface fluid lining the alveoli. Here, in the presence of surfactant proteins and calcium, the phospholipids are arranged into a **lattice** (meshwork) structure called **tubular myelin.** Tubular myelin is in turn converted into surfactant in the form of a **film** that spreads over the entire surface of alveoli.

Most of the surfactant is absorbed into the type II alveolar cells, catabolized and the products are loaded into lamellar bodies for recycling.

Factors necessary for the formation and spreading of surfactant

Formation of surfactant requires many substances. Formation of tubular myelin requires DPPC, PG and the hydrophobic proteins, SP-B and SP-C. Formation of surfactant film requires SP-B, SP-C and PG.

Type II alveolar epithelial cells occupy only about 5% of alveolar surface. However, the surfactant must spread over the entire alveolar surface. It is facilitated by PG and calcium ions.

Glucocorticoids play important role in the formation of surfactant.

Functions of surfactant

1. Surfactant reduces the **surface tension** in the alveoli of lungs and prevents **collapsing tendency** of lungs.

Surfactant acts by the following mechanism:

Phospholipid molecule in the surfactant has two portions. One portion of the molecule is **hydrophilic.** This portion dissolves in water and lines the alveoli. Other portion is **hydrophobic** and it is directed towards the alveolar air. This surface of the phospholipid along with other portion spreads over the alveoli and reduces the surface tension. SP-B and SP-C play active role in this process.

2. Surfactant is responsible for stabilization of the alveoli, which is necessary to withstand the collapsing tendency.

3. It plays an important role in the inflation of lungs after birth. In fetus, the secretion of surfactant begins after the 3rd month. Until birth, the lungs are solid and not expanded. Soon after birth, the first breath starts because of the stimulation of respiratory centers by hypoxia and hypercapnea. Although the respiratory movements are attempted by the infant, the lungs tend to collapse repeatedly. And, the presence of surfactant in the alveoli prevents the lungs from collapsing.

4. Another important function of surfactant is its role in defense within the lungs against infection and inflammation. Hydrophilic proteins SP-A and SP-D destroy the bacteria and viruses by means of opsonization. These two proteins also control the formation of inflammatory mediators.

Effect of deficiency of surfactant – respiratory distress syndrome

Absence of surfactant in infants, causes collapse of lungs and the condition is called respiratory distress syndrome or hyaline membrane disease. Deficiency of surfactant occurs in adults also and it is called **adult respiratory distress syndrome (ARDS).**

In addition, the deficiency of surfactant increases the susceptibility for bacterial and viral infections.

■ RESPIRATORY PRESSURES

Two types of pressures are exerted in the thoracic cavity and lungs during process of respiration:
1. Intrapleural pressure or intrathoracic pressure
2. Intra-alveolar pressure or intrapulmonary pressure.

■ INTRAPLEURAL PRESSURE

Definition

Intrapleural pressure is the pressure existing in pleural cavity, that is, in between the visceral and parietal layers of pleura. It is exerted by the suction of the fluid that lines the pleural cavity (Fig. 120.1). It is also called

intrathoracic pressure since it is exerted in the whole of thoracic cavity.

Normal Values

Respiratory pressures are always expressed in relation to atmospheric pressure, which is 760 mm Hg. Under physiological conditions, the intrapleural pressure is always negative.

Normal values are:
1. At the end of normal inspiration:
   –6 mm Hg (760 – 6 = 754 mm Hg)
2. At the end of normal expiration:
   –2 mm Hg (760 – 2 = 758 mm Hg)
3. At the end of forced inspiration:
   –30 mm Hg
4. At the end of forced inspiration with closed glottis (Müller maneuver):
   –70 mm Hg
5. At the end of forced expiration with closed glottis (Valsalva maneuver):
   +50 mm Hg.

Cause for Negativity of Intrapleural Pressure

Pleural cavity is always lined by a thin layer of fluid that is secreted by the visceral layer of pleura. This fluid is constantly pumped from the pleural cavity into the lymphatic vessels. Pumping of fluid creates the negative pressure in the pleural cavity.

Intrapleural pressure becomes positive in **Valsalva maneuver** (Chapter 104) and in some pathological conditions such as pneumothorax, hydrothorax, hemothorax and pyothorax.

Measurement

Intrapleural pressure is measured by direct method and indirect method. In the direct method, the intrapleural pressure is determined by introducing a needle into the pleural cavity and connecting the needle to a mercury manometer. In indirect method, intrapleural pressure is measured by introducing the esophageal balloon, which is connected to a manometer. Intrapleural pressure is considered as equivalent to the pressure existing in the esophagus.

Significance of Intrapleural Pressure

Throughout the respiratory cycle intrapleural pressure remains lower than intra-alveolar pressure. This keeps the lungs always inflated.

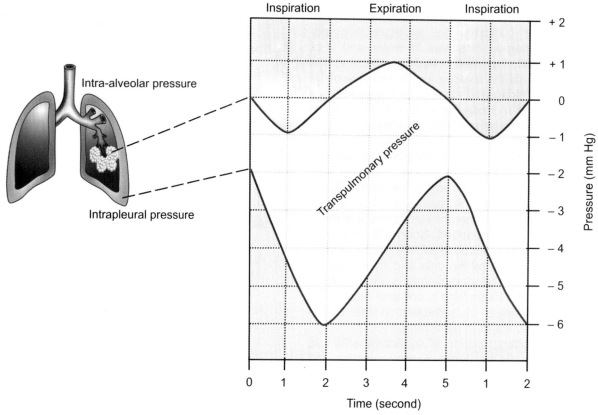

FIGURE 120.1: Changes in respiratory pressures during inspiration and expiration. '0' indicates the normal atmospheric pressure (760 mm Hg).

Intrapleural pressure has two important functions:
1. It prevents the collapsing tendency of lungs
2. Because of the negative pressure in thoracic region, larger veins and vena cava are enlarged, i.e. dilated. Also, the negative pressure acts like suction pump and pulls the venous blood from lower part of body towards the heart against gravity. Thus, the intrapleural pressure is responsible for venous return. So, it is called the **respiratory pump** for venous return (Chapter 98).

■ INTRA-ALVEOLAR PRESSURE

Definition

Intra-alveolar pressure is the pressure existing in the alveoli of the lungs. It is also known as **intrapulmonary pressure.**

Normal Values

Normally, intra-alveolar pressure is equal to the atmospheric pressure, which is 760 mm Hg. It becomes negative during inspiration and positive during expiration.

Normal values are:
1. During normal inspiration:
   −1 mm Hg (760 − 1 = 759 mm Hg)
2. During normal expiration:
   +1 mm Hg (760 + 1 = 761 mm Hg)
3. At the end of inspiration and expiration:
   Equal to atmospheric pressure (760 mm Hg)
4. During forced inspiration with closed glottis (Müller maneuver): −80 mm Hg
5. During forced expiration with closed glottis (Valsalva maneuver): +100 mm Hg.

Measurement

Intra-alveolar pressure is measured by using plethysmograph (Chapter 121).

Significance of Intra-alveolar Pressure

1. Intra-alveolar pressure causes flow of air in and out of alveoli. During inspiration, the intra-alveolar pressure becomes negative, so the atmospheric air enters the alveoli. During

expiration, intra-alveolar pressure becomes positive. So, air is expelled out of alveoli.
2. Intra-alveolar pressure also helps in exchange of gases between the alveolar air and the blood.

Transpulmonary Pressure

Transpulmonary pressure is the pressure difference between intra-alveolar pressure and intrapleural pressure. It is the measure of elastic forces in lungs, which is responsible for collapsing tendency of lungs.

■ COMPLIANCE

■ DEFINITION

Compliance is the ability of the lungs and thorax to expand or it is the **expansibility** of lungs and thorax. It is defined as the change in volume per unit change in the pressure.

Significance of Determining Compliance

Determination of compliance is useful as it is the measure of stiffness of lungs. Stiffer the lungs, less is the compliance.

■ NORMAL VALUES

Compliance is expressed by two ways:
1. In relation to intra-alveolar pressure
2. In relation to intrapleural pressure.

Compliance in Relation to Intra-alveolar Pressure

Compliance is the volume increase in lungs per unit increase in the intra-alveolar pressure.
1. Compliance of lungs and thorax together:
    130 mL/1 cm H_2O pressure
2. Compliance of lungs alone:
    220 mL/1 cm H_2O pressure.

Compliance in Relation to Intrapleural Pressure

Compliance is the volume increase in lungs per unit decrease in the intrapleural pressure.
1. Compliance of lungs and thorax together:
    100 mL/1 cm H_2O pressure
2. Compliance of lungs alone:
    200 mL/1 cm H_2O pressure.
    Thus, if lungs could be removed from thorax, the expansibility (compliance) of lungs alone will be doubled. It is because of the absence of inertia and restriction exerted by the structures of thoracic cage, which interfere with expansion of lungs.

Specific Compliance

The term specific compliance is introduced to assess the stiffness of lung tissues more accurately. Specific compliance is the compliance per liter of lung volume. It is usually reported for expiration at functional residual capacity. It is the compliance divided by functional residual capacity.

$$\text{Specific compliance of lungs} = \frac{\text{Compliance of lungs}}{\text{Functional residual capacity}}$$

Functional residual capacity is the volume of air present in lungs at the end of normal expiration.

■ TYPES OF COMPLIANCE

Compliance is of two types:
1. Static compliance
2. Dynamic compliance.

1. Static Compliance

Static compliance is the compliance measured under **static conditions,** i.e. by measuring pressure and volume when breathing does not take place (see below). Static compliance is the pressure required to overcome the elastic resistance of respiratory system for a given tidal volume under zero flow (static) condition.

2. Dynamic Compliance

Dynamic compliance is the compliance measured during **dynamic conditions,** i.e. during breathing.

Static Compliance Vs Dynamic Compliance

In healthy subjects, there is little difference between static and dynamic compliance. In patients with stiff lungs, the dynamic compliance decreases while little change occurs in the static compliance.

■ MEASUREMENT OF COMPLIANCE

Measurement of Static Compliance

To measure the static compliance, the subject is asked to inspire air periodically at regular steps from a spirometer. In each step, a known volume of air is inspired. At the end of each step, intrapleural pressure is measured by means of an **esophageal balloon.** Then, the air is expired in steps until the volume returns to original preinspiratory level. Intrapleural pressure is measured at the end of each step.

Values of volume and pressure are plotted to obtain a curve, which is called **pressure-volume curve.** From this curve compliance can be calculated. This curve also shows the difference in inspiration and expiration (Fig. 120.2).

Measurement of Dynamic Compliance

Dynamic compliance is measured during normal breathing. It is measured by determining the lung volume and esophageal pressure (intrapleural pressure) at the end of inspiration and expiration when the lungs are apparently stationary.

■ APPLIED PHYSIOLOGY

Increase in Compliance

Compliance increases due to loss of elastic property of lung tissues, which occurs both in physiological and pathological conditions:
1. Physiological condition: Old age
2. Pathological condition: Emphysema (Fig. 120.3).

Decrease in Compliance

Compliance decreases in several pathological conditions such as:
1. Deformities of thorax like kyphosis and scoliosis (Chapter 68)
2. Fibrotic pleurisy (inflammation of pleura resulting in fibrosis)
3. Paralysis of respiratory muscles
4. Pleural effusion (Chapter 127)
5. Abnormal thorax such as pneumothorax, hydrothorax, hemothorax and pyothorax (Chapter 127).

■ WORK OF BREATHING

Work of breathing is the work done by respiratory muscles during breathing to overcome the resistance in thorax and respiratory tract.

■ WORK DONE BY RESPIRATORY MUSCLES

During respiratory processes, inspiration is active process and the expiration is a passive process. So, during quiet breathing, respiratory muscles perform the work only during inspiration and not during expiration.

■ UTILIZATION OF ENERGY

During the work of breathing, the energy is utilized to overcome three types of resistance:

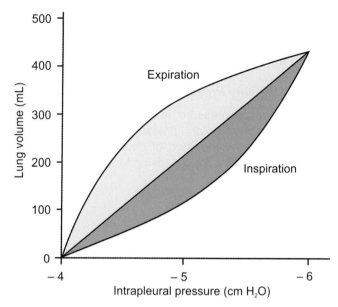

FIGURE 120.2: Pressure-volume curve

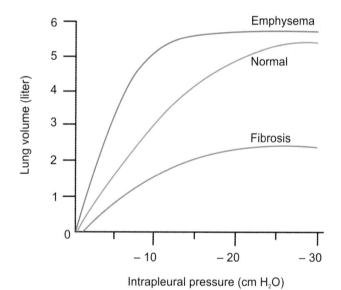

FIGURE 120.3: Variations in lung compliance

1. Airway resistance
2. Elastic resistance of lungs and thorax
3. Non-elastic viscous resistance.

1. Airway Resistance

Airway resistance is the resistance offered to the passage of air through respiratory tract. Resistance increases during bronchiolar constriction, which in-

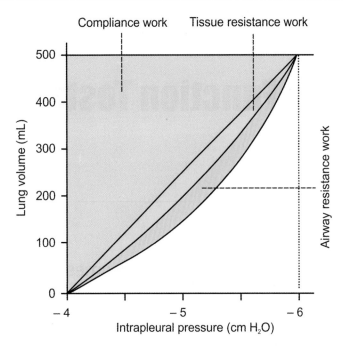

FIGURE 120.4: Work of breathing

creases the work done by the muscles during breathing. **Work done** to overcome the airway resistance is called **airway resistance work.**

2. *Elastic Resistance of Lungs and Thorax*

Energy is required to expand lungs and thorax against the elastic force. Work done to overcome this elastic resistance is called **compliance work.**

3. *Non-elastic Viscous Resistance*

Energy is also required to overcome the viscosity of lung tissues and tissues of thoracic cage. Work done to overcome this viscous resistance is called **tissue resistance work.**

Above factors are explained by the curve that shows the relation between lung volume and pleural pressure (Fig. 120.4).

Pulmonary Function Tests

- ■ INTRODUCTION
- ■ LUNG VOLUMES
- ■ LUNG CAPACITIES
- ■ MEASUREMENT OF LUNG VOLUMES AND CAPACITIES
- ■ MEASUREMENT OF FUNCTIONAL RESIDUAL CAPACITY AND RESIDUAL VOLUME
- ■ VITAL CAPACITY
- ■ FORCED EXPIRATORY VOLUME OR TIMED VITAL CAPACITY
- ■ RESPIRATORY MINUTE VOLUME
- ■ MAXIMUM BREATHING CAPACITY OR MAXIMUM VENTILATION VOLUME
- ■ PEAK EXPIRATORY FLOW RATE
- ■ RESTRICTIVE AND OBSTRUCTIVE RESPIRATORY DISEASES

■ INTRODUCTION

Pulmonary function tests or lung function tests are useful in assessing the **functional status** of the respiratory system both in physiological and pathological conditions. Lung function tests are based on the measurement of volume of air breathed in and out in quiet breathing and forced breathing. These tests are carried out mostly by using spirometer.

■ TYPES OF LUNG FUNCTION TESTS

Lung function tests are of two types:
1. Static lung function tests
2. Dynamic lung function tests.

Static Lung Function Tests

Static lung function tests are based on **volume of air that flows** into or out of lungs. These tests do not depend upon the rate at which air flows.

Static lung function tests include static lung volumes and static lung capacities.

Dynamic Lung Function Tests

Dynamic lung function tests are based on time, i.e. the **rate at which air flows** into or out of lungs. These tests include forced vital capacity, forced expiratory volume, maximum ventilation volume and peak expiratory flow.

Dynamic lung function tests are useful in determining the severity of obstructive and restrictive lung diseases.

■ LUNG VOLUMES

Static lung volumes are the volumes of air breathed by an individual. Each of these volumes represents the volume of air present in the lung under a specified static condition (specific position of thorax).

Static lung volumes are of four types:
1. Tidal volume
2. Inspiratory reserve volume
3. Expiratory reserve volume
4. Residual volume.

■ TIDAL VOLUME

Tidal volume (TV) is the volume of air breathed in and out of lungs in a single normal quiet respiration. Tidal volume signifies the normal depth of breathing.

Normal Value

500 mL (0.5 L).

■ INSPIRATORY RESERVE VOLUME

Inspiratory reserve volume (IRV) is an additional volume of air that can be inspired forcefully after the end of normal inspiration.

Normal Value

3,300 mL (3.3 L).

■ EXPIRATORY RESERVE VOLUME

Expiratory reserve volume (EVR) is the additional volume of air that can be expired out forcefully, after normal expiration.

Normal Value

1,000 mL (1 L).

■ RESIDUAL VOLUME

Residual volume (RV) is the volume of air remaining in lungs even after forced expiration. Normally, lungs cannot be emptied completely even by forceful expiration. Some quantity of air always remains in the lungs even after the forced expiration.

Residual volume is significant because of two reasons:
1. It helps to aerate the blood in between breathing and during expiration
2. It maintains the contour of the lungs.

Normal Value

1,200 mL (1.2 L)

■ LUNG CAPACITIES

Static lung capacities are the combination of two or more lung volumes.
   Static lung capacities are of four types:
1. Inspiratory capacity
2. Vital capacity
3. Functional residual capacity
4. Total lung capacity.

■ INSPIRATORY CAPACITY

Inspiratory capacity (IC) is the maximum volume of air that is inspired after normal expiration (end expiratory position). It includes tidal volume and inspiratory reserve volume (Fig. 121.1).

$$IC = TV + IRV$$
$$= 500 + 3,300 = 3,800 \text{ mL}$$

■ VITAL CAPACITY (VC)

Vital capacity (VC) is the maximum volume of air that can be expelled out forcefully after a deep (maximal) inspiration. VC includes inspiratory reserve volume, tidal volume and expiratory reserve volume.

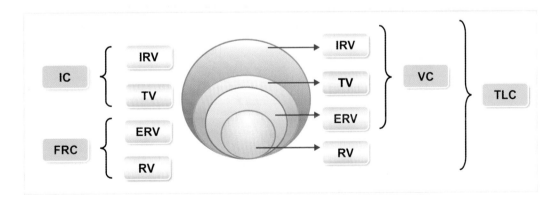

FIGURE 121.1: Lung volumes and capacities. TV = Tidal volume, IRV = Inspiratory reserve volume, ERV = Expiratory reserve volume, RV = Residual volume, IC = Inspiratory capacity, FRC = Functional residual capacity, VC = Vital capacity, TLC = Total lung capacity.

VC = IRV + TV + ERV
      = 3,300 + 500 + 1,000 = 4,800 mL

Vital capacity is significant physiologically and its determination is useful in clinical diagnosis as explained later in this chapter.

■ FUNCTIONAL RESIDUAL CAPACITY

Functional residual capacity (FRC) is the volume of air remaining in lungs after normal expiration (after normal tidal expiration). Functional residual capacity includes expiratory reserve volume and residual volume.

FRC = ERV + RV
     = 1,000 + 1,200 = 2,200 mL

■ TOTAL LUNG CAPACITY

Total lung capacity (TLC) is the volume of air present in lungs after a deep (maximal) inspiration. It includes all the volumes.

TLC = IRV + TV + ERV + RV
     = 3,300 + 500 + 1,000 + 1,200 = 6,000 mL

■ MEASUREMENT OF LUNG VOLUMES AND CAPACITIES

Spirometry is the method to measure lung volumes and capacities. Simple instrument used for this purpose is called **spirometer**. Modified spirometer is known as **respirometer**. Nowadays **plethysmograph** is also used to measure lung volumes and capacities.

■ SPIROMETER

Spirometer is made up of metal and it contains two chambers namely outer chamber and inner chamber (Fig. 121.2). Outer chamber is called the **water chamber** because it is filled with water. A **floating drum** is immersed in the water in an inverted position. Drum is counter balanced by a **weight**. Weight is attached to the top of the inverted drum by means of string or chain. A **pen with ink** is attached to the counter weight. Pen is made to write on a **calibrated paper,** which is fixed to a recording device.

Inner chamber is inverted and has a small hole at the top. A long metal tube passes through the inner

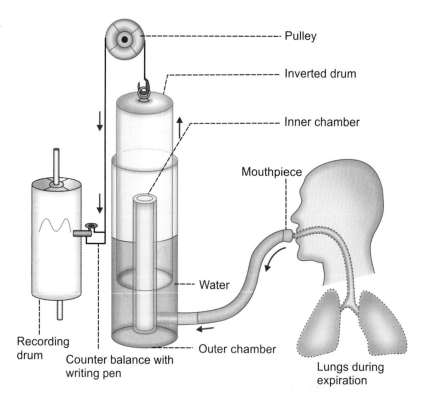

FIGURE 121.2: Spirometer. During expiration, the air enters the spirometer from lungs. Inverted drum moves up and the pen draws a downward curve on the recording drum.

chamber from the bottom towards the top. Upper end of this tube reaches the top portion of the inner chamber. Then the tube passes through a hole at the top of inner chamber and penetrates into outer water chamber above the level of water. A **rubber tube** is connected to the outer end of the metal tube. At the other end of this rubber tube, a mouthpiece is attached. Subject respires through this mouthpiece by closing the nose with a **nose clip.**

When the subject breathes with spirometer, during expiration, drum moves up and the counter weight comes down. Reverse of this occurs when the subject breathes the air from the spirometer, i.e. during inspiration. Upward and downward movements of the counter weight are recorded in the form of a graph. Upward deflection of the curve in the graph shows inspiration and the downward deflection denotes expiration.

Spirometer is used only for a **single breath.** Repeated cycles of respiration cannot be recorded by using this instrument because carbon dioxide accumulates in the spirometer and oxygen or fresh air cannot be provided to the subject.

Respirometer

Respirometer is the modified spirometer. It has provision for removal of carbon dioxide and supply of oxygen.

Carbon dioxide is removed by placing soda lime inside the instrument. Oxygen is supplied to the instrument from the oxygen cylinder, by a suitable valve system.

Oxygen is filled in the inverted drum above water level and the subject can breathe in and out with instrument for about 6 minutes and recording can be done continuously.

Spirogram

Spirogram is the graphical record of lung volumes and capacities using spirometer. Upward deflection of the spirogram denotes inspiration and the downward curve indicates expiration (Fig. 121.3). In order to determine the lung volumes and capacities, following four levels are to be noted in spirogram:
1. Normal end expiratory level
2. Normal end inspiratory level
3. Maximum expiratory level
4. Maximum inspiratory level.

■ COMPUTERIZED SPIROMETER

Computerized spirometer is the solid state electronic equipment. It does not contain a drum or water chamber. Subject has to respire into a sophisticated transducer, which is connected to the instrument by means of a cable.

Disadvantages of Spirometry

By using simple spirometer, respirometer or computerized spirometer, not all the lung volumes and lung capacities can be measured.

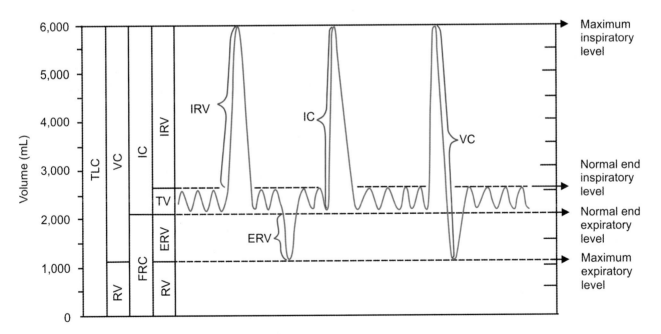

FIGURE 121.3: Spirogram. TV = Tidal volume, IRV = Inspiratory reserve volume, ERV = Expiratory reserve volume, RV = Residual volume, IC = Inspiratory capacity, FRC = Functional residual capacity, VC = Vital capacity, TLC = Total lung capacity.

Volume, which cannot be measured by spirometry, is the **residual volume.** Capacities, which include residual volume also cannot be measured. Capacities that include residual volume are **functional residual capacity** and **total lung capacity.**

Volume and capacities, which cannot be measured by spirometry, are measured by **nitrogen washout technique** or **helium dilution technique** or by **body plethysmograph.**

■ PLETHYSMOGRAPHY

Plethysmography is a technique used to measure all the lung volumes and capacities. It is explained later.

■ MEASUREMENT OF FUNCTIONAL RESIDUAL CAPACITY AND RESIDUAL VOLUME

Residual volume and the functional residual capacity cannot be measured by spirometer and can be determined by three methods:

1. Helium dilution technique
2. Nitrogen washout method
3. Plethysmography.

■ 1. HELIUM DILUTION TECHNIQUE

Procedure to Measure Functional Residual Capacity

Respirometer is filled with air containing a known quantity of **helium.** Initially, the subject breathes normally. Then, after the end of expiration, subject breathes from respirometer. Helium from respirometer enters the lungs and starts mixing with air in lungs. After few minutes of breathing, concentration of helium in the respirometer becomes equal to concentration of helium in the lungs of subject. It is called the equilibration of helium. After **equilibration of helium** between respirometer and lungs, concentration of helium in respirometer is determined (Fig. 121.4).

Functional residual capacity is calculated by the formula:

$$FRC = \frac{V(C_1 - C_2)}{C_2}$$

Where,
C_1 = Initial concentration of helium in the respirometer
C_2 = Final concentration of helium in the respirometer
V = Initial volume of air in the respirometer.

Measured Values

For example, the following data of a subject are obtained from the experiment:

1. Initial volume of air in respirometer = 5 L (5,000 mL)
2. Initial concentration of helium in respirometer = 15%
3. Final concentration of helium in respirometer = 10%.

Calculation

From the above data, the functional residual capacity of the subject is calculated in the following way:

$$FRC = \frac{V(C_1 - C_2)}{C_2}$$

$$FRC = \frac{5,000(15/100 - 10/100)}{10/100} \text{ mL}$$

$$= \frac{5,000(5/100)}{10/100} \text{ mL}$$

$$= \frac{5,000 \times 5}{10} \text{ mL}$$

$$= 2,500 \text{ mL}$$

Thus, the functional residual capacity in this subject is 2,500 mL.

Procedure to Measure Residual Volume

To determine functional residual capacity, the subject starts breathing with respirometer after the end of normal expiration. To measure residual volume, the subject should start breathing from the respirometer after forced expiration.

■ 2. NITROGEN WASHOUT METHOD

Normally, concentration of nitrogen in air is 80%. So, if total quantity of nitrogen in the lungs is measured, the volume of air present in lungs can be calculated.

Procedure to Measure Functional Residual Capacity

Subject is asked to breathe normally. At the end of normal expiration, the subject inspires **pure oxygen** through a valve and expires into a Douglas bag. This procedure is repeated for 6 to 7 minutes, until the **nitrogen** in lungs is displaced by oxygen. Nitrogen comes to the **Douglas bag.** Afterwards, following factors are measured to calculate functional residual capacity.

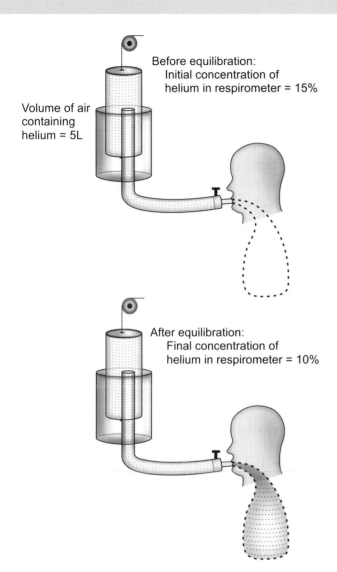

Before equilibration:
Initial concentration of
helium in respirometer = 15%

Volume of air
containing
helium = 5L

After equilibration:
Final concentration of
helium in respirometer = 10%

FIGURE 121.4: Measurement of functional residual
capacity by using helium

Calculation

i. Volume of air collected in Douglas bag
ii. Concentration of nitrogen in Douglas bag.
    By using the data, the functional residual capacity is
calculated by using the formula:

$$FRC = \frac{C_1 \times V}{C_2}$$

Where,
V = Volume of air collected
C_1 = Concentration of nitrogen in the collected
air
C_2 = Normal concentration of nitrogen in the
air.

Measured Values

For example, the following data are obtained from the
experiment with a subject:

   i. Volume of air collected   = 40 L (40,000 mL)
  ii. Concentration of nitrogen   = 5%
     in the collected air
 iii. Normal concentration of   = 80%
     nitrogen in the air.

Calculation

From the above data, the functional residual capacity of
the subject is calculated in the following way:

$$FRC = \frac{C_1 \times V}{C_2}$$

$$FRC = \frac{5/100 \times 40,000}{80/100} \ mL$$

$$= \frac{5 \times 40,000}{80} \ mL$$

$$= 2,500 \ mL.$$

Thus, functional residual capacity in this subject is
2,500 mL.

Procedure to Measure Residual Volume

To measure the functional residual capacity, the subject
starts inhaling pure oxygen after the end of normal
expiration and to determine the residual volume, the
subject starts breathing pure oxygen after forceful
expiration.

■ 3. PLETHYSMOGRAPHY

Plethysmography is a technique to study the variations
in the size or volume of a part of the body such as
limb. **Plethysmograph** is the instrument used for this
purpose. Whole body plethysmograph is the instrument
used to measure the lung volumes including residual
volume.

Plethysmography is based on **Boyle's law of gas,**
which states that the volume of a sample of gas is
inversely proportional to the pressure of that gas at
constant temperature.

Subject sits in an airtight chamber of the whole
body plethysmograph and breathes normally through
a mouthpiece connected to a flow transducer called
pneumotachograph. It detects the volume changes

during different phases of respiration. After normal breathing for few minutes, the subject breathes rapidly with maximum force. During maximum expiration, the lung volume decreases very much. But volume of gas in the chamber increases with decrease in pressure. By measuring the volume and pressure changes inside the chamber, volume of lungs is calculated by using the formula:

$$P_1 \times V = P_2 (V - \Delta V)$$

Where,

P_1 and P_2 = Pressure changes

V = Functional residual capacity.

■ VITAL CAPACITY

■ DEFINITION

Vital capacity is the maximum volume of air that can be expelled out of lungs forcefully after a maximal or deep inspiration.

■ LUNG VOLUMES INCLUDED IN VITAL CAPACITY

Vital capacity includes inspiratory reserve volume, tidal volume and expiratory reserve volume.

■ NORMAL VALUE

VC = IRV + TV + ERV
= 3,300 + 500 + 1,000 = 4,800 mL.

■ VARIATIONS OF VITAL CAPACITY

Physiological Variations

1. *Sex:* In females, vital capacity is less than in males
2. *Body built:* Vital capacity is slightly more in heavily built persons
3. *Posture:* Vital capacity is more in standing position and less in lying position
4. *Athletes:* Vital capacity is more in athletes
5. *Occupation:* Vital capacity is decreased in people with sedentary jobs. It is increased in persons who play musical wind instruments such as bugle and flute.

Pathological Variations

Vital capacity is decreased in the following respiratory diseases:

1. Asthma
2. Emphysema
3. Weakness or paralysis of respiratory muscle
4. Pulmonary congestion
5. Pneumonia
6. Pneumothorax
7. Hemothorax
8. Pyothorax
9. Hydrothorax
10. Pulmonary edema
11. Pulmonary tuberculosis.

Measurement

Vital capacity is measured by spirometry. The subject is asked to take a deep inspiration and expire forcefully.

■ FORCED VITAL CAPACITY

Forced vital capacity (FVC) is the volume of air that can be exhaled forcefully and rapidly after a maximal or deep inspiration. It is a dynamic lung capacity.

Normally FVC is equal to VC. However in some pulmonary diseases, FVC is decreased.

■ FORCED EXPIRATORY VOLUME OR TIMED VITAL CAPACITY

■ DEFINITION

Forced expiratory volume (FEV) is the volume of air, which can be expired forcefully in a given unit of time (after a deep inspiration). It is also called timed vital capacity or forced expiratory vital capacity (FEVC). It is a dynamic lung volume.

FEV_1 = Volume of air expired forcefully in 1 second

FEV_2 = Volume of air expired forcefully in 2 seconds

FEV_3 = Volume of air expired forcefully in 3 seconds.

■ NORMAL VALUES

Forced expiratory volume in persons with normal respiratory functions is as follows:

FEV_1 = 83% of total vital capacity

FEV_2 = 94% of total vital capacity

FEV_3 = 97% of total vital capacity

After 3rd second = 100% of total vital capacity.

■ SIGNIFICANCE OF DETERMINING FEV

Vital capacity may be almost normal in some of the respiratory diseases. However, the FEV has great diagnostic value, as it is decreased significantly in some respiratory diseases.

It is very much decreased in obstructive diseases like asthma and emphysema. It is slightly reduced in some restrictive respiratory diseases like fibrosis of lungs (Fig. 121.5).

■ RESPIRATORY MINUTE VOLUME

■ DEFINITION

Respiratory minute volume (RMV) is the volume of air breathed in and out of lungs every minute. It is the product of tidal volume (TV) and respiratory rate (RR).

$$RMV = TV \times RR$$
$$= 500 \times 12 = 6,000 \text{ mL.}$$

■ NORMAL VALUE

Normal respiratory minute volume is 6 L.

■ VARIATIONS

Respiratory minute volume increases in physiological conditions such as voluntary hyperventilation, exercise and emotional conditions. It is reduced in respiratory diseases.

■ MAXIMUM BREATHING CAPACITY OR MAXIMUM VENTILATION VOLUME

■ DEFINITION

Maximum breathing capacity (MBC) is the maximum volume of air, which can be breathed in and out of lungs by forceful respiration (hyperventilation: increase in rate and force of respiration) per minute. It is also called maximum ventilation volume (MVV).

MBC is a dynamic lung capacity and it is reduced in respiratory diseases.

■ NORMAL VALUE

In healthy adult male, it is 150 to 170 L/minute and in females, it is 80 to 100 L/minute.

■ MEASUREMENT

Subject is asked to breathe forcefully and rapidly with a **respirometer** for 15 seconds. Volume of air inspired and expired is measured from the spirogram. From this value, the MBC is calculated for 1 minute.

For example, MBC in 12 seconds = 32 L

$$\text{MBC per minute} = \frac{32}{12} \times 60 \text{ L}$$
$$= 160 \text{ L}$$

■ PEAK EXPIRATORY FLOW RATE

■ DEFINITION

Peak expiratory flow rate (PEFR) is the maximum rate at which the air can be expired after a deep inspiration.

■ NORMAL VALUE

In normal persons, it is 400 L/minute.

■ MEASUREMENT

Peak expiratory flow rate is measured by using **Wright peak flow meter** or a mini peak flow meter.

■ SIGNIFICANCE OF DETERMINING PEFR

Determination of PEFR rate is useful for assessing the respiratory diseases especially to differentiate the obstructive and restrictive diseases. Generally, PEFR is reduced in all type of respiratory disease. However, reduction is more significant in the obstructive diseases than in the restrictive diseases.

Thus, in restrictive diseases, the PEFR is 200 L/minute and in obstructive diseases, it is only 100 L/minute.

■ RESTRICTIVE AND OBSTRUCTIVE RESPIRATORY DISEASES

Diseases of respiratory tract are classified into two types:
1. Restrictive respiratory disease
2. Obstructive respiratory disease.

These two types of respiratory diseases are determined by lung functions tests, particularly FEV.

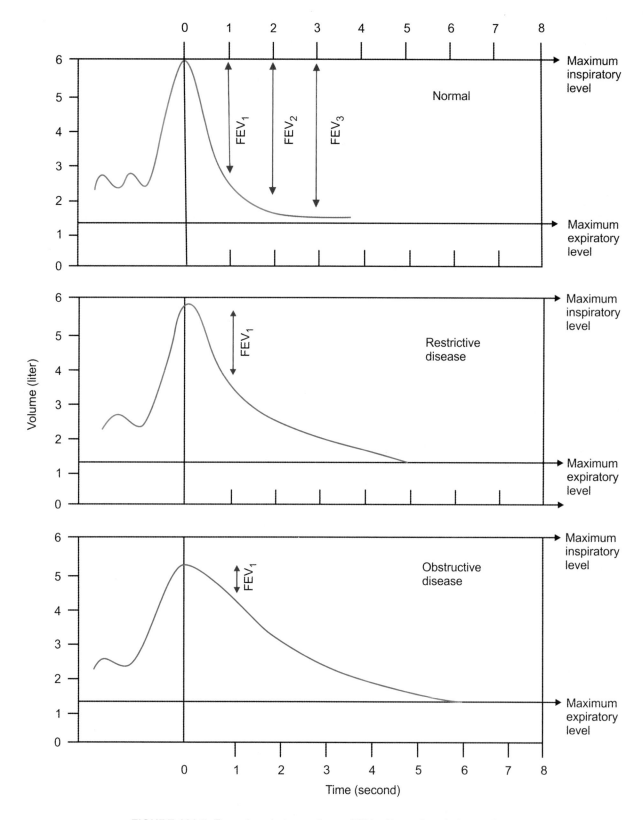

FIGURE 121.5: Forced expiratory volume. FEV = Forced expiratory volume.

TABLE 121.1: Restrictive and obstructive respiratory diseases

Type	Disease	Structures involved
Restrictive respiratory diseases	Polio myelitis	CNS
	Myasthenia gravis	CNS and thoracic cavity
	Flail chest (broken ribs)	Thoracic cavity
	Paralysis of diaphragm	CNS
	Spinal cord diseases	CNS
	Pleural effusion	Thoracic cavity
Obstructive respiratory diseases	Asthma Chronic bronchitis Emphysema Cystic fibrosis	Lower respiratory tract
	Laryngotracheobronchitis Epiglottis Tumors Severe cough and cold with phlegm	Upper respiratory tract

■ RESTRICTIVE RESPIRATORY DISEASE

Restrictive respiratory disease is the abnormal respiratory condition characterized by difficulty in inspiration. Expiration is not affected. Restrictive respiratory disease may be because of abnormality of lungs, thoracic cavity or/and nervous system.

■ OBSTRUCTIVE RESPIRATORY DISEASE

Obstructive respiratory disease is the abnormal respiratory condition characterized by difficulty in expiration.

Obstructive and respiratory diseases are listed in Table 121.1.

Ventilation

- **VENTILATION**
- **PULMONARY VENTILATION**
  - **DEFINITION**
  - **NORMAL VALUE AND CALCULATION**
- **ALVEOLAR VENTILATION**
  - **DEFINITION**
  - **NORMAL VALUE AND CALCULATION**
- **DEAD SPACE**
  - **DEFINITION**
  - **TYPES**
  - **NORMAL VALUE**
  - **MEASUREMENT**
- **VENTILATION-PERFUSION RATIO**
  - **DEFINITION**
  - **NORMAL VALUE AND CALCULATION**
  - **SIGNIFICANCE**
  - **WASTED AIR AND WASTED BLOOD**
  - **VARIATIONS**

■ VENTILATION

In general, the word 'ventilation' refers to circulation of replacement of air or gas in a space. In respiratory physiology, ventilation is the rate at which air enters or leaves the lungs. Ventilation in **respiratory physiology** is of two types:

1. Pulmonary ventilation
2. Alveolar ventilation.

■ PULMONARY VENTILATION

■ DEFINITION

Pulmonary ventilation is defined as the volume of air moving in and out of respiratory tract in a given unit of time during quiet breathing. It is also called **minute ventilation** or **respiratory minute volume** (RMV).

Pulmonary ventilation is a cyclic process, by which fresh air enters the lungs and an equal volume of air leaves the lungs.

■ NORMAL VALUE AND CALCULATION

Normal value of pulmonary ventilation is 6,000 mL (6 L)/minute. It is the product of tidal volume (TV) and the rate of respiration (RR).

It is calculated by the formula:

Pulmonary ventilation
= Tidal volume × Respiratory rate
= 500 mL × 12/minute
= 6,000 mL/minute.

■ ALVEOLAR VENTILATION

■ DEFINITION

Alveolar ventilation is the amount of air utilized for gaseous exchange every minute.

Alveolar ventilation is different from pulmonary ventilation. In pulmonary ventilation, 6 L of air moves in and out of respiratory tract every minute. But the whole volume of air is not utilized for exchange of gases. Volume of air subjected for exchange of gases is the alveolar ventilation. Air trapped in the respiratory passage (dead space) does not take part in gaseous exchange.

■ NORMAL VALUE AND CALCULATION

Normal value of alveolar ventilation is 4,200 mL (4.2 L)/minute.

It is calculated by the formula:

Alveolar ventilation
= (Tidal volume – Dead space) x Respiratory rate
= (500 – 150) mL × 12/minute
= 4,200 mL (4.2 L)/minute.

■ DEAD SPACE

■ DEFINITION

Dead space is defined as the part of the respiratory tract, where gaseous exchange does not take place. Air present in the dead space is called dead space air.

■ TYPES OF DEAD SPACE

Dead space is of two types:
1. Anatomical dead space
2. Physiological dead space.

Anatomical Dead Space

Anatomical dead space extends from nose up to terminal bronchiole. It includes nose, pharynx, trachea, bronchi and branches of bronchi up to terminal bronchioles. These structures serve only as the passage for air movement. Gaseous exchange does not take place in these structures.

Physiological Dead Space

Physiological dead space includes anatomical dead space plus two additional volumes.

Additional volumes included in physiological dead space are:
1. Air in the alveoli, which are **non-functioning**. In some respiratory diseases, alveoli do not function because of dysfunction or destruction of alveolar membrane.
2. Air in the alveoli, which do not receive adequate blood flow. Gaseous exchange does not take place during inadequate blood supply.

These two additional volumes are generally considered as wasted ventilation.

Wasted ventilation and wasted air

Wasted ventilation is the volume of air that ventilates physiological dead space. Wasted air refers to air that is not utilized for gaseous exchange. Dead space air is generally considered as wasted air.

■ NORMAL VALUE OF DEAD SPACE

Volume of normal dead space is 150 mL. Under normal conditions, physiological dead space is equal to anatomical dead space. It is because, all the alveoli are functioning and all the alveoli receive adequate blood flow in normal conditions.

Physiological dead space increases during respiratory diseases, which affect the pulmonary blood flow or the alveoli.

■ MEASUREMENT OF DEAD SPACE – NITROGEN WASHOUT METHOD

Dead space is measured by single breath nitrogen washout method. The subject respires normally for few minutes. Then, he takes a sudden inhalation of pure oxygen.

Oxygen replaces the air in dead space (air passage), i.e. the dead space air contains only oxygen and it pushes the other gases into alveoli.

Now, the subject exhales through a nitrogen meter. Nitrogen meter shows the concentration of nitrogen in expired air continuously.

First portion of expired air comes from upper part of respiratory tract or air passage, which contains only oxygen. Next portion of expired air comes from the alveoli, which contains nitrogen. Now, the nitrogen meter shows the nitrogen concentration, which rises sharply and reaches the plateau soon. By using data obtained from nitrogen meter, a graph is plotted. From this graph, the dead space is calculated (Fig. 122.1).

The graph has two areas, area without nitrogen and area with nitrogen. Area of the graph is measured by a planimeter or by computer. Area without nitrogen indicates dead space air.

It is calculated by the formula:

$$\text{Dead space} = \frac{\text{Area without } N_2}{\text{Area with } N_2 + \text{Area without } N_2} \times \text{Volume of expired air}$$

For example, in a subject:
Area with nitrogen   = 70 sq cm
Area without nitrogen   = 30 sq cm
Volume of air expired   = 500 mL

$$\text{Dead space} = \frac{30}{70+30} \times 500$$

$$= \frac{30}{100} \times 500$$

$$= 150 \text{ mL.}$$

■ VENTILATION-PERFUSION RATIO

■ DEFINITION

Ventilation-perfusion ratio is the ratio of alveolar ventilation and the amount of blood that perfuse the alveoli.

It is expressed as V_A/Q. V_A is alveolar ventilation and Q is the blood flow (perfusion).

■ NORMAL VALUE AND CALCULATION

Normal Value

Normal value of ventilation-perfusion ratio is about 0.84.

Calculation

Alveolar ventilation is calculated by the formula:

$$\text{Ventilation-perfusion ratio} = \frac{\text{Alveolar ventilation}}{\text{Pulmonary blood flow}}$$

$$\begin{aligned}\text{Alveolar ventilation} &= (\text{Tidal volume} - \text{Dead space}) \times \\ &\quad\text{Respiratory rate} \\ &= (500-150)\text{ mL} \times 12/\text{minute} \\ &= 4{,}200 \text{ mL/minute}\end{aligned}$$

$$\begin{aligned}\text{Blood flow through alveoli} \\ (\text{Pulmonary blood flow}) &= 5{,}000 \text{ mL/minute}\end{aligned}$$

Therefore,

$$\text{Ventilation-perfusion ratio} = \frac{4{,}200}{5{,}000}$$

$$= 0.84$$

■ SIGNIFICANCE OF VENTILATION-PERFUSION RATIO

Ventilation-perfusion ratio signifies the gaseous exchange. It is affected if there is any change in alveolar ventilation or in blood flow.
Ventilation without perfusion = dead space
Perfusion without ventilation = shunt

■ WASTED AIR AND WASTED BLOOD

Ventilation-perfusion ratio is not perfect because of existence of two factors on either side of alveolar membrane.

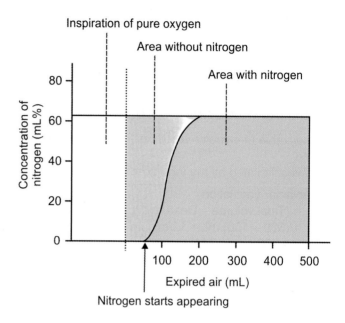

FIGURE 122.1: Measurement of dead space

These factors are:
1. Physiological dead space, which includes wasted air (see above)
2. Physiological shunt, which includes wasted blood (Chapter 119).

■ VARIATIONS IN VENTILATION-PERFUSION RATIO

Physiological Variation

1. Ratio increases, if ventilation increases without any change in blood flow
2. Ratio decreases, if blood flow increases without any change in ventilation
3. In sitting position, there is reduction in blood flow in the upper part of the lungs (zone 1) than in the lower part (zone 3). Therefore, in zone 1 of lungs ventilation-perfusion ratio increases three times. At the same time, in zone 3 of the lungs, because of increased blood flow ventilation-perfusion ratio decreases (Chapter 119).

Pathological Variation

In chronic obstructive pulmonary diseases (COPD), ventilation is affected because of obstruction and destruction of alveolar membrane. So, ventilation-perfusion ratio reduces greatly.

Inspired Air, Alveolar Air and Expired Air

Chapter **123**

- ■ **INSPIRED AIR**
  - ■ DEFINITION
  - ■ COMPOSITION
- ■ **ALVEOLAR AIR**
  - ■ DEFINITION
  - ■ COMPOSITION
  - ■ RENEWAL
  - ■ METHOD OF COLLECTION
- ■ **EXPIRED AIR**
  - ■ DEFINITION
  - ■ COMPOSITION
  - ■ METHOD OF COLLECTION

■ INSPIRED AIR

■ DEFINITION

Inspired air is the atmospheric air, which is inhaled during inspiration.

■ COMPOSITION

Composition of inspired air is given in Table 123.1.

■ ALVEOLAR AIR

■ DEFINITION

Alveolar air is the air present in alveoli of lungs. Its composition is given in Table 123.1.

Alveolar Air Vs Inspired Air

Alveolar air is different from inspired air in four ways:

TABLE 123.1: Composition of inspired air, alveolar air and expired air

Air	Inspired (atmospheric) air		Alveolar air		Expired air	
Gas	Content (mL%)	Partial pressure (mm Hg)	Content (mL%)	Partial pressure (mm Hg)	Content (mL%)	Partial pressure (mm Hg)
Oxygen	20.84	159.00	13.60	104.00	15.70	120.00
Carbon dioxide	0.04	0.30	5.30	40.00	3.60	27.00
Nitrogen	78.62	596.90	74.90	569.00	74.50	566.00
Water vapor, etc.	0.50	3.80	6.20	47.00	6.20	47.00
Total	100.00	760.00	100.00	760.00	100.00	760.00

1. Alveolar air is partially replaced by the atmospheric air during each breath
2. Oxygen diffuses from the alveolar air into pulmonary capillaries constantly
3. Carbon dioxide diffuses from pulmonary blood into alveolar air constantly
4. Dry atmospheric air is humidified, while passing through respiratory passage before entering the alveoli (Table 123.1).

■ COMPOSITION

Composition of alveolar air is given in Table 123.1.

■ RENEWAL

Alveolar air is constantly renewed. Rate of renewal is slow during normal breathing. During each breath, out of 500 mL of tidal volume only 350 mL of air enters the alveoli and the remaining quantity of 150 mL (30%) becomes dead space air. Hence, the amount of alveolar air replaced by new atmospheric air with each breath is only about 70% of the total alveolar air.

Thus,

$$\text{Alveolar air} = \frac{350}{500} \times 100 = 70\%$$

Slow renewal of alveolar air is responsible for prevention of sudden changes in concentration of gases in the blood.

■ METHOD OF COLLECTION

Alveolar air is collected by using **Haldane-Priestely tube.** This tube consists of a canvas rubber tube, which is 1 m long and having a diameter of 2.5 cm. It is opened on both ends.

A mouthpiece is fitted at one end of the tube. Near the mouthpiece, there is a side tube, which is fixed with a sampling tube. Mouthpiece and the side tube are interconnected by means of a three-way cock. By keeping the mouthpiece in the mouth, the subject makes a forceful expiration through the mouthpiece. Alveolar air is expired at the end of forced expiration. So, by using the three-way cock, the last portion of expired air (alveolar air) is collected in the sampling tube.

■ EXPIRED AIR

■ DEFINITION

Expired air is the amount of air that is exhaled during expiration. It is a combination of dead space air and alveolar air.

■ COMPOSITION

Concentration of gases in expired air is somewhere between inspired air and alveolar air. Composition of expired air is given in Table 123.1 along with composition of inspired air and alveolar air.

■ METHOD OF COLLECTION

Expired air is collected by using **Douglas bag.**

Exchange of Respiratory Gases

■ INTRODUCTION

Oxygen is essential for the cells. Carbon dioxide, which is produced as waste product in the cells must be expelled from the cells and body. Lungs serve to exchange these two gases with blood.

■ EXCHANGE OF RESPIRATORY GASES IN LUNGS

In the lungs, exchange of respiratory gases takes place between the alveoli of lungs and the blood. Oxygen enters the blood from alveoli and carbon dioxide is expelled out of blood into alveoli. Exchange occurs through **bulk flow diffusion** (Chapter 3).

Exchange of gases between blood and alveoli takes place through respiratory membrane. Refer Chapter 118 for details.

■ RESPIRATORY MEMBRANE

Respiratory membrance is a membranous structure through which exchange of respiratory gases takes place. It is formed by **epithelium** of respiratory unit and **endothelium** of pulmonary capillary. Epithelium of respiratory unit is a very thin layer (Chapter 118). Since, the capillaries are in close contact with this membrane, alveolar air is in close proximity to capillary blood. This facilitates gaseous exchange between air and blood (Fig. 124.1).

Respiratory membrane is formed by different layers of structures belonging to the alveoli and capillaries.

Layers of Respiratory Membrane

Different layers of respiratory membrane from within outside are given in Table 124.1.

In spite of having many layers, respiratory membrane is very thin with an average thickness of 0.5 μ. Total surface area of the respiratory membrane in both the lungs is about 70 square meter.

Average diameter of pulmonary capillary is only 8 μ, which means that the RBCs with a diameter of 7.4 μ actually squeeze through the capillaries. Therefore, the membrane of RBCs is in close contact with capillary wall. This facilitates quick exchange of oxygen and carbon dioxide between the blood and alveoli.

■ DIFFUSING CAPACITY

Diffusing capacity is defined as the volume of gas that diffuses through the respiratory membrane each minute for a pressure gradient of 1 mm Hg.

TABLE 124.1: Layers of respiratory membrane

Portion	Layers
Alveolar portion	1. Monomolecular layer of surfactant, which spreads over the surface of alveoli 2. Thin fluid layer that lines the alveoli 3. Alveolar epithelial layer, which is composed of thin epithelial cells resting on a basement membrane
Between alveolar and capillary portions	4. An interstitial space
Capillary portion	5. Basement membrane of capillary 6. Capillary endothelial cells

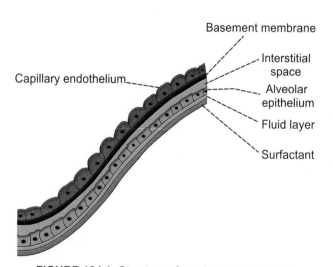

FIGURE 124.1: Structure of respiratory membrane

Diffusing Capacity for Oxygen and Carbon Dioxide

Diffusing capacity for oxygen is 21 mL/minute/1 mm Hg. Diffusing capacity for carbon dioxide is 400 mL/minute/1 mm Hg. Thus, the diffusing capacity for carbon dioxide is about 20 times more than that of oxygen.

Factors Affecting Diffusing Capacity

1. Pressure gradient

Diffusing capacity is **directly proportional** to pressure gradient. Pressure gradient is the difference between the partial pressure of a gas in alveoli and pulmonary capillary blood (see below). It is the major factor, which affects the diffusing capacity.

2. Solubility of gas in fluid medium

Diffusing capacity is **directly proportional** to solubility of the gas. If the solubility of a gas is more in the fluid medium, a large number of molecules dissolve in it and diffuse easily.

3. Total surface area of respiratory membrane

Diffusing capacity is **directly proportional** to surface area of respiratory membrane. Surface area of respiratory membrane in each lung is about 70 sq m. If the total surface area of respiratory membrane decreases, the diffusing capacity for the gases is decreased. Diffusing capacity is decreased in emphysema in which many of the alveoli are collapsed because of heavy smoking or oxidant gases.

4. Molecular weight of the gas

Diffusing capacity is **inversely proportional** to molecular weight of the gas. If the molecular weight is more, the density is more and the rate of diffusion is less.

5. Thickness of respiratory membrane

Diffusion is **inversely proportional** to the thickness of respiratory membrane. More the thickness of respiratory membrane less is the diffusion. It is because the distance through which the diffusion takes place is long. In conditions like fibrosis and edema, the diffusion rate is reduced, because the thickness of respiratory membrane is increased.

Relation between Diffusing Capacity and Factors Affecting it

Relation between diffusing capacity and the factors affecting it is expressed by the following formula:

$$DC \; \infty \; \frac{Pg \times S \times A}{Mw \times D}$$

DC = Diffusing capacity
Pg = Pressure gradient
S = Solubility of gas
A = Surface area of respiratory membrane
Mw = Molecular weight
D = Thickness of respiratory membrane.

■ DIFFUSION COEFFICIENT AND FICK LAW OF DIFFUSION

Diffusion Coefficient

Diffusion coefficient is defined as a constant (a factor of proportionality), which is the measure of a substance diffusing through the concentration gradient. It is also known as **diffusion constant.** It is related to size and shape of the molecules of the substance.

Fick Law of Diffusion

Diffusion is well described by Fick law of diffusion. According to this law, amount of a substance crossing a given area is directly proportional to the area available for diffusion, concentration gradient and a constant known as diffusion coefficient.

Thus,

Amount diffused = Area × Concentration gradient × Diffusion coefficient

Formula of Fick law:

$$J = -D \times A \times \frac{dc}{dx}$$

Where,

J = Amount of substance diffused
D = Diffusion coefficient
A = Area through which diffusion occurs
dc/dx = Concentration gradient.

Negative sign in the formula indicates that diffusion occurs from region of higher concentration to region of lower concentration. Diffusion coefficient reduces when the molecular size of diffusing substance is increased. It increases when the size is decreased, i.e. the smaller molecules diffuse rapidly than the larger ones.

■ DIFFUSION OF OXYGEN

Diffusion of Oxygen from Atmospheric Air into Alveoli

Partial pressure of oxygen in the atmospheric air is 159 mm Hg and in the alveoli, it is 104 mm Hg. Because of

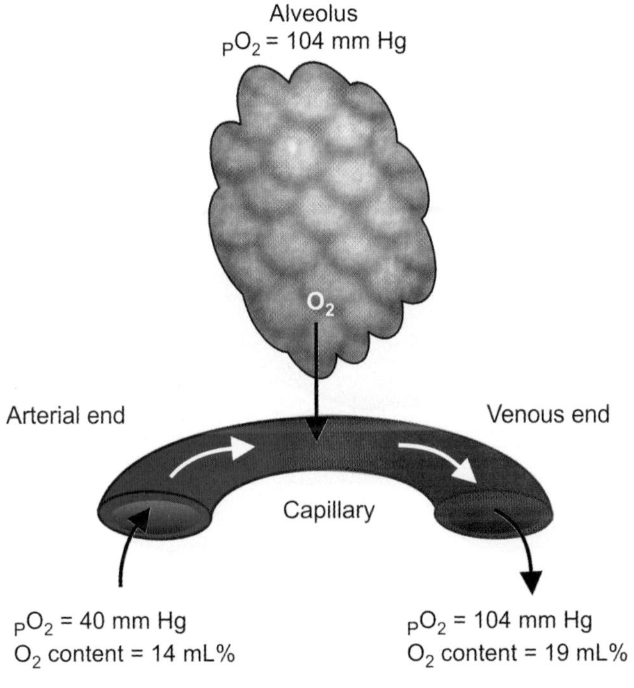

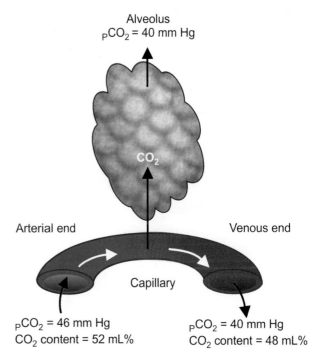

FIGURE 124.2: Diffusion of oxygen from alveolus to pulmonary capillary

Alveolus
pO_2 = 104 mm Hg

O_2

Arterial end

Venous end

Capillary

pO_2 = 40 mm Hg
O_2 content = 14 mL%

pO_2 = 104 mm Hg
O_2 content = 19 mL%

FIGURE 124.3: Diffusion of carbon dioxide from pulmonary capillary to alveolus

Alveolus
pCO_2 = 40 mm Hg

CO_2

Arterial end

Venous end

Capillary

pCO_2 = 46 mm Hg
CO_2 content = 52 mL%

pCO_2 = 40 mm Hg
CO_2 content = 48 mL%

TABLE 124.2: Partial pressure and content of oxygen and carbon dioxide in alveoli, capillaries and tissue

Gas	Arterial end of pulmonary capillary	Alveoli	Venous end of pulmonary capillary	Arterial end of systemic capillary	Tissue	Venous end of systemic capillary
pO_2 (mm Hg)	40	104	104	95	40	40
Oxygen content (mL%)	14	–	19	19	–	14
pCO_2 (mm Hg)	46	40	40	40	46	46
Carbon dioxide content (mL%)	52	–	48	48	–	52

the pressure gradient of 55 mm Hg, oxygen easily enters from atmospheric air into the alveoli (Table 124.2).

Diffusion of Oxygen from Alveoli into Blood

When blood passes through pulmonary capillary, RBC is exposed to oxygen only for 0.75 second at rest and only for 0.25 second during severe exercise. So, diffusion of oxygen must be quicker and effective. Fortunately, this is possible because of pressure gradient.

Partial pressure of oxygen in the pulmonary capillary is 40 mm Hg and in the alveoli, it is 104 mm Hg. Pressure gradient is 64 mm Hg. It facilitates the diffusion of oxygen from alveoli into the blood (Fig. 124.2).

■ DIFFUSION OF CARBON DIOXIDE

Diffusion of Carbon Dioxide from Blood into Alveoli

Partial pressure of carbon dioxide in alveoli is 40 mm Hg whereas in the blood it is 46 mm Hg. Pressure gradient

of 6 mm Hg is responsible for the diffusion of carbon dioxide from blood into the alveoli (Fig. 124.3).

Diffusion of Carbon Dioxide from Alveoli into Atmospheric Air

In atmospheric air, partial pressure of carbon dioxide is very insignificant and is only about 0.3 mm Hg whereas, in the alveoli, it is 40 mm Hg. So, carbon dioxide enters passes to atmosphere from alveoli easily.

■ EXCHANGE OF RESPIRATORY GASES AT TISSUE LEVEL

Oxygen enters the cells of tissues from blood and carbon dioxide is expelled from cells into the blood.

■ DIFFUSION OF OXYGEN FROM BLOOD INTO THE TISSUES

Partial pressure of oxygen in venous end of pulmonary capillary is 104 mm Hg. However, partial pressure of

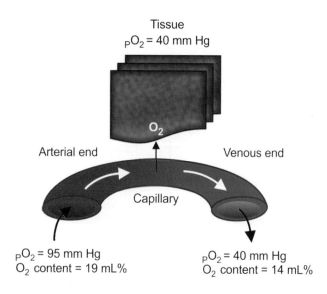

FIGURE 124.4: Diffusion of oxygen from capillary to tissue

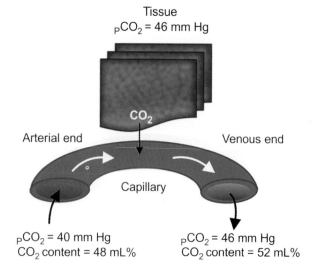

FIGURE 124.5: Diffusion of carbon dioxide from tissue to capillary

oxygen in the arterial end of systemic capillary is only 95 mm Hg. It may be because of physiological shunt in lungs. Due to **venous admixture** in the **shunt** (Chapter 119), 2% of blood reaches the heart without being oxygenated.

Average oxygen tension in the tissues is 40 mm Hg. It is because of continuous metabolic activity and constant utilization of oxygen. Thus, a pressure gradient of about 55 mm Hg exists between capillary blood and the tissues so that oxygen can easily diffuse into the tissues (Fig. 124.4).

Oxygen content in arterial blood is 19 mL% and in the venous blood, it is 14 mL%. Thus, the diffusion of oxygen from blood to tissues is 5 mL/100 mL of blood.

■ DIFFUSION OF CARBON DIOXIDE FROM TISSUES INTO THE BLOOD

Due to continuous metabolic activity, carbon dioxide is produced constantly in the cells of tissues. So, the partial pressure of carbon dioxide is high in the cells and is about 46 mm Hg. Partial pressure of carbon dioxide in arterial blood is 40 mm Hg. Pressure gradient of 6 mm Hg is responsible for the diffusion of carbon dioxide from tissues to the blood (Figs. 124.5 and 124.6).

Carbon dioxide content in arterial blood is 48 mL%. And in the venous blood, it is 52 mL%. So, the diffusion of carbon dioxide from tissues to blood is 4 mL/100 mL of blood (Fig. 124.5).

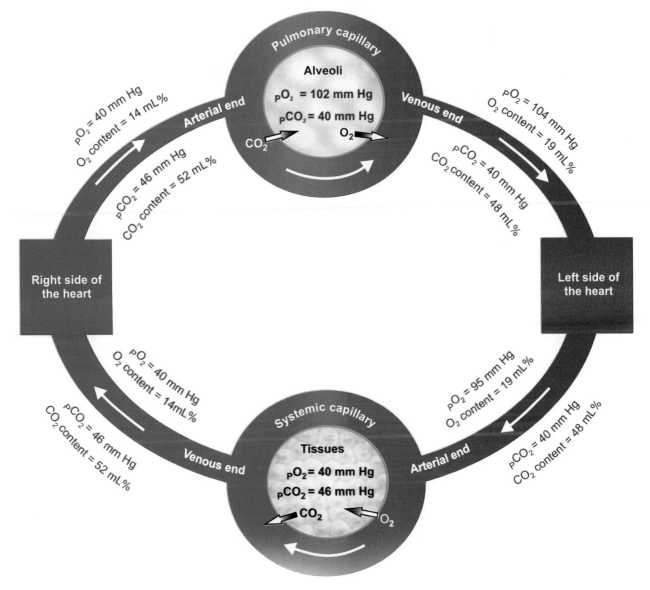

FIGURE 124.6: Partial pressure and content of oxygen and carbon dioxide in blood, alveoli and tissues

■ RESPIRATORY EXCHANGE RATIO

■ DEFINITION

Respiratory exchange ratio (R) is the ratio between the net output of carbon dioxide from tissues to simultaneous net uptake of oxygen by the tissues.

$$R = \frac{CO_2 \text{ output}}{O_2 \text{ uptake}}$$

■ NORMAL VALUES

Value of R depends upon the type of food substance that is metabolized.

When a person utilizes only carbohydrates for metabolism, R is 1.0. That means during carbohydrate metabolism, the amount of carbon dioxide produced in the tissue is equal to the amount of oxygen consumed.

If only fat is used for metabolism, the R is 0.7. When fat is utilized, oxygen reacts with fats and a large portion of oxygen combines with hydrogen ions to form water instead of carbon dioxide. So, the carbon dioxide output is less than the oxygen consumed. And the R is less.

If only protein is utilized, R is 0.803.

However, when a balanced diet containing average quantity of proteins, carbohydrates and lipids is utilized, the R is about 0.825. In steady conditions, respiratory exchange ratio is equal to respiratory quotient.

■ RESPIRATORY QUOTIENT

■ DEFINITION

Respiratory quotient is the molar ratio of carbon dioxide production to oxygen consumption. It is used to determine the utilization of different foodstuffs.

■ NORMAL VALUE

For about 1 hour after meals the respiratory quotient is 1.0. It is because usually, immediately after taking meals, only the carbohydrates are utilized by the tissues. During the metabolism of carbohydrates, one molecule of carbon dioxide is produced for every molecule of oxygen consumed by the tissues. Respiratory quotient is 1.0, which is equal to respiratory exchange ratio.

After utilization of all the carbohydrates available, body starts utilizing fats. Now the respiratory quotient becomes 0.7. When the proteins are metabolized, it becomes 0.8.

During exercise, the respiratory quotient increases (Chapter 132).

Transport of Respiratory Gases

- ■ INTRODUCTION
- ■ TRANSPORT OF OXYGEN
  - ■ AS SIMPLE SOLUTION
  - ■ IN COMBINATION WITH HEMOGLOBIN
  - ■ OXYGEN-HEMOGLOBIN DISSOCIATION CURVE
- ■ TRANSPORT OF CARBON DIOXIDE
  - ■ AS DISSOLVED FORM
  - ■ AS CARBONIC ACID
  - ■ AS BICARBONATE
  - ■ AS CARBAMINO COMPOUNDS
  - ■ CARBON DIOXIDE DISSOCIATION CURVE

■ INTRODUCTION

Blood serves to transport the respiratory gases. Oxygen, which is essential for the cells is transported from alveoli of lungs to the cells. Carbon dioxide, which is the waste product in cells is transported from cells to lungs.

■ TRANSPORT OF OXYGEN

Oxygen is transported from alveoli to the tissue by blood in two forms:

1. As simple physical solution
2. In combination with hemoglobin.

Partial pressure and content of oxygen in arterial blood and venous blood are given in Table 125.1.

TABLE 125.1: Gases in arterial and venous blood

Gas		Arterial blood	Venous blood
Oxygen	Partial pressure (mm Hg)	95	40
	Content (mL%)	19	14
Carbon dioxide	Partial pressure (mm Hg)	40	46
	Content (mL%)	48	52

■ AS SIMPLE SOLUTION

Oxygen dissolves in water of plasma and is transported in this **physical form.** Amount of oxygen transported in this way is very negligible. It is only 0.3 mL/100 mL of plasma. It forms only about 3% of total oxygen in blood. It is because of poor solubility of oxygen in water content of plasma. Still, transport of oxygen in this form becomes important during the conditions like muscular exercise to meet the excess demand of oxygen by the tissues.

■ IN COMBINATION WITH HEMOGLOBIN

Oxygen combines with hemoglobin in blood and is transported as **oxyhemoglobin.** Transport of oxygen in this form is important because, maximum amount (97%) of oxygen is transported by this method.

Oxygenation of Hemoglobin

Oxygen combines with hemoglobin only as a physical combination. It is only **oxygenation** and not **oxidation.** This type of combination of oxygen with hemoglobin has got some advantages. Oxygen can be readily released from hemoglobin when it is needed.

Hemoglobin accepts oxygen readily whenever the partial pressure of oxygen in the blood is more. Hemoglobin gives out oxygen whenever the partial pressure of oxygen in the blood is less.

Oxygen combines with the iron in heme part of hemoglobin. Each molecule of hemoglobin contains 4 atoms of iron. Iron of the hemoglobin is present in ferrous form. Each iron atom combines with one molecule of oxygen. After combination, iron remains in ferrous form only. That is why the combination of oxygen with hemoglobin is called oxygenation and not oxidation.

Oxygen Carrying Capacity of Hemoglobin

Oxygen carrying capacity of hemoglobin is the amount of oxygen transported by 1 gram of hemoglobin. It is 1.34 mL/g.

Oxygen Carrying Capacity of Blood

Oxygen carrying capacity of blood refers to the amount of oxygen transported by blood. Normal hemoglobin content in blood is 15 g%.

Since oxygen carrying capacity of hemoglobin is 1.34 mL/g, blood with 15 g% of hemoglobin should carry 20.1 mL% of oxygen, i.e. 20.1 mL of oxygen in 100 mL of blood.

But, blood with 15 g% of hemoglobin carries only 19 mL% of oxygen, i.e. 19 mL of oxygen is carried by 100 mL of blood (Table 125.1). Oxygen carrying capacity of blood is only 19 mL% because the hemoglobin is not fully saturated with oxygen. It is saturated only for about 95%.

Saturation of Hemoglobin with Oxygen

Saturation is the state or condition when hemoglobin is unable to hold or carry any more oxygen. Saturation of hemoglobin with oxygen depends upon partial pressure of oxygen. And it is explained by oxygen-hemoglobin dissociation curve.

■ OXYGEN-HEMOGLOBIN DISSOCIATION CURVE

Oxygen-hemoglobin dissociation curve is the curve that demonstrates the relationship between partial pressure of oxygen and the percentage saturation of hemoglobin with oxygen. It explains hemoglobin's affinity for oxygen.

Normally in the blood, hemoglobin is saturated with oxygen only up to 95%. Saturation of hemoglobin with oxygen depends upon the partial pressure of oxygen. When the partial pressure of oxygen is more,

hemoglobin accepts oxygen and when the partial pressure of oxygen is less, hemoglobin releases oxygen.

Method to Plot Oxygen-hemoglobin Dissociation Curve

Ten flasks or tonometers are taken. Each one is filled with a known quantity of blood with known concentration of hemoglobin. Blood in each tonometer is exposed to oxygen at different partial pressures. Tonometer is rotated at a constant temperature till the blood takes as much of oxygen as it can. Then, blood is analyzed to measure the percentage saturation of hemoglobin with oxygen. Partial pressure of oxygen and saturation of hemoglobin are plotted to obtain the oxygen-hemoglobin dissociation curve.

Normal Oxygen-hemoglobin Dissociation Curve

Under normal conditions, oxygen-hemoglobin dissociation curve is 'S' shaped or **sigmoid shaped** (Fig.125.1). Lower part of the curve indicates dissociation of oxygen from hemoglobin. Upper part of the curve indicates the uptake of oxygen by hemoglobin depending upon partial pressure of oxygen.

P_{50}

P_{50} is the partial pressure of oxygen at which hemoglobin saturation with oxygen is 50%. When the partial pressure of oxygen is 25 to 27 mm Hg, the hemoglobin is

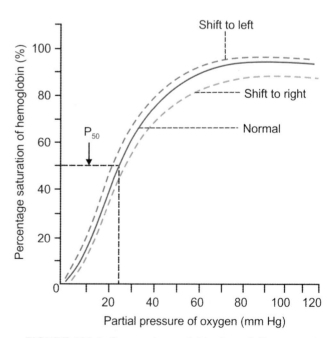

FIGURE 125.1: Oxygen-hemoglobin dissociation curve

saturated to about 50%. That is, the blood contains 50% of oxygen. At 40 mm Hg of partial pressure of oxygen, the saturation is 75%. It becomes 95% when the partial pressure of oxygen is 100 mm Hg.

Factors Affecting Oxygen-hemoglobin Dissociation Curve

Oxygen-hemoglobin dissociation curve is shifted to left or right by various factors:

1. Shift to left indicates acceptance (**association**) of oxygen by hemoglobin
2. Shift to right indicates **dissociation** of oxygen from hemoglobin.

1. Shift to right

Oxygen-hemoglobin dissociation curve is shifted to right in the following conditions:

   i. Decrease in partial pressure of oxygen
   ii. Increase in partial pressure of carbon dioxide (Bohr effect)
   iii. Increase in hydrogen ion concentration and decrease in pH (acidity)
   iv. Increased body temperature
   v. Excess of 2,3-diphosphoglycerate (DPG) in RBC. It is also called 2,3-biphosphoglycerate (BPG). DPG is a byproduct in Embden-Meyerhof pathway of carbohydrate metabolism. It combines with β-chains of hemoglobin. In conditions like muscular exercise and in high attitude, the DPG increases in RBC. So, the oxygen-hemoglobin dissociation curve shifts to right to a great extent.

2. Shift to left

Oxygen-hemoglobin dissociation curve is shifted to left in the following conditions:

   i. In fetal blood because, fetal hemoglobin has got more affinity for oxygen than the adult hemoglobin
   ii. Decrease in hydrogen ion concentration and increase in pH (alkalinity).

Bohr Effect

Bohr effect is the effect by which presence of carbon dioxide decreases the affinity of hemoglobin for oxygen. Bohr effect was postulated by **Christian Bohr** in 1904. In the tissues, due to continuous metabolic activities, the partial pressure of carbon dioxide is very high and the partial pressure of oxygen is low.

Due to this pressure gradient, carbon dioxide enters the blood and oxygen is released from the blood to the tissues. Presence of carbon dioxide decreases the affinity of hemoglobin for oxygen. It enhances further release of oxygen to the tissues and oxygen-dissociation curve is shifted to right.

Factors influencing Bohr effect

All the factors, which shift the oxygen-dissociation curve to right (mentioned above) enhance the Bohr effect.

■ TRANSPORT OF CARBON DIOXIDE

Carbon dioxide is transported by the blood from cells to the alveoli.

Carbon dioxide is transported in the blood in four ways:

1. As dissolved form (7%)
2. As carbonic acid (negligible)
3. As bicarbonate (63%)
4. As carbamino compounds (30%).

■ AS DISSOLVED FORM

Carbon dioxide diffuses into blood and dissolves in the fluid of plasma forming a simple solution. Only about 3 mL/100 mL of plasma of carbon dioxide is transported as dissolved state. It is about 7% of total carbon dioxide in the blood.

■ AS CARBONIC ACID

Part of dissolved carbon dioxide in plasma combines with the water to form carbonic acid. Transport of carbon dioxide in this form is negligible.

■ AS BICARBONATE

About 63% of carbon dioxide is transported as bicarbonate. From plasma, carbon dioxide enters the RBCs. In the RBCs, carbon dioxide combines with water to form carbonic acid. The reaction inside RBCs is very rapid because of the presence of carbonic anhydrase. This enzyme accelerates the reaction. Carbonic anhydrase is present only inside the RBCs and not in plasma. That is why carbonic acid formation is at least 200 to 300 times more in RBCs than in plasma.

Carbonic acid is very unstable. Almost all carbonic acid (99.9%) formed in red blood corpuscles, dissociates into bicarbonate and hydrogen ions. Concentration of bicarbonate ions in the cell increases more and more. Due to high concentration, bicarbonate ions diffuse through the cell membrane into plasma.

Chloride Shift or Hamburger Phenomenon

Chloride shift or Hamburger phenomenon is the exchange of a chloride ion for a bicarbonate ion across RBC membrane. It was discovered by **Hartog Jakob Hamburger** in 1892.

Chloride shift occurs when carbon dioxide enters the blood from tissues. In plasma, plenty of sodium chloride is present. It dissociates into sodium and chloride ions (Fig. 125.2). When the negatively charged bicarbonate ions move out of RBC into the plasma, the negatively charged chloride ions move into the RBC in order to maintain the **electrolyte equilibrium (ionic balance).**

Anion exchanger 1 (band 3 protein), which acts like antiport pump in RBC membrane is responsible for the exchange of bicarbonate ions and chloride ions. Bicarbonate ions combine with sodium ions in the plasma and form sodium bicarbonate. In this form, it is transported in the blood.

Hydrogen ions dissociated from carbonic acid are buffered by hemoglobin inside the cell.

Reverse Chloride Shift

Reverse chloride shift is the process by which chloride ions are moved back into plasma from RBC shift. It occurs in lungs. It helps in elimination of carbon dioxide from the blood. Bicarbonate is converted back into carbon dioxide, which has to be expelled out. It takes place by the following mechanism:

When blood reaches the alveoli, sodium bicarbonate in plasma dissociates into sodium and bicarbonate ions. Bicarbonate ion moves into the RBC. It makes chloride ion to move out of the RBC into the plasma, where it combines with sodium and forms sodium chloride.

Bicarbonate ion inside the RBC combines with hydrogen ion forms carbonic acid, which dissociates into water and carbon dioxide. Carbon dioxide is then expelled out.

■ AS CARBAMINO COMPOUNDS

About 30% of carbon dioxide is transported as carbamino compounds. Carbon dioxide is transported in blood in combination with hemoglobin and plasma proteins. Carbon dioxide combines with hemoglobin to form carbamino hemoglobin or carbhemoglobin. And it combines with plasma proteins to form carbamino proteins. Carbamino hemoglobin and carbamino proteins are together called carbamino compounds.

Carbon dioxide combines with proteins or hemoglobin with a loose bond so that, carbon dioxide is easily released into alveoli, where the partial pressure of carbon dioxide is low. Thus, the combination of carbon dioxide with proteins and hemoglobin is a reversible one. Amount of carbon dioxide transported in combination with plasma proteins is very less compared to the amount transported in combination with hemoglobin. It is because the quantity of proteins in plasma is only half of the quantity of hemoglobin.

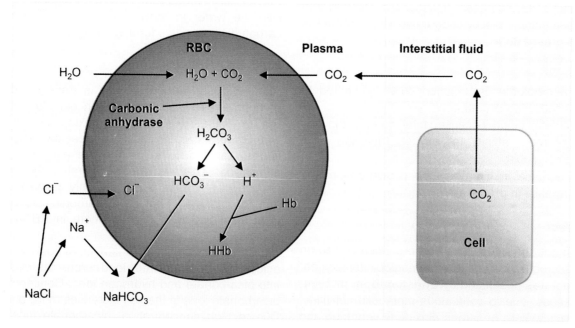

FIGURE 125.2: Transport of carbon dioxide in blood in the form of bicarbonate and chloride shift

■ CARBON DIOXIDE DISSOCIATION CURVE

Carbon dioxide is transported in blood as physical solution and in combination with water, plasma proteins and hemoglobin. The amount of carbon dioxide combining with blood depends upon the partial pressure of carbon dioxide.

Carbon dioxide dissociation curve is the curve that demonstrates the relationship between the partial pressure of carbon dioxide and the quantity of carbon dioxide that combines with blood.

Normal Carbon Dioxide Dissociation Curve

Normal carbon dioxide dissociation curve shows that the carbon dioxide content in the blood is 48 mL% when the partial pressure of carbon dioxide is 40 mm Hg and it is 52 mL% when the partial pressure of carbon dioxide is 48 mm Hg. Carbon dioxide content becomes 70 mL% when the partial pressure is about 100 mm Hg (Fig. 125.3).

Haldane Effect

Haldane effect is the effect by which combination of oxygen with hemoglobin displaces carbon dioxide from hemoglobin. It was first described by **John Scott Haldane** in 1860. Excess of oxygen content in blood causes shift of the carbon dioxide dissociation curve to right.

Causes for Haldane effect

Due to the combination with oxygen, hemoglobin becomes strongly acidic. It causes displacement of carbon dioxide from hemoglobin in two ways:

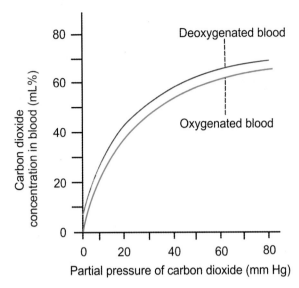

FIGURE 125.3: Carbon dioxide dissociation curve

1. Highly acidic hemoglobin has low tendency to combine with carbon dioxide. So, carbon dioxide is displaced from blood.
2. Because of the acidity, hydrogen ions are released in excess. Hydrogen ions bind with bicarbonate ions to form carbonic acid. Carbonic acid in turn dissociates into water and carbon dioxide. Carbon dioxide is released from blood into alveoli.

Significance of Haldane effect

Haldane effect is essential for:
1. Release of carbon dioxide from blood into the alveoli of lungs
2. Uptake of oxygen by the blood.

Regulation of Respiration

Chapter

126

■ INTRODUCTION
■ NERVOUS MECHANISM
   ■ RESPIRATORY CENTERS
   ■ MEDULLARY CENTERS
   ■ PONTINE CENTERS
   ■ CONNECTIONS OF RESPIRATORY CENTERS
   ■ INTEGRATION OF RESPIRATORY CENTERS
   ■ FACTORS AFFECTING RESPIRATORY CENTERS
■ CHEMICAL MECHANISM
   ■ CENTRAL CHEMORECEPTORS
   ■ PERIPHERAL CHEMORECEPTORS

■ INTRODUCTION

Respiration is a reflex process. But it can be controlled voluntarily for a short period of about 40 seconds. However, by practice, breathing can be withheld for a long period. At the end of that period, the person is forced to breathe.

Respiration is subjected to variation, even under normal physiological conditions. For example, emotion and exercise increase the rate and force of respiration. But the altered pattern of respiration is brought back to normal, within a short time by some regulatory mechanisms in the body.

Normally, quiet regular breathing occurs because of two regulatory mechanisms:
1. Nervous or neural mechanism
2. Chemical mechanism.

■ NERVOUS MECHANISM

Nervous mechanism that regulates the respiration includes:
1. Respiratory centers
2. Afferent nerves
3. Efferent nerves.

■ RESPIRATORY CENTERS

Respiratory centers are group of neurons, which control the rate, rhythm and force of respiration. These centers are bilaterally situated in reticular formation of the brainstem (Fig. 126.1). Depending upon the situation in brainstem, the respiratory centers are classified into two groups:
 A. Medullary centers consisting of
   1. Dorsal respiratory group of neurons
   2. Ventral respiratory group of neurons
 B. Pontine centers
   3. Apneustic center
   4. Pneumotaxic center.

■ MEDULLARY CENTERS

1. *Dorsal Respiratory Group of Neurons*

Situation

Dorsal respiratory group of neurons are diffusely situated in the nucleus of **tractus solitarius** which is present in the upper part of the medulla oblongata (Fig. 126.1). Usually, these neurons are collectively called **inspiratory center.**

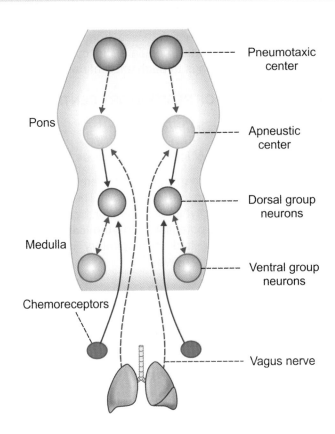

FIGURE 126.1: Nervous regulation of respiration.
Solid green line = Stimulation, Dotted red line = Inhibition.

All the neurons of dorsal respiratory group are **inspiratory neurons** and generate **inspiratory ramp** by the virtue of their **autorhythmic property** (Table 126.1).

Function

Dorsal group of neurons are responsible for basic rhythm of respiration (see below for details).

Experimental evidence

Electrical stimulation of these neurons in animals by using needle electrode causes contraction of inspiratory muscles and **prolonged inspiration.**

2. *Ventral Respiratory Group of Neurons*

Situation

Ventral respiratory group of neurons are present in **nucleus ambiguous** and **nucleus retroambiguous.** These two nuclei are situated in the medulla oblongata, anterior and lateral to the nucleus of tractus solitarius. Earlier, the ventral group neurons were collectively called **expiratory center.**

Ventral respiratory group has both **inspiratory** and **expiratory neurons.** Inspiratory neurons are found in the central area of the group. Expiratory neurons are in the caudal and rostral areas of the group.

Function

Normally, ventral group neurons are inactive during quiet breathing and become active during forced breathing. During forced breathing, these neurons stimulate both inspiratory muscles and expiratory muscles.

Experimental evidence

Electrical stimulation of the inspiratory neurons in ventral group causes contraction of inspiratory muscles and prolonged inspiration. Stimulation of expiratory neurons causes contraction of expiratory muscles and **prolonged expiration.**

■ PONTINE CENTERS

3. *Apneustic Center*

Situation

Apneustic center is situated in the reticular formation of lower pons.

Function

Apneustic center increases depth of inspiration by acting directly on dorsal group neurons.

Experimental evidence

Stimulation of apneustic center causes **apneusis.** Apneusis is an abnormal pattern of respiration, charac-

TABLE 126.1: Medullary centers

Features	Dorsal group	Ventral group
Situation	Diffusely situated in nucleus of tractus solitarius	In nucleus ambiguous and nucleus retroambiguous
Type of neurons	Inspiratory neurons	Inspiratory and expiratory neurons
Function	Always active Generate inspiratory ramp Has autorhythmic property	Inactive during quiet breathing Active during forced breathing

terized by prolonged inspiration followed by short, inefficient expiration.

4. Pneumotaxic Center

Situation

Pneumotaxic center is situated in the dorsolateral part of **reticular formation** in **upper pons.** It is formed by neurons of medial **parabrachial** and **subparabrachial nuclei.** Subparabrachial nucleus is also called **ventral parabrachial** or **Kölliker-Fuse nucleus.**

Function

Primary function of pneumotaxic center is to control the medullary respiratory centers, particularly the dorsal group neurons. It acts through apneustic center. Pneumotaxic center inhibits the apneustic center so that the dorsal group neurons are inhibited. Because of this, inspiration stops and expiration starts. Thus, pneumotaxic center influences the switching between inspiration and expiration.

Pneumotaxic center increases respiratory rate by reducing the duration of inspiration.

Experimental evidence

Stimulation of pneumotaxic center does not produce any typical effect, except slight **prolongation of expiration,** by inhibiting the dorsal respiratory group of neurons through apneustic center. Destruction or inactivation of pneumotaxic center results in apneusis.

■ CONNECTIONS OF RESPIRATORY CENTERS

Efferent Pathway

Nerve fibers from respiratory centers leave the brainstem and descend in anterior part of lateral columns of spinal cord.

These nerve fibers terminate on motor neurons in the anterior horn cells of cervical and thoracic segments of spinal cord. From motor neurons of spinal cord, two sets of nerve fibers arise:
1. Phrenic nerve fibers (C3 to C5), which supply the diaphragm
2. Intercostal nerve fibers (T1 to T11), which supply the external intercostal muscles.

Vagus nerve also contains some efferent fibers from the respiratory centers.

Afferent Pathway

Respiratory centers receive afferent impulses from:
1. Peripheral chemoreceptors and baroreceptors via branches of glossopharyngeal and vagus nerves

2. Stretch receptors of lungs via vagus nerve.

By receiving afferent impulses from these receptors, respiratory centers modulate the movements of thoracic cage and lungs through efferent nerve fibers.

■ INTEGRATION OF RESPIRATORY CENTERS

Role of Medullary Centers

Rhythmic discharge of inspiratory impulses

Dorsal respiratory group of neurons are responsible for the normal rhythm of respiration. These neurons maintain the normal rhythm of respiration by discharging impulses (action potentials) **rhythmically.** These impulses are transmitted to respiratory muscles by phrenic and intercostal nerves.

Inspiratory ramp

Inspiratory ramp is the pattern of impulse discharge from dorsal respiratory group of neurons. These impulses are characterized by steady increase in amplitude of the action potential. Impulse discharge from these neurons is not sudden and it is also not uniform.

Inspiratory ramp signals

To start with, the amplitude of action potential is low. It is due to the activation of only few neurons. Later, more and more neurons are activated, leading to gradual increase in the amplitude of action potential in a ramp fashion. Impulses of this type discharged from dorsal group of neurons are called inspiratory ramp signals.

Ramp signals are not produced continuously but only for a period of 2 seconds, during which inspiration occurs. After 2 seconds, ramp signals stop abruptly and do not appear for another 3 seconds. Switching off the ramp signals causes expiration. At the end of 3 seconds, inspiratory ramp signals reappear in the same pattern and the cycle is repeated.

Normally, during inspiration, dorsal respiratory group neurons inhibit expiratory neurons of ventral group. During expiration, the expiratory neurons inhibit the dorsal group neurons. Thus, the medullary respiratory centers control each other.

Significance of inspiratory ramp signals

Significance of inspiratory ramp signals is that there is a slow and steady inspiration, so that the filling of lungs with air is also steady.

Role of Pontine Centers

Pontine respiratory centers regulate the medullary centers. Apneustic center accelerates the activity of dorsal group of neurons and the stimulation of this center causes prolonged inspiration.

Pneumotaxic center inhibits the apneustic center and restricts the duration of inspiration.

Pre-Bötzinger Complex

Pre-Bötzinger complex (**pre-BötC**) is an **additional respiratory center** found in animals. It is formed by a group of neurons called **pacemaker neurons,** located in the ventrolateral part of medulla. Pacemaker neurons generate the rhythmic respiratory impulses. Medullary centers send nerve fibers into this complex. Exact functioning mechanism of this complex is not known.

■ FACTORS AFFECTING RESPIRATORY CENTERS

Respiratory centers regulate the respiratory movements by receiving impulses from various sources in the body.

1. Impulses from Higher Centers

Higher centers alter the respiration by sending impulses directly to dorsal group of neurons. Impulses from anterior cingulate gyrus, genu of corpus callosum, olfactory tubercle and posterior orbital gyrus of cerebral cortex inhibit respiration. Impulses from motor area and Sylvian area of cerebral cortex cause **forced breathing.**

2. Impulses from Stretch Receptors of Lungs: Hering-Breuer Reflex

Hering-Breuer reflex is a **protective reflex** that restricts inspiration and prevents overstretching of lung tissues. It is initiated by the stimulation of stretch receptors of air passage.

Stretch receptors are the receptors which give response to stretch of the tissues. These receptors are situated on the wall of the bronchi and bronchioles.

Expansion of lungs during inspiration stimulates the stretch receptors. Impulses from stretch receptors reach the dorsal group neurons via vagal afferent fibers and inhibit them. So, inspiration stops and expiration starts (Fig. 126.2). Thus, the overstretching of lung tissues is prevented.

However, Hering-Breuer reflex does not operate during quiet breathing. It operates, only when the tidal volume increases beyond 1,000 mL.

Hering-Breuer inflation reflex and deflation reflex

The above mentioned reflex is called **Hering-Breuer inflation reflex** since it restricts the inspiration and

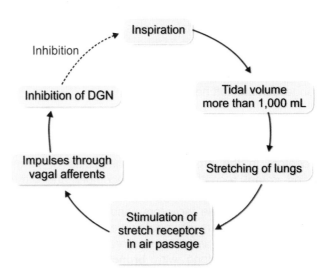

FIGURE 126.2: Hering-Breuer inflation reflex. DGN = Dorsal respiratory group of neurons. Dashed red arrow indicates inhibition.

limits the overstretching of lung tissues. Reverse of this reflex is called **Hering-Breuer deflation reflex** and it takes place during expiration. During expiration, as the stretching of lungs is absent, deflation occurs.

3. Impulses from 'J' Receptors of Lungs

'J' receptors are **juxtacapillary receptors** which are present on the wall of the alveoli and have close contact with the pulmonary capillaries. **AS Paintal** discovered that these receptors are the sensory nerve endings of vagus. Nerve fibers from these receptors are non-myelinated and belong to C type. Few receptors are found on the wall of the bronchi.

Conditions when 'J' receptors are stimulated

i.   Pulmonary congestion
ii. Pulmonary edema
iii. Pneumonia
iv. Over inflation of lungs
v.   Microembolism in pulmonary capillaries
vi. Stimulation by exogenous and endogenous chemical substances such as histamine, halothane, bradykinin, serotonin and phenyldiguanide.

Effect of stimulation of 'J' receptors

Stimulation of the 'J' receptors produces a reflex response, which is characterized by **apnea**. Apnea is followed by hyperventilation, bradycardia, hypotension and weakness of skeletal muscles.

Role of 'J' receptors in physiological conditions is not clear. However, these receptors are responsible for hyperventilation in patients affected by pulmonary congestion and left heart failure.

4. Impulses from Irritant Receptors of Lungs

Besides stretch receptors, there is another type of receptors in the bronchi and bronchioles of lungs, called irritant receptors. Irritant receptors are stimulated by irritant chemical agents such as ammonia and sulfur dioxide. These receptors send afferent impulses to respiratory centers via vagal nerve fibers.

Stimulation of irritant receptors produces **reflex hyperventilation** along with **bronchospasm**. Hyperventilation along with bronchospasm prevents further entry of harmful agents into the alveoli.

5. Impulses from Baroreceptors

Baroreceptors or **pressoreceptors** are the receptors which give response to change in blood pressure. Refer Chapter 101 for details of baroreceptors.

Function

Baroreceptors in carotid sinus and arch of aorta give response to increase in blood pressure. Whenever arterial blood pressure increases, baroreceptors are activated and send inhibitory impulses to vasomotor center in medulla oblongata. This causes decrease in blood pressure and inhibition of respiration. However, in physiological conditions, the role of baroreceptors in regulation of respiration is insignificant.

6. Impulses from Chemoreceptors

Chemoreceptors play an important role in the chemical regulation of respiration. Details of chemoreceptors and chemical regulation of respiration are explained later in this Chapter.

7. Impulses from Proprioceptors

Proprioceptors are the receptors which give response to change in the position of body. These receptors are situated in joints, tendons and muscles. Proprioceptors are stimulated during the muscular exercise and send impulses to brain, particularly cerebral cortex, through somatic afferent nerves. Cerebral cortex in turn causes hyperventilation by sending impulses to medullary respiratory centers.

8. Impulses from Thermoreceptors

Thermoreceptors are cutaneous receptors, which give response to change in the environmental temperature. Thermoreceptors are of two types, namely receptors for cold and receptors for warmth. When body is exposed to cold or when cold water is applied over the body, cold receptors are stimulated and send impulses to cerebral cortex via somatic afferent nerves. Cerebral cortex in turn, stimulates the respiratory centers and causes hyperventilation.

9. Impulses from Pain Receptors

Pain receptors are those which give response to pain stimulus. Whenever pain receptors are stimulated, the impulses are sent to cerebral cortex via somatic afferent nerves. Cerebral cortex in turn, stimulates the respiratory centers and causes hyperventilation (Fig. 126.3).

■ CHEMICAL MECHANISM

Chemical mechanism of regulation of respiration is operated through the chemoreceptors. Chemoreceptors are the sensory nerve endings, which give response to changes in chemical constituents of blood.

Changes in Chemical Constituents of Blood which Stimulate Chemoreceptors

1. Hypoxia (decreased pO_2)
2. Hypercapnea (increased pCO_2)
3. Increased hydrogen ion concentration.

Types of Chemoreceptors

Chemoreceptors are classified into two groups:
1. Central chemoreceptors
2. Peripheral chemoreceptors.

■ CENTRAL CHEMORECEPTORS

Central chemoreceptors are the chemoreceptors present in the brain.

Situation

Central chemoreceptors are situated in deeper part of medulla oblongata, close to the dorsal respiratory group of neurons. This area is known as **chemosensitive area** and the neurons are called chemoreceptors. Chemoreceptors are in close contact with blood and cerebrospinal fluid.

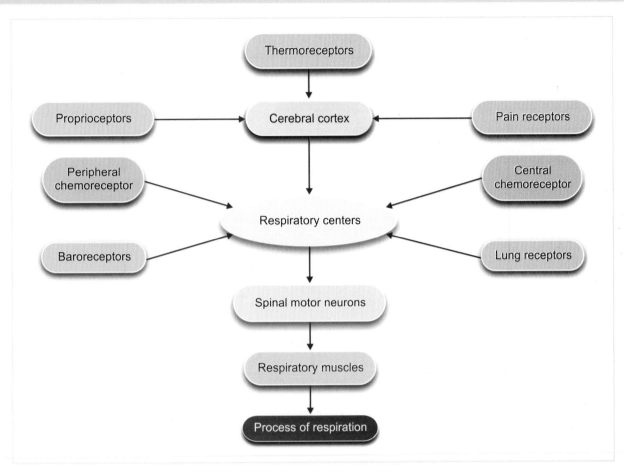

FIGURE 126.3: Factors affecting respiratory centers

Mechanism of Action

Central chemoreceptors are connected with respiratory centers, particularly the dorsal respiratory group of neurons through synapses. These chemoreceptors act slowly but effectively. Central chemoreceptors are responsible for 70% to 80% of increased ventilation through chemical regulatory mechanism.

Main stimulant for central chemoreceptors is the increased hydrogen ion concentration. However, if hydrogen ion concentration increases in the blood, it cannot stimulate the central chemoreceptors because, the hydrogen ions from blood cannot cross the **blood-brain barrier** and **blood-cerebrospinal fluid barrier.**

On the other hand, if carbon dioxide increases in the blood, it can easily cross the blood-brain barrier and blood-cerebrospinal fluid barrier and enter the interstitial fluid of brain or the cerebrospinal fluid. There, the carbon dioxide combines with water to form carbonic acid. Since carbonic acid is unstable, it immediately dissociates into hydrogen ion and bicarbonate ion (Fig. 126.4).

$$CO_2 + H_2O \rightarrow H_2CO_3 \rightarrow H^+ + HCO_3^-$$

Hydrogen ions stimulate the central chemoreceptors. From chemoreceptors, the excitatory impulses are sent to dorsal respiratory group of neurons, resulting in increased ventilation (increased rate and force of breathing). Because of this, excess carbon dioxide is washed out and respiration is brought back to normal. Lack of oxygen does not have significant effect on the central chemoreceptors, except that it generally depresses the overall function of brain.

■ **PERIPHERAL CHEMORECEPTORS**

Peripheral chemoreceptors are the chemoreceptors present in carotid and aortic region. Refer Chapter 101 for details.

Mechanism of Action

Hypoxia is the most potent stimulant for peripheral chemoreceptors. It is because of the presence of

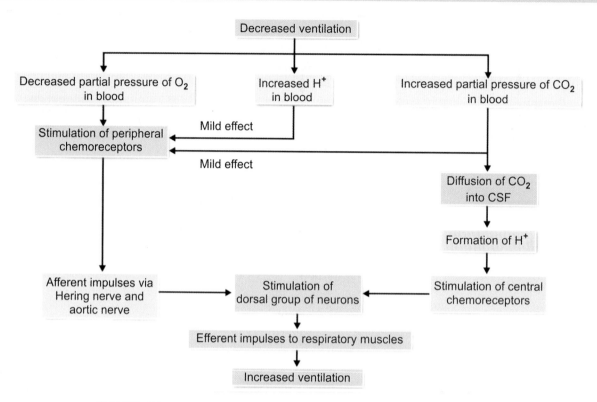

FIGURE 126.4: Chemical regulation of respiration. CSF = Cerebrospinal fluid.

oxygen sensitive potassium channels in the glomus cells of peripheral chemoreceptors.

Hypoxia causes closure of oxygen sensitive potassium channels and prevents potassium efflux. This leads to depolarization of **glomus cells** (receptor potential) and generation of action potentials in nerve ending.

These impulses pass through aortic and Hering nerves and excite the dorsal group of neurons. Dorsal group of neurons in turn, send excitatory impulses to respiratory muscles, resulting in increased ventilation. This provides enough oxygen and rectifies the lack of oxygen.

In addition to hypoxia, peripheral chemoreceptors are also stimulated by hypercapnea and increased hydrogen ion concentration. However, the sensitivity of peripheral chemoreceptors to hypercapnea and increased hydrogen ion concentration is mild.

Disturbances of Respiration

■ INTRODUCTION

Normal respiratory pattern is called **eupnea.** Respiratory pattern is altered by many ways. Altered patterns of respiration are:

1. *Tachypnea:* Increase in the rate of respiration
2. *Bradypnea:* Decrease in the rate of respiration
3. *Polypnea:* Rapid, shallow breathing resembling panting in dogs. In this type of breathing, only the rate of respiration increases but the force does not increase significantly.
4. *Apnea:* Temporary arrest of breathing
5. *Hyperpnea:* Increase in pulmonary ventilation due to increase in rate or force of respiration. Increase in rate and force of respiration occurs after exercise. It also occurs in abnormal conditions like fever or other disorders.
6. *Hyperventilation:* Abnormal increase in rate and force of respiration, which often leads to dizziness and sometimes chest pain
7. *Hypoventilation:* Decrease in rate and force of respiration
8. *Dyspnea:* Difficulty in breathing
9. *Periodic breathing:* Abnormal respiratory rhythm.

■ APNEA

■ DEFINITION

Apnea is defined as the **temporary arrest** of breathing. Literally, apnea means absence of breathing. Apnea can also be produced voluntarily, which is called **breath holding** or **voluntary apnea.**

■ APNEA TIME

Breath holding time is known as apnea time. It is about 40 to 60 seconds in a normal person, after a deep inspiration.

■ CONDITIONS WHEN APNEA OCCURS

1. *Voluntary Effort*

Arrest of breathing by voluntary effort is known as **voluntary apnea** or **breath holding.** Breath holding time can be increased beyond 40 to 60 seconds by practice, exercise, willpower and yoga.

At the end of voluntary apnea, the subject is forced to breathe, which is called the **breaking point.** It is because of the accumulation of carbon dioxide in blood, which stimulates the respiratory centers. Besides increased carbon dioxide content in blood, hypoxia and increased hydrogen ion concentration are also responsible for stimulation of respiratory centers. Apnea is always followed by hyperventilation.

2. *Apnea after Hyperventilation*

Apnea occurs after hyperventilation. It is due to lack of carbon dioxide. During hyperventilation, more carbon dioxide is washed out. So, partial pressure of carbon dioxide in the blood decreases and the number of stimuli to the respiratory centers also decreases, leading to apnea. During apnea, carbon dioxide accumulates in the blood. When partial pressure of carbon dioxide increases, the respiratory centers are stimulated and respiration starts.

3. *Deglutition Apnea*

Arrest of breathing during deglutition is known as deglutition **(swallowing)** apnea. It occurs reflexly during pharyngeal stage of deglutition. When the bolus is pushed into esophagus from pharynx during pharyngeal stage of deglutition, there is possibility for bolus to enter the respiratory passage through larynx, causing serious consequences like choking. This is prevented by deglutition apnea, during which the larynx is closed by backward movement of epiglottis (Chapter 43).

4. *Vagal Apnea*

Vagal apnea is an **experimental apnea,** which is produced by the stimulation of vagus nerve in animals. Stimulation of vagus nerve causes apnea by inhibiting the inspiratory center.

5. *Adrenaline Apnea*

Adrenaline apnea is the apnea that occurs after injection of adrenaline. Administration of adrenaline produces marked increase in arterial blood pressure. It stimulates the baroreceptors, which in turn reflexly inhibit vasomotor center and the respiratory centers, causing fall in blood pressure and apnea.

■ CLINICAL CLASSIFICATION OF APNEA

Clinically, apnea is classified into three types:
1. Obstructive apnea
2. Central apnea
3. Mixed apnea.

1. *Obstructive Apnea*

Obstructive apnea occurs because of obstruction in the respiratory tract. Respiratory tract obstruction is mainly due to excess tissue growth like tonsils and adenoids. Common obstructive apnea is the sleep apnea.

Sleep apnea

Sleep apnea is the temporary stoppage of breathing that occurs repeatedly during sleep. It is also called **sleep disordered breathing** (SDB). It commonly affects overweight people.

Major cause for sleep apnea is obstruction of upper respiratory tract by excess tissue growth in airway, like enlarged tonsils and large tongue.

Characteristic feature of sleep apnea is loud **snoring.** Snoring without sleep apnea is called **simple** or **primary snoring.** But snoring with sleep apnea is serious and it may become life threatening. If left unnoticed, it may lead to hypertension, heart failure and stroke (refer Chapter 160 for sleep apnea syndrome).

2. *Central Apnea*

Central apnea occurs due to brain disorders, especially when the respiratory centers are affected. It is seen in premature babies. Typical feature of central apnea is a short pause in between breathing.

3. *Mixed Apnea*

Mixed apnea is a combination of central and obstructive apnea. It is usually seen in **premature babies** and in **full-term born infants.** Main reason for mixed apnea is the abnormal control of breathing due to immature or underdeveloped brain or respiratory system.

■ HYPERVENTILATION

■ DEFINITION

Hyperventilation means increased pulmonary ventilation due to forced breathing. It is also called **over ventilation.** In hyperventilation, both rate and force of breathing are increased and a large amount of air moves in and out of lungs. Thus, pulmonary ventilation is increased to a great extent. Very often, hyperventilation leads to dizziness, discomfort and chest pain.

■ CONDITIONS WHEN HYPERVENTILATION OCCURS

Hyperventilation mostly occurs in conditions like exercise when partial pressure of carbon dioxide (pCO_2) is increased. Excess of carbon dioxide stimulates the respiratory centers. Voluntarily also, hyperventilation can be produced. It is called voluntary hyperventilation.

■ EFFECTS OF HYPERVENTILATION

During hyperventilation, excessive carbon dioxide is washed out. In blood, the partial pressure of carbon dioxide is reduced. It causes suppression of respiratory centers, resulting in **apnea.** Apnea is followed by Cheyne-Stokes type of periodic breathing. After a period of **Cheyne-Stokes breathing,** normal respiration is restored (Fig. 127.1).

■ HYPOVENTILATION

■ DEFINITION

Hypoventilation is the decrease in pulmonary ventilation caused by decrease in rate or force of breathing. Thus, the amount of air moving in and out of lungs is reduced.

■ CONDITIONS WHEN HYPOVENTILATION OCCURS

Hypoventilation occurs when respiratory centers are suppressed or by administration of some drugs. It occurs during partial paralysis of respiratory muscles also.

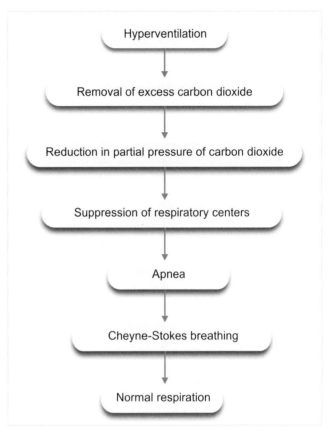

FIGURE 127.1: Effects of hyperventilation

■ EFFECTS OF HYPOVENTILATION

Hypoventilation results in development of hypoxia along with hypercapnea. It increases the rate and force of respiration, leading to dyspnea. Severe conditions result in lethargy, coma and death (Fig. 127.2).

■ HYPOXIA

■ DEFINITION

Hypoxia is defined as reduced availability of oxygen to the tissues. The term anoxia refers to absence of oxygen. In olden days, the term anoxia was in use. Since there is no possibility for total absence of oxygen in living conditions, use of this term is abandoned.

■ CLASSIFICATION AND CAUSES OF HYPOXIA

Four important factors which leads to hypoxia are:
1. Oxygen tension in arterial blood
2. Oxygen carrying capacity of blood
3. Velocity of blood flow
4. Utilization of oxygen by the cells.

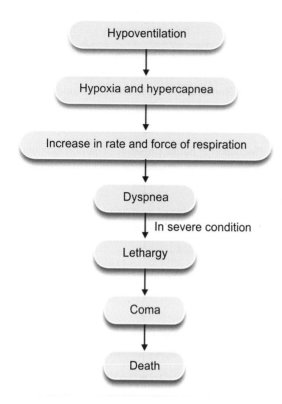

FIGURE 127.2: Effects of hypoventilation

On the basis of above factors, hypoxia is classified into four types:
1. Hypoxic hypoxia
2. Anemic hypoxia
3. Stagnant hypoxia
4. Histotoxic hypoxia.

Each type of hypoxia may be acute or chronic. Simultaneously, two or more types of hypoxia may be present.

1. Hypoxic Hypoxia

Hypoxic hypoxia means decreased oxygen content in blood. It is also called arterial hypoxia.

Causes for hypoxic hypoxia

Hypoxic hypoxia is caused by four factors.
  i. Low oxygen tension in inspired (atmospheric) air, which does not provide enough oxygen
 ii. Respiratory disorders associated with decreased pulmonary ventilation, which does not allow intake of enough oxygen
iii. Respiratory disorders associated with inadequate oxygenation in lungs, which does not allow diffusion of enough oxygen

 iv. Cardiac disorders, in which enough blood is not pumped to transport oxygen.

i. *Low oxygen tension in inspired air*

Oxygen tension in inspired air is reduced in the following conditions:
  a. High altitude
  b. While breathing air in closed space
  c. While breathing gas mixture containing low partial pressure of oxygen (PO_2).

Because of these conditions, required quantity of oxygen cannot enter the lungs.

ii. *Respiratory disorders associated with decreased pulmonary ventilation*

Pulmonary ventilation decreases in the following conditions:
  a. Obstruction of respiratory passage as in asthma
  b. Nervous and mechanical hindrance to respiratory movements as in poliomyelitis
  c. Depression of respiratory centers as in brain tumors
  d. Pneumothorax.

In these conditions, even though enough oxygen is available in the atmosphere, it cannot reach the lungs.

iii. *Respiratory disorders associated with inadequate oxygenation of blood in lungs*

Inadequate oxygenation of blood in lungs occurs in the following conditions:
  a. Impaired alveolar diffusion as in emphysema
  b. Presence of non-functioning alveoli as in fibrosis
  c. Filling of alveoli with fluid as in pulmonary edema, pneumonia, pulmonary hemorrhage
  d. Collapse of lungs as in bronchiolar obstruction
  e. Lack of surfactant
  f. Abnormal pleural cavity such as pneumothorax, hydrothorax, hemothorax and pyothorax
  g. Increased venous admixture as in the case of bronchiectasis.

In these conditions, in spite of oxygen availability and entrance of oxygen into the alveoli, it cannot diffuse into the blood.

iv. *Cardiac disorders*

In congestive heart failure, oxygen availability and diffusion are normal, but the blood cannot be pumped from heart properly.

Characteristic features of hypoxic hypoxia

Hypoxic hypoxia is characterized by reduced oxygen tension in arterial blood. All other features remain normal (Table 127.1).

2. Anemic Hypoxia

Anemic hypoxia is the condition characterized by the inability of blood to carry enough amount of oxygen. Oxygen availability is normal. But the blood is not able to take up sufficient amount of oxygen due to anemic condition.

Causes for anemic hypoxia

Any condition that causes anemia can cause anemic hypoxia. It is caused by the following conditions:
  i. Decreased number of RBCs
  ii. Decreased hemoglobin content in the blood
  iii. Formation of altered hemoglobin
  iv. Combination of hemoglobin with gases other than oxygen and carbon dioxide.

i. Decreased number of RBCs

RBC decreases in conditions like bone marrow diseases, hemorrhage, etc.

ii. Decreased hemoglobin content in the blood

Conditions which decrease the RBC count or change the structure, shape and size of RBC (microcytes, macrocytes, spherocytes, sickle cells, poikilocytes, etc.) can decrease the hemoglobin content in blood.

iii. Formation of altered hemoglobin

Poisoning with chlorates, nitrates, ferricyanides, etc. causes oxidation of iron into ferric form and the hemoglobin is known as **methemoglobin.** Methemoglobin cannot combine with oxygen. Thus, the quantity of hemoglobin available for oxygen transport is decreased (Chapter 11).

iv. Combination of hemoglobin with gases other than oxygen and carbon dioxide

When hemoglobin combines with carbon monoxide, hydrogen sulfide or nitrous oxide, it looses the capacity to transport oxygen (Chapter 11).

Characteristic features of anemic hypoxia

Anemic hypoxia is characterized by decreased oxygen carrying capacity of blood. All other features remain normal (Table 127.1).

3. Stagnant Hypoxia

Stagnant hypoxia is the hypoxia caused by decreased velocity of blood flow. It is otherwise called hypokinetic hypoxia.

Causes for stagnant hypoxia

Stagnant hypoxia occurs mainly due to reduction in velocity of blood flow. Velocity of blood flow decreases in the following conditions:
  i. Congestive cardiac failure
  ii. Hemorrhage
  iii. Surgical shock
  iv. Vasospasm
  v. Thrombosis
  vi. Embolism.

Characteristic features of stagnant hypoxia

Stagnant hypoxia is characterized by decreased velocity of blood flow. All other features remain normal (Table 127.1).

4. Histotoxic Hypoxia

Histotoxic hypoxia is the type of hypoxia produced by the inability of tissues to utilize oxygen.

Causes for histotoxic hypoxia

Histotoxic hypoxia occurs due to cyanide or sulfide poisoning. These poisonous substances destroy the

TABLE 127.1: Characteristic features of different types of hypoxia

Features	Hypoxic hypoxia	Anemic hypoxia	Stagnant hypoxia	Histotoxic hypoxia
1. PO_2 in arterial blood	Reduced	Normal	Normal	Normal
2. Oxygen carrying capacity of blood	Normal	Reduced	Normal	Normal
3. Velocity of blood flow	Normal	Normal	Reduced	Normal
4. Utilization of oxygen by tissues	Normal	Normal	Normal	Reduced
5. Efficacy of oxygen therapy	100%	75%	< 50%	Not useful

cellular oxidative enzymes and there is a complete paralysis of **cytochrome oxidase system.** So, even if oxygen is supplied, the tissues are not in a position to utilize it.

Characteristic features of histotoxic hypoxia

Histotoxic hypoxia is characterized by inability of tissues to utilize oxygen even if it is delivered. All other features remain normal (Table 127.1).

■ EFFECTS OF HYPOXIA

Acute and severe hypoxia leads to unconsciousness. If not treated immediately, brain death occurs. Chronic hypoxia produces various symptoms in the body.

Effects of hypoxia are of two types:
1. Immediate effects
2. Delayed effects.

Immediate Effects

i. Effects on blood

Hypoxia induces secretion of **erythropoietin** from kidney. Erythropoietin increases production of RBC. This in turn, increases the oxygen carrying capacity of blood.

ii. Effects on cardiovascular system

Initially, due to the reflex stimulation of cardiac and vasomotor centers, there is an increase in rate and force of contraction of heart, cardiac output and blood pressure. Later, there is reduction in the rate and force of contraction of heart. Cardiac output and blood pressure are also decreased.

iii. Effects on respiration

Initially, respiratory rate increases due to chemoreceptor reflex. Because of this, large amount of carbon dioxide is washed out leading to **alkalemia.** Later, the respiration tends to be **shallow and periodic.** Finally, the rate and force of breathing are reduced to a great extent due to the failure of respiratory centers.

iv. Effects on digestive system

Hypoxia is associated with loss of appetite, nausea and vomiting. Mouth becomes dry and there is a feeling of thirst.

v. Effects on kidneys

Hypoxia causes increased secretion of erythropoietin from the juxtaglomerular apparatus. And **alkaline urine** is excreted.

vi. Effects on central nervous system

In mild hypoxia, the symptoms are similar to those of **alcoholic intoxication.**

Individual is depressed, apathetic with general loss of self control. The person becomes talkative, quarrelsome, ill-tempered and rude. The person starts shouting, singing or crying.

There is disorientation and loss of discriminative ability and loss of power of judgment. Memory is impaired. Weakness, lack of coordination and fatigue of muscles are common in hypoxia.

If hypoxia is acute and severe, there is a sudden loss of consciousness. If not treated immediately, **coma** occurs, which leads to **death.**

Delayed Effects of Hypoxia

Delayed effects appear depending upon the length and severity of the exposure to hypoxia.

The person becomes highly irritable and develops the symptoms of mountain sickness, such as nausea, vomiting, depression, weakness and fatigue.

■ TREATMENT FOR HYPOXIA – OXYGEN THERAPY

Best treatment for hypoxia is oxygen therapy, i.e. treating the affected person with oxygen. Pure oxygen or oxygen combined with another gas is administered.

Oxygen therapy is carried out by two methods:
1. By placing the patient's head in a 'tent' containing oxygen
2. By allowing the patient to breathe oxygen either from a mask or an intranasal tube.

Depending upon the situation, oxygen therapy can be given either under normal atmospheric pressure or under high pressure (hyperbaric oxygen).

In Normal Atmospheric Pressure

With normal atmospheric pressure, i.e. at one atmosphere (760 mm Hg), administration of pure oxygen is well tolerated by the patient for long hours. However, after 8 hours or more, lung tissues show fluid effusion and edema. Other tissues are not affected very much because of **hemoglobin-oxygen buffer system.**

In High Atmospheric Pressure – Hyperbaric Oxygen

Hyperbaric oxygen is the pure oxygen with high atmospheric pressure of 2 or more than 2 atmosphere. Hyperbaric oxygen therapy with 2 to 3 atmosphere is tolerated by the patient for about 5 hours. During this period, the dissolved form of oxygen increases in arterial blood because the oxygen carrying capacity of hemoglobin is limited. At this level, tissue oxygen tension also increases to about 200 mm Hg. However, tissues tolerate the high partial pressure of oxygen, without much adverse effects. But, oxygen toxicity develops when pure oxygen is administered for long periods. Refer oxygen toxicity below.

Efficacy of Oxygen Therapy in Different Types of Hypoxia

Oxygen therapy is the best treatment for hypoxia. But it is not effective equally in all types of hypoxia. Value of oxygen therapy depends upon the type of hypoxia. So, before deciding the oxygen therapy, one should recall the physiological basis of different types of hypoxia.

In hypoxic hypoxia, the oxygen therapy is 100% useful. In anemic hypoxia, oxygen therapy is moderately effective to about 70%. In stagnant hypoxia, the effectiveness of oxygen therapy is less than 50%. In histotoxic hypoxia, the oxygen therapy is not useful at all. It is because, even if oxygen is delivered, the cells cannot utilize oxygen.

■ OXYGEN TOXICITY (POISONING)

■ DEFINITION AND CAUSE

Oxygen toxicity is the increased oxygen content in tissues, beyond certain critical level. It is also called oxygen poisoning. It occurs because of breathing pure oxygen with a high pressure of 2 to 3 atmosphere (hyperbaric oxygen). In this condition, an excess amount of oxygen is transported in plasma as dissolved form because oxygen carrying capacity of hemoglobin is limited to 1.34 mL/g.

■ EFFECTS OF OXYGEN TOXICITY

1. Lung tissues are affected first with tracheobronchial irritation and pulmonary edema
2. Metabolic rate increases in all the body tissues and the tissues are burnt out by excess heat. Heat also destroys **cytochrome system,** leading to damage of tissues.
3. When brain is affected, first hyperirritability occurs. Later, it is followed by increased muscular twitching, ringing in ears and dizziness.
4. Finally, the toxicity results in convulsions, coma and death.

■ HYPERCAPNEA

■ DEFINITION

Hypercapnea is the increased carbon dioxide content of blood.

■ CONDITIONS WHEN HYPERCAPNEA OCCURS

Hypercapnea occurs in conditions, which leads to blockage of respiratory pathway, as in case of asphyxia. It also occurs while breathing the air containing excess carbon dioxide content.

■ EFFECTS OF HYPERCAPNEA

1. *Effects on Respiration*

During hypercapnea, the respiratory centers are stimulated excessively. It leads to dyspnea.

2. *Effects on Blood*

The pH of blood reduces and blood becomes acidic.

3. *Effects on Cardiovascular System*

Hypercapnea is associated with tachycardia and increased blood pressure. There is flushing of skin due to peripheral vasodilatation.

4. *Effects on Central Nervous System*

During hypercapnea, the nervous system is also affected, resulting in headache, depression and laziness. These symptoms are followed by muscular rigidity, fine tremors and generalized convulsions. Finally, giddiness and loss of consciousness occur.

■ HYPOCAPNEA

■ DEFINITION

Hypocapnea is the decreased carbon dioxide content in blood.

■ CONDITIONS WHEN HYPOCAPNEA OCCURS

Hypocapnea occurs in conditions associated with hypoventilation. It also occurs after prolonged hyperventilation, because of washing out of excess carbon dioxide.

■ EFFECTS OF HYPOCAPNEA

1. *Effects on Respiration*

Respiratory centers are depressed, leading to decreased rate and force of respiration.

2. *Effects on Blood*

The pH of blood increases, leading to respiratory alkalosis. Calcium concentration decreases. It causes tetany, which is characterized by **neuromuscular hyperexcitability** and **carpopedal spasm.**

3. *Effects on Central Nervous System*

Dizziness, mental confusion, muscular twitching and loss of consciousness are the common features of hypocapnea.

■ ASPHYXIA

■ DEFINITION

Asphyxia is the condition characterized by combination of **hypoxia** and **hypercapnea,** due to obstruction of air passage.

■ CONDITIONS WHEN ASPHYXIA OCCURS

Axphyxia develops in conditions characterized by acute obstruction of air passage such as:
1. Strangulation
2. Hanging
3. Drowning, etc.

■ EFFECTS OF ASPHYXIA

Effects of asphyxia develop in three stages:
1. Stage of hyperpnea
2. Stage of convulsions
3. Stage of collapse.

1. *Stage of Hyperpnea*

Hyperpnea is the first stage of asphyxia. It extends for about 1 minute. In this stage, breathing becomes deep and rapid. It is due to the powerful stimulation of respiratory centers by excess of carbon dioxide. Hyperpnea is followed by **dyspnea** and **cyanosis.** Eyes become more prominent.

2. *Stage of Convulsions*

Stage of convulsions is characterized mainly by convulsions (uncontrolled involuntary muscular contractions).

Duration of this stage is less than 1 minute. Hypercapnea acts on brain and produces the following effects:
   i. Violent expiratory efforts
   ii. Generalized convulsions
   iii. Increase in heart rate
   iv. Increase in arterial blood pressure
   v. Loss of consciousness.

3. *Stage of Collapse*

Stage of collapse lasts for about 3 minutes. Severe hypoxia produces the following effects during this stage:
   i. Depression of centers in brain and disappearance of convulsions
   ii. Development of respiratory gasping occurs. During respiratory gasping, there is stretching of the body with opening of mouth, as if gasping for breath.
   iii. Dilatation of pupils
   iv. Decrease in heart rate
   v. Loss of all reflexes.
   Duration between the gasps is gradually increased and finally death occurs.
   All together, asphyxia extends only for 5 minutes. The person can survive only by timely help such as relieving the respiratory obstruction, good aeration, etc.

■ DYSPNEA

■ DEFINITION

Dyspnea means difficulty in breathing. It is otherwise called the air hunger. Normally, the breathing goes on without consciousness. When breathing enters the consciousness and produces discomfort, it is called dyspnea. Dyspnea is also defined 'as a consciousness of necessity for increased respiratory effort'.

■ DYSPNEA POINT

Dyspnea point is the level at which there is increased ventilation with severe breathing discomfort. The normal person is not aware of any increase in breathing until the pulmonary ventilation is doubled. The real discomfort develops when ventilation increases by 4 or 5 times.

■ CONDITIONS WHEN DYSPNEA OCCURS

Physiologically, dyspnea occurs during severe muscular exercise. The pathological conditions when dyspnea occurs are:

1. *Respiratory Disorders*

Dyspnea occurs in the respiratory disorders, characterized by mechanical or nervous hindrance to respiratory movements and obstruction in any part of respiratory tract. Thus, dyspnea occurs in:

 i. Pneumonia
 ii. Pulmonary edema
 iii. Pulmonary effusion
 iv. Poliomyelitis
 v. Pneumothorax
 vi. Severe asthma, etc.

2. *Cardiac Disorders*

Dyspnea is common in left ventricular failure and decompensated mitral stenosis.

3. *Metabolic Disorders*

Metabolic disorders, which cause dyspnea are diabetic acidosis, uremia and increased hydrogen ion concentration.

■ DYSPNEIC INDEX

Dyspneic index is the index between breathing reserve and maximum breathing capacity (MBC). Breathing reserve is the balance (difference) between MBC and respiratory minute volume (RMV).

For example, in a normal subject, MBC is 116 L and RMV is 6 L.

$$\text{Dyspneic index} = \frac{MBC - RMV}{MBC} \times 100$$

$$= \frac{116 - 6}{116} \times 100$$

$$= 94.8\%.$$

Dyspnea develops when the dyspneic index decreases below 60%.

■ PERIODIC BREATHING

■ DEFINITION AND TYPES

Periodic breathing is the abnormal or uneven respiratory rhythm. It is of two types:
1. Cheyne-Stokes breathing
2. Biot breathing.

■ CHEYNE-STOKES BREATHING

Features of Cheyne-Stokes Breathing

Cheyne-Stokes breathing is the periodic breathing characterized by rhythmic hyperpnea and apnea. It is the most common type of periodic breathing. It is marked by two alternate patterns of respiration:
 i. Hyperpneic period
 ii. Apneic period.

Hyperpneic period – waxing and waning of breathing

To begin with, the breathing is shallow. Force of respiration increases gradually and reaches the maximum (hyperpnea). Then, it decreases gradually and reaches minimum and is followed by apnea. Gradual increase followed by gradual decrease in force of respiration is called **waxing** and **waning** of breathing (Fig. 127.3).

Apneic period

When, the force of breathing is reduced to minimum, cessation of breathing occurs for a short period. It is again followed by hyperpneic period and the cycle is repeated. Duration of one cycle is about 1 minute. Sometimes, waxing and waning of breathing occurs without apnea.

Causes for Waxing and Waning

Initially, during forced breathing, large quantity of carbon dioxide is washed out from blood. When partial pressure of carbon dioxide decreases, respiratory centers become inactive. It causes apnea. During

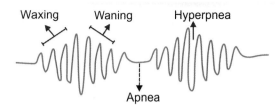

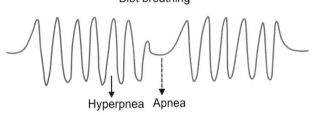

FIGURE 127.3: Periodic breathing

apnea, there is accumulation of carbon dioxide **(hypercapnea)** and reduction in oxygen tension **(hypoxia)**. Now, the respiratory centers are activated, resulting in gradual increase in the force of breathing. When the force of breathing reaches maximum, the cycle is repeated (Fig. 127.4).

Conditions when Cheyne-Stokes Breathing Occurs

Cheyne-Stokes breathing occurs in both physiological and pathological conditions.

Physiological conditions when Cheyne-Stokes breathing occurs

   i. During deep sleep
  ii. In high altitude
 iii. After prolonged voluntary hyperventilation
  iv. During hibernation in animals
   v. In newborn babies
  vi. After severe muscular exercise.

Pathological conditions when Cheyne-Stokes breathing occurs

   i. During increased intracranial pressure
  ii. During advanced cardiac diseases, leading to cardiac failure

 iii. During advanced renal diseases, leading to uremia
  iv. Poisoning by narcotics
   v. In premature infants.

■ BIOT BREATHING

Features of Biot Breathing

Biot breathing is another form of periodic breathing characterized by period of **apnea** and **hyperpnea.** Waxing and waning of breathing do not occur (Fig. 127.2). After apneic period, hyperpnea occurs abruptly.

Causes of Abrupt Apnea and Hyperpnea

Due to apnea, carbon dioxide accumulates and it stimulates the respiratory centers, leading to hyperventilation. During hyperventilation, lot of carbon dioxide is washed out. So, the respiratory centers are not stimulated and apnea occurs.

Conditions when Biot Breathing Occurs

Biot breathing does not occur in physiological conditions. It occurs only in pathological conditions. It occurs in conditions involving nervous disorders due to lesions or injuries to brain.

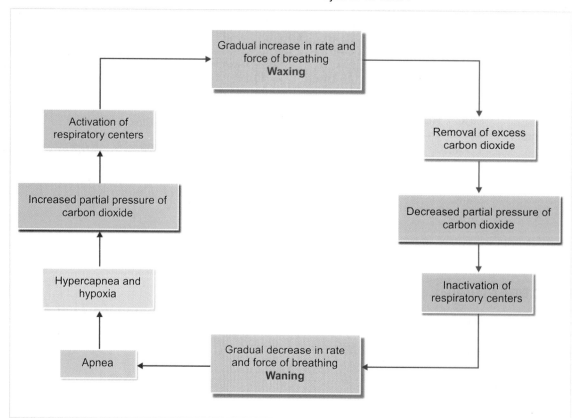

FIGURE 127.4: Cycle of waxing and waning

■ CYANOSIS

■ DEFINITION

Cyanosis is defined as the diffused **bluish coloration** of skin and mucus membrane. It is due to the presence of large amount of **reduced hemoglobin** in the blood. Quantity of reduced hemoglobin should be at least 5 to 7 g/dL in the blood to cause cyanosis.

■ DISTRIBUTION OF CYANOSIS

When it occurs, cyanosis is distributed all over the body. But, it is more marked in certain regions where the skin is thin. These areas are lips, cheeks, ear lobes, nose and fingertips above the base of the nail.

■ CONDITIONS WHEN CYANOSIS OCCURS

1. Any condition which leads to arterial hypoxia and stagnant hypoxia. Cyanosis does not occur in anemic hypoxia because the hemoglobin content itself is less. It does not occur in histotoxic hypoxia because of tissue damage.
2. Conditions when altered hemoglobin is formed. Due to poisoning, hemoglobin is altered into methemoglobin or sulfhemoglobin, which causes cyanosis. The **cyanotic discoloration** is due to the dark color of these compounds only and not due to reduced hemoglobin.
3. Conditions like polycythemia when blood flow is slow. During polycythemia, because of increased RBC count, the viscosity of blood is increased and it leads to **sluggishness of blood** flow. So the quantity of deoxygenated blood increases, which causes **bluish discoloration of skin.**

■ CYANOSIS AND ANEMIA

Cyanosis usually occurs only when the quantity of reduced hemoglobin is about 5 g/dL to 7 g/dL. But, in anemia, the hemoglobin content itself is less. So, cyanosis cannot occur in anemia.

■ CARBON MONOXIDE POISONING

■ INTRODUCTION

Carbon monoxide is a **dangerous gas** since it causes death. This gas was used by Greeks and Romans for the **execution of criminals.** Carbon monoxide causes more deaths than any other gases.

■ SOURCES OF CARBON MONOXIDE

Common sources for carbon monoxide are exhaust of gasoline engines, coal mines, gases from guns, deep wells and underground drainage system (Chapter 11).

■ TOXIC EFFECTS OF CARBON MONOXIDE

Carbon monoxide is a dangerous gas because it displaces oxygen from hemoglobin, by binding with same site in hemoglobin for oxygen. So, oxygen transport and oxygen carrying capacity of the blood are decreased.

Hemoglobin has got 200 times more affinity for carbon monoxide than for oxygen. So, even with low partial pressure of 0.4 mm Hg of carbon monoxide in alveoli, 50% of hemoglobin is saturated with it. It can be dangerous if the partial pressure increases to 0.6 mm Hg, (1/1,000 of volume concentration in air). Presence of carboxyhemoglobin decreases the release of oxygen from hemoglobin and the oxygen-hemoglobin dissociation curve shifts to left.

It is still more dangerous because, during carbon monoxide poisoning, the partial pressure of oxygen in blood may normal in spite of low oxygen content of blood. So, the regular feedback stimulation of respiratory centers by hypoxia does not take place because of normal partial pressure of oxygen.

However, low oxygen content in blood affects the brain, resulting in unconsciousness. The condition becomes fatal if immediate treatment is not given.

Carbon monoxide is toxic to the **cytochrome system** in cells also.

■ SYMPTOMS OF CARBON MONOXIDE POISONING

Symptoms of carbon monoxide poisoning depend upon its concentration:

1. While breathing air with 1% of carbon monoxide, saturation of hemoglobin with carbon monoxide becomes 15% to 20%. **Mild symptoms like headache** and **nausea** appear.
2. While breathing air containing carbon monoxide more than 1%, the saturation becomes 30% to 40%. It causes **convulsions, cardiorespiratory arrest, loss of consciousness** and **coma.**
3. When hemoglobin saturation is above 50%, death occurs.

■ TREATMENT FOR CARBON MONOXIDE POISONING

Treatment for carbon monoxide poisoning includes:
1. Immediate termination of exposure to carbon monoxide
2. Providing adequate ventilation and artificial respiration
3. Administration of 100% oxygen if possible. It is to replace carbon monoxide
4. Administration of air with few percent of carbon dioxide, if possible. It is done to stimulate the respiratory centers.

■ ATELECTASIS

■ DEFINITION

Atelectasis refers to partial or complete **collapse of lungs.** When a large portion of lung is collapsed, the partial pressure of oxygen is reduced in blood, leading to respiratory disturbances.

■ CAUSES

1. Deficiency or inactivation of surfactant. It causes collapse of lungs due to increased surface tension, which leads to respiratory distress syndrome.
2. Obstruction of a bronchus or a bronchiole. In this condition, the alveoli attached to the bronchus or bronchiole are collapsed.
3. Presence of air **(pneumothorax),** fluid **(hydrothorax),** blood **(hemothorax)** or pus **(pyothorax)** in the pleural space.

■ EFFECTS

Effects of atelectasis are decreased partial pressure of oxygen, leading to dyspnea.

■ PNEUMOTHORAX

■ DEFINITION

Pneumothorax is the presence of air in pleural space. Intrapleural pressure, which is always negative, becomes positive in pneumothorax and it causes collapse of lungs.

■ CAUSES

Air enters the pleural cavity because of damage of chest wall or lungs during accidents, bullet injury or stab injury.

■ TYPES AND EFFECTS

Pneumothorax is of three types:
1. Open pneumothorax
2. Closed pneumothorax
3. Tension pneumothorax.

1. *Open Pneumothorax*

After the injury, an open communication is developed between pleural cavity and exterior. It is known as open pneumothorax. Air enters the pleural cavity during inspiration and comes out during expiration. Collapse of lungs causes hypoxia, hypercapnea, dyspnea, cyanosis and asphyxia.

2. *Closed Pneumothorax*

During a mild injury, air enters into the pleural cavity and then the hole in the pleura is sealed and closed. It is called the closed pneumothorax. It does not produce hypoxia. Air from the pleural cavity is absorbed slowly.

3. *Tension Pneumothorax*

During injuries, sometimes the tissues over the hole in the chest wall or the lungs behave like a fluttering valve. It permits entrance of air into pleural cavity during inspiration but prevents the exit of air during expiration, due to its valvular nature. Because of this, the intrapleural pressure increases above atmospheric pressure. This condition is very fatal, since it results in collapse of the whole lung.

■ PNEUMONIA

■ DEFINITION

Pneumonia is the **inflammation** of lung tissues, followed by the accumulation of blood cells, fibrin and exudates in the alveoli. Affected part of the lungs becomes **consolidated.**

■ CAUSES

Inflammation of lung is caused by:
1. Bacterial or viral infection
2. Inhaling noxious chemical substance.

■ TYPES

Pneumonia is of two types, namely **lobar pneumonia** and **lobular pneumonia.** When it is lobular and associated with inflammation of bronchi, it is known as **bronchopneumonia.**

■ EFFECTS

Following are the effects of pneumonia:
1. Fever
2. Compression of chest and chest pain
3. Shallow breathing
4. Cyanosis
5. Sleeplessness (insomnia)
6. Delirium.

Delirium

Delirium is the extreme mental condition that is caused by cerebral hypoxia.

Features of delirium

i. Confused mental state (confused way of thought and speech)
ii. Illusion (misinterpretation of a sensory stimulus)
iii. Hallucination (feeling of sensations such as touch, pain, taste, smell, etc. without any stimulus)
iv. Disorientation (loss of ability to recognize place, time and other persons)
v. Hyperexcitability
vi. Loss of memory.

■ BRONCHIAL ASTHMA

■ DEFINITION

Bronchial asthma is the respiratory disease characterized by difficult breathing with **wheezing.** Wheezing refers to **whistling type** of respiration. It is due to bronchiolar constriction, caused by spastic contraction of smooth muscles in bronchioles, leading to obstruction of air passage. Obstruction is further exaggerated by the edema of mucus membrane and accumulation of mucus in the lumen of bronchioles.

■ CAUSES

1. *Inflammation of air passage:* Leukotrienes released from eosinophils and mast cells during inflammation cause bronchospasm.
2. *Hypersensitivity of afferent glossopharyngeal and vagal ending in larynx and afferent trigeminal endings in nose:* Hypersensitivity of these nerve endings is produced by some allergic substances like foreign proteins.
3. *Pulmonary edema and congestion of lungs caused by left ventricular failure:* Asthma developed due to this condition is called cardiac asthma.

■ FEATURES

Asthma is a **paroxysmal** (sudden) **disorder** because the attack commences and ends abruptly. During the attack, the difficulty is felt both during inspiration and expiration. Bronchioles have inherent tendency to dilate during inspiration and constrict during expiration. So, more difficulty is experienced during expiration. During expiration, great effort is exerted by all the expiratory muscles causing compression of chest. There is severe contraction of abdominal muscles also. So, air from lungs is pushed through the constricted bronchioles, producing a whistling sound.

Because of difficulty during expiration, the lungs are not deflated completely, so that the residual volume and functional residual capacity are increased.

There is reduction in:
i. Tidal volume
ii. Vital capacity
iii. Forced expiratory volume in 1 second (FEV1)
iv. Alveolar ventilation
v. Partial pressure of oxygen in blood.

Carbon dioxide accumulates, resulting in acidosis, dyspnea and cyanosis.

■ PULMONARY EDEMA

■ DEFINITION

Pulmonary edema is the accumulation of serous fluid in the alveoli and the interstitial tissue of lungs.

■ CAUSES

1. Increased pulmonary capillary pressure due to left ventricular failure or mitral valve disease
2. Pneumonia
3. Breathing harmful chemicals like chlorine or sulfur dioxide.

■ EFFECTS

Effects of pulmonary edema are severe dyspnea, cough with frothy bloodstained expectoration, cyanosis and cold extremities.

Chronic interstitial edema leads to asthma. Alveolar edema is fatal and causes sudden death due to suffocation.

■ PLEURAL EFFUSION

■ DEFINITION

Pleural effusion is the accumulation of large amount of fluid in the pleural cavity.

■ CAUSES

1. Blockage of lymphatic drainage
2. Excessive transudation of fluid from pulmonary capillaries due to increased pulmonary capillary pressure caused by left ventricular failure
3. Inflammation of pleural membrane which damages the capillary membrane, allowing leakage of fluid and plasma proteins into the pleural cavity.

■ FEATURES

Pleural effusion causes atelectasis, leading to dyspnea and other respiratory disturbances.

■ PULMONARY TUBERCULOSIS

■ DEFINITION

Tuberculosis is the disease caused by **tubercle bacilli.** This disease can affect any organ in the body. However, the lungs are affected more commonly. Infected tissue is invaded by macrophages and later it becomes fibrous. Affected tissue is called **tubercle.**

■ FEATURES

Initially, alveoli in the affected part become non-functioning, due to thickness of respiratory membrane. If a large part of lungs is involved, the diffusing capacity is very much reduced. In severe conditions, the destruction of the lung tissue is followed by formation of large **abscess cavities.**

■ EMPHYSEMA

■ DEFINITION AND CAUSES

Emphysema is one of the obstructive respiratory diseases in which lung tissues are extensively damaged. Damage of lung tissues results in loss of alveolar walls. Because of this, the elastic recoil of lungs is also lost.

Emphysema is caused by:
1. Cigarette smoking
2. Exposure to oxidant gases
3. Untreated bronchitis.

■ DEVELOPMENT OF EMPHYSEMA

1. Smoke or oxidant gases irritate the bronchi and bronchioles, leading to chronic infection

2. It increases the mucus secretion from the respiratory epithelial cells causing obstruction of air passage
3. Cilia of respiratory epithelial cells are partially paralyzed and the movement is very much reduced. Because of this, the mucus cannot be removed from the respiratory passage.
4. Destruction of alveolar mucus membrane
5. Destruction of elastic tissues occur. Normally, there is loss of some elastic tissues because of the proteolytic enzyme called **elastase.** But, that is very much negligible. Moreover, liver produces **elastase inhibitors** especially, **α_1-antitrypsin,** which prevents the destruction of elastic tissues. But, due to heavy smoking or because of constant exposure to oxidant gases, the pulmonary alveolar macrophages increase in number. Macrophages release a chemical substance, which attracts a large number of leukocytes. Leukocytes release proteases including elastase, which destroy the elastic tissues of the lungs.

■ EFFECTS OF EMPHYSEMA

1. Airway resistance increases several times due to the bronchiolar obstruction. So, the movement of air through the respiratory passage becomes very difficult. It is more pronounced during expiration.
2. Due to the destruction of alveolar membrane and elastic tissues, the lungs become loose and floppy. So, the diffusing capacity reduces to a great extent. However, lung compliance increases (Chapter 120) and the aeration of blood is impaired. Enough oxygen cannot diffuse into blood and carbon dioxide cannot diffuse out.
3. Obstruction also affects ventilation-perfusion ratio, resulting in poor aeration of blood
4. Due to the destruction of lung tissues, the number of pulmonary capillaries also decreases. It increases the pulmonary vascular resistance, leading to pulmonary hypertension.
5. Over the years, chronic emphysema could lead to hypoxia and hypercapnea. It will finally cause prolonged and severe air hunger (dyspnea), leading to death.

High Altitude and Space Physiology

Chapter 128

■ HIGH ALTITUDE
■ BAROMETRIC PRESSURE AND PARTIAL PRESSURE OF OXYGEN AT DIFFERENT ALTITUDES
■ CHANGES IN THE BODY AT HIGH ALTITUDE
  ■ EFFECTS OF HYPOXIA
  ■ EFFECTS OF EXPANSION OF GASES ON THE BODY
  ■ EFFECTS OF REDUCED ATMOSPHERIC TEMPERATURE
  ■ EFFECTS OF LIGHT RAYS
■ MOUNTAIN SICKNESS
  ■ DEFINITION
  ■ SYMPTOMS
  ■ TREATMENT
■ ACCLIMATIZATION
  ■ DEFINITION
  ■ CHANGES DURING ACCLIMATIZATION
■ AVIATION PHYSIOLOGY
  ■ ACCELERATIVE FORCE
  ■ GRAVITATIONAL FORCE
  ■ EFFECTS OF GRAVITATIONAL FORCES ON THE BODY
  ■ PREVENTION OF EFFECTS OF G FORCES ON THE BODY
■ SPACE PHYSIOLOGY
  ■ EFFECTS OF TRAVEL BY SPACECRAFT

■ HIGH ALTITUDE

High altitude is the region of earth located at an altitude of above 8,000 feet from mean sea level. People can ascend up to this level, without any adverse effect. Different altitudes are given in Table 128.1.

Characteristic feature of high altitude is the **low barometric pressure.** However, amount of oxygen available in the atmosphere is same as that of sea level. Due to low barometric pressure, partial pressure of gases, particularly oxygen proportionally decreases. It leads to hypoxia.

Carbon dioxide in high altitude is very much negligible and it does not create any problem.

TABLE 128.1: Different altitudes

Altitude	Feet	Meter
High altitude	8,000 to 13,000	2,500 to 4,000
Very high altitude	13,000 to 18,000	4,000 to 5,500
Extreme altitude	> 18,000	> 5,500

■ BAROMETRIC PRESSURE AND PARTIAL PRESSURE OF OXYGEN AT DIFFERENT ALTITUDES

Barometric pressure decreases at different altitudes. Accordingly, partial pressure of oxygen also decreases and produces various effects on the body. Barometric pressure and partial pressure of oxygen at different altitudes and their common effects on the body are given in Table 128.2.

CHANGES IN THE BODY AT HIGH ALTITUDE

When a person is exposed to high altitude, particularly by rapid ascent, the various systems in the body cannot cope with lowered oxygen tension and effects of hypoxia start. Besides hypoxia, some other factors are also responsible for the changes in functions of the body at high altitude.

Factors Affecting Physiological Functions at High Altitude

1. Hypoxia
2. Expansion of gases
3. Fall in atmospheric temperature
4. Light rays.

EFFECTS OF HYPOXIA

Refer Chapter 127 for effects of hypoxia.

EFFECTS OF EXPANSION OF GASES ON THE BODY

Volume of gases increases when the barometric pressure is reduced. So at high altitude, due to the decreased barometric pressure, volume of all gases increases in atmospheric air, as well as in the body.

At the sea level with atmospheric pressure of 760 mm Hg, if the volume of gas is 1 liter, at the height of 18,000 feet (where atmospheric pressure is 379 mm Hg), it becomes 2 liter. And it becomes 3 liter, at the height of 30,000 feet (where atmospheric pressure is 226 mm Hg).

Expansion of gases in GI tract causes painful distention of stomach and intestine. It is minimized by supporting the abdomen with a belt or by evacuation of the gases. Expansion of gases also destroys the alveoli.

During very rapid ascent from sea level to over 30,000 feet height, the gases evolve as bubbles, particularly nitrogen, resulting in decompression sickness. Refer Chapter 129 for details of decompression sickness.

TABLE 128.2: Barometric pressure, partial pressure of oxygen and common effects at different altitudes

Altitude (feet)	Barometric pressure (mm Hg)	Partial pressure of oxygen (mm Hg)	Common effects
Sea level	760	159	–
5,000	600	132	No hypoxia
10,000	523	110	Mild symptoms of hypoxia start appearing

15,000	400	90	Moderate hypoxia develops with following symptoms:
			– Reduction in visual acuity
			– Effects on mental functions:
			  – Improper judgment and
			  – Feeling of over confidence

20,000	349	73	Severe hypoxia appears with cardiorespiratory symptoms such as – Increase in heart rate and cardiac output – Increase in respiratory rate and respiratory minute volume This is the highest level for permanent inhabitants
25,000	250	62	This is the critical altitude for survival – Hypoxia becomes severe – Breathing oxygen becomes essential
29,628	235	49	This is the height of Mount Everest
30,000	226	47	Symptoms become severe even with oxygen
50,000	87	18	Hypoxia becomes more severe even with pure oxygen

■ EFFECTS OF REDUCED ATMOSPHERIC TEMPERATURE

Environmental temperature falls gradually at high altitudes. The temperature decreases to about 0°C at the height of 10,000 feet. It becomes –22°C at the height of 20,000 feet. At the altitude of 40,000 feet, the temperature falls to –44°C. Injury due to cold or frostbite occurs if the body is not adequately protected by warm clothing.

■ EFFECTS OF LIGHT RAYS

Skin becomes susceptible for injury due to many harmful rays like **ultraviolet rays** of sunlight. Moreover, the sunrays reflected by the snow might injure the retina of the eye, if it is not protected with suitable tinted glasses.

Severity of all these effects depends upon the speed at which one ascends in high altitude. The effects are comparatively milder or moderate in slow ascent and are severe in rapid ascent.

■ MOUNTAIN SICKNESS

■ DEFINITION

Mountain sickness is the condition characterized by adverse effects of hypoxia at high altitude. It is commonly developed in persons going to high altitude for the first time. It occurs within a day in these persons, before they get acclimatized to the altitude.

■ SYMPTOMS

In mountain sickness, the symptoms occur mostly in digestive system, cardiovascular system, respiratory system and nervous system. Symptoms of mountain sickness are:

1. Digestive System

Loss of appetite, nausea and vomiting occur because of expansion of gases in GI tract.

2. Cardiovascular System

Heart rate and force of contraction of heart increases.

3. Respiratory System

Pulmonary blood pressure increases due to increased blood flow. Blood flow increases because of vasodilatation induced by hypoxia. Increased pulmonary blood pressure results in pulmonary edema, which casus breathlessness.

4. Nervous System

Symptoms occuring in nervous system are headache, depression, disorientation, irritability, lack of sleep, weakness and fatigue. These symptoms are developed because of **cerebral edema.** Sudden exposure to hypoxia in high altitude causes vasodilatation in brain. **Autoregulation** mechanism of cerebral blood flow fails to cope with hypoxia. It leads to an increased capillary pressure and leakage of fluid from capillaries into the brain tissues.

■ TREATMENT

Symptoms of mountain sickness disappear by breathing oxygen.

■ ACCLIMATIZATION

■ DEFINITION

Acclimatization refers to the adaptations or the adjustments by the body in high altitude. While staying at high altitudes for several days to several weeks, a person slowly gets adapted or adjusted to the low oxygen tension, so that hypoxic effects are reduced. It enables the person to ascent further.

■ CHANGES DURING ACCLIMATIZATION

Various changes that take place during acclimatization help the body to cope with adverse effects of hypoxia at high altitude. Following changes occur in the body during acclimatization:

1. Changes in Blood

During acclimatization, RBC count increases and packed cell volume rises from normal value of 45% to about 59%. Hemoglobin content in the blood rises from 15 g% to 20 g%. So, the oxygen carrying capacity of the blood is increased. Thus, more oxygen can be carried to tissues, in spite of hypoxia. Increase in packed cell volume and hemoglobin content is due to erythropoietin actions.

Increase in RBC count, packed cell volume and hemoglobin content is due to erythropoietin, that is released from juxtaglomerular apparatus of kidney.

2. Changes in Cardiovascular System

Overall activity of cardiovascular system is increased in high altitude. There is an increase in rate and force of contraction of the heart and cardiac output. Vascularity in the body is increased due to vasodilatation induced by hypoxia. So, blood flow to vital organs such as heart, brain, muscles, etc. increases.

3. *Changes in Respiratory System*

i. *Pulmonary ventilation*

Pulmonary ventilation increases up to 65%. This is the **immediate compensation** for hypoxia in high altitude and this alone helps the person to ascend several thousand feet. Increase in pulmonary ventilation is due to the stimulation of chemoreceptors (Chapter 126).

ii. *Pulmonary hypertension*

Increased cardiac output increases the pulmonary blood flow that leads to pulmonary hypertension. It is very common even in persons acclimatized to high altitude. In some of these persons, pulmonary hypertension is associated with right ventricular hypertrophy.

iii. *Diffusing capacity of gases*

Due to increased pulmonary blood flow and increased ventilation, diffusing capacity of gases increases in alveoli. It enables more diffusion of oxygen in blood.

4. *Changes in Tissues*

Both in human beings and animals residing at high altitudes permanently, the cellular oxidative enzymes involved in metabolic reactions are more than the inhabitants at sea level.

Even when a sea level inhabitant stays at high altitude for certain period, the amount of oxidative enzymes is not increased. So, the elevation in the amount of oxidative enzymes occurs only in fully acclimatized persons. An increase in the number of mitochondria is observed in these persons.

■ AVIATION PHYSIOLOGY

Aviation physiology is the study of physiological responses of the body in **aviation environment.**

Flying exerts great effects on the body through **accelerative forces** and **gravitational forces,** which are developed during the **flight maneuvering.** Pilots and other crew members of aircraft are trained to overcome the effects of these forces.

■ ACCELERATIVE FORCE

Acceleration means change in velocity. Flying straight in horizontal plane with constant velocity has minimum effects on the body. However, changes in velocity produce severe physiological effects. Accelerative forces are developed in the flight during linear, radial or centripetal and angular acceleration.

■ GRAVITATIONAL FORCE

Gravitational force (G force) is the major factor that develops accelerative force. **G force** and the direction in which body receives the force are responsible for physiological changes in the body during acceleration.

Force or pull of gravity upon the body is expressed in **G unit.** On the earth, this pull is responsible for body weight. Force of gravity while sitting, standing or lying position is considered to be equal to body weight and it is referred as 1 G. G unit increases in acceleration. If we say that G unit increases to 5 G during acceleration, it means that the force of gravity on body at that moment is equal to five times the body weight.

While traveling in an airplane, elevator or a car, if there is a sudden change in speed or direction, passengers are thrown or centrifuged in the opposite direction. It is because of change in the G unit. G unit may increase or decrease. Increase in G unit is called positive G and decrease in G unit is called **negative G. Positive G** occurs while increasing the speed (acceleration). Negative G occurs while decreasing the speed (slowing down; deceleration). G unit is altered during the change in direction also.

While flying, both positive G and negative G cause physiological changes in the body.

■ EFFECTS OF GRAVITATIONAL FORCES ON THE BODY

Effects of Positive G

Major effects of positive G during acceleration are on the blood circulation. When G unit increases to about 4 to 5 G, blood is pushed toward the lower parts of the body including abdomen. So the cardiac output decreases, resulting in reduced blood supply to the brain and eyes. Decreased blood flow in turn, decreases oxygen supply (hypoxia) to the head and leads to following disturbances:

1. *Grayout*

Grayout is the **graying of vision** that occurs when blood flow to eyes starts diminishing. It occurs because the retina is more sensitive to hypoxia than brain. Though physical impairment does not occur, grayout is considered as a warning for decreased blood flow to head.

2. Blackout

Blackout is the complete **loss of vision** that occurs when retinal function is affected by hypoxia. Consciousness and muscular activities are still retained. But it indicates the risk of loss of consciousness.

3. Loss of consciousness

When force increases beyond 5 G, hypoxia reaches the critical level and causes loss of consciousness. It may be associated with convulsions. Unconscious state may last for about 15 seconds. After recovery from unconsciousness, the person needs another 10 to 15 minutes for orientation. If the affected person happens to be a lone pilot, then he will loose control over his aircraft.

4. Fracture of bones

When force increases to about 20 G, bones, particularly the spine, becomes susceptible for fracture even during sitting posture.

Effects of Negative G

Negative G develops while flying downwards (inverted flying). It causes the following disturbances:

1. Hyperemia

When the force decreases to –4 to –6 G, **hyperemia** (abnormal increase in blood flow) occurs in head because the blood is pushed towards head. Sometimes the blood accumulates in head, resulting in **brain edema.** There is congestion, flushing of face and mild headache. Negative G at this level is tolerable and the effects are only momentary. Brain also can withstand hyperemia in such conditions.

2. Redout and headache

Redout is the **blurring of vision** and sudden reddening of visual field, caused by engorgement of blood vessels in head. When the negative G reaches to about –15 G to –20 G, there is dilatation and congestion of blood vessels in head and eyes, resulting in redout and headache. Blood vessels in brain may not be affected much because of CSF. When blood accumulates in brain, there is simultaneous pooling of CSF in cranium. The high pressure exerted by CSF acts as a cushion (buffer) and protects the blood vessels of brain.

3. Loss of consciousness

High negative G affects the body by other means. It increases the pressure in the blood vessels of chest and neck. It causes bradycardia or irregular heartbeat, which adds to stagnation of blood in head. All these factors ultimately lead to unconsciousness.

■ PREVENTION OF EFFECTS OF G FORCES ON THE BODY

Body can be protected from the effects of G forces, particularly positive G by the following methods:

1. By Using Abdominal Belts

Pooling of blood in the abdominal blood vessels is prevented by using abdominal belt and leaning forward while sitting in the aircraft. This procedure postpones grayout or blackout.

2. By Using Anti-G Suit

Anti-G suit exerts a positive pressure on lower limbs and abdomen and prevents the pooling of blood in lower part of the body.

■ SPACE PHYSIOLOGY

Space physiology is the study of physiological responses of the body in space and spacecrafts.

Major differences between the environments of earth and space are atmosphere, radiation and gravity. These three factors challenge the human survival in space. Atmospheric factors include atmospheric pressure, temperature, humidity and gas composition.

Spacecraft or **spacelab** is provided with stable and sophisticated environmental control system, which maintains all the atmospheric factors close to earth's environment. **Astronauts** also wear **launch and entry suit (LES).** LES is a pressurized suit that protects the body from space environment.

Another factor which affects the body in the space is **weightlessness.** Weightlessness is because of absence of gravity (microgravity).

■ EFFECTS OF TRAVEL BY SPACECRAFT

While traveling by spacecraft, the astronauts experience some intense symptoms only during blast off, due to acceleration and during landing because of deceleration. Otherwise, the accelerative forces are least while traveling in a spacecraft, since the spacecraft cannot make rapid changes in speed or direction like an aircraft.

Most of the physiological changes occur due to weightlessness in space travel. These changes are responsible for the adaptation of astronaut's body to space environment. Further, problems develop only when they return to earth. They require a longtime to readapt to earth environment.

Effects of weightlessness in spacecraft are:

1. Effects on Cardiovascular Systems and Kidneys

Cardiovascular changes are due to the fluid shift. Due to absence of gravity, blood moves from lower part to upper part of the body (upper trunk and head). It causes **enlargement of heart** to cope up with increased blood flow. In addition, there is an accumulation of other body fluids in upper part. Now, the compensatory mechanism in the body interprets the increase in blood and other fluids as a serious threat and starts correcting it by excreting large amount of fluid through kidneys. It causes decrease in blood volume and the heart need not pump the blood against gravity in space. So, initially enlarged heart starts shrinking slowly and becomes small. Thus during the initial fluid shift, astronauts experience dizziness or feeling of fainting.

Along with water, kidneys excrete electrolytes also. Because of this, osmolarity of body fluids is not altered. So the thirst center is not stimulated and the astronauts do not feel thirsty during space travel.

2. Effects on Blood

Plasma volume decreases due to excretion of fluid through urine. RBC count also decreases and it is called space anemia.

3. Effects on Musculoskeletal System

Because of microgravity in space, the muscles need not support the body against gravity. Astronauts move by floating instead of using their legs. This leads to decrease in muscle mass and muscle strength. **Endurance** of the muscles also decreases. Bones become weak. **Osteoclastic activity** increases during space travel. Calcium removed from bone is excreted through urine.

4. Effects on Immune System

Space travel causes suppression of immune system in the body.

5. Space Motion Sickness

After obtaining weightlessness, some astronauts develop space motion sickness. It is characterized by nausea, vomiting, headache and malaise (generalized feeling of discomfort or lack of well-being or illness that is associated with sensation of exhaustion). It persists for two or three days and then disappears. It is thought that the motion sickness occurs due to abnormal stimulation of vestibular apparatus and fluid shift.

Deep Sea Physiology

- ■ INRODUCTION
- ■ BAROMETRIC PRESSURE AT DIFFERENT DEPTHS
- ■ EFFECT OF HIGH BAROMETRIC PRESSURE – NITROGEN NARCOSIS
  - ■ MECHANISM
  - ■ SYMPTOMS
  - ■ PREVENTION
  - ■ TREATMENT
- ■ DECOMPRESSION SICKNESS
  - ■ DEFINITION
  - ■ CAUSE
  - ■ SYMPTOMS
  - ■ PREVENTION
  - ■ TREATMENT
- ■ SCUBA

■ INTRODUCTION

In high altitude, the problem is with **low atmospheric (barometric) pressure.** In deep sea or mines, the problem is with **high barometric pressure.** Increased pressure creates two major problems:

1. Compression effect on the body and internal organs
2. Decrease in volume of gases.

■ BAROMETRIC PRESSURE AT DIFFERENT DEPTHS

At sea level, the barometric pressure is 760 mm Hg, which is referred as 1 atmosphere. At the depth of every 33 feet (about 10 m), the pressure increases by 1 atmosphere. Thus, at the depth of 33 feet, the pressure is 2 atmospheres. It is due to the air above water and the weight of water itself. Pressure at different depths is given in Table 129.1.

■ EFFECT OF HIGH BAROMETRIC PRESSURE – NITROGEN NARCOSIS

Narcosis refers to unconsciousness or **stupor** produced by drugs. Stupor refers to lethargy with suppression of sensations and feelings. Nitrogen narcosis means narcotic effect produced by nitrogen at high pressure.

Nitrogen narcosis is common in deep sea divers, who breathe **compressed air** (air under high pressure). Breathing compressed air is essential for a deep sea diver or an underwater tunnel worker. It is to equalize the surrounding high pressure acting on thoracic wall and abdomen.

Eighty percent of the atmospheric air is nitrogen. Being an inert gas, it does not produce any known effect on the functions of the body at normal atmospheric pressure (sea level). When a person breathes **pressurized air** as in deep sea, the **narcotic effect** of nitrogen appears. It produces an altered mental state, similar to **alcoholic intoxication.**

TABLE 129.1: Barometric pressure and its effects at different depth

Depth (feet)	Atmospheric pressure (mm Hg)	Effects on the subject
Sea level	1	–
33	2	–
66	3	–
100	4	Symptoms of nitrogen narcosis appear
133	5	Lack of concentration Becomes jovial and careless
166	6	Starts feeling drowsy
200	7	Feels fatigued, weak and careless
233	8	Looses power of judgment Unable to do skilled work
266	9	Becomes unconscious
Barometric pressure: 1 atmosphere = 760 mm Hg		

■ MECHANISM

Nitrogen is soluble in fat. During compression by high barometric pressure in deep sea, nitrogen escapes from blood vessels and gets dissolved in the fat present in various parts of the body, especially the neuronal membranes. Dissolved nitrogen acts like an **anesthetic agent** suppressing the neuronal excitability. Nitrogen remains in dissolved form in the fat till the person remains in the deep sea.

■ SYMPTOMS

1. First symptom starts appearing at a depth of 120 feet. The person becomes very jovial, careless and does not understand the seriousness of the conditions.
2. At the depth of 150 to 200 feet, the person becomes drowsy
3. At 200 to 250 feet depth, the person becomes extremely fatigued and weak. There is loss of concentration and judgment. Ability to perform skilled work or movements is also lost.
4. Beyond the depth of 250 feet, the person becomes unconscious.

■ PREVENTION

Nitrogen narcosis can be prevented by mixing **helium** with oxygen. Helium is used as a substitute for nitrogen, to dilute oxygen during deep water diving. Helium also produces some effects like nausea and dizziness. But, the adverse effects of helium are less severe than nitrogen narcosis.

Nitrogen narcosis may be prevented by limiting the depth of dives. Effects of nitrogen narcosis may also be minimized by safe diving procedures such as proper maintenance of equipments and less work effort. In addition, alcohol consumption should be avoided 24 hours before diving.

■ TREATMENT

Symptoms of nitrogen narcosis completely disappear when the diver returns to a depth of 60 feet. There is no need for any further treatment since nitrogen narcosis does not have any hangover effect. However, the physician should be consulted if the diver loses consciousness.

■ DECOMPRESSION SICKNESS

■ DEFINITION

Decompression sickness is the disorder that occurs when a person returns rapidly to normal surroundings (atmospheric pressure) from the area of high atmospheric pressure like deep sea. It is also known as **dysbarism, compressed air sickness, caisson disease, bends** or **diver's palsy.**

■ CAUSE

High barometric pressure at deep sea leads to compression of gases in the body. Compression reduces the volume of gases.

Among the respiratory gases, oxygen is utilized by tissues. Carbon dioxide can be expired out. But, nitrogen, which is present in high concentration, i.e. 80% is an inert gas. So, it is neither utilized nor expired. When nitrogen is compressed by high atmospheric pressure in deep sea, it escapes from blood vessels and enters the organs. As it is fat soluble, it gets dissolved in the fat of the tissues and tissue fluids. It is very common in the brain tissues.

As long as the person remains in deep sea, nitrogen remains in solution and does not cause any problem. But, if the person ascends rapidly and returns to atmospheric pressure, decompression sickness occurs.

Due to sudden return to atmospheric pressure, the nitrogen is decompressed and escapes from the tissues at a faster rate. Being a gas, it forms **bubbles** while escaping rapidly. The bubbles travel through blood vessels and ducts. In many places, the bubbles obstruct the blood flow and produce air **embolism,** leading to decompression sickness.

Underground tunnel workers who use the **caissons** (pressurized chambers) also develop decompression **(caisson disease)** sickness. Pressure in the chamber is increased to prevent the entry of water inside. Decompression sickness also occurs in a person who ascends up rapidly from sea level in an airplane without any precaution.

■ SYMPTOMS

Symptoms of decompression sickness are mainly due to the escape of nitrogen from tissues in the form of bubbles.

Symptoms are:
1. Severe pain in tissues, particularly the joints, produced by nitrogen bubbles in the myelin sheath of sensory nerve fibers
2. Sensation of numbness, tingling or pricking (paresthesia) and itching
3. Temporary paralysis due to nitrogen bubbles in the myelin sheath of motor nerve fibers
4. Muscle cramps associated with severe pain
5. Occlusion of coronary arteries followed by coronary ischemia, caused by bubbles in the blood

6. Occlusion of blood vessels in brain and spinal cord also
7. Damage of tissues of brain and spinal cord because of obstruction of blood vessels by the bubbles
8. Dizziness, paralysis of muscle, shortness of breath and choking occur
9. Finally, fatigue, unconsciousness and death.

■ PREVENTION

Decompression sickness is prevented by proper precautionary measures. While returning to mean sea level, the ascent should be very slow with short stay at regular intervals. **Stepwise ascent** allows nitrogen to come back to the blood, without forming bubbles. It prevents the decompression sickness.

■ TREATMENT

If a person is affected by decompression sickness, first recompression should be done. It is done by keeping the person in a **recompression chamber.** Then, he is brought back to atmospheric pressure by reducing the pressure slowly.

Hyperbaric oxygen therapy may be useful.

■ SCUBA

SCUBA (self-contained underwater breathing apparatus) is used by the deep sea divers and the underwater tunnel workers, to prevent the ill effects of increased barometric pressure in deep sea or tunnels.

This instrument can be easily carried and it contains air cylinders, valve system and a mask. By using this instrument, it is possible to breathe air or gas mixture without high pressure. Also, because of the valve system, only the amount of air necessary during inspiration enters the mask and the expired air is expelled out of the mask.

Disadvantage of this instrument is that the person using this can remain in the sea or tunnel only for a short period. Especially, beyond the depth of 150 feet, the person can stay only for few minutes.

Effects of Exposure to Cold and Heat

- ■ **EFFECTS OF EXPOSURE TO COLD**
  - ■ **HEAT PRODUCTION**
  - ■ **PREVENTION OF HEAT LOSS**
- ■ **EFFECTS OF EXPOSURE TO SEVERE COLD**
  - ■ **LOSS OF TEMPERATURE REGULATING CAPACITY**
  - ■ **FROSTBITE**
- ■ **EFFECTS OF EXPOSURE TO HEAT**
  - ■ **HEAT EXHAUSTION**
  - ■ **DEHYDRATION EXHAUSTION**
  - ■ **HEAT CRAMPS**
  - ■ **HEATSTROKE – SUNSTROKE**

■ EFFECTS OF EXPOSURE TO COLD

During exposure to cold, the body temperature is maintained by two mechanisms (Chapter 63).

1. Heat production
2. Prevention of heat loss.

■ HEAT PRODUCTION

When body is exposed to cold, heat is produced by the following activities:

1. By Accelerating Metabolic Activities

Heat gain center in hypothalamus is stimulated during exposure to cold. It activates the sympathetic centers, which cause secretion of adrenaline and noradrenaline. These hormones, especially adrenaline increase heat production by accelerating cellular metabolic activities.

2. By Shivering

Shivering is the increased **involuntary muscular activity** with slight vibration of the body in response to fear, onset of fever or exposure to cold. Shivering occurs when the body temperature falls to about 25°C (77°F). Primary motor center for shivering is situated in posterior

hypothalamus near the wall of the III ventricle. During exposure to cold, heat gain center activates the motor center and shivering occurs. Enormous heat is produced during shivering due to severe muscular activities.

■ PREVENTION OF HEAT LOSS

When the body is exposed to cold, heat gain center in the posterior nucleus of hypothalamus is stimulated. It activates the sympathetic centers in posterior hypothalamus, resulting in cutaneous vasoconstriction and decrease in blood flow. Due to decrease in cutaneous blood flow, sweat secretion is decreased and heat loss is prevented.

■ EFFECTS OF EXPOSURE TO SEVERE COLD

Exposure of body to severe cold leads to death, if quick remedy is not provided. The survival time depends upon environmental temperature.

If a person is exposed to ice cold water, i.e. 0°C for 20 to 30 minutes, the body temperature falls below 25°C (77°F) and the person can survive if he is placed immediately in hot water tub with a temperature of 43°C

(110°F). Survival time at 9°C (28°F) is about 1 hour and at 15.5°C (60°F) it is about 5 hours.

Effects of exposure of body to extreme cold are:
1. Loss of temperature regulating capacity
2. Frostbite.

■ LOSS OF TEMPERATURE REGULATING CAPACITY

Temperature regulating capacity of hypothalamus is affected when the body temperature decreases to about 34.4°C (94°F). Hypothalamus totally looses the power of temperature regulation when body temperature falls below 25°C (77°F). Shivering does not occur.

In addition to loss of hypothalamic function, the metabolic activities are also suppressed. **Sleep or coma** develops due to depression of central nervous system.

■ FROSTBITE

Frostbite is the freezing of surface of the body when it is exposed to cold. It occurs due to sluggishness of blood flow. Most commonly, the exposed areas such as ear lobes and digits of hands and feet are affected. Frostbite is common in mountaineers. Prolonged exposure will lead to permanent damage of the cells, followed by **thawing** and **gangrene** (death and decay of tissues) formation.

■ EFFECTS OF EXPOSURE TO HEAT

Effects of exposure to heat are:
1. Heat exhaustion
2. Dehydration exhaustion
3. Heat cramps
4. Heatstroke (sunstroke).

■ HEAT EXHAUSTION

Heat exhaustion is the body's response to excess loss of water and salt through sweat, caused by exposure to hot environmental conditions. In fact, it is the warning that body is getting too hot. Heat exhaustion results in loss of consciousness and collapse. Before the loss of consciousness, following warning signs appear in the body:
  i. Increased heart rate
 ii. Increased cardiac output
iii. Dilatation of cutaneous blood vessels
 iv. Increased moisture of the body
  v. Fall in blood pressure
 vi. Weakness and uneasiness
vii. Mild dyspnea.

■ DEHYDRATION EXHAUSTION

Prolonged exposure to heat results in dehydration. It is due to excessive sweating. Dehydration leads to fall in cardiac output and blood pressure. Collapse occurs if treatment is not given immediately.

■ HEAT CRAMPS

Severe painful cramps occur due to reduction in the quantity of salts and water as a result of increased sweating, during continuous exposure to heat.

■ HEATSTROKE – SUNSTROKE

Heatstroke

Heatstroke is an abnormal type of **hyperthermia** that occurs during exposure to extreme heat. It is characterized by increase in body temperature above 41°C (106°F), accompanied by some physical and neurological symptoms. Compared to other effects of exposure to heat such as heat exhaustion and heat cramps, heatstroke is very severe and often becomes fatal if not treated immediately. Hypothalamus loses the power of regulating body temperature.

Sunstroke

Sunstroke is the hyperthermia caused by prolonged exposure to sun during summer in desert or tropical areas.

Persons Susceptible to Heatstroke or Sunstroke

People more susceptible to heatstroke or sunstroke are:
  i. Infants
 ii. Old people with renal, cardiac or pulmonary disorders
iii. People doing physical labor under sun
 iv. Sportsmen involved in continuous sports activities without break.

Features

Common features of heatstroke or sunstroke are:
  i. Nausea and vomiting
 ii. Dizziness
iii. Headache
 iv. Abdominal pain
  v. Difficulty in breathing
 vi. Vertigo

vii. Confusion

viii. Muscle cramps and convulsions

ix. Paralysis

x. Unconsciousness.

If immediate and vigorous treatment is not given, damage of brain tissues occurs, resulting in coma and death.

Heatstroke and Humidity

Development of heatstroke depends upon humidity of the environment. If the environmental air is completely dry, exposure of body for several hours even to a temperature of 54.4°C (130°F) does not cause heatstroke. If air is 100% humid, even the temperature of 41°C (106.8°F) causes heatstroke.

Prevention

Heatstroke or sunstroke can be avoided by the following measures:

i. Avoiding dehydration by taking plenty of fluids such as water or sports drinks

ii. Taking frequent breaks during work or sports activity

iii. Wearing light clothes with hat.

Treatment

Person affected by heatstroke or sunstroke must be treated before the damage of organs. The subject should be immediately moved from hot environment and **hospitalized** as soon as possible. Immediate cooling of the body is the usual treatment. The person must be immersed in **cold water** or cold water may be sprayed on the skin. If water supply is not sufficient, cooling the head and neck of the subject should be done first. **Ice cubes** can be rubbed on head and neck. Ice packs must be kept under armpits and groin. Cooling efforts should be continued till the body temperature falls to about 35°C.

Artificial Respiration

- ■ **CONDITIONS WHEN ARTIFICIAL RESPIRATION IS REQUIRED**
- ■ **METHODS OF ARTIFICIAL RESPIRATION**
  - ■ **MANUAL METHODS**
  - ■ **MECHANICAL METHODS**

■ CONDITIONS WHEN ARTIFICIAL RESPIRATION IS REQUIRED

Artificial respiration is required whenever there is an arrest of breathing, without cardiac failure. Arrest of breathing occurs in the following conditions:

1. Accidents
2. Drowning
3. Gas poisoning
4. Electric shock
5. Anesthesia.

Stoppage of oxygen supply for 5 minutes causes irreversible changes in tissues of brain, particularly tissues of cerebral cortex. So, artificial respiration (resuscitation) must be started quickly without any delay, before the development of cardiac failure.

Purpose of artificial respiration is to ventilate the alveoli and to stimulate the respiratory centers.

■ METHODS OF ARTIFICIAL RESPIRATION

Methods of artificial respiration are of two types:

1. Manual methods
2. Mechanical methods.

■ MANUAL METHODS

Manual methods of **resuscitation** can be applied quickly without waiting for the availability of any mechanical aids.

Affected person must be provided with clear air. Clothes around neck and chest regions must be loosened. Mouth, face and throat should be cleared of mucus, saliva, foreign particles, etc. Tongue must be drawn forward and it must be prevented from falling posteriorly, which may cause airway obstruction.

Manual methods are of two types:

i. Mouth-to-mouth method
ii. Holger Nielsen method.

Mouth-to-mouth Method

The subject is kept in supine position and the **resuscitator** (person who give resuscitation) kneels at the side of the subject. By keeping the thumb on subject's mouth, the lower jaw is pulled downwards. Nostrils of the subject are closed with thumb and index finger of the other hand.

Resuscitator then takes a deep breath and exhales into the subject's mouth forcefully. Volume of exhaled air must be twice the normal tidal volume. This expands the subject's lungs. Then, the resuscitator removes his mouth from that of the subject. Now, a passive expiration occurs in the subject due to elastic recoil of the lungs. This procedure is repeated at a rate of 12 to 14 times a minute, till normal respiration is restored.

Mouth-to-mouth method is the most effective manual method because, carbon dioxide in expired air of the resuscitator can directly stimulate the respiratory centers and facilitate the onset of respiration. Only disadvantage is that the close contact between the mouths of resuscitator and subject may not be acceptable for various reasons.

Holger Nielsen Method or Back Pressure Arm Lift Method

Subject is placed in prone position with head turned to one side. Hands are placed under the cheeks with flexion at elbow joint and abduction of arms at the shoulders. Resuscitator kneels beside the head of the subject. By placing the palm of the hands over the back of the subject, the resuscitator bends forward with straight arms (without flexion at elbow) and applies pressure on the back of the subject.

Weight of the resuscitator and pressure on back of the subject compresses his chest and expels air from the lungs. Later, the resuscitator leans back. At the same time, he draws the subject's arm forward by holding it just above elbow.

This procedure causes expansion of thoracic cage and flow of air into the lungs. The movements are repeated at the rate of 12 per minute, till the normal respiration is restored.

■ MECHANICAL METHODS

Mechanical methods of artificial respiration become necessary when the subject needs artificial respiration for long periods. It is essential during the respiratory failure due to paralysis of respiratory muscles or any other cause.

Mechanical methods are of two types:
  i. Drinker method
  ii. Ventilation method.

Drinker Method

The machine used in this method is called **iron lung chamber** or **tank respirator.** The equipment has an airtight chamber, made of iron or steel. Subject is placed inside this chamber with the head outside the chamber.

By means of some pumps, the pressure inside the chamber is made positive and negative alternately. During the negative pressure in the chamber, the subject's thoracic cage expands and inspiration occurs and during positive pressure the expiration occurs.

By using tank respirator, the patient can survive for a longer time, even up to the period of one year till the natural respiratory functions are restored.

Ventilation Method

A rubber tube is introduced into the trachea of the patient through the mouth. By using a pump, air or oxygen is pumped into the lungs with pressure intermittently. When air is pumped, inflation of lungs and inspiration occur. When it is stopped, expiration occurs and the cycle is repeated. Apparatus used for ventilation is called **ventilator** and it is mostly used to treat acute respiratory failure.

Ventilator is of two types:
  a. Volume ventilator
  b. Pressure ventilator.

Volume ventilator

By volume ventilator, a constant volume of air is pumped into the lungs of patients intermittently with minimum pressure.

Pressure ventilator

By pressure ventilator, air is pumped into the lungs of subject with constant high pressure.

Effects of Exercise on Respiration

- ■ INTRODUCTION
- ■ EFFECTS OF EXERCISE ON RESPIRATION
    - ■ PULMONARY VENTILATION
    - ■ DIFFUSING CAPACITY FOR OXYGEN
    - ■ CONSUMPTION OF OXYGEN
    - ■ OXYGEN DEBT
    - ■ VO$_2$ MAX
    - ■ RESPIRATORY QUOTIENT

■ INTRODUCTION

Muscular exercise brings about a lot of changes on various systems of the body. Degree of changes depends upon the severity of exercise. Refer Chapter 117 for types and severity of exercise.

■ EFFECTS OF EXERCISE ON RESPIRATION

■ EFFECT ON PULMONARY VENTILATION

Pulmonary ventilation is the amount of air that enters and leaves the lungs in 1 minute. It is the product of tidal volume and respiratory rate. It is about 6 liter/minute, with a normal tidal volume of 500 mL and respiratory rate of 12/minute.

During exercise, hyperventilation, which includes increase in rate and force of respiration occurs. In moderate exercise, respiratory rate increases to about 30/minute and tidal volume increases to about 2,000 mL. Thus, the pulmonary ventilation increases to about 60 L/minute during moderate exercise. In severe muscular exercise, it rises still further up to 100 L/minute.

Factors increasing pulmonary ventilation during exercise

1. Higher centers
2. Chemoreceptors

3. Proprioceptors
4. Body temperature
5. Acidosis.

1. *Higher Centers*

Rate and depth of respiration increase during the onset of exercise. Sometimes, before starting the exercise, thought or anticipation of exercise itself increases the rate and force of respiration. It is a **psychic phenomenon** due to the activation of higher centers like Sylvian cortex and motor cortex of brain. Higher centers, in turn accelerate the respiratory processes by stimulating respiratory centers.

2. *Chemoreceptors*

Chemoreceptors which are stimulated by exercise-induced hypoxia and hypercapnea, send impulses to the respiratory centers. Respiratory centers, in turn increase the rate and force of respiration. Chemoreceptors are described in detail in Chapter 126.

3. *Proprioceptors*

Proprioceptors, which are activated during exercise, send impulses to cerebral cortex through the somatic afferent nerves. Cerebral cortex, in turn causes hyperventilation by sending impulses to the medullary respiratory centers. Refer Chapter 156 for proprioceptors.

4. *Body Temperature*

Body temperature which increases by muscular activity, increases the ventilation by stimulating the respiratory centers.

5. *Acidosis*

Acidosis developed during exercise also stimulates the respiratory centers, resulting in hyperventilation.

■ EFFECT ON DIFFUSING CAPACITY FOR OXYGEN

Diffusing capacity for oxygen is about 21 mL/minute at resting condition. It rises to 45 to 50 mL/minute during moderate exercise because of increased blood flow through pulmonary capillaries.

■ EFFECT ON CONSUMPTION OF OXYGEN

Oxygen consumed by the tissues, particularly the skeletal muscles is greatly enhanced during exercise. Because of vasodilatation in muscles during exercise, more amount of blood flows through the muscles and more amount of oxygen diffuses into the muscles from blood. The amount of oxygen utilized by the muscles is directly proportional to the amount of oxygen available.

■ EFFECT ON OXYGEN DEBT

Oxygen debt is the extra amount of oxygen required by the muscles during recovery from severe muscular exercise. After a period of severe muscular exercise, amount of oxygen consumed is greatly increased. Oxygen required is more than the quantity available to the muscle. This much of oxygen is required not only for the activity of the muscle but also for reversal of some metabolic processes such as:

1. Reformation of glucose from lactic acid, accumulated during exercise
2. Resynthesis of ATP and creatine phosphate
3. Restoration of amount of oxygen dissociated from hemoglobin and myoglobin.

Thus, for the above reversal phenomena, an extra amount of oxygen must be made available in the body after severe muscular exercise. Oxygen debt is about six times more than the amount of oxygen consumed under resting conditions.

■ EFFECT ON VO$_2$ MAX

VO$_2$ max is the amount of oxygen consumed under maximal aerobic metabolism. It is the product of maximal cardiac output and maximal amount of oxygen consumed by the muscle.

In a normal active and healthy male, the VO$_2$ max is 35 to 40 mL/kg body weight/minute. In females, it is 30 to 35 mL/kg body weight/minute. During exercise, VO$_2$ max increases by 50%.

■ EFFECT ON RESPIRATORY QUOTIENT

Respiratory quotient is the molar ratio of carbon dioxide production to oxygen consumption. Refer Chapter 124 for details.

Respiratory quotient in resting condition is 1.0 and during exercise it increases to 1.5 to 2. However, at the end of exercise, the respiratory quotient reduces to 0.5.

QUESTIONS IN RESPIRATORY SYSTEM AND ENVIRONMENTAL PHYSIOLOGY

■ LONG QUESTIONS

1. Describe the various movements of thoracic cage and lungs during respiration.
2. Describe in detail the pulmonary circulation.
3. Give the definition and normal values of lung volumes and lung capacities and explain the measurement of the same.
4. Explain the transport of oxygen in blood.
5. Explain the transport of carbon dioxide in blood.
6. Describe the nervous regulation of respiration.
7. Describe the chemical regulation of respiration.
8. What is hypoxia? Describe the types, causes and effects of hypoxia. Add a note on oxygen therapy.
9. Describe the changes in the body at high altitude and explain the acclimatization.
10. Describe in detail the respiratory and cardio-vascular changes during exercise.

■ SHORT QUESTIONS

1. Respiratory unit.
2. Respiratory membrane.
3. Non-respiratory functions of respiratory tract.
4. Physiological shunt.
5. Characteristic features of pulmonary circulation.
6. Collapsing tendency of lungs.
7. Surfactant.
8. Respiratory pressures.
9. Compliance.
10. Work of breathing.
11. Spirometry.
12. Measurement of functional residual capacity.
13. Measurement of residual volume.
14. Vital capacity.
15. MBC or MVV.
16. Forced expiratory volume.
17. Plethysmography.
18. Peak expiratory flow rate.
19. Alveolar ventilation.
20. Dead space.
21. Ventilation perfusion ratio.
22. Respiratory quotient or respiratory exchange ratio.
23. Alveolar air.
24. Oxygen hemoglobin dissociation curve.
25. Carbon dioxide dissociation curve.
26. Bohr effect.
27. Haldane effect.
28. Chloride shift.
29. Diffusing capacity.
30. Exchange of gases between alveoli and blood.
31. Exchange of gases between blood and tissues.
32. Respiratory centers.
33. Inspiratory ramp.
34. Hering-Breuer reflex.
35. Receptors of lungs taking part in control of breathing.
36. Chemoreceptors.
37. Apnea.
38. Hypoxia.
39. Hyperventilation and hypoventilation.
40. Hypercapnea and hypocapnea.
41. Asphyxia.
42. Dyspnea.
43. Periodic breathing.
44. Cyanosis.
45. Oxygen toxicity (poisoning).
46. Carbon monoxide poisoning.
47. Pneumothorax.
48. Pneumonia.
49. Pulmonary edema.
50. Mountain sickness.
51. Acclimatization.
52. Effect of G force.
53. Decompression sickness.
54. Nitrogen narcosis.
55. Effects of sudden exposure to cold.
56. Effects of sudden exposure to heat.
57. Heatstroke or sunstroke.
58. Artificial respiration.
59. Respiratory changes during exercise.
60. Oxygen debt.
61. VO_2 max.
62. Fetal respiration and first breath.

Section

10

Nervous System

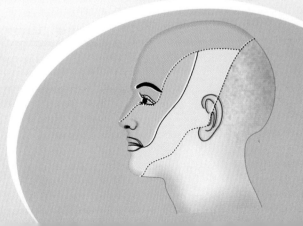

Introduction to Nervous System

> ■ DIVISIONS OF NERVOUS SYSTEM
> ■ CENTRAL NERVOUS SYSTEM
> ■ PERIPHERAL NERVOUS SYSTEM

■ DIVISIONS OF NERVOUS SYSTEM

Nervous system controls all the activities of the body. It is quicker than other control system in the body, namely endocrine system. Primarily, nervous system is divided into two parts:
1. Central nervous system
2. Peripheral nervous system.

■ CENTRAL NERVOUS SYSTEM

Central nervous system (CNS) includes **brain** and **spinal cord.** It is formed by **neurons** and supporting cells called **neuroglia.** Structures of brain and spinal cord are arranged in two layers, namely **gray matter** and **white matter.** Gray matter is formed by nerve cell bodies and the proximal parts of nerve fibers, arising from nerve cell body. White matter is formed by remaining parts of nerve fibers.

In brain, white matter is placed in the inner part and gray matter is placed in the outer part. In spinal cord, white matter is in the outer part and gray matter is in the inner part.

Brain is situated in the **skull.** It is continued as spinal cord in the **vertebral canal** through the **foramen magnum** of the skull bone. Brain and spinal cord are surrounded by three layers of **meninges** called the outer **dura mater,** middle **arachnoid mater** and inner **pia mater.**

The space between arachnoid mater and pia mater is known as **subarachnoid space.** This space is filled with a fluid called cerebrospinal fluid. Brain and spinal cord are actually suspended in the **cerebrospinal fluid.** Important parts of brain and segments of spinal cord are shown in Figure 133.1.

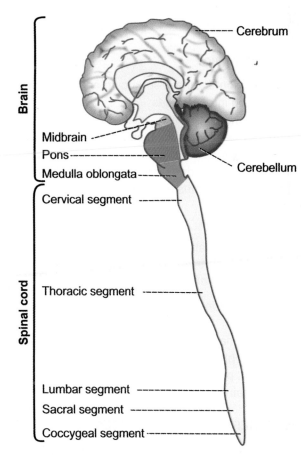

FIGURE 133.1: Parts of central nervous system

Parts of Brain

Brain consists of three major divisions:
1. Prosencephalon

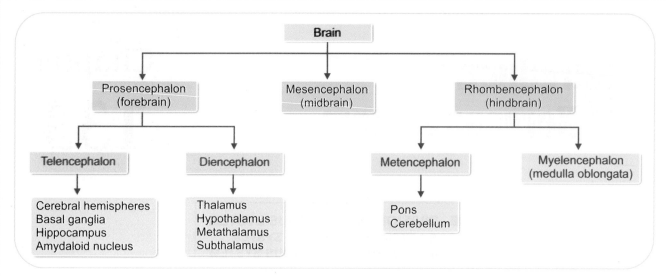

FIGURE 133.2: Parts of brain

2. Mesencephalon
3. Rhombencephalon

1. *Prosencephalon*

Prosencephalon is otherwise known as **forebrain**. It is further divided into two parts:

i. Telencephalon, which includes cerebral hemispheres, basal ganglia, hippocampus and amygdaloid nucleus

ii. Diencephalon, consisting of thalamus, hypothalamus, metathalamus and subthalamus.

2. *Mesencephalon*

Mesencephalon is also known as **midbrain.**

3. *Rhombencephalon*

Rhombencephalon or **hindbrain** is subdivided into two portions:

i. Metencephalon, formed by pons and cerebellum
ii. Myelencephalon or medulla oblongata (Fig. 133.2).
   Midbrain, pons and medulla oblongata are together called the brainstem.

■ PERIPHERAL NERVOUS SYSTEM

Peripheral nervous system (PNS) is formed by neurons and their processes present in all regions of the body. It consists of cranial nerves, arising from brain and spinal nerves, arising from the spinal cord. It is again divided into two subdivisions:

1. Somatic nervous system
2. Autonomic nervous system.

1. *Somatic Nervous System*

Somatic nervous system is concerned with **somatic functions.** It includes the nerves supplying the skeletal muscles. Somatic nervous system is responsible for muscular activities and movements of the body (Fig. 133.3).

2. *Autonomic Nervous System*

Autonomic nervous system is concerned with regulation of **visceral** or **vegetative functions.** So, it is otherwise called **vegetative** or **involuntary nervous system.** Autonomic nervous system consists of two divisions, sympathetic division and parasympathetic division.

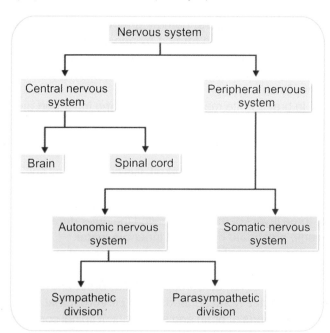

FIGURE 133.3: Organization of nervous system

Neuron

- ■ INTRODUCTION
- ■ CLASSIFICATION
  - ■ DEPENDING UPON THE NUMBER OF POLES
  - ■ DEPENDING UPON THE FUNCTION
  - ■ DEPENDING UPON THE LENGTH OF AXON
- ■ STRUCTURE
  - ■ NERVE CELL BODY
  - ■ DENDRITE
  - ■ AXON
  - ■ MYELIN SHEATH
  - ■ NEURILEMMA
- ■ NEUROTROPHINS – NEUROTROPHIC FACTORS
  - ■ NERVE GROWTH FACTOR
  - ■ OTHER NEUROTROPHINS

■ INTRODUCTION

Neuron or **nerve cell** is defined as the structural and functional unit of nervous system. Neuron is similar to any other cell in the body, having nucleus and all the organelles in cytoplasm. However, it is different from other cells by two ways:

1. Neuron has branches or processes called **axon** and **dendrites**
2. Neuron does not have centrosome. So, it cannot undergo division.

■ CLASSIFICATION OF NEURON

Neurons are classified by three different methods.
A. Depending upon the number of poles
B. Depending upon the function
C. Depending upon the length of axon.

■ DEPENDING UPON THE NUMBER OF POLES

Based on the number of poles from which the nerve fibers arise, neurons are divided into three types:

1. Unipolar neurons
2. Bipolar neurons
3. Multipolar neurons.

1. *Unipolar Neurons*

Unipolar neurons are the neurons that have only **one pole.** From a single pole, both axon and dendrite arise (Fig. 134.1). This type of nerve cells is present only in embryonic stage in human beings.

2. *Bipolar Neurons*

Neurons with **two poles** are known as bipolar neurons. Axon arises from one pole and dendrites arise from the other pole.

3. *Multipolar Neurons*

Multipolar neurons are the neurons which have **many poles.** One of the poles gives rise to axon and all other poles give rise to dendrites.

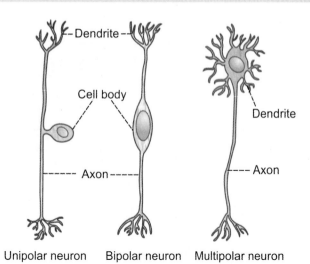

Unipolar neuron   Bipolar neuron   Multipolar neuron

FIGURE 134.1: Types of neuron

■ DEPENDING UPON THE FUNCTION

On the basis of function, nerve cells are classified into two types:
1. Motor or efferent neurons
2. Sensory or afferent neurons.

1. *Motor or Efferent Neurons*

Motor or efferent neurons are the neurons which carry the **motor impulses** from central nervous system to peripheral effector organs like muscles, glands, blood vessels, etc. Generally, each motor neuron has a long axon and short dendrites.

2. *Sensory or Afferent Neurons*

Sensory or afferent neurons are the neurons which carry the **sensory impulses** from periphery to central nervous system. Generally, each sensory neuron has a short axon and long dendrites.

■ DEPENDING UPON THE LENGTH OF AXON

Depending upon the length of axon, neurons are divided into two types:
1. Golgi type I neurons
2. Golgi type II neurons.

1. *Golgi Type I Neurons*

Golgi type I neurons have **long axons.** Cell body of these neurons is in different parts of central nervous system and their axons reach the remote peripheral organs.

2. *Golgi Type II Neurons*

Neurons of this type have **short axons.** These neurons are present in cerebral cortex and spinal cord.

■ STRUCTURE OF NEURON

Neuron is made up of three parts:
1. Nerve cell body
2. Dendrite
3. Axon.

Dendrite and axon form the **processes** of neuron (Fig. 134.2). Dendrites are **short processes** and the axons are **long processes**. Dendrites and axons are usually called **nerve fibers.**

■ NERVE CELL BODY

Nerve cell body is also known as **soma** or **perikaryon.** It is irregular in shape. Like any other cell, it is constituted by a mass of cytoplasm called neuroplasm, which is covered by a cell membrane. The cytoplasm contains a large nucleus, Nissl bodies, neurofibrils, mitochondria and Golgi apparatus. Nissl bodies and neurofibrils are found only in nerve cell and not in other cells.

Nucleus

Each neuron has one nucleus, which is centrally placed in the nerve cell body. Nucleus has one or two prominent nucleoli. Nucleus does not contain centrosome. So, the nerve cell cannot multiply like other cells.

Nissl Bodies

Nissl bodies or **Nissl granules** are small basophilic granules found in cytoplasm of neurons and are named after the discoverer. These bodies are present in soma and dendrite but not in axon and **axon hillock.** Nissl bodies are called **tigroid substances**, since these bodies are responsible for tigroid or spotted appearance of soma after suitable staining. Dendrites are distinguished from axons by the presence of Nissl granules under microscope.

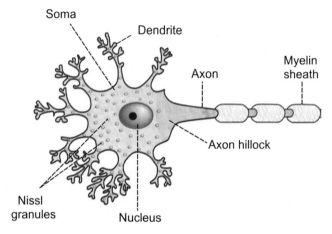

FIGURE 134.2: Structure of a neuron

Nissl bodies are membranous organelles containing ribosomes. So, these bodies are concerned with synthesis of proteins in the neurons. Proteins formed in soma are transported to the axon by axonal flow.

Number of Nissl bodies varies with the condition of the nerve. During fatigue or injury of the neuron, these bodies fragment and disappear by a process called **chromatolysis.** Granules reappear after recovery from fatigue or after regeneration of nerve fibers.

Neurofibrils

Neurofibrils are thread-like structures present in the form of network in the soma and the nerve processes. Presence of neurofibrils is another characteristic feature of the neurons. The neurofibrils consist of microfilaments and microtubules.

Mitochondria

Mitochondria are present in soma and in axon. As in other cells, here also mitochondria form the powerhouse of the nerve cell, where ATP is produced (Chapter 1).

Golgi Apparatus

Golgi apparatus of nerve cell body is similar to that of other cells. It is concerned with processing and packing of proteins into granules (Chapter 1).

■ DENDRITE

Dendrite is the **branched process** of neuron and it is branched repeatedly. Dendrite may be present or absent. If present, it may be one or many in number. Dendrite has Nissl granules and neurofibrils.

Dendrite transmits impulses towards the nerve cell body. Usually, the dendrite is shorter than axon.

■ AXON

Axon is the **longer process** of nerve cell. Each neuron has only one axon. Axon arises from axon hillock of the nerve cell body and it is devoid of Nissl granules. Axon extends for a long distance away from the nerve cell body. Length of longest axon is about 1 meter.

Axon transmits impulses away from the nerve cell body.

Organization of Nerve

Each nerve is formed by many bundles or groups of nerve fibers. Each bundle of nerve fibers is called a **fasciculus.**

Coverings of Nerve

The whole nerve is covered by tubular sheath, which is formed by a areolar membrane. This sheath is called **epineurium.** Each fasciculus is covered by **perineurium** and each nerve fiber (axon) is covered by **endoneurium** (Fig. 134.3).

Internal Structure of Axon – Axis Cylinder

Axon has a long central core of cytoplasm called **axoplasm.** Axoplasm is covered by the tubular sheath-like membrane called **axolemma.** Axolemma is the continuation of the cell membrane of nerve cell body. Axoplasm along with axolemma is called the **axis cylinder** of the nerve fiber (Fig. 134.4).

Axoplasm contains mitochondria, neurofibrils and axoplasmic vesicles. Because of the absence of Nissl bodies in the axon, proteins necessary for the nerve fibers are synthesized in the soma and not in axoplasm. After synthesis, the protein molecules are transported from soma to axon, by means of **axonal flow.** Some neurotransmitter substances are also transported by axonal flow from soma to axon.

Axis cylinder of the nerve fiber is covered by a membrane called **neurilemma** (see below).

Non-myelinated Nerve Fiber

Nerve fiber described above is the non-myelinated nerve fiber, which is not covered by myelin sheath.

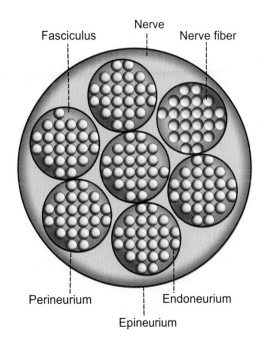

FIGURE 134.3: Cross section of a nerve

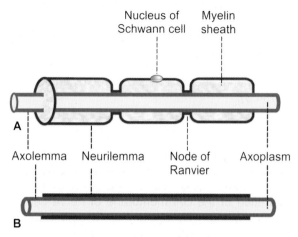

Nucleus of Schwann cell   Myelin sheath

A

Axolemma   Neurilemma   Node of Ranvier   Axoplasm

B

FIGURE 134.4: A. Myelinated nerve fiber;
B. Non-myelinated nerve fiber.

Myelinated Nerve Fiber

Nerve fiber which is insulated by myelin sheath is called myelinated nerve fibers.

■ MYELIN SHEATH

Myelin sheath is a thick lipoprotein sheath that insulates the myelinated nerve fiber. Myelin sheath is not a continuous sheath. It is absent at regular intervals. The area where myelin sheath is absent is called **node of Ranvier.** Segment of the nerve fiber between two nodes is called **internode.** Myelin sheath is responsible for white color of nerve fibers.

Chemistry of Myelin Sheath

Myelin sheath is formed by concentric layers of proteins, alternating with lipids. The lipids are cholesterol, lecithin and cerebroside (sphingomyelin).

Formation of Myelin Sheath – Myelinogenesis

Formation of myelin sheath around the axon is called the myelinogenesis. It is formed by **Schwann cells** in neurilemma. In the peripheral nerve, the myelinogenesis starts at 4th month of intrauterine life. It is completed only in the second year after birth.

Before myelinogenesis, Schwann cells of the neurilemma are very close to axolemma, as in the case of unmyelinated nerve fiber. The membrane of the Schwann cell is double layered.

Schwann cells wrap up and rotate around the axis cylinder in many concentric layers. The concentric layers fuse to produce myelin sheath but cytoplasm of the cells is not deposited. Outermost membrane of Schwann cell remains as neurilemma. Nucleus of these cells remains in between myelin sheath and neurilemma.

Functions of Myelin Sheath

1. *Faster conduction*

Myelin sheath is responsible for faster conduction of impulse through the nerve fibers. In myelinated nerve fibers, the impulses jump from one node to another node. This type of transmission of impulses is called **saltatory conduction** (Chapter 136).

2. *Insulating capacity*

Myelin sheath has a high insulating capacity. Because of this quality, myelin sheath restricts the nerve impulse within single nerve fiber and prevents the stimulation of neighboring nerve fibers.

■ NEURILEMMA

Neurilemma is a thin membrane, which surrounds the axis cylinder. It is also called **neurilemmal sheath** or **sheath of Schwann.** It contains Schwann cells, which have flattened and elongated nuclei. Cytoplasm is thin and modified to form the thin sheath of neurilemma.

One nucleus is present in each internode of the axon. Nucleus is situated between myelin sheath and neurilemma.

In non-myelinated nerve fiber, the neurilemma surrounds axolemma continuously. In myelinated nerve fiber, it covers the myelin sheath. At the node of Ranvier (where myelin sheath is absent), neurilemma invaginates and runs up to axolemma in the form of a finger-like process.

Functions of Neurilemma

In non-myelinated nerve fiber, the neurilemma serves as a covering membrane. In myelinated nerve fiber, it is necessary for the formation of myelin sheath (myelinogenesis). Neurilemma is absent in central nervous system. So, the neuroglial cells called **oligodendroglia** are responsible for myelinogenesis in central nervous system.

■ NEUROTROPHINS – NEUROTROPHIC FACTORS

Neurotrophins or neurotrophic factors are the protein substances, which play an important role in growth and functioning of nervous tissue.

Source of Secretion

Neurotrophins are secreted by many tissues in the body, particularly muscles, neuroglial cells called astrocytes and neurons.

Functions

Neurotrophins:
1. Facilitate initial growth and development of nerve cells in central and peripheral nervous system
2. Promote survival and repair of the nerve cells
3. Play an important role in the maintenance of nervous tissue and neural transmission.

Recently, it is found that neurotrophins are capable of making the damaged neurons regrow their processes *in vitro* and in animal models. This indicates the possibilities of reversing the devastating symptoms of nervous disorders like **Parkinson disease** and **Alzheimer disease.**

Commercial preparations of neurotrophins are used for the treatment of some neural diseases.

Mode of Action

Neurotrophins act via neurotrophin receptors, which are situated at the nerve terminals and nerve cell body. Neurotrophins bind with receptors and initiate the phosphorylation of tyrosine kinase.

Types

Nerve growth factor (NGF) was the first protein substance identified as neurotrophin. Now, many types of neurotophic factors are identified.

■ NERVE GROWTH FACTOR

Nerve growth factor (NGF) is a neurotrophin found in many peripheral tissues.

Chemistry

NGF is a peptide with 118 amino acids. Each molecule of NGF is made up of two α-subunits, two β-subunits and two γ-subunits. Only the β-subunits have nerve growth-stimulating activity.

Functions

1. NGF promotes early growth and development of neurons. Its major action is on sympathetic and sensory neurons, particularly the neurons concerned with pain. Because of its major action on sympathetic neurons, it is also called **sympathetic NGF.** NGF also promotes the growth of cholinergic neurons in cerebral hemispheres.
2. Commercial preparation of NGF extracted from snake venom and submaxillary glands of male mouse is used to treat sympathetic neuron diseases.

3. NGF plays an important role in treating many nervous disorders such as Alzheimer disease, neuron degeneration in aging and neuron regeneration in spinal cord injury.

■ OTHER NEUROTROPHINS

1. Brain-derived Neurotrophic Growth Factor

Brain-derived neurotrophic growth factor (BDGF) was first discovered in the brain of pig. Now it is found in human brain and human sperm. BDGF promotes the survival of sensory and motor neurons, arising from embryonic neural crest. It also protects the sensory neurons in peripheral nervous system and motor neurons of pyramidal system. It enhances the growth of cholinergic, dopaminergic and optic nerves. It is suggested that BDGF may regulate synaptic transmission.

Commercial preparation is used to treat **motor neuron diseases.**

2. Ciliary Neurotrophic Factor (CNTF)

CNTF is secreted in peripheral nerves, ocular muscles and cardiac muscle. It protects neurons of ciliary ganglion and motor neurons.

3. Glial Cell Line-derived Neurotrophic Factor (GNDF)

GDNF is found in neuroglial cells. It has a potent protective action on dopaminergic neurons. It is used for the treatment of **Parkinson disease.**

4. Fibroblast Growth Factor (FGF)

FGF was first discovered as growth factor promoting the fibroblastic growth. It is also known to protect the neurons.

5. Neurotrophin-3 (NT-3)

Neurotrophin-3 (NT-3) acts on γ-motor neurons, sympathetic neurons and neurons from sensory organs. It also regulates the release of neurotransmitter from neuromuscular junction.

NT-3 is useful for the treatment of motor axonal neuropathy and diabetic neuropathy.

Recently, few more substances belonging to the neurotrophin family such as NT-4, NT-5 and leukemia-inhibiting factor are identified. NT-4 and NT-5 act on sympathetic neurons, sensory neurons and motor neurons.

Classification of Nerve Fibers

> ■ BASIS OF CLASSIFICATION
> ■ DEPENDING UPON STRUCTURE
> ■ DEPENDING UPON DISTRIBUTION
> ■ DEPENDING UPON ORIGIN
> ■ DEPENDING UPON FUNCTION
> ■ DEPENDING UPON SECRETION OF NEUROTRANSMITTER
> ■ DEPENDING UPON DIAMETER AND CONDUCTION OF IMPULSE

■ BASIS OF CLASSIFICATION

Nerve fibers are classified by six different methods. The basis of classification differs in each method. Different methods of classification are listed in Box 135.1.

BOX 135.1: Different methods to classify nerve fibers

Classification of nerve fibers
1. Depending upon structure
2. Depending upon distribution
3. Depending upon origin
4. Depending upon function
5. Depending upon secretion of neurotransmitter
6. Depending upon diameter and conduction of impulse (Erlanger-Gasser classification)

■ 1. DEPENDING UPON STRUCTURE

Based on structure, nerve fibers are classified into two types:

i. *Myelinated Nerve Fibers*

Myelinated nerve fibers are the nerve fibers that are covered by **myelin sheath.**

ii. *Non-myelinated Nerve Fibers*

Non-myelinated nerve fibers are the nerve fibers which are not covered by myelin sheath.

■ 2. DEPENDING UPON DISTRIBUTION

Nerve fibers are classified into two types, on the basis of distribution:

i. *Somatic Nerve Fibers*

Somatic nerve fibers supply the **skeletal muscles** of the body.

ii. *Visceral or Autonomic Nerve Fibers*

Autonomic nerve fibers supply the various **internal organs** of the body.

■ 3. DEPENDING UPON ORIGIN

On the basis of origin, nerve fibers are divided into two types:

i. *Cranial Nerve Fibers*

Nerve fibers arising from **brain** are called cranial nerve fibers.

ii. *Spinal Nerve Fibers*

Nerve fibers arising from **spinal cord** are called spinal nerve fibers.

■ 4. DEPENDING UPON FUNCTION

Functionally, nerve fibers are classified into two types:

i. Sensory Nerve Fibers

Sensory nerve fibers carry sensory impulses from different parts of the body to the central nervous system. These nerve fibers are also known as **afferent nerve fibers.**

ii. Motor Nerve Fibers

Motor nerve fibers carry motor impulses from central nervous system to different parts of the body. These nerve fibers are also called **efferent nerve fibers.**

■ 5. DEPENDING UPON SECRETION OF NEUROTRANSMITTER

Depending upon the neurotransmitter substance secreted, nerve fibers are divided into two types:

i. Adrenergic Nerve Fibers

Adrenergic nerve fibers secrete **noradrenaline.**

ii. Cholinergic Nerve Fibers

Cholinergic nerve fibers secrete **acetylcholine.**

■ 6. DEPENDING UPON DIAMETER AND CONDUCTION OF IMPULSE (ERLANGER-GASSER CLASSIFICATION)

Erlanger and Gasser classified the nerve fibers into three major types, on the basis of **diameter** (thickness) of the fibers and velocity of **conduction of impulses:**

TABLE 135.1: Types of nerve fibers

Type	Diameter (μ)	Velocity of conduction (meter/second)
A alpha	12 to 24	70 to 120
A beta	6 to 12	30 to 70
A gamma	5 to 6	15 to 30
A delta	2 to 5	12 to 15
B	1 to 2	3 to 10
C	< 1.5	0.5 to 2

i. Type A nerve fibers
ii. Type B nerve fibers
iii. Type C nerve fibers.

Among these fibers, type A nerve fibers are the thickest fibers and type C nerve fibers are the thinnest fibers. Type C fibers are also known as Type IV fibers. Except type C fibers, all the nerve fibers are myelinated.

Type A nerve fibers are divided into four types:

a. Type A alpha or Type I nerve fibers
b. Type A beta or Type II nerve fibers
c. Type A gamma nerve fibers
d. Type A delta or Type III nerve fibers.

Velocity of Impulse

Velocity of impulse through a nerve fiber is directly proportional to the thickness of the fiber. Different types of nerve fibers along with diameter and velocity of conduction are given in Table 135.1.

Properties of Nerve Fibers

Chapter
136

+--+
| ■ **EXCITABILITY** |
| ■ **ACTION POTENTIAL OR NERVE IMPULSE** |
| ■ **ELECTROTONIC POTENTIAL OR LOCAL POTENTIAL** |
| ■ **VOLTAGE CLAMPING** |
| ■ **CONDUCTIVITY** |
| ■ **MECHANISM OF CONDUCTION OF ACTION POTENTIAL** |
| ■ **CONDUCTION THROUGH MYELINATED NERVE FIBER –** |
| **SALTATORY CONDUCTION** |
| ■ **REFRACTORY PERIOD** |
| ■ **TYPES OF REFRACTORY PERIOD** |
| ■ **SUMMATION** |
| ■ **ADAPTATION** |
| ■ **INFATIGABILITY** |
| ■ **ALL-OR-NONE LAW** |
+--+

■ EXCITABILITY

Excitability is defined as the **physiochemical change** that occurs in a tissue when stimulus is applied.

Stimulus is defined as an external agent, which produces excitability in the tissues. Different types of stimulus, qualities of stimulus and strength-duration curve are explained in Chapter 30. **Chronaxie** is an important parameter to determine the condition of nerve fiber. Clinically, the damage of nerve fiber is determined by measuring the chronaxie. It is measured by chronaxie meter.

Nerve fibers have a low threshold for excitation than the other cells.

Response Due to Stimulation of Nerve Fiber

When a nerve fiber is stimulated, based on the strength of stimulus, two types of response develop:

1. *Action potential or nerve impulse*

Action potential develops in a nerve fiber when it is stimulated by a stimulus with adequate strength. Adequate strength of stimulus, necessary for producing the

action potential in a nerve fiber is known as **threshold** or **minimal stimulus.** Action potential is propagated.

2. *Electrotonic potential or local potential*

When the stimulus with **subliminal strength** is applied, only electrotonic potential develops and the action potential does not develop. Electrotonic potential is non-propagated.

Cathelectrotonic and Anelectrotonic Potentials

While recording electrical potential in a nerve fiber, two electrodes, namely **cathode** and **anode** are used. The potential change that is produced at cathode is called cathelectrotonic potential. The potential that is developed at anode is known as anelectrotonic potential.

Only the cathelectrotonic potential can be transformed into electrotonic potential or action potential.

■ ACTION POTENTIAL OR NERVE IMPULSE

Action potential in a nerve fiber is similar to that in a muscle, except for some minor differences (Table 136.1). Action potential in a skeletal muscle fiber is described in Chapter 31.

TABLE 136.1: Differences between electrical potential in nerve fiber and muscle fiber

Event	Nerve fiber	Skeletal muscle fiber
Resting membrane potential	–70 mV	–90 mV
Firing level	–55 mV	–75 mV
End of depolarization	+35 mV	+55 mV

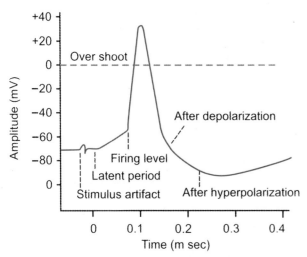

FIGURE 136.1: Action potential in nerve fiber

Resting membrane potential in the nerve fiber is –70 mV. The firing level is at –55 mV. Depolarization ends at +35 mV (Fig. 136.1). Usually, the action potential starts in the initial segment of nerve fiber.

Properties of Action Potential

Properties of action potential are given in Chapter 31.

■ ELECTROTONIC POTENTIAL OR LOCAL POTENTIAL

Electrotonic potential or local potential is a non-propagated **local response** that develops in the nerve fiber when a subliminal stimulus is applied. Subliminal or subthreshold stimulus does not produce action potential. But, it alters the resting membrane potential and produces **slight depolarization** for about 7 mV. This slight depolarized state is called electrotonic potential. Firing level is reached only if depolarization occurs up to 15 mV. Then only action potential can develop.

Electrotonic potential is a **graded potential** (Refer to Chapter 31).

Properties of Electrotonic Potential

1. Electrotonic potential is **non-propagated**
2. It does not obey **all-or-none law.** If the intensity of the stimulus is increased gradually every time, there is increase in the amplitude till the firing level is reached, i.e. at 15 mV.

■ VOLTAGE CLAMPING

The term 'voltage clamping' refers to an experimental method that uses electrodes to alter and control the membrane potential. Voltage clamp technique is a modified **patch clamp technique** (Chapter 31) applied to nerve fibers. It is used to measure the ionic current across the membrane of nerve fiber by fixing the membrane potential at a desired voltage.

Principle of Voltage Clamping

Normally, the voltage-gated ion channels open and close in response to positive or negative charge within the cell. In order to understand the movement of ions across the membrane (ion flux), it would be necessary to eliminate the other variable, i.e. the differences in the membrane potential. It is because of two reasons:

1. Both the ion flux and membrane potential are inter-related
2. Differences in membrane potential would lead to differences in ion flux.

So the membrane potential is fixed (clamped) at a specific level by using voltage clamp. It allows study of the ion flux through ionic channels at specific membrane potentials.

Equipment for Voltage Clamping

Voltage clamp equipment has three units:

1. Recording amplifier
2. Current generator
3. Feedback amplifier.

1. Recording amplifier measures the voltage of membrane potential. Two recording electrodes namely, the **extracelluar electrode** and **intracellular electrode** are connected to this amplifier. Extracellular electrode is placed on the outer surface of the nerve membrane and the intracellular electrode is inserted into the nerve fiber.

2. Current generator or **signal generator** is used to control the resting membrane potential of the nerve fiber. The current signals generated by this instrument are passed into the nerve fiber through a current electrode.

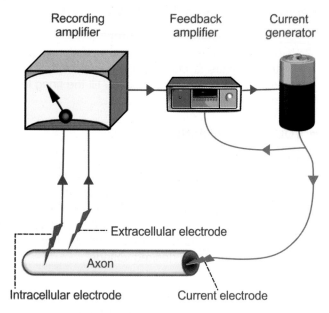

Recording amplifier   Feedback amplifier   Current generator

Extracellular electrode

Axon

Intracellular electrode   Current electrode

FIGURE 136.2: Voltage clamping

3. Feedback amplifier receives feedback inputs from recording amplifier and current generator and accordingly modifies the current signals that are sent into the nerve fiber (Fig. 136.2).

Thus, by voltage clamping, it is possible to maintain the constant membrane potential at a desired voltage.

Nerve Fibers Used for Voltage Clamping

Earlier, the voltage clamp tests were done on the giant axon of the squid *Loligo,* whose size facilitates such tests. Then the investigations were done on the neurons of small mammals. Nowadays, the tests are done on the human nerve fibers obtained from surgical procedures.

■ CONDUCTIVITY

Conductivity is the ability of nerve fibers to transmit the impulse from the area of stimulation to the other areas. Action potential is transmitted through the nerve fiber as nerve impulse. Normally in the body, the action potential is transmitted through the nerve fiber in only one direction. However, in experimental conditions when, the nerve is stimulated, the action potential travels through the nerve fiber in either direction.

■ MECHANISM OF CONDUCTION OF ACTION POTENTIAL

Depolarization occurs first at the site of stimulation in the nerve fiber. It causes depolarization of the neighboring

areas. Like this, depolarization travels throughout the nerve fiber. Depolarization is followed by repolarization.

■ CONDUCTION THROUGH MYELINATED NERVE FIBER – SALTATORY CONDUCTION

Saltatory conduction is the form of conduction of nerve impulse in which, the impulse jumps from **one node to another.** Conduction of impulse through a myelinated nerve fiber is about 50 times faster than through a non-myelinated fiber. It is because the action potential jumps from one node to another node of Ranvier instead of travelling through the entire nerve fiber (Fig. 136.3).

Mechanism of Saltatory Conduction

Myelin sheath is not permeable to ions. So, the entry of sodium from extracellular fluid into nerve fiber occurs only in the node of Ranvier, where the myelin sheath is absent. It causes depolarization in the node and not in the internode. Thus, depolarization occurs at successive

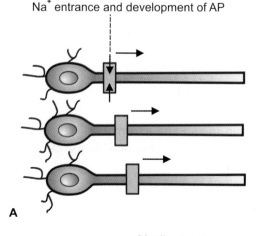

Na^+ entrance and development of AP

A

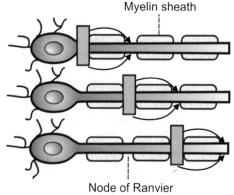

Myelin sheath

Node of Ranvier

B

FIGURE 136.3: Mode of conduction through nerve fibers A. Non-myelinated nerve fiber: continuous conduction. B. Myelinated nerve fiber: saltatory conduction (impulse jumps from node to node). AP = Action potential.

nodes. So, the action potential jumps from one node to another. Hence, it is called saltatory conduction (saltare = jumping).

■ REFRACTORY PERIOD

Refractory period is the period at which the nerve does not give any response to a stimulus.

■ TYPES OF REFRACTORY PERIOD

Refractory period is of two types:

1. *Absolute Refractory Period*

Absolute refractory period is the period during which the nerve does not show any response at all, whatever may be the strength of stimulus.

2. *Relative Refractory Period*

It is the period, during which the nerve fiber shows response, if the strength of stimulus is increased to maximum.

Absolute refractory period corresponds to the period from the time when firing level is reached till the time when one third of repolarization is completed. Relative refractory period extends through rest of the repolarization period.

■ SUMMATION

When one subliminal stimulus is applied, it does not produce any response in the nerve fiber because, the subliminal stimulus is very weak. However, if two or more subliminal stimuli are applied within a short interval of about 0.5 millisecond, the response is produced. It is because the subliminal stimuli are summed up together to become strong enough to produce the response. This phenomenon is known as summation.

■ ADAPTATION

While stimulating a nerve fiber continuously, the excitability of the nerve fiber is greater in the beginning. Later the response decreases slowly and finally the nerve fiber does not show any response at all. This phenomenon is known as adaptation or **accommodation.**

Cause for Adaptation

When a nerve fiber is stimulated continuously, depolarization occurs continuously. Continuous depolarization inactivates the sodium pump and increases the efflux of potassium ions.

■ INFATIGABILITY

Nerve fiber cannot be fatigued, even if it is stimulated continuously for a long time. The reason is that nerve fiber can conduct only one action potential at a time. At that time, it is completely refractory and does not conduct another action potential.

■ ALL-OR-NONE LAW

All-or-none law states that when a nerve is stimulated by a stimulus it gives maximum response or does not give response at all. Refer Chapter 90 for more details on all-or-none law.

Degeneration and Regeneration of Nerve Fibers

■ INTRODUCTION

When a nerve fiber is injured, various changes occur in the nerve fiber and nerve cell body. All these changes are together called the **degenerative changes.**

Causes for Injury

Injury to nerve fiber occurs due to following causes:
1. Obstruction of blood flow
2. Local injection of toxic substances
3. Crushing of nerve fiber
4. Transection of nerve fiber.

■ DEGREES OF INJURY

Sunderland had classified the injury to nerve fibers into five categories depending upon the order of severity.

■ FIRST DEGREE

First degree injury is the most common type of injury to the nerves. It is caused by **applying pressure** over a nerve for a short period leading to occlusion of blood flow and hypoxia.

By first degree of injury, axon is not destroyed but mild demyelination occurs. It is not a true degeneration. Axon looses the function temporarily for a short time, which is called conduction block. The function returns within few hours to few weeks. First degree of injury is called **Seddon neuropraxia.**

■ SECOND DEGREE

Second degree is due to the **prolonged severe pressure,** which causes **Wallerian degeneration** (see below). However, the endoneurium is intact. Repair and restoration of function take about 18 months. Second degree of injury is called **axonotmesis.**

■ THIRD DEGREE

In this case, the **endoneurium** is interrupted. Epineurium and perineurium are intact. After degeneration, the recovery is slow and poor or incomplete. Third, fourth and fifth degrees of injury are called **neurotmesis.**

■ FOURTH DEGREE

This type of injury is more severe. Epineurium and perineurium are also interrupted. Fasciculi of nerve fibers are disturbed and disorganized. Regeneration is poor or incomplete.

■ FIFTH DEGREE

Fifth degree of injury involves **complete transaction** of the nerve trunk with loss of continuity. Useful regeneration is not possible unless the cut ends are rearranged and approximated quickly by surgery.

■ DEGENERATIVE CHANGES IN THE NEURON

Degeneration refers to deterioration or impairment or pathological changes of an injured tissue. When a peripheral nerve fiber is injured, the degenerative changes occur in the nerve cell body and the nerve fiber of same neuron and the adjoining neuron.

Accordingly, degenerative changes are classified into three types:

1. Wallerian degeneration
2. Retrograde degeneration
3. Transneuronal degeneration.

■ WALLERIAN DEGENERATION OR ORTHOGRADE DEGENERATION

Wallerian degeneration is the pathological change that occurs in the distal cut end of nerve fiber (axon). It is named after the discoverer **Waller.** It is also called orthograde degeneration. Wallerian degeneration starts within 24 hours of injury. Change occurs throughout the length of distal part of nerve fiber simultaneously.

Changes in Nerve

i. Axis cylinder swells and breaks up into small pieces. After few days, the broken pieces appear as debris in the space occupied by axis cylinder (Fig. 137.1).
ii. Myelin sheath is slowly disintegrated into fat droplets. The changes in myelin sheath occur from 8th to 35th day.
iii. Neurilemmal sheath is unaffected, but the Schwann cells multiply rapidly. Macrophages invade from outside and remove the debris of axis cylinder and fat droplets of disintegrated myelin sheath. So, the neurilemmal tube becomes empty. Later it is filled by the cytoplasm of Schwann cell. All these

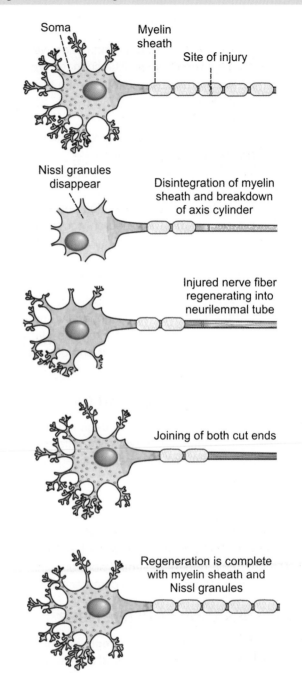

FIGURE 137.1: Degeneration and regeneration of nerve fiber

changes take place for about 2 months from the day of injury.

■ RETROGRADE DEGENERATION

Retrograde degeneration is the pathological changes, which occur in the nerve cell body and axon proximal to the cut end.

Changes in Nerve Cell Body

Changes in the nerve cell body commence within 48 hours after the section of nerve. The changes are:

i. First, the Nissl granules disintegrate into fragments by chromatolysis
ii. Golgi apparatus is disintegrated
iii. Nerve cell body swells due to accumulation of fluid and becomes round
iv. Neurofibrils disappear followed by displacement of the nucleus towards the periphery
v. Sometimes, the nucleus is extruded out of the cell. In this case, death of the neuron occurs and regeneration of the injured nerve is not possible.

Changes in Axon Proximal to Cut End

In the axon, changes occur only up to first node of Ranvier from the site of injury. Degenerative changes that occur in proximal cut end of axon are similar to those changes occurring in distal cut end of the nerve fiber.

■ TRANSNEURONAL DEGENERATION

If an afferent nerve fiber is cut, the degenerative changes occur in the neuron with which the afferent nerve fiber synapses. It is called transneuronal degeneration.

Examples:
i. Chromatolysis in the cells of lateral geniculate body occurs due to sectioning of optic nerve
ii. Degeneration of cells in dorsal horn of spinal cord occurs when the posterior nerve root is cut
iii. Degeneration of cells in ventral horn of spinal cord occurs when there is tumor in cerebral cortex.

■ REGENERATION OF NERVE FIBER

The term regeneration refers to **regrowth** of lost or destroyed part of a tissue. The injured and degenerated nerve fiber can regenerate. It starts as early as 4th day after injury, but becomes more effective only after 30 days and is completed in about 80 days.

■ CRITERIA FOR REGENERATION

Regeneration is possible only if certain criteria are fulfilled by the degenerated nerve fiber:

1. Gap between the cut ends of the nerve should not exceed 3 mm
2. Neurilemma should be present; as neurilemma is absent in CNS, the regeneration of nerve does not occur in CNS
3. Nucleus must be intact; if it is extruded from nerve cell body, the nerve is atrophied and the regeneration does not occur
4. Two cut ends should remain in the same line. Regeneration does not occur if any one end is moved away.

■ STAGES OF REGENERATION

1. First, some pseudopodia like extensions grow from the proximal cut end of the nerve. These extensions are called **fibrils** or **regenerative sprouts.** The number of fibrils is up to 100.
2. Fibrils move towards the distal cut end of the nerve fiber
3. Some of the fibrils enter the **neurilemmal tube** of distal end and form axis cylinder
4. Schwann cells line up in the neurilemmal tube and actually guide the fibrils into the tube. Schwann cells also synthesize nerve growth factors, which attract the fibrils form proximal segment.
5. Axis cylinder is fully established inside the neurilemmal tube. These processes are completed in about 3 months after injury.
6. Myelin sheath is formed by Schwann cells slowly. Myelination is completed in 1 year.
7. Diameter of the nerve fiber gradually increases. However, the degenerated nerve fiber obtains only 80% of original diameter. Newly formed internodes are also shorter than the original ones.
8. In the nerve cell body, first the Nissl granules appear followed by Golgi apparatus
9. Cell looses the excess fluid; nucleus occupies the central portion
10. Though anatomical regeneration occurs in the nerve, functional recovery occurs after a long period.

Neuroglia

- ■ DEFINITION
- ■ CLASSIFICATION
- ■ CENTRAL NEUROGLIAL CELLS
  - ■ ASTROCYTES
  - ■ MICROGLIA
  - ■ OLIGODENDROCYTES
- ■ PERIPHERAL NEUROGLIAL CELLS
  - ■ SCHWANN CELLS
  - ■ SATELLITE CELLS

■ DEFINITION

Neuroglia or glia (glia = glue) is the **supporting cell** of the nervous system. Neuroglial cells are **non-excitable** and do not transmit nerve impulse (action potential). So, these cells are also called **non-neural cells** or **glial cells.** When compared to the number of neurons, the number of glial cells is 10 to 15 times greater. Neuroglial cells play an important role in the reaction of nerve during infection. Most commonly, neuroglial cells constitute the site of **tumors** in nervous system.

■ CLASSIFICATION OF NEUROGLIAL CELLS

Neuroglial cells are distributed in central nervous system (CNS) as well as peripheral nervous system (PNS). Accordingly the neuroglial cells are classified into two types:

A. Central neuroglial cells
B. Peripheral neuroglial cells.

■ CENTRAL NEUROGLIAL CELLS

Neuroglial cells in CNS are of three types:
1. Astrocytes

2. Microglia
3. Oligodendrocytes.

■ ASTROCYTES

Astrocytes are star-shaped neuroglial cells present in all the parts of the brain (Fig. 138.1). Two types of astrocytes are found in human brain:
   i. Fibrous astrocytes
   ii. Protoplasmic astrocytes.

Fibrous Astrocytes

Fibrous astrocytes occupy mainly the white matter. Few fibrous astrocytes are seen in gray matter also. The processes of these cells cover the nerve cells and synapses. This type of astrocytes play an important role in the formation of **blood-brain barrier** by sending processes to the blood vessels of brain, particularly the capillaries, forming tight junction with capillary membrane. **Tight junction** in turn forms the blood-brain barrier.

Protoplasmic Astrocytes

Protoplasmic astrocytes are present mainly in gray matter. The processes of neuroglia run between nerve cell bodies.

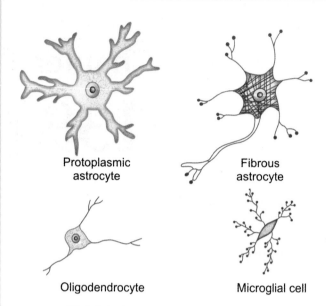

Protoplasmic astrocyte

Fibrous astrocyte

Oligodendrocyte

Microglial cell

FIGURE 138.1: Neuroglial cells in CNS

Functions of Astrocytes

Astrocytes:

  i. Twist around the nerve cells and form the **supporting network** in brain and spinal cord
  ii. Form the **blood-brain barrier** and thereby regulate the entry of substances from blood into brain tissues (Chapter 163)
  iii. Maintain the **chemical environment** of ECF around CNS neurons
  iv. Provide calcium and potassium and regulate neurotransmitter level in synapses
  v. Regulate **recycling of neurotransmitter** during synaptic transmission.

■ MICROGLIA

Microglia are the smallest neuroglial cells. These cells are derived from monocytes and enter the tissues of nervous system from blood. These **phagocytic cells** migrate to the site of infection or injury and are often called the **macrophages of CNS.**

Functions of Microglia

Microglia:

  i. Engulf and destroy the microorganisms and cellular debris by means of **phagocytosis**

  ii. Migrate to the injured or infected area of CNS and act as miniature macrophages.

■ OLIGODENDROCYTES

Oligodendrocytes are the neuroglial cells, which produce myelin sheath around the nerve fibers in CNS. Oligodentrocytes are also called **oligodendroglia.** Oligodendrocytes have only few processes, which are short.

Functions of Oligodendrocytes

Oligodendrocytes:

  i. **Provide myelination** around the nerve fibers in CNS where Schwann cells are absent
  ii. **Provide support** to the CNS neurons by forming a semi-stiff connective tissue between the neurons.

■ PERIPHERAL NEUROGLIAL CELLS

Neuroglial cells in PNS are of two types:
  1. Schwann cells
  2. Satellite cells.

■ SCHWANN CELLS

Schwann cells are the major glial cells in PNS (Refer to Chapter 134).

Functions of Schwann Cells

Schwann cells:

  i. **Provide myelination** (insulation) around the nerve fibers in PNS
  ii. Play important role in **nerve regeneration** (Chapter 137)
  iii. Remove cellular debris during regeneration by their phagocytic activity.

■ SATELLITE CELLS

Satellite cells are the glial cells present on the exterior surface of PNS neurons.

Functions of Satellite Cells

Satellite cells:

  i. Provide **physical support** to the PNS neurons
  ii. Help in regulation of chemical environment of ECF around the PNS neurons.

Receptors

- ■ **DEFINITION**
- ■ **CLASSIFICATION**
  - ■ **EXTEROCEPTORS**
  - ■ **INTEROCEPTORS**
- ■ **PROPERTIES**
  - ■ **SPECIFICITY OF RESPONSE**
  - ■ **ADAPTATION – SENSORY ADAPTATION**
  - ■ **RESPONSE TO INCREASE IN THE STRENGTH OF STIMULUS**
  - ■ **SENSORY TRANSDUCTION**
  - ■ **RECEPTOR POTENTIAL**
  - ■ **LAW OF PROJECTION**

■ DEFINITION

Receptors are sensory (afferent) nerve endings that terminate in periphery as bare **unmyelinated endings** or in the form of specialized **capsulated structures**. Receptors give response to the stimulus. When stimulated, receptors produce a series of impulses, which are transmitted through the afferent nerves.

Biological Transducers

Actually receptors function like a transducer. Transducer is a device, which converts one form of energy into another. So, receptors are often defined as the biological transducers, which convert (transducer) various forms of **energy** (stimuli) in the environment into **action potentials** in nerve fiber.

■ CLASSIFICATION OF RECEPTORS

Generally, receptors are classified into two types:
A. Exteroceptors
B. Interoceptors.

■ EXTEROCEPTORS

Exteroceptors are the receptors, which give response to stimuli arising from **outside the body.**

Exteroceptors are divided into three groups:

1. Cutaneous Receptors or Mechanoreceptors

Receptors situated in the skin are called the cutaneous receptors. Cutaneous receptors are also called mechanoreceptors because of their response to **mechanical stimuli** such as touch, pressure and pain. Touch and pressure receptors give response to **vibration** also. Different types of cutaneous receptors are given in Figure 139.1.

2. Chemoreceptors

Receptors, which give response to **chemical stimuli,** are called the chemoreceptors.

3. Telereceptors

Telereceptors are the receptors that give response to stimuli arising **away from the body.** These receptors are also called the **distance receptors** (Fig. 139.2).

■ INTEROCEPTORS

Interoceptors are the receptors, which give response to stimuli arising from **within the body.**

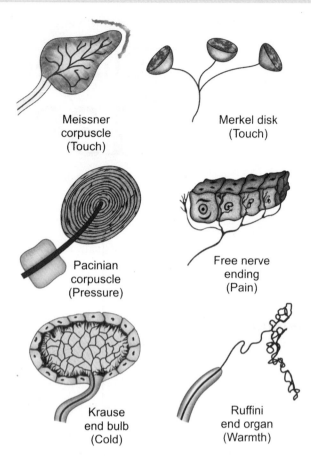

FIGURE 139.1: Cutaneous receptors

Interoceptors are of two types which are as follows:

1. *Visceroceptors*

Receptors situated in the viscera are called visceroceptors. Different visceroceptors are listed in Figure 139.3.

2. *Proprioceptors*

Proprioceptors are the receptors, which give response to **change in the position** of different parts of the body. Proprioceptors are explained in Chapter 156.

■ PROPERTIES OF RECEPTORS

■ 1. SPECIFICITY OF RESPONSE – MÜLLER LAW

Specificity of response or Müller law refers to the response given by a particular type of receptor to a specific sensation. For example, pain receptors give response only to pain sensation. Similarly, temperature receptors give response only to temperature sensation. In addition, each type of sensation depends upon the part of the brain in which its fibers terminate.

Specificity of response is also called **Müller's doctrine** of specific nerve energies.

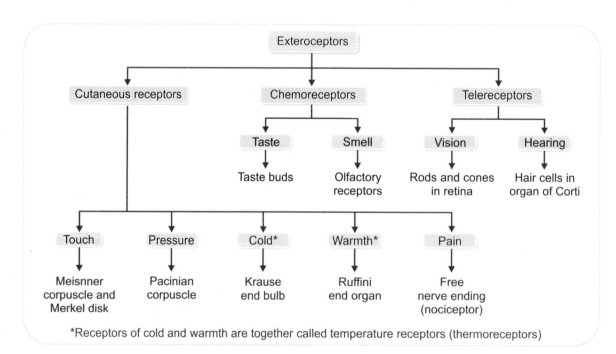

*Receptors of cold and warmth are together called temperature receptors (thermoreceptors)

FIGURE 139.2: Exteroceptors

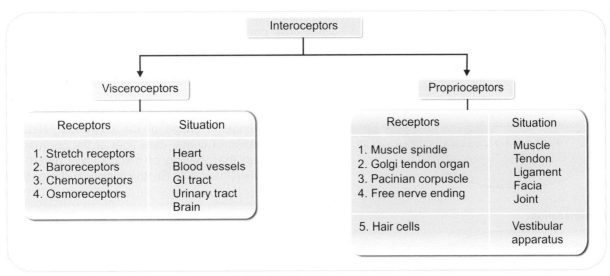

FIGURE 139.3: Interoceptors

■ 2. ADAPTATION – SENSORY ADAPTATION

Adaptation is the decline in discharge of sensory impulses when a receptor is stimulated continuously with constant strength. It is also called sensory adaptation or desensitization.

Depending upon adaptation time, receptors are divided into two types:

  i. **Phasic receptors,** which get adapted rapidly. Touch and pressure receptors are the phasic receptors

  ii. **Tonic receptors,** which adapt slowly. Muscle spindle, pain receptors and cold receptors are the tonic receptors.

■ 3. RESPONSE TO INCREASE IN STRENGTH OF STIMULUS – WEBER-FECHNER LAW

During the stimulation of a receptor, if the response given by the receptor is to be doubled, the strength of stimulus must be increased 100 times. This phenomenon is called Weber-Fechner law, which states that intensity of response (sensation) of a receptor is directly proportional to logarithmic increase in the intensity of stimulus.

Derivation of Weber-Fechner Law

Weber-Fechner law is derived as follows:

$$R = k \log S$$

Where,

  R = Intensity of response (sensation)
  k = Constant
  S = Intensity of stimulus

■ 4. SENSORY TRANSDUCTION

Sensory transduction in a receptor is a process by which the energy (stimulus) in the environment is converted into electrical impulses (action potentials) in nerve fiber (transduction = conversion of one form of energy into another).

When a receptor is stimulated, it gives response by sending information about the stimulus to CNS. Series of events occur to carry out this function such as the development of receptor potential in the receptor cell and development of action potential in the sensory nerve.

Sensory transduction varies depending upon the type of receptor. For example, the chemoreceptor converts chemical energy into action potential in the sensory nerve fiber. Touch receptor converts mechanical energy into action potential in the sensory nerve fiber.

■ 5. RECEPTOR POTENTIAL

Definition

Receptor potential is a **non-propagated** transmembrane potential difference that develops when a receptor is stimulated. It is also called **generator potential.** Receptor potential is short lived and hence, it is called **transient receptor potential.**

Receptor potential is not action potential. It is a graded potential (Chapter 31). It is similar to excitatory postsynaptic potential (EPSP) in synapse, endplate potential in neuromuscular junction and electrotonic potential in the nerve fiber.

Before stimulation

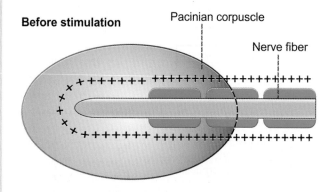

Pacinian corpuscle

Nerve fiber

After stimulation

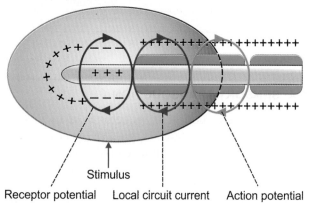

Stimulus

Receptor potential   Local circuit current   Action potential

FIGURE 139.4: Receptor potential in pacinian corpuscle. Receptor potential leads to development of local circuit which spreads up to first node within the capsule. It leads to development of action potential in the first node of nerve fiber.

Properties of Receptor Potential

Receptor potential has two important properties.
  i. Receptor potential is **non-propagated;** it is confined within the receptor itself
  ii. It does not obey **all-or-none law.**

Significance of Receptor Potential

When receptor potential is sufficiently strong (when the magnitude is about 10 mV), it causes development of action potential in the sensory nerve.

Mechanism of Development of Receptor Potential

Pacinian corpuscles are generally used to study the receptor potential because of their large size and anatomical configuration. These corpuscles can be easily dissected from the mesentery of experimental animals. In the pacinian corpuscle, the tip of the nerve fiber is unmyelinated. This unmyelinated nerve tip

extends through the corpuscle as **center core fiber.** The concentric layers of the corpuscle surround the core fiber of the nerve.

Pacinian corpuscles give response to pressure stimulus. When pressure stimulus is applied, the Pacinian corpuscle is compressed. This compression causes elongation or change in shape of the corpuscle. The change in shape of the corpuscle leads to the deformation of center core fiber of the corpuscle. This results in the opening of mechanically gated **sodium channels** (Chapter 3). So, the positively charged sodium

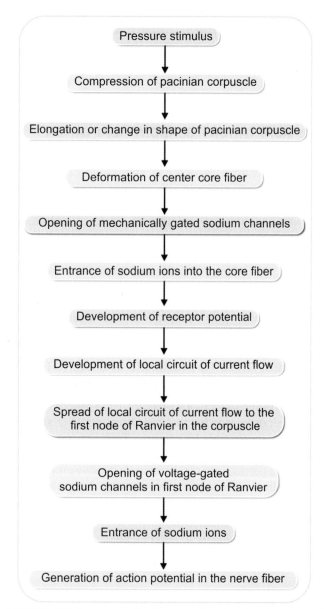

FIGURE 139.5: Schematic diagram showing development of receptor potential and generation of action potential in nerve fiber.

ions enter the interior of core fiber. This produces a **mild depolarization,** i.e. receptor potential (Fig. 139.4).

Generation of Action Potential in the Nerve Fiber

Receptor potential causes development of a **local circuit** of current flow, which spreads along the unmyelinated part of nerve fiber within the corpuscle.

When this local circuit of current reaches the first node of Ranvier within the corpuscle, it causes opening of voltage-gated sodium channels and entrance of sodium ions into the nerve fiber. This leads to the development of action potential in the nerve fiber (Fig. 139.5).

■ 6. LAW OF PROJECTION

When a sensory pathway from receptor to cerebral cortex is stimulated on any particular site along its course, the sensation caused by stimulus is always felt (referred) at the location of receptor, irrespective of site stimulated. This phenomenon is known as law of projection.

Examples of Law of Projection

i. If somesthetic area in right cerebral cortex, which receives sensation from left hand is stimulated, sensations are felt in left hand and not in head.

ii. Sensation complained by amputated patients in the missing limb **(phantom limb)** is the best example of law of projection. For example, if a leg has been amputated, the cut end heals with scar formation. The cut ends of nerve fibers are merged within the scar. If the cut end of sensory fibers are stimulated during movement of thigh, the patient feels as if the sensation is originating from **non-existent leg.** Sometimes, the patient feels pain in non-existent limb. This type of pain is called **phantom limb pain.**

Synapse

- ■ **DEFINITION**
- ■ **CLASSIFICATION**
  - ■ ANATOMICAL CLASSIFICATION
  - ■ FUNCTIONAL CLASSIFICATION
- ■ **FUNCTIONAL ANATOMY**
- ■ **FUNCTIONS**
  - ■ EXCITATORY FUNCTION
  - ■ INHIBITORY FUNCTION
- ■ **PROPERTIES**
  - ■ ONE WAY CONDUCTION – BELL-MAGENDIE LAW
  - ■ SYNAPTIC DELAY
  - ■ FATIGUE
  - ■ SUMMATION
  - ■ ELECTRICAL PROPERTY
- ■ **CONVERGENCE AND DIVERGENCE**
  - ■ CONVERGENCE
  - ■ DIVERGENCE

■ DEFINITION

Synapse is the junction between two neurons. It is not an anatomical continuation. But, it is only a physiological continuity between two nerve cells.

■ CLASSIFICATION OF SYNAPSE

Synapse is classified by two methods:
- A. Anatomical classification
- B. Functional classification.

■ ANATOMICAL CLASSIFICATION

Usually synapse is formed by axon of one neuron ending on the cell body, dendrite or axon of the next neuron. Depending upon **ending of axon,** synapse is classified into three types:
1. **Axoaxonic synapse** in which axon of one neuron terminates on axon of another neuron

2. **Axodendritic synapse** in which the axon of one neuron terminates on dendrite of another neuron
3. **Axosomatic synapse** in which axon of one neuron ends on soma (cell body) of another neuron (Fig. 140.1).

■ FUNCTIONAL CLASSIFICATION

Functional classification of synapse is on the basis of **mode of impulse transmission.** According to this, synapse is classified into two categories:
1. Electrical synapse
2. Chemical synapse.

However, generally the word synapse refers to a chemical synapse.

1. Electrical Synapse

Electrical synapse is the synapse in which the physiological continuity between the presynaptic and the post-

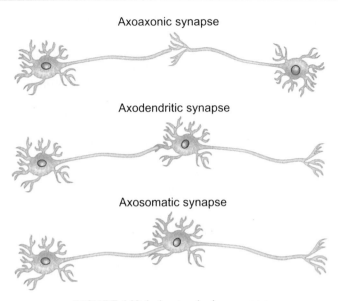

FIGURE 140.1: Anatomical synapses

Axoaxonic synapse

Axodendritic synapse

Axosomatic synapse

synaptic neurons is provided by **gap junction** between the two neurons (Fig. 140.2). There is **direct exchange** of ions between the two neurons through the gap junction. Because of this reason, the action potential reaching the terminal portion of presynaptic neuron directly enters the postsynaptic neuron.

Important feature of electrical synapse is that the synaptic delay is very less because of the direct flow of current. Moreover, the impulse is transmitted in either direction through the electrical synapse.

This type of impulse transmission occurs in some tissues like the cardiac muscle fibers, smooth muscle fibers of intestine and the epithelial cells of lens in the eye.

2. Chemical Synapse

Chemical synapse is the junction between a nerve fiber and a muscle fiber or between two nerve fibers, through which the signals are transmitted by the release of chemical transmitter. In the chemical synapse, there is no continuity between the two neurons because of the presence of a space called **synaptic cleft** between the two neurons. Action potential reaching the presynaptic terminal causes release of neurotransmitter substance from the vesicles of this terminal. Neurotransmitter reaches the postsynaptic neuron through synaptic cleft and causes the production of potential change. Structure and functions of the chemical synapse are given here.

■ FUNCTIONAL ANATOMY OF CHEMICAL SYNAPSE

Functional anatomy of a chemical synapse is shown in Figure 140.3. Neuron from which the axon arises is called the **presynaptic neuron** and the neuron on which the axon ends is called **postsynaptic neuron.** Axon of the presynaptic neuron divides into many small branches before forming the synapse. These branches are known as presynaptic **axon terminals.**

Types of Axon Terminals

1. Terminal knobs

Some of the terminals are enlarged slightly like knobs called **terminal knobs.** Terminal knobs are concerned with excitatory function of the synapse.

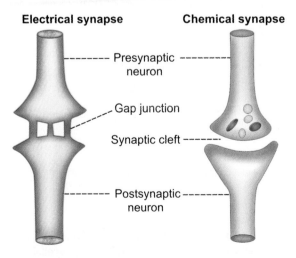

FIGURE 140.2: Electrical and chemical synapse

Electrical synapse   Chemical synapse

Presynaptic neuron
Gap junction
Synaptic cleft
Postsynaptic neuron

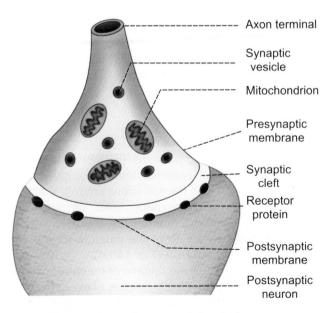

FIGURE 140.3: Structure of chemical synapse

Axon terminal
Synaptic vesicle
Mitochondrion
Presynaptic membrane
Synaptic cleft
Receptor protein
Postsynaptic membrane
Postsynaptic neuron

2. Terminal coils or free endings

Other terminals are wavy or coiled with free ending without the knob. These terminals are concerned with inhibitory function.

Structures of Axon Terminals and Presynaptic Membrane

Presynaptic axon terminal has a definite intact membrane known as **presynaptic membrane.**

Axon terminal has two important structures:

i. **Mitochondria,** which help in the synthesis of neurotransmitter substance
ii. **Synaptic vesicles,** which store neurotransmitter substance.

Synaptic Cleft and Postsynaptic Membrane

Membrane of the postsynaptic neuron is called **postsynaptic membrane.** It contains some **receptor proteins.** Small space in between the presynaptic membrane and the postsynaptic membrane is called **synaptic cleft.** The **basal lamina** of this cleft contains **cholinesterase,** which destroys **acetylcholine.**

■ FUNCTIONS OF SYNAPSE

Main function of the synapse is to transmit the impulses, i.e. action potential from one neuron to another. However, some of the synapses inhibit these impulses. So the impulses are not transmitted to the postsynaptic neuron.

On the basis of functions, synapses are divided into two types:

1. Excitatory synapses, which transmit the impulses (excitatory function)
2. Inhibitory synapses, which inhibit the transmission of impulses (inhibitory function).

■ EXCITATORY FUNCTION

Excitatory Postsynaptic Potential

Excitatory postsynaptic potential (EPSP) is the non-propagated electrical potential that develops during the process of synaptic transmission. When the action potential reaches the presynaptic axon terminal, the voltage-gated **calcium channels** at the presynaptic membrane are opened. Now, the **calcium ions** enter the axon terminal from ECF (Fig. 140.4).

Calcium ions cause the release of neurotransmitter substance from the vesicles by means of **exocytosis.**

Neurotransmitter, which is excitatory in function (excitatory neurotransmitter) passes through presy-

naptic membrane and synaptic cleft and reaches the postsynaptic membrane. Now, the neurotransmitter binds with receptor protein present in postsynaptic membrane to form neurotransmitter-receptor complex. Neurotransmitter-receptor complex causes production of a non-propagated EPSP. Common excitatory neurotransmitter in a synapse is **acetylcholine.**

Mechanism of Development of EPSP

Neurotransmitter-receptor complex causes opening of ligand-gated **sodium channels.** Now, the **sodium ions**

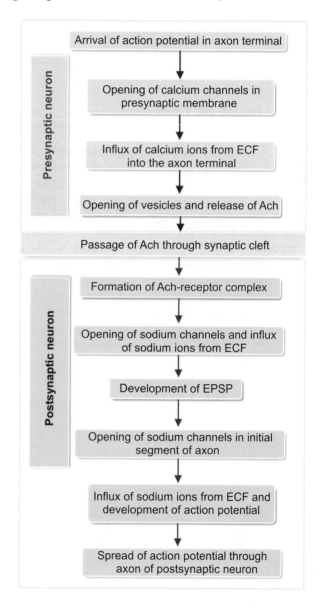

FIGURE 140.4: Sequence of events during synaptic transmission. Ach = Acetylcholine, ECF = Extracellular fluid, EPSP = Excitatory postsynaptic potential.

from ECF enter the cell body of postsynaptic neuron. As the sodium ions are positively charged, resting membrane potential inside the cell body is altered and **mild depolarization** develops. This type of mild depolarization is called EPSP. It is a **local potential** (response) in the synapse.

Properties of EPSP

EPSP is confined only to the synapse. It is a **graded potential** (Chapter 31). It is similar to receptor potential and endplate potential.

EPSP has two properties:
1. It is non-propagated
2. It does not obey all-or-none law.

Significance of EPSP

EPSP is not transmitted into the axon of postsynaptic neuron. However, it causes development of action potential in the axon.

When EPSP is strong enough, it causes the opening of voltage-gated **sodium channels** in the initial segment of axon. Now, due to the entrance of **sodium ions,** the depolarization occurs in the initial segment of axon and thus, the action potential develops. From here, the action potential spreads to other segment of the axon.

■ INHIBITORY FUNCTION

Inhibition of synaptic transmission is classified into five types:
1. Postsynaptic or direct inhibition
2. Presynaptic or indirect inhibition
3. Negative feedback or Renshaw cell inhibition
4. Feedforward inhibition
5. Reciprocal inhibition.

1. Postsynaptic or Direct Inhibition

Postsynaptic inhibition is the type of synaptic inhibition that occurs due to the release of an inhibitory neuro-transmitter from presynaptic terminal instead of an excitatory neurotransmitter substance. It is also called **direct inhibition.** Inhibitory neurotransmitters are gamma-aminobutyric acid **(GABA)**, dopamine and glycine.

Action of GABA – development of inhibitory postsynaptic potential

Inhibitory postsynaptic potential (IPSP) is the electrical potential in the form of **hyperpolarization** that develops during postsynaptic inhibition. Inhibitory neurotransmitter substance acts on postsynaptic membrane by binding with receptor. Transmitter-receptor complex opens the ligand-gated **potassium channels** instead of sodium

channels. Now, the **potassium ions,** which are available in plenty in the cell body of postsynaptic neuron move to ECF. Simultaneously, **chloride channels** also open and chloride ions (which are more in ECF) move inside the cell body of postsynaptic neuron. The exit of potassium ions and influx of chloride ions cause **more negativity** inside, leading to **hyperpolarization.** Hyperpolarized state of the synapse inhibits synaptic transmission (Fig. 140.5).

2. Presynaptic or Indirect Inhibition

Presynaptic inhibition occurs due to the failure of presynaptic axon terminal to release sufficient quantity of excitatory neurotransmitter substance. It is also called indirect inhibition.

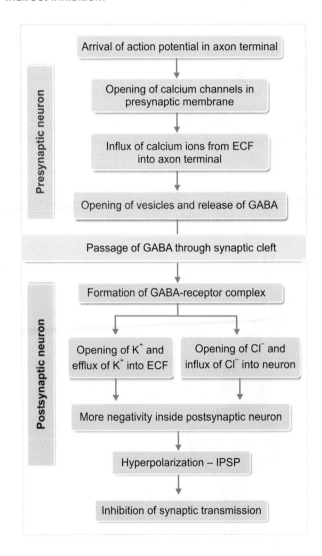

FIGURE 140.5: Sequence of events during postsynaptic inhibition. GABA = Gamma-aminobutyric acid, ECF = Extracellular fluid, IPSP = Inhibitory postsynaptic potential.

Presynaptic inhibition is mediated by axoaxonal synapses. It is prominent in **spinal cord** and regulates the propagation of information to higher centers in brain.

Normally, during synaptic transmission, action potential reaching the presynaptic neuron produces development of EPSP in the postsynaptic neuron. But, in spinal cord, a **modulatory neuron** called **presynaptic inhibitory neuron** forms an axoaxonic synapse with the presynaptic neuron (Fig. 140.6).

This inhibitory neuron inhibits the presynaptic neuron and decreases the magnitude of action potential in presynaptic neuron. The **smaller action potential** reduces **calcium influx.** This in turn decreases the quantity of neurotransmitter released by presynaptic neuron. So the magnitude of EPSP in postsynaptic neuron is decreased resulting in synaptic inhibition.

3. Renshaw Cell or Negative Feedback Inhibition

Negative feedback inhibition is the type of synaptic inhibition, which is caused by Renshaw cells in **spinal cord.** Renshaw cells are small motor neurons present in anterior gray horn of spinal cord (Chapter 143). Anterior nerve root consists of nerve fibers, which leave the spinal cord. These nerve fibers arise from α-motor neurons in anterior gray horn of the spinal cord and reach the effector organ, muscles. Some of the fibers called collaterals fibers terminate on Renshaw cells instead of leaving the spinal cord.

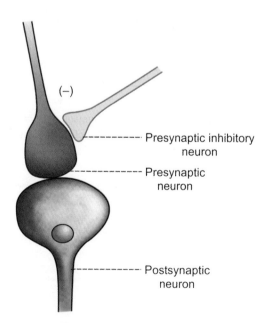

FIGURE 140.6: Presynaptic inhibition

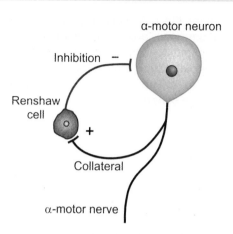

FIGURE 140.7: Renshaw cell inhibition

When motor neurons send motor impulses, some of the impulses reach the Renshaw cell by passing through **collaterals.** Now, the Renshaw cell is stimulated. In turn, it sends inhibitory impulses to α-motor neurons so that, the discharge from motor neurons is reduced (Fig. 140.7).

In this way, Renshaw cell inhibition represents a **negative feedback mechanism.** A Renshaw cell may be supplied by more than one alpha motor neuron collateral and it may synapse on many motor neurons.

4. Feedforward Inhibition

Feedforward synaptic inhibition occurs in **cerebellum** and it controls the **neuronal activity** in cerebellum.

During the process of neuronal activity in cerebellum, stellate cells and basket cells, which are activated by granule cells, inhibit the **Purkinje cells** by releasing **GABA** (Chapter 150). This type of inhibition is called feedforward inhibition.

5. Reciprocal Inhibition

Inhibition of antagonistic muscles when a group of muscles are activated is called reciprocal inhibition. It is because of **reciprocal innervation** (Chapter 142).

Significance of Synaptic Inhibition

Synaptic inhibition in CNS limits the number of impulses going to muscles and enables the muscles to act properly and appropriately. Thus, the inhibition helps to select exact number of impulses and to omit or block the excess ones. When a poison like **strychnine** is introduced into the body, it destroys the inhibitory function at synaptic level resulting in continuous and convulsive contraction even with slight stimulation. In the nervous disorders like **parkinsonism,** the inhibitory system is impaired resulting in rigidity.

■ PROPERTIES OF SYNAPSE

■ 1. ONE WAY CONDUCTION – BELL-MAGENDIE LAW

According to Bell-Magendie law, the impulses are transmitted only in **one direction** in synapse, i.e. from presynaptic neuron to postsynaptic neuron.

■ 2. SYNAPTIC DELAY

Synaptic delay is a short delay that occurs during the transmission of impulses through the synapse. It is due to the time taken for:

   i. Release of neurotransmitter
   ii. Passage of neurotransmitter from axon terminal to postsynaptic membrane
   iii. Action of the neurotransmitter to open the ionic channels in postsynaptic membrane.

Normal duration of synaptic delay is 0.3 to 0.5 millisecond. Synaptic delay is one of the causes for **reaction time** of reflex activity.

Significance of Determining Synaptic Delay

Determination of synaptic delay helps to find out whether the pathway for a reflex is monosynapatic or polysynaptic.

■ 3. FATIGUE

During continuous muscular activity, synapse becomes the seat of fatigue along with **Betz cells** present in motor area of frontal lobe of cerebral cortex (Refer Chapter 30 for details of fatigue). Fatigue at synapse is due to the **depletion of neurotransmitter** substance, acetylcholine.

Depletion of acetylcholine occurs because of two factors:

   i. Soon after the action, acetylcholine is destroyed by acetylcholinesterase
   ii. Due to continuous action, new acetylcholine is not synthesized.

■ 4. SUMMATION

Summation is the fusion of effects or progressive increase in the excitatory postsynaptic potential in postsynaptic neuron when many presynaptic excitatory terminals are stimulated simultaneously or when single presynaptic terminal is stimulated repeatedly. Increased EPSP triggers the axon potential in the initial segment of axon of postsynaptic neuron (Fig.140.8).

Summation is of two types:

i. Spatial Summation

Spatial summation occurs when many presynaptic terminals are stimulated simultaneously.

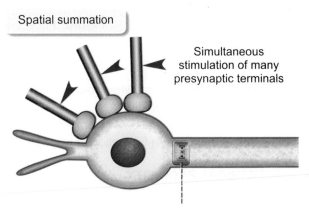

Spatial summation

Simultaneous stimulation of many presynaptic terminals

Action potential in initial segment of postsynaptic neuron

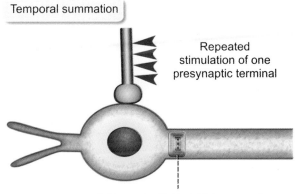

Temporal summation

Repeated stimulation of one presynaptic terminal

Action potential in initial segment of postsynaptic neuron

FIGURE 140.8: Spatial and temporal summation

Convergence   **Divergence**

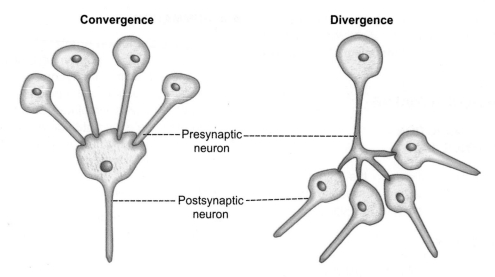

- - - - - - Presynaptic - - - - - - - -
            neuron

- - - - - - - - - - Postsynaptic - - - - - - - -
                    neuron

FIGURE 140.9: Convergence and divergence

ii. *Temporal Summation*

Temporal summation occurs when one presynaptic terminal is stimulated repeatedly.

Thus, both spatial summation and temporal summation play an important role in facilitation of response.

■ 5. ELECTRICAL PROPERTY

Electrical properties of the synapse are the EPSP and IPSP, which are already described in this chapter.

■ CONVERGENCE AND DIVERGENCE

■ CONVERGENCE

Convergence is the process by which many presynaptic neurons terminate on a single postsynaptic neuron (Fig.140.9).

■ DIVERGENCE

Divergence is the process by which one presynaptic neuron terminates on many postsynaptic neurons.

Neurotransmitters

- ■ DEFINITION
- ■ HISTORY
- ■ CRITERIA
- ■ CLASSIFICATION
- ■ TRANSPORT AND RELEASE
- ■ INACTIVATION
- ■ REUPTAKE
- ■ IMPORTANT NEUROTRANSMITTERS
- ■ NEUROMODULATORS
- ■ COTRANSMISSION AND COTRANSMITTERS

■ DEFINITION

Neurotransmitter is a chemical substance that acts as a **mediator** for the transmission of nerve impulse from one neuron to another neuron through a synapse.

■ HISTORY

Existence of neurotransmitter was first discovered by an Austrian scientist named **Otto Loewi** in 1921. He dreamt of an experiment, which he did practically and came out with this discovery.

Loewi Experiment

Otto Loewi used two frogs for this experiment. Heart of frog A was with intact vagus nerve and was placed in a saline-filled chamber. Heart of frog B was denervated and was kept in another saline-filled chamber. Both the chambers were connected in such a way that the fluid from chamber of frog A could flow into the chamber of frog B.

When vagus nerve of frog A was electrically stimulated, slowing of heart rate was observed. After a short delay, the heart rate in frog B also was found to be slowing down. From this observation, Loewi speculated that some chemical substance must have

been released from the vagus nerve of frog A, which was responsible for the slowing down of the heart rate in frog B. He named it as **'vagusstoff'**. Later this chemical substance was considered as a neurotransmitter and called acetylcholine (Ach).

■ CRITERIA FOR NEUROTRANSMITTER

Nowadays, many substances are categorized as neurotransmitters. To consider a substance as a neurotransmitter, it should fulfill certain criteria as given below:

1. It must be found in a neuron
2. It must be produced by a neuron
3. It must be released by a neuron
4. After release, it must act on a target area and produce some biological effect
5. After the action, it must be inactivated.

■ CLASSIFICATION OF NEUROTRANSMITTERS

■ DEPENDING UPON CHEMICAL NATURE

Many substances of different chemical nature are identified as neurotransmitters. Depending upon their chemical nature, neurotransmitters are classified into three groups.

1. Amino Acids

Neurotransmitters of this group are involved in **fast synaptic transmission** and are inhibitory and excitatory in action. GABA, glycine, glutamate (glutamic acid) and aspartate (aspartic acid) belong to this group.

2. Amines

Amines are the modified amino acids. These neurotransmitters involve in **slow synaptic transmission.** These neurotransmitters are also inhibitory and excitatory in action. Noradrenaline, adrenaline, dopamine, serotonin and histamine belong to this group.

3. Others

Some neurotransmitters do not fit into any of these categories. One such substance is acetylcholine. It is formed from the choline and acetyl coenzyme A in the presence of the enzyme called choline acetyltransferase. Another substance included in this category is the soluble gas nitric oxide (NO).

■ DEPENDING UPON FUNCTION

Some of the neurotransmitters cause excitation of postsynaptic neuron while others cause inhibition.

Thus, neurotransmitters are classified into two types:
1. Excitatory neurotransmitters
2. Inhibitory neurotransmitters.

1. Excitatory Neurotransmitters

Excitatory neurotransmitter is a chemical substance, which is responsible for the conduction of impulse from presynaptic neuron to postsynaptic neuron. Neurotransmitter released from the presynaptic axon terminal does not cause development of action potential in the postsynaptic neuron. Rather, it causes some change in the resting membrane potential, i.e. slight depolarization by the opening of sodium channels in the postsynaptic membrane and the influx of sodium ions from ECF. This slight depolarization is called **excitatory postsynaptic potential (EPSP)**. EPSP in turn causes development of action potential in the initial segment of the axon of the postsynaptic neuron (Chapter 140).

TABLE 141.1: Neurotransmitters

Group	Name	Site of secretion	Action
Aminoacids	GABA	Cerebral cortex, cerebellum, basal ganglia, retina and spinal cord	Inhibitory
	Glycine	Forebrain, brainstem, spinal cord and retina	Inhibitory
	Glutamate	Cerebral cortex, brainstem and cerebellum	Excitatory
	Aspartate	Cerebellum, spinal cord and retina	Excitatory
Amines	Noradrenaline	Postganglionic adrenergic sympathetic nerve endings, cerebral cortex, hypothalamus, basal ganglia, brainstem, locus coeruleus and spinal cord	Excitatory and inhibitory
	Adrenaline	Hypothalamus, thalamus and spinal cord	Excitatory and inhibitory
	Dopamine	Basal ganglia, hypothalamus, limbic system, neocortex, retina and sympathetic ganglia	Inhibitory
	Serotonin	Hypothalamus, limbic system, cerebellum, spinal cord, retina, gastrointestinal (GI) tract, lungs and platelets	Inhibitory
	Histamine	Hypothalamus, cerebral cortex, GI tract and mast cells	Excitatory
Others	Nitric oxide	Many parts of CNS, neuromuscular junction and GI tract	Excitatory
	Acetylcholine	Preganglionic parasympathetic nerve endings Postganglionic parasympathetic nerve endings Preganglionic sympathetic nerve endings Postganglionic sympathetic cholinergic nerve endings Neuromuscular junction, cerebral cortex, hypothalamus, basal ganglia, thalamus, hippocampus and amacrine cells of retina	Excitatory

GABA = Gamma-aminobutyric acid, CNS = Central nervous system.

Common excitatory neurotransmitters are **acetylcholine** and **noradrenaline.**

2. *Inhibitory Neurotransmitters*

Inhibitory neurotransmitter is a chemical substance, which inhibits the conduction of impulse from the presynaptic neuron to the postsynaptic neuron (Chapter 140). When it is released from the presynaptic axon terminal due to the arrival of action potential, it causes opening of potassium channels in the postsynaptic membrane and efflux of potassium ions. This leads to hyperpolarization, which is called the **inhibitory postsynaptic potential (IPSP).** When IPSP is developed, the action potential is not generated in the postsynaptic neuron.

Common inhibitory neurotransmitters are **gamma-aminobutyric acid (GABA)** and dopamine.

■ TRANSPORT AND RELEASE OF NEUROTRANSMITTER

Neurotransmitter is produced in the cell body of the neuron and is transported through axon. At the axon terminal, the neurotransmitter is stored in small packets called vesicles. Under the influence of a stimulus, these vesicles open and release the neurotransmitter into synaptic cleft. It binds to specific receptors on the surface of the postsynaptic cell. Receptors are G proteins, protein kinase or ligand-gated receptors.

■ INACTIVATION OF NEUROTRANSMITTER

After the execution of the action, neurotransmitter is inactivated by four different mechanisms:
1. It diffuses out of synaptic cleft to the area where it has no action
2. It is destroyed or disintegrated by specific enzymes
3. It is engulfed and removed by astrocytes (macrophages)
4. It is removed by means of reuptake into the axon terminal.

■ REUPTAKE OF NEUROTRANSMITTER

Reuptake is a process by which the neurotransmitter is taken back from synaptic cleft into the axon terminal after execution of its action. Reuptake process involves a specific carrier protein for each neurotransmitter.

■ IMPORTANT NEUROTRANSMITTERS

Some of the important neurotransmitters are described here. Details of neurotransmitters are given in Tables 141.1 and 141.2.

■ ACETYLCHOLINE

Acetylcholine is a **cholinergic neurotransmitter.** It possesses excitatory function. It produces the excitatory function by opening the ligand-gated sodium channels (Chapters 32 and 140).

Source

Acetylcholine is the transmitter substance at the neuromuscular junction and synapse. It is also released by the following nerve endings:
1. Preganglionic parasympathetic nerve
2. Postganglionic parasympathetic nerve
3. Preganglionic sympathetic nerve
4. Postganglionic sympathetic cholinergic nerves:
   i. Nerves supplying eccrine sweat glands
   ii. Sympathetic vasodilator nerves in skeletal muscle
5. Nerves in amacrine cells of retina
6. Many regions of brain.

Synthesis

Ach is synthesized in the cholinergic nerve endings. Synthesis takes place in axoplasm and Ach is stored in the vesicles. It is synthesized from acetyl coenzyme A (acetyl CoA). It combines with choline in the presence of the enzyme choline acetyltransferase to form Ach.

TABLE 141.2: Excitatory and inhibitory neurotransmitters

Excitatory neurotransmitters	Inhibitory neurotransmitters	Neurotransmitters with excitatory and inhibitory actions
1. Acetylcholine	1. Gamma-aminobutyric acid	1. Noradrenaline
2. Nitric oxide	2. Glycine	2. Adrenaline
3. Histamine	3. Dopamine	
4. Glutamate	4. Serotonin	
5. Aspartate		

Fate

Action of Ach is short lived. Within one millisecond after the release from the vesicles, it is hydrolyzed into acetate and choline by the enzyme **acetylcholinesterase** (Fig. 141.1). This enzyme is present in basal lamina of the synaptic cleft.

Acetylcholine Receptors

There are two types of receptors through which Ach acts on the tissues namely, **muscarinic receptors** and **nicotinic receptors.** Reason for the terminology of these receptors is as follows: Poisonous substance from toadstools called **muscarine,** acts on a specific group of receptors known as muscarinic receptors; similarly, another substance called **nicotine** acts on a specific group of receptors known as nicotinic receptors but Ach acts on both the receptors.

Muscarinic receptors are present in all the organs innervated by the postganglionic fibers of the parasympathetic system and by the sympathetic cholinergic nerves. Nicotinic receptors are present in the synapses between preganglionic and postganglionic neurons of both sympathetic and parasympathetic systems.

Nicotinic receptors are also present in the neuromuscular junction on membrane of skeletal muscle.

■ NORADRENALINE

Noradrenaline is the neurotransmitter in adrenergic nerve fibers. It is released from the following structures:
1. Postganglionic sympathetic nerve endings
2. Cerebral cortex

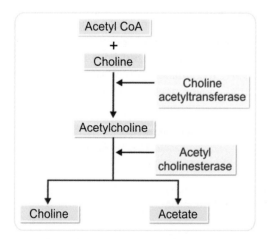

FIGURE 141.1: Synthesis and breakdown of acetylcholine

3. Hypothalamus
4. Basal ganglia
5. Brainstem
6. Locus ceruleus in pons
7. Spinal cord.

In many places, noradrenaline is the **excitatory** chemical mediator and in very few places, it causes **inhibition.** It is believed to be involved in dreams, arousal and elevation of moods. Refer Chapter 71 for the synthesis of noradrenaline.

■ DOPAMINE

Dopamine is secreted by nerve endings in the following areas:
1. Basal ganglia
2. Hypothalamus
3. Limbic system
4. Neocortex
5. Retina
6. Small, intensely fluorescent cells in sympathetic ganglia.

Dopamine possesses **inhibitory** action. Prolactin inhibitory hormone secreted by hypothalamus is considered to be dopamine. Refer Chapter 71 for the synthesis of dopamine.

■ SEROTONIN

Serotonin is otherwise known as **5-hydroxytryptamine** (5-HT). It is synthesized from tryptophan by hydroxylation and decarboxylation. Large amount of serotonin (90%) is found in enterochromatin cells of GI tract. Small amount is found in platelets and nervous system. It is secreted in the following structures:
1. Hypothalamus
2. Limbic system
3. Cerebellum
4. Dorsal raphe nucleus of midbrain
5. Spinal cord
6. Retina
7. GI tract
8. Lungs
9. Platelets.

It is an **inhibitory** substance. It inhibits impulses of pain sensation in posterior gray horn of spinal cord. It is supposed to cause depression of mood and sleep (Chapter 145). Serotonin causes vasoconstriction, platelet aggregation and smooth muscle contraction. It also controls food intake.

■ HISTAMINE

Histamine is secreted in nerve endings of hypothalamus, limbic cortex and other parts of cerebral cortex. It is also secreted by gastric mucosa and mast cells. Histamine is an **excitatory** neurotransmitter. It is believed to play an important role in arousal mechanism.

■ GAMMA-AMINOBUTYRIC ACID

Gamma-aminobutyric acid (GABA) is an **inhibitory** neurotransmitter in synapses particularly in CNS. It is responsible for presynaptic inhibition. It is secreted by nerve endings in the following structures:

1. Cerebral cortex
2. Cerebellum
3. Basal ganglia
4. Spinal cord
5. Retina.

GABA causes synaptic inhibition by opening potassium channels and chloride channels. So, potassium comes out of synapse and chloride enters in (Chapter 140). This leads to hyperpolarization, which is known as inhibitory postsynaptic potential (IPSP).

■ SUBSTANCE P

Substance P is a neuropeptide that acts as a neurotransmitter and as a neuromodulator (see below). Substance P is a polypeptide with 11 amino acid residues. It belongs to a family of 3 related peptides called **neurokinins** or **tachykinins.** The other peptides of this family are neurokinin A and neurokinin B which are not well known like substance P.

Substance P is secreted by the nerve endings (first order neurons) of pain pathway in spinal cord. It is also found in many peripheral nerves, different parts of brain particularly hypothalamus, retina and intestine (Chapter 44).

It mediates **pain sensation.** It is a potent vasodilator in CNS. It is responsible for regulation of anxiety, stress, mood disorders, neurotoxicity, nausea and vomiting.

■ NITRIC OXIDE

Nitric oxide (NO) is a neurotransmitter in the CNS. It is also the important neurotransmitter in the neuromuscular junctions between the inhibitory motor fibers of intrinsic nerve plexus and the smooth muscle fibers of GI tract.

Nitric oxide acts as a mediator for the **dilator effect** of Ach on small arteries. In the smooth muscle fibers of arterioles, NO activates the enzyme guanylyl cyclase, which in turn causes formation of cyclic guanosine monophosphate (cGMP) from GMP. The cGMP is a smooth muscle relaxant and it causes dilatation of arterioles. Thus, NO indirectly causes dilatation of arterioles.

Peculiarity of NO is that it is neither produced by the neuronal cells nor stored in the vesicles. It is produced by **non-neuronal cells** like the endothelial cells of blood vessels. From the site of production, it diffuses into the neuronal and non-neuronal cells where it exerts its action.

■ NEUROMODULATORS

Definition

Neuromodulator is the chemical messenger, which modifies and regulates activities that take place during the synaptic transmission.

These peptides do not propagate nerve impulses like neurotransmitters.

Neuromodulators Vs Neurotransmitters

Neuromodulators are distinct from neurotransmitters. However, both the terms are wrongly interchanged. Neurotransmitters propagate nerve impulses through synapse whereas neuromodulators modify and regulate the activities of synaptic transmission (Table 141.3).

Neurotransmitters are packed in small vesicles in axon terminals only. But neuromodulators are generally

TABLE 141.3: Differences between neurotransmitters and neuromodulators

SI No	Neurotransmitters	Neuromodulators
1	Propagate nerve impulse through synapse	Modify and regulate synaptic transmission
2	Packed in small synaptic vesicles	Packed in large synaptic vesicles
3	Found only in axon terminals	Found in all parts of the body
4	Generally, neuron has only one neurotransmitter	Neuron may have one or more neuromodulators
5	Act by changing the electric potential – depolarization or repolarization	Have diverse actions
6	Chemically, neurotransmitters are amino acids, amine or others	Chemically, neuromodulators are only peptides

packed in large synaptic vesicles, which are present in all parts of neuron like soma, dendrite, axon and nerve endings. Many neurons have one conventional neurotransmitter and one or more neuromodulators.

Few peptides like substance P (see above) act as neurotransmitters and neuromodulators.

Actions of Neuromodulators

Neurotransmitters affect the excitability of other neurons or other tissues (like muscle fiber) by producing **depolarization** or **hyperpolarization** through the receptors of ionic channels. But neuromodulators have diverse actions such as:

1. Regulation of synthesis, breakdown or reuptake of neurotransmitter
2. Excitation or inhibition of membrane receptors by acting independently or together with neurotransmitter
3. Control of gene expression
4. Regulation of local blood flow
5. Promotion of synaptic formation
6. Control of glial cell morphology
7. Regulation of behavior.

Chemistry of Neuromodulators

Generally the neuromodulators are **peptides**. So neuromodulators are often referred as **neuropeptides**. Almost all the peptides found in nervous tissues are neuromodulators.

Types of Neuromodulators

Neuromodulators are classified into two types:

1. Non-opioid peptides
2. Opioid peptides.

■ NON-OPIOID PEPTIDES

Non-opioid neuropeptides act by binding with G-protein coupled receptors. These neuropeptides are also called **non-opioid neuromodulators.** Non-opioid peptides are listed in Table 141.4.

■ OPIOID PEPTIDES

Peptides, which bind to opioid receptors are called **opioid peptides** (Table 141.5). Opioid peptides are also called opioid neuropeptides or opioid neuromodulators. Opioid receptors are the membrane proteins located in nerve endings in brain and GI tract. Opioid receptors are of three types μ, κ and δ. These proteins are called

opioid receptors because of their affinity towards the opiate or morphine, which are derived from opium.

Opium is the juice of white **poppy (Papaver somniferum).** It is used as a narcotic to produce hallucinations and induce sleep. Opiate also induces sleep. **Morphine** is a powerful analgesic (pain reliever). Both opiate and morphine have high medicinal values, but are highly addictive.

These two substances act by binding with the receptor proteins (opioid receptors) for the natural neuropeptides. Natural neuropeptides are called **endogenous opioid peptides.**

Endogenous opioid peptides have opiate like activity and inhibit the neurons in the brain involved in pain sensation.

Opioid peptides are of three types:

i. Enkephalins
ii. Dynorphins
iii. Endorphins.

i. Enkephalins

Enkephalins are the natural opiate peptides recognized first in pig's brain. Derived from the precursor proenkephalin, these peptides are present in the nerve endings in many parts of forebrain, substantia gelatinosa of brainstem, spinal cord and GI tract. Two types of enkephalins are known, **leucine** enkephalin (YGGFL) and **methionine** enkephalin (YGGFM).

ii. Dynorphins

Dynorphins are derived from prodynorphin. Dynorphins are found in hypothalamus, posterior pituitary and duodenum. Dynorphins are of two types, α- and β-dynorphins.

iii. Endorphins

Endorphins are the large peptides derived from the precursor pro-opiomelanocortin. Endorphins are predominant in diencephalic region particularly hypothalamus and anterior and intermediate lobes of pituitary gland. Three types of endorphins are recognized, α-, β- and γ-endorphins.

■ COTRANSMISSION AND COTRANSMITTERS

Cotransmission is the release of many neurotransmitters from a single nerve terminal. Cotransmitters are the

TABLE 141.4: Non-opioid neuromodulators

Name	Site of secretion	Action
Bradykinin	Blood vessels, kidneys	Vasodilator
Substance P	Brain, spinal cord, retina peripheral nerves and intestine	Mediates pain. Regulates anxiety, stress, mood disorders, neurotoxicity, nausea and vomiting. Causes vasodilatation.
Secretin	Cerebral cortex, hypothalamus, thalamus, olfactory bulb, brainstem and small intestine	Inhibits gastric secretion and motility
CCK	Cerebral cortex, hypothalamus, retina and small intestine	Contracts gallbladder Inhibits gastric motility Increases intestinal motility
Gastrin	Hypothalamus, medulla oblongata, posterior pituitary and gastrointestinal (GI) tract	Increases gastric secretion and motility Stimulates islets in pancreas
VIP	Cerebral cortex, hypothalamus, retina and intestine	Causes vasodilatation
Motilin	Cerebral cortex, cerebellum, posterior pituitary and intestine	Stimulates intestinal motility
Neurotensin	Hypothalamus and retina	Inhibits pain sensation Decreases food intake
Vasopressin	Posterior pituitary, medulla oblongata and spinal cord	Causes vasoconstriction
Oxytocin	Posterior pituitary, medulla oblongata and spinal cord	Stimulates milk ejection and uterine contraction
CRH	Hypothalamus	Stimulates release of ACTH
GHRH	Hypothalamus	Stimulates release of growth hormone
GHRP	Hypothalamus	Stimulates release of GHRH
TRH	Hypothalamus, other parts of brain and retina	Stimulates release of thyroid hormones
Somatostatin	Hypothalamus, other parts of brain, substantia gelatinosa and retina	Inhibits growth hormone secretion Decreases food intake
GnRH	Hypothalamus, preganglionic autonomic nerve endings and retina	Inhibits gonadotropin secretion
Endothelin	Posterior pituitary, brainstem and endothelium	Causes vasoconstriction
Angiotensin II	Hypothalamus, brainstem and spinal cord	Causes vasoconstriction
ANP	Hypothalamus, brainstem and heart	Causes vasodilatation Increases sodium excretion
BNP	Hypothalamus and heart	Causes vasodilatation Increases sodium excretion
CNP	Brain, myocardium, endothelium of blood vessels, GI tract and kidneys	Causes vasodilatation Increases sodium excretion
Neuropeptide Y	Medulla, hypothalamus and small intestine	Increases food intake Causes vasoconstriction Increases enteric blood flow
Ghrelin	Hypothalamus, stomach, pituitary, kidney and placenta	Promotes GH release Induces appetite and food intake Stimulates gastric emptying

ACTH = Adrenocorticotropic hormone, ANP = Atrial natriuretic peptide, BNP = Brain natriuretic peptide, CCK = Cholecystokinin. CNP = C-type natriuretic peptide, CRH = Corticotropin-releasing hormone, GHRH = Growth hormone-releasing hormone, GHRP = Growth hormone-releasing polypeptide, GnRH = Gonadotropin-releasing hormone, TRH = Thyrotropin-releasing hormone, VIP = Vasoactive intestinal polypeptide.

TABLE 141.5: Opioid neuromodulators

Name	Site of secretion	Action
Enkephalins	Many parts of brain, substantia gelatinosa and retina	
Dynorphins	Hypothalamus, posterior pituitary and duodenum	Inhibit pain sensation
β-endorphin	Thalamus, hypothalamus, brainstem and retina	

neurotransmitter substances that are released in addition to primary transmitter at the nerve endings.

For many years, it was believed that each neuron releases only one neurotransmitter substance from its terminals. Now it is known that some of the neurons release many neurotransmitter substances. It is also believed that the additional neurotransmitters, i.e. the cotransmitters modulate the effects of primary neuro-transmitters.

Some of the primary neurotransmitters act as co-transmitters in other nerve endings.

Examples of cotransmitters:

1. Calcitonin
2. Dopamine
3. Dynorphin
4. GABA
5. Gene-related peptide
6. Glutamate
7. Glycine
8. Neuropeptide Y
9. Substance P
10. Vasoactive intestinal polypeptide (VIP).

Reflex Activity

■ DEFINITION AND SIGNIFICANCE OF REFLEXES
■ REFLEX ARC
■ CLASSIFICATION OF REFLEXES
■ SUPERFICIAL REFLEXES
■ DEEP REFLEXES
■ VISCERAL REFLEXES
■ PATHOLOGICAL REFLEXES
■ PROPERTIES OF REFLEXES
■ RECIPROCAL INHIBITION AND RECIPROCAL INNERVATION
■ REFLEXES IN MOTOR NEURON LESION

■ DEFINITION AND SIGNIFICANCE OF REFLEXES

Reflex activity is the response to a peripheral nervous stimulation that occurs without our consciousness. It is a type of **protective mechanism** and it protects the body from irreparable damages.

For example, when hand is placed on a hot object, it is withdrawn immediately. When a bright light is thrown into the eyes, eyelids are closed and pupil is constricted to prevent the damage of retina by entrance of excessive light into the eyes.

■ REFLEX ARC

Reflex arc is the anatomical nervous pathway for a reflex action. A simple reflex arc includes five components (Fig. 142.1).

1. Receptor

Receptor is the **end organ,** which receives the stimulus. When receptor is stimulated, impulses are generated in afferent nerve.

2. Afferent Nerve

Afferent or **sensory nerve** transmits sensory impulses from the receptor to center.

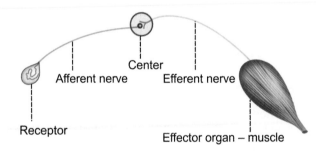

FIGURE 142.1: Simple reflex arc

3. Center

Center receives the sensory impulses via afferent nerve fibers and in turn, it generates appropriate motor impulses. Center is located in the brain or spinal cord.

4. Efferent Nerve

Efferent or **motor nerve** transmits motor impulses from the center to the effector organ.

5. Effector Organ

Effector organ is the structure such as muscle or gland where the activity occurs in response to stimulus.

Afferent and efferent nerve fibers may be connected directly to the center. In some places, one or more neurons are interposed between these nerve fibers and the center. Such neurons are called **connector neurons** or **internuncial neurons** or **interneurons.**

■ CLASSIFICATION OF REFLEXES

Reflexes are classified by six different methods depending upon various factors. Different methods of classification are listed in Box 142.1.

BOX 142.1: Different methods to classify reflexes

Classification of reflexes
1. Depending upon whether inborn or acquired
2. Depending upon situation – anatomical classification
3. Depending upon purpose – physiological classification
4. Depending upon number of synapse
5. Depending upon whether visceral or somatic
6. Depending upon clinical basis

■ 1. DEPENDING UPON WHETHER INBORN OR ACQUIRED REFLEXES

i. *Inborn Reflexes or Unconditioned Reflexes*

Unconditioned reflexes are the **natural reflexes,** which are present since the time of birth, hence the name inborn reflexes. Such reflexes do not require previous learning, training or conditioning. Best example is the secretion of saliva when a drop of honey is kept in the mouth of a newborn baby for the first time. The baby does not know the taste of honey, but still saliva is secreted.

ii. *Acquired Reflexes or Conditioned Reflexes*

Conditioned or acquired reflexes are the reflexes that are developed **after conditioning** or **training.** These reflexes are not inborn but, acquired after birth. Such reflexes need previous learning, training or conditioning. Example is the secretion of saliva by sight, smell, thought or hearing of a known edible substance.

■ 2. DEPENDING UPON SITUATION – ANATOMICAL CLASSIFICATION

In this method, reflexes are classified depending upon the situation of the center.

i. *Cerebellar Reflexes*

Cerebellar reflexes are the reflexes which have their center in **cerebellum.**

ii. *Cortical Reflexes*

Cortical reflexes are the reflexes that have their center in **cerebral cortex.**

iii. *Midbrain Reflexes*

Midbrain reflexes are the reflexes which have their center in **midbrain.**

iv. *Bulbar or Medullary Reflexes*

Bulbar or medullary reflexes are the reflexes which have their center in **medulla oblongata.**

v. *Spinal Reflexes*

Reflexes having their center in the spinal cord are called spinal reflexes. Depending upon the segments involved, spinal reflexes are divided into three groups:

    a. Segmental spinal reflexes
    b. Intrasegmental spinal reflexes
    c. Suprasegmental spinal reflexes.

■ 3. DEPENDING UPON PURPOSE – PHYSIOLOGICAL CLASSIFICATION

In this method, reflexes are classified depending upon the purpose (**functional significance**).

i. *Protective Reflexes or Flexor Reflexes*

Protective reflexes are the reflexes which protect the body from **nociceptic (harmful) stimuli.** These reflexes are also called **withdrawal reflexes** or flexor reflexes. Protective reflexes involve flexion at different joints hence the name flexor reflexes.

ii. *Antigravity Reflexes or Extensor Reflexes*

Antigravity reflexes are the reflexes that protect the body against **gravitational force.** These reflexes are also called the extensor reflexes because, the extensor muscles contract during these reflexes resulting in extension at joints.

■ 4. DEPENDING UPON THE NUMBER OF SYNAPSE

Depending upon the number of synapse in reflex arc, reflexes are classified into two types:

i. *Monosynaptic Reflexes*

Reflexes having only **one synapse** in the reflex arc are called monosynaptic reflexes. Stretch reflex is the best example for monosynaptic reflex and it is elicited due to the stimulation of muscle spindle.

ii. *Polysynaptic Reflexes*

Reflexes having **more than one** synapse in the reflex arc are called polysynaptic reflexes. Flexor reflexes (withdrawal reflexes) are the polysynaptic reflexes.

■ 5. DEPENDING UPON WHETHER SOMATIC OR VISCERAL REFLEXES

i. *Somatic Reflexes*

Somatic reflexes are the reflexes, for which the reflex arc is formed by **somatic nerve fibers.** These reflexes involve the participation of skeletal muscles. And there may be flexion or extension at different joints during these reflexes.

ii. *Visceral or Autonomic Reflexes*

Visceral or autonomic reflexes are the reflexes, for which at least a part of reflex arc is formed by **autonomic nerve fibers.** These reflexes involve participation of smooth muscle or cardiac muscle. Visceral reflexes include pupillary reflexes, gastrointestinal reflexes, cardiovascular reflexes, respiratory reflexes, etc.

Some reflexes like swallowing, coughing or vomiting are considered as visceral reflexes. However, these reflexes involve some participation of skeletal muscles also.

■ 6. DEPENDING UPON CLINICAL BASIS

Depending upon the clinical basis, reflexes are classified into four types:
  i. Superficial reflexes
  ii. Deep reflexes
  iii. Visceral reflexes
  iv. Pathological reflexes.

■ SUPERFICIAL REFLEXES

Superficial reflexes are the reflexes, which are elicited from the surface of the body. Superficial reflexes are of two types: mucus membrane reflexes and skin reflexes.

■ 1. MUCOUS MEMBRANE REFLEXES

Mucous membrane reflexes arise from the mucus membrane. Details of mucus membrane reflexes are listed in Table 142.1.

■ 2. CUTANEOUS REFLEXES OR SKIN REFLEXES

Cutaneous reflexes are elicited from skin by the stimulation of cutaneous receptors. Details of these reflexes are given in Table 142.2.

■ DEEP REFLEXES

Deep reflexes are elicited from deeper structures beneath the skin like tendon. These reflexes are otherwise known as **tendon reflexes.** Details of these are given in Table 142.3.

■ VISCERAL REFLEXES

Visceral reflexes are the reflexes arising from **pupil** and **visceral organs.** Other details of visceral reflexes are already given above.

TABLE 142.1: Superficial mucous membrane reflexes

Reflex	Stimulus	Response	Afferent Nerve	Center	Efferent Nerve
1. Corneal reflex	Irritation of cornea	Blinking of eye (closure of eyelids)	V cranial nerve	Pons	VII cranial nerve
2. Conjunctival reflex	Irritation of conjunctiva	Blinking of eye	V cranial nerve	Pons	VII cranial nerve
3. Nasal reflex (sneezing reflex)	Irritation of nasal mucus membrane	Sneezing	V cranial nerve	Motor nucleus of V cranial nerve	X cranial nerve and upper cervical nerves
4. Pharyngeal reflex	Irritation of pharyngeal mucus membrane	Retching or gagging (opening of mouth)	IX cranial nerve	Nuclei of X cranial nerve	X cranial nerve
5. Uvular reflex	Irritation of uvula	Raising of uvula	IX cranial nerve	Nuclei of X cranial nerve	X cranial nerve

TABLE 142.2: Superficial cutaneous reflexes

Reflex	Stimulus	Response	Center – spinal segments involved
1. Scapular reflex	Irritation of skin at the interscapular space	Contraction of scapular muscles and drawing in of scapula	C5 to T1
2. Upper abdominal reflex	Stroking the abdominal wall below the costal margin	Ipsilateral contraction of abdominal muscle and movement of umbilicus towards the site of stroke	T6 to T9
3. Lower abdominal reflex	Stroking the abdominal wall at umbilical and iliac level	Ipsilateral contraction of abdominal muscle and movement of umbilicus towards the site of stroke	T10 to T12
4. Cremasteric reflex	Stroking the skin at upper and inner aspect of thigh	Elevation of testicles	L1, L2
5. Gluteal reflex	Stroking the skin over glutei	Contraction of glutei	L4 to S1,2
6. Plantar reflex	Stroking the sole	Plantar flexion and adduction of toes	L5 to S2
7. Bulbocavernous reflex	Stroking the dorsum of glans penis	Contraction of bulbocavernosus	S3, S4
8. Anal reflex	Stroking the perianal region	Contraction of anal sphincter	S4, S5

TABLE 142.3: Deep reflexes

Reflex	Stimulus	Response	Center – spinal segments involved
1. Jaw jerk	Tapping middle of the chin with slightly opened mouth	Closure of mouth	Pons – V cranial nerve
2. Biceps jerk	Percussion of biceps tendon	Flexion of forearm	C5, C6
3. Triceps jerk	Percussion of triceps tendon	Extension of forearm	C6 to C8
4. Supinator jerk or radial periosteal reflex	Percussion of tendon over distal end (styloid process) of radius	Supination and flexion of forearm	C7, C8
5. Wrist tendon or finger flexion reflex	Percussion of wrist tendons	Flexion of corresponding finger	C8, T1
6. Knee jerk or patellar tendon reflex	Percussion of patellar ligament	Extension of leg	L2 to L4
7. Ankle jerk or Achilles tendon reflex	Percussion of Achilles tendon	Plantar flexion of foot	L5 to S2

Following are the visceral reflexes:
1. Pupillary reflexes
2. Oculocardiac reflex
3. Carotid sinus reflex.

■ PUPILLARY REFLEXES

Pupillary reflexes are the reflexes in which, the size of pupil is altered.

Pupillary reflexes are:
  i. Light reflex

  ii. Accommodation reflex
  iii. Ciliospinal reflex.

i. *Light Reflex*

When retina of the eye is stimulated by a sudden flash of light, **constriction of pupil occurs.** It is called light reflex.

Light reflex of two types:
  a. Direct light reflex, in which stimulation of retina in one eye by flash of light causes constriction of pupil in the same eye

b. Indirect or consensual light reflex, in which stimulation of retina in one eye by flash of light causes simultaneous constriction of pupil in the other eye also.

ii. *Accommodation Reflex*

While eyes are fixed on a distant object and if another object is brought in front of the eye (near the eye) the vision shifts form **far object** to **near object**. During that time some changes occur in the eyes.

Changes during accommodation reflex are:

a. Constriction of pupil
b. Convergence of eyeball
c. Increase in anterior curvature of lens.

iii. *Ciliospinal Reflex*

Ciliospinal reflex is the **dilatation of pupil** due to stimulation of skin over the neck.

More details of pupillary reflexes are given in Chapter 169.

■ OCULOCARDIAC REFLEX

Oculocardiac reflex is the reflex, in which **heart rate decreases** due to the pressure applied over eyeball.

■ CAROTID SINUS REFLEX

Carotid sinus reflex is the **decrease in heart rate** and blood pressure caused by pressure over carotid sinus in neck due to tight collar.

■ PATHOLOGICAL REFLEXES

Pathological reflexes are the reflexes that are elicited only in pathological conditions. Well-known pathological reflexes are:

1. Babinski sign
2. Clonus
3. Pendular movements.

■ BABINSKI SIGN

Abnormal plantar reflex is called Babinski sign. It is also called Babinski reflex or phenomenon. It is named after the discoverer **Joseph Babinski**. In normal plantar reflex, a gentle scratch over the outer edge of the sole of foot causes plantar flexion and adduction of all toes. But in Babinski sign, there is dorsiflexion of great toe and fanning of other toes.

When Babinski reflex is present, the condition is commonly called Babinski **positive sign** and when it is negative, the condition is called Babinski **negative sign**.

Babinski sign is present in **upper motor neuron lesion**. Physiological conditions when Babinski sign is present are infancy and deep sleep. It is present in infants because of non-myelination of pyramidal tracts.

■ CLONUS

Clonus is a series of rapid and repeated involuntary jerky movements, which occur while eliciting a deep reflex. When a deep reflex is elicited in a normal person, the contractions of a muscle or group of muscles are smooth and continuous. But clonus occurs when the deep reflexes are exaggerated due to hypertonicity of muscles in **pyramidal tract lesion.** Clonus is well seen in calf muscles producing ankle clonus and quadriceps producing patella clonus.

Ankle Clonus

Ankle clonus is the repeated rhythmical contractions of calf muscles caused by sudden dorsiflexion of foot.

Repeated rhythmical contractions of calf muscles lead to a series of rhythmic plantar flexion at ankle joint. Sudden dorsiflexion of foot is done by supporting patient's knee in a slightly flexed position.

Patellar Clonus

Patellar clonus is the rhythmic jerky movements of patella produced by grasping it between thumb and index finger of the examiner and pushing it down forcibly towards the foot. It is caused by clonic contractions of quadriceps muscle.

■ PENDULAR MOVEMENTS

Pendular movements are the slow oscillatory movements (instead of brisk movements) that are developed while eliciting a tendon jerk. Unlike clonus, pendular movements occur because of hypotonicity of muscles. Pendular movements are very common while eliciting the knee jerk or patellar tendon reflex in the patients affected by cerebellar lesion.

A tap on the patellar tendon when leg is hanging freely causes a brisk extension of leg due to the contraction of quadriceps muscle (knee jerk). In normal conditions, after the extension, the leg returns back to resting position immediately. In **cerebellar lesion,** the leg swings forwards and backwards several times before coming to rest. Such movements are similar to movements of **clock's pendulum** hence the name pendular movements.

■ PROPERTIES OF REFLEXES

■ 1. ONE WAY CONDUCTION (BELL-MAGENDIE LAW)

During any reflex activity, impulses are transmitted in only **one direction** through the reflex arc as per Bell-Magendie law. The impulses pass from receptors to center and then from center to effector organ.

■ 2. REACTION TIME

Reaction time is the time interval between application of stimulus and the onset of reflex. It depends upon the length of afferent and efferent nerve fibers, velocity of impulse through these fibers and central delay. Central delay is the delay at the synapse. It is also called **synaptic delay.**

■ 3. SUMMATION

Refer Chapter 140 for details of summation. Summation in reflex action is of two types:

i. *Spatial Summation*

When two afferent nerve fibers supplying a muscle are stimulated separately with subliminal stimulus, there is no response. But the muscle contracts when both the nerve fibers are stimulated together with same strength of stimulus. It is called spatial summation.

ii. *Temporal Summation*

When one nerve fiber is stimulated repeatedly with subliminal stimuli, these stimuli are summed up to give response in the muscle. It is called temporal summation.

Thus, both spatial summation and temporal summation play an important role in the **facilitation of responses** during the reflex activity.

■ 4. OCCLUSION

Occlusion is demonstrated in a flexor reflex involving a muscle, which is innervated by two motor nerves. These nerves can be called A and B. When both the nerves, A and B, are stimulated simultaneously, the tension developed by the muscle is less than the sum of the tension developed when each nerve is stimulated separately.

For example, if nerve A is stimulated alone, the arbitrary unit of tension developed is 9. If the nerve B is stimulated then 9 units of tension is developed. So, the sum of tension developed when the nerves A and B are separately stimulated = 9 + 9 = 18 units (Fig. 142.2).

But, when both A and B are stimulated together, the tension produced is (A + B) = 12 units. Thus, the tension here is less than sum of tension produced when A and B were stimulated separately. This phenomenon is called occlusion. Occlusion is due to the **overlapping** of the nerve fibers during the distribution.

■ 5. SUBLIMINAL FRINGE

In some reflexes involving the muscle with two nerve fibers, the tension developed by simultaneous stimulation of two nerves is greater than the sum of tension produced by the stimulation of these nerves separately.

For example, if nerve A is stimulated alone, the arbitrary unit of tension developed by muscle = 3 units (Fig. 142.3). If nerve B is stimulated alone, the tension produced = 3 units. So, the sum of tension developed, if nerves A and B are stimulated separately = 3 + 3 = 6 units. When both the nerves A and B were stimulated together, the tension developed is (A + B) = 12 units. Thus, the tension here is greater than the sum of tension produced, if A and B are separately stimulated. This phenomenon is called subliminal fringe. It is due to the effect of **spatial summation.**

■ 6. RECRUITMENT

Recruitment is defined as the successive activation of additional motor units with progressive increase in force of muscular contraction.

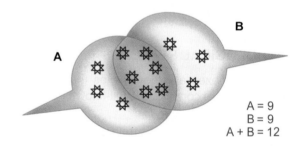

A = 9
B = 9
A + B = 12

FIGURE 142.2: Occlusion

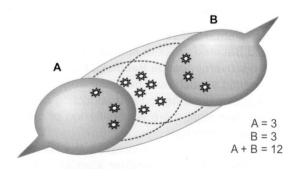

A = 3
B = 3
A + B = 12

FIGURE 142.3: Subliminal fringe

When an excitatory nerve is stimulated for a long time, there is a gradual increase in the response of reflex activities. It is due to the activation of more and more motor neurons. Recruitment is similar to the effect of **temporal summation.**

Indefinite increase in response does not produce unlimited recruitment. A **plateau** is reached. Thus, there is a limit to the number of motor neurons, which are recruited. So, beyond certain limit, the prolongation of stimulation does not increase the response.

■ 7. AFTER DISCHARGE

After discharge is the persistence or continuation of response for some time even after cessation of stimulus. When a reflex action is elicited continuously for sometime and then the stimulation is stopped, the reflex activity (contraction) will be continued for some-time even after the stoppage of the stimulus. It is because of the discharge of impulses from the center even after stoppage of stimulus. Internuncial neurons, which continue to transmit afferent impulses even after stoppage of stimulus are responsible for after discharge.

■ 8. REBOUND PHENOMENON

Reflex activities can be forcefully inhibited for some time. But, when the inhibition is suddenly removed, the reflex activity becomes more forceful than before inhibition. It is called rebound phenomenon. Reason for this state of over excitation is not known.

■ 9. FATIGUE

When a reflex activity is continuously elicited for a long time, the response is reduced slowly and at one stage, the response does not occur. This type of failure to give response to the stimulus is called fatigue. Center or the synapse of the reflex arc is the **first seat** of fatigue.

■ RECIPROCAL INHIBITION AND RECIPROCAL INNERVATION

■ RECIPROCAL INHIBITION

Reciprocal inhibition is one of the important features of both flexor and extensor reflexes. Usually, excitation of one group of muscles is associated with inhibition of another, i.e. antagonistic group of muscles on the same side. For example, when a flexor reflex is elicited, the flexor muscles are excited (contracted) and the extensor muscles are inhibited (relaxed) in that side. This phenomenon is called the reciprocal inhibition.

Reciprocal inhibition occurs because of the reciprocal innervation.

■ RECIPROCAL INNERVATION – SHERRINGTON LAW

Neural mechanism involved in reciprocal inhibition was postulated by **Sherrington.** Hence, it is called Sherrington law of reciprocal innervation. According to this law, the reciprocal inhibition is due to segmental arrangement of afferent and efferent connections in the spinal cord. Afferent nerve fibers, which evoke flexor reflex in a limb, have connections with motor neurons supplying flexors and the motor neurons supplying the extensors of same side. Afferent nerve excites the motor neurons, which supply the flexors.

Simultaneously, it also inhibits the motor neurons supplying extensors through an interneuron. According-ly, the flexor muscles contract and extensor muscles relax resulting in flexion of the limb (Fig. 142.4).

■ CROSSED EXTENSOR REFLEX

Crossed extensor reflex is the withdrawal reflex in which the flexors of the withdrawing limb are excited (contracting) and extensors are inhibited (relaxed), while the opposite occurs in the other limb. For example, while eliciting a flexor reflex activity in a limb, that limb is flexed. Simultaneously the opposite limb is extended.

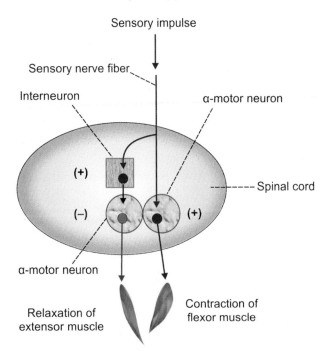

FIGURE 142.4: Reciprocal inhibition
(+) = Excitation. (−) = Inhibition.

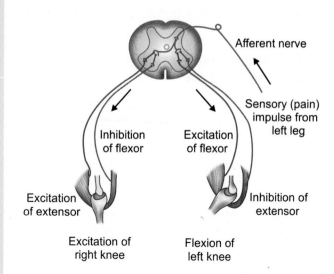

FIGURE 142.5: Crossed extensor reflex. Green lines indicate excitation and red lines indicate inhibition.

Flexors are excited and extensors are inhibited in this limb, but in the opposite limb, the flexors are inhibited and extensors are excited. This type of crossed extensor reflex is because of reciprocal inhibition. It occurs in upper motor neuron lesion.

Crossed extensor reflex is demonstrated in a spinal animal. When one limb of the animal is pinched, it is withdrawn, i.e. flexed. But the opposite limb is extended (Fig. 142.5).

■ SIGNIFICANCE OF RECIPROCAL INHIBITION

Reciprocal inhibition and reciprocal innervation are very important in spinal reflexes, which are involved in **locomotion.** It helps in the forward movement of one limb while causing the backward movement of the opposite limb.

■ REFLEXES IN MOTOR NEURON LESION

■ UPPER MOTOR NEURON LESION

During upper motor neuron lesion, all the superficial reflexes are lost. Deep reflexes are exaggerated and the Babinski sign is positive (Chapter 144).

■ LOWER MOTOR NEURON LESION

During lower motor lesion, all the superficial and deep reflexes are lost (Chapter 144).

Spinal Cord

- ■ INTRODUCTION
- ■ GRAY MATTER
- ■ WHITE MATTER
- ■ TRACTS IN SPINAL CORD
- ■ ASCENDING TRACTS
- ■ DESCENDING TRACTS
- ■ APPLIED PHYSIOLOGY

■ INTRODUCTION

Situation and Extent

Spinal cord lies loosely in the **vertebral canal.** It extends from **foramen magnum** where it is continuous with medulla oblongata, above and up to the lower border of first lumbar vertebra below.

Coverings

Spinal cord is covered by sheaths called **meninges,** which are membranous in nature. Meninges are **dura mater, pia mater** and **arachnoid mater.** These coverings continue as coverings of brain. Meninges are responsible for protection and nourishment of the nervous tissues.

Shape and Length

Spinal cord is cylindrical in shape. Length of the spinal cord is about 45 cm in males and about 43 cm in females.

Enlargements

Spinal cord has two spindle-shaped swellings, namely **cervical** and **lumbar enlargements.** These two portions of spinal cord innervate upper and lower extremities respectively.

Conus Medullaris and Filum Terminale

Below the lumbar enlargement, spinal cord rapidly narrows to a cone-shaped termination called **conus medullaris.** A slender non-nervous filament called **filum terminale** extends from conus medullaris downward to the fundus of the dural sac at the level of second sacral vertebra.

Segments

Spinal cord is made up of 31 segments, which are listed in Box 143.1. In fact, spinal cord is a continuous structure. Appearance of the segment is by nerves arising from spinal cord, which are called spinal nerve.

Spinal Nerves

Segments of spinal cord correspond to 31 pairs of spinal nerves in a symmetrical manner. The spinal nerves are listed in Box 143.1.

BOX 143.1: Segments of spinal cord and spinal nerves

Spinal segments/Spinal nerves		
1. Cervical segments/Cervical spinal nerves	=	8
2. Thoracic segments/Thoracic spinal nerves	=	12
3. Lumbar segments/Lumbar spinal nerves	=	5
4. Sacral segments/Sacral spinal nerves	=	5
5. Coccygeal segment/Coccygeal spinal nerves	=	1
Total	=	31

Nerve Roots

Each spinal nerve is formed by an **anterior (ventral) root** and a **posterior (dorsal) root.** Both the roots on either side leave the spinal cord and pass through the corresponding **intervertebral foramina.** The first cervical spinal nerves pass through a foramen between occipital bone and first vertebra, which is called **atlas.** Cervical and thoracic roots are shorter whereas, the lumbar and sacral roots are longer. Long nerves descend in dural sac to reach their respective intervertebral foramina. This bundle of descending roots surrounding the filum terminale resembles the tail of horse. Hence, it is called cauda equina.

Fissure and Sulci

On the anterior surface of spinal cord, there is a deep furrow known as **anterior median fissure.** Depth of this fissure is about 3 mm. Lateral to the anterior median fissure on either side, there is a slight depression called the **anterolateral sulcus.** It denotes the exit of anterior nerve root. On the posterior aspect, there is a depression called **posterior median sulcus.** This sulcus is continuous with a thin glial partition called the **posterior median septum.** It extends inside the spinal cord for about 5 mm and reaches the gray matter.

On either side, lateral to posterior median sulcus, there is **posterior intermediate sulcus.** It is continuous with **posterior intermediate septum,** which extends for about 3 mm into the spinal cord. Lateral to the posterior intermediate sulcus, is the **posterolateral sulcus.** This denotes the entry of posterior nerve root.

Internal Structure of Spinal Cord

Neural substance of spinal cord is divided into inner gray matter and outer white matter (Fig. 143.1).

■ GRAY MATTER OF SPINAL CORD

Gray matter of spinal cord is the collection of nerve cell bodies, dendrites and parts of axons. It is placed centrally in the form of **wings of the butterfly** and it resembles the letter 'H'. Exactly in the center of gray matter, there is a canal called the **spinal canal.**

Ventral and the dorsal portions of each lateral half of gray matter are called ventral (anterior) and dorsal (posterior) gray horns respectively. In addition, the gray matter forms a small projection in between the anterior and posterior horns in all thoracic and first two lumbar segments. It is called the lateral gray horn. Part of the gray matter anterior to central canal is called the **anterior gray commissure** and part of gray matter posterior to the central canal is called **posterior gray commissure.**

Neurons in Gray Matter of Spinal Cord

Gray matter contains two types of multipolar neurons:

1. *Golgi type I neurons*

Golgi type I neurons have **long axons** and are usually found in anterior horns. Axons of these neurons form the long tracts of spinal cord.

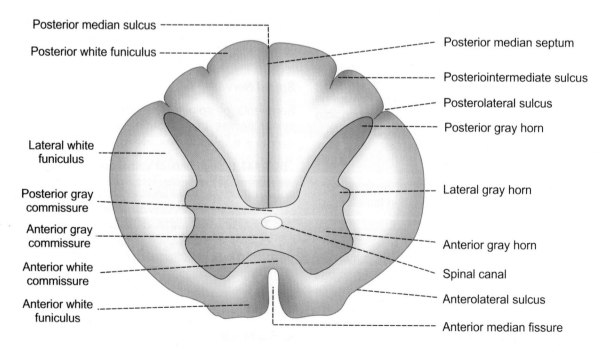

Posterior median sulcus

Posterior white funiculus

Lateral white funiculus

Posterior gray commissure

Anterior gray commissure

Anterior white commissure

Anterior white funiculus

Posterior median septum

Posteriointermediate sulcus

Posterolateral sulcus

Posterior gray horn

Lateral gray horn

Anterior gray horn

Spinal canal

Anterolateral sulcus

Anterior median fissure

FIGURE 143.1: Section of spinal cord: thoracic segment

Golgi type II neurons

Golgi type II neurons have **short axons,** which are found mostly in posterior horns. Axons of these neurons pass towards the anterior horn of same side or opposite side.

Organization of Neurons in Gray Matter

Organization of neurons in the gray matter of spinal cord is described in two methods:
  1. Nuclei or columns
  2. Laminae or layers (Fig. 143.2).

■ NUCLEI

Clusters of neurons are present in the form of nuclei or cell columns in gray matter. Advantage of this method is that different nuclei are easily distinguished. Disadvantage is that some neurons like internuncial neurons, which are outside the distinct nuclei are not included.

Nuclei in Posterior Gray Horn

Posterior gray horn contains the nuclei of sensory neurons, which receive impulses from various receptors of the body through posterior nerve root fibers. There are four types of nuclei of sensory neurons:

1. *Marginal nucleus*

Marginal nucleus is also called **posteromarginal nucleus, marginal zone nucleus** or **border nucleus.** It covers the very tip of posterior gray horn and it is found in all levels of spinal cord.

2. *Substantia gelatinosa of Rolando*

Substantia gelatinosa of Rolando is a cap-like gelatinous material at the apex of posterior horn situated in all levels of spinal cord. It is formed by small neurons.

3. *Chief sensory nucleus or nucleus proprius*

Chief sensory nucleus is situated in the posterior gray horn ventral to substantia gelatinosa. It is a poorly defined cell column located in all segments of spinal cord.

4. *Dorsal nucleus of Clarke*

Clarke nucleus is also called **Clarke column of cells** and it is the collection of well-defined neurons. It occupies the basal portion of posterior horn. This nucleus is found in spinal segments between C8 and L3 only.

Nuclei in Lateral Gray Horn

Lateral gray horn has cluster of neurons called intermediolateral nucleus. The neurons of this nucleus give rise to sympathetic preganglionic fibers, which leave the spinal cord through the anterior nerve root. Intermediolateral nucleus extends between T1 and L2 segments of spinal cord.

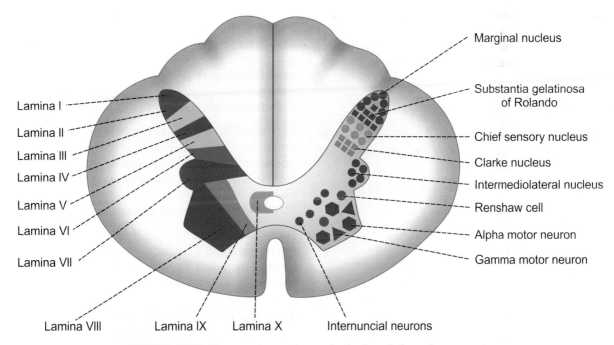

FIGURE 143.2: Neurons in gray horn of spinal cord: thoracic segment

Nuclei in Anterior Gray Horn

Anterior gray horn contains the nuclei of lower motor neurons, which are involved in motor function. These nuclei are present in almost all the levels of spinal cord. Three types of motor neurons are present in lower motor neuron nuclei:

1. Alpha motor neurons

Alpha motor neurons are large and multipolar cells. Axons of these neurons leave the spinal cord through the anterior root and end in groups of skeletal muscle fibers called **extrafusal fibers.**

2. Gamma motor neurons

Gamma motor neurons are smaller cells scattered among alpha motor neurons. These neurons send axons to **intrafusal fibers** of the muscle spindle.

3. Renshaw cells

These cells are also smaller in size. Renshaw cells are the **inhibitory neurons,** which play an important role in **synaptic inhibition** at the spinal cord (Chapter 140).

■ LAMINAE

Neurons of gray matter are distributed in laminae or layers. Each lamina consists of neurons of different size and shape. This cytoarchitectural lamination was identified in 1950 by **Brian Burke** and **Rexed.** He classified the neurons in 10 laminae based on his observation on sections of brain in a neonatal cat. Laminae are also called **Rexed laminae.**

Advantage of this method is that all the neurons of gray horn are included. Disadvantage is that it is difficult to distinguish the laminae from one another.

Laminae in Posterior Gray Horn

Laminae I to VI constitute the posterior gray horn. These laminae contain nuclei of sensory neurons, which are concerned with sensory functions.

Nuclei present in the laminae of posterior gray horn

Marginal nucleus	: Lamina I
Substantial gelatinosa of Rolando	: Laminae II and III
Chief sensory nucleus	: Laminae III, IV and V
Dorsal nucleus of Clarke	: Lamina VI

Lamina in Lateral Gray Horn

Lateral gray horn contains only one lamina, the lamina VII. It contains intermediolateral nucleus.

Laminae in Anterior Gray Horn

Laminae VIII and IX form the anterior gray horn. These laminae contain nuclei of motor neurons, which are concerned with motor functions.

Neurons present in the laminae of anterior gray horn

Motor internuncial neurons, which are also called interneurons	: Lamina VIII
Motor neurons	: Lamina IX

Lamina Around Central Canal

There is only one lamina around the center of the spinal canal, the lamina X. It contains neuroglia, which form the supporting tissue.

■ WHITE MATTER OF SPINAL CORD

White matter of spinal cord surrounds the gray matter. It is formed by the bundles of both myelinated and non-myelinated fibers, but predominantly the myelinated fibers. Anterior median fissure and posterior median septum divide the entire mass of white matter into two lateral halves. The band of white matter lying in front of anterior gray commissure is called **anterior white commissure** (Fig. 143.2).

Each half of the white matter is divided by the fibers of anterior and posterior nerve roots into three white columns or funiculi:

I. Anterior or Ventral White Column

Ventral white column lies between the anterior median fissure on one side and anterior nerve root and anterior gray horn on the other side. It is also called **anterior** or **ventral funiculus.**

II. Lateral White Column

Lateral white column is present between the anterior nerve root and anterior gray horn on one side and posterior nerve root and posterior gray horn on the other side. It is also called **lateral funiculus.**

III. Posterior or Dorsal White Column

Dorsal white column is situated between the posterior nerve root and posterior gray horn on one side and posterior median septum on the other side. It is also called **posterior or dorsal funiculus.**

■ TRACTS IN SPINAL CORD

Groups of nerve fibers passing through spinal cord are known as tracts of the spinal cord. The spinal tracts are

divided into two main groups. They are:
1. Short tracts
2. Long tracts.

1. *Short Tracts*

Fibers of the short tracts connect different parts of spinal cord itself.
Short tracts are of two types:
i. **Association or intrinsic tracts,** which connect adjacent segments of spinal cord on the same side
ii. **Commissural tracts,** which connect opposite halves of same segment of spinal cord.

2. *Long Tracts*

Long tracts of spinal cord, which are also called **projection tracts,** connect the spinal cord with other parts of central nervous system.
Long tracts are of two types:
i. Ascending tracts, which carry sensory impulses from the spinal cord to brain
ii. Descending tracts, which carry motor impulses from brain to the spinal cord.

■ ASCENDING TRACTS OF SPINAL CORD

Ascending tracts of spinal cord carry the impulses of various sensations to the brain.
Pathway for each sensation is formed by two or three groups of neurons, which are:
1. First order neurons
2. Second order neurons
3. Third order neurons.

First Order Neurons

First order neurons receive sensory impulses from the receptors and send them to sensory neurons present in the posterior gray horn of spinal cord through their fibers. Nerve cell bodies of these neurons are located in the **posterior nerve root ganglion.**

Second Order Neurons

Second order neurons are the sensory neurons present in the posterior gray horn. Fibers from these neurons form the ascending tracts of spinal cord. These fibers carry sensory impulses from spinal cord to different brain areas below cerebral cortex **(subcortical areas)** such as thalamus.
All the ascending tracts are formed by fibers of second order neurons of the sensory pathways except the ascending tracts in the posterior white funiculus, which are formed by the fibers of first order neurons.

Third Order Neurons

Third order neurons are in the **subcortical areas.** Fibers of these neurons carry the sensory impulses from subcortical areas to cerebral cortex.
Ascending tracts situated in different white funiculi are listed in Table 143.1 and their features are given in Table 143.2.

■ 1. ANTERIOR SPINOTHALAMIC TRACT

Anterior spinothalamic tract is formed by the fibers of second order neurons of the pathway for **crude touch sensation** (Figs. 143.3 and 143.4).

Situation

Anterior spinothalamic tract is situated in **anterior white funiculus** near the periphery.

Origin

Fibers of anterior spinothalamic tract arise from the neurons of **chief sensory nucleus** of posterior gray horn, which form the **second order neurons** of the crude touch pathway. First order neurons are situated in the posterior nerve root ganglia. These neurons receive the impulses of crude touch sensation from the pressure receptors. Axons of the first order neurons reach the chief sensory nucleus through the posterior nerve root.

Course

Anterior spinothalamic tract contains **crossed fibers.** After taking origin, these fibers cross obliquely in the anterior white commissure and enter the anterior white column of opposite side. Here, the fibers ascend through other segments of spinal cord and brainstem (medulla, pons and midbrain) and reach thalamus.

TABLE 143.1: List of ascending tracts of spinal cord

White column	Tract
Anterior white column	1. Anterior spinothalamic tract
Lateral white column	1. Lateral spinothalamic tract 2. Ventral spinocerebellar tract 3. Dorsal spinocerebellar tract 4. Spinotectal tract 5. Fasiculus dorsolateralis 6. Spinoreticular tract 7. Spino-olivary tract 8. Spinovestibular tract
Posterior white column	1. Fasciculus gracilis 2. Fasciculus cuneatus 3. Comma tract of Schultze

TABLE 143.2: Ascending tracts of spinal cord

Situation	Tract	Origin	Course	Termination	Function
Anterior white column	1. Anterior spinothalamic tract	Chief sensory nucleus	Crossing in spinal cord Forms spinal lemniscus	Ventral posterolateral nucleus of thalamus	Crude touch sensation
Lateral white column	1. Lateral spinothalamic tract	Substantia gelatinosa	Crossing in spinal cord Forms spinal lemniscus	Ventral posterolateral nucleus of thalamus	Pain and temperature sensations
	2. Ventral spinocerebellar tract	Marginal nucleus	Crossing in spinal cord	Anterior lobe of cerebellum	Subconscious kinesthetic sensations
	3. Dorsal spinocerebellar tract	Clarke nucleus	Uncrossed fibers	Anterior lobe of cerebellum	Subconscious kinesthetic sensations
	4. Spinotectal tract	Chief sensory nucleus	Crossing in spinal cord	Superior colliculus	Spinovisual reflex
	5. Fasciculus dorsolateralis	Posterior nerve root ganglion	Component of lateral spinothalamic tract	Substantia gelatinosa	Pain and temperature sensations
	6. Spinoreticular tract	Intermediolateral cells	Crossed and uncrossed fibers	Reticular formation of brainstem	Consciousness and awareness
	7. Spino-olivary tract	Non-specific	Uncrossed fibers	Olivary nucleus	Proprioception
	8. Spinovestibular tract	Non-specific	Crossed and uncrossed fibers	Lateral vestibular nucleus	Proprioception
Posterior white column	1. Fasciculus gracilis	Posterior nerve root ganglia	Uncrossed fibers No synapse in spinal cord	Nucleus gracilis in medulla	Tactile sensation Tactile localization Tactile discrimination Vibratory sensation Conscious kinesthetic sensation Stereognosis
	2. Fasciculus cuneatus	Posterior nerve root ganglia	Uncrossed fibers No synapse in spinal cord	Nucleus cuneatus in medulla	

Descending tracts

Ascending tracts

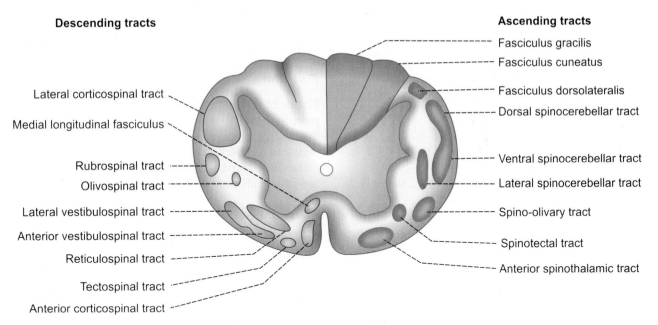

Lateral corticospinal tract

Medial longitudinal fasciculus

Rubrospinal tract

Olivospinal tract

Lateral vestibulospinal tract

Anterior vestibulospinal tract

Reticulospinal tract

Tectospinal tract

Anterior corticospinal tract

Fasciculus gracilis

Fasciculus cuneatus

Fasciculus dorsolateralis

Dorsal spinocerebellar tract

Ventral spinocerebellar tract

Lateral spinocerebellar tract

Spino-olivary tract

Spinotectal tract

Anterior spinothalamic tract

FIGURE 143.3: Tracts of spinal cord

Few fibers of this tract ascend in posterior gray horn for 2 or 3 segments in the same side and then cross over to the anterior white column of opposite side.

While ascending through brainstem, the number of fibers is considerably reduced since some of the fibers form the collaterals and reach the reticular formation of brainstem.

Termination

Fibers of anterior spinothalamic tract terminate in the **ventral posterolateral nucleus** of **thalamus**. Neurons of this thalamic nucleus form third order neurons of the pathway. Fibers from thalamic nucleus carry the impulses to somesthetic area (sensory cortex) of cerebral cortex.

Function

Anterior spinothalamic tract carries impulses of **crude touch** (protopathic) sensation.

Effect of Lesion

Bilateral lesion of this tract leads to loss of crude touch sensation and loss of sensations like itching and tickling. Unilateral lesion of this tract causes **loss of crude touch** sensation in opposite side below the level of lesion (because fibers of this tract cross to the opposite side in spinal cord).

■ 2. LATERAL SPINOTHALAMIC TRACT

Lateral spinothalamic tract is formed by the fibers from second order neurons of the pathway for the sensations of **pain** and **temperature** (Fig. 143.4).

Situation

Lateral spinothalamic tract is situated in the **lateral column** towards medial side, i.e. near the gray matter.

Origin

Fibers of lateral spinothalamic tract take origin from two sources:
  i. Marginal nucleus
  ii. Substantia gelatinosa of Rolando.

Course

Lateral spinothalamic tract has **crossed fibers**. Axons from **marginal nucleus** and **substantia gelatinosa** of **Rolando** cross to the opposite side and reach the lateral column of same segment. Few fibers may ascend one or two segments, then cross to the opposite side and then ascend in the lateral column.

All the fibers pass through medulla, pons and midbrain and reach thalamus along with fibers of anterior spinothalamic tract. Some of the fibers of lateral spinothalamic tract form collaterals and reach the reticular formation of brainstem.

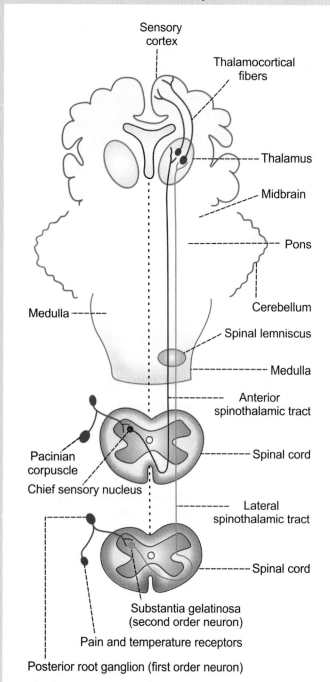

FIGURE 143.4: Spinothalamic tracts and pathways for crude touch, pain and temperature sensations. Anterior spinothalamic tract (red) carries crude touch sensation. Lateral spinothalamic tract (blue) carries pain and temperature sensations.

Fibers of lateral spinothalamic tract form **spinal lemniscus** along with the fibers of anterior spinothalamic tract at the lower part of medulla.

Termination

Fibers of lateral spinothalamic tract terminate in the **ventral posterolateral nucleus** of **thalamus** along with anterior spinothalamic tract fibers. From here, third order neuron fibers run to somesthetic area (sensory cortex) of cerebral cortex.

Function

Fibers of lateral spinothalamic tract carry impulses of **pain** and **temperature** sensations. Fibers arising from this marginal nucleus transmit impulses of fast pain sensation. Fibers arising from substantia gelatinosa of Rolando transmit impulses of slow pain and temperature sensations. Refer Chapter 145 for details of pain fibers.

Effect of Lesion

Bilateral lesion of this tract leads to total loss of pain and temperature sensations on both sides below the level of lesion. Unilateral lesion or sectioning of the lateral spinothalamic tract causes loss of pain **(analgesia)** and temperature **(thermoanesthesia)** below the level of lesion in the opposite side.

■ 3. VENTRAL SPINOCEREBELLAR TRACT

Ventral spinocerebellar tract is also known as **Gower tract, indirect spinocerebellar tract** or **anterior spino-cerebellar tract.** It is constituted by the fibers of second order neurons of the pathway for **subconscious kinesthetic sensation** (Fig. 143.5).

Situation

This tract is situated in **lateral white column** of the spinal cord along the lateral periphery.

Origin

Fibers of this tract arise from the **marginal nucleus** in posterior gray horn. Neurons of marginal nucleus form the second order neurons. Fibers from these neurons make their first appearance in **lower lumbar segments** of spinal cord.

First order neurons are in the posterior root ganglia and receive the impulses of proprioception from the proprioceptors in muscle, tendon and joints. Fibers from neurons of posterior root ganglia reach the marginal cells through posterior nerve root.

Course

Ventral spinocerebellar tract contains both **crossed** and **uncrossed fibers.** Majority of the fibers from the marginal nucleus cross the midline and ascend in lateral white column of opposite side. Some fibers ascend in the lateral white column of the same side also. These nerve fibers ascend through other spinal segments, medulla, pons and midbrain.

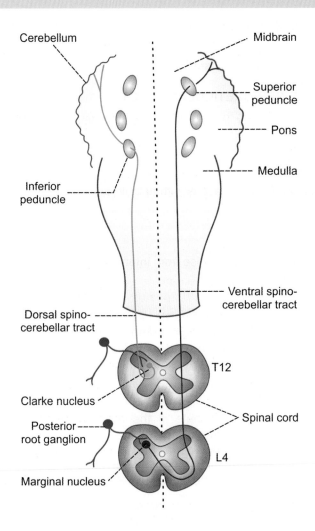

Cerebellum

Midbrain

Superior peduncle

Pons

Medulla

Inferior peduncle

Ventral spino- cerebellar tract

Dorsal spino- cerebellar tract

T12

Clarke nucleus

Spinal cord

Posterior root ganglion

L4

Marginal nucleus

FIGURE 143.5: Spinocerebellar tracts and pathway for subconscious kinesthetic sensation

Finally, the fibers reach the cerebellum through the superior cerebellar peduncle.

Termination

These fibers terminate in the cortex of anterior lobe of **cerebellum.**

Function

Ventral spinocerebellar tract carries the impulses of **subconscious kinesthetic sensation** (proprioceptive impulses from muscles, tendons and joints). Impulses of subconscious kinesthetic sensation are also called **non-sensory impulses.**

Effect of Lesion

Lesion of this tract leads to loss of subconscious kinesthetic sensation in the opposite side.

■ 4. DORSAL SPINOCEREBELLAR TRACT

Dorsal spinocerebellar tract is otherwise called **Flechsig tract, direct spinocerebellar tract** or **posterior spinocerebellar tract.** Like the ventral spinocerebellar tract, this tract is also constituted by the second order neuron fibers of the pathway for subconscious kinesthetic sensation. The first order neurons are in the posterior nerve root ganglia. But, the fibers of this tract are uncrossed (Fig. 143.5).

Situation

Dorsal spinocerebellar tract is situated in the **lateral column** along the posterolateral periphery of spinal cord. It is situated posterior to ventral cerebellar tract and anterior to the entry of posterior nerve root.

Origin

Fibers of this tract originate from the **dorsal nucleus of Clarke** situated in the posterior gray matter of the spinal cord. First appearance of the fibers is in **upper lumbar segments.** From lower lumbar and sacral segments, the impulses are carried upwards by dorsal nerve roots to upper lumbar segments.

Course

Flechsig tract is formed by **uncrossed fibers.** Axons from neurons in dorsal nucleus of Clarke (second order neurons) reach lateral column of same side. Then, these fibers ascend through other spinal segments and reach medulla oblongata. From here, the fibers reach cerebellum through inferior cerebellar peduncle.

Termination

Fibers of this tract end in the cortex of anterior lobe of **cerebellum** along with ventral spinocerebellar tract fibers.

Function

Along with ventral spinocerebellar tract, the dorsal spinocerebellar tract carries the impulses of **subconscious kinesthetic sensation,** which are known as **non-sensory impulses.**

Effect of Lesion

Unilateral loss of the subconscious kinesthetic sensation occurs in lesion of this tract on the same side, as this tract has uncrossed fibers.

■ 5. SPINOTECTAL TRACT

Spinotectal tract is considered as a component of anterior spinothalamic tract. It is constituted by the fibers of second order neurons.

Situation

Spinotectal tract occupies the lateral side of **lateral white column,** anterior to lateral spinothalamic tract. It is bound anteriorly by anterior nerve root.

Origin

Fibers of this tract originate from the **chief sensory nucleus** (like anterior spinothalamic tract). First appearance of the fibers is in upper lumbar segments. This tract is very prominent in the cervical segments.

Course

Spinotectal tract contains **crossed fibers.** After taking origin, the fibers cross to opposite side through anterior white commissure to the lateral column. Then, these fibers ascend to the midbrain along with anterior spinothalamic tract.

Termination

Fibers of spinotectal tract end in the **superior colliculus** of tectum in midbrain.

Function

Spinotectal tract is concerned with **spinovisual reflex.**

■ 6. FASCICULUS DORSOLATERALIS

Fasciculus dorsolateralis is otherwise called **tract of Lissauer.** It is considered as a component of lateral spinothalamic tract. And, it is constituted by the fibers of first order neurons.

Situation

Lissauer tract is situated in the **lateral white column** between the periphery of spinal cord and tip of posterior gray horn.

Origin

Lissauer tract is formed by fibers arising from the **cells of posterior root ganglia** and enters the spinal cord through lateral division of posterior nerve root.

Course

Lissauer tract contains **uncrossed fibers.** After entering spinal cord, the fibers pass upwards or downwards for few segments on the same side and synapse with cells of substantia gelatinosa of Rolando. Axons from these cells (second order neurons) join the lateral spinothalamic tract.

Function

Fibers of the dorsolateral fasciculus carry impulses of **pain** and **thermal sensations.**

■ 7. SPINORETICULAR TRACT

Spinoreticular tract is formed by the fibers of second order neurons.

Situation

Spinoreticular tract is situated in **anterolateral white column.**

Origin

Fibers of this tract arise from **intermediolateral nucleus.**

Course

Spinoreticular tract consists of **crossed** and **uncrossed** fibers. After taking origin, some of the fibers cross the midline and then ascend upwards. Remaining fibers ascend up in the same side without crossing.

Termination

All the fibers terminate in the reticular formation of brainstem by three ways:

  i. Some fibers terminate in **nucleus reticularis gigantocellularis** and **lateral reticular nucleus** of medulla in the same side. Some fibers terminate in the nuclei present in the opposite side.
 ii. Some fibers terminate in **nucleus reticularis pontis caudalis** of the pons in the same side or opposite side
iii. Very few fibers terminate in midbrain.

Function

Fibers of the spinoreticular tract are the components of ascending reticular activating system and are concerned with consciousness and awareness.

■ 8. SPINO-OLIVARY TRACT

Spino-olivary tract is situated in anterolateral part of white column. Origin of the fibers of this tract is not specific. However, the fibers terminate in olivary nucleus of medulla oblongata. From here, the neurons project into cerebellum. This tract is concerned with **proprioception.**

■ 9. SPINOVESTIBULAR TRACT

Spinovestibular tract is situated in the **lateral white column** of the spinal cord. Fibers of this tract arise from all the segments of spinal cord and terminate on the **lateral vestibular nucleus**. This tract is also concerned with **proprioception**.

■ 10. FASCICULUS GRACILIS (TRACT OF GOLL) AND

■ 11. FASCICULUS CUNEATUS (TRACT OF BURDACH)

Fasciculus gracilis and fasciculus cuneatus are together called **ascending posterior column tracts**. These tracts are formed by the fibers from posterior root ganglia. Thus, both the tracts are constituted by the fibers of **first order neurons** of sensory pathway (Fig. 143.6).

Situation

Tracts of Goll and Burdach are situated in **posterior white column** of spinal cord hence the name posterior column tracts. In the cervical and upper thoracic segments of spinal cord, the posterior white column is divided by posterior intermediate septum into medial fasciculus gracilis and lateral fasciculus cuneatus.

Thus, the fasciculus gracilis is situated medially in between posterior median sulcus and posterior median septum on one side and posterior intermediate sulcus and posterior intermediate septum on the other side. Fasciculus cuneatus is situated laterally. It is bound medially by posterior intermediate septum and sulcus and laterally by posterior gray horn, tract of Lissauer and posterior nerve root.

Origin

Fibers of these two tracts are the axons of **first order neurons**. Cell body of these neurons is in the **posterior root ganglia** and their fibers form the medial division (bundle) of posterior nerve root.

Course

After entering spinal cord, the fibers ascend through the **posterior white column**. These fibers do not synapse in the spinal cord. Some fibers of medial division of posterior nerve root descend through posterior white column in the form of **fasciculus interfascicularis** or **comma tract of Schultze**.

Fasciculus gracilis contains the fibers from **lower extremities** and **lower parts of the body**, i.e. from sacral, lumbar and lower thoracic ganglia of posterior nerve root. Fasciculus cuneatus contains fibers from **upper part of the body**, i.e. from upper thoracic and cervical ganglia of posterior nerve root.

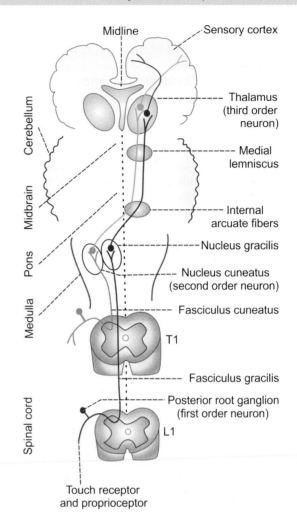

FIGURE 143.6: Ascending tracts in posterior white column of spinal cord and pathway for – 1. Fine touch sensation, 2. Tactile localization, 3. Tactile discrimination, 4. Vibratory sensation, 5. Conscious kinesthetic sensation, 6. Stereognosis.

Termination

Tracts of Goll and Burdach terminate in the medulla oblongata. Fibers of fasciculus gracilis terminate in the **nucleus gracilis** and the fibers of fasciculus cuneatus terminate in the **nucleus cuneatus**. Neurons of these medullary nuclei form the second order neurons.

Axons of second order neurons form the **internal arcuate fibers**. Internal arcuate fibers from both sides cross the midline forming **sensory decussation** and then ascend through pons and midbrain as **medial lemniscus**. Fibers of medial lemniscus terminate in **ventral posterolateral nucleus of thalamus**. From here, fibers of the third order neurons relay to **sensory area of cerebral cortex**.

Functions

Tracts of the posterior white column convey impulses of following sensations:

    i. **Fine** (epicritic) **tactile sensation**

    ii. **Tactile localization** (ability to locate the area of skin where the tactile stimulus is applied with closed eyes)

    iii. **Tactile discrimination** or two point discrimination (ability to recognize the two stimuli applied over the skin simultaneously with closed eyes)

    iv. **Sensation of vibration** (ability to perceive the vibrations from a vibrating tuning fork placed over bony prominence conducted to deep tissues through skin). It is the synthetic sense (Chapter 144) produced by combination of touch and pressure sensations.

    v. **Conscious kinesthetic sensation** (sensation or awareness of various muscular activities in different parts of the body)

    vi. **Stereognosis** (ability to recognize the known objects by touch with closed eyes). It is also a synthetic sense produced by combination of touch and pressure sensations.

Effect of Lesion

Lesion of nerve fibers in tracts of Goll and Burdach or lesion in the posterior white column leads to the following symptoms on the same side below the lesion:

    i. Loss of fine tactile sensation; however, crude touch sensation is normal

    ii. Loss of tactile localization

    iii. Loss of two point discrimination

    iv. Loss of sensation of vibration

    v. **Astereognosis** (inability to recognize known objects by touch while closing the eyes)

    vi. Lack of ability to differentiate the weight of different objects

    vii. Loss of proprioception (inability to appreciate the position and movement of different parts of the body)

    viii. **Sensory ataxia** or posterior column ataxia (condition characterized by uncoordinated, slow and clumsy voluntary movements because of the loss of proprioception).

■ 12. COMMA TRACT OF SCHULTZE

Comma tract of schultze is also called fasciculus interfascicularis. It is situated in between tracts of Goll and Burdach. This tract is formed by the short descending fibers, arising from the medial division of posterior nerve root. These fibers are also considered as the descending branches of the tracts of Goll and Burdach. Function of this tract is to establish intersegmental communications and to form short reflex arc.

■ DESCENDING TRACTS OF SPINAL CORD

Descending tracts of the spinal cord are formed by motor nerve fibers arising from brain and descend into the spinal cord. These tracts carry motor impulses from brain to spinal cord.

    Descending tracts of spinal cord are of two types:

A. Pyramidal tracts

B. Extrapyramidal tracts.

    Descending tracts are listed in Table 143.3 and their features given in Table 143.4.

■ PYRAMIDAL TRACTS

Pyramidal tracts were the first tracts to be found in man. Pyramidal tracts of spinal cord are the descending tracts concerned with voluntary motor activities of the body. These tracts are otherwise known as **corticospinal tracts.** There are two corticospinal tracts, the anterior corticospinal tract and lateral corticospinal tract. While running from cerebral cortex towards spinal cord, the fibers of these two tracts give the appearance of a **pyramid** on the upper part of anterior surface of medulla oblongata hence the name pyramidal tracts (Fig. 143.7).

Nerve Fibers

All the fibers of the pyramidal tracts are present since birth. However, myelination of these fibers is completed in about 2 years after birth. The pyramidal tracts on each side have more than a million fibers. About 70% of the fibers are large myelinated fibers having a diameter of 4 to 22 micron.

TABLE 143.3: List of descending tracts of spinal cord

Type	Tract
Pyramidal tracts	1. Anterior corticospinal tract 2. Lateral corticospinal tract
Extrapyramidal tracts	1. Medial longitudinal fasciculus 2. Anterior vestibulospinal tract 3. Lateral vestibulospinal tract 4. Reticulospinal tract 5. Tectospinal tract 6. Rubrospinal tract 7. Olivospinal tract

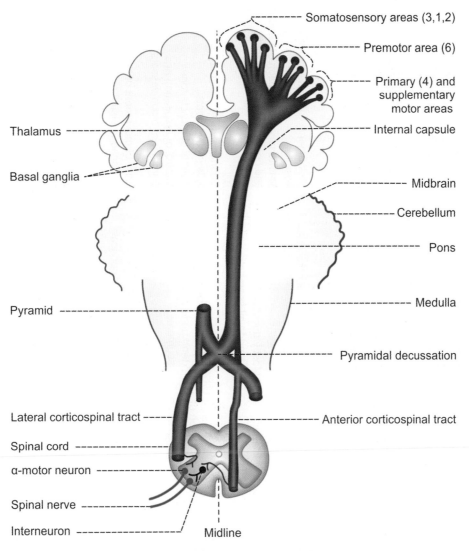

Somatosensory areas (3,1,2)

Premotor area (6)

Primary (4) and
supplementary
motor areas

Thalamus

Internal capsule

Basal ganglia

Midbrain

Cerebellum

Pons

Medulla

Pyramid

Pyramidal decussation

Lateral corticospinal tract

Anterior corticospinal tract

Spinal cord

α-motor neuron

Spinal nerve

Interneuron

Midline

FIGURE 143.7: Pyramidal tracts

Large fibers of pyramidal tracts have the tendency to disappear at old age. Since these tracts are concerned with control of voluntary movements, the disappearance of the fibers of pyramidal tracts causes automatic **shivering** movements in old age.

Fibers of pyramidal tracts are the axons of upper motor neurons.

Origin

Fibers of pyramidal tracts arise from following cells or areas of cerebral cortex:

1. **Giant cells** or **Betz cells** or pyramidal cells in precentral gyrus of the motor cortex. These cells are situated in area 4 (primary motor area) of frontal lobe.

2. Other areas of motor cortex namely, premotor area (area 6) and supplementary motor areas

3. Other parts of frontal lobe

4. Somatosensory areas of parietal lobe.

It is believed that 30% of pyramidal fibers arise from primary motor area (area 4) and supplementary motor areas, another 30% from premotor area (area 6) and the remaining 40% of fibers arise from somatosensory areas. All the above fibers form fibers of upper motor neurons of motor pathway.

Course

Corona radiata

After taking origin, the nerve fibers run downwards in a diffused manner through white matter of cerebral hemisphere and converge in the form of a fan-like structure along with ascending fibers, which project from thalamus to cerebral cortex. This fan-like structure

TABLE 143.4: Descending tracts of spinal cord

	Tract	Situation	Origin	Course	Function
Pyramidal Tracts	1. Anterior corticospinal tract	Anterior white column	Betz cells and other cells of motor area	Uncrossed fibers	i. Control of voluntary movements
	2. Lateral corticospinal tract	Lateral white column	Betz cells and other cells of motor area	Crossed fibers	ii. Form upper motor neurons
Extrapyramidal tracts	1. Medial longitudinal fasciculus	Anterior white column	Vestibular nucleus Reticular formation Superior colliculus and cells of Cajal	Uncrossed fibers Extend up to uppercervical segments	i. Coordination of reflex ocular movements ii. Integration of movements of eyes and neck
	2. Anterior vestibulospinal tract	Anterior white column	Medial vestibular nucleus	Uncrossed fibers Extend up to upper thoracic segments	i. Maintenance of muscle tone and posture ii. Maintenance of position of head and body during acceleration
	3. Lateral vestibulospinal tract	Lateral white column	Lateral vestibular nucleus	Mostly uncrossed Extend to all segments	
	4. Reticulospinal tract	Lateral white fasciculus	Reticular formation of pons and medulla	Mostly uncrossed Extend up to thoracic segments	i. Coordination of voluntary and reflex movements ii. Control of muscle tone iii. Control of respiration and diameter of blood vessels
	5. Tectospinal tract	Anterior white column	Superior colliculus	Crossed fibers Extend up to lower cervical segments	Control of movement of head in response to visual and auditory impulses
	6. Rubrospinal tract	Lateral white column	Red nucleus	Crossed fibers Extend up to thoracic segments	Facilitatory influence on flexor muscle tone
	7. Olivospinal tract	Lateral white column	Inferior olivary nucleus	Mostly crossed Extent – not clear	Control of movements due to proprioception

Termination – fibers of all the tracts terminate in motor neurons situated in the anterior gray horn of spinal cord.

is called corona radiata. Thus, corona radiata contains both ascending fibers from thalamus and descending fibers from cerebral cortex.

Internal capsule

While passing down towards the brainstem the corona radiata converges in the form of internal capsule. It is situated in between thalamus and caudate nucleus on the medial side and lenticular nucleus on the lateral side (Chapter 148).

In pons

The fibers descend down through internal capsule, midbrain and pons. While descending through pons, the fibers are divided into different bundles by the nuclei of pons. At lower border of pons, the fibers are grouped once again into a compact bundle and then descend down into medulla oblongata.

In medulla

This compact bundle of corticospinal fibers gives the appearance of a **pyramid** in the anterior surface of upper part of medulla. So, the corticospinal tracts are called the pyramidal tracts.

At the lower border of medulla, pyramidal tract on each side is divided into two bundles of unequal sizes. About 80% of fibers from each side cross to the opposite side. While crossing the midline, the fibers of both sides form the **pyramidal decussation.**

In spinal cord

Fibers which cross the midline and form pyramidal decussation descend through posterior part of lateral white column of spinal cord. This bundle of crossed fibers is called the **crossed pyramidal tract** or **lateral corticospinal tract** or **indirect corticospinal tract.**

Remaining 20% of fibers do not cross to the opposite side but descend down through the anterior white column of the spinal cord. This bundle of uncrossed fibers is called the **uncrossed pyramidal tract** or **anterior corticospinal tract** or **direct corticospinal tract.** This tract is well marked in cervical region. Since, the fibers of this tract terminate in different segments of spinal cord, this tract usually gets thinner while descending through the successive segments of spinal cord. Fibers of this tract are absent mostly below the mid thoracic level. Before termination, majority of the fibers of this anterior corticospinal tract cross to the opposite side at different levels of spinal cord.

Termination

All the fibers of pyramidal tracts, both crossed and uncrossed fibers, terminate in the motor neurons of anterior gray horn either directly or through internuncial neurons. Pyramidal tract fibers terminate on both **α-motor neurons** and **β-motor neurons.** Axons of the motor neurons leave the spinal cord as spinal nerves through anterior nerve roots and supply the skeletal muscles.

Neurons giving origin to the fibers of pyramidal tract are called the **upper motor neurons.** Anterior motor neurons in the spinal cord are called the **lower motor neurons.**

Function

Pyramidal tracts are concerned with **voluntary movements** of the body. Fibers of the pyramidal tracts transmit motor impulses from motor area of cerebral cortex to the anterior motor neurons of the spinal cord. These two tracts are responsible for fine, skilled movements.

Effects of lesion

Lesion in the neurons of motor cortex and the fibers of pyramidal tracts is called the **upper motor neuron lesion.** In human beings, pure pyramidal tract lesions do not occur. Lesion of pyramidal fibers occurs most commonly in **stroke** (cardiovascular accident) due to hemorrhage and thrombosis. During such lesions, many extrapyramidal fibers are also damaged along with pyramidal fibers. Because of this reason, neurologists often consider the lesion as upper motor neuron lesion and not as pyramidal tract lesion.

Following are the effects of lesion:

1. *Voluntary movements*

Voluntary movements of the body are very much affected. Initially, there is loss of voluntary movements in the extremities. Later, it involves the other parts of the body like hip and shoulder.

2. *Muscle tone*

Muscle tone is increased leading to **spasticity.** Muscles are also paralyzed. This type of paralysis of muscles is called the **spastic paralysis.** The spasticity is due to the failure of inhibitory impulses from upper motor neurons, particularly the neurons of extrapyramidal system to reach the γ-motor neurons in spinal cord.

However, hypotonia occurs in pure pyramidal tract lesion, which is very rare. In monkeys, sectioning of pyramidal tract fibers alone results in **hypotonia.**

3. *Reflexes*

All the superficial reflexes are lost and the deep reflexes are exaggerated. Abnormal plantar reflex called **Babinski sign** is present (Babinski sign positive).

More details of upper motor neuron lesion are given in the next chapter.

Effects of Lesion at Different Levels

Cerebral cortex

Lesion of pyramidal tract fibers in cerebral cortex causes **hypertonia, spasticity** and contralateral monoplegia (paralysis of one limb) or contralateral **hemiplegia** (paralysis of one side of the body).

Internal capsule

Lesion of pyramidal tract fibers at posterior limb of internal capsule results in contralateral **hemiplegia.**

Brainstem

Lesion at brainstem involves not only pyramidal tract fibers but also other structures such as VI and VII cranial nerve nuclei. So the lesion results in contralateral **hemiparesis** (weakness of muscles in one side of the body) along with VI and VII cranial nerve palsies.

Spinal cord

Unilateral lesion of lateral corticospinal fibers at upper cervical segment causes ipsilateral **hemiplegia** and bilateral lesion causes **quadriplegia** (paralysis of all four limbs) and paralysis of respiratory muscles.

Bilateral lesion of these fibers in thoracic and lumbar segments results in **paraplegia** (paralysis of both lower limbs) without paralysis of respiratory muscles.

■ EXTRAPYRAMIDAL TRACTS

Descending tracts of spinal cord other than pyramidal tracts are called extrapyramidal tracts. Extrapyramidal tracts are listed in Table 143.3.

■ 1. MEDIAL LONGITUDINAL FASCICULUS

Situation

Medial longitudinal fasciculus descends through posterior part of **anterior white column** of the spinal cord.

Origin

Actually, this tract is the extension of medial longitudinal fasciculus of brainstem. Fibers of this tract take origin from four different areas in brainstem:

   i. Vestibular nuclei
   ii. Reticular formation
   iii. Superior colliculus
   iv. Interstitial cells of Cajal.

Course

After entering the spinal cord from the brainstem, the fibers of medial longitudinal fasciculus descend through posterior part of anterior white column of the same side. In the spinal cord, this tract is well defined only in upper cervical segments. Below this level, the fibers run along with the fibers of anterior vestibulospinal tract.

Extent

Fibers of this tract extend up to the **upper cervical segments** of spinal cord.

Termination

Fibers of this tract terminate in anterior motor neurons of the spinal cord along with fibers of anterior vestibulospinal tract either directly or through internuncial neurons.

Function

Medial longitudinal fasciculus helps in the coordination of **reflex ocular movements** and the integration of ocular and neck movements.

Effects of Lesion

Reflex ocular movements and reflex neck movements are affected in the lesion of this tract.

■ 2. ANTERIOR VESTIBULOSPINAL TRACT

Situation

Anterior vestibulospinal tract is situated in the **anterior white column,** along the periphery of spinal cord lateral to tectospinal tract.

Origin

Fibers of this tract arise from medial vestibular nucleus in medulla oblongata. In fact, anterior vestibulospinal tract is the extension of medial longitudinal fasciculus. Most of the fibers are uncrossed.

Extent

Fibers run up to **thoracic segments** of spinal cord.

Course

Fibers of this tract run down from medulla into the anterior column of spinal cord along the periphery. All the fibers are uncrossed.

Termination

Along with fibers of lateral vestibulospinal tract, the fibers of this tract terminate in anterior motor neurons directly or through internuncial neurons.

Function

Function of this tract is explained along with the function of lateral vestibulospinal tract.

■ 3. LATERAL VESTIBULOSPINAL TRACT

Situation

Lateral vestibulospinal tract occupies the anterior part of **lateral white column** of spinal cord.

Origin

Fibers of this tract take origin from the **lateral vestibular nucleus** in medulla. This nucleus is also called Deiter nucleus.

Extent

Fibers of this tract are present **throughout the spinal cord.**

Course

From Deiter nucleus, most of the fibers descend directly through lateral column. Very few fibers cross to the opposite side before descending.

Termination

Fibers of this tract terminate in the anterior motor neuron, either directly or via internuncial neurons.

Functions

Vestibular nuclei receive impulses concerned with muscle tone and posture from vestibular apparatus and cerebellum. Vestibular nuclei in turn convey the impulses to different parts of the body through the anterior and lateral vestibulospinal tracts.

Vestibulospinal tracts are concerned with adjustment of **position of head and body** during angular and linear acceleration.

Effect of Lesion

Adjustment of head and body becomes difficult during acceleration when the vestibulospinal tracts are affected by lesion.

■ 4. RETICULOSPINAL TRACT

Situation

Reticulospinal tract is situated in the **anterior white column,** posterior to anterior vestibulospinal tract.

Origin

Fibers of this tract arise from the **reticular formation** of pons and medulla. Pontine reticular fibers are uncrossed (direct) and descend in medial part of anterior column. Fibers from medullary reticular formation are predominantly uncrossed and only few fibers are crossed. These fibers descend in lateral part of anterior column and to some extend in the anterior part of lateral column.

Extent

Fibers of reticulospinal tract extend up to **thoracic segments.**

Termination

Fibers of reticulospinal tract terminate in gamma motor neurons of anterior gray horn through the internuncial neuron.

Functions

Reticulospinal tract is concerned with control of **movements** and maintenance of **muscle tone,** respiration and diameter of blood vessels. Pontine and medullary fibers have opposite effects on these functions, which are given in Table 143.5.

TABLE 143.5: Functions of pontine and medullary reticulospinal fibers

Function	Pontine reticular fibers	Medullary reticular fibers
Control of voluntary and reflex movements	Facilitation	Inhibition
Control of muscle tone through gamma motor neurons	Facilitation	Inhibition
On respiration	Favor expiration	Favor inspiration
On blood vessels	Cause vasoconstriction	Cause vasodilatation

Effect of Lesion

Lesion of reticulospinal tract causes disturbances in respiration, blood pressure, movements of body and muscle tone.

■ 5. TECTOSPINAL TRACT

Situation

Tectospinal tract is situated in the **anterior white column** of spinal cord.

Origin

Nerve fibers of this tract arise from **superior colliculus** of midbrain.

Extent

Tectospinal tract extends only up to **lower cervical segments.**

Course

After taking origin from superior colliculus, the fibers cross the midline in dorsal tegmental decussation and descend in anterior column.

Termination

Fibers of tectospinal tract terminate in the anterior motor neurons of spinal cord, directly or via internuncial neurons.

Function

Tectospinal tract is responsible for the **movement of head** in response to visual and auditory stimuli.

■ 6. RUBROSPINAL TRACT

Situation

Rubrospinal tract is situated in the **lateral white column** of spinal cord.

Origin

Fibers of this tract arise from large cells (nucleus magnocellularis) of **red nucleus** in midbrain.

Extent

Nerve fibers of this tract appear in the spinal cord only **up to thoracic segments.**

Course

After arising from the red nucleus, the fibers cross the midline in ventral tegmental decussation and descend into spinal cord through the reticular formation of pons and medulla.

Termination

Fibers of rubrospinal tract end in the anterior motor neurons of the spinal cord via internuncial neurons.

Function

Rubrospinal tract exhibits facilitatory influence upon **flexor muscle tone.**

■ 7. OLIVOSPINAL TRACT

Situation

Olivospinal tract is present in **lateral white column** of spinal cord.

Origin

The nerve fibers of the olivospinal tract take origin from the **inferior olivary nucleus,** which is present in the medulla oblongata.

Termination

Fibers of this tract terminate in the anterior motor neurons of spinal cord.

Function

Functions of the olivospinal tract are not known clearly. It is believed that this tract is involved in **reflex movements** arising from the proprioceptors.

■ APPLIED PHYSIOLOGY

Spinal cord injury leads to either temporary or permanent dysfunction. Dysfunction of spinal cord occurs because of:
1. Direct injury due to bullet firing or accidents (on road, in working place, during communal violence, etc.)
2. Compression by bone fragments, hematoma or disk material
3. Ischemia due to rupture of spinal arteries.
   During mechanical injury, spinal cord may be cut into two or one lateral half of the spinal cord may be damaged or diffused crushing of several segments of spinal cord may also occur.

Accordingly, dysfunction of spinal cord is classified into four types:

A. Complete transection
B. Incomplete transection
C. Hemisection
D. Diseases of spinal cord.

■ COMPLETE TRANSECTION OF SPINAL CORD

Complete transection of spinal cord occurs due to:

1. Bullet injury, which causes dislocation of spinal cord
2. Accidents, which cause dislocation of spinal cord or occlusion of blood vessels.

Complete transection causes immediate **loss of sensation** and **voluntary movement** below the level of lesion. In quick transection of spinal cord, the patient feels himself cut into two. For a while, his mind remains clear but he feels as if his lower part of the body below the injury does not exist. It is because his higher centers remain unaffected but the spinal centers below the level of injury loose the function.

Then the effects (symptoms) of complete transection of spinal cord start appearing. Effects occur in three stages:

1. Stage of spinal shock
2. Stage of reflex activity
3. Stage of reflex failure.

1. Stage of Spinal Shock

Stage of spinal shock is the first stage of effects that occurs immediately after injury. It is also called **stage of flaccidity.** Following are the signs and symptoms that develop during this stage:

i. Paralysis of limbs

Paralysis occurs in two limbs or in all four limbs. Paralysis of limbs depends upon the level of Injury:

   a. Injury at the cervical region of the spinal cord leads to the paralysis of all the four limbs. Paralysis of all the four limbs is called **quadriplegia** or **tetraplegia**
   b. Injury at the thoracic, lumbar or sacral segments including cauda equina and conus medullaris causes paralysis of lower limbs. Paralysis of lower limbs is called **paraplegia.**

ii. Flaccid paralysis

Paralyzed muscles become flaccid, i.e. loose stiffness because of loss of tone. This type of paralysis is called **flaccid paralysis.**

iii. Loss of reflexes

All the reflexes are lost because of the injury to anterior and posterior nerve roots.

iv. Loss of sensations

All the sensations are lost because of the injury to posterior nerve roots and sensory neurons in the posterior gray horn.

v. Effect on visceral organs

Some of the visceral organs are also affected; especially, urinary bladder and rectum are paralyzed.

vi. Heart rate

Heart rate is decreased and pulse becomes weak and thready.

vii. Venous return

Venous return is very much decreased. Venous return depends upon the muscle tone during resting condition. During activity it depends upon contraction of skeletal muscle (muscle pump, refer to Chapter 98). But, in complete transection of spinal cord, muscle tone is lost and flaccid paralysis occurs. This leads to decrease in venous return.

In addition, the limbs are immobile and smooth muscles of blood vessels loose the tone. So, the blood gets accumulated in blood vessels of limbs, particularly in lower limbs. And, the lower limbs become **cold and blue.**

viii. Effect on blood pressure

Effect on blood pressure depends upon the level of injury:

   a. *Lesion anywhere below L2 segment*
      Blood pressure is not affected much because the sympathetic vasoconstrictor fibers leave the spinal cord between T1 and L2 segments.
   b. *Lesion at or above T1 segment*
      All the sympathetic vasoconstrictor fibers leaving the spinal cord from T1 and L2 segments are transected and are completely cut off from higher medullary cardiovascular centers, which regulate the blood pressure. So the blood pressure falls drastically. Mean arterial pressure falls below 40 mm Hg.

Severity of complete transection depends upon the level of lesion. Complete transection at the level of cervical region can be very fatal. Because, the diaphragm and other respiratory muscles are cut off from respiratory centers. It causes paralysis of respiratory muscles leading to sudden arrest of breathing.

The **crushing injury** at sacral segments of spinal cord results in atonic bladder and loss of micturition reflex (Chapter 57).

In human beings, the stage of spinal shock lasts for about 3 weeks. In animals the duration of spinal shock varies in different species. In amphibians like frog, it lasts only for few minutes. In mammals like dogs and cats, it lasts for few hours. In monkeys, it lasts for few days.

2. Stage of Reflex Activity

Stage of reflex activity is also called **stage of recovery.** After 3 weeks period, depending largely upon the general health of the patient, the reflex activity begins to return to the isolated segments of spinal cord below the level of lesion.

Developments taking place in this stage

i. First, the functional activities return to smooth muscles
ii. Next, the sympathetic tone to blood vessels returns. As the neurons in gray horn act independently of vasomotor center, the tone in blood vessels is restored and the blood pressure is also restored to its normal level.
iii. Lastly, after another 3 months, the tone in skeletal muscle returns. Tone returns to flexor muscles first. So, the flexor muscles of lower limb become less flabby and offer some resistance to the toes. Though the tonicity is returned, it is not complete even in flexor muscles. So, the muscles remain hypotonic.

   Limbs in this condition tend to adopt a position of slight flexion and the paralysis is therefore called the **paraplegia in flexion.** Limbs cannot support weight of the body.
iv. After few weeks, when tone returns to more muscles, reflex movements can occur. Flexor reflexes appear first. To elicit the flexor reflex, a painful stimulus is required. First reflex, which usually appears, is the **Babinski reflex.**
v. After a variable period of 1 to 5 weeks of reappearance of flexor reflexes, the extensor reflexes return. Initially, knee jerk returns and then the ankle jerk.
vi. In some cases, a widespread reaction can be elicited by scratching the skin over the lower limbs or the anterior abdominal wall, depending upon the level of lesion. This reaction constitutes the spasm in flexor muscles of both the lower limbs, evacuation of urinary bladder and profuse sweating. This is known as the **mass reflex.**

3. Stage of Reflex Failure

Though the reflex movements return, muscles below the level of injury have less power and less resistance. Usually, general condition of the patient starts deteriorating. General infection or **toxemia** becomes common. Due to this, the failure of reflex function develops. The reflexes become more difficult to elicit. The threshold for stimulus increases. Mass reflex is abolished and the muscles become extremely **flaccid** and undergo **wasting.**

■ INCOMPLETE TRANSECTION OF SPINAL CORD

If spinal cord is gravely injured, but does not suffer complete division, the condition is called as incomplete transection.

Symptoms of Incomplete Transection

After incomplete transection of the spinal cord, all the three stages of complete transection occur.
1. Stage of spinal shock
2. Stage of reflex activity
3. Stage of reflex failure.

1. Stage of Spinal Shock

Features are similar to those of complete transection.

2. Stage of Reflex Activity

Features of this stage:
i. Tone returns to extensor muscles first and not to the flexor muscles. This is because, in incomplete transection, some of the descending fibers in lateral column of cord, especially vestibulospinal and reticulospinal tracts may escape the injury. So, some connections persist between brainstem and spinal cord. Fibers of vestibulospinal and reticulospinal tracts mainly reinforce the activity of extensor motor neurons.

   Because of this, there is extensor hypertonia and so, the lower limbs are extended at hip and knee with toes pointing slightly downwards. This condition is known as **paraplegia in extension.**
ii. Stretch reflex reappears first. Flexor reflexes return later. **Philipson reflex (clasp-knife reflex)** can be elicited.
iii. In the upper limb, some resistance is offered when the arm is flexed at elbow joint passively. That is, the arm cannot be flexed. This resistance is offered because of the stretch reflex developed in the triceps muscle. However, if forearm is flexed forcefully, the resistance to flexion is abolished

suddenly, leading to quick flexion of arm. This is called the **Philipson reflex** or **clasp-knife reflex.**

iv. Mass reflex, which is produced in complete transection, does not occur in incomplete transection of spinal cord.

3. *Stage of Reflex Failure*

Features are similar to those of complete transection.

■ HEMISECTION OF SPINAL CORD – BROWN-SÉQUARD SYNDROME

Lesion involving one lateral half of the spinal cord is called hemisection (Fig. 143.8). It can occur due to injury during accidents. It can also be produced experimentally in animals.

Symptoms of Hemisection of Spinal Cord

Signs and symptoms, which occur after hemisection of the spinal cord, constitute Brown-Séquard syndrome.

If the hemisection is due to injury, spinal shock occurs immediately. Muscles loose the tone and become flaccid. The reflexes are abolished. In case the patient survives, this stage gradually passes off and certain signs and symptoms develop. Effects are seen below the level of lesion and at the level of lesion. Effects in these areas differ on the same side and opposite side. There are changes in sensory and motor functions.

■ EFFECTS OF HEMISECTION OF SPINAL CORD BELOW THE LEVEL OF LESION

On the Same Side

Sensory changes

1. On the same side below the level of lesion, following sensations are lost because these sensations are carried by the **uncrossed fibers** of tracts of Goll and Burdach:
   i. Fine touch
   ii. Tactile localization
   iii. Tactile discrimination
   iv. Sensation of vibration
   v. Conscious kinesthetic sensation
   vi. Stereognosis.
2. Some sensations are not affected because these sensations are carried by **crossed fibers** of spinothalamic tracts. These sensations are:
   i. Crude touch
   ii. Pain
   iii. Temperature.

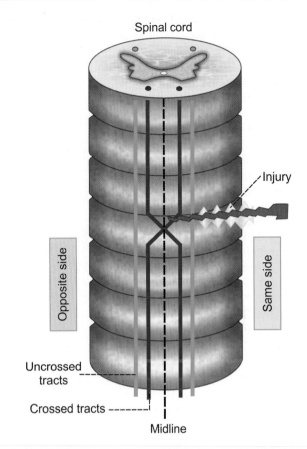

FIGURE 143.8: Hemisection of spinal cord (Brown-Séquard syndrome). Below the level of lesion: same side = loss of sensations carried by uncrossed fibers, opposite side = loss of sensations carried by crossed fibers. At the level of lesion: same side = complete anesthesia, opposite side = loss of sensations carried by crossed fibers.

Motor changes

Motor changes resemble the effects of upper motor neuron lesion (Chapter 144).
1. Muscle tone increases, leading to spastic paralysis
2. Rigidity of limbs occurs
3. Muscle wastage does not occur
4. Superficial reflexes are lost
5. Babinski sign is positive
6. Deep reflexes are exaggerated
7. Fall in blood pressure because of loss of vasomotor tone.

On the Opposite Side

Sensory changes

1. On the opposite side, below the level of lesion, the following sensations are lost completely because, these sensations are carried by **crossed spinothalamic tracts:**

TABLE 143.6: Effects of hemisection (Brown-Séquard syndrome) of spinal cord

Level	Same side		Opposite side	
	Sensory changes	**Motor changes**	**Sensory changes**	**Motor changes**
Below the level of lesion	**Sensations lost** *Sensations carried by uncrossed tracts:* 1. Fine touch 2. Tactile localization 3. Tactile discrimination 4. Vibration sense 5. Conscious kinesthetic sensation 6. Stereognosis **Sensations retained** *Sensations carried by crossed tracts:* 1. Crude touch 2. Pain 3. Temperature	**Upper motor neuron lesion type** 1. Increased tone 2. Spastic paralysis 3. Loss of superficial reflexes 4. Exaggeration of deep reflexes 5. Babinski positive sign 6. Rigidity in the limbs 7. No muscular wastage	**Sensations lost** *Sensations carried by crossed tracts:* 1. Crude touch 2. Pain 3. Temperature **Sensations retained** *Sensations carried by uncrossed tracts:* 1. Fine touch 2. Tactile localization 3. Tactile discrimination 4. Vibration sense 5. Conscious kinesthetic sensation 6. Stereognosis	**No paralysis** *If it occurs:* 1. Very mild 2. Resembles upper motor neuron lesion type
At the level of lesion	**Complete anesthesia**	**Lower motor neuron lesion type** 1. Loss of muscle tone 2. Flaccid paralysis 3. Loss of all reflexes 4. Wastage of muscle 5. Loss of vasomotor tone	**Sensations lost** *Sensations carried by crossed tracts:* 1. Crude touch 2. Pain 3. Temperature **Sensations retained** *Sensations carried by uncrossed tracts:* 1. Fine touch 2. Tactile localization 3. Tactile discrimination 4. Vibration sense 5. Conscious kinesthetic sensation 6. Stereognosis	**No paralysis** *If it occurs:* 1. Very mild 2. Resembles lower motor neuron lesion type

   i. Crude touch
  ii. Pain
 iii. Temperature.
2. Following sensations are not affected because, these sensations are carried by **uncrossed tracts** of Goll and Burdach:
   i. Fine touch
  ii. Tactile localization
 iii. Tactile discrimination
 iv. Sensation of vibration
  v. Conscious kinesthetic sensation
 vi. Stereognosis.

Motor changes

Mostly there may not be any paralysis of muscles. If it occurs, it would be mild as only a few fibers of

pyramidal tract are affected. This is because pyramidal fibers cross to the opposite side. Paralysis is of **upper motor neuron lesion** type.

Thus, during hemisection of spinal cord, motor loss is extensive and sensory loss is less below the level of lesion on the same side. On the opposite side, sensory loss is extensive and motor loss is less.

■ EFFECTS OF HEMISECTION OF SPINAL CORD AT THE LEVEL OF LESION

On the Same Side

Sensory changes

On the same side at the level of hemisection, there is complete anesthesia. That is, all the sensations are lost

(Table 143.6). This is because of complete destruction of the posterior nerve root.

Motor changes

Effects of **lower motor neuron lesion** occur because the motor neurons and their fibers leaving the spinal cord are affected.

Motor changes of lower motor neuron lesion are:

1. Muscles loose the tone and become flaccid and paralyzed. This type of paralysis with loss of muscle tone is called flaccid paralysis.
2. All the reflexes are lost
3. Muscles degenerate and undergo wasting due to loss of tone
4. Vasomotor tone is lost.

On the Opposite Side

Sensory changes

1. There is loss of pain, temperature and crude touch sensations because the **crossed spinothalamic tracts** are affected
2. But tracts of Goll and Burdach are not affected. So, the sensations carried by these two tracts are not affected.

Motor changes

No motor change occurs. If it occurs, it is very mild and is similar to the effects of **lower motor neuron lesion** (Chapter 144).

■ DISEASES OF SPINAL CORD

1. Syringomyelia

Syringomyelia is spinal cord disorder characterized by the presence of **fluid-filled cavities** in the spinal cord. Gray matter around the central canal is the most affected part. So the sensory disturbances are more pronounced than the motor disturbances.

Cause

Stringomyelia occurs due to the over growth of neuroglial cells in spinal cord accompanied by cavity formation and accumulation of fluid. Initially, a cavity appears in gray matter near the central canal of spinal cord. In later stages, the cavity extends and involves the surrounding white matter to a variable degree.

The disease usually starts in one or two segments. Then, it extends up and down for considerable distances. Lower cervical and upper thoracic regions are affected the most.

Features

Characteristic features of this disease are the loss of pain and temperature sensations and muscular weakness. Severity of the loss of sensations depends upon the extent of disease in spinal cord.

Symptoms of syringomyelia:

1. If disease is only **around central canal,** there is loss of temperature, pain and crude touch sensations only. It is due to lesion of the fibers crossing through the anterior gray commissure. Fine touch sensation is not affected because the fibers of fine touch pathway are in the posterior white column.
2. If lesion is **unilateral,** effect occurs only on the same side
3. If disease extends to **posterior gray horn,** all the sensations are lost. Due to loss of pain and temperature sensations, the affected part is not withdrawn either reflexly or consciously from a painful stimulus. So, the affected persons become prone for injuries. Since, the injury is not perceived it leads to severe damage to the tissues.
4. If **anterior gray horn** is affected, there is flaccid paralysis of muscles. In later stages, both pyramidal and extrapyramidal tracts are also involved, if the disease spreads to white matter. It causes spastic paralysis of limbs, especially in lower limbs, resulting in **spastic paraplegia.** Weakness and **wasting** of small muscle of limbs occur. **Winging of scapula** and **scoliosis** (lateral curvature of spine) develops.

2. Tabes Dorsalis

Tabes dorsalis is another disease of the spinal cord. It is a slowly progressive nervous disorder affecting both the motor and sensory functions of spinal cord.

Cause

It occurs due to the degeneration of posterior (sensory) nerve roots. It usually occurs in **syphilis.**

Posterior nerve roots are affected proximal to the posterior root ganglia. Ganglia are not affected. Among the fibers of posterior root, the fibers of lateral division are affected much. Reason for this type of selective degeneration is not known.

Along with lateral fibers of posterior root, the fibers in posterior white column of spinal cord are also affected.

Features

In tabes dorsalis, both sensory and motor functions are affected. Following are the features:

Sensations

1. During the onset of degenerative changes, there is exaggeration of pain sensation
2. Then, there is impairment and loss of all sensations
3. Loss of sensations, particularly pain sensation leads to deformities of joint. There is no proper support and movements at the joints become uncontrolled. It is called **Charcot joint.**
4. Joints enlarge due to inflammation by the development of osteoarthritis.

Reflexes

Both superficial and deep reflexes are lost in tabes dorsalis mostly because of loss of sensations.

Voluntary movements

There is lack of coordination of movements **(ataxia).** Normal movements like walking also become clumsy. The gait is awkward. Every movement of the limb is exaggerated while walking. Patient keeps the leg apart, raises the leg very high and stamps it down forcibly. This is called **stamping gait.**

Urinary bladder

If sacral segments are affected in tabes dorsalis, the smooth muscles of the urinary bladder become hypotonic. Micturition reflexes are lost. And the urinary bladder becomes **atonic bladder** (Chapter 57).

3. Multiple Sclerosis

Multiple sclerosis (MS) is a chronic and progressive inflammatory disease characterized by demyelination in brain and spinal cord. It affects the myelinated nerve fibers of brain, spinal cord and optic nerve and causes gradual destruction of myelin sheath **(demyelination).** When the disease progresses, there is transection of axons in patches throughout brain and spinal cord. The term sclerosis refers to scars (scleroses) in the myelin sheath.

Cause

Cause of multiple sclerosis is unknown. It is hypothesized that multiple sclerosis occurs due to combination and interaction of environmental factors (chemicals, bacteria and virus) and genetic factors resulting in abnormal reactions of immune system. During the process, the immune system attacks the myelin sheath.

Signs and symptoms

Initial attack by multiple sclerosis is often mild or asymptomatic. As the disease progresses variety of symptoms start appearing. Symptoms become severe during further progress of the disease.

Common initial symptoms:

1. Mild disturbance in the sensations on face, arms and legs
2. Weakness and disturbances in maintenance of posture
3. Double vision followed by partial blindness.

Other symptoms when the disease progresses:

1. Tremor, fatigue and muscle spasms
2. Speech difficulty
3. Difficulty in performing day-to-day activities
4. Bowel problems
5. Bladder dysfunction
6. Emotional outbursts like anxiety, anger and frustration
7. Short-term memory loss
8. Complete blindness
9. Development of suicidal tendency.

4. Disk Prolapse

Intervertebral or **spinal disk** is the cartilagenous structure of vertebral column that separates each vertebra. It is made up of a tough outer fibrous layer and a soft inner part. Inner part acts as a shock absorber and cushions the vertebrae while moving. A small gap in between the adjacent vertebrae allows nerve roots to enter or leave the spinal cord.

Rupture of disk is called disk prolapse. During disk prolapse, the soft inner material bulges out through a weak area in the hard outer layer. The bulged disk material may irritate or compress or damage the nerve root that passes through the gap between the vertebrae. Severity of the condition depends upon the degree of bulging.

Causes

1. Injury to spinal cord, neck or back
2. Heavy weight lifting
3. Sitting for a long time
4. Sudden violent twisting of the body involving spine
5. Aging: Because of gradual degeneration of disk with age. After about 30 years of age, the disk starts dehydrating. So it is more susceptible for rupture at the age of 30 to 40 years.

Symptoms

Symptoms of disk prolapse include pain and weakness in the area of prolapse. Most common area of disk prolapse is the lower part of vertebral column. If it compresses the sciatic nerve, the symptoms become more severe. Pain spreads down the back of leg to ankle, heel or toes of foot. Lower limb cannot be lifted sometimes. There is numbness and tingling in the affected region. Sitting for long period aggravates the pain and develops other symptoms such as sneezing, coughing or voiding of urine. Prolonged compression of sciatic nerve leads to weakness of leg muscles.

Next common area of disk prolapse is the neck. In this case, the pain is felt in neck, shoulder blade and armpit. If the nerves supplying upper limbs are compressed, the pain spreads through the arm up to the fingers. It also causes stiffness, weakness or tingling in the upper limbs. Even the movements of fingers or arm are restricted.

Somatosensory System and Somatomotor System

- **■ SOMATOSENSORY SYSTEM**
  - ■ DEFINITION AND TYPES OF SENSATIONS
  - ■ TYPES OF SOMATIC SENSATIONS
  - ■ SENSORY PATHWAYS
  - ■ SENSORY FIBERS OF TRIGEMINAL NERVE
  - ■ LEMNISCUS
  - ■ APPLIED PHYSIOLOGY
- **■ SOMATOMOTOR SYSTEM**
  - ■ MOTOR ACTIVITIES OF THE BODY
  - ■ SOMATOMOTOR SYSTEM
  - ■ SPINAL CORD AND CRANIAL NERVE NUCLEI
  - ■ CEREBRAL CORTEX
  - ■ CEREBELLUM
  - ■ BASAL GANGLIA
  - ■ CLASSIFICATION OF MOTOR PATHWAYS
  - ■ UPPER MOTOR NEURON AND LOWER MOTOR NEURON
  - ■ APPLIED PHYSIOLOGY

■ SOMATOSENSORY SYSTEM

■ DEFINITION AND TYPES OF SENSATIONS

Somatosensory system is defined as the sensory system associated with different parts of the body.

Sensations are of two types:
1. Somatic sensations
2. Special sensations.

1. *Somatic Sensations*

Somatic sensations are the sensations arising from skin, muscles, tendons and joints. These sensations have **specific receptors,** which respond to a particular type of stimulus.

2. *Special Sensations*

Special sensations are the **complex sensations** for which the body has some **specialized sense organs.**

These sensations are usually called special senses. Sensations of vision, hearing, taste and smell are the special sensations.

This chapter deals with somatic sensations.

■ TYPES OF SOMATIC SENSATIONS

Generally, somatic sensations are classified into three types:
1. Epicritic sensations
2. Protopathic sensations
3. Deep sensations.

1. *Epicritic Sensations*

Epicritic sensations are the mild or light sensations. Such sensations are perceived more accurately.

Epicritic sensations are:

i. Fine touch or tactile sensation (Chapter 143)
ii. Tactile localization (Chapter 143)

iii. Tactile discrimination (Chapter 143)
iv. Temperature sensation with finer range between 25°C and 40°C.

2. Protopathic Sensations

Protopathic sensations are the **crude sensations.** These sensations are primitive type of sensations.

Protopathic sensations are:

i. Pressure sensation (Chapter 143)
ii. Pain sensation (Chapter 143)
iii. Temperature sensation with a wider range, i.e. above 40°C and below 25°C.

3. Deep Sensations

Deep sensations are sensations arising from deeper structures beneath the skin and visceral organs.

Deep sensations are:

i. **Sensation of vibration** or **pallesthesia,** which is the combination of touch and pressure sensation (Chapter 143)
ii. **Kinesthetic sensation** or **kinesthesia:** Sensation of position and movements of different parts of the body. This sensation arises from the proprioceptors present in muscles, tendons, joints and ligaments. Proprioceptors are the receptors, which give response during various movements of a joint.
   Kinesthetic sensation is of two types:
   a. **Conscious kinesthetic sensation** (Chapter 143)

b. **Subconscious kinesthetic** sensation (Chapter 143). Impulses of this sensation are called non-sensory impulses.
iii. **Visceral sensations** arising from viscera (Fig. 144.1).

Synthetic Senses

Synthetic senses are the sensations synthesized at cortical level, by integration of impulses of basic sensations. Two or more basic sensations are combined in some of the synthetic senses. Best examples of synthetic senses are vibratory sensation, stereognosis and two-point discrimination.

■ SENSORY PATHWAYS

Nervous pathways of sensations are called the sensory pathways. These pathways carry the impulses from receptors in different parts of the body to centers in brain.

Sensory pathways are of two types:
1. Pathways of somatosensory system
2. Pathways of viscerosensory system.

Pathways of somatosensory system convey the information from sensory receptors in skin, skeletal muscles and joints. Pathways of this system are constituted by somatic nerve fibers called somatic afferent nerve fibers.

Pathways of viscerosensory system convey the information from receptors of the viscera. Pathways of this system are constituted by visceral or autonomic fibers.

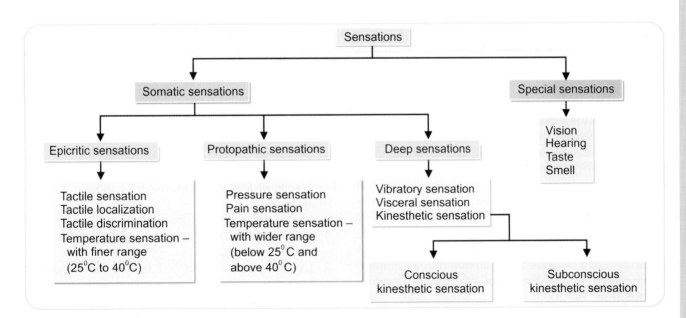

FIGURE 144.1: Classification of sensations

This chapter deals mainly with the somatosensory system.

Somatosensory Pathways

Each sensory pathway is constituted by two or three groups of neurons:
  i. First order neurons
  ii. Second order neurons
  iii. Third order neurons.

Details of these neurons are given in Chapter 143. Pathways of some sensations like kinesthetic sensation have only first and second order neurons.

Details of pathways are given in Table 144.1. Diagrams of pathways are given in Chapter 143, along with ascending tracts of spinal cord.

■ SENSORY FIBERS OF TRIGEMINAL NERVE

Trigeminal nerve carries somatosensory information from face, teeth, periodontal tissues (tissues around teeth), oral cavity, nasal cavity, cranial dura mater and major part of scalp to sensory cortex. It also conveys proprioceptive impulses from the extrinsic muscles of the eyeball.

Origin

Sensory fibers of trigeminal nerve arise from the trigeminal ganglion situated near temporal bone. Peripheral processes of neurons in this ganglion form three divisions of trigeminal nerve, namely ophthalmic, mandibular and maxillary divisions. Cutaneous distribution of the three divisions of trigeminal nerve is shown in Figure 144.2.

Central processes from neurons of trigeminal ganglion enter pons in the form of sensory root.

Termination

After reaching the pons, fibers of sensory root divide into two groups, namely descending fibers and ascending fibers. Descending fibers terminate on primary sensory nucleus and spinal nucleus of trigeminal nerve. Primary sensory nucleus is situated in pons. Spinal nucleus of trigeminal nerve is situated below the primary sensory nucleus and extends up to the upper segments of spinal cord.

Ascending fibers of sensory root terminate in the mesencephalic nucleus of trigeminal nerve, situated in brainstem above the level of primary sensory nucleus (Fig. 144.3).

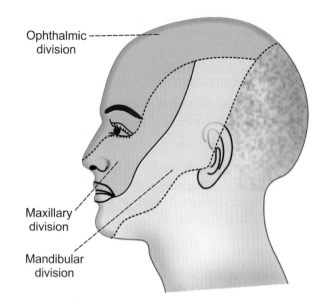

FIGURE 144.2: Cutaneous distribution (sensory) of the three divisions of trigeminal nerve

Central Connections

Majority of fibers from the primary sensory nucleus and spinal nucleus of trigeminal nerve ascend in the form of trigeminal lemniscus and terminate in ventral posteromedial nucleus of thalamus in the opposite side. Remaining fibers from these two nuclei terminate on the thalamic nucleus of same side. From thalamus, the fibers pass via superior thalamic radiation and reach the somatosensory areas of cerebral cortex.

Primary sensory nucleus and spinal nucleus of trigeminal nerve relay the sensations of touch, pressure, pain and temperature from the regions mentioned above.

Fibers from mesencephalic nucleus form the trigeminocerebellar tract that enters spinocerebellum via the superior cerebellar peduncle of the same side. This nucleus conveys proprioceptive impulses from facial muscles, muscles of mastication and ocular muscles.

■ LEMNISCUS

Lemniscus or fillet is the prominent bundle of sensory nerves in brain.

Lemniscus is of four types:
1. **Spinal lemniscus** formed by spinothalamic tracts in medulla oblongata
2. **Lateral lemniscus** formed by the fibers carrying sensation of hearing from cochlear nuclei to inferior colliculus and medial geniculate body

TABLE 144.1: Sensory pathways

Sensation	Receptor	First order neuron in	Second order neuron in	Third order neuron in	Center
Fine touch Tactile localization Tactile discrimination Vibratory sensation Stereognosis	Meissner corpuscles and Merkel disc	Posterior nerve root ganglion – Fibers form Fasciculus gracilis and Fasciculus cuneatus	Nucleus gracilis and Nucleus cuneatus – Fibers form internal arcuate fibers	Ventral posterolateral nucleus of thalamus	Sensory cortex
Pressure Crude touch	Pacinian corpuscle	Posterior nerve root ganglion	Chief sensory nucleus – Fibers form anterior spinothalamic tract	Ventral posterolateral nucleus of thalamus	Sensory cortex
Temperature	Warmth – Ruffini end bulb Cold – Krause end bulb	Posterior nerve root ganglion	Substantia gelatinosa – Fibers form lateral spinothalamic tract	Ventral posterolateral nucleus of thalamus	Sensory cortex
Conscious kinesthetic sensation	Proprioceptors – Muscle spindle Golgi tendon apparatus	Posterior nerve root ganglion – Fibers form Fasciculus gracilis and Fasciculus cuneatus	Nucleus gracilis and Nucleus cuneatus – Fibers form internal arcuate fibers	Ventral posterolateral nucleus of thalamus	Sensory cortex
Subconscious kinesthetic sensation	Proprioceptors – Muscle spindle Golgi tendon apparatus	Posterior nerve root ganglion	Nucleus of Clarke and Marginal nucleus – Fibers form dorsal and ventral spinocerebellar tracts	—	Anterior lobe of cerebellum
Pain	Free nerve endings	Posterior nerve root ganglion Fast pain – A δ-fibers Slow pain – C fibers	Fast pain – marginal nucleus in spinal cord Slow pain – substantia gelatinosa of Rolando Fibers form lateral spinothalamic tract	Ventral posterolateral nucleus of thalamus, reticular formation and midbrain	Sensory cortex

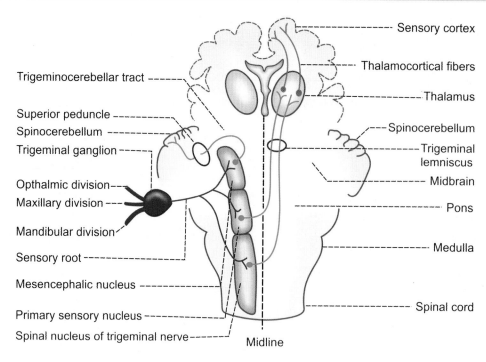

Trigeminocerebellar tract

Superior peduncle

Spinocerebellum

Trigeminal ganglion

Opthalmic division

Maxillary division

Mandibular division

Sensory root

Mesencephalic nucleus

Primary sensory nucleus

Spinal nucleus of trigeminal nerve

Midline

Sensory cortex

Thalamocortical fibers

Thalamus

Spinocerebellum

Trigeminal lemniscus

Midbrain

Pons

Medulla

Spinal cord

FIGURE 144.3: Diagrammatic representation of trigeminal pathway. Trigeminal lemniscus carries impulses of touch, pressure, pain and temperature sensations to somatosensory cortex. Trigeminocerebellar tract carries proprioceptive impulses to spinocerebellum.

3. **Medial lemniscus** formed by fibers arising from nucleus cuneatus and nucleus gracilis
4. **Trigeminal lemniscus** formed by fibers from sensory nuclei of trigeminal nerve. This lemniscus carries general senses from head, neck, face, mouth, eyeballs and ears.

■ APPLIED PHYSIOLOGY

Lesions or other nervous disorders in sensory pathway affect the sensory functions of the body. The effects are given in Table 144.2.

■ SOMATOMOTOR SYSTEM

■ MOTOR ACTIVITIES OF THE BODY

Motor activities of the body depend upon different groups of tissues of the body.

Motor activities are divided into two types:

1. Activities of skeletal muscles, which are involved in posture and movement
2. Activities of smooth muscles, cardiac muscles and other tissues, which are involved in the functions of various visceral organs.

Activities of skeletal muscles (voluntary functions) are controlled by somatomotor system, which is constituted by the somatic motor nerve fibers. Activities of tissues or visceral organs (involuntary functions) are controlled by visceral or autonomic nervous system, which is constituted by the sympathetic and parasympathetic systems. Autonomic nervous system is described in Chapter 164.

This chapter deals with somatomotor system.

■ SOMATOMOTOR SYSTEM

Movements of the body depend upon different groups of skeletal muscles. Various types of movements or motor activities brought about by these muscles are:

1. Execution of smooth, precise and accurate voluntary movements
2. Coordination of movements responsible for skilled activities
3. Coordination of movements responsible for the maintenance of posture and equilibrium.

Voluntary actions and postural movements are carried out by not only the simple contraction and relaxation of skeletal muscles but also the adjustments of tone in these muscles. The execution,

TABLE 144.2: Effects of disorders of sensory pathways

No	Condition	Definition
1.	Anesthesia	Loss of all sensations
2.	Hyperesthesia	Increased sensitivity to sensory stimuli
3.	Hypoesthesia	Reduction in sensitivity to stimuli
4.	Hemiesthesia	Loss of all sensations in one side of body
5.	Paresthesia	Abnormal sensations such as tingling, burning, prickling and numbness
6.	Hemiparesthesia	Abnormal sensations in one side of body
7.	Dissociated anesthesia	Loss of some sensations while other sensations are intact
8.	General anesthesia	Loss of all sensations with loss of consciousness produced by anesthetic agents
9.	Local anesthesia	Loss of sensations in a restricted area of the body
10.	Spinal anesthesia	Loss of sensations due to spinal cord lesion or anesthetic agents injected beneath the coverings of spinal cord
11.	Tactile anesthesia	Loss of tactile sensations
12.	Tactile hyperesthesia	Increased sensitivity to tactile stimuli
13.	Analgesia	Loss of pain sensation
14.	Hyperalgesia	Increased sensitivity to pain stimulus
15.	Paralgesia	Abnormal pain sensation
16.	Thermoanesthesia or thermanesthesia or thermanalgesia	Loss of thermal sensation
17.	Pallanesthesia	Loss of sensation of vibration
18.	Astereognosis	Loss of ability to recognize known object with closed eyes due to loss of cutaneous sensations
19.	Illusion	Mental depression due to misinterpretation of a sensory stimulus
20.	Hallucination	Feeling of a sensation without any stimulus

planning, coordination and adjustments of movements of the body are under the influence of different parts of nervous system, which are together called motor system. Sensory system of the body also plays a vital role in the control of movements.

Spinal reflexes are responsible for most of the movements concerned with voluntary actions and posture. Stimulation of receptor activates the motor neuron in spinal cord, leading to the contraction of muscle innervated by spinal motor neuron. Apart from these reflexes, signals for voluntary motor activities are also sent from different areas of the brain, particularly the cerebral cortex to spinal motor neurons.

Coordination and control of movements initiated by cerebral cortex depends upon two factors:
1. Feedback signals from proprioceptors in muscle and other sensory receptors
2. Interaction of other parts of brain such as brainstem, cerebellum and basal ganglia.

Thus, the motor system includes spinal cord and its nerves, cranial nerves, brainstem, cerebral cortex, cerebellum and basal ganglia. Neuronal circuits between these parts of nervous system, which are responsible for the motor activities are called the motor pathways. Classification of motor pathways is given in the later part of this chapter because the knowledge of role of different parts of nervous system is essential to understand the classification of the motor pathways.

■ **SPINAL CORD AND CRANIAL NERVE NUCLEI**

Motor Neurons

Activities of skeletal muscles are executed by the impulses discharged from alpha motor neurons situated in ventral (anterior) gray horn of spinal cord and nuclei of many of the cranial nerves present in brainstem.

Alpha motor neurons in the spinal cord, which innervate the **extrafusal fibers** of skeletal muscles are responsible for the contraction of muscles in upper limbs, trunk and lower part of the body. The **gamma motor neurons,** which innervate the **intrafusal fibers** of muscle, are responsible for the maintenance of muscle tone.

Motor neurons of the cranial nerve nuclei situated in brainstem send their signals to the muscles of neck and upper part of trunk via cranial nerves.

Final Common Pathway

Activities of a particular skeletal muscle depend upon the excitation of alpha motor neuron (also known as **lower motor neuron**) in the spinal cord or cranial nerve nuclei. This is the only pathway, through which the signals from other parts of nervous system reach the muscles (Fig. 144.4). Hence, the alpha motor neurons are called **'final common pathway'** of motor system.

Functions of Motor Neurons

Motor neurons responsible for the contraction of skeletal muscles are arranged topographically in the ventral gray horn of spinal cord. Neurons situated in the medial part of ventral gray horn innervate the muscles near midline of the body called **axial muscles** and muscles in the proximal portions of limbs called **proximal muscles.** These two types of muscles are involved in the adjustment of posture and gross movement. Motor neurons in lateral part of ventral gray horn innervate the muscles in distal portions of the limbs called **distal muscles.** Distal muscles are involved in the well coordinated skilled voluntary movements.

Motor neurons in cranial nerve nuclei of brainstem innervate the extrinsic muscles of eyeball and muscles of face, tongue, neck and upper part of trunk. These muscles are concerned with ocular movements and movements of facial expressions, chewing, swallowing and movements of head and shoulder. Motor neurons are situated in the nuclei of cranial nerves III, IV, V, VI, VII, IX, X, XI and XII.

■ CEREBRAL CORTEX

Cortical areas concerned with origin of motor signals are the primary motor area, premotor area and supplementary motor area in frontal lobe and sensory area in the parietal lobe. Details of the cortical areas are given in Chapter 152.

Cortical areas send their output signals to spinal cord via corticospinal tracts and to brainstem via corticobulbar tracts. About 30% of the fibers forming corticospinal and corticobulbar tracts take their origin from primary and supplementary motor cortex, 30% from premotor area and remaining 40% from parietal lobe particularly from somatosensory area.

■ CEREBELLUM

Cerebellum plays an important role in planning, programming and integrating the skilled voluntary movements. It is also concerned with the maintenance of muscle tone, posture and equilibrium. Cerebellum

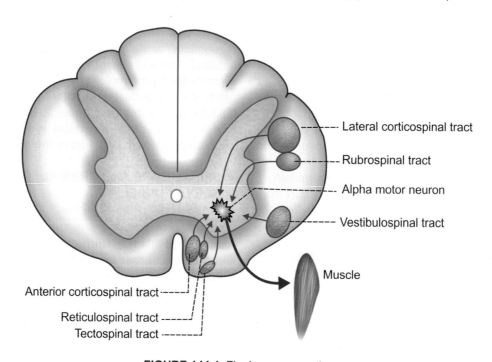

FIGURE 144.4: Final common pathway

receives impulses from proprioceptors of muscle, vestibular apparatus, cerebral cortex, brainstem and basal ganglia. It interprets these impulses and sends signals to motor cortex, reticular formation and nuclei of brainstem.

Role of cerebellum in motor functions is described in detail in Chapter 150.

■ BASAL GANGLIA

Basal ganglia play an important role in the coordination of skilled movements, regulation of automatic associated movements and control of muscle tone by sending output signals to motor cortex, reticular formation and spinal cord. Functions of basal ganglia are explained in Chapter 151.

■ CLASSIFICATION OF MOTOR PATHWAYS

There are two methods to classify the motor pathways. In the first method of classification, motor pathways are divided into pyramidal and extrapyramidal tracts. In the second method, motor pathways are classified into lateral and medial systems.

Pyramidal and Extrapyramidal Pathways

Motor pathways are classified into pyramidal and extrapyramidal tracts, depending upon the situation of their fibers in medulla oblongata.

Pyramidal tracts

Pyramidal tracts are those fibers which form the pyramids in upper part of medulla. Pyramidal tracts are the anterior and lateral corticospinal tracts. These tracts control the **voluntary movements** of the body (Chapter 143).

Extrapyramidal tracts

Motor pathways other than pyramidal tracts are known as extrapyramidal tracts.

Extrapyramidal tracts are:
1. Medial longitudinal fasciculus
2. Anterior and lateral vestibulospinal tracts
3. Reticulospinal tract
4. Tectospinal tract
5. Reticulospinal tract
6. Rubrospinal tract
7. Olivospinal tract.

Extrapyramidal tracts are concerned with the regulation of tone, posture and equilibrium (Chapter 143).

Lateral and Medial Motor Systems

Depending upon the location or termination, motor pathways are divided into two categories, namely the lateral system or pathway and the medial system or pathway. Lateral motor system is phylogenetically new and medial motor system is old.

Lateral motor system

Fibers of this system terminate on motor neurons situated in lateral part of ventral gray horn in spinal cord (directly or via interneurons) and on equivalent motor neurons of cranial nerve nuclei in brainstem.

Components of lateral system:

1. Lateral corticospinal tract, which arises from different areas of cerebral cortex and terminates in the alpha motor neurons situated in lateral part of ventral gray horn of spinal cord. Other details of this tract are given in Chapter 143.
2. Rubrospinal tract, which arises from red nucleus in midbrain (Chapter 143)
3. Part of corticobulbar tract, which arises from different areas of frontal and parietal lobes of cerebral cortex along with corticospinal tracts. Part of corticobulbar tract belonging to lateral motor system terminates on the nucleus of hypoglossal nerve and motor nucleus of facial nerve. Fibers from hypoglossal nerve innervate the muscles of tongue. Fibers from motor nucleus of facial nerve innervate the muscles of lower part of face.

Functions of lateral motor system:

1. Lateral corticospinal tract activates the muscles of distal portions of limbs and regulates the skilled voluntary movements
2. Rubrospinal tract facilitates the tone in the muscles, particularly the flexor muscles
3. Corticobulbar fibers of lateral system are concerned with the movements of expression in lower part of face and movements of tongue.

Medial motor system

Fibers of medial motor system terminate on motor neurons situated in the medial part of ventral gray horn of spinal cord (via interneurons) and on equivalent motor neurons of cranial nerve nuclei, situated in the brainstem.

Components of medial motor system:

1. Anterior corticospinal tract, which arises from different areas of cerebral cortex and terminates in the alpha motor neurons situated in medial part of ventral gray horn of spinal cord (Chapter 143).

2. Part of corticobulbar fibers of medial system, which arises from different areas of frontal and parietal lobes of cerebral cortex along with corticospinal tracts. Fibers of corticobulbar tract belonging to medial motor system innervate the muscles of trunk and limbs, muscles of jaw and muscles of upper part of face.
3. Lateral and medial vestibulospinal tracts that arise from lateral vestibular nucleus and medial vestibular nucleus, respectively (Chapter 143)
4. Reticulospinal tract, which arises from reticular formation in brainstem (Chapter 143)
5. Tectospinal tract, which takes origin from superior colliculus of midbrain (Chapter 143).

Functions of medial motor system:

1. Anterior corticospinal tract is responsible for the maintenance of posture and equilibrium
2. Fibers of corticobulbar tract belonging to medial motor system, innervating muscles of upper part of trunk are involved in the maintenance of posture and equilibrium. Fibers innervating muscles of jaw and face are involved in the movements of chewing and movements of eyebrow.
3. Vestibulospinal tract is concerned with the adjustment of position of head and body during angular and linear acceleration
4. Pontine fibers of reticulospinal tract facilitate the tone of extensor muscles and regulate the postural reflexes. However, medullary fibers of this tract inhibit the tone of the muscles involved in postural movements.
5. Tectospinal tract is responsible for the movement of head in response to visual and auditory stimuli.

■ UPPER MOTOR NEURON AND LOWER MOTOR NEURON

Neurons of the motor system are divided into upper motor neurons and lower motor neurons, depending upon their location and termination.

Upper Motor Neuron

Upper motor neurons are the neurons in higher centers of brain, which control the lower motor neurons.

Upper motor neurons are of three types:
1. Motor neurons in cerebral cortex. Fibers of these neurons form corticospinal (pyramidal) and corticobulbar tracts.
2. Neurons in basal ganglia and brainstem nuclei
3. Neurons in cerebellum.

Motor neurons in cerebral cortex, which give origin to pyramidal tracts belong to the pyramidal system and the remaining motor neurons belong to extrapyramidal system.

Some controversy exists in including the neurons of extrapyramidal system under the category of upper motor neurons. However, considering in terms of the definition, neurons other than lower motor neurons are to be named as upper motor neurons.

Lower Motor Neuron

Lower motor neurons are the anterior gray horn cells in spinal cord and motor neurons of cranial nerve nuclei, situated in brainstem, which innervate the muscles directly.

Thus, the lower motor neurons constitute 'final common pathway' of motor system. Lower motor neurons are under the influence of upper motor neurons.

TABLE 144.3: Effects of upper motor neuron lesion and lower motor neuron lesion

	Effects	Upper motor neuron lesion	Lower motor neuron lesion
Clinical observation	1. Muscle tone	Hypertonia	Hypotonia
	2. Paralysis	Spastic type of paralysis	Flaccid type of paralysis
	3. Wastage of muscle	Wastage of muscle occurs	Wastage of muscle occurs
	4. Superficial reflexes	Lost	Lost
	5. Plantar reflex	Abnormal plantar reflex – Babinski sign	Absent
	6. Deep reflexes	Exaggerated	Lost
	7. Clonus	Present	Absent
Clinical confirmation	8. Electrical activity	Normal	Absent
	9. Muscles affected	Groups of muscles are affected	Individual muscles are affected
	10. Fascicular twitch in EMG	Absent	Present

TABLE 144.4: Types of paralysis

Paralysis	Parts of the body affected	Causes
Monoplegia	Paralysis of one limb	Isolated damage of central nervous system or peripheral nervous system
Diplegia	Paralysis of both the upper limbs or both the lower limbs	Isolated damage of brain
Hemiplegia	Paralysis of upper limb and lower limb on one side of the body	Lesion in motor cortex and corticospinal tracts in posterior limb of internal capsule on the side opposite to the paralysis
Paraplegia	Paralysis of lower half of the body	Injury to lower part of spinal cord
Quadriplegia or tetraplegia	Paralysis of all the four limbs	Injury to upper part of spinal cord (shoulder level or above, at which the motor nerves of upper limbs leave the spinal cord)

■ APPLIED PHYSIOLOGY

Effects of Motor Neuron Lesions

Effects of lesions of upper motor neurons and lower motor neurons are given in Table 144.3. Effects of lower motor neuron lesion are the loss of muscle tone and flaccid paralysis.

Effects of upper motor neuron lesion depends upon the type of neuron involved. Effects of upper motor neuron lesion are:

1. Lesion in pyramidal system causes **hypertonia** and **spastic paralysis.** Spastic paralysis involves only one group of muscles, particularly the extensor muscles.
2. Lesion in basal ganglia produces hypertonia and **rigidity** involving both flexor and extensor muscles

3. Lesion in cerebellum causes hypotonia, muscular weakness and incoordination of movements.

Paralysis

Paralysis is defined as the complete loss of strength and functions of muscle group or a limb.

Causes for paralysis

Common causes for paralysis are trauma, tumor, stroke, cerebral palsy (condition caused by brain injury immediately after birth), multiple sclerosis (Chapter 143) and neurodegenerative diseases.

Types of paralysis

Paralysis of muscles in the body depends upon type and location of motor neurons affected by the lesion. Different types of paralysis are given in Table 144.4.

Physiology of Pain

Chapter

145

- ■ INTRODUCTION
- ■ BENEFITS OF PAIN SENSATION
- ■ COMPONENTS OF PAIN SENSATION
- ■ PATHWAYS OF PAIN SENSATION
  - ■ FROM SKIN AND DEEPER STRUCTURES
  - ■ FROM FACE
  - ■ FROM VISCERA
  - ■ FROM PELVIC REGION
- ■ VISCERAL PAIN
  - ■ CAUSES OF VISCERAL PAIN
- ■ REFERRED PAIN
  - ■ DEFINITION
  - ■ EXAMPLES OF REFERRED PAIN
  - ■ MECHANISM OF REFERRED PAIN
- ■ NEUROTRANSMITTERS INVOLVED IN PAIN SENSATION
- ■ ANALGESIA SYSTEM
  - ■ ANALGESIC PATHWAY
- ■ GATE CONTROL THEORY
- ■ APPLIED PHYSIOLOGY

■ INTRODUCTION

Pain is defined as an unpleasant and emotional experience associated with or without actual tissue damage. Pain sensation is described in many ways like sharp, pricking, electrical, dull ache, shooting, cutting, stabbing, etc. Often it induces crying and fainting.

Pain is produced by real or potential injury to the body. Often it is expressed in terms of injury. For example, pain produced by fire is expressed as burning sensation; pain produced by severe sustained contraction of skeletal muscles is expressed as cramps.

Pain may be acute or chronic. **Acute pain** is a sharp pain of short duration with easily identified cause. Often it is localized in a small area before spreading to neighboring areas. Usually it is treated by medications. **Chronic pain** is the intermittent or constant pain with

different intensities. It lasts for longer periods. It is somewhat difficult to treat chronic pain and it needs professional expert care.

■ BENEFITS OF PAIN SENSATION

Pain is an important sensory symptom. Though it is an unpleasant sensation, it has protective or survival benefits such as:

1. Pain gives warning signal about the existence of a problem or threat. It also creates awareness of injury.
2. Pain prevents further damage by causing reflex withdrawal of the body from the source of injury
3. Pain forces the person to rest or to minimize the activities thus enabling rapid healing of injured part
4. Pain urges the person to take required treatment to prevent major damage.

■ COMPONENTS OF PAIN SENSATION

Pain sensation has two components:
1. Fast pain
2. Slow pain.

Fast pain is the first sensation whenever a pain stimulus is applied. It is experienced as a bright, sharp and localized pain sensation. Fast pain is followed by the slow pain, which is experienced as a dull, diffused and unpleasant pain.

Receptors for both the components of pain are same, i.e. the free nerve endings. But, afferent nerve fibers are different. Fast pain sensation is carried by Aδ fibers and slow pain sensation is carried by C type of nerve fibers.

■ PATHWAYS OF PAIN SENSATION

Pain sensation from various parts of body is carried to brain by different pathways which are:
1. Pathway from skin and deeper structures
2. Pathway from face
3. Pathway from viscera
4. Pathway from pelvic region.

■ 1. FROM SKIN AND DEEPER STRUCTURES

Receptors

Receptors of pain sensation are the free nerve endings, which are distributed throughout the body.

First Order Neurons

First order neurons are the cells in posterior nerve root ganglia, which receive the impulses of pain sensation from pain receptors through their dendrites. These impulses are transmitted to spinal cord through the axons of these neurons.

Fast pain fibers

Fast pain sensation is carried by Aδ type afferent fibers which synapse with neurons of **marginal nucleus** in the posterior gray horn.

Slow pain fibers

Slow pain sensation is carried by C type afferent fibers, which synapse with neurons of **substantia gelatinosa** of Rolando in the posterior gray horn (Fig. 143.4).

Second Order Neurons

Neurons of marginal nucleus and substantia gelatinosa of Rolando form the second order neurons. Fibers from these neurons ascend in the form of the lateral spinothalamic tract.

Fast pain fibers

Fibers of fast pain arise from neurons of marginal nucleus. Immediately after taking origin, the fibers cross the midline via anterior gray commissure, reach the lateral white column of the opposite side and ascend. These fibers form the neospinothalamic fibers in lateral spinothalamic tract. These nerve fibers terminate in **ventral posterolateral nucleus** of thalamus. Some of the fibers terminate in ascending reticular activating system of brainstem.

Slow pain fibers

Fibers of slow pain, which arise from neurons of substantia gelatinosa, cross the midline and run along the fibers of fast pain as **paleospinothalamic fibers** in lateral spinothalamic tract. One fifth of these fibers terminate in ventral posterolateral nucleus of thalamus. Remaining fibers terminate in any of the following areas:
   i. Nuclei of reticular formation in brainstem
   ii. Tectum of midbrain
   iii. Gray matter surrounding aqueduct of Sylvius.

Third Order Neurons

Third order neurons of pain pathway are the neurons in:
   i. Thalamic nucleus
   ii. Reticular formation
   iii. Tectum
   iv. Gray matter around aqueduct of Sylvius.

Axons from these neurons reach the sensory area of cerebral cortex (Fig. 145.2). Some fibers from reticular formation reach hypothalamus.

Center for Pain Sensation

Center for pain sensation is in postcentral gyrus of parietal cortex. Fibers reaching hypothalamus are concerned with arousal mechanism due to pain stimulus.

■ 2. FROM FACE

Pain sensation from face is carried by trigeminal nerve (Chapter 144).

■ 3. FROM VISCERA

Pain sensation from thoracic and abdominal viscera is transmitted by sympathetic (thoracolumbar) nerves. Pain from esophagus, trachea and pharynx is carried by vagus and glossopharyngeal nerves.

■ 4. FROM PELVIC REGION

Pain sensation from deeper structures of pelvic region is conveyed by sacral parasympathetic nerves.

■ VISCERAL PAIN

Pain from viscera is unpleasant. It is poorly localized.

■ CAUSES OF VISCERAL PAIN

1. *Ischemia*

Substances released during ischemic reactions such as bradykinin and proteolytic enzymes stimulate the pain receptors of viscera.

2. *Chemical Stimuli*

Chemical substances like acidic gastric juice, leak from ruptured ulcers into peritoneal cavity and produce pain.

3. *Spasm and Overdistention of Hollow Organs*

Spastic contraction of smooth muscles in gastrointestinal tract and other hollow organs of viscera cause pain by stimulating the free nerve endings. Overdistention of hollow organs also causes pain.

■ REFERRED PAIN

■ DEFINITION

Referred pain is the pain that is perceived at a site adjacent to or away from the site of origin. Deep pain and some visceral pain are referred to other areas. But, superficial pain is not referred.

■ EXAMPLES OF REFERRED PAIN

1. Cardiac pain is felt at inner part of left arm and left shoulder (Fig. 145.1)
2. Pain in ovary is referred to umbilicus
3. Pain from testis is felt in abdomen
4. Pain in diaphragm is referred to shoulder
5. Pain in gallbladder is referred to epigastric region
6. Renal pain is referred to loin.

■ MECHANISM OF REFERRED PAIN

Dermatomal Rule

According to dermatomal rule, pain is referred to a structure, which is developed from the same **dermatome** from which the pain producing structure is developed.

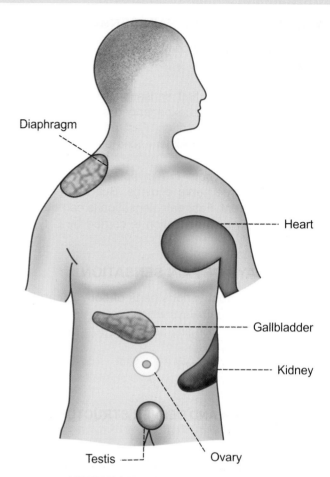

FIGURE 145.1: Sites of referred pain

A dermatome includes all the structures or parts of the body, which are innervated by afferent nerve fibers of one dorsal root. For example, the heart and inner aspect of left arm originate from the same dermatome. So, the pain in heart is referred to left arm.

■ NEUROTRANSMITTERS INVOLVED IN PAIN SENSATION

Glutamate and substance P are the neurotransmitters secreted by pain nerve endings. Aδ afferent fibers, which transmit impulses of fast pain secrete glutamate. The C type fibers, which transmit impulses of slow pain secrete substance P.

■ ANALGESIA SYSTEM

Analgesia system means the pain control system. Body has its own analgesia system in brain, which provides a short-term relief from pain. It is also called

endogenous analgesic system. Analgesia system has got its own pathway through which it blocks the synaptic transmission of pain sensation in spinal cord and thus attenuates the experience of pain. In fact analgesic drugs such as opioids act through this system and provide a controlled pain relief.

■ ANALGESIC PATHWAY

Analgesic pathway that interferes with pain transmission is often considered as descending pain pathway, the ascending pain pathway being the afferent fibers that transmit pain sensation to the brain (Fig. 145.2).

Role of Analgesic Pathway in Inhibiting Pain Transmission

1. Fibers of analgesic pathway arise from frontal lobe of cerebral cortex and hypothalamus
2. These fibers terminate in the gray matter surrounding the third ventricle and aqueduct of Sylvius (periaqueductal gray matter)
3. Fibers from here descend down to brainstem and terminate on:
   i. **Nucleus raphe magnus,** situated in reticular formation of lower pons and upper medulla
   ii. **Nucleus reticularis,** paragigantocellularis situated in medulla
4. Fibers from these reticular nuclei descend through lateral white column of spinal cord and reach the synapses of the neurons in afferent pain pathway situated in anterior gray horn
   Synapses of the afferent pain pathway are between:
   i. Aδ type afferent fibers and neurons of marginal nucleus
   ii. C type afferent fibers and neurons of substantia gelatinosa of Rolando.
5. At synaptic level, analgesic fibers release neurotransmitters and inhibit the pain transmission before being relayed to brain.

Neurotransmitters of Analgesic Pathway

Neurotransmitters released by the fibers of analgesic pathway are serotonin and opiate receptor substances namely enkephalin, dynorphin and endorphin.

■ GATE CONTROL THEORY

Psychologist **Ronald Melzack** and the anatomist **Patrick Wall** proposed the gate control theory for pain in 1965 to explain the pain suppression.

According to them, the pain stimuli transmitted by afferent pain fibers are blocked by gate mechanism

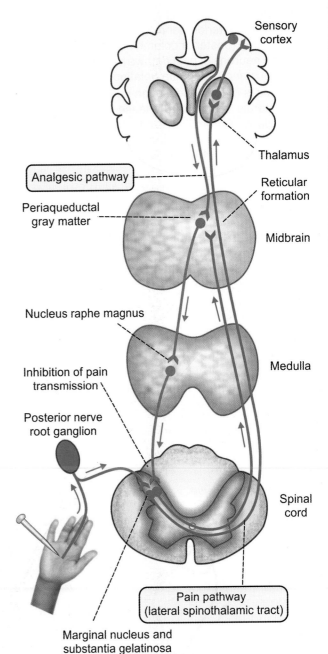

FIGURE 145.2: Pain pathway and analgesic pathway

located at the posterior gray horn of spinal cord. If the gate is opened, pain is felt. If the gate is closed, pain is suppressed.

Mechanism of Gate Control at Spinal Level

1. When pain stimulus is applied on any part of body, besides pain receptors, the receptors of other sensations such as touch are also stimulated

2. When all these impulses reach the spinal cord through posterior nerve root, the fibers of touch sensation (posterior column fibers) send collaterals to the neurons of pain pathway, i.e. cells of marginal nucleus and substantia gelatinosa
3. Impulses of touch sensation passing through these collaterals inhibit the release of glutamate and substance P from the pain fibers
4. This closes the gate and the pain transmission is blocked (Fig. 145.3).

Role of Brain in Gate Control Mechanism

According to Melzack and Wall, brain also plays some important role in the gate control system of the spinal cord as follows:
1. If the gates in spinal cord are not closed, pain signals reach thalamus through lateral spinothalamic tract
2. These signals are processed in thalamus and sent to sensory cortex

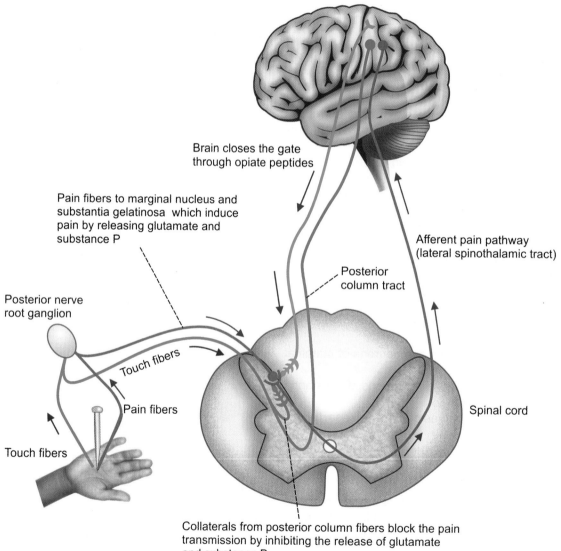

Brain closes the gate through opiate peptides

Pain fibers to marginal nucleus and substantia gelatinosa which induce pain by releasing glutamate and substance P

Afferent pain pathway (lateral spinothalamic tract)

Posterior column tract

Posterior nerve root ganglion

Touch fibers

Pain fibers

Touch fibers

Spinal cord

Collaterals from posterior column fibers block the pain transmission by inhibiting the release of glutamate and substance P

FIGURE 145.3: Gate control system

3. Perception of pain occurs in cortical level in context of the person's emotional status and previous experiences
4. The person responds to the pain based on the integration of all these information in the brain. Thus, the brain determines the severity and extent of pain.
5. To minimize the severity and extent of pain, brain sends message back to spinal cord to close the gate by releasing pain relievers such as opiate peptides
6. Now the pain stimulus is blocked and the person feels less pain.

Significance of Gate Control

Thus, gating of pain at spinal level is similar to pre-synaptic inhibition. It forms the basis for relief of pain through rubbing, massage techniques, application of ice packs, acupuncture and electrical analgesia. All these techniques relieve pain by stimulating the re-lease of endogenous pain relievers (opioid peptides), which close the gate and block the pain signals.

■ APPLIED PHYSIOLOGY

1. Analgesia

Analgesia means loss of pain sensation.

2. Hyperalgesia

Hyperalgesia is defined as the increased sensitivity to pain sensation.

3. Paralgesia

Abnormal pain sensation is called paralgesia.

Brainstem

```
■ INTRODUCTION
■ MEDULLA OBLONGATA
■ PONS
■ MIDBRAIN
    ■ TECTUM
    ■ CEREBRAL PEDUNCLES
```

■ INTRODUCTION

Brainstem is the part of brain formed by medulla oblongata, pons and midbrain. Brainstem contains ascending and descending tracts between brain and spinal cord. It also contains many centers for regulation of vital functions in the body.

■ MEDULLA OBLONGATA

Medulla oblongata or medulla is the lowermost part of brain. It is situated below pons and is continued downwards as spinal cord. Medulla forms the main pathway for ascending and descending tracts of the spinal cord. It also has many important centers which control the vital functions.

1. Respiratory Centers

Dorsal and ventral group of neurons form the medullary respiratory centers, which maintain normal rhythmic respiration.

2. Vasomotor Center

Vasomotor center controls blood pressure and heart rate.

3. Deglutition Center

Deglutition center regulates the pharyngeal and eso-phageal stages of deglutition.

4. Vomiting Center

Vomiting center induces vomiting during irritation or inflammation of gastrointestinal (GI) tract.

5. Superior and Inferior Salivatory Nuclei

Salivatory nuclei control the secretion of **saliva.**

6. Cranial Nerve Nuclei

Nuclei of 12th, 11th, 10th and some nuclei of 8th and 5th cranial nerves are located in the medulla oblongata. 12th cranial (hypoglossal) nerve controls the movements of **tongue.** 11th cranial (accessory) nerve controls the movements of **shoulder** and 10th cranial (vagus) nerve controls almost all the **vital functions** in the body, viz. cardiovascular system, respiratory system, GI system, etc. 8th cranial nerve (the cochlear division of this nerve), which has the relay in medulla oblongata, is concerned with the auditory function.

7. Vestibular Nuclei

Vestibular nuclei contain the second order neurons of vestibular nerve. There are four vestibular nuclei, situated in the rostral part of medulla and caudal part of pons, namely superior, medial, lateral and inferior vestibular nuclei. Medial and inferior vestibular nuclei extend into medulla.

All the medullary centers and nuclei of cranial nerves are controlled by higher centers, situated in cerebral cortex and hypothalamus.

■ PONS

Pons forms a bridge between medulla and midbrain.

Functions of Pons

1. Axons of pontine nuclei join to form the middle cerebellar peduncle or the brachium pontis. Pons forms the pathway that connects cerebellum with cerebral cortex.
2. Pyramidal tracts pass through the pons
3. Medial lemniscus is joined by the fibers of 10th, 9th, 7th and 5th cranial nerves in pons
4. Nuclei of 8th, 7th, 6th and 5th cranial nerves are located in pons
5. Pons contains the pneumotaxic and apneustic centers for regulation of respiration
6. It also contains the vestibular nuclei, which are already mentioned in medulla oblongata.

■ MIDBRAIN

Midbrain lies between pons and diencephalon. It consists of two parts:
A. Tectum
B. Cerebral peduncles.

■ TECTUM

Tectum is formed by two structures:
1. Superior colliculus
2. Inferior colliculus.

1. Superior Colliculus

Superior colliculus is a small structure and is an important center for reflexes. Through tectospinal tract, superior colliculus controls the **movements** of the eyes, head, trunk and limbs, in response to visual impulses. Efferent fibers from superior colliculus going to the nucleus of III cranial (oculomotor) nerve cause constriction of pupil during light reflex. Thus, it forms the center for **light reflex.** Superior colliculus also receives afferents from optic tract, which helps in the integration of **optical and postural reflexes.**

2. Inferior Colliculus

Inferior colliculus consists of single layer of neurons to which the lateral lemniscus (auditory fibers) synapses.

Inferior colliculus is the center for auditory reflexes. Stimulation of this also produces reflex vocalization.

■ CEREBRAL PEDUNCLES

Cerebral peduncles include:
1. Basis pedunculi
2. Substantia nigra
3. Tegmentum, which includes red nucleus.

1. Basis Pedunculus

Basis pedunculus consists of pyramidal tract fibers in the middle, temporopontine fibers laterally and frontopontine fibers medially.

2. Substantia Nigra

Substantia nigra is situated below the red nucleus. Substantia nigra is considered as one of the components of basal ganglia (Chapter 151).

3. Tegmentum

Tegmentum lies dorsal to substantia nigra and is actually the upward continuation of the reticular formation in pons. Tegmentum comprises three decussations and red nucleus.

Decussations in tegmentum

i. **Superior cerebellar peduncle,** which is formed by fibers between cerebellum and other parts of CNS. These fibers are predominantly efferent fibers from dentate nucleus of cerebellum; few fibers are from other cerebellar nuclei such as nucleus globosus and nucleus emboliformis.
ii. **Forel decussation,** which is due to the crossing of rubrospinal tracts from either side
iii. **Meynert decussation,** which is due to the crossing of medial longitudinal bundle that is formed by efferent fibers of 3rd, 4th and 6th cranial nerves.

Red Nucleus

Red nucleus is a large oval or round mass of gray matter, extending between the superior colliculus and hypothalamus.

Parts of red nucleus

Red nucleus has two parts:
1. **Nucleus magnocellularis,** which is formed by large cells. Fibers from this form the rubrospinal and rubrobulbar tracts.

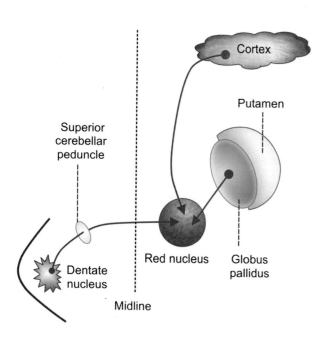

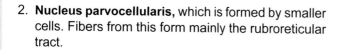

FIGURE 146.1: Afferent connections of red nucleus

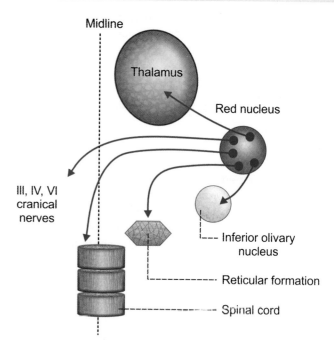

FIGURE 146.2: Efferent connections of red nucleus

2. **Nucleus parvocellularis,** which is formed by smaller cells. Fibers from this form mainly the rubroreticular tract.

Connections of red nucleus

Afferent connections: Red nucleus receives fibers from:
1. Nucleus parvocellularis, which receives fibers from motor cortex (area 6) – corticorubral fibers (Fig. 146.1)
2. Nucleus magnocellularis, which receives fibers from motor cortex (area 6) – pallidorubral fibers
3. Nucleus magnocellularis, which receives fibers from dentate nucleus (of opposite side) – cerebellorubral or dentatorubral tract.

Efferent connections: Red nucleus sends efferent fibers to various parts of brain and spinal cord:
1. Rubrospinal tract to spinal cord (Fig. 146.2)
2. Rubrobulbar tract to medulla
3. Rubroreticular fibers to reticular formation
4. Rubrothalamic tract to lateral ventral nucleus of thalamus
5. Rubro-olivary tract to inferior olivary nucleus
6. Fibers to nuclei of 3rd, 4th and 6th cranial nerves.

Functions of red nucleus

1. *Control of muscle tone:* Because of its connections with cerebellum, vestibular apparatus and skeletal muscle, the red nucleus plays an important role in facilitating the muscle tone.
2. *Control of complex muscular movements:* Red nucleus controls the complex muscular movements. It plays an important role in the integration of various impulses received from many important areas of brain.
3. *Control of righting reflexes:* Red nucleus is the center for all righting reflexes except optical righting reflexes (Chapter 157).
4. *Control of movements of eyeball:* Through its efferent connections with nuclei of 3rd, 4th and 6th cranial nerves, red nucleus plays an important role in the control of ocular movements (Chapter 165).
5. *Control of skilled movements:* Red nucleus plays an important role in controlling the skilled muscular movements by its connections with spinal cord and cerebral cortex.

Thalamus

■ INTRODUCTION

Thalamus is a large ovoid mass of gray matter, situated bilaterally in **diencephalon.** Both thalami form 80% of diencephalon. Thalami on both sides are connected in their rostral portions by means of an **intermediate mass.** Caudal portions are more widely separated by corpora quadrigemina.

■ THALAMIC NUCLEI

Thalamic nuclei are classified by two methods:
A. Anatomical classification
B. Physiological classification.

■ ANATOMICAL CLASSIFICATION

Thalamus on each side is divided into five main nuclear groups by 'Y'-shaped internal medullary lamina.

1. Midline nuclei
2. Intralaminar nuclei
3. Medial mass of nuclei
4. Lateral mass of nuclei
5. Posterior group of nuclei.

1. *Midline Nuclei*

Midline nuclei are a group of small nuclei, situated on the medial surface of thalamus near the midline (Fig. 147.1).

2. *Intralaminar Nuclei*

Intralaminar nuclei are smaller nuclei present in the medullary septum of thalamus.

3. *Medial Mass of Nuclei*

Medial mass of nuclei are situated medial to septum and it comprises two nuclei:
i. Anterior nucleus
ii. Dorsomedial nucleus.

4. *Lateral Mass of Nuclei*

This group of nuclei are situated lateral to septum. Lateral mass of nuclei are again divided into two subgroups:
i. Dorsal group of lateral mass with two nuclei:
   a. Dorsolateral nucleus
   b. Posterolateral nucleus
ii. Ventral group of lateral mass with three nuclei:
   a. Ventral anterior nucleus
   b. Ventral lateral nucleus
   c. Ventral posterior nucleus. It consists of two parts:
      • Ventral posterolateral nucleus
      • Ventral posteromedial nucleus.

5. *Posterior Group of Nuclei*

Posterior group of nuclei are the continuation of lateral mass of nuclei. It has two subgroups:

i. Pulvinar
ii. Metathalamus which consists of two structures:
   a. Medial geniculate body
   b. Lateral geniculate body.

Thalamic reticular nucleus

Thalamus also includes thalamic reticular nucleus, which is a thin layer of neurons covering the lateral aspect of thalamus. It is separated from thalamus by external medullary lamina. It receives information from reticular formation, cerebral cortex and other thalamic and sends inhibitory signals to other thalamic nuclei.

■ PHYSIOLOGICAL CLASSIFICATION

On the basis of functions and their projections, thalamic nuclei are classified into five groups. This type of classification is also called **Bondok classification**. Five groups of thalamic nuclei are:
1. Specific sensory relay nuclei
2. Specific motor nuclei
3. Association or less specific nuclei
4. Non-specific nuclei
5. Limbic system nuclei.

Nuclei and their functions of each group are given in Table 147.1.

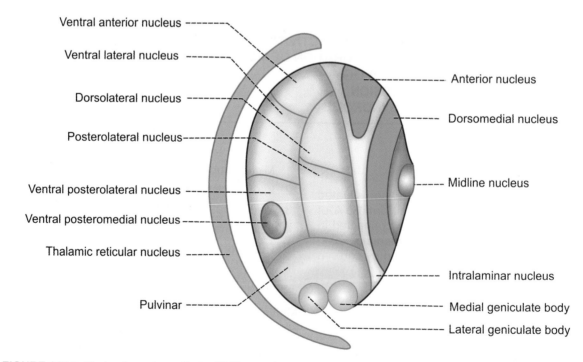

FIGURE 147.1: Thalamic nucleus. Red = Midline nucleus, Yellow = Intralaminar nuclei, Green = Medial mass of nuclei, Blue = Lateral mass of nuclei, Pink = Posterior group of nuclei.

TABLE 147.1: Bondok classification of thalamic nuclei

Group	Nuclei	Functions
1. Specific sensory relay nuclei	i. Ventral posterior nucleus ii. Medical geniculate body iii. Lateral geniculate body	Project sensory signals to distinct (specific) areas of cerebral cortex
2. Specific nuclei	i. Ventral anterior nucleus ii. Ventral lateral nucleus	Receive signals controlling motor activities from cerebellum and corpus striatum and send these signals to motor areas in the cerebral cortex to complete the feedback system of motor control mechanism
3. Association or less specific nuclei	i. Dorsolateral nucleus ii. Posterolateral nucleus iii. Pulvinar	Send information to association areas of cerebral cortex
4. Non-specific nuclei	i. Midline nuclei ii. Intralaminar nuclei iii. Reticular nucleus	Project signals to diffused areas of cerebral cortex
5. Limbic system nuclei	i. Anterior nucleus ii. Dorsolateral nucleus	Project into limbic cortex

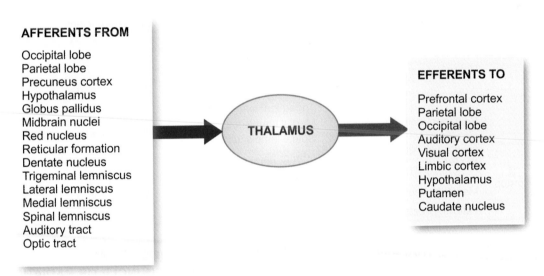

AFFERENTS FROM

Occipital lobe
Parietal lobe
Precuneus cortex
Hypothalamus
Globus pallidus
Midbrain nuclei
Red nucleus
Reticular formation
Dentate nucleus
Trigeminal lemniscus
Lateral lemniscus
Medial lemniscus
Spinal lemniscus
Auditory tract
Optic tract

THALAMUS

EFFERENTS TO

Prefrontal cortex
Parietal lobe
Occipital lobe
Auditory cortex
Visual cortex
Limbic cortex
Hypothalamus
Putamen
Caudate nucleus

FIGURE 147.2: Connections of thalamus

■ CONNECTIONS OF THALAMIC NUCLEI

Connections of different groups of nuclei are given in Table 147.2 and Figure 147.2.

■ THALAMIC RADIATIONS

Thalamic radiation is the collection of nerve fibers connecting thalamus and cerebral cortex. It contains both thalamocortical and corticothalamic fibers. All these fibers between thalamus and cerebral cortex pass through internal capsule.

Fibers of thalamic radiation are divided into four groups, which are called **thalamic peduncles** or **thalamic stalks.** Thalamic peduncles are:

1. Anterior (frontal) thalamic peduncle or radiation
2. Superior (centroparietal) thalamic peduncle or radiation
3. Posterior (occipital) thalamic peduncle or radiation
4. Inferior (temporal) thalamic peduncle or radiation.

TABLE 147.2: Connections of different nuclear groups of thalamus

Nuclei		Afferent fibers from	Efferent fibers to
1. Midline nuclei		Globus pallidus Hypothalamus Cerebral cortex Midbrain nuclei Reticular formation	Different areas of cerebral cortex
2. Intralaminar nuclei		Reticular formation Trigeminal lemniscus Lateral lemniscus	Cerebral cortex Putamen Caudate nucleus Other thalamic nuclei
3. Medial mass	Anterior nucleus	Mamillary body	Limbic cortex
	Dorsomedial nucleus	Hypothalamus	Limbic cortex Putamen Caudate nucleus Hypothalamus
4. Lateral mass	Dorsolateral nucleus	Precuneus cortex	Precuneus cortex
	Posterolateral nucleus	Parietal lobe	Parietal lobe
	Ventral anterior nucleus	Globus pallidus	Putamen Caudate nucleus Premotor cortex
	Ventral lateral nucleus	Globus pallidus Dentate nucleus Red nucleus	Putamen Caudate nucleus Precentral cortex
	Posterior ventral nucleus	Trigeminal lemniscus Medial lemniscus Spinal lemniscus	Hypothalamus Cerebral cortex – areas 3, 1, 2, 5, 7
5. Posterior group	Pulvinar	Inferior parietal lobe Occipital lobe – areas 18, 19	Inferior parietal lobe Occipital lobe – areas 18, 19
	Medial geniculate body	Auditory tract	Auditory cortex
	Lateral geniculate body	Optic tract	Visual cortex

■ ANTERIOR (FRONTAL) THALAMIC PEDUNCLE OR RADIATION

Anterior thalamic peduncle connects the frontal lobe of cerebral cortex with medial and lateral thalamic nuclei. It contains mostly motor nerve fibers.

■ SUPERIOR (CENTROPARIETAL) THALAMIC PEDUNCLE OR RADIATION

Fibers of this peduncle connect postcentral gyrus (somesthetic area) of parietal lobe and adjacent area in frontal cortex with lateral mass of thalamic nuclei. It contains mainly the sensory fibers.

■ POSTERIOR (OCCIPITAL) THALAMIC PEDUNCLE OR RADIATION

Posterior thalamic peduncle connects occipital lobe of cerebral cortex with pulvinar and lateral geniculate body. It contains the nerve fibers concerned with vision.

■ INFERIOR (TEMPORAL) THALAMIC PEDUNCLE OR RADIATION

Fibers of this peduncle connect temporal lobe and insula with pulvinar and medial geniculate body. This peduncle contains the nerve fibers concerned with hearing.

■ FUNCTIONS OF THALAMUS

Thalamus is primarily concerned with **somatic functions** and it plays little role in the visceral functions. Following are the various functions of thalamus:

■ 1. RELAY CENTER

Thalamus forms the relay center for the sensations. Impulses of almost all the sensations reach the thalamic nuclei, particularly in the ventral posterolateral nucleus. After being processed in the thalamus, the impulses are carried to cerebral cortex through thalamocortical fibers.

■ 2. CENTER FOR PROCESSING OF SENSORY INFORMATION

Thalamus forms the major center for processing the sensory information. All the peripheral sensory impulses reaching thalamus are integrated and modified before being sent to specific areas of cerebral cortex. This function of thalamus is usually called the processing of sensory information.

Functional Gateway for Cerebral Cortex

Almost all the sensations are processed in thalamus before reaching cerebral cortex. Very little information of somatosensory function is sent directly to cerebral cortex without being processed by the thalamic nuclei. Because of this function, thalamus is usually called 'functional gateway' for cerebral cortex.

■ 3. CENTER FOR DETERMINING QUALITY OF SENSATIONS

Thalamus is also the center for determining the quality of sensations, i.e. to determine the affective nature of sensations. Usually the sensations have two qualities:
  i. Discriminative nature
  ii. Affective nature.

i. Discriminative Nature

Discriminative nature is the ability to recognize the type, location and other details of the sensations and it is the function of cerebral cortex.

ii. Affective Nature

Affective nature is the capacity to determine whether a sensation is pleasant or unpleasant and agreeable or disagreeable. Determining the affective nature of sensations is the function of thalamus.

■ 4. CENTER FOR SEXUAL SENSATIONS

Thalamus forms the center for perception of sexual sensations.

■ 5. ROLE IN AROUSAL AND ALERTNESS REACTIONS

Because of its connections with nuclei of reticular formation, thalamus plays an important role in arousal and alertness reactions.

■ 6. CENTER FOR REFLEX ACTIVITY

Since the sensory fibers relay here, thalamus forms the center for many reflex activities.

■ 7. CENTER FOR INTEGRATION OF MOTOR ACTIVITY

Through the connections with cerebellum and basal ganglia, thalamus serves as a center for integration of motor functions.

■ APPLIED PHYSIOLOGY

■ THALAMIC LESION

Thalamic lesion occurs mainly because of blockage (due to thrombosis) in thalamogeniculate branch of posterior cerebral artery. Mostly, posteroventral nuclei of thalamus are affected because the thalamogeniculate branch of posterior cerebral artery supplies this part of thalamus. Lesion of thalamus leads to a condition called thalamic syndrome.

■ THALAMIC SYNDROME

Thalamic syndrome is the neurological disease caused by infarction of posteroventral part of thalamus. It is a rare disease and it has many names. Synonyms of thalamic syndrome are listed in Box 147.1.

BOX 147.1: Synonyms of thalamic syndrome

1. Dejerine-Roussy syndrome
2. Thalamic hyperesthetic anesthesia
3. Thalamic pain syndrome
4. Central pain syndrome
5. Central poststroke pain syndrome
6. Posterior thalamic syndrome
7. Retrolenticular syndrome

In thalamic syndrome, whole body becomes hypersensitive to pain. Effects of thalamic lesion occur in the contralateral (opposite) side.

Following are the symptoms of thalamic syndrome:

1. *Loss of Sensations*

Loss of all sensations **(anesthesia)** occurs as the sensory relay system in thalamus is affected.

2. *Astereognosis*

Astereognosis is the loss of ability to recognize a known object by touch with closed eyes. It is due to the loss of tactile and kinesthetic sensations in thalamic syndrome.

3. *Ataxia*

Ataxia refers to incoordination of voluntary movements. It occurs due to loss of kinesthetic sensation. This type of ataxia due to loss of sensation is called **sensory ataxia.** It is very common in thalamic syndrome.

4. *Thalamic Phantom Limb*

The patient is unable to locate the position of a limb with closed eyes. The patient may search for the limb in air or may have the illusion that the limb is lost. This is called thalamic phantom limb.

5. *Anosognosia*

Anosognosia is the lack of awareness or denial of existance of a neurological defect or general illness or any disability.

6. *Spontaneous Pain and Thalamic Over-reaction*

Spontaneous pain occurs often. Pain stimulus is felt more acutely than in normal conditions **(hyperalgesia).** Pain may be so intense, that it even resists the action of powerful sedatives like morphine. Threshold for pain is very much reduced. Even the light touch may be unpleasant. Sometimes, the patient feels pain even in the absence of pain stimulus. It becomes worst in conditions such as emotional disturbance and exposure to cold or heat. Pain is due to over activity of medial mass of nuclei of thalamus, which escape the lesion.

Abnormal reaction to various stimuli is called thalamic over-reaction.

7. *Involuntary Movements*

Thalamic syndrome is always associated with some involuntary motor movements.

Athetosis

Athetosis means slow writhing and twisting movements.

Chorea

Chorea means quick, jerky, involuntary movements.

Intention tremor

Tremor is defined as rapid alternate rhythmic and involuntary movement of flexion and extension in the joints of fingers and wrist or elbow. Intention tremor is the tremor that develops while attempting to do any voluntary act. Intention tremor is the common feature of thalamic syndrome.

8. *Thalamic Hand or Athetoid Hand*

Athetoid hand is the abnormal attitude of hand in thalamic lesion. It is characterized by moderate flexion at wrist and hyperextension of all fingers.

Internal Capsule

Chapter 148

- ■ DEFINITION
- ■ SITUATION
- ■ DIVISIONS
    - ■ ANTERIOR LIMB
    - ■ POSTERIOR LIMB
    - ■ GENU
    - ■ CAUDAL PORTION
- ■ APPLIED PHYSIOLOGY – EFFECT OF LESIONS
    - ■ IN ANTERIOR LIMB
    - ■ IN POSTERIOR LIMB
    - ■ IN GENU
    - ■ IN CAUDAL PORTION

■ DEFINITION

Internal capsule is the broad and compact band of afferent and efferent fibers connecting cerebral cortex with brainstem and spinal cord. Cerebral cortex is connected with brainstem and spinal cord by both afferent and efferent fibers. Fibers arising from different parts of cerebral cortex descend down into white matter of cerebral hemispheres in the form of radiating mass of fibers called corona radiata. While passing down towards the brainstem, corona radiata converges in the form of internal capsule.

Fibers from spinal cord and brainstem reach cerebral cortex in the same route. A large portion of internal capsule is formed by thalamic radiation.

■ SITUATION

Internal capsule is situated in between thalamus and caudate nucleus on the medial side and lenticular nucleus on the lateral side.

■ DIVISIONS

Internal capsule has two limbs, the anterior and posterior limbs. In between these two limbs, lies the genu of internal capsule. Distal end of posterior limb is continued

as the caudal portion of internal capsule (Fig. 148.1). Nerve fibers of each division are given in Table 148.1.

■ ANTERIOR LIMB

Anterior limb of internal capsule is short and lies between lenticular and caudate nuclei.

■ POSTERIOR LIMB

Posterior limb is long and situated between thalamus and lenticular nucleus.

■ GENU

Genu is situated between the anterior and the posterior limbs.

■ CAUDAL PORTION

Caudal portion is otherwise known as **retrolenticular portion** of internal capsule.

■ APPLIED PHYSIOLOGY – EFFECT OF LESIONS OF INTERNAL CAPSULE

Lesion of internal capsule is caused by thrombosis or hemorrhage in branches of middle cerebral arteries.

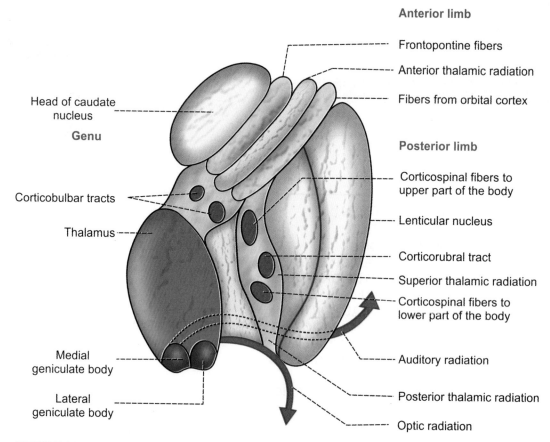

FIGURE 148.1: Components of internal capsule. Pink = Descending fibers, Blue = Ascending fibers.

The effects of lesion depend upon the part of internal capsule involved.

TABLE 148.1: Fibers of internal capsule

Division	Nerve fibers present
1. Anterior limb	1. Anterior thalamic radiation 2. Prefrontal corticopontine (frontopontine) tract 3. Fibers from orbital cortex to hypothalamus
2. Posterior limb	1. Corticospinal tracts 2. Superior thalamic radiation 3. Frontal corticopontine tract
3. Genu	Corticobulbar tract
4. Caudal portion	Posterior thalamic radiation

■ IN ANTERIOR LIMB

Anterior limb contains thalamocortical and frontopontine fibers. Lesion in this limb causes widespread **disability** in the body. Both motor and sensory functions are lost.

■ IN POSTERIOR LIMB

Lesion in posterior limb affects the sensory fibers (thalamocortical fibers). So, it causes:
1. Contralateral **hemianesthesia** (loss of sensation in opposite side of the body)
2. Contralateral **hemihyperesthesia** (abnormal sensation in opposite side of the body)
3. **Hemiplegia** (paralysis of upper and lower limbs in one side of the body).

Hemianesthesia and hemiparesthesia occur because of lesion of superior thalamic radiation. Hemiplegia is due to injury of corticospinal tracts.

■ IN GENU

Lesion in genu causes alteration in **motor activities** in opposite side due to damage of corticobulbar fibers.

■ IN CAUDAL PORTION

Lesion in this portion of internal capsule causes contralateral **hemianesthesia.** It also produces **hemianopia** and **deafness,** because of the involvement of the auditory and visual fibers.

Hypothalamus

■ INTRODUCTION

Hypothalamus is a diencephalic structure. It is situated just below thalamus in the ventral part of **diencephalon.** It is formed by groups of nuclei, scattered in the walls and floor of third ventricle. It extends from optic chiasma to mamillary body.

■ NUCLEI OF HYPOTHALAMUS

Nuclei of hypothalamus are divided into three groups:
1. Anterior or preoptic group
2. Middle or tuberal group
3. Posterior or mamillary group.

Nuclei of each group are listed in Table 149.1 and represented diagrammatically in Figure 149.1.

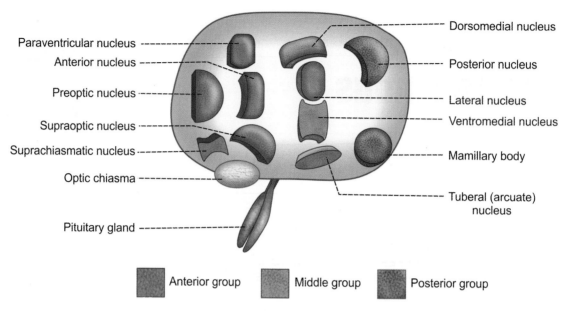

FIGURE 149.1: Nuclei of hypothalamus

TABLE 149.1: Nuclei of hypothalamus

Anterior or Preoptic group	Middle or Tuberal group	Posterior or Mamillary group
1. Preoptic nucleus	1. Dorsomedial nucleus	1. Posterior nucleus
2. Paraventricular nucleus	2. Ventromedial nucleus	2. Mamillary body
3. Anterior nucleus	3. Lateral nucleus	
4. Supraoptic nucleus	4. Arcuate (tuberal) nucleus	
5. Suprachiasmatic nucleus		

■ CONNECTIONS OF HYPOTHALAMUS

■ AFFERENT CONNECTIONS TO HYPOTHALAMUS

1. *Medial forebrain bundle:* From rhinencephalon (limbic cortex) to preoptic nucleus, lateral nucleus and mamillary body
2. *Fornix:* From hippocampus to mamillary body
3. *Stria terminalis:* From amygdaloid to preoptic nucleus
4. *Corticohypothalamic fibers:* From prefrontal area (8) and precentral area (6) of cerebral cortex to the supraoptic and paraventricular nuclei of hypothalamus
5. *Pallidohypothalamic fibers:* From globus pallidus to diffused areas of hypothalamus
6. *Thalamohypothalamic fibers:* From dorsomedial and midline nuclei of thalamus to diffused areas of hypothalamus
7. *Reticulohypothalamic fibers:* From reticular formation of brainstem to diffused areas of hypothalamus

8. *Retinohypothalamic fibers:* Fibers from retina to supraoptic, suprachiasmatic and ventromedial nuclei of hypothalamus (Fig. 149.2).

■ EFFERENT CONNECTIONS FROM HYPOTHALAMUS

1. *Mamillothalamic tract:* From mamillary body to anterior thalamic nuclei
2. *Mamillotegmental tract:* From mamillary body to the tegmental nuclei of midbrain
3. *Periventricular fibers:* Fibers from posterior, supraoptic and tuberal nuclei of hypothalamus pass through periventricular gray matter and reach the following:
   i. Reticular formation in brainstem and spinal cord
   ii. Dorsomedial nucleus of thalamus
   iii. Frontal lobe of cerebral cortex
4. *Hypothalamohypophyseal tract:* From supraoptic and paraventricular nuclei of hypothalamus to posterior pituitary.

■ FUNCTIONS OF HYPOTHALAMUS

Hypothalamus is the important part of brain, concerned with **homeostasis** of the body. It regulates many vital functions of the body like endocrine functions, visceral functions, metabolic activities, hunger, thirst, sleep, wakefulness, emotion, sexual functions, etc. (Table 149.2).

■ 1. SECRETION OF POSTERIOR PITUITARY HORMONES

Hypothalamus is the site of secretion for the posterior pituitary hormones. **Antidiuretic hormone** (ADH) and **oxytocin** are secreted by supraoptic and paraventricular nuclei. These two hormones are transported by means of axonic or axoplasmic flow through the fibers of hypothalamohypophyseal tracts to posterior pituitary. Refer Chapter 66 for details.

■ 2. CONTROL OF ANTERIOR PITUITARY

Hypothalamus controls the secretions of anterior pituitary gland by secreting **releasing hormones** and **inhibitory hormones.** It secretes seven hormones.

   i. Growth hormone-releasing hormone (GHRH)
   ii. Growth hormone-releasing polypeptide (GHRP)
   iii. Growth hormone-inhibiting hormone (GHIH) or somatostatin
   iv. Thyrotropin-releasing hormone (TRH)
   v. Corticotropin-releasing hormone (CRH)
   vi. Gonadotropin-releasing hormone (GnRH)
   vii. Prolactin-inhibiting hormone (PIH).

These hormones are secreted by discrete areas of hypothalamus and transported to anterior pituitary by the **hypothalamohypophyseal portal blood vessels.** Refer Chapter 66 for details.

■ 3. CONTROL OF ADRENAL CORTEX

Anterior pituitary regulates adrenal cortex by secreting **adrenocorticotropic hormone** (ACTH). ACTH secretion is in turn regulated by corticotropin-releasing hormone (CRH), which is secreted by the paraventricular nucleus of hypothalamus (Refer Chapter 70 for details).

■ 4. CONTROL OF ADRENAL MEDULLA

Dorsomedial and posterior hypothamic nuclei are excited by emotional stimuli. These hypothalamic nuclei, in turn, send impulses to adrenal medulla through sympathetic fibers and cause release of **catecholamines,** which are essential to cope up with emotional stress (Chapter 71).

■ 5. REGULATION OF AUTONOMIC NERVOUS SYSTEM

Hypothalamus controls autonomic nervous system (ANS). Sympathetic division of ANS is regulated by posterior and lateral nuclei of hypothalamus. Parasympathetic division of ANS is controlled by anterior group of nuclei. The effects of cerebral cortex on ANS are executed through hypothalamus (Chapter 164).

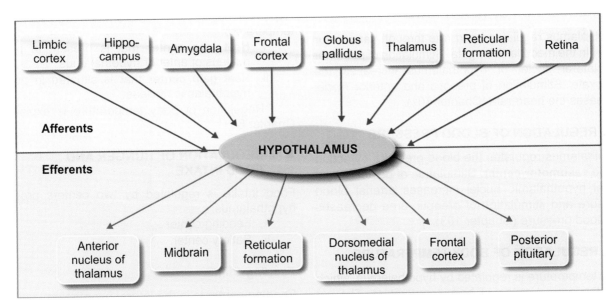

FIGURE 149.2: Connections of hypothalamus

TABLE 149.2: Functions of hypothalamus

Functions	Action/Center	Nuclei/Parts involved
1. Control of anterior pituitary	Releasing hormones Inhibiting hormones	Discrete areas
2. Secretion of posterior pituitary hormones	Oxytocin Antidiuretic hormone (ADH)	Paraventricular nucleus Supraoptic nucleus
3. Control of adrenal cortex	Corticotropin-releasing hormone (CRH)	Paraventricular nucleus
4. Control of adrenal medulla	Catecholamines during emotion	Posterior and dorsomedial nuclei
5. Regulation of autonomic nervous system (ANS)	Sympathetic Parasympathetic	Posterior and lateral nuclei Anterior nuclei
6. Regulation of heart rate	Acceleration Inhibition	Posterior and lateral nuclei Preoptic and anterior nuclei
7. Regulation of blood pressure	Pressor effect Depressor effect	Posterior and lateral nuclei Preoptic area
8. Regulation of body temperature	Heat gain center Heat loss center	Posterior hypothalamus Anterior hypothalamus
9. Regulation of hunger and food intake	Feeding center Satiety center	Lateral nucleus Ventromedial nucleus
10. Regulation of water intake	Thirst center Water retention by ADH	Lateral nucleus Supraoptic nucleus
11. Regulation of sleep and wakefulness	Sleep Wakefulness	Anterior hypothalamus Mamillary body
12. Regulation of behavior and emotion	Reward center Punishment center	Ventromedial nucleus Posterior and lateral nuclei
13. Regulation of sexual function	Sexual cycle	Arcuate and posterior nuclei
14. Regulation of response to smell	Autonomic responses	Posterior hypothalamus
15. Role in circadian rhythm	Rhythmic changes	Suprachiasmatic nucleus

■ 6. REGULATION OF HEART RATE

Hypothalamus regulates heart rate through **vasomotor center** in the medulla oblongata. Stimulation of posterior and lateral nuclei of hypothalamus increases the heart rate. Stimulation of preoptic and anterior nuclei decreases the heart rate (Chapter 101).

■ 7. REGULATION OF BLOOD PRESSURE

Hypothalamus regulates the blood pressure by acting on the **vasomotor center.** Stimulation of posterior and lateral hypothalamic nuclei increases arterial blood pressure and stimulation of preoptic area decreases the blood pressure (Chapter 103).

■ 8. REGULATION OF BODY TEMPERATURE

Body temperature is regulated by hypothalamus, which sets the normal range of body temperature. The set point, under normal physiological conditions is 37°C.

Hypothalamus has two centers which regulate the body temperature:

    i. **Heat loss center** that is present in preoptic nucleus of anterior hypothalamus

    ii. **Heat gain center** that is situated in posterior hypothalamic nucleus.

Regulation of body temperature is explained in Chapter 63.

■ 9. REGULATION OF HUNGER AND FOOD INTAKE

Food intake is regulated by two centers present in hypothalamus:

    i. Feeding center

    ii. Satiety center.

Feeding Center

Feeding center is in the lateral hypothalamic nucleus. In experimental conditions, stimulation of this center in animals leads to uncontrolled hunger and increased food intake **(hyperphagia),** resulting in obesity. Destruction of feeding center leads to loss of appetite **(anorexia)** and the animal refuses to take food.

Normally, feeding center is always active. That means, it has the tendency to induce food intake always.

Satiety Center

Satiety center is in the ventromedial nucleus of the hypothalamus. Stimulation of this nucleus in animals causes total loss of appetite and cessation of food intake. Destruction of satiety center leads to **hyperphagia** and the animal becomes obese. This type of obesity is called **hypothalamic obesity.**

Satiety center plays an important role in the regulation of food intake by temporary inhibition of feeding center after food intake.

Mechanism of Regulation of Food Intake

Under normal physiological conditions, appetite and food intake are well balanced and continues in a cyclic manner. Feeding center and satiety center of hypothalamus are responsible for the regulation of appetite and food intake. These centers are regulated by the following mechanisms:

i. Glucostatic mechanism
ii. Lipostatic mechanism
iii. Peptide mechanism
iv. Hormonal mechanism
v. Thermostatic mechanism.

i. Glucostatic Mechanism

Cells of satiety center function as **glucostats** or **glucose receptors,** which are stimulated by increased blood glucose level.

While taking food, blood glucose level increases. Slowly the glucostats are stimulated and satiety center is activated. At one stage, it develops the feeling of 'fullness'. Now, the satiety center inhibits the feeding center and stops the food intake.

After few hours of food intake, the blood glucose level decreases and satiety center becomes inactive. So, the feeding center is no longer inhibited. Now it becomes active and increases the appetite and induces food intake. After taking food, once again blood glucose level increases and the cycle is repeated (Fig. 149.3).

However, glucostats do not give response to very high level of glucose in blood **(hyperglycemia).** So, in conditions like diabetes, hyperglycemia fails to stimulate the satiety center. The satiety center does not inhibit the feeding center, so the frequency of food intake increases (polyphagia).

ii. Lipostatic Mechanism

Leptin is a peptide secreted by **adipocytes** (cells of adipose tissue). It plays an important role in controlling the food intake and adipose tissue volume. Details of leptin are given in Chapter 73.

When the volume of adipose tissues increases, adipocytes secrete and release a large quantity of leptin into the blood. While circulating through brain, leptin crosses the blood-brain barrier and enters hypothalamus.

In hypothalamus, leptin inhibits the feeding center, resulting in loss of appetite and stoppage of food intake. It is suggested that the cells present in blood-brain barrier contain many receptor-like proteins, which are responsible for the transport of leptin across the barrier.

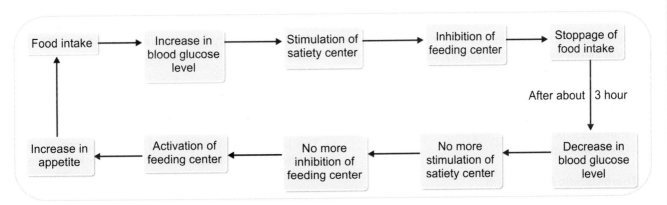

FIGURE 149.3: Glucostatic mechanism

Mode of action of leptin

Leptin acts through some specific neuropeptides in hypothalamus, such as:

a. Neuropeptide Y: It is secreted in small intestine, medulla and hypothalamus. Normally, this peptide stimulates the food intake. But, leptin inhibits neuropeptide Y, leading to stoppage of food intake. Refer Chapters 44 and 141 for details of neuropeptide Y.

b. *Pro-opiomelanocortin (POMC):* It is secreted from anterior pituitary. It is also secreted from hypothalamus, lungs, GI tract and placenta. Normally, it inhibits food intake. Leptin stimulates the secretion of POMC.

Leptin receptor

Many leptin receptors are identified. However, leptin acts via **'LepRb'**, which is the only active receptor present in many nuclei of hypothalamus.

iii. *Peptide Mechanism*

Some peptides regulate the food intake either by stimulating or inhibiting the feeding center, directly or indirectly. The important one among the peptides is ghrelin.

Ghrelin is secreted in stomach (Chapter 44) during fasting. It directly stimulates the feeding center and increases the appetite and food intake. Besides ghrelin, several other peptides are involved in the regulation of food intake.

Peptides, which increase the food intake:

a. Ghrelin
b. Neuropeptide Y.

Peptides, which decrease the food intake:

a. Leptin
b. Peptide YY.

iv. *Hormonal Mechanism*

Some endocrine hormones and GI hormones inhibit the food intake by acting through hypothalamus.

Hormones which inhibit the food intake:

a. Somatostatin
b. Oxytocin
c. Glucagon
d. Pancreatic polypeptide
e. Cholecystokinin.

v. *Thermostatic Mechanism*

Food intake is inversely proportional to body temperature. So in fever, the food intake is decreased. Exact mechanism of this fact is not known. It is suggested that the **preoptic thermoreceptors** (see above) may act via feeding center. The cytokines are also suggested to play a role in decreasing the appetite during fever.

■ 10. REGULATION OF WATER BALANCE

Hypothalamus regulates water content of the body by two mechanisms:

i. Thirst mechanism
ii. Antidiuretic hormone (ADH) mechanism.

i. *Thirst Mechanism*

Thirst center is in the lateral nucleus of hypothalamus. There are some **osmoreceptors** in the areas adjacent to thirst center. When the ECF volume decreases, the osmolality of ECF is increased. If the osmolarity increases by 1% to 2%, the osmoreceptors are stimulated. Osmoreceptors in turn, activate the **thirst center** and thirst sensation is initiated. Now, the person feels thirsty and drinks water. Water intake increases the ECF volume and decreases the osmolality (Fig. 149.4).

ii. *ADH Mechanism*

Simultaneously, when the volume of ECF decreases with increased osmolality, the supraoptic nucleus is stimulated and ADH is released. ADH causes **retention of water** by facultative reabsorption in the renal tubules. It increases the ECF volume and brings the osmolality back to the normal level. On the contrary, when ECF volume is increased, the supraoptic nucleus is not stimulated and ADH is not secreted. In the absence of ADH, more amount of water is excreted through urine and the volume of ECF is brought back to normal.

■ 11. REGULATION OF SLEEP AND WAKEFULNESS

Mamillary body in the posterior hypothalamus is considered as the **wakefulness center.** Stimulation of mamillary body causes wakefulness and its lesion leads to sleep. Stimulation of anterior hypothalamus also leads to sleep.

■ 12. ROLE IN BEHAVIOR AND EMOTIONAL CHANGES

The behavior of animals and human beings is mostly affected by two responding systems in hypothalamus and other structures of limbic system. These two systems act opposite to one another.

The responding systems are concerned with the affective nature of sensations, i.e. whether the sensations

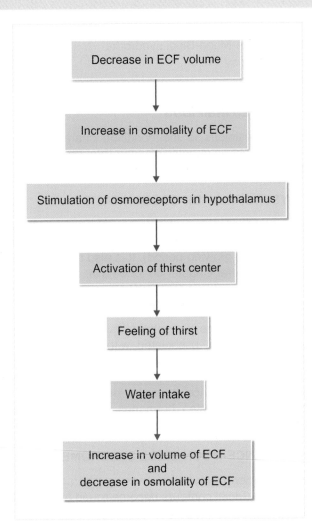

FIGURE 149.4: Thirst mechanism. ECF = Extracellular fluid.

are pleasant or painful. These two qualities are called the reward (satisfaction) and punishment (aversion or avoidance). Hypothalamus has two centers for behaviorial and emotional changes. They are:

  i. Reward center
  ii. Punishment center.

Reward Center

Reward center is situated in medial forebrain bundle and ventromedial nucleus of hypothalamus. Electrical stimulation of these areas in animals pleases or satisfies the animals.

Punishment Center

Punishment center is situated in posterior and lateral nuclei of hypothalamus. Electrical stimulation of these nuclei in animals leads to pain, fear, defense, escape reactions and other elements of punishment.

Role of Reward and Punishment Centers

The importance of the reward and punishment centers lies in the behavioral pattern of the individuals. Almost all the activities of day-to-day life depend upon reward and punishment. While doing something, if the person is rewarded or feels satisfied, he or she continues to do so. If the person feels punished or unpleasant, he or she stops doing so. Thus, these two centers play an important role in the development of the behavioral pattern of a person.

Rage

Rage refers to violent and aggressive emotional expression with extreme anger. It can be developed in animals by stimulating the punishment centers in posterior and lateral hypothalamus. The reactions of rage are expressed by developing a defense posture, which includes:

  i. Extension of limbs
  ii. Lifting of tail
  iii. Hissing and spitting
  iv. Piloerection
  v. Wide opening of eyeballs
  vi. Dilatation of pupil
  vii. Severe savage attack even by mild provocation.

Sham Rage

Sham rage means false rage. It is an extreme emotional condition that resembles rage and occurs in some pathological conditions in humans.

In physiological conditions, the animals and human beings maintain a balance between the rage and its opposite state. This balanced condition is called the **calm emotional state.** A major irritation may make a person to loose the temper. However, the minor irritations are usually ignored or overcome. It is because of inhibitory influence of cerebral cortex on hypothalamus. But the calm emotional state is altered during brain lesions. In some cases, even a mild stimulus evokes sham rage. It can occur in decorticated animal also.

Sham rage is due to release of hypothalamus from the inhibitory influence of cortical control.

■ 13. REGULATION OF SEXUAL FUNCTION

In animals, hypothalamus plays an important role in maintaining the sexual functions, especially in females. A decorticate female animal will have regular estrous cycle, provided the hypothalamus is intact. In human beings also, hypothalamus regulates the sexual functions by secreting gonadotropin-releasing hormones. Arcuate and posterior hypothalamic nuclei are involved in the regulation of sexual functions.

■ 14. ROLE IN RESPONSE TO SMELL

Posterior hypothalamus along with other structures like hippocampus and brainstem nuclei are responsible for the autonomic responses of body to olfactory stimuli. The responses include feeding activities and emotional responses like fear, excitement and pleasure.

■ 15. ROLE IN CIRCADIAN RHYTHM

Circadian rhythm is the regular recurrence of physiological processes or activities, which occur in cycles of 24 hours. It is also called diurnal rhythm. The term circadian is a Latin word, meaning 'around the day'.

Circadian rhythm develops in response to recurring daylight and darkness. The cyclic changes taking place in various physiological processes are set by means of a hypothetical internal clock that is often called **biological clock.**

Suprachiasmatic nucleus of hypothalamus plays an important role in setting the biological clock by its connection with retina via retinohypothalamic fibers. Through the efferent fibers, it sends circadian signals to different parts and maintains the circadian rhythm of sleep, hormonal secretion, thirst, hunger, appetite, etc.

Whenever body is exposed to a new pattern of daylight or darkness rhythm, the biological clock is reset, provided the new pattern is regular. Accordingly, the circadian rhythm also changes.

■ APPLIED PHYSIOLOGY – DISORDERS OF HYPOTHALAMUS

The lesion of hypothalamus occurs due to tumors, encephalitis and ischemia. Following features develop in hypothalamic lesion:
1. Disturbances in carbohydrate and fat metabolisms, when lateral, arcuate and ventromedial nuclei are involved in lesion
2. Disturbance in sleep due to lesion in mamillary body and anterior hypothalamus
3. Disturbance in sympathetic or parasympathetic function occurs due to lesion in posterior, lateral and anterior nuclei
4. Emotional manifestations, leading to sham rage due to lesion in ventromedial and posterolateral parts
5. Disturbance in sexual functions due to the lesion in midhypothalamus.

One or more of the above features can become prominent, resulting in some clinical manifestations such as:
1. Diabetes insipidus
2. Dystrophia adiposogenitalis

3. Kallmann syndrome
4. Laurence-Moon-Biedl syndrome
5. Narcolepsy
6. Cataplexy.

■ DIABETES INSIPIDUS

Diabetes insipidus is the condition characterized by excretion of large quantity of water through urine. Refer Chapter 66 for details.

■ DYSTROPHIA ADIPOSOGENITALIS

This condition is characterized by obesity and sexual infantilism, associated with dwarfism (if the condition occurs during growing period). It is also called **Fröhlich syndrome.** Refer Chapter 66 for details.

■ KALLMANN SYNDROME

Kallmann syndrome is a genetic disorder characterized by hypogonadism, associated with **anosmia** (loss of olfactory sensation) or **hyposmia** (decreased olfactory sensation). It is also called **hypogonadotropic hypogonadism,** since it occurs due to deficiency of gonadotropin-releasing hormones, secreted by hypothalamus. Refer Chapter 66 for details.

■ LAURENCE-MOON-BIEDL SYNDROME

This disorder of hypothalamus is characterized by moon face (facial contours become round by hiding the bony structures), obesity, **polydactylism** (having one or more extra fingers or toes), mental retardation and hypogenitalism.

■ NARCOLEPSY

Narcolepsy is a hypothalamic disorder with abnormal sleep pattern. There is a sudden attack of uncontrollable desire for sleep and the person suddenly falls asleep. It occurs in the daytime.

The sleep may resemble the normal sleep. The duration of sleep is very short. It may be from few seconds to 20 minutes. In night, sleep may be normal but is often disturbed or there may be insomnia (loss of sleep).

■ CATAPLEXY

Cataplexy is the sudden uncontrolled outbursts of emotion associated with narcolepsy. Due to emotional outburst like anger, fear or excitement, the person becomes completely exhausted with muscular weakness. The attack is brief and last for few seconds to a few minutes. Consciousness is not lost.

Cerebellum

Chapter 150

- **PARTS**
  - **VERMIS**
  - **CEREBELLAR HEMISPHERES**
- **DIVISIONS**
  - **ANATOMICAL DIVISIONS**
  - **PHYLOGENETIC DIVISIONS**
  - **FUNCTIONAL DIVISIONS**
- **FUNCTIONAL ANATOMY**
  - **GRAY MATTER**
  - **CEREBELLAR NUCLEI**
  - **WHITE MATTER**
- **VESTIBULOCEREBELLUM**
  - **COMPONENTS**
  - **CONNECTIONS**
  - **FUNCTIONS**
- **SPINOCEREBELLUM**
  - **COMPONENTS**
  - **CONNECTIONS**
  - **FUNCTIONS**
- **CORTICOCEREBELLUM**
  - **COMPONENTS**
  - **CONNECTIONS**
  - **AFFERENT-EFFERENT CIRCUIT**
  - **FUNCTIONS**
- **APPLIED PHYSIOLOGY – CEREBELLAR LESIONS**
  - **DISTURBANCES IN TONE AND POSTURE**
  - **DISTURBANCES IN EQUILIBRIUM**
  - **DISTURBANCES IN MOVEMENTS**

■ PARTS OF CEREBELLUM

Cerebellum consists of a narrow, worm-like central body called **vermis** and two lateral lobes, the right and left **cerebellar hemispheres** (Fig. 150.1).

■ VERMIS

Vermis of cerebellum is formed by nine parts. Part of vermis on the upper surface of cerebellum is known as **superior vermis** and the part on lower surface of cerebellum is called **inferior vermis.**

Parts of superior vermis and inferior vermis are listed in Table 150.1.

Nodulus is continued on either side as an elongated and somewhat lobulated structure called flocculus. Nodulus and **flocculi** are together called **flocculonodular lobe.** On either side of pyramid, there is another extension named paraflocculus.

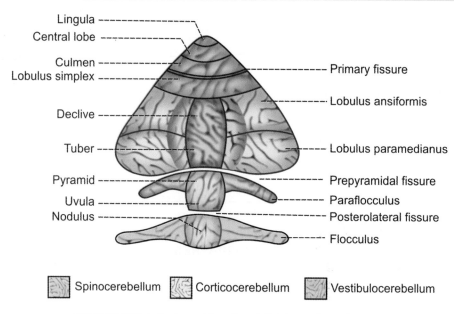

Lingula
Central lobe
Culmen
Lobulus simplex
Declive
Tuber
Pyramid
Uvula
Nodulus

Primary fissure
Lobulus ansiformis
Lobulus paramedianus
Prepyramidal fissure
Paraflocculus
Posterolateral fissure
Flocculus

Spinocerebellum   Corticocerebellum   Vestibulocerebellum

FIGURE 150.1: Parts and functional divisions of cerebellum

TABLE 150.1: Parts of superior and inferior vermis

Superior vermis	Inferior vermis
1. Lingula	6. Tuber
2. Central lobe	7. Pyramid
3. Culmen	8. Uvula
4. Lobulus simplex	9. Nodulus
5. Declive	

Fissures Present Over the Surface of Vermis

1. Primary fissure between culmen and lobulus simplex
2. Prepyramidal fissure between tuber and pyramid
3. Posterolateral fissure between uvula and nodulus.

■ CEREBELLAR HEMISPHERES

Cerebellar hemispheres are the extended portions on either side of vermis.

Each hemisphere has two portions:
1. **Lobulus ansiformis** or **ansiform lobe,** which is the larger portion of cerebellar hemisphere
2. **Lobulus paramedianus** or **paramedian lobe,** which is the smaller portion of cerebellar hemisphere.

■ DIVISIONS OF CEREBELLUM

Division of cerebellum into different major parts is done by three methods:
A. Anatomical divisions
B. Phylogenetic divisions
C. Physiological or functional divisions.

■ ANATOMICAL DIVISIONS

On structural basis, the whole cerebellum is divided into three portions:
1. Anterior lobe
2. Posterior lobe
3. Flocculonodular lobe.

1. *Anterior Lobe*

Anterior lobe includes lingula, central lobe and culmen. It is separated from posterior lobe by primary fissure.

2. *Posterior Lobe*

Posterior lobe consists of lobulus simplex, declive, tuber, pyramid, uvula, paraflocculi and the two portions of hemispheres, viz. ansiform lobe and paramedian lobe.

3. *Flocculonodular Lobe*

Flocculonodular lobe includes nodulus and the lateral extension on either side called flocculus. It is separated from rest of the cerebellum by posterolateral fissure.

■ PHYLOGENETIC DIVISIONS

Depending upon phylogeny, the cerebellum is divided into two divisions:
1. Paleocerebellum
2. Neocerebellum.

1. *Paleocerebellum*

Paleocerebellum is the phylogenetically oldest part of cerebellum. It includes two divisions:

    i. **Archicerebellum,** which includes flocculo-nodular lobe

    ii. **Paleocerebellum proper,** which includes lingula, central lobe, culmen, lobulus simplex, pyramid, uvula and paraflocculi.

2. *Neocerebellum*

Neocerebellum is the phylogenetically newer portion of cerebellum. It includes declive, tuber and the two portions of cerebellar hemispheres, viz. lobulus ansiformis and lobulus paramedianus.

■ PHYSIOLOGICAL OR FUNCTIONAL DIVISIONS

Based on functions, the cerebellum is divided into three divisions:

1. Vestibulocerebellum
2. Spinocerebellum
3. Corticocerebellum.

1. *Vestibulocerebellum*

Vestibulocerebellum includes flocculonodular lobe that forms the archicerebellum.

2. *Spinocerebellum*

Spinocerebellum includes lingula, central lobe, culmen, lobulus simplex, declive, tuber, pyramid, uvula and paraflocculi and medial portions of lobulus ansiformis and lobulus paramedianus.

3. *Corticocerebellum*

Corticocerebellum includes lateral portions of lobulus ansiformis and lobulus paramedianus.

■ FUNCTIONAL ANATOMY OF CEREBELLUM

Cerebellum is made up of outer gray matter or **cerebellar cortex** and an inner **white matter.** White matter is formed by afferent and efferent nerve fibers of cerebellum. Gray masses called **cerebellar nuclei** are located within the white matter.

■ GRAY MATTER

Gray matter or cerebellar cortex is made up of structures arranged in three layers (Fig. 150.2).

Each layer of gray matter is uniform in structure and thickness, throughout the cerebellum.

    Layers of gray matter:

1. Outer molecular or plexiform layer
2. Intermediate Purkinje layer
3. Inner granular layer.

1. *Molecular or Plexiform Layer*

Molecular or plexiform layer is the outermost layer of cortex having the cells arranged in two strata. Superficial stratum contains few star-shaped cells known as **stellate cells.** Deep stratum contains **basket cells.** In addition to stellate and basket cells, the molecular layer contains the following structures:

    i. **Parallel fibers,** which are the axons of granule cells, present in granular layer

    ii. Terminal portions of **climbing fibers** (afferents from medulla)

    iii. Dendrites of **Purkinje cells** and **Golgi cells.**

Cell junctions in molecular layer

Molecular layer contains the following cellular junctions:

    i. Dendrites of stellate cells and basket cells synapse with parallel fibers, which are the axons of granule cells

    ii. Axons of stellate cells end on the dendrites of Purkinje cells. However, the axon of basket cell descends down into the Purkinje layer and forms the transverse fiber, that ends on the soma of Purkinje cells.

    iii. Dendrites of Purkinje cells synapse with climbing fibers and parallel fibers

    iv. Dendrites of Golgi cells situated in inner granular layer enter the molecular layer and end on parallel fibers.

2. *Purkinje Layer*

Purkinje layer is situated in between outer molecular layer and inner granular layer. It is the thinnest layer, having a single layer of flask-shaped **Purkinje cells.** Purkinje cells are the largest neurons in the body. Dendrites of these cells ascend through the entire thickness of molecular layer and arborize there. These dendrites terminate either on climbing fibers or the parallel fibers. Axons of the basket cells form the transverse fibers, which descend down and end on the soma of Purkinje cells. Axons of Purkinje cells descend into the white matter and terminate on the cerebellar nuclei and vestibular nuclei via cerebellovestibular tract.

    Purkinje cells are termed as **'final common path' of cerebellar cortex.** It is because the impulses from

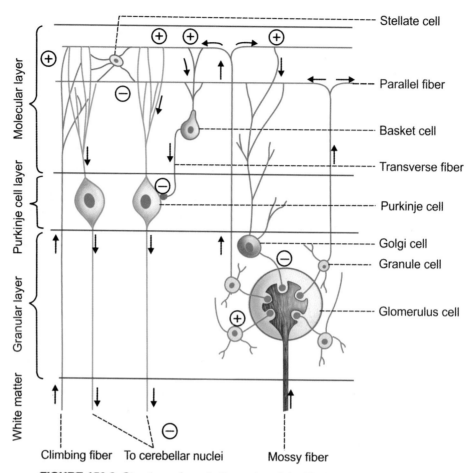

FIGURE 150.2: Structure of cerebellar cortex. (+) = Excitation, (−) = Inhibition.

different parts of cerebellar cortex are transmitted to other parts of brain only through Purkinje cells.

3. Granular Layer

Granular layer is the innermost layer of cerebellar gray matter and it is in between Purkinje layer and the cerebellar white matter. It is formed by interneurons called **granule cells** and **Golgi cells.** Total number of interneurons in this layer is about half the number of all neurons in the whole nervous system.

Axon of granule cell ascends into molecular layer and forms the parallel fiber, which synapses with dendrites of Purkinje cells, stellate cells, basket cells and Golgi cells. Dendrites of granule cells and the axon and few dendrites of a Golgi cell synapse with **Mossy fiber.** The synaptic area of these cells is called **glomerulus** and it is encapsulated by the processes of **glial cells.**

Afferent Fibers to Cerebellar Cortex

Cerebellar cortex receives afferent signals from other parts of brain through two types of nerve fibers:

1. Climbing fibers
2. Mossy fibers.

1. Climbing fibers

Climbing fibers arise from the neurons of inferior olivary nucleus, situated in medulla and reach the cerebellum via **olivocerebellar tract. Inferior olivary nucleus** relays the output signals from motor areas of cerebral cortex and the proprioceptive signals from different parts of the body to the cerebellar cortex via climbing fibers. Proprioceptive impulses from different parts of the body reach the inferior olivary nucleus through spinal cord and vestibular system.

After reaching the cerebellum, the climbing fibers ascend into molecular layer and terminate on the dendrites of Purkinje cells. While passing through cerebellum, climbing fibers of olivocerebellar tract send collaterals to cerebellar nuclei. So, impulses from cerebral cortex and proprioceptors of the body are conveyed not only to cerebellar cortex, but also to the cerebellar nuclei through the climbing fibers. Each climbing fiber innervates one single Purkinje cell.

2. *Mossy fibers*

Unlike climbing fibers, the mossy fibers have many sources of origin, namely motor areas of cerebral cortex, pons, medulla and spinal cord. Fibers arising from all these areas send collaterals to cerebellar nuclei before reaching the cerebellar cortex. So, like climbing fibers, mossy fibers also convey afferent impulses to both cerebellar nuclei and cerebellar cortex. Some of the mossy fibers arise from cerebellar nuclei.

Mossy fibers reach the granular layer of cerebellar cortex and divide into many terminals. Each terminal enters a specialized structure called glomerulus and ends in a large expanded structure that forms the central portion of the glomerulus. Dendrites of granule cells and axon and dendrites of Golgi cells synapse on the mossy fiber giving a thick bushy appearance. The word '**mossy**' refers to the appearance of a plant called **moss,** which grows into dense clumps and hence, these fibers are called mossy fibers.

Neuronal Activity in Cerebellar Cortex and Nuclei

Functions of cerebellum are executed mainly by the impulses discharged from cerebellar nuclei. However, cerebellar cortex controls the discharge from nuclei constantly via the fibers of Purkinje cells. It is done in accordance with the signals received by cerebellar cortex from different parts of the brain and body via climbing and mossy fibers.

Entire process involves a series of neuronal activity:

1. Climbing fibers excite the Purkinje cells directly and cerebellar nuclei via collaterals, by releasing **aspartate.** Excitatory effect of climbing fiber on Purkinje cell is very strong because each climbing fiber ends on a single Purkinje cell (Table 150.2).
2. Mossy fibers excite the Purkinje cells indirectly. In the glomeruli, mossy fibers release glutamate and excite the granule cells and Golgi cells. Collaterals of mossy fibers activate the cerebellar nuclei also by **glutamate.**
3. Granule cells, which are activated by mossy fibers in turn, excite the Purkinje cells, stellate cells and the basket cells through the parallel fibers.

Neurotransmitter utilized by granule cells is **glutamate** or **aspartate.** Granule cells are the only excitatory cells in cerebellar cortex, while all other cells are inhibitory in function. Each mossy fiber innervates many Purkinje cells indirectly via granule cells. So, the excitatory effect of mossy fibers on Purkinje cells is weak.

4. Stellate cells and basket cells, which are activated by granule cells, inhibit the Purkinje cells by releasing GABA. This type of inhibition is called feed forward inhibition (Chapter 140).
5. Golgi cell that is activated by mossy fibers, in turn, provides feedback inhibition to granule cells by releasing **GABA,** i.e. it inhibits the transmission of impulse from mossy fiber to granule cell
6. Cerebellar nuclei are excited by collaterals from climbing and mossy fibers. In turn, the nuclei send excitatory impulses to thalamus and different nuclei in brainstem.
7. However, signals discharged from Purkinje cells inhibit cerebellar nuclei via GABA. Purkinje cells

TABLE 150.2: Interneuronal activity in cerebellum

Neuron	Action on	Action	Neurotransmitter
Climbing fibers	Purkinje cells and Cerebellar nuclei	Excitation	Aspartate
Mossy fibers	Granule cells Golgi cells and Cerebellar nuclei	Excitation	Glutamate
Granule cells	Purkinje cells Stellate cells Basket cells	Excitation	Glutamate/Aspartate
Stellate cells	Purkinje cells	Inhibition	GABA
Basket cells	Purkinje cells	Inhibition	GABA
Golgi cells	Granule cells	Inhibition	GABA
Purkinje cells	Cerebellar nuclei Vestibular nuclei	Inhibition	GABA

GABA = Gamma aminobutyric acid

inhibit the activities of vestibular nuclei also. Thus, it is clear that the cerebellar cortex plays an important role in modulating the excitatory signals of following pathways:

    i. From cerebellar nuclei to cerebral cortex via thalamus
   ii. From final common motor pathway via brainstem and spinal cord.

Because of this activity of cerebellar cortex, movements of body are well organized and coordinated.

■ CEREBELLAR NUCLEI

Cerebellar nuclei are the masses of gray matter scattered in the white matter of cerebellum. There are four nuclei on either side (Fig. 150.3).

1. Fastigial Nucleus

Fastigial nucleus is also known as **nucleus fastigi.** Phylogenetically, it is the oldest cerebellar nucleus. It is placed near the midline on the roof of IV ventricle.

2. Globosus Nucleus

Globosus nucleus is situated lateral to nucleus fastigi. This is also known as **nucleus globosus.**

3. Emboliform Nucleus

Emboliform nucleus is also called **nucleus emboli-formis.** This nucleus is below the nucleus fastigi and nucleus globosus.

4. Dentate Nucleus

Dentate nucleus is also called **nucleus dentatus.** It is the largest cerebellar nucleus. As it is crenated, it is called dentate nucleus. It is situated lateral to all the other nuclei.

■ WHITE MATTER OF CEREBELLUM

White matter of cerebellum is formed by afferent and efferent nerve fibers. These nerve fibers are classified into three groups.

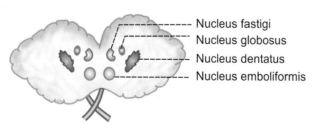

FIGURE 150.3: Cerebellar nuclei

1. Association fibers

Association fibers connect different regions of same cerebellar hemisphere.

2. Commissural fibers

Commissural fibers connect the areas of both halves of cerebellar cortex.

3. Projection fibers

Projection fibers are the afferent and efferent nerve fibers which connect cerebellum with other parts of central nervous system. Projection fibers of cerebellum are arranged in three bundles (Fig. 150.4):

    i. Inferior cerebellar peduncles between cerebellum and medulla oblongata
   ii. Middle cerebellar peduncles between cerebellum and pons
  iii. Superior cerebellar peduncles between cerebellum and midbrain.

i. Inferior Peduncles

Inferior cerebellar peduncles are otherwise called **restiform bodies** and contain predominantly afferent fibers. These nerve fibers transmit the impulses from tactile receptors, proprioceptors and receptors in vestibular apparatus to cerebellum.

ii. Middle Peduncles

Middle cerebellar peduncles are otherwise called **brachia pontis.** These penduncles contain predominantly, the afferent fibers. Most of the fibers of the middle cerebellar peduncles are commissural fibers, which connect the areas of both the halves of cerebellar cortex.

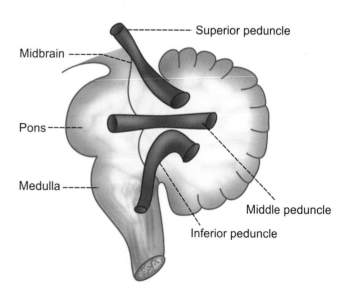

FIGURE 150.4: Cerebellar peduncles

iii. *Superior Peduncles*

Superior cerebellar peduncles are otherwise called the **brachia conjunctivae** and contain predominantly, efferent fibers.

■ VESTIBULOCEREBELLUM (ARCHICEREBELLUM)

Vestibulocerebellum is connected with the **vestibular apparatus** and so it is known as vestibulocerebellum. Since vestibulocerebellum is the phylogenetically oldest part of cerebellum, it is also called **archicerebellum.** It is concerned with the maintenance of posture and equilibrium.

■ COMPONENTS

Vestibulocerebellum includes the **flocculonodular lobe** that is formed by the **nodulus** of vermis and its lateral extensions called **flocculi** (Fig. 150.1 and Table 150.3).

Uvula of vermis is also considered as the part of vestibulocerebellum by some physiologists.

■ CONNECTIONS

Afferent Connections

Vestibulocerebellar tract

Vestibulocerebellar tract is formed by the fibers arising from the vestibular nuclei, situated in pons and medulla. It passes through the inferior cerebellar peduncle of the same side and reaches the cerebellar nuclei,

nucleus globosus, nucleus emboliformis and nucleus fastigi (Fig. 150.5). Fibers from these nuclei, reach the vestibulocerebellum (flocculonodular node).

Vestibular nuclei in turn, receive fibers from vestibular apparatus situated in the inner ear, through vestibular division of cochlear (VIII cranial) nerve.

Efferent Connections

1. *Cerebellovestibular tract*

Fibers of cerebellovestibular tract arise from the flocculonodular lobe, pass through the inferior cerebellar peduncle of the same side and terminate on the vestibular nuclei in brainstem.

Fibers from vestibular nuclei form medial and lateral vestibulospinal tracts, which terminate on the medial group of alpha motor neurons in the spinal cord. This pathway forms the part of medial system of motor pathway (extrapyramidal system).

2. *Fastigiobulbar tract*

Fibers of fastigiobulbar tract arise from fastigial nucleus, pass through inferior cerebellar peduncle of the same side and terminate on vestibular nuclei and reticular formation in medulla oblongata.

From vestibular nuclei, vestibulospinal tracts (mentioned above) arise and terminate on alpha motor neurons. From reticular formation, reticulospinal tract arises and terminates on gamma motor neurons in the spinal cord forming the part of medial motor system (extrapyramidal system).

TABLE 150.3: Components and connections of functional divisions of cerebellum

Division	Components	Afferent connections	Efferent connections
Vestibulocerebellum	Flocculonodular lobe (nodulus and flocculi)	Vestibulocerebellar tract	1. Cerebellovestibular tract 2. Fastigiobulbar tract
Spinocerebellum	Lingula Central lobe Culmen Lobulus simplex Declive Tuber Pyramid Uvula Paraflocculi and Medial portions of cerebral hemispheres	1. Dorsal spinocerebellar tract 2. Ventral spinocerebellar tract 3. Cuneocerebellar tract 4. Olivocerebellar tract 5. Pontocerebellar tract 6. Tectocerebellar tract 7. Trigeminocerebellar tract	1. Fastigiobulbar tract 2. Cerebelloreticular tract 3. Cerebello-olivary tract
Corticocerebellum	Lateral portions of cerebral hemispheres	1. Pontocerebellar tract 2. Olivocerebellar tract	1. Dentatothalamic tract 2. Dentatorubral tract

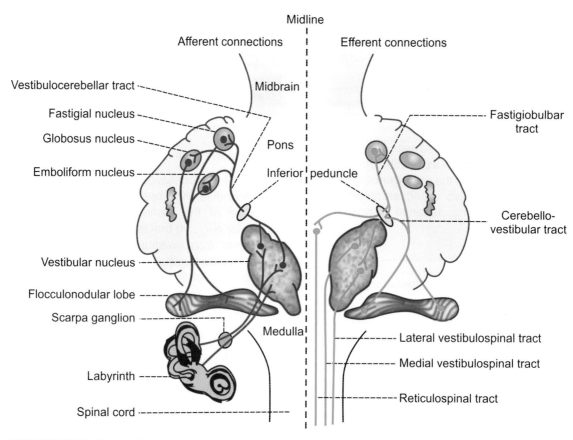

FIGURE 150.5: Connections of vestibulocerebellum. Red = Affernt connections, Blue = Efferent connections.

■ FUNCTIONS

Vestibulocerebellum regulates **tone, posture** and **equilibrium** by receiving impulses from vestibular apparatus. Vestibular apparatus sends information regarding gravity, linear movement and angular acceleration to vestibulocerebellum through vestibulocerebellar tract. Vestibulocerebellum, in turn, sends signals to spinal cord via vestibulospinal and reticulospinal tracts.

Mechanism of Action of Vestibulocerebellum

Normally, vestibular nuclei **facilitate the movements** of trunk, neck and limbs through vestibulospinal tracts and alpha motor neurons. Medullary reticular formation **inhibits the muscle tone** through reticulospinal tract and gamma motor neurons.

However, vestibulocerebellum inhibits both vestibular nuclei and medullary reticular formation. As a result, the **movements** of neck, trunk and limbs are **checked** and the **muscle tone increases.** Because of these effects, any disturbance in posture and equilibrium is corrected.

In the lesion of vestibulocerebellum, there is a reduction in muscle tone (hypotonia) and failure to maintain posture and equilibrium.

■ SPINOCEREBELLUM (PALEOCEREBELLUM)

Spinocerebellum is connected with spinal cord and hence the name. It forms the major **receiving area** of cerebellum for sensory inputs. It is concerned with the maintenance of muscle tone and anticipatory adjustment of muscle contraction during movement. Spinocerebellum is also phylogenetically older part of cerebellum. It is otherwise called **paleocerebellum.**

■ COMPONENTS

Spinocerebellum consists of medial portions of **cerebellar hemisphere,** paraflocculi and the parts of vermis, viz. lingula, central lobe, culmen, lobulus simplex, declive, tuber, pyramid and uvula (Fig. 150.1 and Table 150.3). However, some physiologists do not consider uvula as a part of spinocerebellum.

■ CONNECTIONS

Afferent Connections

1. Dorsal spinocerebellar tract

Dorsal spinocerebellar tract arises from Clarke's column of cells in the dorsal gray horn of spinal cord. It is uncrossed tract and reaches the spinocerebellum through the inferior peduncle of same side (Fig. 150.6). This tract conveys the proprioceptive information from the limbs of same side regarding the position and movements.

2. Ventral spinocerebellar tract

Fibers of ventral spinocerebellar tract arise from the marginal cells in the dorsal gray horn of spinal cord. After taking the origin, the fibers cross the midline, ascend in the opposite side and reach the spinocerebellum through superior cerebellar peduncle. This tract conveys the information about the position and movements of opposite limbs to spinocerebellum.

3. Cuneocerebellar tract

Cuneocerebellar tract arises from accessory cuneate nucleus, situated lateral to cuneate nucleus in medulla. It reaches the spinocerebellum through the inferior cerebellar peduncle of the same side. This tract conveys the proprioceptive impulses from upper limb, upper trunk and neck to spinocerebellum.

4. Olivocerebellar tract

Olivocerebellar tract is formed by climbing fibers arising from the inferior olivary nucleus in medulla. After taking origin, these fibers cross the midline and reach

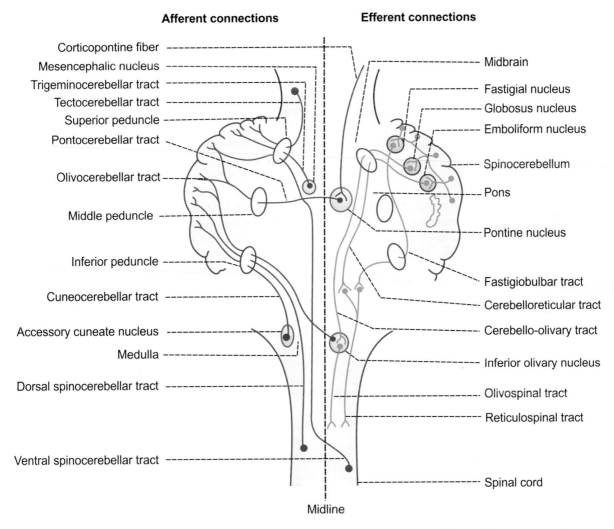

FIGURE 150.6: Connections of spinocerebellum. Red = Afferent connections, Blue = Efferent connections.

the spinocerebellum through the inferior cerebellar peduncle of the opposite side. This tract also gives collaterals to cerebellar nuclei, particularly the globosus nucleus and emboliform nucleus. Inferior olivary nucleus receives afferent fibers from three sources:

i. Brainstem nuclei of same side
ii. Spinal cord through spino-olivary tract of same side
iii. Cerebral cortex of opposite side.

Olivocerebellar tract conveys proprioceptive impulses from the body and output signals from cerebral cortex to spinocerebellum.

5. Pontocerebellar tract

Pontocerebellar tract arises from pontine nuclei, crosses the midline and reaches the spinocerebellum through the middle cerebellar peduncle of opposite side. Pontine nuclei receive afferents from cerebral cortex. Pontocerebellar tract conveys the information to spinocerebellum about the motor signals discharged from cerebral cortex.

6. Tectocerebellar tract

Tectocerebellar tract arises from superior and inferior colliculi of tectum in midbrain. It reaches the spinocerebellum through superior cerebellar peduncle of the same side. This tract carries visual impulses from superior colliculus and auditory impulses from inferior colliculus to spinocerebellum.

7. Trigeminocerebellar tract

Trigeminocerebellar tract is formed by the fibers arising from mesencephalic nucleus of trigeminal nerve. It reaches the spinocerebellum via superior cerebellar peduncle of same side. This tract conveys proprioceptive information from jaw muscles and temporomandibular joint to spinocerebellum. It also carries the sensory impulses from the periodontal tissues (tissues around the teeth) to spinocerebellum.

Efferent Connections

Cortex of spinocerebellum is projected into the nuclei fastigi, emboliformis and globosus of cerebellum. Fibers from these nuclei pass through following tracts:

1. Fastigiobulbar tract

Fastigiobulbar tract arises from fastigial nucleus, passes through superior cerebellar peduncle of same side and ends in the reticular formation.

2. Cerebelloreticular tract

Fibers of cerebelloreticular tract arise from the emboliform and globosus nuclei, pass through superior

cerebellar peduncle of same side and terminate in the reticular formation.

From reticular formation, reticulospinal tract arise and terminate on the gamma motor neurons of spinal cord.

3. Cerebello-olivary tract

Cerebello-olivary tract arises from the emboliform and globosus nuclei and reaches the inferior olivary nucleus of the same side by passing through the superior cerebellar peduncle. From olivary nucleus, the olivospinal tract arises and fibers of this tract end on the alpha motor neurons of spinal cord.

■ FUNCTIONS

Spinocerebellum regulates **tone, posture** and **equilibrium** by receiving sensory impulses form tactile receptors, proprioceptors, visual receptors and auditory receptors.

Spinocerebellum is the **receiving area** for tactile, proprioceptive, auditory and visual impulses. It also receives the cortical impulses via pontine nuclei. Tactile and proprioceptive impulses are localized in the spinocerebellum. **Localization** of tactile and proprioceptive impulses in spinocerebellum is determined by stimulating the tactile receptors and the proprioceptors and by recording the electrical responses in different parts of spinocerebellum. The different parts of the body are represented in the spinocerebellum in the following manner:

Lingula	:	Coccygeal region
Central lobe	:	Hind limb
Culmen	:	Forelimb
Lobulus simplex	:	Face and head.

In cerebral cortex, different parts of the body are represented in an inverted manner. But in cerebellum, different parts are represented in upright manner.

Spinocerebellum regulates the postural reflexes by modifying muscle tone. It facilitates the discharge from gamma motor neurons in spinal cord via cerebello-vestibulospinal and cerebello-reticulospinal fibers. Increased discharge from gamma motor neurons **increases the muscle tone.** Lesion, destruction or abolishing the function of spinocerebellum by cooling, causes stoppage of discharge from gamma motor neurons, resulting in hypotonia and disturbances in posture.

Spinocerebellum also receives impulses from optic and auditory pathway and helps in adjustment of posture and equilibrium in response to visual and auditory impulses.

■ CORTICOCEREBELLUM (NEOCEREBELLUM)

Corticocerebellum is the largest part of cerebellum. Because of its connection with cerebral cortex, it is called corticocerebellum or **cerebrocerebellum.** It is phylogenetically newer part of cerebellum. So, it is also called **neocerebellum.** It is concerned with planning, programming and coordination of skilled movements.

■ COMPONENTS

Corticocerebellum includes the lateral portions of cerebellar hemispheres (Fig. 150.1 and Table 150.3).

■ CONNECTIONS

Afferent Connections

1. *Pontocerebellar tract*

Pontocerebellar tract arises from pontine nuclei, crosses the midline and enters corticocerebellum via middle cerebellar peduncle (Fig. 150.7). It is the largest tract in the body having about 20 million nerve fibers.

Pontocerebellar tract is also called the corticopontocerebellar circuit. Because, it receives signals from motor area of cerebral cortex and conveys those signals to corticocerebellum. It helps the cerebellum in planning the movements initiated by the cerebral cortex.

2. *Olivocerebellar tract*

Olivocerebellar tract arises from the inferior olivary nucleus situated in medulla. It crosses the midline and enters corticocerebellum via inferior cerebellar peduncle of the opposite side. There it terminates on the dentate nucleus and cerebellar cortex. This tract is formed by climbing fibers.

Inferior olivary nucleus receives impulses from brainstem, spinal cord and cerebral cortex and conveys these impulses to the corticocerebellum through the olivocerebellar tract.

Efferent Connections

Output signals from corticocerebellum are relayed mainly through the dentate nucleus. Fibers from dentate nucleus pass through superior cerebellar peduncle, cross the midline and form decussation with the fibers of opposite side. After forming the decussation, these fibers divide into two tracts:
1. Dentatothalamic tract
2. Dentatorubral tract.

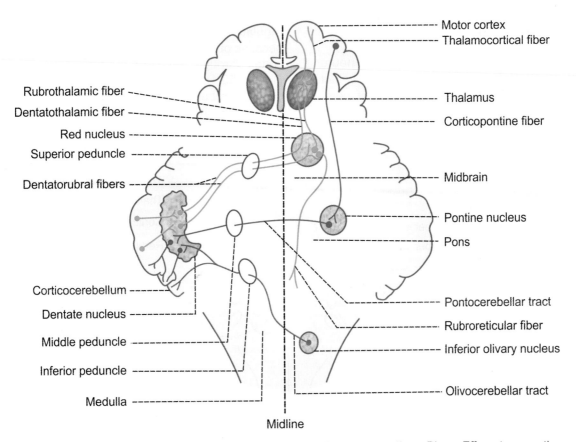

FIGURE 150.7: Connections of corticocerebellum. Red = Afferent connections, Blue = Efferent connections.

1. *Dentatothalamic tract*

After crossing, some of the fibers pass through red nucleus without having any synapse and terminate in lateral ventral nucleus of thalamus. Tract formed by these fibers is called dentatothalamic tract. Thalamus in turn, projects into the motor area of cerebral cortex via thalamocortical fibers.

2. *Dentatorubral tract*

Remaining fibers terminate in the red nucleus of opposite side as dentatorubral tract. Three tracts arise from red nucleus:

   i. Rubrothalamic tract: From red nucleus, this tract ascends and terminates in lateral ventral nucleus of thalamus. From here, thalamocortical fibers arise and reach the cerebral cortex.

  ii. Rubroreticular tract: It descends down and ends in reticular formation. Reticular formation projects into spinal cord via reticulospinal tract.

 iii. Rubrospinal tract: Red nucleus also projects directly into spinal cord through rubrospinal tract.

■ AFFERENT-EFFERENT CIRCUIT (CEREBRO-CEREBELLO-CEREBRAL CONNECTIONS)

Afferent-efferent circuit is an important neuronal pathway, involved in cerebellar control of voluntary movements, initiated by the motor area of cerebral cortex. This pathway includes two tracts:

1. Cerebropontocerebellar tract
2. Dentatorubrothalamocortical tract.

1. *Cerebropontocerebellar Tract*

Fibers from motor areas 4 and 6 in frontal lobe of cerebral cortex enter the pontine nuclei. These fibers are called corticopontine fibers (Figs. 150.8 and 150.9). From pontine nuclei, the pontocerebellar fibers arise and pass through middle cerebellar peduncle of the opposite side and terminate in the cerebellar cortex. This pathway is called the cerebropontocerebellar tract.

2. *Dentatorubrothalamocortical Tract*

Cerebellar cortex is, in turn, connected to the dentate nucleus. Fibers from the dentate nucleus pass via superior cerebellar peduncle and end in red nucleus of opposite side. These fibers are called dentatorubral fibers. From red nucleus, the rubrothalamic fibers go to thalamus. Thalamus is connected to areas 4 and 6 in motor cortex of cerebrum by thalamocortical fibers. This pathway is called dentatorubrothalamocortical tract.

■ FUNCTIONS

Corticocerebellum is concerned with the **integration** and **regulation** of well-coordinated **muscular activities.** It is because of its afferent-efferent connection with cerebral cortex through the cerebro-cerebello-cerebral circuit (Table 150.4). Apart from its connections with cerebral cortex, cerebellum also receives feedback signals from the muscles through the nerve fibers of proprioceptors.

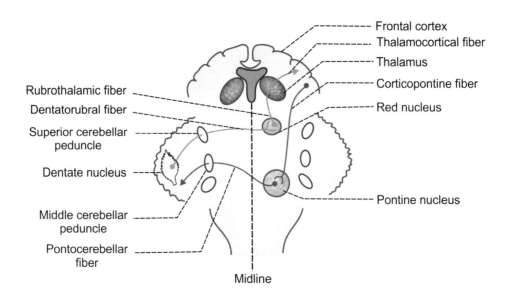

FIGURE 150.8: Cerebro-cerebello-cerebral circuit

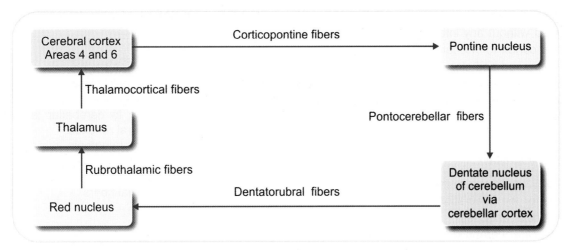

FIGURE 150.9: Schematic representation of cerebro-cerebello-cerebral circuit

TABLE 150.4: Functions of cerebellum

	Functions	Division of cerebellum involved
1. Regulation of tone, posture and equilibrium	By receiving impulses from vestibular apparatus	Vestibulocerebellum
	By receiving impulses from proprioceptors in muscles, tendons and joints, tactile receptors, visual receptors and auditory receptors	Spinocerebellum
2. Regulation of coordinated movements	i. Damping action ii. Control of ballistic movements iii. Timing and programming the movements iv. Servomechanism v. Comparator function	Corticocerebellum (Neocerebellum)

Mechanism of Action of Corticocerebellum

1. Damping action

Damping action refers to prevention of exaggerated muscular activity. This helps in making the voluntary movements smooth and accurate. All the voluntary muscular activities are initiated by motor areas of cerebral cortex. Simultaneously, corticocerebellum receives impulses from motor cortex as well as feedback signals from the muscles, as soon as the muscular activity starts.

Corticocerebellum, in turn, sends information (impulses) to cerebral cortex to discharge only appropriate signals to the muscles and to cut off any extra impulses. Because of this damping action of corticocerebellum, the exaggeration of muscular activity is prevented and the movements become smooth and accurate. Literally, the word damping means any effect that decreases the amplitude of mechanical oscillation.

2. Control of ballistic movements

Ballistic movements are the rapid alternate movements, which take place in different parts of the body while doing any skilled or trained work like typing, cycling, dancing, etc. Corticocerebellum plays an important role in preplanning the ballistic movements during learning process.

3. Timing and programming the movements

Corticocerebellum plays an important role in timing and programming the movements, particularly during learning process. While using a typewriter or while doing any other fast-skilled work, a chain of movements occur rapidly in a sequential manner. During the learning process of these skilled works, corticocerebellum plans the various sequential movements. It also plans schedule of time duration of each movement and the time interval between movements. All the information from corticocerebellum are communicated to **sensory motor area** of cerebral cortex and stored in the form of memory. So, after the learning process is over, these activities are executed easily and smoothly in a sequential manner.

4. Servomechanism

Servomechanism is the correction of any disturbance or interference while performing skilled work. Once the skilled works are learnt, the sequential movements are executed without any interruption. Cerebellum lets the cerebral cortex to discharge the signals, which are already programed and stored at sensory motor cortex and does not interfere much. However, if there is any disturbance or interference, the corticocerebellum immediately influences the cortex and corrects the movements.

5. Comparator function

Comparator function of the corticocerebellum is responsible for the integration and coordination of the various muscular activities.

On one side, cerebellum receives the information from cerebral cortex, regarding the cortical impulses which are sent to the muscles. On the other side, it receives the feedback information (proprioceptive impulses) from muscles, regarding their actions under the instruction of cerebral cortex.

By receiving the messages from both ends, corticocerebellum compares the cortical commands for muscular activity and the actual movements carried out by the muscles. If any correction is to be done, then, corticocerebellum sends instructions (impulses) to the motor cortex.

Accordingly, cerebral cortex corrects or modifies the signals to muscles, so that the movements become accurate, precise and smooth. This function of corticocerebellum is known as comparator function.

Simultaneously, it also receives impulses from tactile receptors, eye and ear. Such additional information facilitates the comparator function of corticocerebellum.

■ APPLIED PHYSIOLOGY – CEREBELLAR LESIONS

Cerebellar lesions may be due to tumor, abscess or an injury. Excess alcohol ingestion also leads to cerebellar lesions. Loss of functions of cerebellum also occurs due to degenerative changes in cerebellar cortex, cerebellar nuclei, cerebellar peduncles and spinocerebellar tracts.

In general, during cerebellar lesions, there are disturbances in posture, equilibrium and movements. In unilateral lesion, symptoms appear on the affected side because cerebellum controls the same (**ipsilateral**) side of the body.

Most of the disturbances are due to the damage to corticocerebellum (neocerebellum) because in human beings, it is larger than other divisions.

■ DISTURBANCES IN TONE AND POSTURE

1. Atonia or Hypotonia

Atonia is the loss of tone and hypotonia is reduction in tone of the muscle. Cerebellar lesion causes atonia or hypotonia, depending upon the severity of the lesion. Atonia or hypotonia due to cerebellar lesion causes disturbances in the postural reflexes.

Cause for atonia or hypotonia during cerebellar lesion is the loss of facilitatory impulses to gamma motor neurons in the spinal cord via cerebello-vestibulospinal and cerebello-reticulospinal fibers.

2. Attitude

Attitude of the body changes in unilateral lesion of the cerebellum. Changes in the attitude are:
  i. Rotation of head towards the opposite side (unaffected side)
  ii. Lowering of shoulder on the same side
  iii. Abduction of leg on the affected side. Leg is rotated outward.
  iv. Weight of the body is thrown on leg of unaffected side. So, trunk is bent with concavity towards the affected side.

3. Deviation Movement

Deviation movement is the lateral deviation of arms when both the arms are stretched and held in front of the body, with closed eyes. In bilateral lesion, both the arms deviate and in unilateral lesion, arm of the affected side deviates.

4. Effect on Deep Reflexes

Pendular movements (Chapter 142) occur while eliciting a tendon jerk. These movements are very common while eliciting the knee jerk or patellar tendon reflex in the patients affected by cerebellar lesion.

A tap on the patellar tendon when leg is hanging freely causes a brisk extension of leg due to the contraction of quadriceps muscle. In normal conditions, after extension, the leg returns back to resting position immediately. In cerebellar lesion, the leg shows pendular movements.

■ DISTURBANCES IN EQUILIBRIUM

While Standing

While standing, the legs are spread to provide a broad base and the body sways side-to-side with oscillations of the head.

While Moving – Gait

Gait means manner of walking. In cerebellar lesion, a staggering, reeling and **drunken-like gait** is observed.

■ DISTURBANCES IN MOVEMENTS

1. *Ataxia:* Lack of coordination of movements.
2. *Asynergia:* Lack of coordination between different groups of muscles such as protagonists, antagonists and synergists.
3. *Asthenia:* Weakness, easy fatigability and slowness of muscles.
4. *Dysmetria:* Inability to check exact strength and duration of muscular contractions required for any voluntary act. While reaching for an object, the arm may overshoot (past pointing) or it may fall short of the object. Overshooting is called **hypermetria** and falling short is known as **hypometria.**
5. *Intention tremor:* Tremor that occurs while attempting to do any voluntary act. Refer Chapter 147 for details of tremor.
6. *Astasia:* Unsteady voluntary movements.
7. *Nystagmus:* To and fro movement of eyeball is called nystagmus. Details of nystagmus are given in Chapter 158.
8. *Rebound phenomenon:* When the patient attempts to do a movement against resistance and if the resistance is suddenly removed, the limb moves forcibly in the direction in which the attempt was made. It is called rebound phenomenon. It is due to the absence of breaking action of antagonistic muscle.
9. *Dysarthria:* Disturbance in speech. It is due to the incoordination of various muscles and structures involved in speech.
10. *Adiadochokinesis:* Ability to do rapid alternate successive movements such as supination and pronation of arm is called **diadochokinesis.** Inability to do rapid alternate successive movements is called adiadochokinesis. It is a common feature of cerebellar lesion. It is also called **dysdiadochokinesia.**

Basal Ganglia

■ INTRODUCTION

Basal ganglia are the scattered **masses of gray matter** submerged in subcortical substance of cerebral hemisphere (Fig. 151.1). Basal ganglia form the part of **extrapyramidal system,** which is concerned with motor activities.

■ COMPONENTS OF BASAL GANGLIA

Basal ganglia include three primary components:
1. Corpus striatum
2. Substantia nigra
3. Subthalamic nucleus of Luys.

■ CORPUS STRIATUM

Corpus striatum is a mass of gray matter situated at the base of cerebral hemispheres in close relation to thalamus (Fig. 151.2). Corpus striatum is incompletely divided into two parts by internal capsule:
    i. Caudate nucleus
    ii. Lenticular nucleus.

i. *Caudate Nucleus*

Caudate nucleus is an elongated arched gray mass, lying medial to internal capsule. Throughout its length, the caudate nucleus is related to lateral ventricle. Caudate nucleus has a head portion and a tail portion.

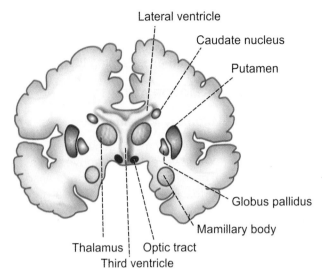

FIGURE 151.1: Basal ganglia

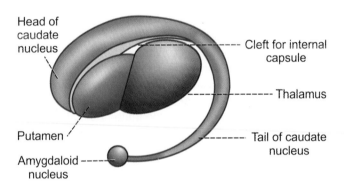

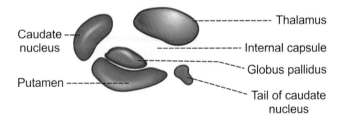

FIGURE 151.2: Corpus striatum

Head is bulged into lateral ventricle and situated rostral to thalamus. The tail is long and arched. It extends along the dorsolateral surface of thalamus and ends in amygdaloid nucleus.

ii. *Lenticular Nucleus*

Lenticular nucleus is a wedge-shaped gray mass, situated lateral to internal capsule. A vertical plate of white matter called **external medullary lamina,** divides lenticular nucleus into two portions:

a. Outer putamen
b. Inner globus pallidus.

Putamen and caudate nucleus are the phylogenetically newer parts of corpus striatum and these two parts are together called **neostriatum** or **striatum.** Globus pallidus is phylogenetically older part of corpus striatum. And, it is called **pallidum** or **paleostriatum.** Globus pallidus has two parts, an outer part and an inner part.

■ SUBSTANTIA NIGRA

Substantia nigra is situated below red nucleus. It is made up of large pigmented and small non-pigmented cells. The pigment contains high quantity of iron.

■ SUBTHALAMIC NUCLEUS OF LUYS

Subthalamic nucleus is situated lateral to red nucleus and dorsal to substantia nigra.

■ CONNECTIONS OF BASAL GANGLIA

Afferent and efferent connections of corpus striatum (Figs. 151.3 and 151.4), substantia nigra and subthalamic nucleus of Luys are given in Table 151.1.

In addition to afferent and efferent connections, different components of corpus striatum of the same side are interconnected by intrinsic fibers.

1. Putamen to globus pallidus
2. Caudate nucleus to globus pallidus
3. Caudate nucleus to putamen.

Different components of corpus striatum in each side are connected to those of the opposite side by commissural fibers.

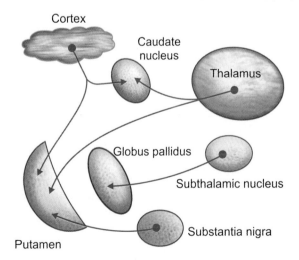

FIGURE 151.3: Afferent connections of corpus striatum

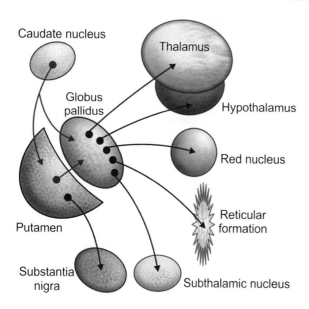

FIGURE 151.4: Efferent and intrinsic connections of corpus striatum

FUNCTIONS OF BASAL GANGLIA

Basal ganglia form the part of **extrapyramidal system,** which is concerned with integration and regulation motor activities. Various functions of basal ganglia are:

■ 1. CONTROL OF MUSCLE TONE

Basal ganglia control the muscle tone. In fact, gamma motor neurons of spinal cord are responsible for development of tone in the muscles (Chapter 157). Basal ganglia **decrease** the **muscle tone** by inhibiting gamma motor neurons through descending inhibitory reticular system in brainstem. During the lesion of basal ganglia, muscle tone increases leading to rigidity.

■ 2. CONTROL OF MOTOR ACTIVITY

i. *Regulation of Voluntary Movements*

Movements during voluntary motor activity are initiated by cerebral cortex. However, these movements are controlled by basal ganglia, which are in close association with cerebral cortex. During lesions of basal ganglia, the control mechanism is lost and so the movements become inaccurate and awkward.

Basal ganglia control the motor activities because of the nervous (neuronal) circuits between basal ganglia and other parts of the brain involved in motor activity. Neuronal circuits arise from three areas of the cerebral cortex:

a. Premotor area
b. Primary motor area
c. Supplementary motor area (Chapter 152).

All these nerve fibers from cerebral cortex reach the caudate nucleus. From here, the fibers go to putamen. Some of the fibers from cerebral cortex go directly to putamen also. Putamen sends fibers to globus pallidus. Fibers from here run towards the thalamus, subthalamic nucleus of Luys and substantia nigra. Subthalamic nucleus and substantia nigra are in turn, projected into thalamus. Now, the fibers from thalamus are projected back into primary motor area and other two motor areas, i.e. premotor area and supplementary motor area.

TABLE 151.1: Connections of basal ganglia

Component	Afferent connections from	Efferent connections to
Corpus striatum	1. Thalamic nuclei to caudate nucleus and putamen 2. Cerebral cortex to caudate nucleus and putamen 3. Substantia nigra to putamen 4. Subthalamic nucleus to globus pallidus	1. Thalamic nuclei 2. Subthalamic nucleus 3. Red nucleus 4. Substantia nigra 5. Hypothalamus 6. Reticular formation (Most of the fibers leave from globus pallidus)
Substantia nigra	1. Putamen 2. Frontal lobe of cerebral cortex 3. Superior colliculus 4. Mamillary body of hypothalamus 5. Medial and lateral lemnisci 6. Red nucleus	Putamen
Subthalamic nucleus of Luys	Globus pallidus	1. Globus pallidus 2. Red nucleus

ii. *Regulation of Conscious Movements*

Fibers between cerebral cortex and caudate nucleus are concerned with regulation of conscious movements. This function of basal ganglia is also known as the **cognitive control** of activity. For example, when a stray dog barks at a man, immediately the person, understands the situation, turns away and starts running.

iii. *Regulation of Subconscious Movements*

Cortical fibers reaching putamen are directly concerned with regulation of some subconscious movements, which take place during trained motor activities, i.e. skilled activities such as writing the learnt alphabet, paper cutting, nail hammering, etc.

■ 3. CONTROL OF REFLEX MUSCULAR ACTIVITY

Some reflex muscular activities, particularly **visual** and **labyrinthine reflexes** are important in maintaining the posture. Basal ganglia are responsible for the coordination and integration of impulses for these reflex activities.

During lesion of basal ganglia, the postural movements, especially the visual and labyrinthine reflexes become abnormal. These abnormal movements are associated with rigidity. Rigidity is because of the loss of inhibitory influence from the cerebral cortex on spinal cord via basal ganglia.

■ 4. CONTROL OF AUTOMATIC ASSOCIATED MOVEMENTS

Automatic associated movements are the movements in the body, which take place along with some motor activities. Examples are the swing of the arms while walking, appropriate facial expressions while talking or doing any work. Basal ganglia are responsible for the automatic associated movements.

Lesion in basal ganglia causes absence of these automatic associated movements, resulting in **poverty of movements.** Face without appropriate expressions while doing any work is called **mask-like face.** Body without associated movements is called **statue-like body.**

■ 5. ROLE IN AROUSAL MECHANISM

Globus pallidus and red nucleus are involved in arousal mechanism because of their connections with reticular formation. Extensive lesion in globus pallidus causes drowsiness, leading to sleep.

■ 6. ROLE OF NEUROTRANSMITTERS IN THE FUNCTIONS OF BASAL GANGLIA

Functions of basal ganglia on motor activities are executed by some neurotransmitters released by nerve endings within basal ganglia. Following neurotransmitters are released in basal ganglia (Table 151.2):

1. Dopamine released by dopaminergic fibers from substantia nigra to corpus striatum (putamen and caudate nucleus: dopaminergic nigrostriatal fibers): deficiency of dopamine leads to parkinsonism
2. Gamma-aminobutyric acid (GABA) secreted by intrinsic fibers of corpus striatum and substantia nigra
3. Acetylcholine released by fibers from cerebral cortex to caudate nucleus and putamen
4. Substance P released by fibers from globus pallidus reaching substantia nigra
5. Enkephalins released by fibers from globus pallidus reaching substantia nigra
6. Noradrenaline secreted by fibers between basal ganglia and reticular formation
7. Glutamic acid secreted by fibers from subthalamic nucleus to globus pallidus and substantia nigra.

Among these neurotransmitters, dopamine and GABA are inhibitory neurotransmitters. So, the fibers

TABLE 151.2: Neurotransmitters involved in the functions of basal ganglia

Neurotransmitter	Released by	Action
1. Dopamine	Fibers from substantia nigra to corpus striatum	Inhibition
2. Gamma aminobutyric acid	Intrinsic fibers of corpus striatum and substantia nigra	Inhibition
3. Acetylcholine	Fibers from cerebral cortex to caudate nucleus and putamen	Excitation
4. Substance P	Fibers from globus pallidus reaching substantia nigra	Excitation
5. Enkephalins	Fibers from globus pallidus reaching substantia nigra	Excitation
6. Noradrenaline	Fibers between basal ganglia and reticular formation	Excitation
7. Glutamic acid	Fibers from subthalamic nucleus to globus pallidus and substantia nigra	Excitation

releasing dopamine and GABA are inhibitory fibers. All other neurotransmitters have excitatory function.

■ APPLIED PHYSIOLOGY –
DISORDERS OF BASAL GANGLIA

■ 1. PARKINSON DISEASE

Parkinson disease is a slowly progressive degenerative disease of nervous system associated with destruction of brain cells, which produce dopamine. It is named after the discoverer **James Parkinson**. It is also called **parkinsonism** or **paralysis agitans**. Great boxer Mohammed Ali is affected by parkinsonism because of repeated blows he might have received on head resulting in damage of brain cells producing dopamine.

Causes of Parkinson Disease

Parkinson disease occurs due to lack of **dopamine** caused by damage of basal ganglia. It is mostly due to the destruction of **substantia nigra** and the **nigrostriatal pathway,** which has dopaminergic fibers. Damage of basal ganglia usually occurs because of the following causes:

　i.　Viral infection of brain like encephalitis
　ii.　Cerebral arteriosclerosis
　iii.　Injury to basal ganglia
　iv.　Destruction or removal of dopamine in basal ganglia. It occurs mostly due to long-term treatment with antihypertensive drugs like reserpine. Parkinsonism due to the drugs is known as **drug-induced parkinsonism.**
　v.　Unknown causes: Parkinsonism can occur because of the destruction of basal ganglia due to some unknown causes. This type of parkinsonism is called **idiopathic parkinsonism.**

Signs and Symptoms of Parkinson Disease

Parkinson disease develops very slowly and the early signs and symptoms may be unnoticed for months or even for years. Often the symptoms start with a mild noticeable tremor in just one hand. When the tremor becomes remarkable the disease causes slowing or freezing of movements followed by rigidity.

　Following are the common signs and symptoms of Parkinson disease:

i. Tremor

Refer Chapter 147 for details of tremor. In Parkinson disease, the tremor occurs during rest. But it disappears while doing any work. So, it is called **static tremor** or **resting tremor.** It is also called **drum-beating tremor,** as the movements are similar to beating a drum. Thumb moves rhythmically over the index and middle fingers. These movements are called **pill-rolling movements.**

ii. Slowness of movements

Over the time, movements start slowing down **(bradykinesia)** and it takes a long time even to perform a simple task. Gradually the patient becomes unable to initiate the voluntary activity **(akinesia)** or the voluntary movements are reduced **(hypokinesia).** It is because of hypertonicity of the muscles.

iii. Poverty of movements

Poverty of movements is the loss of all automatic associated movements. Because of absence of the automatic associate movements, the body becomes **statue-like.** The face becomes **mask-like,** due to absence of appropriate expressions like blinking and smiling.

iv. Rigidity

Stiffness of muscles occurs in limbs resulting in rigidity of limbs. The muscular stiffness occurs because of increased muscle tone which is due to the removal of inhibitory influence on gamma motor neurons. It affects both flexor and extensor muscles equally. So, the limbs become more **rigid like pillars.** The condition is called **lead-pipe rigidity.** In later stages the rigidity extends to neck and trunk.

v. Gait

Gait refers to manner of walking. The patient looses the normal gait. Gait in Parkinson disease is called **festinant gait.** The patient walks quickly in short steps by bending forward as if he is going to catch up the center of gravity.

vi. Speech problems

Many patients develop speech problems. They may speak very softly or sometimes rapidly. The words are repeated many times. Finally, the speech becomes slurred and they hesitate to speak.

vii. Emotional changes

The persons affected by Parkinson disease are often upset emotionally.

viii. Dementia

In later stages, some patients develop dementia (Chapter 162).

Treatment for Parkinson Disease

As Parkinson disease is due to lack of dopamine caused by damage of dopaminergic fibers, it is treated by **dopamine injection.**

Dopamine does not cross the blood-brain barrier. So, another substance called **levodopa** (L-dopa) which crosses the blood-brain barrier is injected. L-dopa moves into the brain and there it is converted into dopamine. Since, L-dopa can be converted into dopamine in liver, some side effects occur due to excess dopamine content in liver and blood. So, along with L-dopa, another substance called **carbidopa** is administered. Carbidopa prevents the conversion of L-dopa into dopamine and carbidopa cannot pass through blood-brain barrier. Thus, L-dopa moves into the brain tissues and is converted into dopamine.

Some of the symptoms of Parkinson disease such as tremor are abolished by **surgical destruction** of basal ganglia or thalamic nuclei.

■ 2. WILSON DISEASE

Wilson disease is an inherited disorder characterized by excess of copper in the body tissues. It is also known as **progressive hepatolenticular degeneration.** This disease develops due to damage of the lenticular nucleus particularly, putamen.

In Wilson disease, copper is deposited in the liver, brain, kidneys and eyes. **Copper deposits** cause damage of tissues. And the affected organs stop functioning.

In addition to symptoms of Parkinson disease, **liver failure** and damage to the central nervous system are the most predominant effects of this disorder. Wilson disease is fatal if not treated early.

■ 3. CHOREA

Chorea is an abnormal involuntary movement. Chorea means **rapid jerky movements.** It mostly involves the limbs. Chorea is due to the lesion in caudate nucleus and putamen.

■ 4. ATHETOSIS

Athetosis is another type of abnormal involuntary movement, which refers to slow **rhythmic and twisting movements.** It is because of the lesion in caudate nucleus and putamen.

■ 5. CHOREOATHETOSIS

Choreoathetosis is the condition characterized by aimless involuntary muscular movements. It is due to combined effects of chorea and athetosis.

■ 6. HUNTINGTON CHOREA

Huntington disease is an inherited progressive neural disorder due to the degeneration of neurons secreting GABA in corpus striatum and substantia nigra. This disease starts mostly in middle age. It is characterized by chorea, hypotonia and dementia. In severe cases bilateral wasting of muscles occurs. It is otherwise called **Huntington disease, chronic progressive chorea, degenerative chorea** or **hereditary chorea.**

■ 7. HEMIBALLISMUS

Hemiballismus is a disorder characterized by violent involuntary abnormal movements on one side of the body involving mostly the arm. While walking, the arm swings widely. These movements are called the **flinging movements.** These movements are due to the **release phenomenon** because of the absence of inhibitory influence on movements. Hemiballismus occurs due to degeneration of subthalamic nucleus of Luys.

■ 8. KERNICTERUS

Kernicterus is a form of brain damage in infants caused by **severe jaundice.** Basal ganglia are the mainly affected parts of brain. Refer Chapter 21 for details.

Cerebral Cortex

Chapter
152

■ INTRODUCTION

Cerebral cortex is also called **pallidum** and it consists of two hemispheres. Surface area of cerebral cortex in human beings is 2.2 sq m.

Both the **cerebral hemispheres** are separated by a deep **vertical fissure** (deep furrow or groove). The separation is complete anteriorly and posteriorly. But in middle portion, the fissure extends only up to corpus callosum. **Corpus callosum** is the broad band of commissural fibers, connecting the two hemispheres.

Surface of the cerebral cortex is characterized by complicated pattern of sulci (singular = sulcus) and gyri (singular = gyrus). Sulcus is a slight depression or groove and gyrus is a raised ridge.

■ HISTOLOGY OF CEREBRAL CORTEX

■ LAYERS OF CEREBRAL CORTEX

Cerebral cortex consists of **gray matter** that surrounds the deeper **white matter.** It is formed by different types of nerve cells along with their processes and neuroglia. It is not uniform throughout. It is thickest, i.e. 4.5 cm at the precentral gyrus and thinnest at frontal and occipital poles. According to **Economo,** the cerebral cortex is formed by six layers of structures. Following are the layers from outside to inside:

1. *Molecular or Plexiform Layer*

Molecular layer has few small fusiform cells. It also contains dendrites or axons from cells of deeper layers.

2. *External Granular Layer*

External granular layer consists of large number of closely packed small cells, which are round, polygonal or triangular in shape. Dendrites of these cells pass into molecular layer. Axons end in the deeper layers. Some axons enter white substance of the hemisphere.

3. *Outer Pyramidal Layer*

Outer pyramidal layer is formed by **pyramidal cells,** which are of two sizes. Medium sized pyramidal cells are in the outer portion and larger pyramidal cells are in deeper portion.

4. *Internal Granular Layer*

Like external granular layer, this layer also has closely packed smaller cells, which are **stellate type.** But, the nerve fibers are more in this layer than in external granular layer. This layer contains many **horizontal fibers,** which appear as a white strip known as **outer strip.**

5. *Ganglionic Layer or Internal Pyramidal Layer*

Ganglionic layer or internal pyramidal layer consists of **pyramidal cells** of graded sizes. It is well developed in the precentral (motor) cortex. Pyramidal cells in this region are otherwise known as **Betz cells** or **giant cells.** This layer also contains **cells of Martinotti.** Martinotti cells are peculiar in that their axons pass outward towards the surface of the cortex.

6. *Fusiform Cell Layer*

Fusiform cell layer is in contact with white matter of cerebral hemisphere. It is composed of closely packed small spindle-shaped cells.

■ PARTS OF CEREBRAL CORTEX

Cerebral cortex is divided into two parts based on phylogeny (evolutionary development of a species):
1. Neocortex
2. Allocortex.

1. *Neocortex*

Neocortex is the phylogenetically new structure of cerebral cortex. It is also called **isocortex** or **neopallium.**

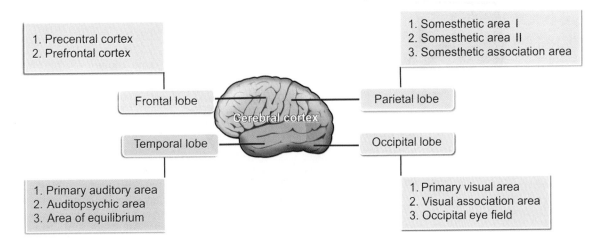

FIGURE 152.1: Parts of cerebral cortex

This part forms the major portion of cerebral cortex.

Part of the cerebral cortex that has all six layers of structures is called neocortex.

2. *Allocortex*

Allocortex is the phylogenetically oldest structure of cerebral cortex. It has less than six layers of structures. It is divided into two divisions namely, **archicortex** and **paleocortex,** which form the parts of **limbic system** (Chapter 153).

■ LOBES OF CEREBRAL CORTEX

In each hemisphere, there are three surfaces lateral, medial and inferior surfaces. **Neocortex** of each cerebral hemisphere consists of four lobes (Figs. 152.1 to 152.3):

1. Frontal lobe
2. Parietal lobe
3. Occipital lobe
4. Temporal lobe.

Lobes of each hemisphere are demarcated by four main fissures and sulci:

1. **Central sulcus** or **Rolandic fissure** between frontal and parietal lobes

2. **Parieto-occipital sulcus** between parietal and occipital lobe
3. **Sylvian fissure** or **lateral sulcus** between parietal and temporal lobes
4. **Callosomarginal fissure** between temporal lobe and limbic area.

■ CEREBRAL DOMINANCE

Cerebral dominance is defined as the dominance of one cerebral hemisphere over the other in the control of cerebral functions. Both the cerebral hemispheres are not functionally equivalent. Some functional asymmetries are well known.

■ CEREBRAL DOMINANCE AND HANDEDNESS

Cerebral dominance is related to handedness, i.e. preference of the individual to use right or left hand. More than 90% of people are **right handed.** In these individuals, the left hemisphere is dominant and it controls the analytical process and language related functions such as speech, reading and writing. Hence, left hemisphere of these persons is called **dominant or categorical hemisphere.**

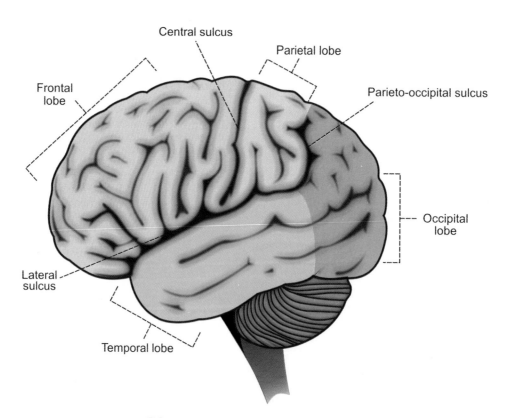

FIGURE 152.2: Lobes of cerebral cortex

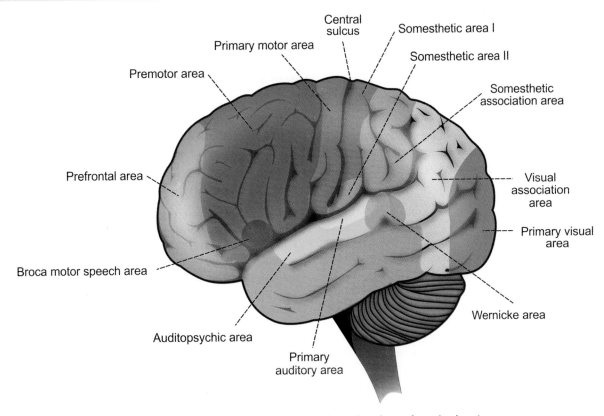

FIGURE 152.3: Functional regions on lateral surface of cerebral cortex

Right hemisphere is called **representational hemisphere** since it is associated with artistic and visuospatial functions like judging the distance, determining the direction, recognizing the tones, etc.

Lesion in dominant hemisphere leads to language disorders. Lesion in representational hemisphere causes only mild effects like astereognosis.

Left hemisphere is the dominant hemisphere in about 75% of the right-handed persons. In the remaining left-handed persons, right hemisphere controls the language function. Some of these persons do not have dominant hemisphere.

■ BRODMANN AREAS

Brodmann area is a region of cerebral cortex defined on the basis of its **cytoarchitecture.** Cytoarchitecture means organization of cells. Brodmann areas were originally defined and numbered in 1909 by **Korbinian Brodmann** depending upon the laminar organization of neurons in the cortex. Some of these areas were given specific names based on their functions. During the period of a century Brodmann areas had been extensively discussed and renamed.

■ FRONTAL LOBE OF CEREBRAL CORTEX

Frontal lobe forms one third of the cortical surface. It extends from frontal pole to the central sulcus and limited below by the lateral sulcus. Frontal lobe of cerebral cortex is divided into two parts:

A. Precentral cortex, which is situated posteriorly
B. Prefrontal cortex, which is situated anteriorly.

■ PRECENTRAL CORTEX

Precentral cortex forms the posterior part of frontal lobe. It includes the lip of central sulcus, whole of precentral gyrus and posterior portions of superior, middle and inferior frontal gyri. It also extends to the medial surface.

This part of cerebral cortex is also called excito-motor cortex or area, since the stimulation of different points in this area causes activity of discrete skeletal muscle. Precentral cortex is further divided into three functional areas (Fig. 152.3):

1. Primary motor area
2. Premotor area
3. Supplementary motor area.

1. *Primary Motor Area*

Primary motor area extends throughout the precentral gyrus and the adjoining lip of central sulcus. Areas 4 and 4S are present here.

Structure of primary motor area

Though this area has all the six layers, the granular layer is thin. Special structural feature of this layer is the presence of **giant pyramidal cells** called **Betz cells** in ganglionic layer.

Connections of primary motor area

Efferent connections

i. Fibers of pyramidal tracts arise from the Betz cells. These fibers synapse with motor neurons in anterior gray horn of opposite side (few fibers reach the same side motor neurons) in spinal cord
ii. Frontopontine fibers from this area reach pontine nuclei of same side
iii. Fibers are also projected to corpus striatum, red nucleus, thalamus, subthalamus and reticular formation
iv. Association fibers connect the primary motor area to other areas of cortex.

Afferent connections

Primary motor area receives fibers from dentate nucleus (cerebellum) via red nucleus and thalamus.

Functions of primary motor area

Primary motor area is concerned with initiation of voluntary movements and speech.

Area 4

It is a tapering strip of area situated in precentral gyrus of frontal lobe. Broad end lies superiorly at the upper border of hemisphere and most of the efferent fibers of primary motor area arise from this area (Figs. 152.4 and 152.5).

Function of area 4

Area 4 is the center for movement, as it sends all efferent (corticospinal) fibers of primary motor area. Through the fibers of corticospinal tracts, area 4 activates the lower motor neurons in the spinal cord. It activates both **α-motor neurons** and **γ-motor neurons** simultaneously by the process called **coactivation** (Chapter 157).

Activation of α-motor neurons causes contraction of **extrafusal fibers** of the muscles. Activation of γ-motor neurons causes contraction of **intrafusal fibers** leading to increase in muscle tone.

Effect of stimulation of area 4

Electrical stimulation of area 4 causes discrete **isolated movements** in the opposite side of the body. The groups of muscles or single isolated muscle may be activated depending upon the area stimulated.

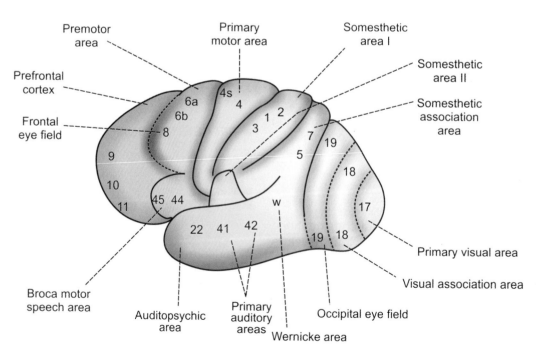

FIGURE 152.4: Lateral surface of cerebral cortex

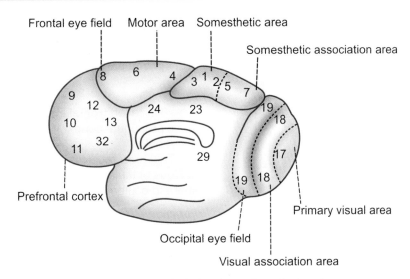

Frontal eye field   Motor area   Somesthetic area

Somesthetic association area

Prefrontal cortex

Occipital eye field

Visual association area

Primary visual area

FIGURE 152.5: Medial surface of cerebral cortex

Localization – homunculus

Muscles of various parts of the body are represented in area 4 in an **inverted way** from medial to lateral surface. Lower parts of body are represented in medial surface and upper parts of the body are represented in the lateral surface.

Order of representation from medial to lateral surface: Toes, ankle, knee, hip, trunk, shoulder, arm, elbow, wrist, hand fingers and face. However, parts of the face are not represented in inverted manner (Fig. 152.6).

Area 4 is concerned with contraction of discrete muscles. It sends motor signals to the facial muscles of both sides (bilateral) and the other muscles of the opposite side (contralateral).

Effect of lesion of area 4

Effect of lesion or ablation of area 4 differs in different species. In cats, the ability to walk is not affected. In monkeys, there is contralateral flaccid paralysis, hypotonia and loss of reflexes. Myotatic reflexes reappear in a short time. Recovery occurs only in proximal parts of limbs but the digits remain permanently paralyzed.

In man, the symptoms are severe than in monkeys. In unilateral lesion, paralysis occurs in **contralateral side.** Complete paralysis is rare. If both sides are affected, the effect is more severe. Recovery occurs very slowly. During recovery, upper parts of body recover first.

If area 4 is affected along with area 6, the effect is very severe, causing **hemiplegia** with **spastic paralysis.** Hemiplegia means the paralysis in one half of the body. In spastic paralysis, the muscles undergo spastic contraction due to increased muscle tone.

Area 4S

Area 4S is called **suppressor area.** It forms a narrow strip anterior to area 4. It scrutinizes and suppresses the extra impulses produced by area 4 and inhibits exaggeration of movements.

2. *Premotor Area*

Premotor area includes areas 6, 8, 44 and 45. The premotor area is anterior to primary motor area in the precentral cortex. The premotor area is concerned with control of postural movements by sending motor signals to **axial muscles** (muscles near the midline of the body).

Structure of premotor area

Premotor area is similar to primary motor area in structure except for the absence of giant pyramidal cells in ganglionic layer.

Area 6

Area 6 is in the posterior portions of superior, middle and inferior frontal gyri. It is subdivided into 6a and 6b. It gives origin to some of the pyramidal tract fibers. The other connections are similar to those of area 4.

Functions of area 6

Area 6 has two functions:

   i. It is concerned with **coordination of movements** initiated by area 4. It helps to make the skilled movements more accurate and smooth.

   ii. It is believed to be the **cortical center** for **extra-pyramidal system.**

occur; but the movements become awkward. It also produces **grasping reflexes.** Lesion involving areas 6 and area 4 produces severe symptoms of **hemiplegia** with **spastic paralysis.**

Area 8

Area 8 is called **frontal eye field.** It lies anterior to area 6 in the precentral cortex. It is concerned with movements of eyeball.

This area receives afferent fibers from dorsomedial nucleus of thalamus and occipital lobe. It sends efferent fibers to oculomotor nuclei in tegmentum of midbrain.

Function of area 8

Frontal eye field is concerned with **conjugate movement** of eyeballs (Chapter 165). This area initiates voluntary scanning movements of eyeballs and it is independent of visual stimuli. It is also responsible for opening and closing of eyelids, pupillary dilatation and lacrimation.

Effect of stimulation of area 8

Stimulation of this area causes conjugate movements of eyeballs to the opposite side.

Effect of lesion of area 8

Lesion of this area turns the eyes to the affected side. Conjugate movements of eyes are lost. However, pupils and eyelids are not affected. In animals, while walking, circular movements occur towards the affected side.

Broca area

Broca area is the **motor area for speech.** It includes areas 44 and 45. Broca area is present in left hemisphere (dominant hemisphere) of right-handed persons and in the right hemisphere of left-handed persons. It is a special region of premotor cortex situated in inferior frontal gyrus. Area 44 is situated in pars triangularis and 45 in pars opercularis of this gyrus.

Function of Broca area

Broca area is responsible for movements of tongue, lips and larynx, which are involved in **speech.**

Effect of lesion of Broca area

Lesion in Broca area leads to **aphasia** (Chapter 162).

3. Supplementary Motor Area

Supplementary motor area is situated in medial surface of frontal lobe rostral to primary motor area. Various motor movements are elicited by electrical stimulation of this area like raising the contralateral arm, turning the head and eye and movements of synergistic muscles of trunk and legs.

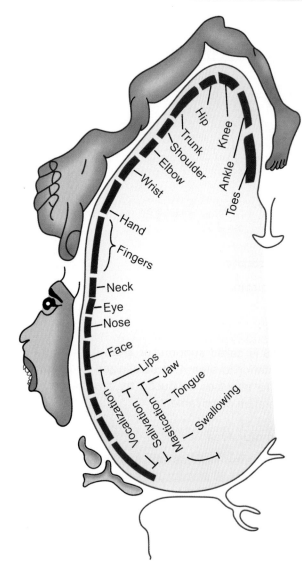

FIGURE 152.6: Topographical arrangement (homunculus) of motor areas in cerebral cortex

Effect of stimulation of area 6

Electrical stimulation of area 6a in human being causes the same effects as the stimulation of area 4. However, the stimulus must be stronger to evoke response from area 6. The effects of stimulation of this area are:
  i. Stimulation of area 6a causes **generalized pattern of movements** like rotation of head, eyes and trunk towards the opposite side
  ii. Stimulation of 6b produces rhythmic, **complex coordinated movements** involving the muscles of face, buccal cavity, larynx and pharynx.

Effect of lesion of area 6

Lesion or removal of area 6 in monkeys leads to loss of skilled movements. After the lesion, the recovery may

Function of supplementary motor area

Exact function of this area is not understood clearly. It is suggested that it is concerned with **coordinated skilled movements.**

Effect of lesion of supplementary motor area

During lesion in this area of human being, the head and eyeballs turn towards the affected side.

Destruction of this area in monkeys causes weak grasping reflexes in contralateral side and bilateral hypertonia of shoulder muscles. But, paralysis is not noticed.

■ PREFRONTAL CORTEX OR ORBITOFRONTAL CORTEX

Prefrontal cortex is the anterior part of frontal lobe of cerebral cortex, in front of areas 8 and 44. It occupies the medial, lateral and inferior surfaces and includes orbital gyri, medial frontal gyrus and the anterior portions of superior, middle and inferior frontal gyri.

Areas present in prefrontal cortex are 9, 10, 11, 12, 13, 14, 23, 24, 29 and 32. Areas 12, 13, 14, 23, 24, 29 and 32 are in medial surface (Table 152.1). Areas 9, 10 and 11 are in lateral surface.

Connections of Prefrontal Cortex

Afferent fibers

Afferent fibers of prefrontal cortex come from:
1. Dorsomedial nucleus of thalamus
2. Hypothalamus
3. Corpus striatum
4. Amygdala
5. Midbrain.

Areas 23, 24, 29 and 32 receive fibers from anterior nucleus of thalamus. Area 32 receives fibers from suppressor area of precentral cortex also.

Efferent fibers

Efferent fibers are projected to:
1. Thalamus
2. Hypothalamus
3. Tegmentum
4. Caudate nucleus
5. Pons
6. Temporal lobe of cerebral cortex.

Area 13, along with hippocampus, uncus and amygdala sends fibers to mamillary body of hypothalamus via fornix. This area is concerned with **emotional reactions.**

Functions of Prefrontal Cortex

Earlier, this area was considered as inexcitable to electrical stimulation. Hence, it was called the **silent area** or **association area**. But, now it is known that the stimulation of this area with low voltage electrical stimulus causes changes in the activity of digestive, cardiovascular, respiratory and excretory systems and other autonomic functions. It also causes fear. Various functions of prefrontal cortex are:
1. It forms the center for the higher functions like emotion, learning, memory and social behavior. **Short-term memories** are registered here.
2. It is the center for **planned actions**
3. This area is the **seat of intelligence;** so, it is also called the **organ of mind**
4. It is responsible for the **personality** of the individuals
5. Prefrontal cortex is responsible for the various **autonomic changes** during emotional conditions, because of its connections with hypothalamus and brainstem.

Effect of Lesion of Prefrontal Cortex

Bilateral lesion or removal of prefrontal cortex in human beings does not cause paralysis. It causes lack of initiation and loss of mental alertness. Very little or no change occurs in memory, judgment and intelligence.

■ APPLIED PHYSIOLOGY – FRONTAL LOBE SYNDROME

Injury or ablation of prefrontal cortex leads to a condition called frontal lobe syndrome.

Features of this syndrome are:
1. **Emotional instability:** There is lack of restraint, leading to hostility, aggressiveness and restlessness
2. **Lack of concentration** and lack of fixing attention
3. There is **lack of initiation** and difficulty in planning any course of action
4. Impairment of **recent memory** occurs. However, the memory of remote events is not lost.
5. Loss of **moral and social sense** is common and there is loss of love for family and friends
6. There is failure to realize the seriousness of the condition. The subject has the sense of well-being and also has **flight of ideas.**
7. Apart from mental defects, there are some functional abnormalities also:
   i. **Hyperphagia** (increased food intake)
   ii. Loss of control over sphincter of the urinary bladder or rectum
   iii. Disturbances in orientation
   iv. Slight tremor.

TABLE 152.1: Areas and connections of frontal lobe

Areas		Afferent fibers from	Efferent fibers to
Precentral cortex	Primary motor areas 4, 4s	1. Cerebellum (Dentate nucleus – via red nucleus) 2. Thalamus	1. Corticospinal tract 2. Pons 3. corpus striatum 4. Red nucleus 5. Thalamus 6 Subthalamus 7. Reticular formation
	Premotor areas 6, 8, 44, 45		
	Supplementary area		
Prefrontal cortex	Areas 9, 10, 11, 12, 13, 14, 29, 23, 24, 32	1. Thalamus 2. Hypothalamus 3. Corpus striatum 4. Amygdala 5. Midbrain	1. Thalamus 2. Hypothalamus 3. Tegmentum 4. Caudate nucleus 5. Temporal lobe

■ PARIETAL LOBE

Parietal lobe extends from central sulcus and merges with occipital lobe behind and temporal lobe below. This lobe is separated from occipital lobe by parieto-occipital sulcus and from temporal lobe by Sylvian sulcus. Parietal lobe is divided into three functional areas:

A. Somesthetic area I
B. Somesthetic area II
C. Somesthetic association area.

In addition to these three areas, a part of sensory motor area is also situated in parietal lobe (see below).

■ SOMESTHETIC AREA I

Somesthetic area I is also called **somatosensory area** I or primary somesthetic or primary sensory area. It is present in the posterior lip of central sulcus, in the postcentral gyrus and in the paracentral lobule.

Areas of Somesthetic Area I

Somesthetic area I has three areas, which are called areas 3, 1 and 2. Anterior part of this forms area 3 and posterior part forms areas 1 and 2.

Connections of Somesthetic Area I

Somesthetic area I receives sensory fibers from thalamus via parietal part of thalamic radiation.

Localization – Homunculus

Different sensory areas of the body are represented in postcentral gyrus (primary sensory area) in an **inverted manner** as in the motor area. Toes are represented in lowest part of medial surface, legs at the upper border of hemispheres, then from above downwards knee, thigh, hip, trunk, upper limb, neck and face. Representation of face is not inverted. Representation of parts of face from above downwards is eyelids, nose, cheek, upper lip and lower lip (Fig. 152.7).

Functions of Somesthetic Area I

1. Somesthetic area I is responsible for perception and integration of **cutaneous** and **kinesthetic sensations.** It receives sensory impulses from cutaneous receptors (touch, pressure, pain, temperature) and proprioceptors of opposite side through thalamic radiation. Area 1 is concerned with sensory perception. Areas 3 and 2 are involved in the integration of these sensations.
2. This area sends **sensory feedback** to the premotor area
3. This area is also concerned with the movements of head and eyeballs
4. Discriminative functions: In addition to perception of cutaneous and kinesthetic sensation, this area is also responsible for recognizing the **discriminative features** of sensations.
   Discriminative functions are:
   i. Spatial recognition: Tactile localization, two point discrimination and recognition of position and passive movements of limbs
   ii. Recognition of intensity of different stimuli
   iii. Recognition of similarities and differences between the stimuli.

Effect of Stimulation of Somesthetic Area I

Electrical stimulation of somesthetic area I produces vague sensations like numbness and tingling.

Effects of Lesion of Somesthetic Area I

If lesion occurs only in the sensory area without involvement of thalamus, the sensations are still perceived.

with perception of sensation. Thus, the sensory parts of body have two representations, in somesthetic area I and area II.

■ SOMESTHETIC ASSOCIATION AREA

Somesthetic association area is situated posterior to postcentral gyrus, above the auditory cortex and in front of visual cortex. It has two areas, 5 and 7.

Functions of Somesthetic Association Area

Somesthetic association area is concerned with synthesis of various sensations perceived by somesthetic area I. Thus, the somesthetic association area forms the center for combined sensations like stereognosis. Lesion of this area causes astereognosis.

Sensory Motor Area

Sensory area of cortex is not limited to postcentral gyrus in parietal lobe. It extends anteriorly into motor area in precentral gyrus of frontal lobe. Similarly, the motor area is extended from precentral gyrus posteriorly into postcentral gyrus.

Thus, the precentral and postcentral gyri are knit together by association neurons and are functionally inter-related. So, this area is called sensory motor area.

Function of sensory motor area is to store the timing and programming of various sequential movements of complicated skilled movements, which are planned by neocerebellum (Table 152.2).

■ APPLIED PHYSIOLOGY

Lesion or ablation of parietal lobe (sensory cortex) results in the following disturbances:
1. Contralateral disturbance of cutaneous sensations
2. Disturbances in kinesthetic sensations
3. Loss of tactile localization and discrimination.

■ TEMPORAL LOBE

Temporal lobe of cerebral cortex includes three functional areas (Table 152.3):
A. Primary auditory area
B. Secondary auditory area or auditopsychic area
C. Area for equilibrium.

■ PRIMARY AUDITORY AREA

Primary auditory area includes:
1. Area 41
2. Area 42
3. Wernicke area.

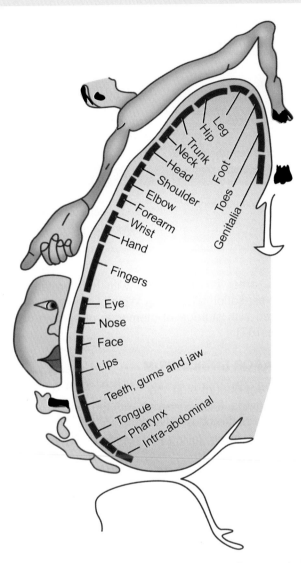

FIGURE 152.7: Topographical arrangement (homunculus) of sensory areas in cerebral cortex

But, the discriminative functions are lost. If thalamus also is affected by lesion, there is loss of sensations in the opposite side of the body.

■ SOMESTHETIC AREA II

Somesthetic area II is situated in postcentral gyrus below the area of face of somesthetic area I. A part of this is buried in Sylvian sulcus. It is also known as secondary somesthetic area or somatosensory area II.

Functions of Somesthetic Area II

Somesthetic area II receives sensory impulses from somesthetic area I and from thalamus directly. Though the exact role of this area is not clear, it is concerned

TABLE 152.2: Areas and connections of parietal lobe

Areas	Afferent fibers from	Efferent fibers to
Somesthetic area I – 3, 1, 2 (Primary somesthetic area)	Thalamus	Premotor area
Somesthetic area II	Somesthetic area I Thalamus	Motor area
Somesthetic association areas 5, 7	Somesthetic area I	Somesthetic area I

TABLE 152.3: Areas and connections of temporal lobe

Areas	Afferent fibers from	Efferent fibers to
Primary auditory areas 41, 42, Wernicke area	1. Medial geniculate body via auditory radiation 2. Pulvinar	1. Medial geniculate body 2. Pulvinar
Auditopsychic area 22		
Area for equilibrium		

Areas 41 and 42 are situated in anterior transverse gyrus and lateral surface of superior temporal gyrus. Wernicke area is in upper part of superior temporal gyrus posterior to areas 41 and 42.

Connections of Primary Auditory Area

Afferent connections

Primary auditory are receives afferent fibers from:
1. Medial geniculate body via auditory radiation
2. Pulvinar of thalamus.

Efferent connections

This area sends efferent fibers to:
1. Medial geniculate body
2. Pulvinar.

Functions of Primary Auditory Area

Primary auditory area is concerned with perception of auditory impulses, analysis of pitch and determination of intensity and source of sound.

Areas 41 and 42 are concerned only with the **perception** of auditory sensation (sound). Wernicke area is responsible for the **interpretation** of auditory sensation. It carries out this function with the help of secondary auditory area (area 22). Wernicke area is also responsible for understanding the auditory information about any word and sending the information to Broca area (Chapter 162).

■ **SECONDARY AUDITORY AREA**

Secondary auditory area occupies the superior temporal gyrus. It is also called or **auditopsychic area** or **auditory association** area. It includes area 22.

This area is concerned with interpretation of auditory sensation along with Wernicke area. It is also concerned with storage of memories of spoken words (Chapter 162).

■ **AREA FOR EQUILIBRIUM**

Area for equilibrium is in the posterior part of superior temporal gyrus. It is concerned with the maintenance of equilibrium of the body. Stimulation of this area causes dizziness, swaying, falling and feeling of rotation.

■ **APPLIED PHYSIOLOGY – TEMPORAL LOBE SYNDROME**

Temporal lobe syndrome is otherwise known as **Kluver-Bucy syndrome.** It is observed in animals, particularly monkeys after the bilateral ablation of temporal lobe along with amygdala and uncus. It occurs in human beings during bilateral lesions of these structures.

Manifestations of this syndrome are:
1. **Aphasia** (disturbance in speech: Chapter 162)
2. Auditory disturbances such as frequent attacks of tinnitus, auditory hallucinations with sounds like buzzing, ringing or humming. **Tinnitus** means noise in the ear. **Hallucination** means feeling of a particular type of sensation without any stimulus.
3. Disturbances in smell and taste sensations
4. Dreamy states: The patients are not aware of their own activities and have the feeling of unreality
5. **Visual hallucinations** associated with hemianopia.

■ **OCCIPITAL LOBE**

Occipital lobe is called the **visual cortex.** Areas and connections of occipital lobe is given in Table 152.4.

TABLE 152.4: Areas and connections of occipital lobe

Areas	Afferent fibers from	Efferent fibers to
Primary visual area – 17		
Visual association area – 18	Lateral geniculate body	Superior colliculus Lateral geniculate body
Occipital eye field – 19		

■ AREAS OF VISUAL CORTEX

Occipital lobe consists of three functional areas:
1. Primary visual area (area 17)
2. Secondary visual area or visuopsychic area (area 18)
3. Occipital eye field (area 19).

Connections of Occipital Lobe

Occipital lobe receives afferent fibers from lateral geniculate body. It sends efferent fibers to superior colliculus and lateral geniculate body.

Functions of Occipital Lobe

1. Primary visual area (area 17) is concerned with **perception** of visual sensation
2. Secondary visual area (area 18) is concerned with **interpretation** of visual sensation and storage of memories of visual symbols (Chapter 162)
3. Occipital eye field (area 19) is concerned with reflex **movement of eyeballs.** It is also concerned with associated movements of eyeballs while following a moving object. (Table 152.5).

■ APPLIED PHYSIOLOGY

Lesion in the upper or lower part of visual cortex results in hemianopia. Bilateral lesion leads to total blindness. Refer Chapter 168 for details.

■ METHODS TO STUDY CORTICAL CONNECTIONS AND FUNCTIONS

■ BY CUTTING OR DESTRUCTION OF NERVE CELL

1. If the nerve cell body is destroyed, degenerative changes occur throughout the axon arising from it. By using **Marchi staining** technique, course of the nerve fiber could be traced. If any part of motor area is destroyed, the degeneration of the fibers in the pyramidal tracts can be traced. If arm fibers are involved, the degeneration occurs up to lower cervical and upper thoracic level.

2. If an axon is cut, the nerve cell body (from which the axon arises) undergoes **chromatolysis**. If any fiber in pyramidal tract is cut, the chromatolysis occurs in nerve cell body situated in motor cortex.

Thus, this method is used to study connections and localization in motor cortex. It is also used for the study of connections of different parts of cerebral cortex.

■ BY RECORDING ELECTRICAL ACTIVITY – EVOKED POTENTIAL

When an impulse passes through a nerve, its route and the termination can be determined by recording the electrical potentials using microelectrodes at different points along the course of the nerve fiber. This method is used to trace certain pathways from or to the cortex, particularly auditory pathway and pyramidal tract.

Evoked Potential

Evoked potential is the electrical potential or electrical response in a neuron or group of neurons in the brain produced by an external stimulus. It is also called **evoked cortical potential.**

When any receptor of skin or a sense organ (eye or ear) is stimulated, the impulses pass through the afferents and reach cerebral cortex. By using scalp electrodes, the potentials developed in cortical areas can be recorded. This method is used to determine the functions of various cortical areas. It is also used to map out the cortical representation of body (localization) for sensory function.

Evoked potential is recorded by placing the exploring electrode on the surface of the head over the primary cortical area of the particular sensation. Indifferent electrode is placed on a distant area of head. In human beings small disk like electrodes are placed on different areas of head by using a tape or washable paste. Electrode cap, which is placed over the head can also be used.

Analysis and interpretation of the potential is done by computer. Evoked potential is characterized by two types of response.

TABLE 152.5: Functions of cortical lobes

Lobe				Functions
Frontal lobe	Precentral cortex	Primary motor area	Area 4	Initiates of movements
			Area 4S	Inhibits exaggeration of movements initiated by area 4
		Premotor area	Area 6	Coordinates movements initiated by area 4 Acts as higher center for extrapyramidal system
			Area 8	Frontal eye field Concerned with conjugate movements of eyeballs Concerned with voluntary movements of eyeballs
			Broca area: Areas 44 and 45	Initiates movements involved in speech; motor speech area
		Supplementary motor area	–	Concerned with coordinated skilled movements
	Prefrontal cortex	Areas 9, 10, 11, 12, 13, 14, 23, 24, 29 and 32		Concerned with emotion, learning, memory and social behavior Act as the center for planned actions Form seat of intelligence Initiate autonomic changes during emotional conditions
Parietal lobe	Somesthetic area I	Area 1		Perceives cutaneous and kinesthetic sensations
		Areas 3 and 2		Integrate cutaneous and kinesthetic sensations
		Areas 3, 2 and 1		Send feedback to premotor area Concerned with movements of head and eyeballs Concerned with recognition of discriminative features of sensations
	Somesthetic area II	–		Perceives cutaneous and kinesthetic sensations
	Somesthetic association area	Areas 5 and 7		Synthesize sensations perceived by somesthetic area I (forms the center for combined sensations)
Temporal lobe	Primary auditory area	Areas 41 and 42		Perceive auditory sensation
		Wernicke area		Interprets auditory sensation (along with area 22)
	Secondary auditory area	Area 22		Interprets auditory sensation (along with Wernicke area)
	Area for equilibrium	–		Concerned with maintenance of equilibrium of body
Occipital lobe	Primary visual area	Area 17		Perceives visual sensation
	Secondary visual area	Area 18		Interprets visual sensation
	Occipital eye field	Area 19		Concerned with reflex movement of eyeballs Concerned with associated movements of eyeballs while following a moving object

1. *Primary evoked potential*

When the stimulus is applied to the receptor or sense organ, the primary evoked potential appears after a latent period of 5 to 10 milliseconds. It includes a positive wave followed by a small negative wave. Primary evoked potential is highly localized and appears specifically on the cortical surface where the particular sensory pathway terminates.

2. *Diffuse secondary evoked potential*

Finally another larger and prolonged positive wave called secondary evoked potential is recorded. It is not localized. It appears on the diffused areas of cortex.

Thus, the evoked potential includes P1-N1-P2 sequence, i.e. first positive wave – first negative wave – second positive wave.

Diagnostic Uses of Evoked Potential

An evoked potential test determines the functional status of a nervous pathway. It also measures the time taken by the nerves to respond to stimulation. Intensity of response is also measured. Nerves from different areas of the body may be tested. However, three types of evoked potentials are commonly used in diagnosis.

1. **Visual evoked potential,** which is recorded when the visual receptors are stimulated by looking at a test pattern
2. **Auditory evoked potential** that is recorded when auditory receptors are stimulated by listening to a test sound
3. **Somatosensory evoked potential,** which is recorded when the somatic nerves of the limbs are stimulated by electrical stimulus.

■ BY PHYSIOLOGICAL NEURONOGRAPHY

When a small piece of blotting paper soaked in **strychnine** solution is placed over cerebral cortex, the nerve cells are stimulated by strychnine. The impulses discharged by these nerve cells pass through the axons and reach the termination in other part of cortex or other part of brain. By recording these impulses, the connections of cortex can be studied.

■ BY SCANNING

Nowadays, the functional activities of cerebral cortex or other parts of the brain are determined by scanning. Due to the fast development of technology, many sophisticated scanning methods are being introduced. Three such methods used widely are:

1. Computerized axial tomography (CAT)
2. Positron emission tomography (PET)
3. Magnetic resonance imaging (MRI).

Refer Chapter 109 for details of these scanning methods.

Limbic System

- ■ INTRODUCTION
- ■ COMPONENTS
  - ■ ARCHICORTICAL STRUCTURES
  - ■ PALEOCORTICAL STRUCTURES
  - ■ JUXTALLOCORTICAL STRUCTURES
  - ■ SUBCORTICAL STRUCTURES
- ■ CONNECTIONS
- ■ FUNCTIONS
  - ■ OLFACTION
  - ■ REGULATION OF ENDOCRINE GLANDS
  - ■ REGULATION OF AUTONOMIC FUNCTIONS
  - ■ REGULATION OF FOOD INTAKE
  - ■ CONTROL OF CIRCADIAN RHYTHM
  - ■ REGULATION OF SEXUAL FUNCTION
  - ■ ROLE IN EMOTIONAL STATE
  - ■ ROLE IN MEMORY
  - ■ ROLE IN MOTIVATION

■ INTRODUCTION

Limbic system is a complex system of cortical and subcortical structures that form a **ring** around the hilus of cerebral hemisphere. **Limbus** means ring. It is also known as **limbic lobe.** Earlier, it was called **rhinencephalon.**

In terms of evolutionary development **(phylogeny),** limbic system is one of the oldest parts of the brain and it is related to olfactory lobe. It is found as a prominent structure in fish, amphibians, reptiles and mammals.

Limbic system is primarily related to emotional part of our life and is extensively concerned with memory.

■ COMPONENTS OF LIMBIC SYSTEM

Structures of limbic system are classified into four groups (Fig. 153.1):
 1. Archicortical structures
 2. Paleocortical structures
 3. Juxtallocortical structures
 4. Subcortical structures.

■ ARCHICORTICAL STRUCTURES

Archicortex forms **allocortex** along with **paleocortex** (Chapter 152). Archicortex is the phylogenetically oldest structure. It is concerned with **memory.**

■ PALEOCORTICAL STRUCTURES

Paleocortex is in between archicortex and neocortex. It is concerned with **olfaction.**

■ JUXTALLOCORTICAL STRUCTURES

Juxtallocortex or **mesocortex** is situated between paleo-cortex and neocortex.

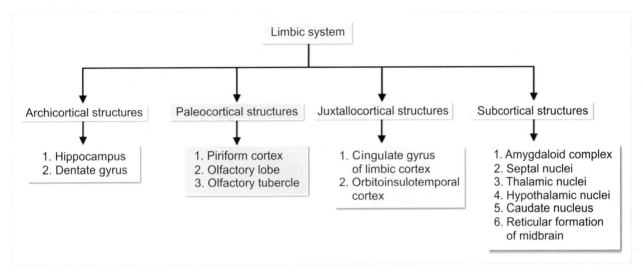

FIGURE 153.1: Components of limbic system

■ SUBCORTICAL STRUCTURES

Structures situated below the level of cortex are called subcortical structures. Limbic system includes six subcortical structures (Figs. 153.1 and 153.2).

■ CONNECTIONS OF LIMBIC SYSTEM

Connections of limbic system are complex. Following are the major (afferent and efferent) connections of limbic system:

1. Fornix: It includes fibers connecting:
   i. Hippocampus and septal nuclei with the mamillary body
   ii. Hippocampus with hypothalamic nuclei.
2. Lateral hypothalamus receives afferent fibers from:
   i. Hippocampus
   ii. Septal nuclei
   iii. Olfactory tubercle
   iv. Head of caudate nucleus
   v. Piriform area
   vi. Periamygdaloid area.
3. Caudate nucleus receives fibers from:
   i. Cingulate gyrus
   ii. Intralaminar nuclei of thalamus.
4. Brainstem reticular formation receives fibers from:
   i. Hippocampus
   ii. Cingulate gyrus.
5. Papez circuit.

Papez Circuit

Papez circuit is the interconnections between various structures of limbic system, which form a complex of closed circuit. This circuit was described by Papez.

Hippocampus is connected to mamillary bodies of hypothalamus via fornix. Mamillary bodies are connected to anterior thalamic nucleus via mamillothalamic tract. Anterior thalamic nucleus is projected into cingulate gyrus through medial thalamocortical fibers. Cingulate gyrus is in turn connected to hippocampus (Fig. 153.3). Papez circuit plays a role in **memory encoding** (Chapter 162).

■ FUNCTIONS OF LIMBIC SYSTEM

■ 1. OLFACTION

Piriform cortex and amygdaloid nucleus form the **olfactory centers.** In lower animals, the amygdaloid nucleus is concerned primarily with olfaction.

■ 2. REGULATION OF ENDOCRINE GLANDS

Hypothalamus plays an important role in regulation of endocrine secretion (Chapter 66).

■ 3. REGULATION OF AUTONOMIC FUNCTIONS

Hypothalamus plays an important role in regulating the autonomic functions (Chapter 149) such as:
   i. Heart rate
   ii. Blood pressure

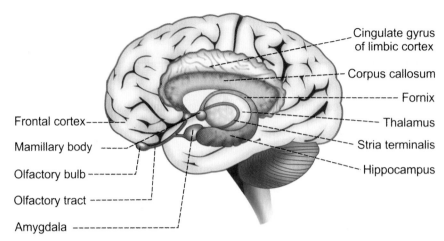

FIGURE 153.2: Major components of limbic system

iii. Water balance

iv. Body temperature.

■ 4. REGULATION OF FOOD INTAKE

Along with amygdaloid complex, the feeding center and satiety center present in hypothalamus regulate food intake (Chapter 149).

■ 5. CONTROL OF CIRCADIAN RHYTHM

Hypothalamus is taking major role in the circadian fluctuations of various physiological activities (Chapter 149).

■ 6. REGULATION OF SEXUAL FUNCTIONS

Hypothalamus is responsible for maintaining sexual functions in both man and animals (Chapter 149).

■ 7. ROLE IN EMOTIONAL STATE

Emotional state of human beings is maintained by hippocampus along with hypothalamus (Chapter 149).

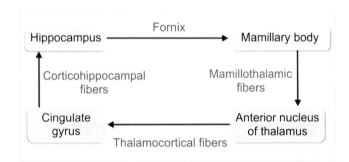

FIGURE 153.3: Papez circuit

■ 8. ROLE IN MEMORY

Hippocampus and Papez circuit play an important role in memory (Chapter 162).

■ 9. ROLE IN MOTIVATION

Reward and punishment centers present in hypothalamus and other structures of limbic system are responsible for motivation and the behavior pattern of human beings (Chapter 149).

Refer Chapter 149 for details of the hypothalamic functions.

Reticular Formation

Chapter 154

- ■ **DEFINITION**
- ■ **SITUATION**
- ■ **ORGANIZATION OF RETICULAR FORMATION**
  - ■ RAPHE GROUP
  - ■ PARAMEDIAN GROUP
  - ■ LATERAL GROUP
  - ■ MEDIAL GROUP
  - ■ INTERMEDIATE GROUP
- ■ **DIVISIONS OF RETICULAR FORMATION**
  - ■ NUCLEI OF MEDULLARY RETICULAR FORMATION
  - ■ NUCLEI OF PONTINE RETICULAR FORMATION
  - ■ NUCLEI OF MIDBRAIN RETICULAR FORMATION
- ■ **CONNECTIONS**
  - ■ AFFERENT CONNECTIONS
  - ■ EFFERENT CONNECTIONS
- ■ **FUNCTIONS**
  - ■ ASCENDING RETICULAR ACTIVATING SYSTEM (ARAS)
  - ■ DESCENDING RETICULAR SYSTEM

■ DEFINITION

Reticular formation is a diffused mass of neurons and nerve fibers, which form an ill-defined meshwork of reticulum in central portion of the brainstem.

■ SITUATION OF RETICULAR FORMATION

Reticular formation is situated in **brainstem**. It extends downwards into spinal cord and upwards up to thalamus and subthalamus.

■ ORGANIZATION OF RETICULAR FORMATION

Reticular formation is constituted by 5 groups of nuclei. All these nuclei are structurally and functionally distinct.

■ 1. RAPHE GROUP

Raphe group of nuclei are situated along the midline of the brainstem forming a continuous column. Raphe nuclei secrete **serotonin** (5-hydroxytryptamine), which is an **inhibitory neurotransmitter.**

■ 2. PARAMEDIAN GROUP

Paramedian group includes nucleus reticularis paramedianus and pontine reticulotegmental nucleus. These nuclei are concerned with **motor functions.**

■ 3. LATERAL GROUP

Lateral group of nuclei are situated in the lateral one third of the tegmentum. It consists of nuclei with small (parvocellular) cells. Neurons of these nuclei receive sensory signals from the cranial nerves, cerebellum and spinal cord.

4. MEDIAL GROUP

Medial group of nuclei are situated in the medial two third of the tegmentum. It consists of nuclei with small cells and giant (gigantocellular) cells. Nuclei of this group form the major output of the reticular formation and send fibers to the hypothalamus, thalamus and spinal cord. These nuclei are associated with **motor functions.**

5. INTERMEDIATE GROUP

Intermediate group of nuclei are present only in the medulla. It is situated between the lateral and medial groups of nuclei. These nuclei are concerned with autonomic regulation of **respiration, heart rate** and **blood pressure.**

■ DIVISIONS OF RETICULAR FORMATION

Reticular formation is divided into three divisions based on the location in brainstem:
  A. Medullary reticular formation
  B. Pontine reticular formation
  C. Midbrain reticular formation.
    Each division of reticular formation has its own collection of nuclei.

■ NUCLEI OF MEDULLARY RETICULAR FORMATION

  1. Lateral reticular nucleus
  2. Ventral reticular nucleus
  3. Dorsal reticular nucleus
  4. Gigantocellular reticular nucleus
  5. Paragigantocellular reticular nucleus
  6. Paramedian reticular nucleus
  7. Parvocellular reticular nucleus
  8. Magnocellular reticular nucleus.

■ NUCLEI OF PONTINE RETICULAR FORMATION

  1. Nucleus reticularis pontis oralis
  2. Nucleus reticularis pontis caudalis
  3. Locus ceruleus nucleus
  4. Subceruleus reticular nucleus
  5. Tegmenti pontis reticular nucleus
  6. Pedunculopontine reticular nucleus
  7. Nucleus reticular cuneiformis.

■ NUCLEI OF MIDBRAIN RETICULAR FORMATION

  1. Red nucleus
  2. Nucleus tegmental pedunculopontis
  3. Nucleus reticular subcuneiformis.

■ CONNECTIONS OF RETICULAR FORMATION

■ AFFERENT CONNECTIONS

Reticular formation receives collaterals from almost all the ascending sensory pathways. It also receives fibers from different parts of the brain (Fig. 154.1):
  1. Optic pathway
  2. Olfactory pathway
  3. Auditory pathway
  4. Taste pathway
  5. Spinal and trigeminal pathways carrying touch sensation
  6. Pathways for pain, temperature, vibration and kinesthetic sensations
  7. Cerebral cortex
  8. Cerebellum
  9. Corpus striatum
  10. Thalamic nuclei.

■ EFFERENT CONNECTIONS

Reticular formation sends fibers to the following parts of central nervous system (Fig. 154.2):
  1. Cerebral cortex
  2. Diencephalon: Thalamus, hypothalamus and subthalamus

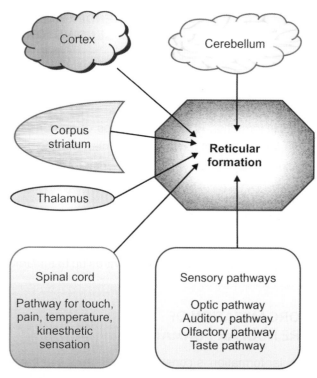

FIGURE 154.1: Afferent connections of reticular formation

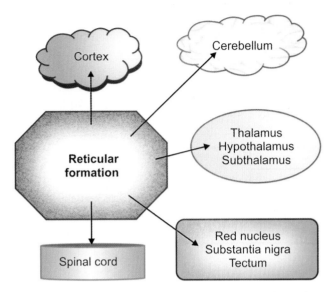

FIGURE 154.2: Efferent connections of reticular formation

3. Midbrain: Red nucleus, tectum and substantia nigra
4. Cerebellum
5. Spinal cord.

■ FUNCTIONS OF RETICULAR FORMATION

Based on functions, reticular formation along with its connections is divided into two systems:
A. Ascending reticular activating system
B. Descending reticular system.

■ ASCENDING RETICULAR ACTIVATING SYSTEM

Ascending reticular activating system **(ARAS)** begins in lower part of brainstem, extends upwards through pons, midbrain, thalamus and finally projects throughout the cerebral cortex. It projects into cerebral cortex in two ways:
1. Via subthalamus
2. Via thalamus.

The ARAS receives fibers from the sensory pathways via long ascending spinal tracts (Fig. 154.3).

Functions of ARAS

1. The ARAS is concerned with **arousal** phenomenon, **alertness,** maintenance of **attention** and **wakefulness.** Hence, it is called ascending reticular activating system. Stimulation of midbrain reticular formation produces wakefulness by **generalized activation** of entire brain including cerebral cortex, thalamus, basal ganglia and brainstem.

Any type of sensory impulses such as impulses of proprioception, pain, auditory, visual, taste and olfactory sensations cause sudden activation of the ARAS producing arousal phenomenon in animals and human beings. Even the impulses of visceral sensations activate this system. Sympathetic stimulation and adrenaline cause arousal by affecting midbrain.

2. The ARAS also causes **emotional reactions**
3. The ARAS plays an important role in regulating the **learning processes** and the development of **conditioned reflexes.**

Mechanism of Action of ARAS

Impulses of all the sensations reach cerebral cortex through two channels:
1. Classical sensory pathways
2. Ascending reticular activating system.

1. Classical or specific sensory pathways

Classical sensory pathways are the pathways, which transmit the sensory impulses from receptors to cerebral cortex via thalamus. Some of the pathways carry impulses of a particular sensation only. For example, auditory stimulus transmitted by auditory pathway reaches the auditory cortex via thalamus and causes perception of sound. Such classical sensory pathways are called specific sensory pathways.

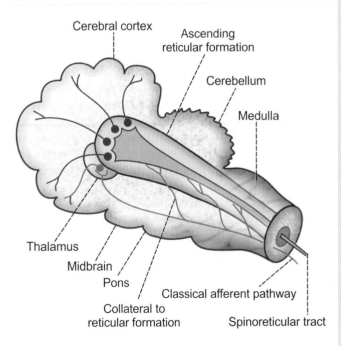

FIGURE 154.3: Ascending reticular formation

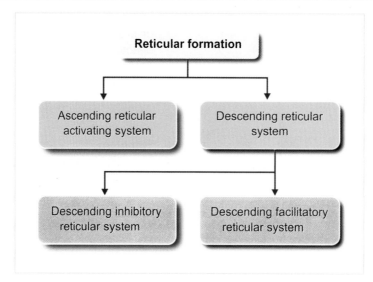

FIGURE 154.4: Functional divisions of reticular formation

2. Ascending reticular activating system
or non-specific sensory pathway

All the sensory pathways send collaterals to ARAS, which is a multisynaptic relay system. These collaterals project in diffused areas of ARAS. So, the sensory impulses transmitted via the collaterals reach different parts of ARAS. It also receives afferents from spinal cord directly in the form of spinoreticular tract. ARAS in turn sends the impulses to almost all the areas of cerebral cortex and other parts of brain. Hence, this pathway is called the non-specific sensory pathway.

Non-specific projection of ARAS into the cortex is responsible for the arousal, alertness and wakefulness. Sensory impulses transmitted directly to cortex via classical pathway causes perception of only the particular sensation. Whereas, the impulses transmitted to cortex via ARAS do not cause the perception of any particular sensation, but cause the generalized activation of almost all the areas of cerebral cortex and other parts of brain. This leads to reactions of arousal, alertness and wakefulness.

The ARAS is in turn controlled by the feedback signals from cerebral cortex. Also, an inhibitory system controls the activities of ARAS. Inhibitory system involves posterior hypothalamus, intralaminar and anterior thalamic nuclei and medullary area at the level of tractus solitarius.

Tumor or lesion in ARAS leads to **sleeping sickness** or **coma.** The impact of head injury on ARAS also causes coma.

■ DESCENDING RETICULAR SYSTEM

Descending reticular system includes reticular formation in brainstem, reticulospinal tract and reticular formation in spiral cord.

It modifies the activities of spinal motor neurons. Functionally, descending reticular system is divided into two subdivisions (Fig. 154.4):
1. Descending facilitatory reticular system
2. Descending inhibitory reticular system.

Descending Facilitatory Reticular System

Descending facilitatory reticular system is present in upper and lateral reticular formation. Its functions are:

i. *Facilitation of somatomotor activities*

  a. Descending facilitatory reticular system maintains muscle tone by exciting the gamma motor neurons in spinal cord; stimulation of this area causes increased muscle tone
  b. It facilitates the movements of the body. Stimulation of this part of reticular system causes exaggerated movements.
  c. It plays a role in wakefulness and alertness by activating the ARAS.

ii. *Facilitation of vegetative functions*

Descending facilitatory reticular system is the center for facilitation of the autonomic functions such as cardiac function, blood pressure, respiration, gastrointestinal function and body temperature.

Descending Inhibitory Reticular System

Descending inhibitory reticular system is located in a small area in lower and medial reticular formation. Its functions are:

i. *Control of somatomotor activities*

   a. Descending inhibitory reticular system plays an important role in the control of muscle tone. By receiving signals from basal ganglia, it inhibits the gamma motor neurons of spinal cord and decreases muscle tone. Stimulation of this area causes decreased muscle tone.

   b. It is responsible for smoothness and accuracy of voluntary movements. It controls the muscular activity by inhibiting the motor neurons of spinal cord.

   c. It also controls the reflex movements.

ii. *Control of vegetative functions*

Descending inhibitory reticular system is the center for inhibition of several autonomic functions such as cardiac function, blood pressure, respiration, gastrointestinal function and body temperature.

Preparations of Animals for Experimental Studies

- ■ INTRODUCTION
- ■ DECORTICATE PREPARATION
- ■ DECEREBRATE PREPARATION
- ■ THALAMIC (MIDBRAIN) PREPARATION
- ■ SPINAL PREPARATION

■ INTRODUCTION

Various functions of nervous system, particularly the maintenance of posture and equilibrium are studied by observing the effects of sections or lesions at different levels of central nervous system in animals. Commonly used animals are monkeys, dogs and cats.

■ DECORTICATE PREPARATION

Decorticate animal is the one **without cerebral cortex.** It is prepared by removing whole cerebral cortex leaving basal ganglia intact. It is also prepared by removing all the connections of cerebral cortex.

Effect of decortication varies with species and the conditions under which the animal is being examined.

In a dog or cat, when the animal is on its feet, posture is normal. Muscle tone is normally distributed and it is present equally in flexor and extensor muscles. Movements during walking can be performed by reflex activity. If the animal is suspended in the air, there is severe hyperextension of all the limbs. In decorticate monkey, the tone is gravely affected. Movements of walking cannot occur by reflex activity.

Effects in Man

In man, decorticate condition is caused by intracranial hemorrhage, head injury, brain abscess or brain tumor. Decorticate condition is called decorticate rigidity.

Decorticate Rigidity

Decorticate rigidity is the abnormal postural changes that involve rigid extension of the lower limbs and flexion of the upper limbs at elbow joint across the chest. Wrists and fingers are also flexed. Posture may develop on one side or both sides of the body.

Effects on Reflexes

Reflexes at the neck level can be elicited. These neck reflexes affect the body also. When the neck is turned to right, there is flexion of the lower and upper limbs on the opposite side. But, on the same side, there is extension of the limbs. It may be due to the cutting or lesion of direct corticospinal tract. Some fibers of corticospinal tract are known to have inhibitory influence on the extensor muscles.

■ DECEREBRATE PREPARATION

It is prepared by removing all **connections of cerebral hemispheres** at the level of midbrain, by sectioning in between the superior colliculus and inferior colliculus. This preparation is characterized by a state of stiffness or rigidity, which is known as **decerebrate rigidity,** resembling the effects of upper motor neuron lesion. This preparation was first done by Nobel laureate, **Sir Charles Sherrington** in cat.

Decerebrate Rigidity

Decerebrate rigidity is the rigid extension of all the limbs due to decerebration. This type of rigidity is well pronounced in the extensor muscles. The term decerebrate rigidity was coined by Sherrington in 1897.

Reason for decerebrate rigidity is the release of the centers, situated below the section, from higher inhibitory controls. The inhibitory area is 4S. It is situated in the motor cortex of cerebrum, just anterior to area 4 and behind area 6. In this area, Betz cells are absent. From here, the fibers are projected to spinal cord via reticular formation. So in decerebration the discharge from neurons of area 4S cannot reach spinal motor neurons. This leads to exaggeration of spinal motor neurons resulting in rigidity.

Decerebrate rigidity is also produced by stopping the blood flow to the forebrain. It is done by occlusion of the common carotid artery and the basilar artery at the center of the pons.

Opisthotonos

In decerebrate animal, the caricature or characteristic posture is the extension of all the four limbs, extension of the tail and arching of the back or hyperextension of the spine. This type of attitude of the animal is called opisthotonos. The animal can stand but, if disturbed, the posture cannot be maintained.

Decerebration in Man

In man, decerebration occurs due to lesion in diencephalon or midbrain.

■ THALAMIC (MIDBRAIN) PREPARATION

In thalamic animal, all the **connections of thalamus** with cerebral cortex are removed by sectioning at the superior border of midbrain. All the fine sensations such as fine touch, tactile discrimination and tactile localization are lost. The conscious kinesthetic sensation is also lost. But, the crude touch, pressure, pain and temperature sensations remain intact.

Righting reflexes are retained. The muscle tone is not affected. Rigidity is absent. But when the animal is held in air, extensor rigidity develops. Coordination of the reflex movements is not lost. However, the exaggeration of movements occurs during emotional states. Abnormal involuntary movements are absent.

■ SPINAL PREPARATION

Complete transection of spinal cord is called spinal preparation. Immediate effect of complete transection of spinal cord is the spinal shock. The animal recovers from the shock after some time. Tone is returned to the flexor muscles. Extensor muscles do not regain the tone or regain it after some time and these muscles attain the flaccidity. It is because the facilitatory impulses from reticular formation are cut off in spinal preparation. Effects of complete transection of spinal cord are given in Chapter 143.

Proprioceptors

- ■ **PROPRIOCEPTORS**
- ■ **MUSCLE SPINDLE**
  - ■ STRUCTURE
  - ■ NERVE SUPPLY
  - ■ FUNCTIONS
- ■ **GOLGI TENDON ORGAN**
  - ■ STRUCTURE
  - ■ NERVE SUPPLY
  - ■ FUNCTIONS
- ■ **PACINIAN CORPUSCLE**
- ■ **FREE NERVE ENDING**

■ PROPRIOCEPTORS

It is necessary to know about the proprioceptors to understand the maintenance of posture and equilibrium, which is explained in the next chapter.

Definition

Proprioceptors are the receptors, which detect and give response to movement and change in position of different parts of the body. These receptors are also called **kinesthetic receptors.**

Situation

Proprioceptors are situated in labyrinth, muscles, tendon of the muscles, joints, ligaments and fascia (Table 156.1).

Different Proprioceptors

1. Muscle spindle
2. Golgi tendon organ
3. Pacinian corpuscle
4. Free nerve ending
5. Proprioceptors in labyrinth.

Proprioceptors in the labyrinth are described in Chapter 158.

TABLE 156.1: Situation of proprioceptors

Proprioceptor	Situation
Muscle spindle	Skeletal muscles
Golgi tendon organ	Tendons
Pacinian corpuscle	Skin Fascia over muscles Tendons Tissues around joint Joint capsule
Free nerve ending	Skin Skeletal muscles Tendons Fascia over muscles Joints
Labyrinthine proprioceptors	Labyrinth

■ MUSCLE SPINDLE

Muscle spindle is a spindle-shaped **proprioceptor** situated in the skeletal muscle. It is formed by modified skeletal muscle fibers called **intrafusal muscle fibers.**

■ STRUCTURE OF MUSCLE SPINDLE

Muscle spindle has a central bulged portion and two tapering ends. Each muscle spindle is formed by 5 to 12

intrafusal muscle fibers. All these fibers are enclosed by a capsule, which is formed by connective tissue. Intrafusal fibers are attached to the capsule on either end. The capsule is attached to either side of extrafusal fibers or the tendon of the muscle. Thus, intrafusal fibers are placed parallel to the extrafusal fibers. Intrafusal fibers are thin and striated (Fig. 156.1).

Central portion of the intrafusal fibers does not contract because it has only few or no actin and myosin filaments. So, this portion acts only as a receptor. Only the end portion of intrafusal fibers can contract. The discharge from gamma motor neurons causes the contraction of intrafusal fibers.

Types of Intrafusal Fibers

Muscle spindle is formed by two types of intrafusal fibers:
1. Nuclear bag fiber
2. Nuclear chain fiber.

1. Nuclear bag fiber

Central portion of this fiber is enlarged like a **bag** and contains many nuclei. Hence, it is called the nuclear bag fiber.

2. Nuclear chain fiber

In nuclear chain fiber, central portion is not bulged and the nuclei are arranged in the center in the form of a chain. Nuclear chain fiber is attached to the side of end portion of nuclear bag fiber.

■ NERVE SUPPLY TO MUSCLE SPINDLE

Muscle spindle is innervated by both sensory and motor nerves. It is the **only receptor** in the body, which has both **sensory** and **motor nerve supply.**

Sensory Nerve Supply

Each muscle spindle receives two types of sensory nerve fibers:
1. Primary sensory nerve fiber
2. Secondary sensory nerve fiber.

1. Primary sensory nerve fiber

Primary sensory nerve fiber belongs to **type Iα (Aα)** nerve fiber. Each sensory (afferent) nerve fiber has two branches. One of the branches supplies the central portion of nuclear bag fiber (Fig. 156.2). The other branch ends in central portion of the nuclear chain fiber. These branches end in the form of rings around central portion of nuclear bag and nuclear chain fibers. Therefore, these nerve endings are called **annulospiral endings.**

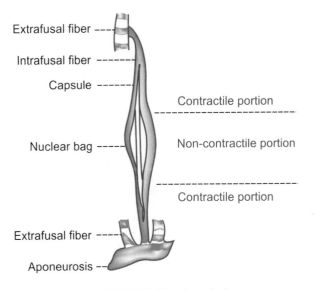

FIGURE 156.1: Muscle spindle

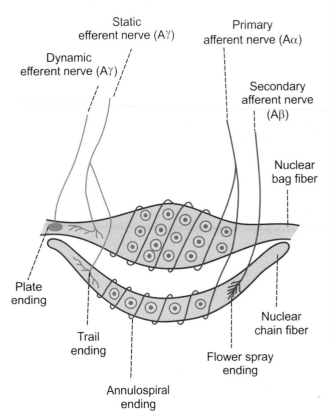

FIGURE 156.2: Nerve supply to muscle spindle. Red = Afferent (sensory) nerve fibers, Blue = Efferent (motor) nerve fibers. Letters in parenthesis indicate the type of nerve fibers.

2. Secondary sensory nerve fiber

Secondary sensory nerve fiber is a **type II (Aβ)** nerve fiber. It innervates only the nuclear chain fiber and ends near the end portion of nuclear chain fiber like the petals of the flower. So, this nerve ending is called **flower spray ending.**

Motor Nerve Supply

Motor (efferent) nerve fiber supplying the muscle spindle belongs to gamma motor neuron **(Aγ) type.**

Motor nerve supply to nuclear bag fiber

Gamma motor nerve fiber supplying the nuclear bag fiber ends as motor end plate. This nerve ending is called **plate ending.** Functionally, it is known as **dynamic gamma efferent** (motor) nerve fiber.

Motor nerve supply to nuclear chain fiber

Gamma motor nerve fiber supplying the nuclear chain fiber divides into many branches, which form a network called **trail ending.** Functionally, it is known as **static gamma efferent** (motor) nerve fiber. Sometimes, it gives a branch to nuclear bag fiber also.

■ FUNCTIONS OF MUSCLE SPINDLE

Muscle spindle gives response to change in the length of the muscle. It detects how much the muscle is being stretched and sends this information to central nervous system (CNS) via sensory nerve fibers. The information is processed in CNS to determine the position of different parts of the body. By detecting the change in length of the muscle, the spindle plays an important role in preventing the overstretching of the muscles.

Muscle spindle has two functions:
1. It forms the receptor organ for stretch reflex
2. It plays an important role in maintaining muscle tone.

1. Role of Muscle Spindle in Stretch Reflex

Stretch reflex

Stretch reflex is the reflex contraction of muscle when it is stretched. It is also called **myotatic reflex.** It is a **monosynaptic reflex** and the quickest of all the reflexes. Extensor muscles, particularly the antigravity muscles exhibit a severe and prolonged contraction during stretch reflex. Stretch reflex plays an important role in maintaining posture.

Muscle spindle as the receptor organ for stretch reflex

Stimulation of muscle spindle elicits the stretch reflex. Intrafusal muscle fibers are situated parallel to the extrafusal muscle fibers and are attached to the tendon of the muscle by means of capsule. So, stretching of the muscle causes **stretching of the muscle spindle** also. This stimulates the muscle spindle and it discharges the sensory impulses. These impulses are transmitted via the primary and secondary sensory nerve fibers to the alpha motor neurons in spinal cord. Alpha motor neurons in turn send motor impulse to muscles through their fibers and cause contraction of extrafusal fibers (Fig. 156.3).

Response of muscle spindle to stretch

When the muscle is stretched, primary sensory nerve fibers from muscle spindle discharge impulses. This response is of two types:
   i. Dynamic response
   ii. Static response.

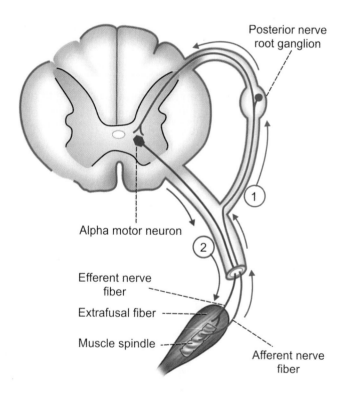

FIGURE 156.3: Stretch reflex. 1. Afferent impulses from muscle spindle of stretched muscle. 2. Efferent impulses from α-motor neurons causing contraction of muscle.

i. *Dynamic response*

Dynamic response is the response in which the primary sensory nerve fibers discharge rapidly. When there is a change in length of the muscle by stretching, primary sensory nerve fibers from nuclear bag fiber start discharging impulses very rapidly. But, the discharge becomes less or nil during continuous stretching of the muscle. Discharge of impulses start only if there is change in degree of stretching of the muscle. Thus, the response depends upon rate of change in length of the muscle.

ii. *Static response*

Static response is the response in which impulses are discharged rapidly and continuously throughout the period of muscle stretch by primary sensory nerve fibers of the nuclear chain fibers.

Thus, the muscle spindle gives response to change in length of the muscle as well as rate of change in length.

Physiologic tremor

Physiologic tremor is the continuous discharge of actions potentials with low voltage and ineffective frequency from primary and secondary sensory nerve fibers of muscle spindle at resting condition. Physiological tremor plays an important role in the feedback regulation of muscle length.

2. *Role of Muscle Spindle in the Maintenance of Muscle Tone*

The state of continuous and partial contraction of the muscle is called muscle tone (Chapter 157). It is due to the continuous discharge of impulses from gamma motor neurons.

Gamma motor neurons innervate the intrafusal fibers. Motor impulses from gamma motor neurons stimulate the intrafusal fibers of muscle spindle, which in turn sends sensory impulses back to spinal cord. Now the alpha motor neurons in spinal cord are activated resulting in contraction of extrafusal fibers of muscle. Refer Chapter 157 for details of this process. When the frequency of discharge from gamma motor neurons increases, activity of muscle spindle is increased and the muscle tone also increases.

■ GOLGI TENDON ORGAN

■ STRUCTURE OF GOLGI TENDON ORGAN

Golgi tendon organ is situated in the **tendon** of skeletal muscle near the attachment of extrafusal

fibers. It is placed in series between the muscle fibers and the tendon. Golgi tendon organ is formed by a group of nerve endings covered by a connective tissue capsule (Fig. 156.4).

■ NERVE SUPPLY TO GOLGI TENDON ORGAN

Sensory nerve fiber supplying the Golgi tendon organ belongs to **Ib type.** The nerve fiber supplying Golgi tendon organ ramifies into many branches. Each branch ends in the form of a knob.

■ FUNCTIONS OF GOLGI TENDON ORGAN

Golgi tendon organ gives response to the change in the force or tension developed in the skeletal muscle during contraction. It is also the receptor for inverse stretch reflex and lengthening reaction and thereby prevents damage of muscle due to overstretching.

1. *Role of Golgi Tendon Organ in Forceful Contraction*

During powerful contraction, tension in the muscles increases and stimulates Golgi tendon organ, which discharges the sensory impulses. Impulses are transmitted by Ib sensory nerve fiber to an inhibitory interneuron in the spinal cord. Interneuron, in turn, causes development of **inhibitory postsynaptic potential** (IPSP) in motor neurons, which supply the muscle. Now, the contraction of the muscle is inhibited.

2. *Role of Golgi Tendon Organ in Inverse Stretch Reflex*

Inverse stretch reflex

Inverse stretch reflex is the sudden decrease in resistance due to relaxation (instead of contraction) when a

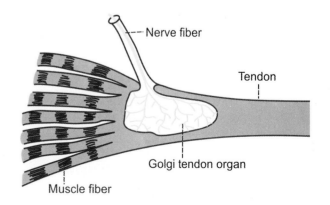

FIGURE 156.4: Golgi tendon apparatus

muscle is stretched excessively. It is also called **inverse myotatic reflex** and it is a **polysynaptic reflex.**

Inverse stretch reflex is actually the inhibition of contraction due to excessive stretching. So, it is also called the **autogenic inhibition.**

Mechanism of inverse stretch reflex

Excessive stretch of the muscle leads to activation of Golgi tendon organ, which send afferent impulses which cause:

i.   Stimulation of inhibitory internuncial neuron, which in turn inhibits alpha motor neuron of the stretched muscle resulting in relaxation
ii. Stimulation of excitatory internuncial neuron, which in turn activates alpha motor neuron of the antagonistic muscle. It leads to contraction of antagonistic muscle and relaxation of stretched muscle.

3. Role of Golgi Tendon Organ in Lengthening Reaction

When tension increases during muscular contraction caused by stretch reflex, the Golgi tendon organ is activated. It causes development of a spinal reaction, which is called the lengthening reaction. It can be demonstrated in a decerebrate preparation.

In **decerebrate rigidity,** the extension of limbs is due to **spastic contraction** of extensor muscles. It is because of increased discharge from gamma motor neurons, which facilitates the **stretch reflex.**

In a decerebrate animal, some resistance is offered when the arm is flexed at elbow joint passively. That is, the arm cannot be flexed easily. This type of resistance is offered because of the stretch reflex developed in the triceps muscle. However, if forearm is flexed forcefully, resistance to flexion is abolished suddenly, leading to quick flexion of arm. It is called the lengthening reaction.

Lengthening reaction is due to the activation of Golgi tendon organ. The sudden flexion of arm is called the **Phillipson reflex** or **clasp knife reflex.**

■ PACINIAN CORPUSCLE

Pacinian corpuscle is a **mechanoreceptor** that senses pressure and vibration. It is situated in the deeper layers of skin. It is also situated in the tissues surrounding the joints such as fascia over the muscle, tendons and joint capsule. Pacinian corpuscles situated in these tissues are responsible for determining the position of joints.

Since pacinian corpuscle is a rapidly adapting receptor **(phasic receptor)** it is very sensitive to quick changes in the position of joints. So it is believed to send information about joint movement to CNS.

■ FREE NERVE ENDING

Free nerve ending is the receptor for pain sensation situated in skin, muscles, tendon, fascia and joints. As it is a slow adapting receptor **(tonic receptor)** it is maximally stimulated at specific joint positions. So it is believed to send information about joint position to CNS.

Posture and Equilibrium

```
■ DEFINITION
■ BASIC PHENOMENA OF POSTURE
    ■ MUSCLE TONE
    ■ STRETCH REFLEX
■ POSTURAL REFLEXES
    ■ CLASSIFICATION OF POSTURAL REFLEXES
    ■ STATIC REFLEXES
    ■ STATOKINETIC REFLEXES
```

■ DEFINITION

Subconscious **adjustment of tone** in different muscles in relation to every movement is known as the **posture.** Significance of posture is to make the movement smooth and accurate and to maintain the line of gravity constant or to keep the body in equilibrium with line of gravity. Posture is not an active movement. It is the **passive movement** associated with **redistribution of tone** in different groups of related muscles.

■ BASIC PHENOMENA OF POSTURE

Basic phenomena for maintenance of posture are muscle tone and stretch reflex.

■ MUSCLE TONE

Definition

Muscle tone is defined as the state of continuous and passive partial contraction of muscle with certain vigor and tension. It is also called **tonus.** It is also defined as resistance offered by the muscle to stretch.

Significance of Muscle Tone

Muscle tone plays an important role in maintenance of posture. Change in muscle tone enables movement of different parts of the body. Muscle tone is present in all the skeletal muscles. However, tone is more in antigravity muscles such as extensors of lower limb, trunk muscles and neck muscles.

Development of Muscle Tone

Gamma motor neurons and muscle spindle are responsible for the development and maintenance of muscle tone.

Muscle tone is purely a reflex process. This reflex is a **spinal segmental reflex.** It is developed by continual synchronous discharge of motor impulses from the gamma motor neurons present in the anterior gray horn of the spinal cord (Figs. 157.1 and 157.2).

Sequence of events

1. Impulses from the gamma motor neurons cause contraction of end portions of intrafusal fibers (stimulus)
2. This stretches and activates the central portion of the intrafusal fibers, which initiates the reflex action for development of muscle tone by discharging the impulses
3. Impulses from the central portion of intrafusal fibers pass through primary sensory nerve fibers (afferent fibers) and reach the anterior gray horn of spinal cord
4. These impulses stimulate the alpha motor neurons in anterior gray horn (center)

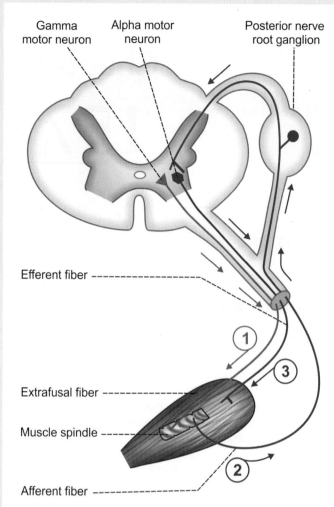

FIGURE 157.1: Development of muscle tone. 1. Impulses from γ-motor neuron stimulate muscle spindle. 2. Afferent impulses from muscle spindle to α-motor neuron. 3. Efferent impulses from α-motor neuron produce contraction of extrafusal fibers and develop muscle tone.

5. Alpha motor neurons in turn, send impulses to extrafusal fibers of the muscle through spinal nerve fibers (efferent fibers)
6. These impulses produce partial contraction of the muscle fibers resulting in development of muscle tone (response).

When the frequency of discharge from gamma motor neurons increases, the activity of muscle spindle is increased and muscle tone also increases.

Stimulation of gamma motor neurons increases the muscle tone. Lesion in gamma motor neurons leads to loss of tone in muscles.

Regulation of Muscle Tone

Though the muscle tone is developed by discharges from gamma motor neurons, it is maintained continuously

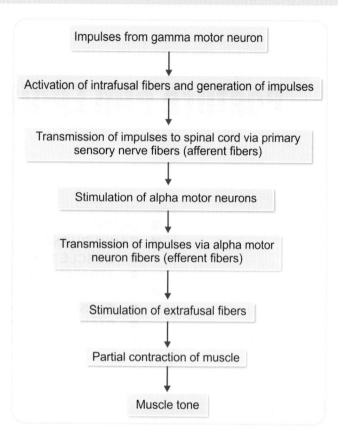

FIGURE 157.2: Schematic diagram showing development of muscle tone

and regulated by some supraspinal centers situated in different parts of brain. Some of these centers increase the muscle tone by sending **facilitatory impulses** while other centers decrease the muscle tone by **inhibitory impulses.**

Supraspinal facilitatory centers

Supraspinal centers, which increase the muscle tone:
1. Motor area 4 in cerebral cortex
2. Cerebellum
3. Descending facilitatory reticular system
4. Red nucleus
5. Vestibular nucleus.

Supraspinal inhibitory centers

Supraspinal centers, which decrease the muscle tone:
1. Suppressor areas of cerebral cortex
2. Basal ganglia
3. Descending inhibitory reticular system.

Role of motor area of cerebral cortex – coactivation

Motor area of cerebral cortex influences the activity of lower motor neurons by sending motor impulses through the pyramidal tract fibers. Motor impulses from cerebral cortex stimulate both α-motor neurons and γ-motor neurons simultaneously. This type of simultaneous stimulation is called coactivation. It is also called **α-γ coactivation.** Stimulation of **α-motor** neurons causes contraction of **extrafusal fibers.** Stimulation of **γ-motor** neurons causes contraction of **intrafusal fibers,** which leads to increase in muscle tone.

Role of cerebellum and basal ganglia

It is interesting to find that cerebellum and basal ganglia influence the muscle tone without sending direct fibers to γ-motor neurons. These parts of brain influence the muscle tone indirectly through brainstem centers.

Role of brainstem centers

Brainstem centers which influence the γ-motor neurons are in reticular formation, red nucleus and vestibular nucleus. These centers modulate the discharge from γ-motor neurons by receiving signals from cerebral cortex, cerebellum and basal ganglia.

Abnormalities

Refer Chapter 34 for details of abnormalities of muscle tone.

■ **STRETCH REFLEX**

Basic reflex involved in maintenance of posture is the stretch reflex, which is described in detail in the previous chapter.

This reflex is normally present and serves particularly to maintain the body in an upright position. Such reflexes are, therefore more pronounced in extensor muscles.

■ **POSTURAL REFLEXES**

Postural reflexes are the reflexes which are responsible for maintenance of posture. Afferent impulses for the maintenance of posture arise from proprioceptors, vestibular apparatus and retina of eye and reach the centers in central nervous system (CNS). The centers, which maintain the posture, are located at different levels of CNS particularly cerebral cortex, cerebellum, brainstem and spinal cord. These centers send motor impulses to the different groups of skeletal muscles so that appropriate movements occur to maintain the posture.

■ **CLASSIFICATION OF POSTURAL REFLEXES**

Postural reflexes are generally classified into two groups:
A. Static reflexes
B. Statokinetic reflexes.

■ **STATIC REFLEXES**

Static reflexes are the postural reflexes that maintain posture at rest. Static reflexes are of four types:
   I.   General static reflexes or righting reflexes
   II. Local static reflexes or supporting reflexes
   III. Segmental static reflexes
   IV. Statotonic or attitudinal reflexes.

I. *General Static Reflexes or Righting Reflexes*

General static reflexes are otherwise called righting reflexes because these reflexes help to maintain an upright position of the body. Righting reflexes help to govern the orientation of the head in space, position of the head in relation to the body and appropriate adjustment of the limbs and eyes in relation to the position of the head, so that upright position of the body is maintained.

When a cat, held with its back downwards, is allowed to fall through the air, it lands upon its paws, with the head and body assuming the normal attitude in a flash. A fish resists any attempt to turn it from its normal position and if it is placed in water upon its back, it flips almost instantly into the normal swimming position. All these actions occur because of the righting reflexes.

Righting reflexes consist of a chain of reactions, which occur one after another in an orderly sequence. Each reflex causes the development of the succeeding one.

Righting reflexes are divided into five types:
   1. Labyrinthine righting reflexes acting on the neck muscles
   2. Neck righting reflexes acting on the body
   3. Body righting reflexes acting on the head
   4. Body righting reflexes acting on the body
   5. Optical righting reflexes.

First four reflexes are easily demonstrated on a thalamic animal or a normal animal, which is blindfolded.

1. *Labyrinthine righting reflexes acting on the neck muscles*

When a **thalamic animal** (rabbit) is suspended by holding at the pelvic region, its head turns up, until it assumes its normal position. It is because of reflexes arising from labyrinth, the sensory organ concerned with equilibrium of head, in regard to the position of the body. Turning the body of animal through air into different positions is followed by compensatory movements of the head. After extirpation of labyrinths, the head shows no compensatory movements when the rabbit is suspended. It hangs simply like that of a dead rabbit.

2. *Neck righting reflexes acting on the body*

It is noticed that during labyrinthine righting reflexes, the head raises up to normal position. It is because of the contraction of neck muscles. Now, the contraction of neck muscles produces proprioceptive impulses, which act on the body and rotate the body in relation to position of head. This reflex is well noticed, if the animal is laid down in resting position upon its side on a table.

3. *Body righting reflexes acting on the head*

Labyrinthine righting reflexes are not the only reflexes acting on neck muscles to cause rotation of head. If the animal is laid down upon its side on a table, the unequal distribution of pressure on that particular side of the body stimulates exteroceptors on the skin. Impulses thus generated by exteroceptors, act on neck muscles and rotate the head.

4. *Body righting reflexes acting on the body*

When the same animal is laid down on the table on its side, with head held down to table, to eliminate labyrinthine and neck righting reflexes, the body attempts to right itself by raising the lower parts. It is because of the impulses from exteroceptors on that side of body acting on the body itself.

5. *Optical righting reflexes*

Optical righting reflexes are initiated through the retinal impulses. Center for optical righting reflexes is in the occipital lobe of cerebral cortex. So, these reflexes are absent in thalamic animal. Optical righting reflexes help to correct the position of the body or head with the help of sight. It is proved in a labyrinthectomized animal. When such an animal is suspended, it rotates its head to normal position with the help of sight. But, the movements of head do not occur if eyes of the animal are closed.

Summary of righting reflexes

Following are the sequential events of righting reflexes:
  i. When the animal is placed upon its back, labyrinthine reflexes acting upon neck muscles turn the head into its normal position in space, in relation to body
 ii. Proprioceptive reflexes of neck muscles then bring the body into its normal position in relation to position of head
iii. When resting upon a rigid support, these reflexes are reinforced by the body righting reflexes on the head as well as on the body
 iv. If the animal happens to be a **labyrinthectomized** one, then it makes an attempt to recover its upright position as a result of operation of the optical righting reaction. If the optical righting reflexes are abolished by covering the eyes, the righting ability is lost.

Optical righting reflexes are also demonstrated in 3 or 4 weeks old baby. When laid down on belly, i.e. prone position, the baby tries to raise the head to a vertical position.

Centers for righting reflexes

Centers for the first four righting reflexes are in **red nucleus** situated in midbrain. Center for optical righting reflexes is in the **occipital lobe** of cerebral cortex (Table 157.1).

II. *Local Static Reflexes or Supporting Reflexes*

Local static reflexes or supporting reactions support the body in different positions against gravity and also protect the limbs against hyperextension or hyperflexion.

Supporting reactions are classified into two types:
1. Positive supporting reflexes
2. Negative supporting reflexes.

1. *Positive supporting reflexes*

Positive supporting reflexes are the reactions, which help to fix the joints and make the limbs rigid like pillars, so that limbs can support the weight of the body against gravity. It is brought about by the simultaneous reflex contractions of both extensor and flexor muscles and other opposing muscles. The impulses for these reflexes arise from proprioceptors present in the muscles, joints and tendons and the exteroceptors, particularly pressure receptors present in deeper layers of the skin of sole. While standing, the positive supporting reflexes are developed in the following manner:
  i. When an animal stands on its limbs, the pressure of the animal's paw upon the ground produces proprioceptive impulses from flexor and extensor muscles of the limbs, particularly in terminal segments of the limbs like digits, ankle or wrist. The proprioceptive impulses cause reflex contraction of the muscles of limbs making the limbs rigid.
 ii. Excessive extension at the joints is checked or guarded by the **myotatic reflexes** setting up in the flexor muscles. When the flexor muscles are simultaneously contracting, extensor muscles cannot be stretched beyond the physiological limits. Similarly, over activity of the flexor muscles is prevented by the **stretch reflexes** developed in the extensor muscles.

TABLE 157.1: Static postural reflexes

Reflex		Center	Animal preparation to demonstrate
General static reflexes (Righting reflexes)	1. Labyrinthine righting reflexes acting on the neck muscles	Red nucleus situated in midbrain	Thalamic or normal blindfolded animal
	2. Neck righting reflexes acting on the body		
	3. Body righting reflexes acting on the head		
	4. Body righting reflexes acting on the body		
	5. Optical righting reflexes	Occipital lobe	Labyrinthectomized animal
Local static reflexes	1. Positive supporting reflexes	Spinal cord	Decorticate animal
	2. Negative supporting reflexes		
Segmental static reflexes	Crossed extensor reflex	Spinal cord	Spinal animals
Statotonic or attitudinal reflexes	1. Tonic labyrinthine and neck reflexes acting on the limbs	Medulla oblongata	Decerebrate animal
	2. Labyrinthine and neck reflexes acting on the eyes		

iii. Impulses arise even from exteroceptors while standing, when the sole remains in contact with the ground. It causes stimulation of the pressure receptors, which are present in deeper layers of the skin. These impulses from pressure receptors reinforce the rigidity of the limbs caused by the proprioceptive impulses.

2. *Negative supporting reflexes*

Relaxation of the muscles and unfixing of the joints enable the limbs to flex and move to a new position. It is called negative supporting reaction. It is brought about by raising the leg off the ground and plantar flexion of toes and ankle. When the leg is lifted off the ground, the exteroceptive impulses are stopped. When the toes and ankle joints are plantar flexed, the stretch stimulus for the plantar muscles is stopped. So, unlocking of the limbs occurs. Moreover, by the plantar flexion of the toes and ankle, the dorsiflexor muscles are stretched, causing relaxation of the extensors and contraction of the flexors of the knee.

The positive and negative supporting reactions are demonstrated well on a **decorticate animal**. The centers for the supporting reflexes are located in the spinal cord.

III. *Segmental Static Reflexes*

Segmental static reflexes are very essential for **walking**. During walking, in one leg, the flexors are active and the extensors are inhibited. On the opposite leg, the flexors are inhibited and extensors are active. Thus, the flexors and extensors of the same limb are not active simultaneously. It is known as **crossed extensor reflex**. It is due to the **reciprocal inhibition** and the neural mechanism responsible for this reflex is called **Sherrington reciprocal innervation**. Refer Chapter 142 for details.

Segmental static reflexes are demonstrated in **spinal animal**. And, the centers for these reflexes are situated in the spinal cord.

IV. *Statotonic or Attitudinal Reflexes*

Statotonic or attitudinal reflexes are developed according to the attitude of the body and are of two types:
1. Tonic labyrinthine and neck reflexes acting on the limbs
2. Labyrinthine and neck reflexes acting on the eyes.

1. *Tonic labyrinthine and neck reflexes acting on the limbs*

Tonic labyrinthine and neck reflexes decrease or increase the tone of the skeletal muscles of the limbs in accordance to the attitude or position of the head. These reflexes are best studied in decerebrate animal. The proprioceptors concerned with these reflexes are in the labyrinthine apparatus. Whenever the position of the head is altered, the receptors present in the labyrinth are stimulated and generate impulses. The impulses are also generated from the neck muscles when the position of the head is altered. The impulses from labyrinth produce the same effect on all the four limbs. But the impulses from neck muscles cause opposite effects in the forelimbs and hind limbs.

The labyrinthine reflexes are particularly effective on extensor muscles. When the head is dorsiflexed, all the four limbs are extended maximally and when the head is ventriflexed, all the four limbs are flexed.

In a labyrinthectomized animal where only neck reflexes are operated, during dorsiflexion of the head, there is extension of the forelimbs and flexion of the hind limbs. The ventriflexion of the head causes flexion of the forelimbs and extension of the hind limbs.

The importance of these reflexes is understood well, while observing the movements during change in the attitude of a normal animal. When an animal turns to one side, the limbs of that side become rigid in order to support the weight of the body. A cat looking upwards, keeps the hind limbs flexed but forelimbs remain extended. It gives a suitable inclination to the back of the animal, which improves the positions of the head and eyes. When the cat looks down, forelimbs are flexed and hind limbs are extended, giving the proper supported inclination at the neck region.

2. *Labyrinthine and neck reflexes acting on the eyes*

According to the changes in the position of the head and neck, the eyes are also moved. These reflexes arise from labyrinth and neck muscles. Turning the head downward causes upward movement of the eyes. The eyes remain in this position as long as the position of the head is retained.

When the head is moved down, the tone in the superior recti and inferior oblique are increased and tone of inferior recti and superior oblique are reduced, so that the eyeballs move upwards. When the head is turned to one side, a corresponding compensatory movement of the eyes occurs.

When the head is turned to one side, the eyes deviate outward or inward in relation to the head. The eyes are moved in a direction opposite to that of the head movement. It is because of external and internal recti.

Centers for statotonic reflexes are present in the medulla oblongata.

■ STATOKINETIC REFLEXES

Statokinetic reflexes are the postural reflexes that maintain posture during movement. These reflexes are concerned with both angular **(rotatory)** and linear **(progressive)** movements. The vestibular apparatus is responsible for these reflexes. So, it is essential to study the structure and functions of vestibular apparatus to understand the statokinetic reflexes. The details of vestibular apparatus are described in Chapter 158.

Vestibular Apparatus

■ INTRODUCTION

Vestibular apparatus is the part of **labyrinth** or **inner ear.** It plays an important role in maintaining posture and equilibrium through **statokinetic reflexes.** Other part of labyrinth is the **cochlea,** which is concerned with sensation of hearing.

■ LABYRINTH

Labyrinth (inner ear) consists of two structures:

1. Bony labyrinth
2. Membranous labyrinth.

■ BONY LABYRINTH

Bony labyrinth is a series of cavities or channels present in the petrous part of temporal bone. Membranous labyrinth is situated inside bony labyrinth. The space between bony labyrinth and membranous labyrinth is filled with a fluid called **perilymph** or **periotic fluid.** This fluid is similar to ECF in composition with large amount of sodium ions. Bony labyrinth encloses membranous labyrinth (Fig. 158.1).

■ MEMBRANOUS LABYRINTH

Membranous labyrinth is formed by membranous tubules and sacs. It consists of two portions:
1. Cochlea, which is concerned with sensation of hearing (Chapter 172)
2. Vestibular apparatus, which is concerned with posture and equilibrium.

Membranous labyrinth is filled with a fluid called **endolymph** or otic **fluid**. Endolymph is similar to ICF in composition. It has large quantity of potassium ions.

■ FUNCTIONAL ANATOMY OF VESTIBULAR APPARATUS

Vestibular apparatus is formed by three semicircular canals and otolith organ (vestibule).

■ SEMICIRCULAR CANALS

Semicircular canals are the tubular structures placed at right angles to each other. Because of this type of arrangement, semicircular canals represent the three

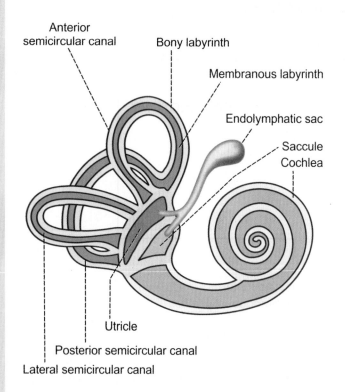

FIGURE 158.1: Labyrinth

axes of rotation, i.e. vertical, anteroposterior and transverse axes. Semicircular canals are named according to the situation as follows:
1. Anterior or superior canal
2. Posterior canal
3. Lateral or horizontal or external canal.

Anterior and posterior canals are situated vertically and the lateral canal is situated in horizontal plane (Fig. 158.2).

When the head is tilted forward at an angle of 30°, lateral canals of both the sides are at horizontal plane parallel to earth with the convexities directed outward and a little backward. Anterior canals are at vertical plane and directed forward and outward at 45°. Posterior canals are also at vertical plane, but directed backward and outward at 45°.

Therefore, the plane of position of anterior canal of one side is parallel to the plane of posterior canal of opposite side.

Ampulla

There are two ends for each semicircular canal. One end is narrow and the other end is enlarged. The enlarged end is called ampulla. Ampulla contains the receptor organ of semicircular canals known as **crista ampullaris**. Ampulla of all the three canals and narrow end of horizontal canal open directly into the **utricle**. The narrow ends of anterior and posterior canals open into utricle jointly, by forming the **common crus**. Thus, all the three semicircular canals open into utricle by means of five openings. Utricle opens into **saccule**.

■ OTOLITH ORGAN OR VESTIBULE

Otolith organ or vestibule is formed by utricle and saccule. Often utricle and saccule are together called **otoliths**. Utricle communicates with saccule through **utriculosaccular duct**. Saccule communicates with cochlear duct through **ductus reuniens**. Another duct called endolymphatic duct arises from **utriculosaccular duct**. It ends in a bag-like structure called **endolymphatic sac**, which lies on the cranial surface of petrous bone.

■ RECEPTOR ORGAN IN VESTIBULAR APPARATUS

Receptor organ in semicircular canal is called **crista ampullaris** and that in otolith organ is called **macula**. These receptor organs contain the **proprioceptors**.

Left side

Posterior canal

Right side

Posterior canal

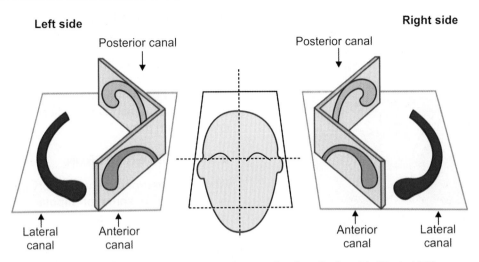

Lateral canal

Anterior canal

Anterior canal

Lateral canal

FIGURE 158.2: Position of semicircular canals when the head is tilted at 30°

■ RECEPTOR ORGAN IN SEMICIRCULAR CANAL – CRISTA AMPULLARIS

Crista ampullaris is a crest-like structure situated inside the ampulla of semicircular canals. The crest is formed by a **receptor epithelium (neuroepithelium),** which consists of hair cells, supporting cells and secreting epithelial cells. The secreting epithelial cells secrete the ground substance, **proteoglycan.** These cells are arranged in **planum semilunatum** (group of epithelial cells) around hair cells (Fig. 158.3).

Hair Cells

Hair cells are the receptor cells (proprioceptors) of crista ampullaris. There are two types of hair cells, type I and type II hair cells. Hair cells of semicircular canals, utricle and saccule receive both afferent and efferent nerve terminals.

Type I hair cells

Type I hair cells are flask shaped. Afferent nerve terminates in the form of a **calyx** that surrounds the cell body. Efferent nerve terminal ends on the surface of calyx.

Type II hair cells

These cells have a cylindrical or test tube shape. Both afferent and efferent nerve fibers terminate on the surface cell body without forming calyx.

Cilia of hair cells

Apex of each hair cell has a **cuticular plate.** From this plate, about 40 to 60 cilia arise, which are called

stereocilia. Each stereocilium is attached at its tip to the neighboring taller one by means of a fine process called tip link. Because of the tip links, all the stereocilia are held together. One of the cilia is very tall, which is named as **kinocilium** (Fig. 158.4).

Cupula

From crista ampullaris, a dome-shaped gelatinous structure extends up to the roof of the ampulla. It is known as **cupula.** Cilia of hair cells are projected into cupula.

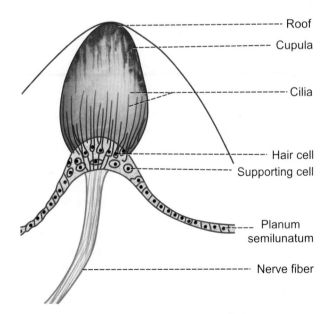

Roof

Cupula

Cilia

Hair cell

Supporting cell

Planum semilunatum

Nerve fiber

FIGURE 158.3: Crista ampullaris

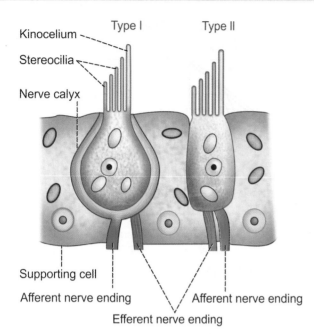

FIGURE 158.4: Hair cells of vestibular apparatus

■ RECEPTOR ORGAN IN OTOLITH ORGAN – MACULA

Receptor organ in otolith organ is called macula. Like crista ampullaris, macula is also formed by neuro-epithelium and supporting cells. Neuroepithelium of macula also has two types of hair cells, the type I and type II hair cells (Fig. 158.5).

Otolith Membrane

Like crista ampullaris, macula is also covered by a gelatinous membrane called otolith membrane. It is a flat structure and not dome shaped like cupula. The **stereocilia** and **kinocelium** of each hair cell are embedded in otolith membrane. Otolith membrane contains some crystals, which are called **ear dust, otoconia** or **statoconia.** Otoconia are mainly constituted by calcium carbonate.

Situation of Macula

Situation of macula is different in utricle and saccule.

Macula in utricle

In utricle, the macula is situated in **horizontal plane,** so that the cilia from hair cells are in **vertical direction.**

Macula in saccule

In the case of saccule, macula is in **vertical plane** and the cilia are in **horizontal direction.**

■ NERVE SUPPLY TO VESTIBULAR APPARATUS

Impulses from the hair cells of crista ampullaris and maculae are transmitted to medulla oblongata and other parts of central nervous system (CNS) through the fibers of vestibular division of vestibulocochlear (VIII cranial) nerve.

■ FIRST ORDER NEURON

First order neurons of the sensory pathway are bipolar in nature. The soma of **bipolar cells** is present in vestibular or Scarpa ganglion, which is situated in the internal auditory meatus. Dendrites of bipolar cells reach the receptor organs, i.e. crista ampullaris and maculae in vestibular apparatus. Branches of the dendrites have close contact with basal part of **hair cells.** Dendrites terminating on type I hair cells are comparatively larger than those ending on type II hair cells.

Axons of the first order neurons (bipolar cells) form **vestibular division** of **vestibulocochlear nerve.** These fibers reach the medulla oblongata and terminate in vestibular nuclei. These nerve fibers are called primary vestibular fibers.

Vestibular Nuclei

There are four vestibular nuclei in the medulla oblongata, viz. superior, inferior, lateral and medial nuclei. Most of the primary vestibular fibers reaching superior and medial nuclei come from crista ampullaris of semicircular canals. Lateral vestibular nucleus receives fibers mainly from maculae of otolith organ and inferior vestibular nucleus receives fibers from both crista ampullaris and maculae.

Efferent nerve fibers to hair cells

Some neurons in vestibular nuclei send efferent fibers, which run back to the hair cells along with primary vestibular fibers (see above). It is believed that these efferent fibers to hair cells provide tonic inhibition of hair cells.

Fibers to Cerebellum

Fibers from some bipolar cells reach cerebellum directly and terminate in **flocculonodular lobe** or the **fastigial nucleus** in cerebellum.

■ SECOND ORDER NEURON

Second order neurons of this pathway are located in the four **vestibular nuclei.** Axons from vestibular nuclei

Macula in saccule (vertically placed)

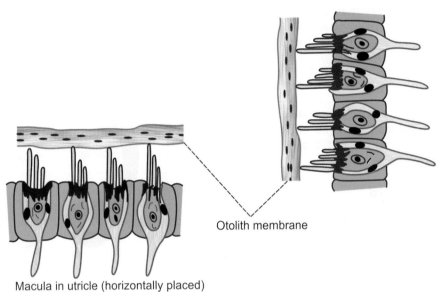

Otolith membrane

Macula in utricle (horizontally placed)

FIGURE 158.5: Macula in otolith organ

form the secondary vestibular fibers. Secondary vestibular fibers form four tracts:
1. Vestibulo-ocular tract
2. Vestibulospinal tract
3. Vestibuloreticular tract
4. Vestibulocerebellar tract.

1. Vestibulo-ocular Tract

Fibers from superior, medial and inferior vestibular nuclei descend downwards for short distance along with vestibulospinal tract. Afterwards, these fibers ascend through the medial longitudinal fasciculus and terminate in the nuclei of III, IV and VI cranial nerves, thus forming vestibulo-ocular tract. This tract is concerned with **movements of eyeballs** in relation to the position of the head.

2. Vestibulospinal Tract

Fibers from lateral nucleus descend downwards and form the vestibulospinal tract. Some fibers from this nucleus ascend upward and join medial longitudinal fasciculus. Fibers of vestibulospinal tract are involved in reflex **movements of head and body** during postural changes.

3. Vestibuloreticular Tract

Some fibers from vestibular nuclei reach the reticular formation of brainstem forming reticulospinal tract.

These fibers are concerned with the **facilitation of muscle tone.**

4. Vestibulocerebellar Tract

Some fibers arising from all four vestibular nuclei form vestibulocerebellar tract and terminate in flocculonodular lobe and fastigial nuclei of cerebellum. This tract is involved in **coordination of movements** according to body position.

■ FUNCTIONS OF VESTIBULAR APPARATUS

Receptors of semicircular canals give response to **rotatory movements** or **angular acceleration** of the head. And receptors of utricle and saccule give response to linear acceleration of head.

Thus, the vestibular apparatus is responsible for detecting the position of head during different movements. It also causes reflex adjustments in the position of eyeball, head and body during postural changes.

■ FUNCTIONS OF SEMICIRCULAR CANALS

Semicircular canals are concerned with **angular (rotatory) acceleration.** Semicircular canals sense the rotational movement. Each semicircular canal is sensitive to rotation in a particular plane.

Superior Semicircular Canal

Superior semicircular canal gives response to rotation in **anteroposterior plane (transverse axis),** i.e. front to back movements like nodding the head while saying 'yes – yes'.

Horizontal Semicircular Canal

Horizontal semicircular canal gives response to rotation in **horizontal plane (vertical axis),** i.e. side to side movements (left to right or right to left) like shaking the head while saying 'no – no'.

Posterior Semicircular Canal

Posterior semicircular canal gives response to rotation in the **vertical plane (anteroposterior axis)** by which head is rotated from shoulder to shoulder.

Mechanism of Stimulation of Receptor Cells in Semicircular Canal

At the beginning of rotation, receptor cells are stimulated by movement of endolymph inside the semicircular canals. However, receptors are stimulated only at the beginning and at the stoppage of rotatory movements. And during rotation at a constant speed, these receptors are not stimulated.

When a person rotates in **clockwise direction** in horizontal plane (vertical axis), horizontal canal moves in clockwise direction. But there is no corresponding movement of **endolymph** inside the canal at the beginning of rotation. Because of the **inertia,** endolymph remains **static.** This phenomenon causes relative displacement of endolymph in the direction opposite to that of the rotation of head. That is, the fluid is pushed in anticlockwise direction.

Thus, in the right horizontal semicircular canal, the endolymph flows towards the ampulla and in the left canal, the fluid moves away from the ampulla (Fig. 158.6).

Movement of **endolymph** in semicircular canal, in turn causes corresponding movement of **gelatinous cupula.** Thus, in the right horizontal canal, the cupula moves towards the ampulla. Whereas in left canal cupula moves away from ampulla. In any semicircular canal, when cupula moves towards the ampulla, **stereocilia** of hair cells are pushed **towards kinocilium** leading to **stimulation of hair cells.** When cupula moves away from ampulla, the stereocilia are pushed away from kinocilium and hair cells are not stimulated.

Thus, at the commencement of rotation in clockwise direction around vertical axis, hair cells at ampulla of

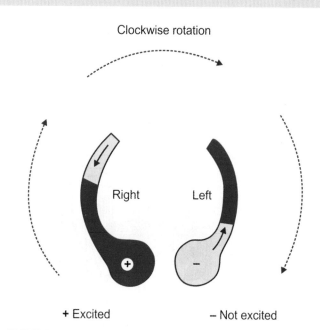

Clockwise rotation

Right   Left

+ Excited   − Not excited

FIGURE 158.6: Movement of fluid and excitation of crista ampullaris in right horizontal semicircular canal during clockwise rotation.

horizontal canal in right ear are stimulated. But, the hair cells in horizontal canal of left ear are not stimulated.

Because of stimulation, the hair cells in right horizontal canal send information (impulses) through sensory nerve fibers to vestibular, cerebellar and reticular centers. Now, these centers send proper instructions to various muscles of the body to maintain equilibrium of the body during angular acceleration (rotation).

On the other hand, rotation in anticlockwise direction causes stimulation of hair cells in ampulla of horizontal canal in left ear only. Hair cells of horizontal canal in right ear are not stimulated. Stimulation of hair cells in left ear is followed by the process as in the case of clockwise rotation.

Electrical Potential in Hair Cells – Mechanotransduction

Mechanotransduction is a type of **sensory transduction** (Chapter 139) in the hair cell (receptor) by which the **mechanical energy** (movement of cilia in hair cell) caused by stimulus is converted into **action potentials** in the vestibular nerve fiber.

Resting membrane potential in hair cells is −60 mV. Movement of stereocilia of hair cells towards kinocilium causes opening of mechanically gated potassium channels (Chapter 3). It is followed by influx of potassium ions from endolymph which contains large amount of potassium ions. Potassium ions cause development of **mild depolarization** in hair cells up to –50 mV. This type of depolarization is called **receptor potential.** Besides potassium ions, calcium ions also enter the hair cells from endolymph.

Receptor potential in hair cells is non-propagative. But, it causes **generation of action potential** in nerve fibers distributed to hair cells. Depolarization of hair cells causes them to release a neurotransmitter, which generates the action potential in the nerve fibers. It is believed that the probable neurotransmitter may be glutamate.

Movement of stereocilia in the opposite direction (away from kinocilium) causes **hyperpolarization** of hair cells. Calcium may play a role in the development of hyperpolarization. Hyperpolarization in hair cells stops generation of action potential in the nerve fibers (Fig. 158.7).

Adaptation of Receptors in Semicircular Canal during Rotation

Hair cells of crista ampullaris generate impulses even at rest. But, the frequency of discharge is very low at resting conditions. It is about 50 to 100 impulses per minute.

At the commencement of rotation, discharge of impulses reaches a higher frequency of 600 to 800 per minute, depending upon the speed of rotation. However, the rapid discharge of impulses lasts only for the first 20 to 25 seconds of rotation. Afterwards, even if rotation continues, the frequency of impulses falls back to the resting level. It is because of the adaptation of receptors during continuous rotation.

Cause for adaptation of receptor cells

At the onset of rotation, endolymph inside the semicircular canal does not move along with semicircular canal because of inertia of the fluid. So semicircular canal moves leaving the endolymph behind, which is like moving in the opposite direction. Now the endolymph is pushed into ampulla towards the utricle. It causes stimulation of hair cells but, after about 20 seconds due to the accumulation of endolymph, a pressure is developed in ampulla. Due to the back pressure, endolymph starts moving away from ampulla, i.e. it starts moving along with semicircular canal at the same speed. It causes adaptation of the hair cells.

Hair cells of crista ampullaris of vertical semicircular canals are stimulated during the rotation of head in anteroposterior or transverse axis. However, the mechanism involved is similar to that of the hair cells of crista ampullaris of horizontal canals.

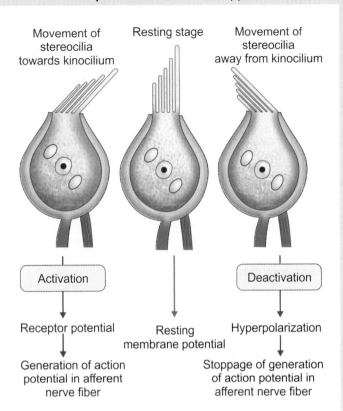

FIGURE 158.7: Mechanotransduction in hair cell of vestibular apparatus. During activation, receptor potential develops in hair cell due to the influx of potassium and calcium ions. Receptor potential causes release of neurotransmitter from hair cell, which induces development of action potential in the afferent nerve fiber.

Nystagmus

Nystagmus is the rhythmic oscillatory involuntary movements of eyeball. It is common during rotation. It is due to the natural stimulatory effect of vestibular apparatus during rotational acceleration. Nystagmus occurs both in physiological and pathological conditions.

Vestibulo-ocular reflex and nystagmus

Nystagmus is a **reflex phenomenon** that occurs in order to maintain the visual fixation. Since the movements of eyeballs occur in response to stimulation of vestibular apparatus this reflex is called **vestibulo-ocular reflex.**

Movement of eyeball during nystagmus

Nystagmus has two components of movement, which occur alternately:

1. Slow component
2. Quick component.

1. *Slow component*

At the beginning of rotation, since eyes are fixed at a particular object (point), eyeballs rotate slowly in the direction opposite to that of rotation of the head. It is called slow component of nystagmus. It is due to vestibulo-ocular reflex. This reflex is because of labyrinthine impulses reaching the ocular muscles via vestibular nuclei and III, IV and V cranial nerves.

2. *Quick component*

When the slow movement of eyeballs is limited, the eyeballs move to a new fixation point in the direction of rotation of head. This movement to a new fixation point occurs with a jerk. So, it is called the quick component. Quick component of nystagmus is due to the activation of some centers in brainstem.

Postrotatory nystagmus

Nystagmus that occurs immediately after stoppage of rotation is called postrotatory nystagmus. It is due to movement of cupula in opposite direction caused by the endolymph, when rotation is stopped. Postrotatory nystagmus can be demonstrated by Barany chair (see below for details).

Postrotatory Reactions

After the end of rotatory movement, two reactions occur:
  1. Feeling of rotation in opposite direction
  2. Postrotatory nystagmus.

1. *Feeling of rotation in the opposite direction*

When rotation in clockwise direction is stopped suddenly, endolymph moves in the direction of rotation in right horizontal semicircular canal although the semicircular canal stops moving. So, cupula moves away from utricle.

However, in the case of left horizontal semicircular canal, endolymph moves into ampulla. There, it pushes cupula towards the utricle and stimulates the hair cells in crista of left canal. It causes feeling of rotation in opposite direction when the rotation is stopped.

2. *Postrotatory nystagmus*

It is already explained above.

Nystagmus in Pathological Conditions

Nystagmus is very common in lesions of cerebellum and lesions of brainstem involving vestibular nuclei or vestibular nerve. It also occurs due to the damage of labyrinth.

■ FUNCTION OF OTOLITH ORGAN

Otolith organ is concerned with linear acceleration and detects acceleration in both horizontal and vertical planes. Utricle responds during horizontal acceleration and saccule responds during vertical acceleration.

Function of Utricle

Position of hair cells of macula helps utricle to respond to horizontal acceleration. In utricle, the macula is situated in horizontal plane with the hair cells in vertical plane (Fig. 158.5). While moving horizontally, because of inertia the otoconia move in opposite direction and pull the cilia of hair cells resulting in stimulation of hair cells.

For example, when the body moves forward, the otoconia fall back in otolith membrane and pull the cilia of hair cells backward. Pulling of cilia causes stimulation of hair cells. Hair cells send information (impulses) to vestibular, cerebellar and reticular centers. These centers in turn send instructions to various muscles to maintain equilibrium of the body during the forward movement.

Function of Saccule

Macula of saccule is situated in vertical plane with the cilia of hair cells in horizontal plane. While moving vertically, as in the case of utricle, otoconia of saccule move in opposite direction and pull the cilia resulting in stimulation of hair cells.

For example, while climbing up, the otoconia move down by pulling the cilia downwards. It stimulates the hair cells, which in turn send information to the brain centers. And the action follows as in the case of movement in horizontal plane.

Role of Otolith Organ in Resting Position

During resting conditions (in the absence of head movement), hair cells are stimulated continuously because of the pulling of **otoconia** by gravitational force. Stimulation of hair cells produces reflex movements of head and limbs for the maintenance of posture in relation to gravity. Because of this function, the receptors of otolith organ are called **gravity receptors.**

■ EFFECTS OF STIMULATION OF SEMICIRCULAR CANALS

Under experimental conditions, semicircular canals can be stimulated by two methods:
  A. Rotational movement
  B. Caloric stimulation.

■ ROTATIONAL MOVEMENT

Semicircular canal can be stimulated by rotational movement with the help of Barany chair.

Barany Chair

Barany chair is a revolving chair. The subject is seated on this chair with the head tilted forward at 30°. Both the eyes are closed. The chair is rotated at a speed of 30 RPM for about 20 seconds and then stopped.

Effects of Stimulation of Semicircular Canals by Rotation

Stimulation of semicircular canals during rotation in Barany chair produces some effects both during rotation and after the end of rotation.

Postrotatory Reactions

Twenty seconds after the stoppage of rotation in Barany chair, following reactions occur:

1. *Postrotatory nystagmus:* Eyes are closed during rotation by Barany chair. When eyes are opened after the sudden stoppage of rotation, nystagmus starts. Postrotatory nystagmus exists for about 30 seconds.
2. *Dizziness:* Immediately after stoppage of rotation, there is a feeling of unsteadiness. It is called the dizziness. Dizziness is associated with feeling of rotation in the opposite direction.
3. *Vertigo:* After the end of rotation, there is a feeling of environment whirling around or, there is a feeling of rotation of the person himself.
4. *Other effects:* Rotation for a longer period causes nausea and vomiting. Blood pressure falls by about 10 to 15 mm Hg. And, heart rate is reduced by 10 to 12 beats per minute.

Reaction during Rotation with Opened Eyes

If Barany chair is rotated with opened eyes, nystagmus occurs continuously throughout the period of rotation.

■ CALORIC STIMULATION

Semicircular canals can be stimulated bypassing hot or cold water into the ear by using a syringe. The transmission of change in temperature into labyrinth alters the specific gravity of endolymph. This in turn causes movement of cupula and stimulation of receptor cells.

Effects of Caloric Stimulation

Stimulation of semicircular canals by thermal stimulus develops nystagmus, vertigo and nausea. During the treatment for ear infection, temperature of fluid instilled into the ear must be equal to body temperature, so that, such symptoms of caloric stimulation are avoided.

■ APPLIED PHYSIOLOGY – EFFECT OF LABYRINTHECTOMY

■ BILATERAL LABYRINTHECTOMY

Removal of labyrinthine apparatus on both sides leads to complete loss of equilibrium.

Equilibrium could be maintained only by visual sensation. Postural reflexes are severely affected. There is loss of hearing sensation too.

■ UNILATERAL LABYRINTHECTOMY

Removal of labyrinthine apparatus on one side causes less effect on postural reflexes. However, severe autonomic symptoms occur. Autonomic symptoms are due to unbalanced generation of impulses from the unaffected labyrinthine apparatus.

Symptoms are nausea, vomiting and diarrhea. During movement, the symptoms become very severe.

The unaffected labyrinthine apparatus starts compensating the loss of functions of affected labyrinth. Hence, the symptoms disappear slowly after a few months.

■ MOTION SICKNESS

■ DEFINITION

Motion sickness is defined as the syndrome of physiological response during movement (travel) to which the person is not adapted. It can occur while traveling in any form of vehicle like automobile, ship, aircraft or spaceship. Motion sickness that occurs while traveling in a watercraft is called seasickness.

■ CAUSE

Motion sickness is due to excessive and repeated stimulation of vestibular apparatus. Excessive and repeated stimulation of vestibular apparatus occurs because of:

1. Rapid and repeated change in rate of motion while traveling
2. Rapid and repeated change in direction.

Psychological factors such as anxiety about the unfamiliar modes of travel may be added up to cause motion sickness.

■ SYMPTOMS

1. Nausea
2. Vomiting
3. Sweating
4. Diarrhea
5. Pallor (paleness)
6. Excess salivation
7. Discomfort
8. Headache
9. Disorientation.

■ PREVENTION

Responses of motion sickness can be prevented by avoiding greasy and bulky food before travel and by taking antiemetic drugs (drugs preventing nausea and vomiting). In experimental animals, motion sickness is abolished by bilateral removal of vestibular apparatus, sectioning of vestibular nerve or ablation of flocculonodular lobe.

Electroencephalogram (EEG)

- ■ INTRODUCTION
- ■ SIGNIFICANCE OF EEG
- ■ METHOD OF RECORDING EEG
- ■ WAVES OF EEG
- ■ EEG DURING SLEEP

■ INTRODUCTION

Electroencephalography is the study of electrical activities of brain. Electroencephalogram (EEG) is the graphical recording of electrical activities of brain. Electrical activity of the brain is complicated when compared to that of a single nerve fiber or neuron. It is due to the involvement of large number of neurons and synapses.

German psychiatrist **Hans Berger** was the first one to analyze the EEG waves systematically and hence the EEG waves are referred as **Berger waves.**

■ SIGNIFICANCE OF EEG

Electroencephalogram is useful in the diagnosis of neurological disorders and sleep disorders. EEG pattern is altered in the following neurological disorders:

1. **Epilepsy,** which occurs due to excessive discharge of impulses from cerebral cortex
2. **Disorders of midbrain** affecting ascending reticular activating system
3. **Subdural hematoma** during which there is collection of blood in subdural space over the cerebral cortex.

■ METHOD OF RECORDING EEG

Electroencephalograph is the instrument used to record EEG. The electrodes called **scalp electrodes** from the instrument are placed over unopened skull or over the brain after opening the skull or by piercing into brain. Electrodes are of two types, unipolar and bipolar electrodes. While using bipolar electrodes, both the terminals are placed in different parts of brain.

When unipolar electrodes are used, the active electrode is placed over cortex and the indifferent electrode is kept on some part of the body away from cortex.

■ WAVES OF EEG

Electrical activity recorded by EEG may have synchronized or desynchronized waves. **Synchronized waves** are the regular and invariant waves, whereas **desynchronized waves** are irregular and variant. In normal persons, EEG has three frequency bands (Fig. 159.1):

1. Alpha rhythm
2. Beta rhythm
3. Delta rhythm.

In addition to these three types of waves, EEG in children shows theta waves.

■ ALPHA RHYTHM

Alpha rhythm consists of rhythmical waves, which appear at a frequency of 8 to 12 waves/second with the amplitude of 50 μV. Alpha waves are **synchronized waves.**

Alpha rhythm is obtained in i**nattentive brain** or **mind** as in drowsiness, light sleep or narcosis with closed eyes. It is abolished by visual stimuli or any other type of stimuli or by mental effort. So, it is diminished when eyes are opened.

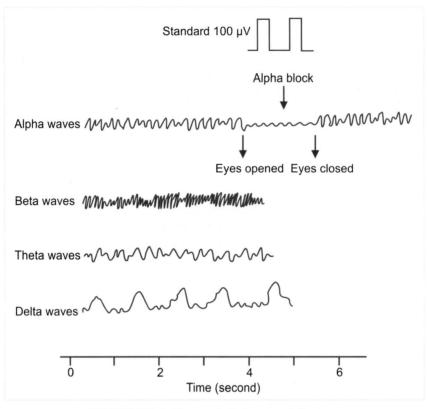

FIGURE 159.1: Waves of electroencephalogram

Waves of alpha rhythm are most marked in parieto-occipital area. Sometimes these waves appear in other areas also.

Alpha Block

Alpha block is the replacement of synchronized alpha waves in EEG by desynchronized and low voltage waves when the eyes are opened. The desynchronized waves do not have specific frequency. It occurs due to any form of sensory stimulation or mental concentration, such as solving arithmetic problems.

Desynchronization is the common term used for replacement of regular alpha waves with irregular low voltage waves. It is due to the loss of synchronized activity in neural elements that are responsible for regular wave pattern.

■ BETA RHYTHM

Beta rhythm includes high frequency waves of 15 to 60 per second but, the amplitude is low, i.e. 5 to 10 μV. Beta waves are **desynchronized waves.** Beta rhythm is recorded during mental activity or mental tension or arousal state. It is not affected by opening the eyes.

During higher mental activity or peak performance state like conscious activity, problem solving and fear, very high frequency waves of 30 to 100 per second

appear. Some controversy exists in naming such waves. Often very high frequency waves are called **gamma rhythm.** However, many scientists consider these waves as beta rhythm.

■ DELTA RHYTHM

Delta rhythm includes waves with low frequency and high amplitude. These waves have the frequency of 1 to 5 per second with the amplitude of 20 to 200 μV. It is common in early childhood during waking hours. In adults, it appears mostly during **deep sleep.**

Presence of delta waves in adults during conditions other than sleep indicates the pathological process in brain like tumor, epilepsy, increased intracranial pressure and mental deficiency or depression. These waves are not affected by opening the eyes.

■ THETA WAVES

Theta waves are obtained generally in children below 5 years of age. These waves are of low frequency and low voltage waves. Frequency of theta waves is 4 to 8 per second and the amplitude is about 10 μV.

■ EEG DURING SLEEP

Changes in the EEG pattern during sleep are described in Chapter 160.

Physiology of Sleep

- ■ DEFINITION
- ■ SLEEP REQUIREMENT
- ■ PHYSIOLOGICAL CHANGES DURING SLEEP
- ■ TYPES OF SLEEP
- ■ STAGES OF SLEEP AND EEG PATTERN
- ■ MECHANISM OF SLEEP
- ■ APPLIED PHYSIOLOGY – SLEEP DISORDERS

■ DEFINITION

Sleep is the natural periodic **state of rest for mind and body** with closed eyes characterized by partial or complete loss of consciousness. Loss of consciousness leads to decreased response to external stimuli and decreased body movements. Depth of sleep is not constant throughout the sleeping period. It varies in different stages of sleep.

■ SLEEP REQUIREMENT

Sleep requirement is not constant. However, average sleep requirement per day at different age groups is:

1. Newborn infants   :   18 to 20 hours
2. Growing children   :   12 to 14 hours
3. Adults   :   7 to   9 hours
4. Old persons   :   5 to   7 hours.

■ PHYSIOLOGICAL CHANGES DURING SLEEP

During sleep, most of the body functions are reduced to basal level. Following are important changes in the body during sleep:

■ 1. PLASMA VOLUME

Plasma volume decreases by about 10% during sleep.

■ 2. CARDIOVASCULAR SYSTEM

Heart Rate

During sleep, the heart rate reduces. It varies between 45 and 60 beats per minute.

Blood Pressure

Systolic pressure falls to about 90 to 110 mm Hg. Lowest level is reached about 4th hour of sleep and remains at this level till a short time before waking up. Then, the pressure commences to rise. If sleep is disturbed by exciting dreams, the pressure is elevated above 130 mm Hg.

■ 3. RESPIRATORY SYSTEM

Rate and force of respiration are decreased. Respiration becomes irregular and **Cheyne-Stokes type** of periodic breathing may develop.

■ 4. GASTROINTESTINAL TRACT

Salivary secretion decreases during sleep. Gastric secretion is not altered or may be increased slightly. Contraction of empty stomach is more vigorous.

■ 5. EXCRETORY SYSTEM

Formation of urine decreases and specific gravity of urine increases.

■ 6. SWEAT SECRETION

Sweat secretion increases during sleep.

■ 7. LACRIMAL SECRETION

Lacrimal secretion decreases during sleep.

■ 8. MUSCLE TONE

Tone in all the muscles of body except ocular muscles decreases very much during sleep. It is called sleep paralysis.

■ 9. REFLEXES

Certain reflexes particularly knee jerk, are abolished. **Babinski sign** becomes positive during deep sleep. Threshold for most of the reflexes increases. Pupils are constricted. Light reflex is retained. Eyeballs move up and down.

■ 10. BRAIN

Brain is not inactive during sleep. There is a characteristic cycle of brain wave activity during sleep with irregular intervals of dreams. Electrical activity in the brain varies with stages of sleep (see below).

■ TYPES OF SLEEP

Sleep is of two types:
1. Rapid eye movement sleep or REM sleep
2. Non-rapid eye movement sleep, NREM sleep or non-REM sleep.

■ 1. RAPID EYE MOVEMENT SLEEP – REM SLEEP

Rapid eye movement sleep is the type of sleep associated with rapid conjugate movements of the eyeballs, which occurs frequently. Though the eyeballs move, the sleep is deep. So, it is also called **para-**doxical sleep. It occupies about 20% to 30% of sleeping period. Functionally, REM sleep is very important because, it plays an important role in consolidation of memory. Dreams occur during this period.

■ 2. NON-RAPID EYE MOVEMENT SLEEP – NREM OR NON-REM SLEEP

Non-rapid eye movement (NREM) sleep is the type of sleep without the movements of eyeballs. It is also called **slow-wave sleep.** Dreams do not occur in this type of sleep and it occupies about 70% to 80% of total sleeping period. Non-REM sleep is followed by REM sleep.

Differences between the two types of sleep are given in Table 160.1.

■ STAGES OF SLEEP AND EEG PATTERN

■ RAPID EYE MOVEMENT SLEEP

During REM sleep, electroencephalogram (EEG) shows irregular waves with high frequency and low amplitude. These waves are **desynchronized waves.**

■ NON-RAPID EYE MOVEMENT SLEEP

The NREM sleep is divided into four stages, based on the EEG pattern. During the stage of wakefulness, i.e. while lying down with closed eyes and relaxed mind, the **alpha waves** of EEG appear. When the person proceeds to drowsy state, the alpha waves diminish (Fig. 160.1).

Stage I: Stage of Drowsiness

Alpha waves are diminished and abolished. EEG shows only **low voltage fluctuations** and **infrequent delta waves.**

Stage II: Stage of Light Sleep

Stage II is characterized by **spindle bursts** at a frequency of 14 per second, superimposed by low voltage **delta waves.**

TABLE 160.1: Rapid eye movement (REM) sleep and non-rapid eye movement (NREM) sleep

Characteristics	REM sleep	Non-REM sleep
1. Rapid eye movement (REM)	Present	Absent
2. Dreams	Present	Absent
3. Muscle twitching	Present	Absent
4. Heart rate	Fluctuating	Stable
5. Blood pressure	Fluctuating	Stable
6. Respiration	Fluctuating	Stable
7. Body temperature	Fluctuating	Stable
8. Neurotransmitter	Noradrenaline	Serotonin

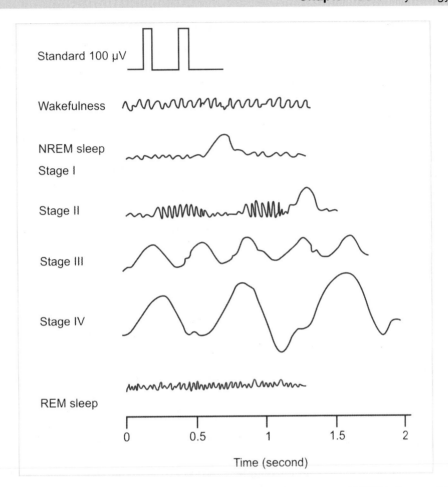

FIGURE 160.1: Electroencephalogram during wakefulness, different stages of NREM sleep and REM sleep.
NREM = Non-rapid eye movement, REM = Rapid eye movement.

Stage III: Stage of Medium Sleep

During this stage, the spindle bursts disappear. Frequency of delta waves decreases to 1 or 2 per second and amplitude increases to about 100 μV.

State IV: Stage of Deep Sleep

Delta waves become more prominent with low frequency and high amplitude.

■ MECHANISM OF SLEEP

Sleep occurs due to the activity of some **sleep-inducing centers** in brain. Stimulation of these centers induces sleep. Damage of sleep centers results in sleeplessness or persistent wakefulness called **insomnia.**

■ SLEEP CENTERS

Complex pathways between the reticular formation of brainstem, diencephalon and cerebral cortex are involved in the onset and maintenance of sleep. However, two centers which induce sleep are located in brainstem:

1. Raphe nucleus
2. Locus ceruleus of pons.

Recently, many more areas that induce sleep are identified in the brain of animals. Inhibition of ascending reticular activating system also results in sleep.

1. Role of Raphe Nucleus

Raphe nucleus is situated in lower pons and medulla. Activation of this nucleus results in non-REM sleep. It is due to release of **serotonin** by the nerve fibers arising from this nucleus. Serotonin induces non-REM sleep.

2. Role of Locus Ceruleus of Pons

Activation of this center produces REM sleep. **Noradrenaline** released by the nerve fibers arising from locus ceruleus induces REM sleep.

*Inhibition of Ascending Reticular
Activating System*

Ascending reticular activating system (ARAS) is responsible for wakefulness because of its afferent and efferent connections with cerebral cortex. Inhibition of ARAS induces sleep. Lesion of ARAS leads to permanent somnolence, i.e. coma.

■ APPLIED PHYSIOLOGY – SLEEP DISORDERS

■ 1. INSOMNIA

Insomnia is the inability to sleep or abnormal wakefulness. It is the most common sleep disorder. It occurs due to systemic illness or mental conditions such as psychiatric problems, alcoholic addiction and drug addiction.

■ 2. HYPERSOMNIA

Hypersomnia is the excess sleep or excess need to sleep. It occurs because of lesion in the floor of the third ventricle, brain tumors, encephalitis, chronic bronchitis and disease of muscles. Hypersomnia also occurs in endocrine disorders such as myxedema and diabetes insipidus.

■ 3. NARCOLEPSY AND CATAPLEXY

Narcolepsy is the sudden attack of **uncontrollable sleep.** Cataplexy is sudden **outburst of emotion.** Both the diseases are due to hypothalamic disorders. Refer Chapter 149 for details.

■ 4. SLEEP APNEA SYNDROME

Sleep apnea is the temporary stoppage of breathing repeatedly during sleep. Sleep apnea syndrome is the disorder that involves fluctuations in the rate and force of respiration during REM sleep with short apneic episode. Apnea is due to decreased stimulation of respiratory centers, arrest of diaphragmatic movements, airway obstruction (Chapter 127) or the combination of all these factors. When breathing stops, the resultant hypercapnia and hypoxia stimulate respiration.

Sleep apnea syndrome occurs in **obesity,** myxedema, enlargement of tonsil and lesion in brainstem. Common features of this syndrome are **loud snoring** (Chapter 127), restless movements, nocturnal insomnia, daytime sleepiness, morning headache and fatigue. In severe conditions, hypertension, right heart failure and stroke occur.

■ 5. NIGHTMARE

Nightmare is a condition during sleep that is characterized by a sense of extreme uneasiness or discomfort or by frightful dreams. Discomfort is felt as of some heavy weight on the stomach or chest or as uncontrolled movement of the body. After a period of extreme anxiety, the subject wakes with a troubled state of mind. It occurs mostly during REM sleep. **Nightmare** occurs due to improper food intake, digestive disorders or nervous disorders. It also occurs during drug withdrawal or alcohol withdrawal.

■ 6. NIGHT TERROR

Night terror is a disorder similar to nightmare. It is common in children. It is also called **pavor nocturnus** or **sleep terror.** The child awakes screaming in a state of fright and semiconsciousness. The child cannot recollect the attack in the morning. Nightmare occurs shortly after falling asleep and during non-REM sleep. There is no psychological disturbance.

■ 7. SOMNAMBULISM

Somnambulism is getting up from bed and walking in the state of sleep. It is also called **walking during sleep** or **sleep walking** (somnus = sleep; ambulare = to walk). It varies from just sitting up in the bed to walking around with eyes open and performing some major complex task. The episode lasts for few minutes to half an hour. It occurs during non-REM sleep. In children, it is associated with bedwetting or night terror without any psychological disturbance. However, in adults it is associated with psychoneurosis.

■ 8. NOCTURNAL ENURESIS

Nocturnal enuresis is the involuntary voiding of urine at bed. It is also called or **bedwetting.** It is common in children. Refer Chapter 57 for details.

■ 9. MOVEMENT DISORDERS DURING SLEEP

Movement disorders occur immediately after falling asleep. **Sleep start** or **hypnic jerk** is the common movement disorder during sleep. It is characterized by sudden jerks of arms or legs. Sleep start is a physiological form of clonus.

Other movement disorders are teeth grinding (bruxism), banging the head and restless moment of arms or legs.

Epilepsy

Chapter 161

- ■ INTRODUCTION
- ■ TYPES OF EPILEPSY
- ■ GENERALIZED EPILEPSY
  - ■ GRAND MAL
  - ■ PETIT MAL
  - ■ PSYCHOMOTOR EPILEPSY
- ■ LOCALIZED EPILEPSY

■ INTRODUCTION

Epilepsy

Epilepsy is a brain disorder characterized by convulsive seizures or loss of consciousness or both.

Convulsion and Convulsive Seizure

Convulsion refers to uncontrolled involuntary muscular contractions. Convulsive seizure means sudden attack of uncontrolled involuntary muscular contractions. It occurs due to **paroxysmal** (sudden and usually recurring periodically) **uncontrolled discharge** of impulses from neurons of brain, particularly cerebral cortex.

Epileptic

Patient affected by epilepsy is called epileptic. The person with epilepsy remains normal in between seizures. Epileptic attack develops only when excitability of the neuron is increased, causing excessive neuronal discharge.

■ TYPES OF EPILEPSY

Epilepsy is divided into two categories:
1. Generalized epilepsy
2. Localized epilepsy.

■ GENERALIZED EPILEPSY

Generalized epilepsy is the type of epilepsy that occurs due to excessive discharge of impulses from all parts of the brain. It is also called general onset seizure or general onset epilepsy.

Generalized epilepsy is subdivided into three types:
1. Grand mal
2. Petit mal
3. Psychomotor epilepsy.

■ GRAND MAL

Grand mal is characterized by sudden loss of consciousness, followed by convulsion. Just before the onset of convulsions, the person feels the warning sensation in the form of some **hallucination.** It is called **epileptic aura.**

Convulsions occur in two stages:
a. Tonic stage
b. Clonic stage.

Tonic Stage

Initially, seizure is characterized by **tonic contractions** of muscle leading to **spasm.** Spasm causes twisting facial features, flexion of arm and extension of lower limbs.

Clonic Stage

Clonic convulsions develop after the tonic stage. This stage is characterized by violent jerky movements of limbs and face due to alternate severe contraction and relaxation of muscles.

At the end of attack, alternative tonic and clonic convulsions are seen. During the entire period of seizure, tongue may be bitten.

Electroencephalogram (EEG) shows fast waves with a frequency of 15 to 30 per second during tonic stage. Slow and large waves appear during clonic phase. After the attack, slow waves are recorded for some time. In between seizures, EEG shows delta waves in all types of epileptics.

Causes of Grand Mal

Cause of grand mal epilepsy is the excess neural activity in all parts of brain. Cause for stoppage of attack is neuronal fatigue. Factors which accelerate the neural activity resulting in grand mal epilepsy are:

   i. Strong emotional stimuli
   ii. Hyperventilation and alkalosis
   iii. Effects of some drugs
   iv. Uncontrolled high fever
   v. Loud noises or bright light
   vi. Traumatic lesions in any part of brain.

■ PETIT MAL

In this type of epilepsy, the person becomes **unconscious** suddenly without any warning. The unconsciousness lasts for a very short period of 3 to 30 seconds. Convulsions do not occur. However, the muscles of face show twitch-like contractions and there is blinking of eyes. Afterwards, the person recovers automatically and becomes normal. Frequency of attack may be once in many months or many attacks may appear in rapid series. It usually occurs in late childhood and disappears completely at the age of 30 or above.

EEG recording shows slow and large waves during the attack. Each wave is followed by a sharp spike. This type of waves appear from recording over any part of the cerebral cortex indicating the involvement of whole brain. Delta waves appear in between the seizures.

Causes of Petit Mal

Cause of petit mal is not known. It occurs in conditions like head injury, stroke, brain tumor and brain infection.

■ PSYCHOMOTOR EPILEPSY

Psychomotor epilepsy is characterized by **emotional outbursts** such as abnormal rage, sudden anxiety, fear or discomfort. There is **amnesia** or a confused mental state for some period. Some persons have the tendency to attack others bodily or rub their own face vigorously. In most cases, the persons are not aware of their activities. Some persons are very well aware of the actions, but still the abnormal actions cannot be controlled.

EEG recordings show low frequency rectangular waves, ranging between 2 and 4 per second.

Causes of Psychomotor Epilepsy

Causes of psychomotor epilepsy are the abnormalities in temporal lobe and tumor in hypothalamus and other regions of limbic system like amygdala and hippocampus.

■ LOCALIZED EPILEPSY

Epilepsy that occurs because of excessive discharge of impulses from one part of brain is called localized epilepsy. It is otherwise known as **local** or **focal epilepsy** or **local seizure.** It involves only a localized area of cerebral cortex or the deeper parts of cerebellum, which are affected by tumor, abscess or vascular defects. The abnormality starts from a particular area and spreads to adjacent areas, developing slow-spreading muscular contractions. Contractions usually start in the mouth region and spread down towards the legs. This type of seizure is also known as **jacksonian epilepsy.**

Causes of Localized Epilepsy

Localized epilepsy is caused by brain tumor.

Higher Intellectual Functions

Chapter

162

- ■ **HIGHER INTELLECTUAL FUNCTIONS**
- ■ **LEARNING**
  - ■ DEFINITION
  - ■ CLASSIFICATION
- ■ **MEMORY**
  - ■ DEFINITION
  - ■ ANATOMICAL BASIS
  - ■ PHYSIOLOGICAL BASIS
  - ■ CHEMICAL OR MOLECULAR BASIS
  - ■ CONSOLIDATION
  - ■ CLASSIFICATION
  - ■ DRUGS FACILITATING MEMORY
  - ■ APPLIED PHYSIOLOGY
- ■ **CONDITIONED REFLEXES**
  - ■ DEFINITION
  - ■ CLASSIFICATION
  - ■ CLASSICAL CONDITIONED REFLEXES
  - ■ TYPES AND PROPERTIES OF CLASSICAL CONDITIONED REFLEXES
  - ■ POSITIVE CONDITIONED REFLEXES
  - ■ NEGATIVE CONDITIONED REFLEXES
  - ■ INSTRUMENTAL OR OPERANT CONDITIONED REFLEXES
  - ■ PHYSIOLOGICAL BASIS OF CONDITIONED REFLEXES
- ■ **SPEECH**
  - ■ DEFINITION
  - ■ MECHANISM
  - ■ DEVELOPMENT
  - ■ NERVOUS CONTROL
  - ■ APPLIED PHYSIOLOGY
  - ■ APHASIA
  - ■ DYSARTHRIA OR ANARTHRIA
  - ■ DYSPHONIA
  - ■ STAMMERING

■ HIGHER INTELLECTUAL FUNCTIONS

Higher intellectual functions are very essential to make up the human mind. These functions are also called **higher brain functions** or **higher cortical functions**. The extensive outer layer of gray matter in cerebral cortex is responsible for higher intellectual functions.

Conditioned reflex forms the basis of all higher intellectual functions.

■ LEARNING

■ DEFINITION

Learning is defined as the process by which new information is acquired. It alters the behavior of a person on the basis of past experience.

■ CLASSIFICATION OF LEARNING

Learning is classified into two types:
1. Non-associative learning
2. Associative learning.

1. *Non-associative Learning*

Non-associative learning involves response of a person to only one type of stimulus. It is based on two factors:
   i. Habituation
   ii. Sensitization.

i. Habituation

Habituation means getting used to something, to which a person is constantly exposed. When a person is exposed to a stimulus repeatedly, he starts ignoring the stimulus slowly. During first experience, the event (stimulus) is novel and evokes a response. However, it evokes less response when it is repeated. Finally, the person is habituated to the event (stimulus) and ignores it.

ii. Sensitization

Sensitization is a process by which the body is made to become more sensitive to a stimulus. It is called **amplification of response.** When a stimulus is applied repeatedly, habituation occurs. But, if the same stimulus is combined with another type of stimulus, which may be pleasant or unpleasant, the person becomes more sensitive to original stimulus.

For example, a woman is sensitized to crying sound of her baby. She gets habituated to different sounds around her and sleep is not disturbed by these sounds. However, she suddenly wakes up when her baby cries because of sensitization to crying sound of the baby.

Thus, sensitization increases the response to an innocuous stimulus when that stimulus is applied after another type of stimulus.

2. *Associative Learning*

Associative learning is a complex process. It involves learning about relations between two or more stimuli at a time. Classic example of associative learning is the conditioned reflex, which is described later in this chapter.

■ MEMORY

■ DEFINITION

Memory is defined as the ability to recall past experience or information. It is also defined as retention of learned materials. There are various degrees of memory. Some memories remain only for few seconds, while others last for hours, days, months or even years together.

■ ANATOMICAL BASIS OF MEMORY

Anatomical basis of memory is the **synapse** in brain. Synapse for memory coding is slightly different from other synapses. Two separate presynaptic terminals are present here. One of the terminals is **primary presynaptic terminal,** which ends on postsynaptic neuron as in conventional synapse. This terminal is called sensory terminal, because sensations are transmitted to the postsynaptic neuron through this terminal (Fig. 162.1).

Other presynaptic terminal ends on the sensory terminal itself. This terminal is called **facilitator terminal.**

When, sensory terminal is stimulated alone without facilitator terminal, the firing from sensory terminal leads to habituation, i.e. the firing decreases slowly. On the other hand, if both the terminals are stimulated, facilitation occurs and the signals remain strong for long period, i.e. for few months to few years.

■ PHYSIOLOGICAL BASIS OF MEMORY

Memory is stored in brain by the alteration of synaptic transmission between the neurons involved in memory.

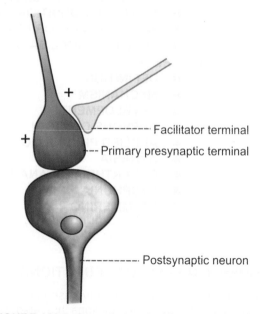

Facilitator terminal

Primary presynaptic terminal

Postsynaptic neuron

FIGURE 162.1: Synaptic terminal for memory encoding

Storage of memory may be facilitated or habituated depending upon many factors, such as neurotransmitter, synaptic transmission, functional status of brain, etc.

Facilitation

Facilitation is the process by which memory storage is enhanced. It involves increase in synaptic transmission and increased postsynaptic activity. Often, facilitation is referred as positive memory.

The process involved in facilitation of memory is called **memory sensitization.**

Habituation

Habituation is the process by which memory storage is **attenuated** (attenuation = decrease in strength, effect or value). It involves reduction in synaptic transmission and slow stoppage of postsynaptic activity. Sometimes, habituation is referred as **negative memory.**

Basis for Short-term Memory

Basic mechanism of memory is the development of new neuronal circuits by the formation of new synapses and facilitation of synaptic transmission. Number of presynaptic terminals and size of the terminals are also increased. This forms the basis of short-term memory.

Basis for Long-term Memory

When neuronal circuit is reinforced by constant activity, memory is consolidated and encoded into different areas of the brain. This encoding makes memory a permanent or a long-term memory.

Sites of Encoding

Hippocampus and Papez circuit (closed circuit between hippocampus, thalamus, hypothalamus and corpus striatum) are the main sites of memory encoding (Chapter 153). Frontal and parietal areas are also involved in memory storage.

Experimental Studies of Memory – Aplysia

Most of the experimental studies of memory and learning are based on the research carried out in the sea hare (sea snail) called *Aplysia*. This animal is useful in brain research because it has a simple uncomplicated nervous system that can be easily approached in living animal with simple dissection. Another advantage of this snail is that the individual nerve cells are large and brightly colored.

Nobel laureate, **Eric Kandel** was the pioneer to use *Aplysia* for the studies of memory and learning.

■ CHEMICAL OR MOLECULAR BASIS OF MEMORY

Memory Engram

Molecular basis of memory can be explained by memory engram. Memory engram is a process by which memory is facilitated and stored in the brain by means of structural and biochemical changes. Often, it is also called **memory trace.**

Molecular Basis of Facilitation

Molecular mechanism of facilitation is given in Figure 162.2. In this process, the neurotransmitter **serotonin** plays major role. Calcium ions increase the release of serotonin, which facilitates the synaptic transmission to a great extent, leading to memory storage.

Molecular Basis of Habituation

Habituation is due to passive closure of calcium channels of terminal membrane. Hence, the release of transmitter decreases, resulting in decrease in number of action potential in the postsynaptic neuron. So, the signals become weak and weakening of signals leads to habituation.

■ CONSOLIDATION OF MEMORY

The process by which a short-term memory is crystallized into a long-term memory is called memory consolidation. Consolidation causes permanent facilitation of synapses. It is possible by rehearsal mechanism, i.e. rehearsal of same information again and again accelerates and potentiates the degree of transfer of short-term memory into long-term memory. This is what happens in memorizing a poem or a phrase.

■ CLASSIFICATION OF MEMORY

Memory is classified by different methods, on the basis of various factors.

Short-term Memories and Long-term Memories

Generally, memory is classified as short-term memory and long-term memory.

1. Short-term memory

Short-term memory is the recalling events that happened very recently, i.e. within hours or days. It is also known as recent memory. For example, telephone number that is known today may be remembered till tomorrow. But if it is not recalled repeatedly, it may be forgotten on the third day.

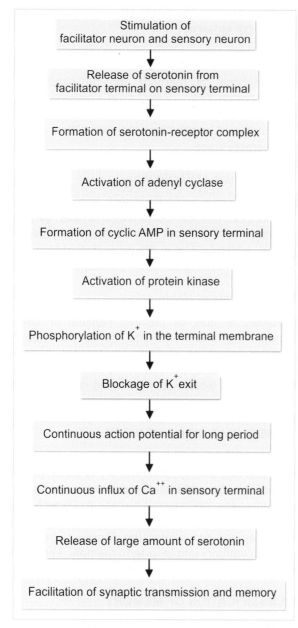

Stimulation of
facilitator neuron and sensory neuron

↓

Release of serotonin from
facilitator terminal on sensory terminal

↓

Formation of serotonin-receptor complex

↓

Activation of adenyl cyclase

↓

Formation of cyclic AMP in sensory terminal

↓

Activation of protein kinase

↓

Phosphorylation of K^+ in the terminal membrane

↓

Blockage of K^+ exit

↓

Continuous action potential for long period

↓

Continuous influx of Ca^{++} in sensory terminal

↓

Release of large amount of serotonin

↓

Facilitation of synaptic transmission and memory

FIGURE 162.2: Memory engram

Short-term memory may be interrupted by many factors such as stress, trauma, drug abuse, etc.

There is another form of short-term memory called **working memory.** It is concerned with recollection of past experience for a very short period, on the basis of which an action is executed.

2. Long-term memory

Long-term memory is the recalling of events of weeks, months, years or sometimes lifetime. It is otherwise called the **remote memory.** Examples are, recalling first

day of schooling, birthday celebration of previous year, picnic enjoyed last week, etc. Long-term memory is more resistant and is not disrupted easily.

Explicit and Implicit Memories

Physiologically, memory is classified into two types, namely explicit memory and implicit memory.

1. Explicit memory

Explicit memory is defined as the memory that involves conscious recollection of past experience. It consists of memories regarding events, which occurred in the external world around us. The information stored may be about a particular event that happened at a particular time and place. Explicit memory is otherwise known as **declarative memory** or **recognition memory.**

Examples of explicit memory are recollection of a birthday party celebrated three days ago, events taken place while taking breakfast, etc.

Explicit memory involves hippocampus and medial part of temporal lobe.

2. Implicit memory

Implicit memory is defined as the memory in which past experience is utilized without conscious awareness. It helps to perform various skilled activities properly. Implicit memory is otherwise known as **non-declarative memory** or **skilled memory.**

Examples of implicit memory are cycling, driving, playing tennis, dancing, typing, etc.

Implicit memory involves the sensory and motor pathways.

Memories Depending upon Duration

Depending upon duration, memory is classified into three types:
1. Sensory memory
2. Primary memory
3. Secondary memory.

1. Sensory memory

Sensory memory is the ability to retain sensory signals in sensory areas of brain, for a very short period of few seconds after the actual sensory experience, i.e. few hundred milliseconds. But, the signals are replaced by new sensory signals in less than 1 second. It is the initial stage of memory. It resembles working memory.

2. Primary memory

Primary memory is the memory of facts, words, numbers, letters or other information retained for few minutes at a time. For example, after searching and finding a telephone number in the directory, we remember the number for a short while. After appreciating beautiful scenery, the details of it could be recalled for some time. Afterwards, it disappears from the memory.

Characteristic feature of this type of memory is that the information is available for recall easily from memory store itself. One need not search or squeeze through the mind, but this memory is easily replaced by new bits of memory, i.e. by looking into another telephone number, the first one may disappear.

3. *Secondary memory*

Secondary memory is the storage of information in brain for a longer period. The information could be recalled after hours, days, months or years. It is also called **fixed memory** or **permanent memory.** It resembles long-term memory.

■ DRUGS FACILITATING MEMORY

Several stimulants for central nervous system are shown to improve learning and memory in animals. Common stimulants are caffeine, physostigmine, amphetamine, nicotine, strychnine and metrazol. All these substances mentioned above facilitate the consolidation of memory.

■ APPLIED PHYSIOLOGY – ABNORMALITIES OF MEMORY

1. *Amnesia*

Loss of memory is known as amnesia. Amnesia is classified into two types:
   i. Anterograde amnesia: Failure to establish new long-term memories. It occurs because of lesion in hippocampus.
   ii. Retrograde amnesia: Failure to recall past remote long-term memory. It occurs in temporal lobe syndrome.

2. *Dementia*

Dementia is the progressive deterioration of intellect, emotional control, social behavior and motivation associated with loss of memory. It is an age-related disorder. Usually, it occurs above the age of 65 years. When it occurs under the age of 65, it is called **presenile dementia.**

Causes

Dementia occurs due to many reasons. Most common cause of dementia is Alzheimer disease. In about 75% of cases, dementia is due to this disease (given below). Other common causes of dementia are hydrocephalus, Huntington chorea, Parkinson disease, viral encephalitis, HIV infection, hypothyroidism, hypoparathyroidism, Cushing syndrome, alcoholic intoxication, poisoning by high dose of barbiturate, carbon monoxide, heavy metals, etc.

Clinical features

Common features are loss of recent memory, lack of thinking and judgment and personality changes. As the disease progresses, psychiatric features begin to appear. Motor functions are also affected. Finally, the patient has to lead a vegetative life without any thinking power. The person is speechless and is unable to understand anything.

There is no effective treatment for this disorder. Physostigmine, which inhibits cholinesterase causes moderate improvement.

3. *Alzheimer Disease*

Alzheimer disease is a progressive neurodegenerative disease. It is due to degeneration, loss of function and death of neurons in many parts of brain, particularly cerebral hemispheres, hippocampus and pons. There is reduction in the synthesis of most of the neurotransmitters, especially acetylcholine. Synthesis of acetylcholine decreases due to lack of enzyme choline acetyltransferase. Norepinephrine synthesis decreases because of degeneration of locus ceruleus. Dementia is the common feature of this disease.

■ CONDITIONED REFLEXES

■ DEFINITION

Conditioned reflex is the acquired reflex that requires learning, memory and recall of previous experience. It is acquired after birth and it forms the basis of learning.

Conditioned reflex is different from unconditioned reflex (Table 162.1). Unconditioned reflex is the inborn reflex, which does not need previous experience.

TABLE 162.1: Conditioned reflex Vs unconditioned reflex

Conditioned reflex	Unconditioned reflex
Acquired after birth	Inborn reflex
Needs previous experience	Does not need previous experience
Involves learning and memory	Does not involve learning and memory
Elicited by conditioned stimulus	Elicited by unconditioned stimulus

■ CLASSIFICATION OF CONDITIONED REFLEXES

Conditioned reflexes are classified into two types:
  A. Classical conditioned reflexes
  B. Instrumental conditioned reflexes.

■ CLASSICAL CONDITIONED REFLEXES

Classical conditioned reflexes are those reflexes, which are established by a **conditioned stimulus,** followed by an **unconditioned stimulus.**

Method of Study – Pavlov's Bell-Dog Experiments

Various types of classical conditioned reflexes and their properties are demonstrated by the classical bell-dog experiments (salivary secretion experiments), done by **Ivan Pavlov** and his associates.

In dogs, the duct of parotid gland or submandibular gland was taken outside through cheek or chin respectively and the saliva was collected by some special apparatus. Apparatus consisted of a funnel, which is sealed over the opening of the duct. Salivary secretion was measured in drops by means of an electrical recorder.

■ TYPES AND PROPERTIES OF CLASSICAL CONDITIONED REFLEXES

Classical conditioned reflexes are classified into two groups according to the properties of reflexes, namely excitation or inhibition:
  I. Positive or excitatory conditioned reflexes
  II. Negative conditioned reflexes.

■ POSITIVE CONDITIONED REFLEXES (EXCITATION OF CONDITIONED REFLEXES)

Types of positive conditioned reflexes:
  1. Primary conditioned reflex
  2. Secondary conditioned reflex
  3. Tertiary conditioned reflex.

1. Primary Conditioned Reflex

Primary conditioned reflex is the reflex developed with one unconditioned stimulus and one conditioned stimulus. This reflex is established in the following way. The animal is fed with food (unconditioned stimulus). Simultaneously a flash of light (conditioned stimulus) is also shown. Both the stimuli are repeated for some days. After the development of reflex, the flash of light (conditioned stimulus) alone causes salivary secretion without food (unconditioned stimulus).

2. Secondary Conditioned Reflex

Secondary conditioned reflex is the reflex developed with one unconditioned stimulus and two conditioned stimuli. After establishment of a conditioned reflex with one conditioned stimulus, another conditioned stimulus is applied along with the first one. For example, the animal is fed with food (unconditioned reflex) and simultaneously a flash of light **(first conditioned stimulus)** and a bell sound **(second conditioned stimulus)** are applied. After development of the reflex, bell sound (second conditioned stimulus) alone can cause salivary secretion (Fig. 162.3).

3. Tertiary Conditioned Reflex

In this reflex, a **third conditioned stimulus** is added and the reflex is established. But, the reflex with more than three conditioned stimuli is not possible. Many types of conditioned stimuli associated with sight and hearing were employed by Pavlov.

■ NEGATIVE CONDITIONED REFLEXES (INHIBITION OF CONDITIONED REFLEXES)

The established conditioned reflexes can be inhibited by some factors. The inhibition is of two types:
  1. External or indirect inhibition
  2. Internal or direct inhibition.

1. External or Indirect Inhibition

Established conditioned reflex is inhibited by some form of stimulus, which is quite different from the conditioned stimulus. It is not related to conditioned stimulus.

For example, some disturbing factors like sudden entrance of a stranger, sudden noise or a strong smell can abolish the conditioned reflex and inhibit salivary secretion. This extra stimulus evokes the animal's curiosity and distracts the attention. According to Pavlov, it evokes an investigatory reflex. If the extra (inhibitory) stimulus is repeated for some time, its inhibitory effect gets weakened or abolished.

2. Internal or Direct Inhibition

There are four ways in which the established conditioned reflex is abolished by direct or internal factors, which are related to the conditioned stimulus.
  i. Extinction of conditioned reflex
  ii. Conditioned inhibition
  iii. Inhibition by delay or delayed conditioned reflex
  iv. Differential inhibition.

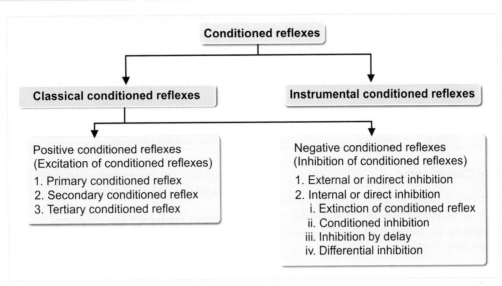

FIGURE 162.3: Conditioned reflexes

i. Extinction of conditioned reflex

Extinction is the failure of conditioned reflex. It occurs if an established conditioned reflex is not reinforced by unconditioned stimulus. After establishing a conditioned reflex, the conditioned stimulus must be coupled with unconditioned stimulus now and then, i.e. the conditioned stimulus must be reinforced by unconditioned stimulus. If a conditioned stimulus is given repeatedly several times, without reinforcing it by unconditioned stimulus, there is failure of conditioned reflex. However, the reflex is not abolished if the unconditioned reflex is also used in between.

ii. Conditioned inhibition

Conditioned inhibition is the failure of conditioned reflex due to introduction of an unknown (new) conditioned stimulus. When a conditioned stimulus like flash of light is effective, if another conditioned stimulus like a bell sound is applied along with this stimulus suddenly, the response does not occur. Of course, if these two conditioned stimuli are given with unconditioned stimulus (food) repeatedly, the secondary conditioned reflex is developed.

iii. Inhibition by delay or delayed conditioned reflex

Inhibition by delay is the absence of response or delayed response that occurs while eliciting a conditioned reflex by delaying the unconditioned stimulus. While establishing a conditioned reflex, the conditioned stimulus (light or sound) must be followed by unconditioned stimulus (food) immediately. If the unconditioned stimulus is applied after a long period, response may be absent or delayed. The reflex is called delayed conditioned reflex.

iv. Differential inhibition

Differential inhibition is the failure of conditioned reflex that occurs when the conditioned stimulus is altered. When an animal is trained or conditioned for a particular type of conditioned stimulus and if this stimulus is altered even slightly, the response does not occur. The animal is able to discriminate the difference. For example, the alteration in frequency of sound or intensity of light abolishes the conditioned reflex (Table 162.2).

■ INSTRUMENTAL OR OPERANT CONDITIONED REFLEXES

Instrumental conditioned reflexes are those reflexes in which the behavior of the person is instrumental. This type of reflexes is developed by the conditioned stimulus, followed by a reward or a punishment. The instrumental conditioned reflexes are also called **operant conditioned reflexes** or **Skinner conditioning.**

During the development of this type of reflexes, the animal is taught to perform some task, in order to obtain a reward or to avoid a punishment. Accordingly, the instrumental conditioned reflexes are of several types, such as:

1. Conditioned avoidance reflex
2. Food avoidance reflex
3. Conditioned reward reflex.

Conditioned Avoidance Reflex

Conditioned avoidance reflex is the reflex by which the animal is trained to avoid an electric shock, by pressing a bar.

TABLE 162.2: Causes for inhibition of conditioned reflex

Type of inhibition		Cause
External inhibition		Disturbing factors like a stranger, noise or strong smell
Internal inhibition	Extinction of conditioned reflex	Failure to reinforce the conditioned reflex by unconditioned stimulus
	Conditioned inhibition	Introduction of unknown (new) conditioned stimulus
	Inhibition by delay	Delay in applying unconditioned stimulus
	Differential inhibition	Alteration of conditioned stimulus

Food Avoidance Conditioning

If an animal is given a tasty food along with injection of a drug, which produces nausea or sickness, the animal starts avoiding or hating that food. It is called **food aversion conditioning.**

Conditioned Reward Reflex

If the animal is rewarded by a banana by pressing a bar, the animal repeatedly presses the bar. It is the conditioned reward reflex.

Instrumental conditioned reflexes play an important role during the learning processes of a child. These conditioned reflexes are also responsible for the behavior pattern of an individual.

■ PHYSIOLOGICAL BASIS OF CONDITIONED REFLEXES

Learning and memory form the physiological basis of conditioned reflexes.

■ SPEECH

■ DEFINITION

Speech is defined as the expression of thoughts by production of articulate sound, bearing a definite meaning. It is one of the highest functions of brain.

When a sound is produced verbally, it is called the speech. If it is expressed by visual symbols, it is known as writing. If visual symbols or written words are expressed verbally, that becomes reading.

■ MECHANISM OF SPEECH

Speech depends upon coordinated activities of central speech apparatus and peripheral speech apparatus. **Central speech apparatus** consists of higher centers, i.e. the cortical and subcortical centers. **Peripheral speech apparatus** includes larynx or sound box, pharynx, mouth, nasal cavities, tongue and lips. All the structures of peripheral speech apparatus function in coordination with respiratory system, with the influences of motor impulses from respective motor areas of the cerebral cortex.

■ DEVELOPMENT OF SPEECH

First Stage

First stage in the development of speech is the association of certain words with visual, tactile, auditory and other sensations, aroused by objects in the external world. Association of words with other sensations is stored as memory.

Second Stage

New neuronal circuits are established during the development of speech. When a definite meaning has been attached to certain words, pathway between the auditory area (Heschl area; area 41) and motor area for the muscles of articulation, which helps in speech (Broca area 44) is established. The child attempts to formulate and pronounce the learnt words.

Role of Cortical Areas in the Development of Speech

Development of speech involves integration of three important areas of cerebral cortex:
1. Wernicke area
2. Broca area
3. Motor area.

Role of Wernicke area – Speech understanding

Understanding of speech begins in Wernicke area that is situated in upper part of temporal lobe. It sends fibers to Broca area through a tract called arcuate fasciculus. Wernicke area is responsible for understanding the visual and auditory information required for the production of words. After understanding the words, it sends the information to Broca area.

Role of Broca area – Speech synthesis

Speech is synthesized in the Broca area. It is situated adjacent to the motor area, responsible for the movements of tongue, lips and larynx, which are necessary for speech. By receiving information required for production of words from Wernicke area, the Broca area develops the pattern of motor activities required to verbalize the words. The pattern of motor activities is sent to motor area.

Role of motor area – Activation of peripheral speech apparatus

By receiving the pattern of activities from Broca area, motor area activates the peripheral speech apparatus. It results in initiation of movements of tongue, lips and larynx required for speech.

Later, when the child is taught to read, auditory speech is associated with visual symbols (area 18). Then, there is an association of the auditory and visual areas with the motor area for the muscles of hand. Now, the child is able to express auditory and visual impressions in the form of written words.

■ NERVOUS CONTROL OF SPEECH

Speech is an integrated and a well-coordinated motor phenomenon. So, many parts of cortical and subcortical areas are involved in the mechanism of speech.

Subcortical areas concerned with speech are controlled by cortical areas of dominant hemisphere. In about 95% of human beings, the left cerebral hemisphere is functionally dominant and those persons are right handed. Following are the motor and sensory cortical areas concerned with speech.

A. *Motor Areas*

1. *Broca area*

Broca area is also called **speech center,** motor speech area or lower frontal area. It includes areas 44 and 45. These areas are situated in lower part of lateral surface of prefrontal cortex.

Broca area controls the movements of structures (tongue, lips and larynx) involved in vocalization.

2. *Upper frontal motor area*

Upper frontal motor area is situated in paracentral gyrus over the medial surface of cerebral hemisphere. It controls the coordinated movements involved in writing.

B. *Sensory Areas*

1. *Secondary auditory area*

Secondary auditory area or auditopsychic area includes area 22. It is situated in the superior temporal gyrus. It is concerned with the **interpretation of auditory sensation** and storage of memories of spoken words.

2. *Secondary visual area*

Secondary visual area or **visuopsychic area** includes area 18. It is present in angular gyrus of the parietal cortex. This area is concerned with the **interpretation of visual sensation** and storage of memories of the visual symbols.

C. *Wernicke Area*

Wernicke area is situated in the upper part of temporal lobe. This area is responsible for the **interpretation of auditory sensation.** It also plays an important role in speech. It is responsible for understanding the auditory information about any word and sending the information to Broca area (Table 162.3).

■ APPLIED PHYSIOLOGY – DISORDERS OF SPEECH

Speech disorder is a communication disorder characterized by disrupted speech. It is of four types:

   I. Aphasia
  II. Anarthria or dysarthria
 III. Dysphonia
 IV. Stammering.

■ APHASIA

Aphasia is defined as the loss or impairment of speech due to brain damage (in Greek, aphasia = without speech). It is an acquired disorder and it is distinct from developmental disorders of speech or other speech disorders like dysarthria. Aphasia is not due to paralysis of muscles of articulation. It is due to damage of speech centers.

Damage of speech centers impairs the expression and understanding of spoken words. It also affects reading and writing. Speech function is localized to left hemisphere in most of the people.

Aphasia may be associated with other speech disorders, which also occur due to brain damage.

Causes for Aphasia

Usually aphasia occurs due to damage of one or more speech centers, which are situated in cerebral cortex (Table 162.4). Damage of speech centers occurs due to:

  1. Stroke
  2. Head injury
  3. Severe blow to head
  4. Cerebral tumors
  5. Brain infections
  6. Degenerative diseases.

TABLE 162.3: Role of cortical areas in control of speech

Cortical areas		Function
Motor areas	Broca area: Areas 44 and 45	Controls movement of structures involved in speech
	Upper frontal motor area	Controls movements involved in writing
Sensory areas	Secondary auditory area: Area 22	Concerned with interpretation of auditory sensation Concerned with storage of memories of spoken words
	Secondary visual area: Area 18	Concerned with interpretation of visual sensation Concerned with storage of memories of visual symbols
Wernicke area		Concerned with interpretation of auditory sensation Concerned with understanding auditory information and sending it to Broca area

TABLE 162.4: Features and causes of different types of aphasia

Type of aphasia	Features	Cause
Broca aphasia	Non-fluent speech problem	Lesion in left frontal lobe
Wernicke aphasia	Speech without any meaning	Lesion in left temporal lobe
Global aphasia	Combined features of Broca aphasia and Wernicke aphasia	Widespread lesion in speech areas of left cerebral hemisphere
Nominal aphasia	Inability to name the familiar objects	Lesion in posterior temporal and inferior parietal gyri
Motor aphasia	Difficulty in uttering individual words	Defect in pathway between left speech center and precentral cortex
Auditory aphasia	Inability to understand spoken words	Lesion in secondary auditory area
Visual aphasia	Inability to understand written symbols	Lesion in secondary visual area
Agraphia	Inability to write	Defect in pathway between cortical areas concerned with writing

Usually, in conditions like head injury, aphasia occurs suddenly and in conditions like infections or cerebral tumors, it develops slowly. In children, traumatic aphasia can develop by exposure to a horrifying event, without any brain damage. It may be cured with psychological treatment.

Types of Aphasia

Aphasia is classified by different methods. The simple and convenient clinical classification divides aphasia into five types:
1. Broca aphasia
2. Wernicke aphasia
3. Global aphasia
4. Nominal aphasia
5. Other types of aphasia.

1. Broca aphasia

Broca aphasia is the **non-fluent speech problem.** It occurs due to lesion in left frontal lobe of cerebral cortex. It is also known as expressive aphasia or anter-ior aphasia. The affected persons do not complete the sentences because of their inability to construct the sentences. They often talk in short phrases by omitting small words such as 'and', 'is', 'for', etc. They make great efforts even to initiate speech.

Persons with Broca aphasia are able to understand spoken or written words. Often, they are affected by weakness or paralysis of right arm or leg. It is due to damage of frontal lobe, which is also responsible for motor activities.

2. Wernicke aphasia

Wernicke aphasia is the speech without any meaning. It is also called receptive aphasia or posterior aphasia. Wernicke aphasia occurs due lesion in left temporal lobe. It is characterized by fluent speech. The affected persons speak long sentences but without any meaning. They use incorrect or non-existent words and cannot speak sensibly. This type of speech is known as jargon speech.

These individuals are unable to understand others' speech. Because of this weakness, they are unaware of their own mistakes while speaking. Often, they are mistaken as psychiatric patients.

Wernicke aphasia is not associated with paralysis or weakness of muscles because, the injury does not involve the centers concerned with movements.

3. Global aphasia

Global aphasia is the type of aphasia characterized by combined features of Broca aphasia and Wernicke aphasia. It is due to widespread lesion in speech areas caused by infarction of left cerebral hemisphere. It is the most common type of aphasia. The affected persons can neither speak nor understand the spoken words. They cannot read and write also. So they have severe communication problems.

4. Nominal aphasia

Nominal aphasia is the speech disorder characterized by inability in naming the familiar objects. It is also called **anomic aphasia** or **amnesic aphasia.** It is due to lesion in posterior temporal and inferior parietal gyri.

5. Other types of aphasia

i. *Motor aphasia:* It is the speech disorder caused by the defect in the pathway between left speech areas and excitomotor or precentral cortex (Chapter 152). It is also known as **verbal aphasia** or **dyspraxia** or **apraxia of speech.** It is characterized by difficulty in uttering individual words due to lack of coordination between central speech apparatus (higher cortical centers) and peripheral speech apparatus. The affected persons are able to decide what to talk. But they cannot pronounce all the words. They are able to pronounce only few monosyllables such as 'yes' or 'no'.

ii. *Sensory aphasia:* It is the inability to understand words or symbols. It is of two types:

a. *Auditory aphasia:* Inability to understand the spoken words. It is also called **word deafness.** It is due to the lesion in secondary auditory area.

b. *Visual aphasia:* Inability to understand written symbols (difficulty in reading). It is also called **word blindness** or **dyslexia** and it occurs due to the lesion in secondary visual area.

iii. *Agraphia:* Agraphia means inability to write. There is no defect in the muscles of the hand concerned with writing. The subject can read and speak. Agraphia is due to the defect in the connection between the cortical areas concerned with writing. Agraphia differs from dysgraphia, which is characterized by distorted writing or writing incorrect letters.

Head's Classification of Aphasia

Henry Head was the pioneer scientist in the field of speech disorders and he was the first one to classify aphasia. In 1926, he classified aphasia into four types. Head's classification of aphasia is given in Table 162.5.

■ DYSARTHRIA OR ANARTHRIA

The term dysarthria refers to disturbed articulation. Anarthria means inability to speak. Dysarthria or anarthria is defined as the difficulty or inability to speak because of paralysis or ataxia of muscles involved in articulation. Psychic aspect of speech is not affected. The spoken and written words are understood.

Causes of Dysarthria

Dysarthria is caused by damage of brain or the nerves that control the muscles involved in speech. It occurs in conditions like stroke, brain injury, degenerative disease like Parkinson disease and Huntington disease.

■ DYSPHONIA

Dysphonia is a voice disorder. Often, it is characterized by hoarseness and a sore or a dry throat. Hoarseness means the difficulty in producing sound while trying to speak or a change in the pitch or loudness of voice. The voice may be weak, breathy, scratchy or husky.

Causes of Dysphonia

1. Trauma of vocal cords
2. Paralysis of vocal cords
3. Lumps (nodules) on vocal cords
4. Inflammation of larynx
5. Hypothyroidism
6. Stress (psychological dysphonia).

TABLE 162.5: Head's classification of aphasia

Type of aphasia	Features
Verbal aphasia	Inability in formation of words
Syntactical aphasia	Inability to arrange words in proper sequence
Semantic aphasia	Inability to recognize the significance of words
Nominal aphasia	Inability to name the familiar objects

■ STAMMERING

Stammering or **shuttering** is a speech disorder characterized by hesitations and involuntary repetitions of certain syllables or words. It is also described as a speech disorder in which normal flow of speech is disturbed by repetitions, prolongations or abnormal block or stoppage of sound and syllables. It is due to the neurological incoordination of speech and it is common in children.

Stammering is associated with some unusual facial and body movements. Exact cause for stammering is not known. It is thought that stammering may be due to genetic factors, brain damage, neurological disorders or anxiety.

Cerebrospinal Fluid (CSF)

Chapter 163

■ INTRODUCTION

Cerebrospinal fluid (CSF) is the clear, colorless and transparent fluid that circulates through **ventricles** of brain, **subarachnoid space** and **central canal** of spinal cord. It is a part of extracellular fluid (ECF).

■ PROPERTIES AND COMPOSITION OF CEREBROSPINAL FLUID

Properties

Volume	:	150 mL (100 mL to 200 mL)
Rate of formation	:	0.3 mL per minute
Specific gravity	:	1.005
Reaction	:	Alkaline.

Composition

Composition of CSF is given in Figure 163.1. Since CSF is a part of ECF, it contains more amount of sodium than potassium. CSF also contains some lymphocytes. CSF secreted by ventricle does not contain any cell. Lymphocytes are added when CSF flows in the spinal cord.

■ FORMATION OF CEREBROSPINAL FLUID

■ SITE OF FORMATION

CSF is formed by **choroid plexuses,** situated within the ventricles. Choroid plexuses are tuft of capillary projections present inside the ventricles and are covered by pia mater and ependymal covering. A large amount of CSF is formed in the lateral ventricles.

■ MECHANISM OF FORMATION

CSF is formed by the process of **secretion** that involves **active transport mechanism.** Formation of CSF does not involve ultrafiltration or dialysis.

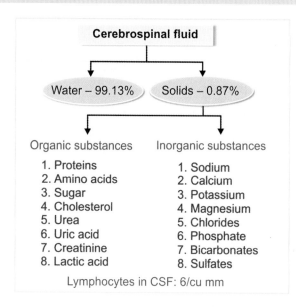

FIGURE 163.1: Composition of cerebrospinal fluid

■ SUBSTANCES AFFECTING THE FORMATION OF CSF

1. Pilocarpine, ether and extracts of pituitary gland stimulate the secretion of CSF by stimulating choroid plexus
2. Injection of isotonic saline also stimulates CSF formation
3. Injection of hypotonic saline causes greater rise in capillary pressure and intracranial pressure and fall in osmotic pressure, leading to increase in CSF formation
4. Hypertonic saline decreases CSF formation and decreases the CSF pressure. The increased intracranial pressure is reduced by injection of 30% to 35% of sodium chloride or 50% sucrose.

■ CIRCULATION OF CEREBROSPINAL FLUID

Major quantity of CSF is formed in **lateral ventricles** and enters third ventricle by passing through **foramen of Monro** (Figs. 163.2 and 163.3). From here, it passes to **fourth ventricle** through **aqueductus Sylvius.** From fourth ventricle, CSF enters the **cisterna magna** and **cisterna lateralis** through **foramen of Magendie** (central opening) and **foramen of Luschka** (lateral opening).

From cisterna magna and cisterna lateralis, CSF circulates through **subarachnoid space** over spinal cord and cerebral hemispheres. It also flows into **central canal** of spinal cord.

■ ABSORPTION OF CEREBROSPINAL FLUID

CSF is mostly absorbed by the **arachnoid villi** into **dural sinuses** and **spinal veins.** Small amount is absorbed along the **perineural spaces** into **cervical lymphatics** and into the **perivascular spaces.**

The mechanism of absorption is by filtration due to pressure gradient between hydrostatic pressure in the subarachnoid space fluid and the pressure that exists in the dural sinus blood. Colloidal substances pass slowly and crystalloids are absorbed rapidly.

Normally, about 500 mL of CSF is formed everyday and an equal amount is absorbed.

■ PRESSURE EXERTED BY CEREBROSPINAL FLUID

Pressure exerted by CSF in man varies in different position, viz.

Lateral recumbent position	: 10 to 18 cm of H_2O
Lying position	: 13 cm of H_2O
Sitting position	: 30 cm of H_2O

Certain events like coughing and crying increase the pressure by decreasing absorption. Compression of internal jugular vein also raises the CSF pressure.

■ FUNCTIONS OF CEREBROSPINAL FLUID

1. Protective Function

CSF acts as fluid buffer and protects the brain from shock. Since, the specific gravity of brain and CSF is more or less same, brain floats in CSF. When head receives a blow, CSF acts like a cushion and prevents the movement of brain against the skull bone and thereby, prevents the damage of brain.

However, if the head receives a severe blow, the brain moves forcefully and hits against the skull bone, leading to the damage of brain tissues. Brain strikes against the skull bone at a point opposite to the point where the blow was applied. So, this type of damage to the brain is known as **countercoup injury.**

2. Regulation of Cranial Content Volume

Regulation of cranial content volume is essential because, brain may be affected if the volume of cranial content increases. It happens in cerebral hemorrhage and brain tumors.

Increase in cranial content volume is prevented by greater absorption of CSF to give space for the increasing cranial contents.

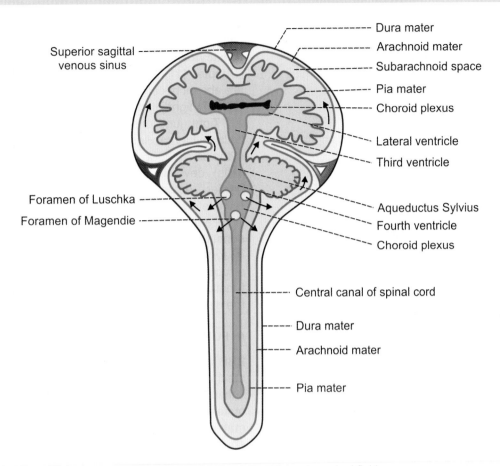

FIGURE 163.2: Circulation of cerebrospinal fluid

3. *Medium of Exchange*

CSF is the medium through which many substances, particularly nutritive substances and waste materials are exchanged between blood and brain tissues.

■ COLLECTION OF CEREBROSPINAL FLUID

CSF is collected either by **cisternal puncture** or **lumbar puncture.** In cisternal puncture, the CSF is collected by passing a needle between the occipital bone and atlas, so that it enters cisterna magna. In lumbar puncture, the lumbar puncture needle is introduced into subarachnoid space in lumbar region, between the third and fourth lumbar spines.

■ LUMBAR PUNCTURE

Posture of Body for Lumbar Puncture

The reclining body is bent forward, so as to flex the vertebral column as far as possible. Then the body is brought near edge of a table. The highest point of iliac crest is determined by palpation. A line is drawn on the back of the subject by joining the highest points of **iliac crests** of both sides. Opposite to midplane, this line crosses the fourth lumbar spine.

After determining the area of fourth lumbar spine, third lumbar spine is palpated. The needle is introduced into subarachnoid space by passing through soft tissue space between the two spines.

Reasons for selecting this site

1. Spinal cord will not be injured, because, it terminates below the lower border of the first lumbar vertebra. Cauda equina may be damaged. But it is regenerated.
2. Subarachnoid space is wider in this site. It is because the pia mater is reduced very much.

Uses of Lumbar Puncture

Lumbar puncture is used for:
1. Collecting CSF for diagnostic purposes
2. Injecting drugs (intrathecal injection) for spinal anesthesia, analgesia and chemotherapy
3. Measuring the pressure exerted by CSF.

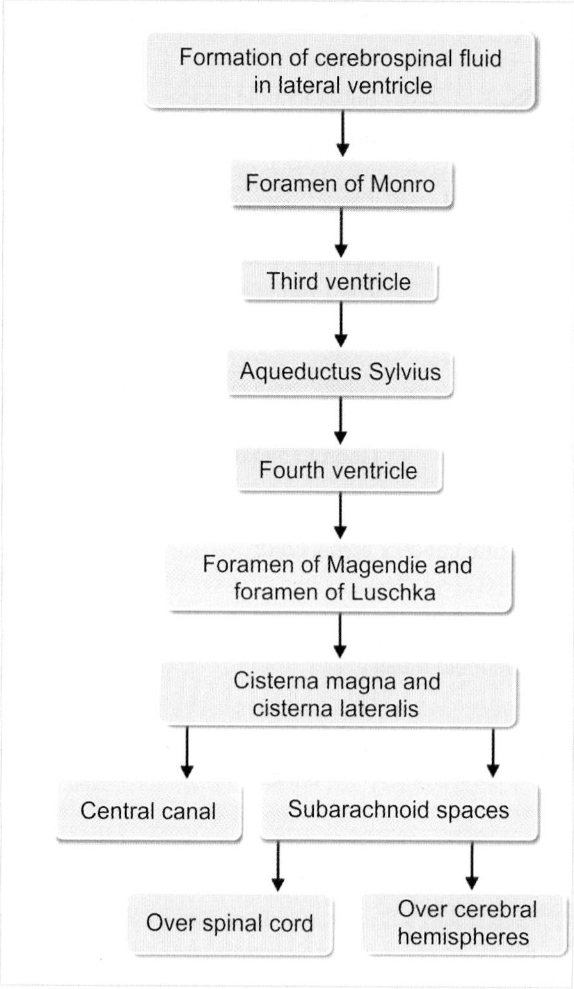

Formation of cerebrospinal fluid in lateral ventricle
Foramen of Monro
Third ventricle
Aqueductus Sylvius
Fourth ventricle
Foramen of Magendie and foramen of Luschka
Cisterna magna and cisterna lateralis
Central canal
Subarachnoid spaces
Over spinal cord
Over cerebral hemispheres

FIGURE 163.3: Cerebrospinal fluid circulation

■ BLOOD-BRAIN BARRIER

Blood-brain barrier (BBB) is a neuroprotective structure that prevents the entry of many substances and pathogens into the brain tissues from blood.

It was observed more than 50 years ago, that when **trypan blue,** the acidic dye was injected into living animals, all the tissues of body were stained by it, except the brain and spinal cord. This observation suggested that there was a hypothetical barrier, which prevented the diffusion of trypan blue into the brain tissues from the capillaries. This barrier was named as blood-brain barrier (BBB). It exists in the capillary membrane of all parts of the brain, except in some areas of hypothalamus.

■ STRUCTURE OF BLOOD-BRAIN BARRIER

Tight junctions in the endothelial cells of brain capillaries are responsible for BBB mechanism.

In capillaries of other organs, adjacent endothelial cells leave the cleft called **fenestra,** which allows **transcytosis** of several substances through endothelium (Chapter 111). However, in capillaries of brain, fenestra are absent because, the endothelial cells fuse with each other by tight junctions (Fig. 163.4).

Tight junctions are formed between endothelial cells of the capillaries at childhood. At the same time, cytoplasmic foot processes of astrocytes (neuroglial cells) develop around capillaries and reinforce the barrier. Astocytes envelop the vasculature almost completely.

Pericytes also form the important cellular constituent of BBB. These cells play an important role in formation and maintenance of tight junction and structural stability of the barrier. In brain, pericytes function as macrophages and play an important role in the defense.

■ FUNCTIONS OF BLOOD-BRAIN BARRIER

BBB acts as both a mechanical barrier and transport mechanisms. It prevents potentially harmful chemical substances and permits metabolic and essential materials into the brain tissues. By preventing injurious materials and organisms, BBB provides healthy environment for the nerve cells of brain.

Substances which can Pass through Blood-Brain Barrier

1. Oxygen
2. Carbon dioxide
3. Water
4. Glucose
5. Amino acids
6. Electrolytes
7. Drugs such as L-dopa, 5-hydroxytryptamine sulfonamides, tetracycline and many lipid-soluble drugs
8. Lipid-soluble anesthetic gases such as ether and nitrous oxide
9. Other lipid-soluble substances.

Substances which cannot Pass through Blood-Brain Barrier

1. Injurious chemical agents
2. Pathogens such as bacteria
3. Drugs such as Penicillin and the catecholamines. Dopamine also cannot pass through BBB. So, parkinsonism is treated with L-dopa, instead of dopamine.

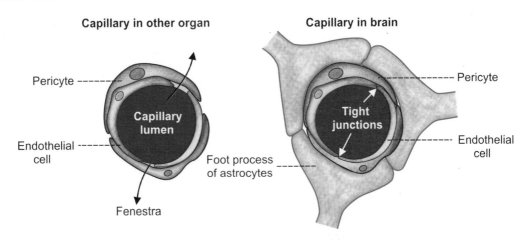

FIGURE 163.4: Blood-brain barrier

4. Bile pigments: However, since the barrier is not well developed in infants, the bile pigments enter the brain tissues. During **jaundice** in infants, the bile pigments enter brain and causes damage of **basal ganglia,** leading to **kernicterus** (refer Chapter 21 for details).

■ BLOOD-CEREBROSPINAL FLUID BARRIER

Blood-CSF barrier is the barrier between blood and cerebrospinal fluid that exists at the choroid plexus. The function of this barrier is similar to that of BBB. It does not allow the movement of many substances from blood to cerebrospinal fluid. It allows the movement of only those substances which are allowed by BBB.

■ APPLIED PHYSIOLOGY – HYDROCEPHALUS

Abnormal accumulation of CSF in the skull, associated with enlargement of head is called hydrocephalus. During obstruction of any foramen, through which CSF escapes, the ventricular cavity dilates and this condition is called **internal hydrocephalus.** It is also known as **non-communicating** hydrocephalus.

On the other hand, if the arachnoid villi are blocked, **external** or **communicating hydrocephalus** occurs.

Hydrocephalus along with increased intracranial pressure causes headache and vomiting. In severe conditions, it leads to atrophy of brain, mental weakness and convulsions.

Autonomic Nervous System (ANS)

- ■ INTRODUCTION
- ■ SYMPATHETIC DIVISION
- ■ PARASYMPATHETIC DIVISION
- ■ FUNCTIONS
- ■ NEUROTRANSMITTERS
- ■ SYMPATHOMIMETIC DRUGS
- ■ SYMPATHETIC BLOCKERS
- ■ PARASYMPATHOMIMETIC DRUGS
- ■ PARASYMPATHETIC BLOCKERS
- ■ GANGLIONIC BLOCKERS

■ INTRODUCTION

Autonomic nervous system (ANS) is primarily concerned with regulation of visceral or vegetative functions of the body. So, it is also called **vegetative** or **involuntary nervous system.**

■ DIVISIONS OF ANS

From anatomical and physiological point of view, ANS is divided into two divisions:

1. Sympathetic division
2. Parasympathetic division.

   Differences and comparison between both the divisions of ANS are given in Tables 164.1 and 164.2.

■ SYMPATHETIC DIVISION

Sympathetic division is otherwise called **thoracolumbar outflow** because, the preganglionic neurons are situated in lateral gray horns of 12 thoracic and first two lumbar segments of spinal cord. Fibers arising from here are known as preganglionic fibers. Preganglionic fibers leave the spinal cord through anterior nerve root and white rami communicantes and terminate in the postganglionic neurons, which are situated in the sympathetic ganglia.

Sympathetic division supplies smooth muscle fibers of all the visceral organs such as blood vessels, heart, lungs, glands, gastrointestinal organs, etc.

■ SYMPATHETIC GANGLIA

Ganglia of sympathetic division are classified into three groups:

- A. Paravertebral or sympathetic chain ganglia
- B. Prevertebral or collateral ganglia
- C. Terminal or peripheral ganglia.

A. *Paravertebral or Sympathetic Chain Ganglia*

Paravertebral or sympathetic chain ganglia are arranged in a segmental fashion along the anterolateral surface of vertebral column. Ganglia on either side of the spinal cord are connected with each other by longitudinal fibers, to form the **sympathetic chains** (Fig. 164.1). Both the chains extend from skull to coccyx.

Ganglia of the sympathetic chain (trunk) on each side are divided into four groups:

1. Cervical ganglia : 8 in number
2. Thoracic ganglia : 12 in number
3. Lumbar ganglia : 5 in number
4. Sacral ganglia : 5 in number.

TABLE 164.1: Actions of sympathetic and parasympathetic divisions of autonomic nervous system

Effector organ		Sympathetic division	Parasympathetic division
1. Eye	Ciliary muscle	Relaxation	Contraction
	Pupil	Dilatation	Constriction
2. Lacrimal glands		Decrease in secretion	Increase in secretion
3. Salivary glands		Decrease in secretion and vasoconstriction	Increase in secretion and vasodilatation
4. Gastrointestinal tract	Motility	Inhibition	Acceleration
	Secretion	Decrease	Increase
	Sphincters	Constriction	Relaxation
	Smooth muscles	Relaxation	Contraction
5. Gallbladder		Relaxation	Contraction
6. Urinary bladder	Detrusor muscle	Relaxation	Contraction
	Internal sphincter	Constriction	Relaxation
7. Sweat glands		Increase in secretion	–
8. Heart – rate and force		Increase	Decrease
9. Blood vessels		Constriction of all blood vessels, except those in heart and skeletal muscle	Dilatation
10. Bronchioles		Dilatation	Constriction

1. *Cervical ganglia*

Eight cervical ganglia are arranged in three groups:

  i. *Superior cervical ganglion:* It is formed by the fusion of upper four cervical ganglia. It is the largest ganglion of ANS. It receives preganglionic fibers from first thoracic spinal segment (T1) via white rami. Postganglionic fibers from this ganglion, supply the blood vessels, glands, etc. Superior cervical ganglion also sends some fibers to heart through superior cervical sympathetic nerve and cardiac plexus.

  ii. *Middle cervical ganglion:* It is formed by fifth and sixth cervical ganglia. Preganglionic fibers arise from T1 segment. Postganglionic fibers from here supply the sweat glands, thyroid gland and parathyroid glands. It also sends fibers to heart via middle cervical sympathetic nerve and cardiac plexus.

  iii. *Inferior cervical ganglion:* This ganglion is formed by the fusion of seventh and eighth cervical ganglia. First thoracic ganglion fuses with inferior cervical ganglion, forming stellate ganglion. It receives preganglionic fibers from T1 segment. It sends postganglionic fibers to heart through inferior cervical sympathetic nerve and cardiac plexus. Postganglionic fibers also form the plexus around subclavian artery and its branches.

2. *Thoracic ganglia*

There are 12 thoracic ganglia on each side and these ganglia are evenly spaced. Thoracic ganglia receive preganglionic fibers from the thoracic segments of spinal cord. Postganglionic fibers from thoracic ganglia are distributed to **visceral organs** in the **thorax** and **abdomen.**

3. *Lumbar ganglia*

There are 5 lumbar ganglia. Preganglionic fibers for these ganglia arise from first and second lumbar spinal segments (L1 and L2) and reach the lumbar ganglia. From here, the fibers extend down to sacral ganglia also. Postganglionic fibers from these ganglia supply the abdominal and **pelvic organs.**

4. *Sacral ganglia*

There are 5 sacral ganglia, which receive the preganglionic fibers from L1 and L2 segments. Postganglionic fibers from sacral ganglia innervate the **blood vessels** and **sweat glands** in the lower limb.

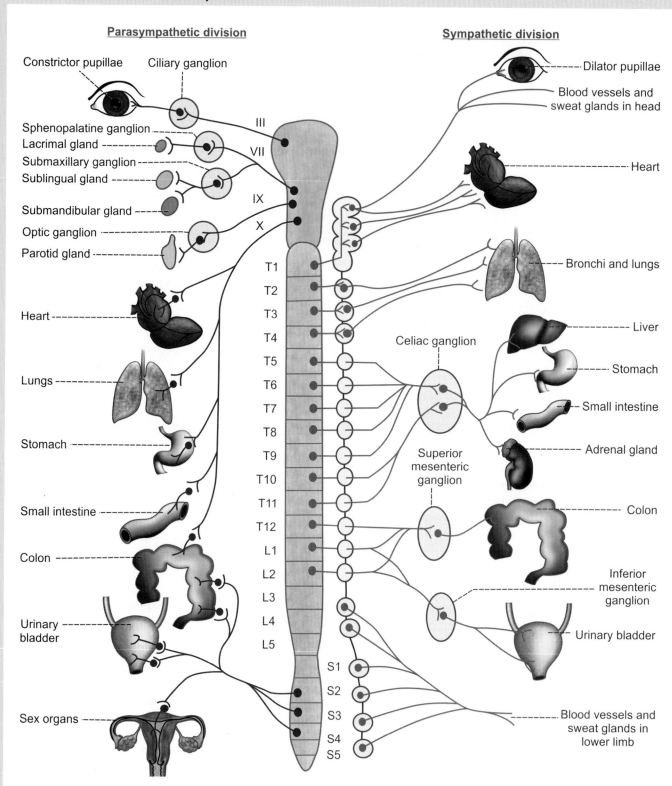

FIGURE 164.1: Autonomic nervous system

TABLE 164.2: Classical comparison of sympathetic and parasympathetic divisions of autonomic nervous system

Features	Sympathetic division	Parasympathetic division
1. Location of preganglionic neuron	Thoracolumbar segments of spinal cord	Nuclei of III, VII, IX and X cranial nerves and sacral (S2 to S4) segments of spinal cord
2. Location of postganglionic neuron	Away from target organ	Near or in the target organ
3. Length of preganglionic fibers	Relatively short	Relatively long
4. Length of postganglionic fibers	Relatively long	Relatively short
5. Preganglionic neurotransmitter	Acetylcholine	Acetylcholine
6. Postganglionic neurotransmitter	Noradrenaline	Acetylcholine

Below the sacral level, both the sympathetic trunks converge and fuse upon the anterior surface of coccyx and form a terminal swelling. This terminal swelling is known as **coccygeal ganglion.** Unpaired coccygeal ganglion is also called **ganglion impar.** It receives preganglionic fibers from L1 and L2 segments. Postganglionic fibers from here are distributed to the abdominal viscera and pelvic region.

B. *Prevertebral or Collateral Ganglia*

Prevertebral ganglia are situated in thorax, abdomen and pelvis, in relation to aorta and its branches.

Prevertebral ganglia are:
1. Celiac ganglion
2. Superior mesenteric ganglion
3. Inferior mesenteric ganglion.

Prevertebral ganglia receive preganglionic fibers from T5 to L2 segments. Postganglionic fibers from these ganglia supply the visceral organs of thorax, abdomen and pelvis.

C. *Terminal or Peripheral Ganglia*

Terminal ganglia are situated within or close to structures innervated by them. Heart, bronchi, pancreas and urinary bladder are innervated by the terminal ganglia.

Sympathoadrenergic System

Sympathoadrenergic system is a functional and phylogenetic unit that includes sympathetic division and adrenal medulla. Adrenal medulla is a modified sympathetic ganglion. Since adrenal medulla and sympathetic division develop from the same neural crest, their secretions and functions are almost the same. Any increase in sympathetic activity increases the secretion of catecholamines from adrenal medulla (refer Chapter 71).

■ PARASYMPATHETIC DIVISION

Parasympathetic division of ANS is otherwise called the **craniosacral outflow** because, the fibers of this division arise from brain and sacral segments of spinal cord.

■ CRANIAL OUTFLOW OR CRANIAL PORTION OF PARASYMPATHETIC DIVISION

Cranial outflow or cranial portion of parasympathetic division arises from brainstem. It innervates the blood vessels of head and neck and many thoracoabdominal visceral organs. Cranial outflow includes the following cranial nerves:
1. Oculomotor (III) nerve
2. Facial (VII) nerve
3. Glossopharyngeal (IX) nerve
4. Vagus (X) nerve.

Preganglionic fibers of these cranial nerves arise from neurons situated at two different levels:
1. Tectal or midbrain outflow (III cranial nerve)
2. Bulbar level or bulbar outflow (VII, IX and X cranial nerves).

Preganglionic fibers are longer and reach the postganglionic neurons, which are situated within the organs or close to the organs innervated by these nerves. Preganglionic fibers are myelinated, but the postganglionic fibers are non-myelinated.

1. *Tectal or Midbrain Outflow*

Group of cells forming **Edinger-Westphal nucleus** of III cranial nerve gives rise to tectal fibers. Fibers from this nucleus end in ciliary ganglion. Postganglionic fibers from here supply the sphincter pupillae and ciliary muscle.

2. *Bulbar Level or Bulbar Outflow*

Preganglionic fibers are the fibers of VII, IX and X cranial nerves, which arise from the nuclei present in the medulla oblongata.

Fibers of VII cranial nerve supply the lacrimal, nasal, submaxillary and sublingual glands. Preganglionic fibers of this nerve end in sphenopalatine ganglion and submaxillary ganglion. Postganglionic fibers from sphenopalatine ganglion supply lacrimal and nasal glands. Postganglionic fibers from submaxillary ganglion supply sublingual and submaxillary glands.

Fibers of IX cranial nerve supply the parotid gland. Preganglionic fibers synapse with neurons of otic ganglion. Postganglionic fibers from otic ganglion supply the parotid gland.

Fibers of X cranial nerve supply visceral organs of the body. Preganglionic fibers terminate in the ganglia, which are situated on or near the organs. Postganglionic fibers from the ganglia supply the organs. Vagus nerve supplies almost all the organs in the thorax and abdomen, but not the pelvic organs.

■ SACRAL OUTFLOW OR SACRAL PORTION OF PARASYMPATHETIC DIVISION

Sacral outflow or sacral portion of parasympathetic division arises from the sacral segments of spinal cord. It innervates smooth muscles forming the walls of viscera and the glands such as large intestine, liver, spleen, kidneys, bladder, genitalia, etc.

Preganglionic fibers arise from anterior gray horn cells of 2nd, 3rd and 4th (from 1st also in some cases) sacral segments of spinal cord and form the pelvic nerve (nervi erigens). Fibers end on postganglionic neurons, which are situated on or near the visceral organs. Fibers from postganglionic neurons supply descending colon, rectum, urinary bladder, internal sphincter, urethra and accessory sex organs.

Sacral parasympathetic fibers supply those visceral organs which are not supplied by vagus.

■ FUNCTIONS OF ANS

Autonomic nervous system is concerned with the regulation of functions, which are beyond voluntary control. By controlling the various vegetative functions, ANS plays an important role in maintaining constant internal environment (homeostasis).

Almost all the visceral organs are supplied by both sympathetic and parasympathetic divisions of ANS and the two divisions produce antagonistic effects on each organ. When the fibers of one division supplying to an organ is sectioned or affected by lesion, the effects of fibers from other division on the organ become more prominent.

Actions of the sympathetic and parasympathetic fibers on various structures are given in Table 164.1.

■ NEUROTRANSMITTERS OF ANS

Different nerve fibers of ANS execute the functions by releasing some neurotransmitter substances (Table 164.2).

■ SYMPATHETIC FIBERS

1. *Preganglionic fibers:* Acetylcholine (Ach)
2. *Postganglionic noradrenergic fibers:* Noradrenaline
3. *Postganglionic cholinergic fibers:* Ach

Postganglionic sympathetic cholinergic nerve fibers supply sweat glands and blood vessels in heart and in skeletal muscle.

■ PARASYMPATHETIC FIBERS

1. Preganglionic fibers: Ach
2. Postganglionic fibers: Ach

Catecholamines

Synthesis and the metabolism of catecholamines are explained in Chapter 71.

Acetylcholine

Refer Chapter 141 for details of acetylcholine.

Receptors of Neurotransmitter

Adrenergic receptors: Details are given in Chapter 71.
Acetylcholine receptors: Details are given in Chapter 141.

■ SYMPATHOMIMETIC DRUGS

Sympathomimetic drugs or **adrenaline-like** drugs are the drugs, which produce the effects of sympathetic stimulation. Adrenaline and noradrenaline produced in the body act only for a short duration of about 1 to 2 minutes. Whereas, sympathomimetic drugs injected intravenously act for a longer period of about 30 minutes to 2 hours. Sympathomimetic drugs are:

Drugs Stimulating the Receptors Directly

1. Phenylephrine (alpha receptors)
2. Isoproterenol (beta receptors)
3. Albuterol (beta-2 receptors).

Drugs Inducing the Release of Noradrenaline

1. Ephedrine
2. Tyramine
3. Amphetamine.

■ SYMPATHETIC BLOCKERS

Sympathetic blockers are the drugs that prevent actions of sympathetic neurotransmitter. Sympathetic blockers act on all levels. Actions of blocking agents are given in Table 164.3.

TABLE 164.3: Actions of sympathetic blocking agents

Blocking agent	Action
1. Reserpine	Prevention of synthesis and storage of noradrenaline
2. Quanethidine	Prevention of release of noradrenaline
3. Phenoxybenzamine	Blockage of alpha adrenergic receptors
4. Phentolamine	Blockage of alpha adrenergic receptors
5. Metaprolal	Blockage of beta adrenergic receptors
6. Hexamethonium	Blockage of transmission of nerve impulse through sympathetic ganglia

■ PARASYMPATHOMIMETIC DRUGS

Parasympathomimetic drugs or Ach-like drugs are drugs, which produce the effects of parasympathetic stimulation. Ach produced in the body acts only for a short period, whereas the injected Ach acts for a long time. Similarly, parasympathomimetic drugs also exhibit their actions for a longer time. Parasympathomimetic drugs are:

1. *Drugs which Act on Muscarinic Receptors*

Pilocarpine and **methacholine** produce their effects by acting on the **muscarinic receptors.**

2. *Drugs which Prolong the Action of Ach*

Action of Ach can be prolonged by preventing its destruction. Drugs like **neostigmine** and **physostigmine** inhibit the activity of acetylcholinesterase and so the Ach is not destroyed quickly.

■ PARASYMPATHETIC BLOCKERS

Parasympathetic blockers are drugs, which prevent the actions of parasympathetic neurotransmitter. The drugs atropine, homatropine and scopolamine inhibit the actions of Ach by blocking the muscarinic receptors.

■ GANGLIONIC BLOCKERS

Ganglionic blockers are the drugs that prevent the transmission of impulses from preganglionic neurons to postganglionic neurons. Tetraethyl ammonium ion, hexamethonium ion and pentolinium are some of the ganglionic blockers. These drugs block both sympathetic and parasympathetic ganglia. However, ganglionic blockers are commonly used to block sympathetic ganglia, rather than the parasympathetic ganglia because sympathetic blockade overshadows the parasympathetic blockade.

QUESTIONS IN NERVOUS SYSTEM

■ LONG QUESTIONS

1. What is neuron? Describe the structure of neuron and the properties of nerve fibers.
2. What are receptors? Classify them and explain their properties.
3. What is synapse? Explain the structure, functions and properties of synapse.
4. Define and classify reflex action. Explain reflex arc and the properties of reflexes.
5. Name the ascending tracts of the spinal cord and explain spinothalamic tracts.
6. What are the tracts of spinal cord? Describe the spinocerebellar tracts.
7. Give an account of tracts in the posterior white funiculus of spinal cord.
8. Enumerate the descending tracts of spinal cord. Describe in detail the pyramidal tracts. Write a note on the effects of upper and lower motor neuron lesions.
9. Write in detail, about the effects of complete and incomplete transection of spinal cord.
10. What are the thalamic nuclei? Describe the connections, functions and effects of lesions of thalamus.
11. Name the hypothalamic nuclei. Explain the connections, functions and effects of lesions of hypothalamus.
12. Explain the different parts of cerebellum? Enumerate the functions of cerebellum. Write a note on cerebellar lesions.
13. Explain the connections, functions and effects of lesions of corticocerebellum (neocerebellum).
14. Explain the connections, functions and effects of lesions of spinocerebellum (paleocerebellum).
15. Explain the connections, functions and effects of lesions of vestibulocerebellum (archicerebellum).
16. What are the components of basal ganglia? Give an account of connections, functions and disorders of basal ganglia.
17. What are the various lobes of cerebral cortex? Describe their functions. Add a note on frontal lobe syndrome.
18. Classify the components of limbic system. Explain the functions of limbic system.
19. What is reticular formation? Describe the connections and the functions of reticular formation.
20. Give an account of postural reflexes.
21. Explain the role of vestibular apparatus in the maintenance of equilibrium.

■ SHORT QUESTIONS

1. Structure of neuron.
2. Myelin sheath.
3. Neurotrophins.
4. Nerve growth factor.
5. Classification of nerve fibers.
6. Properties of nerve fibers.
7. Action potential in nerve fiber.
8. Voltage clamping.
9. Saltatory conduction.
10. Degeneration of nerve fiber.
11. Wallerian degeneration.
12. Regeneration of nerve fiber.
13. Neuroglia.
14. Exteroceptors.
15. Mechanoceptors.
16. Generator (receptor) potential.
17. Sensory transduction.
18. Synapse.
19. Synaptic transmission.
20. Synaptic inhibition/IPSP.
21. Synaptic potentials/EPSP.
22. Neurotransmitters.
23. Neuromodulators.
24. Opioid peptides.
25. Reflex arc.
26. Properties of reflexes.
27. Superficial reflexes.
28. Deep reflexes.
29. Babinski sign.
30. Spinothalamic tracts.
31. Spinocerebellar tracts.
32. Tracts of Goll and Burdach.
33. Pyramidal tracts.
34. Extrapyramidal tracts.
35. Upper motor neuron lesion.
36. Lower motor neuron lesion.
37. Complete transection of spinal cord.
38. Incomplete transection of spinal cord.
39. Brown-Sèquard syndrome/Hemisection of spinal cord.
40. Syringomyelia.
41. Tabes dorsalis.
42. Pathway for fine touch sensations.
43. Pathway for pressure sensation.
44. Pathway for temperature sensations.
45. Pathway for conscious kinesthetic sensations.
46. Pathway for subconscious kinesthetic sensations.
47. Pathway for pain sensations.

48. Pain sensation.
49. Referred pain.
50. Gate theory.
51. Functions of thalamus.
52. Thalamic lesions.
53. Internal capsule.
54. Functions of hypothalamus.
55. Regulation of food intake.
56. Disorders of hypothalamus.
57. Rage and sham rage.
58. Corticocerebellum (neocerebellum).
59. Spinocerebellum (paleocerebellum).
60. Corpus striatum.
61. Red nucleus.
62. Functions of basal ganglia.
63. Effects of lesions of basal ganglia.
64. Parkinson disease.
65. Prefrontal lobe of cerebral cortex.
66. Motor areas of cerebral cortex.
67. Frontal lobe of cerebral cortex.
68. Parietal lobe (or sensory areas) of cerebral cortex.
69. Frontal lobe syndrome.
70. Klüver-Bucy syndrome.
71. Localization of cortical connections.
72. Papez circuit.
73. Functions of limbic system.
74. ARAS.
75. Decerebrate rigidity.
76. Proprioceptors.
77. Muscle spindle.
78. Stretch reflex.
79. Reciprocal innervation.
80. Crossed extensor reflex.
81. Clasp-knife reflex.
82. Righting reflexes.
83. Semicircular canal.
84. Otolith organ.
85. Crista ampullaris.
86. Effects of stimulation of semicircular canals.
87. Nystagmus.
88. Motion sickness.
89. EEG.
90. Epilepsy.
91. EEG pattern during sleep.
92. Physiological changes during sleep.
93. REM and non-REM sleep.
94. Sleep disorders.
95. Learning.
96. Memory.
97. Classical conditioned reflexes.
98. Properties of conditioned reflexes.
99. Speech.
100. Speech disorders.
101. Aphasia.
102. CSF.
103. Blood-brain barrier.
104. Craniosacral outflow.
105. Thoracolumbar outflow.
106. Role of ANS in the regulation of cardiovascular functions.
107. Role of ANS in the regulation of gastrointestinal activity.
108. Neurotransmitters of ANS.
109. Functions of sympathetic division of ANS.
110. Functions of parasympathetic division of ANS.

Section

11

Special Senses

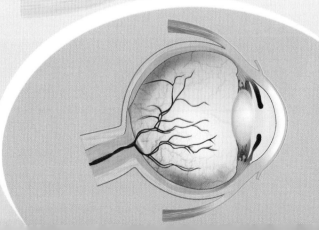

Structure of the Eye

■ SPECIAL SENSES

Special senses or special sensations are the complex sensations which involve specialized sense organs. These sensations are different from somatic sensations that arise from skin, muscles, tendons and joints (Chapter 144).

Special senses are:
1. Sensation of vision
2. Sensation of hearing
3. Sensation of taste
4. Sensation of smell.

■ FUNCTIONAL ANATOMY OF THE EYEBALL

■ MORPHOLOGY

Human eyeball **(bulbus oculi)** is approximately globe shaped, with a diameter of about 24 mm. It is slightly flattened from above downwards. Eyeball is made up of two segments, an anterior part and a posterior part. Anterior part is small and forms one sixth of the eyeball. Posterior part is larger and forms five sixth of the eyeball. Radius of this part is about 8 mm. Posterior wall of this part is lined by the light-sensitive structure called **retina.**

Center of anterior curvature of the eyeball is called **anterior pole** and the center of posterior curvature is called **posterior pole.** Line joining both the poles is called **optic axis.** The line joining a point in cornea, little medial to anterior pole and fovea centralis, situated lateral to posterior pole is known as **visual axis.** Light rays pass through the visual axis of eyeball (Fig. 165.1). Optic nerve leaves the eye, little medial to posterior pole.

■ ORBITAL CAVITY

Except anterior one sixth, the eyeball is situated in a bony cavity known as **orbital cavity** or **eye socket.** A thick layer of areolar tissue is interposed between bone and eyeball. It serves as a cushion to protect the eyeball from external force. Eyeballs are attached to orbital cavity by the **ocular muscles.**

■ EYELIDS

Eyelids protect the eyeball from foreign particles coming in contact with its surface and cutoff the light during sleep. Eyelids are opened and closed voluntarily, as well as by reflex action.

Margins of eyelids have sensitive hair called the **cilia.** Each cilium arises from a follicle, which is surrounded by a sensory nerve plexus. When dust particle comes in contact with cilia, these sensory nerves are activated, resulting in rapid blinking of eyelids. It prevents the dust particles from reaching the eyeball. There are about 100 to 150 cilia in the upper eyelid and about 50 to 75 cilia in the lower eyelid. **Meibomian glands** and some **sebaceous glands** are also found in the eyelids. These glands open into the follicles of cilia. Infection of these glands leads to the development of common **eye sty.**

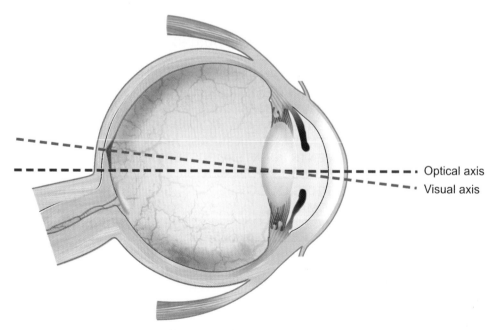

- - Optical axis
- - Visual axis

FIGURE 165.1: Optical and visual axis

Opening between the two eyelids is called **palpebral fissure.** In adults, it is about 25 mm long. Its width is about 12 mm to 15 mm, when opened.

■ CONJUNCTIVA

Conjunctiva is a thin mucus membrane, which covers the exposed part of eye. After covering the anterior surface, conjunctiva is reflected into the inner surfaces of eyelids. Part of conjunctiva covering the eyeball is called **bulbar portion.** Part covering the eyelid is called **palpebral portion.** During closure or opening of eyelids, the opposed portions of conjunctiva slide over each other. Surface of conjunctiva is lubricated by thin film of tear secreted by lacrimal gland.

■ LACRIMAL GLAND AND TEAR

Lacrimal gland is situated in the shelter of bone, forming upper and outer border of wall of the eye socket. From lacrimal gland, **tear** flows over the surface of conjunctiva and drains into nose via **lacrimal ducts, lacrimal sac** and **nasolacrimal duct.** Tear is a hypertonic fluid. Due to its continuous washing and lubrication, the conjunctiva is kept moist and is protected from infection. Tear also contains **lysozyme** that kills bacteria. Secretion of tears is controlled by the parasympathetic fibers of facial (VII cranial) nerve.

■ WALL OF THE EYEBALL

Wall of the eyeball is composed of three layers:
A. Outer layer, which includes cornea and sclera
B. Middle layer, which includes choroid, ciliary body and iris
C. Inner layer, the retina.

■ OUTER LAYER OR TUNICA EXTERNA OR TUNICA FIBROSA

Outer layer preserves the shape of the eyeball. Posterior five sixth of this coat is opaque and it is called the sclera. Anterior one sixth is transparent and is known as cornea.

1. *Sclera*

Sclera is the tough white fibrous outer layer of eyeball, that covers posterior five sixth of the eye. Anteriorly it is continuous with cornea (Fig. 165.2).

Sclera is formed by white fibrous tissues and elastic fibers. Posterior part of sclera, where it is pierced by the optic nerve is thin with perforations. It is named as **lamina cribrosa.**

2. *Cornea*

Cornea is the transparent convex anterior portion of the outer layer of eyeball, which covers the iris and pupil.

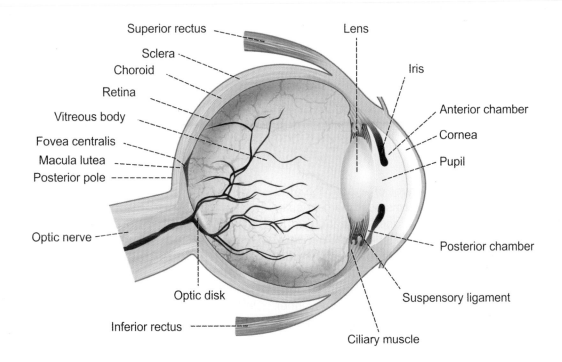

Superior rectus — Sclera — Choroid — Retina — Vitreous body — Fovea centralis — Macula lutea — Posterior pole — Optic nerve — Optic disk — Inferior rectus — Lens — Iris — Anterior chamber — Cornea — Pupil — Posterior chamber — Suspensory ligament — Ciliary muscle

FIGURE 165.2: Structure of eyeball

It forms the anterior one sixth of outer layer and it is continuous with sclera.

Though cornea is transparent, it does not appear transparent. It appears in different colors such as blue, green, brown, grey and black. It is because of the color of iris, which is present just behind the cornea. Sclera overlaps cornea at its periphery and appears in front as white of the eye. Diameter of cornea is about 12 mm horizontally and 11 mm vertically.

Cornea is formed by five layers:
  i. Layer of stratified epithelium
  ii. Bowman membrane or anterior elastic lamina
  iii. Substantia proper
  iv. Descemet layer or posterior elastic lamina
  v. Layer of endothelial cells.

Cornea has a refractory index of 1.376. It is very sensitive to pain, touch, pressure and cold. Center of cornea is more sensitive to pain because of rich supply of free nerve endings. Normally, cornea is not vascularized. Therefore, it derives its nourishment mainly from aqueous humor. However, in some pathological conditions, cornea becomes vascularized.

The transitional part of outer layer between sclera and cornea is called **limbus.** It is about 1 mm width. Blood vessels are seen only at the limbus. These blood vessels form **superficial marginal plexus** in limbus.

■ MIDDLE LAYER OR TUNICA MEDIA OR TUNICA VASCULOSA

Middle layer surrounds the eyeball completely, except for a small opening in front known as pupil.

This layer comprises of three structures:
1. Choroid
2. Ciliary body
3. Iris.

1. *Choroid*

Choroid is the thin vascular layer of eyeball situated between sclera and retina. It forms posterior five sixth of middle layer. Choroid is extended anteriorly up to the insertion of ciliary muscle (the level of **ora serrata**). Choroid is separated from sclera by perichoroidal space. Anteriorly, this space is limited by the insertion of ciliary muscle into sclera. Posteriorly, this space ends at a short distance from the optic nerve. Inner surface of choroid faces the pigment epithelium (innermost layer) of retina.

Choroid is composed of rich capillary plexus, numerous small arteries and veins.

2. *Ciliary Body*

Ciliary body is the thickened anterior part of middle layer of eye, situated between choroid and iris. It is situated in front of ora serrata. It is in the form of a ring. Its outer surface is separated from sclera by **perichoroidal space.** Inner surface of ciliary body faces the vitreous body and lens. **Suspensory ligaments** from the lens are attached to the ciliary body. Anterior surface of ciliary body faces towards the center of cornea. From the surface, the iris arises (Fig. 165.3).

Ciliary body has three parts:
  i. **Orbiculus ciliaris:** It is continuous with choroid and it forms the posterior two third of ciliary body. It is about 4 mm broad.
  ii. **Ciliary body proper:** It is made up of two sets of ciliary muscles, namely outer longitudinal and inner circular muscles. Ciliary muscles are innervated by the parasympathetic fibers of oculomotor nerve.
  iii. **Ciliary processes:** Ciliary processes are the finger-like projections from inner surface of ciliary body. There are about 70 ciliary processes, projecting towards the central axis of eye to form radial fringes called **corona ciliaris.**

3. *Iris*

Iris is a thin colored curtain-like structure of eyeball, located in front of the lens. It forms a thin circular diaphragm with a circular opening in the center called **pupil.**

Iris is formed by muscles:
  i. **Constrictor pupillae** or **iris sphincter** muscle or pupillary constrictor muscle: It is formed by circular muscle fibers. Contraction of this muscle causes constriction of pupil.
  ii. **Dilator pupillae** or **pupillary dilator muscle:** It is formed by radial muscle fibers. Contraction of this muscle causes dilatation of pupil.

Activities of these muscles increase or decrease the diameter of pupil and regulate the amount of light entering the eye. Thus, iris acts like the diaphragm of a camera.

Iris separates the space between cornea and lens into two chambers, namely **anterior** and **posterior chambers.** Both the chambers communicate with each other through pupil. Lateral border of anterior chamber is angular in shape. It is called **iris angle** or **angle of anterior chamber.**

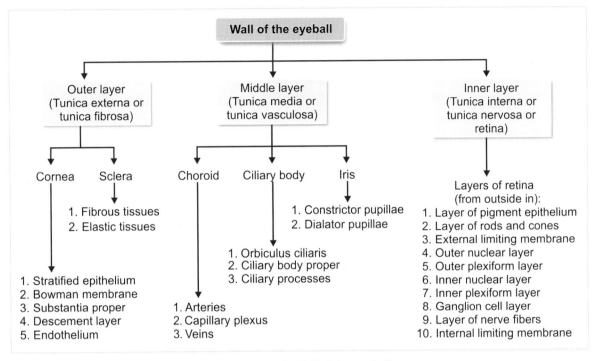

FIGURE 165.3: Wall of the eyeball

■ INNER LAYER OR TUNICA INTERNA OR TUNICA NERVOSA OR RETINA

Retina is a delicate light-sensitive membrane that forms the innermost layer of eyeball. It extends from the margin of **optic disk** to just behind **ciliary body.** Here, it ends abruptly as a dentated border known as ora serrata. Retina has the receptors of vision. Structurally, retina is made up of 10 layers (Fig. 165.4).

Layers of retina from outside in:

1. Layer of pigment epithelium
2. Layer of rods and cones
3. External limiting membrane
4. Outer nuclear layer
5. Outer plexiform layer
6. Inner nuclear layer
7. Inner plexiform layer
8. Ganglion cell layer
9. Layer of nerve fibers
10. Internal limiting membrane.

1. *Layer of Pigment Epithelium*

Layer of pigment epithelium is the outermost layer situated adjacent to choroid. It is a single layer of hexagonal epithelial cells. Outer portion of epithelial cells (towards choroid), contains nucleus and moderate number of round pigment granules. Inner portion has plenty of needle-shaped dark **pigment granules.** Many protoplasmic extensions arise from the inner surface of cells and pass between rods and cones. Cytoplasmic processes also contain dark pigment granules. The pigment present in this layer is a **melanin** called **fuscin.**

Pigment epithelial layer absorbs light and prevents reflection of light rays back from retina. If light rays are reflected back by retina, image becomes blurred. Epithelial cells store **vitamin A** (retinol) and remove the debris from rod cells and cone cells by phagocytic action.

2. *Layer of Rods and Cones*

Layer of rods and cones lies between pigment epithelial layer and external limiting membrane. Rods and cones are the light-sensitive portions of visual receptor cells, namely rod cells and cone cells. Receptor cells are arranged in a parallel fashion and are perpendicular to the inner surface of the eyeball. Structure of rod cell and cone cell is explained in the next chapter.

3. *External Limiting Membrane*

External limiting membrane is a thin layer, formed by the chief supporting elements of retina called the **Müller fibers.**

4. *Outer Nuclear Layer*

Outer nuclear layer is formed by the fibers and granules of rods and cones. **Granules** of rods and cones contain

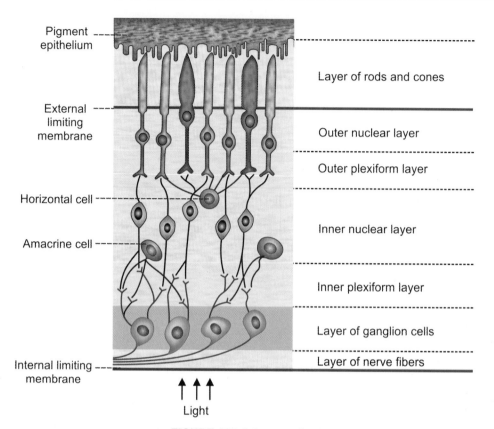

Pigment epithelium

Layer of rods and cones

External limiting membrane

Outer nuclear layer

Outer plexiform layer

Horizontal cell

Inner nuclear layer

Amacrine cell

Inner plexiform layer

Layer of ganglion cells

Layer of nerve fibers

Internal limiting membrane

Light

FIGURE 165.4: Layers of retina

nucleus. Nuclei of rods are smaller and round and the nuclei of cones are larger and oval in shape.

5. Outer Plexiform Layer

Outer plexiform layer contains reticular meshwork, formed by terminal fibers of rods and cones and dendrites from **bipolar cells,** situated in the inner nuclear layer.

6. Inner Nuclear Layer

Inner nuclear layer contains small oval-shaped, flattened **bipolar cells.** Axons of bipolar cells go inside and synapse with dendrites of **ganglionic cells** in the inner plexiform layer. Dendrites synapse with fibers of rods and cones in the **outer plexiform layer.** This layer also contains nuclei of **Müller supporting fibers** and some association neurons called **horizontal cells** and **amacrine** cells.

7. Inner Plexiform Layer

Inner plexiform layer of retina consists of synapses between dendrites of ganglionic cells and axons of bipolar cells. It also contains processes from amacrine cells.

8. Ganglion Cell Layer

Multipolar cells are present in this layer. Some cells are large and are called **giant ganglion cells.** Other cells are smaller called **midget ganglion cells.** Axons from ganglion cells are in the inner surface of the retina. These axons form the optic nerve. Dendrites of ganglion cells synapse with axons of bipolar cells in the inner plexiform layer. Retinal blood vessels are also present in this layer.

9. Layer of Nerve Fibers

Layer of nerve fibers is formed by non-myelinated axons of ganglionic cells. After taking origin, the axons run horizontally to a short distance. Afterwards, the fibers converge towards the **optic disk** and form the **optic nerve.** Neuroglial cells, **Müller cells** and retinal blood vessels are also present in this layer.

10. Internal Limiting Membrane

Internal limiting membrane is the innermost layer of retina and it separates retina from the vitreous body. It is a hyaline membrane, formed by the opposition of expanded ends of Müller fibers.

■ FUNDUS OCULI

Fundus oculi is the posterior part of interior eyeball. It is also called **fundus** (Fig. 165.5). In living subjects, fundus is examined by **ophthalmoscope.**

Fundus has two important structures:
1. Optic disk
2. Macula lutea with fovea centralis.

■ OPTIC DISK – BLIND SPOT

Optic disk is a pale disk, situated near the center of the posterior wall of eyeball. It is also called **optic papilla.** It is formed by the convergence of axons from ganglion cells, while forming the optic nerve. Optic disk contains all the layers of retina, except rods and cones. Therefore, it is insensitive to light, i.e. the object is not seen if the image falls upon this area. Because of this, the optic disk is known as blind spot.

■ MACULA LUTEA

Macula lutea is a small yellowish area, situated a little lateral to the optic disk in retina. It is also called **yellow spot.** Yellow color of macula lutea is due to the presence of a yellow pigment. Macula lutea has **fovea centralis** in its center.

Fovea Centralis

Fovea centralis is a minute depression in the center of macula lutea. Here, all the layers of retina are very thin. Diameter of fovea is only about 0.5 mm. Fovea is the region of most acute vision because it contains only cones.

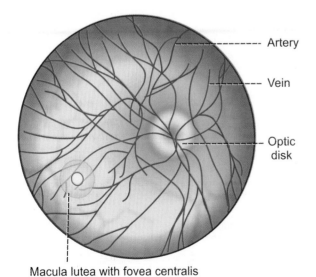

Macula lutea with fovea centralis

FIGURE 165.5: Fundus oculi

Foveal Vision and Extrafoveal vision

When one looks at an object, eyeballs are directed towards the object, so that, the image of that object falls on fovea of each eye and the person can see the object very clearly. It is known as **foveal vision.**

Vision in other parts of retina is called peripheral or **extrafoveal vision.** It is less sensitive and enables the subject to gain only a dim and an ill-defined impression of surroundings.

Degeneration of macula lutea leads to blindness.

■ INTRAOCULAR FLUID

Intraocular fluid (fluid in eyeball) is responsible for the maintenance of shape of the eyeball.

Intraocular fluid is of two types:
1. Vitreous humor
2. Aqueous humor.

■ VITREOUS HUMOR

Vitreous humor is a viscous fluid present behind lens, in the space between lens and retina. It is also known as vitreous body. It is a highly viscous and gelatinous substance that is formed by a fine fibrillar network of proteoglycan molecules. Major substances in vitreous humor are albumin and hyaluronic acid. These substances enter vitreous body from blood, by means of diffusion.

Vitreous humor helps to maintain the shape of eyeball.

■ AQUEOUS HUMOR

Aqueous humor is a thin fluid present in front of retina. It fills the space between lens and cornea. This space is divided into **anterior and posterior chambers** by iris. Both the chambers communicate with each other through **pupil.**

Properties of Aqueous Humor

Volume	: 0.13 mL
Reaction and pH	: Alkaline with a pH of 7.5
Viscosity	: 1.029
Refractory index	: 1.34.

Composition of Aqueous Humor

Composition of aqueous humor is given in Figure 165.6.

Formation of Aqueous Humor

Aqueous humor is formed by **ciliary processes.** It is formed from plasma within capillary network of ciliary

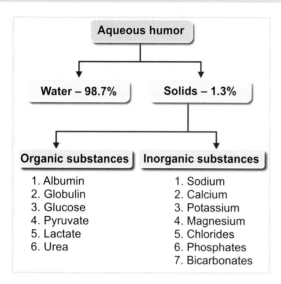

FIGURE 165.6: Composition of aqueous humor

process by diffusion, ultrafiltration and active transport through the epithelial cells lining the ciliary processes. After formation, aqueous humor reaches the posterior chamber by passing through the suspensory ligaments. From here, it reaches the anterior chamber via pupil.

Formation of aqueous humor is a continuous process. Rate of formation is about 2 to 3 μL per minute. Amount of aqueous humor in anterior chamber is about 230 μL to 250 μL and in posterior chamber it is about 50 μL to 60 μL.

Drainage of Aqueous Humor

From anterior chamber, the aqueous humor passes into the angle between cornea and iris called **limbus.** From here, it passes through meshwork of **trabeculae** situated near the junction of iris and cornea. Then it flows through **canal of Schlemm** and reaches the venous system via **anterior ciliary vein** (Fig. 165.7).

Functions of Aqueous Humor

Aqueous humor

i. Maintains the shape of eyeball
ii. Maintains the intraocular pressure
iii. Provides nutrients, oxygen and electrolytes to avascular structures such as lens and cornea
iv. Removes the metabolic end products from lens and cornea.

■ INTRAOCULAR PRESSURE

Intraocular pressure is the measure of fluid pressure in eye, exerted by aqueous humor. Normal intraocular pressure varies between 12 and 20 mm Hg.

Measurement of intraocular pressure is an important part of eye examination. It is measured by **tonometer.** When intraocular pressure increases to about 60 to 70 mm Hg, **glaucoma** occurs. Refer Applied Physiology in this chapter for details.

■ LENS

Lens of the eyeball is **crystalline** in nature. It is situated behind the pupil. It is a biconvex, transparent and elastic structure. It is avascular and receives its nutrition mainly from the aqueous humor.

Lens refracts light rays and helps to focus the image of the objects on retina. Focal length of human lens is 44 mm and its refractory power is 23 D.

Lens is supported by the **suspensory ligaments (zonular fibers),** which are attached with ciliary bodies.

■ STRUCTURE OF THE LENS

Lens is formed of three components:
1. Capsule
2. Anterior epithelium
3. Lens substance.

1. Capsule

Capsule is a highly elastic membrane that covers the lens.

2. Anterior Epithelium

Anterior epithelium is a single layer of cuboidal epithelial cells, situated beneath the capsule. At the margins, epithelial cells are elongated. Epithelial cells give rise to lens fibers present in the lens substance.

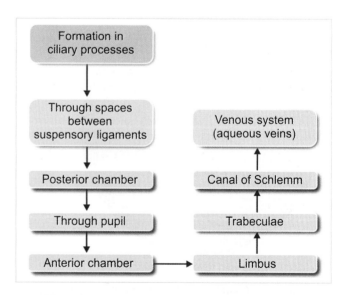

FIGURE 165.7: Circulation and drainage of aqueous humor

3. *Lens Substance*

Lens is formed by long lens fibers derived from anterior epithelium. Lens fibers are prismatic in nature and are arranged in concentric layers.

■ CHANGES IN THE LENS DURING OLD AGE

Elastic property of lens is decreased in old age due to the physical changes in lens and its capsule. It causes **presbyopia** (Chapter 171).

In old age, lens becomes opaque and this condition is called **cataract.** Refer Applied Physiology in this chapter for details.

■ OCULAR MUSCLES

■ MUSCLES OF THE EYEBALL

Muscles of the eyeball are of two types:
A. Intrinsic muscles
B. Extrinsic muscles.

Intrinsic Muscles

Intrinsic muscles are formed by smooth muscle fibers and are controlled by autonomic nerves.
Intrinsic muscles of eye are:
1. Constrictor papillae
2. Dilator papillae
3. Ciliary muscle.

Actions of constrictor pupillae and dilator pupillae are already explained along with iris. Contraction of ciliary muscle increases the anterior curvature of lens during accommodation (Chapter 169).

Extrinsic Muscles

In general, the term 'ocular muscles' refers to extrinsic muscles of the eyeball. Extrinsic muscles are formed by skeletal muscle fibers and are controlled by the somatic nerves. Eyeball moves within the orbit by six extrinsic skeletal muscles (Fig. 165.8). One end of each muscle is attached to the eyeball and the other end to the wall of orbital cavity. There are four straight muscles (rectus) and two oblique muscles.
Extrinsic muscles are:
1. Superior rectus
2. Inferior rectus
3. Medial or internal rectus
4. Lateral or external rectus
5. Superior oblique
6. Inferior oblique.

■ INNERVATION OF OCULAR MUSCLES

Innervation of Intrinsic Muscles

Intrinsic muscles of eyeball are innervated by both sympathetic and parasympathetic divisions of **autonomic nervous system.**

Parasympathetic nerve fibers

Parasympathetic preganglionic fibers arise from **Edinger-Westphal nucleus** of III cranial nerve. After passing through III cranial nerve, these fibers synapse with postganglionic neurons in **ciliary ganglion.** Postganglionic fibers arising from here pass through **ciliary nerves** and innervate the **ciliary muscle** and **constrictor pupillae.** Stimulation of parasympathetic nerve fibers causes contraction of ciliary muscle and constrictor pupillae.

Sympathetic nerve fibers

Sympathetic preganglionic nerve fibers arise from lateral horn of first thoracic segment of spinal cord, pass through **sympathetic chain** and synapse with neurons of **superior cervical sympathetic ganglion.** Postganglionic fibers arising from this ganglion, run along with carotid artery and its branches, to reach the intrinsic muscles of the eyeball. Stimulation of sympathetic nerve fibers causes relaxation of **ciliary muscle** and contraction of **dilator pupillae.**

Innervation of Extrinsic Muscles

Extrinsic muscles of eyeball are innervated by **somatic motor nerve fibers.** Somatic nerve fibers arise from cranial nerve nuclei in brainstem and reach the ocular muscles via three cranial nerves:
1. Oculomotor (third) nerve
2. Trochlear (fourth) nerve
3. Abducent (sixth) nerve.

1. *Oculomotor Nerve*

Oculomotor nerve supplies:
i. Superior rectus
ii. Inferior rectus.
iii. Medial rectus (internal rectus)
iv. Inferior oblique.

2. *Trochlear Nerve*

Trochlear nerve supplies the superior oblique.

3. *Abducent Nerve*

Abducent nerve supplies the lateral rectus (external rectus).

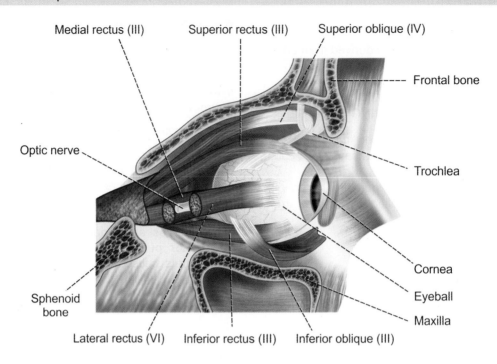

Medial rectus (III)   Superior rectus (III)   Superior oblique (IV)

Frontal bone

Optic nerve

Trochlea

Cornea

Eyeball

Maxilla

Sphenoid
bone

Lateral rectus (VI)   Inferior rectus (III)   Inferior oblique (III)

FIGURE 165.8: Extrinsic muscles of eyeball.
Numbers in parenthesis indicate the cranial nerve supplying the muscle.

■ OCULAR MOVEMENTS

Eyeball moves or rotates within the orbital socket in any of the three primary axes, namely vertical, transverse and anteroposterior axis (Fig. 165.9 and Table 165.1).

■ MOVEMENTS IN VERTICAL AXIS

Movements of eyeball in vertical axis or in horizontal plane are of two types:

1. *Abduction or Lateral Movement or Outward Movement*

Abduction of eyeball is due to the contraction of **lateral rectus** mainly. It is supported by the two oblique muscles.

2. *Adduction or Medial Movement or Inward Movement*

Adduction of the eyeball occurs because of the action of **medial or internal rectus,** along with action of superior rectus and inferior rectus.

■ MOVEMENTS IN TRANSVERSE AXIS

Movements of eyeball in transverse axis or in sagittal plane are of two types:

1. *Elevation or Upward Movement*

Elevation of eyeball occurs because of the contraction of **superior rectus** and **inferior oblique muscles.**

2. *Depression or Downward Movement*

Depression of eyeball is brought out by **inferior rectus** and **superior oblique.**

■ MOVEMENTS IN ANTEROPOSTERIOR AXIS

Movements of eyeball in anteroposterior axis or in the frontal plane are called **torsion** or **wheel movements.** Torsion movements are two types, namely extorsion and intorsion.

1. *Extorsion*

During extorsion, the eyeball is rotated in such a way that the cornea turns in upward and outward direction. This movement is due to contraction of **inferior oblique** and **inferior rectus.**

2. *Intorsion*

During intorsion, the eyeball is rotated so that, the cornea moves in downward and inward direction. It is produced by the contraction of **superior oblique** and **superior rectus muscles.**

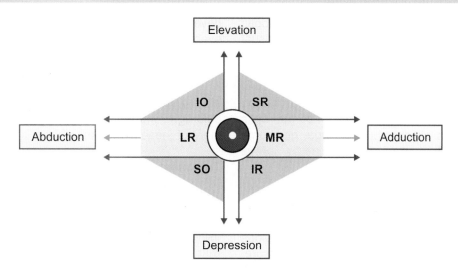

FIGURE 165.9: Diagram showing the movements of right eye. MR = Medial rectus, SO = Superior oblique, LR = Lateral rectus, IO = Inferior oblique, SR = Superior rectus, IR = Inferior rectus.

TABLE 165.1: Muscles taking part in ocular movements

Movement	Primary muscle	Secondary muscle
1. Abduction	Lateral rectus	Superior oblique Inferior oblique
2. Adduction	Medial rectus	Superior rectus Inferior rectus
3. Elevation	Superior rectus	Inferior oblique
4. Depression	Inferior rectus	Superior oblique
5. Extorsion	Inferior oblique	Inferior rectus
6. Intorsion	Superior oblique	Superior rectus

■ SIMULTANEOUS MOVEMENTS OF BOTH EYEBALLS

Simultaneous movements of both eyeballs are of four types:

1. Conjugate Movement

Conjugate movement is the movement of both eyeballs in the same direction. Visual axes of both eyes remain parallel. It is due to contraction of **medial rectus** of one eye and **lateral rectus** of the other eye.

2. Disjugate Movement

Disjugate movement is the movement of both eyeballs in opposite direction. There are two types of disjugate movement, namely convergence and divergence.

Convergence

Convergence is the movement of both eyeballs towards nose. It is due to simultaneous contraction of medial rectus and simultaneous relaxation of lateral rectus of both eyes. Visual axes move close to each other. Convergence of eyeballs occurs during accommodation.

Divergence

Divergence is the movement of both eyeballs towards temporal side. It is due to the simultaneous contraction of lateral rectus and simultaneous relaxation of medial rectus of both eyes. Visual axes of the eyes move away from each other.

3. Pursuit Movement

Pursuit movement is the movement of eyeballs along with object, when eyeballs follow a moving object.

4. Saccadic Movement

Saccadic movement is the quick jerky movement of both eyeballs when the fixation of eyes **(gaze)** is shifted from one object to another object. It is also called **optokinetic movement.**

■ APPLIED PHYSIOLOGY

■ GLAUCOMA

Glaucoma is a group of diseases characterized by increased intraocular pressure, which causes damage of optic nerve, resulting in blindness.

In glaucoma, the drainage of aqueous humor through trabeculae is blocked, resulting in increased intraocular pressure. When the intraocular pressure rises above 60 mm Hg, the optic nerve fibers at the optic disk are compressed. Initially it decreases the visual field (loss of peripheral vision), which eventually leads to total blindness.

However, with early treatment, often the eyes may be protected against serious vision loss. Untreated glaucoma leads to permanent damage of the optic nerve and results in blindness. In old age, glaucoma occurs due to the obstruction of trabeculae by fibrous structures.

Types of Glaucoma

Elevation of intraocular pressure causing glaucoma can occur at any stage of life. Congenital glaucoma develops in babies born with increased intraocular pressure. Glaucoma in infants is called **infantile glaucoma.** When it occurs in childhood, it is known as **juvenile glaucoma.**

Generally glaucoma is divided into two types:
1. Primary open-angle glaucoma
2. Primary angle-closure glaucoma.

1. Primary open-angle glaucoma (POAG)

POAG is the most common type of glaucoma and it accounts for about 80% of all cases of glaucoma. The term open-angle refers to drainage system, which is responsible for draining the aqueous humor from the eye. Actually, in POAG there is no visible obstruction in the drainage system. Still intraocular pressure increases, causing damage to optic nerve. Exact cause of POAG is not known yet. It is suggested that a microscopic (minute) blockage in drainage system beyond limbus may obstruct the flow of aqueous humor. It causes a gradual increase in intraocular pressure.

2. Primary angle-closure glaucoma (PACG)

PACG is characterized by visible obstruction of drainage system for aqueous humor. Iris is pushed against cornea, preventing the drainage of aqueous humor. Intraocular pressure rises over the period of few hours.

Causes of Glaucoma

Major cause of glaucoma is the blockage in drainage system of aqueous humor in trabeculae, resulting in increased intraocular pressure. Glaucoma also develops secondary to other disorders, which affect the eyes. Common causes of secondary glaucoma are diabetes, inflammation or injury to eye and excess use of drugs such as corticosteroid.

Symptoms of Glaucoma

Primary open-angle glaucoma is a **silent chronic disease** without any early symptoms. Symptoms that develop in later stages include heaviness around eyeball, headache and rapid reduction in visual acuity and visual field.

Early symptoms of angle-closure glaucoma are severe pain in eye or eyebrow, headache, nausea, blurred vision and rainbow halo (colored rings) around bulb light. Immediate care should be taken if two or more of these symptoms appear together.

Treatment for Glaucoma

Treatment does not cure the disease but can prevent further damage of optic nerve. Treatment is aimed at lowering the intraocular pressure. It is achieved by using eye drops or medicines alone or in combination with laser treatment. If intraocular pressure cannot be controlled by these methods, surgery is required.

■ CATARACT

Cataract is the **opacity** or cloudiness in the natural lens of the eye. It is the major cause of blindness worldwide. When lens becomes cloudy, light rays cannot pass through it easily and vision is blurred. Cataract develops in old age after 55 to 60 years.

Lens is situated within the sealed capsule. Old cells die and accumulate within the capsule. Over years, the accumulation of cells is associated with accumulation of fluid and denaturation of proteins in lens fibers, causing cloudiness of lens and blurred image.

Causes of Cataract

In addition to age, cataract develops due to many other causes such as:
1. Eye injuries
2. Previous eye surgery
3. Diseases such as diabetes, Wilson disease and hypocalcemia
4. Long-term use of drugs such as steroids, diuretics and tranquilizers
5. Long-term unprotected exposure to sunlight
6. Alcoholism
7. Family history
8. Diet containing large quantity of salt.

Symptoms of Cataract

Common symptoms of cataract:
1. Glare
2. Painless blurred vision
3. Poor night vision
4. Diplopia in affected eye
5. Need for a bright light while reading
6. Fading of colors.

Treatment for Cataract

Surgery is the only treatment for cataract. During surgery, cloudy lens is removed from the eye through a surgical incision. The natural lens is replaced with a permanent, clear and plastic **intraocular lens** (IOL) implant. Different procedures are followed to remove the cloudy lens.

Common methods are:

1. Extracapsular extraction

Extracapsular extraction is rather an old technique. A 12 mm incision is made in the eye under an operating microscope, to remove the lens as a whole. Posterior capsule of lens is left in place to hold the IOL implant. Multiple sutures are required to seal the eye after surgery. Sutures must be perfect; otherwise astigmatism may develop.

2. Phacoemulsification

Phacoemulsification (Phaco) is the current technique. **Phaco** is the procedure in which cataract is broken into smaller fragments by **ultrasonic vibrations.** It is done through a small (3 mm) incision. An ultrasound (or laser) probe is used to break the lens material without damaging the capsule. Lens fragments are aspirated out of the eye. A foldable IOL is then introduced through the incision. After entering the eye, the lens unfolds to take position inside the capsule. No sutures are needed, as the incision is self-sealing.

Visual Process

Chapter
166

■ INTRODUCTION

Visual process is the series of actions that take place during visual perception. During visual process, image of an object seen by the eyes is focused on retina, resulting in production of visual perception of that object.

When the image of an object in environment is focused on retina, the energy in visual spectrum is converted into electrical potentials (impulses) by rods and cones of retina through some chemical reactions. Impulses from rods and cones reach the cerebral cortex through optic nerve and the sensation of vision is produced in cerebral cortex. Thus, process of visual sensation is explained on the basis of image formation and neural, chemical and electrical phenomena.

■ IMAGE FORMING MECHANISM

While looking at an object, light rays from that object are refracted and brought to a focus upon retina. Image of the object falls on the retina in an inverted position and reversed side to side. Inspite of this, the object is seen in an upright position. It is because of the role played by cerebral cortex.

Light rays are refracted by the lens and cornea. **Refractory power** is measured in **diopter** (D). A diopter is the reciprocal of focal length expressed in meters.

Focal length of cornea is 24 mm and refractory power is 42 D. Focal length of lens is 44 mm and refractory power is 23 D.

■ NEURAL BASIS OF VISUAL PROCESS

Retina contains the **visual receptors** (Fig. 166.1), which are also called light sensitive receptors, **photoreceptors** or **electromagnetic receptors.** Visual receptors are rods and cones. There are about 6 million cones and 12 million rods in the human eye. Distribution of the rods and cones varies in different areas of retina. Fovea has only cones and no rods. While proceeding from fovea towards the periphery of retina, the rods increase and the cones decrease in number. At the periphery of the retina, only rods are present and cones are absent.

■ STRUCTURE OF ROD CELL

Rod cells are cylindrical structures with a length of about 40 to 60 μ and a diameter of about 2 μ.

Each rod is composed of four structures:
1. Outer segment
2. Inner segment
3. Cell body
4. Synaptic terminal.

1. *Outer Segment*

Outer segment of rod cell is long and slender. So it gives the rod-like appearance. It is in close contact with the pigmented epithelial cells. Outer segment of rod cell is formed by the modified cilia and it contains a pile of freely floating flat **membranous disks.** There are about 1,000 disks in each rod. Disks in rod cells are closed structures and contain the photosensitive pigment, the **rhodopsin.**

Rhodopsin is synthesized in inner segments and inserted into newly formed membranous disks at the inner portion of outer segment. New disks push the older disks towards outer tip. Older disks are engulfed (by phagocytosis) from tip of the outer segment by cells of pigment epithelial layer. Thus, outer segment of rod cell is constantly renewed by the formation of new disks. Rate of formation of new disks is 3 or 4 per hour.

2. *Inner Segment*

Inner segment is connected to outer segment by means of modified **cilium.** Inner segment contains many types of organelles with large number of mitochondria.

3. *Cell Body*

A slender fiber called rod fiber arises from inner segment of the rod cell and passes to outer nuclear layer through external limiting membrane. In outer nuclear layer, the enlarged portion of this fiber forms the cell body or rod granule that contains the nucleus.

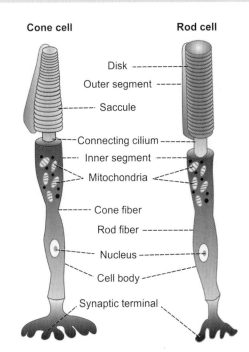

FIGURE 166.1: Structure of visual receptors

4. *Synaptic Terminal*

A thick fiber arising from the cell body passes to outer plexiform layer and ends in a small and enlarged synaptic terminal or body. Synaptic terminal of the rods synapses with dendrites of **bipolar cells** and **horizontal cells.** Synaptic vesicles present in the synaptic terminal contain neurotransmitter, **glutamate.**

■ STRUCTURE OF CONE CELL

Cone cell is the visual receptor with length of 35 μ to 40 μ and a diameter of about 5 μ. Generally, the cone cell is flask shaped. Shape and length of the cone vary in different parts of the retina. Cones in the fovea are long, narrow and almost similar to rods. Near the periphery of retina, cones are short and broad.

Like rods, cones are also formed by four parts:
1. Outer segment
2. Inner segment
3. Cell body
4. Synaptic terminal.

1. *Outer Segment*

Outer segment is small and conical. It does not contain separate membranous disks as in rods. In cone, the infoldings of cell membrane form **saccules,** which are the counterparts of rod disks.

Photopigment of cone is synthesized in the inner segment and incorporated into the folding of surface membrane forming **saccule.** Renewal of outer segment of cone is a slow process and it differs from that in rods. It occurs at many sites of the outer segment of cone.

2. Inner Segment

In cones also, the inner segment is connected to outer segment by a modified cilium as in the case of rods. Though various types of organelles are present in this segment, the number of mitochondria is more.

3. Cell Body

Cone fiber arising from inner segment is thick and it enters the inner nuclear layer through external limiting membrane. In the inner nuclear layer, cone fiber forms the cell body or cone granule that possesses nucleus.

4. Synaptic Terminal

Fiber from cell body of cone leaves the inner nuclear layer and enters outer flexiform layer. Here, it ends in the form of an enlarged synaptic terminal or body. Synaptic vesicle present in the synaptic terminal of cone cell also possesses the neurotransmitter, glutamate.

■ FUNCTIONS OF RODS AND CONES

Functions of Rods

Rods are very sensitive to light and have a **low threshold.** So, the rods are responsible for **dim light vision** or **night vision** or **scotopic vision.** But, rods do not take part in resolving the details and boundaries of objects (visual acuity) or the color of the objects (color vision). Vision by rod is black, white or in the combination of black and white namely, grey. Therefore, the colored objects appear faded or greyish in twilight.

Functions of Cones

Cones have high threshold for light stimulus. So, the cones are sensitive only to bright light. Therefore, cone cells are called receptors of **bright light vision** or **daylight vision** or **photopic vision.** Cones are also responsible for **acuity of vision** and the **color vision** (Table 166.1).

Achromatic Interval

When an object is placed in front of a person in a dark room, he cannot see any object. When there is slight illumination, the person can see the objects but without color. It is because, at this level, only rods are stimulated. When, the illumination is increased, the threshold for cones is reached. Now, the person can see the objects in finer details and in color. Interval between the threshold for rods and cones, i.e. interval from when an object is first seen and the time when that object is seen with color is called **achromatic interval.**

■ CHEMICAL BASIS OF VISUAL PROCESS

Photosensitive pigments present in rods and cones are concerned with chemical basis of visual process. Chemical reactions involved in these pigments lead to the development of electrical activity in retina and generation of impulses (action potentials), which are transmitted through optic nerve. Photochemical changes in the visual receptor cells are called **Wald visual cycle.**

■ RHODOPSIN

Rhodopsin or visual purple is the photosensitive pigment of rod cells. It is present in membranous disks located in outer segment of rod cells.

Chemistry of Rhodopsin

Rhodopsin is a conjugated protein with a molecular weight of 40,000. It is made up of a protein called **opsin** and a **chromophore.** Opsin present in rhodopsin is known as **scotopsin.** Chromophore is a chemical substance that develops color in the cell. Chromophore present in the rod cells is called **retinal.** Retinal is the aldehyde of **vitamin A** or retinol.

Retinal is derived from food sources and it is not synthesized in the body. It is derived from carotinoid substances like **β-carotene** present in carrots.

Retinal is present in the form of **11-*cis* retinal** known as **retinine 1.** Retinine 1 is present in human eyes. It is different from retinine 2 that is present in the eyes of some animals. Significance of 11-*cis* form of retinal is that, only in this form it combines with scotopsin to synthesize rhodopsin.

Photochemical Changes in Rhodopsin – Wald Visual Cycle

When retina is isolated and examined in dark, the rods appear in red because of rhodopsin. During exposure to light, rhodopsin is bleached and the color becomes yellow. When rhodopsin absorbs the light that falls on retina, it is split into retinine and the protein called **opsin** through various intermediate photochemical reactions (Fig. 166.2).

TABLE 166.1: Rods versus cones

Features	Rods	Cones
Number in each eye	12 million	6 million
Length	40 to 60 µ	35 to 40 µ
Diameter	2 µ	5 µ
Shape	Cylindrical	Flask shaped
Outer segment	Long and slender	Small and conical
Sensitivity to light	More sensitive	Sensitive only to bright light
Threshold	Low	High
Type of vision responsible for	Dim light vision or night vision or scotopic vision	Bright light vision or day light vision or photopic vision
Acuity of vision	Not responsible	Responsible
Color vision	Not responsible	Responsible
Photosensitive pigment	Rhodopsin	Porphyropsin or iodopsin or cyanopsin

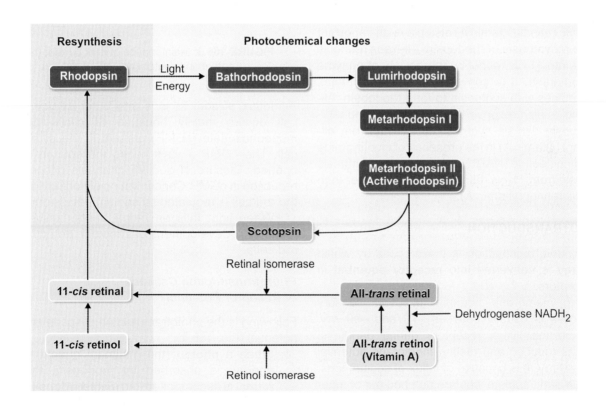

FIGURE 166.2: Photochemical changes and resynthesis of rhodopsin (Wald visual cycle).
NADH$_2$ = Reduced nicotinamide adenine dinucleotide.

Following changes occur due to absorption of light energy by rhodopsin:

1. First, **rhodopsin** is decomposed into **bathorhodopsin** that is very unstable
2. Bathorhodopsin is converted into **lumirhodopsin**
3. Lumirhodopsin decays into **metarhodopsin I**
4. Metarhodopsin I is changed to **metarhodopsin II**
5. Metarhodopsin II is split into **scotopsin** and **all-*trans* retinal**
6. All-*trans* retinal is converted into **all-*trans* retinol (vitamin A)** by the enzyme dehydrogenase in the presence of reduced nicotinamide adenine dinucleotide (NADH$_2$).

Metarhodopsin is usually called **activated rhodopsin** since it is responsible for development of receptor potential in rod cells.

Resynthesis of Rhodopsin

First, the all-*trans* retinal derived from metarhodopsin II is converted into 11-*cis* retinal by the enzyme **retinal isomerase**. 11-*cis* retinal immediately combines with scotopsin to form rhodopsin.

All-*trans* retinol (vitamin A) also plays an important role in the resynthesis of rhodopsin. All-*trans* retinol is converted into 11-*cis* retinol by the activity of enzyme retinol isomerase. It is converted into 11-*cis* retinal, which combines with scotopsin to form rhodopsin. All-*trans* retinol is also reconverted into all-*trans* retinal.

Rhodopsin can be synthesized directly from all-*trans* retinol (vitamin A) in the presence of nicotinamide adenine dinucleotide (NADH$_2$). However, the synthesis of rhodopsin from 11-*cis* retinal (retinine) is faster than from 11-*cis* retinol (vitamin A).

■ PHOTOTRANSDUCTION

Visual or phototransduction is the process by which **light energy** is converted into **receptor potential** in visual receptors.

Resting membrane potential in other sensory receptor cells is usually between −70 and −90 mV. However, in the visual receptors during darkness, negativity is reduced and resting membrane potential is about −40 mV. It is because of influx of sodium ions. Normally in dark, sodium ions are pumped out of inner segments of rod cell to ECF. However, these sodium ions leak back into the rod cells through membrane of outer segment and reduce the **electronegativity** inside rod cell (Fig. 166.3). Thus, **sodium influx** maintains a decreased negative potential up to −40 mV. This potential is constant and it is also called **dark current**.

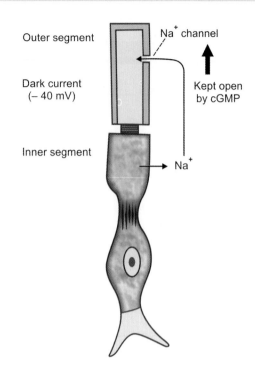

FIGURE 166.3: Maintenance of dark current (resting potential) in outer segment of rod cell

Influx of sodium ions into outer segment of rod cell occurs mainly because of cyclic guanosine monophosphate (cGMP) present in the cytoplasm of cell. The cGMP always keeps the sodium channels opened. Closure of sodium channels occurs due to reduction in cGMP. Concentration of sodium ions inside the rod cell is regulated by sodium potassium pump.

When light falls on retina, rhodopsin is excited leading to development of receptor potential in the rod cells.

Phototransduction Cascade of Receptor Potential

Following is the phototransduction cascade of receptor potential (Fig. 166.4):

1. When a **photon** (the minimum quantum of light energy) is absorbed by rhodopsin, the **11-*cis* retinal** is decomposed into **metarhodopsin** through few reactions mentioned earlier. Metarhodopsin II is considered as the active form of rhodopsin. It plays an important role in the development of receptor potential.
2. Metarhodopsin II activates a **G protein** called **transducin** that is present in rod disks

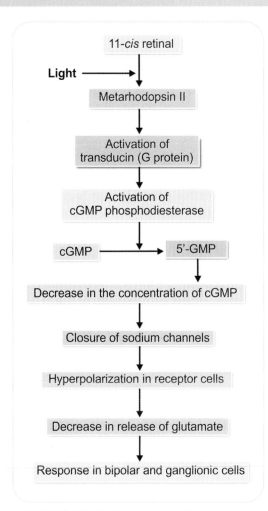

FIGURE 166.4: Phototransduction cascade.
cGMP = Cyclic guanosine monophosphate.

3. Activated transducin activates the enzyme called cyclic guanosine monophosphate phosphodiesterase **(cGMP phosphodiesterase),** which is also present in rod disks
4. Activated cGMP phosphodiesterase hydrolyzes cGMP to 5'-GMP
5. Now, the concentration of cGMP is reduced in rod cell
6. Reduction in concentration of cGMP immediately causes closure of sodium channels in the membrane of visual receptors
7. Sudden closure of sodium channels prevents entry of sodium ions leading to **hyperpolarization.** The potential reaches –70 to –80 mV. It is because of sodium-potassium pump.

Thus, the process of receptor potential in visual receptors is unique in nature. When other sensory receptors are excited, the electrical response is in the form of **depolarization (receptor potential).** But, in visual receptors, the response is in the form of **hyperpolarization.**

Significance of Hyperpolarization

Hyperpolarization in visual receptor cells reduces the release of synaptic transmitter glutamate. It leads to development of response in bipolar cells and ganglionic cells so that, the action potentials are transmitted to cerebral cortex via optic pathway.

■ PHOTOSENSITIVE PIGMENTS IN CONES

Photosensitive pigment in cone cells is of three types, namely **porphyropsin, iodopsin** and **cyanopsin.** Only one of these pigments is present in each cone. Photopigment in cone cell also is a conjugated protein made up of a protein and chromophore. Protein in cone pigment is called **photopsin,** which is different from scotopsin, the protein part of rhodopsin. However, chromophore of cone pigment is the retinal that is present in rhodopsin. Each type of cone pigment is sensitive to a particular light and the maximum response is shown at a particular light and wave-length. Details are given in the Table 166.2.

Various processes involved in phototransduction in cone cells are similar to those in rod cells.

■ DARK ADAPTATION

Definition

Dark adaption is the process by which the person is able to see the objects in dim light. If a person enters a dim-lighted room (darkroom) from a bright-lighted area, he is blind for some time, i.e. he cannot see any object. After sometime his eyes get adapted and he starts seeing the objects slowly. Maximum duration for dark adaptation is about 20 minutes.

Causes for Dark Adaptation

Dark adaptation is due to the following changes in eyeball:

1. *Increased sensitivity of rods as a result of resynthesis of rhodopsin*

Time required for dark adaptation is partly determined by the time for resynthesis of rhodopsin. In bright light, most of the pigment molecules are bleached (broken down). But in dim light, it requires some time for regeneration of certain amount of rhodopsin, which is necessary for optimal rod function.

Dark adaptation occurs in cones also.

2. *Dilatation of pupil*

Dilatation of pupil during dark adaptation allows more and more light to enter the eye.

TABLE 166.2: Sensitivity of cone pigments

Pigment	Sensitive to	Wavelength of maximum response
Porphyropsin	Red	665 nm
Iodopsin	Green	535 nm
Cyanopsin	Blue	445 nm

Radiologists, aircraft pilots and others, who need maximal visual sensitivity in dim light, wear **red glass** before entering dim-lighted area, because red light of spectrum stimulates the rods slightly while the cones are allowed to function well. Thus, the person wearing **red goggles** can see well in bright-lighted area and also can see the objects clearly, as soon as he enters the dim-lighted area.

Dark Adaptation Curve

Dart adaptation curve is the curve that demonstrates the relationship between threshold of light stimulus (illumination) and time spent in dark.

Procedure

Experiment to obtain dark adaptation curve is done in a completely dark room. First, the subject is exposed to a bright light in order to bleach (breakdown) most of the photopigment in retina. The subject looks directly at a bright flashing light with a wavelength of 420 nm against dark background for about 5 to 7 minutes.

Then the bright light is switched off and the subject is in dark. Now a small dim light (stimulus) is produced. Immediately, the absolute threshold (minimum strength of stimulus; minimum intensity of light stimulus) for detecting this dim light is determined by adjusting the intensity of light (illumination). Time interval between the switching off bright light and detection of dim light is noted. After a short time, absolute threshold is measured again and elapsed time is noted. This procedure is repeated for about 30 minutes.

When the experiment is completed, results are plotted and the dark adaptation curve is obtained.

Parts of dark adaptation curve

Dark adaptation curve is **biphasic**. First part of the curve represents threshold of photopic vision, which indicates the cone adaptation. Second part of the curve represents threshold of scotopic vision, which indicates the rod adaptation (Fig. 166.5).

Cone adaptation

This first phase is rapid and it is completed in 8 to 10 minutes. During this period the threshold decreases by 2 to 3 log units. That is the sensitivity of the eye in dark room increases by 1,000 times within 8 to 10 minutes. By this time, the cones get adapted.

Rod-cone break

After the first phase, there is a sudden change in slope of the curve and this point of curve is called rod-cone break. Rod-cone break represents the point where rod sensitivity begins to exceed cone sensitivity and the remaining part of the curve is determined by the continuing adaptation of rods.

During this phase the threshold decreases further by 5 to 6 log units. That is the sensitivity of eye in dark room increases by 100,000 to 1,000,000 times within 20 to 30 minutes. By this time, rods get adapted completely.

■ LIGHT ADAPTATION

Rod adaptation

Second phase of the curve is slow. During this phase, there is a gradual decrease in the threshold and it is completed in 20 to 30 minutes.

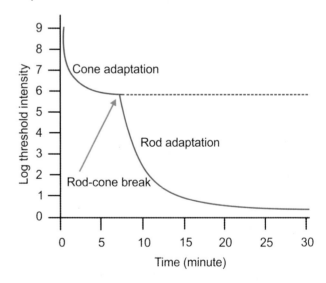

FIGURE 166.5: Dark adaptation curve. During cone adaptation, threshold decreases by 3 logs and sensitivity of the eyes increases 1,000 times. During rod adaptation, threshold decreases by 6 logs and sensitivity of the eyes increases by 1,000,000.

Definition

Light adaptation is the process in which eyes get adapted to increased illumination. When a person enters a bright-lighted area from a dim-lighted area, he feels discomfort due to the dazzling effect of bright light. After some time, when the eyes become adapted to light, he sees the objects around him without any discomfort. It is the mere disappearance of dark adaptation. Maximum period for light adaptation is about 5 minutes.

Causes of Light Adaptation

There are two causes of light adaptation:

1. *Reduced sensitivity of rods*

During light adaptation, the sensitivity of rods decreases. It is due to the breakdown of rhodopsin.

2. *Constriction of pupil*

Constriction of pupil reduces the quantity of light rays entering the eye.

■ NIGHT BLINDNESS

Definition

Night blindness is defined as the loss of vision when light in the environment becomes dim. It is otherwise called **nyctalopia** or **defective dim light** (scotopic) **vision.**

Causes of Night Blindness

Night blindness is due to the deficiency of **vitamin A,** which is essential for the function of rods.

Deficiency of vitamin A occurs because of following causes:

1. Diet containing less amount of vitamin A
2. Decreased absorption of vitamin A from intestine.

Vitamin A deficiency causes defective cone function. Prolonged deficiency leads to anatomical changes in rods and cones and finally the degeneration of other retinal layers occurs. So, retinal function can be restored, only if treatment is given with vitamin A before the visual receptors start degenerating.

■ ELECTRICAL BASIS OF VISUAL PROCESS – ELECTRORETINOGRAM

■ DEFINITION

Electroretinogram (ERG) is the record of electrical activity in retina. When light rays stimulate the retina, a characteristic sequence of potential changes occurs, which can be recorded in the form of ERG. This diagnostic procedure is useful in determining retinal disorders such as **cone dystrophy** (degeneration of cones) and **retinitis pigmentosa** (hyperactivity of the pigmented retinal epithelial cells, leading to damage of photoreceptors and blindness).

■ METHOD OF RECORDING ERG

Electroretinogram is recorded by using a **galvanometer** or a suitable recording device. Recording electrode is placed on the cornea of eye in its usual forward up looking position. Indifferent electrode is placed over any moist surface of body, like inside the mouth.

■ WAVES OF ELECTRORETINOGRAM

Electroretinogram has 4 waves namely 'A', 'B', 'C' and 'D' (Fig. 166.6). 'A' is the only negative wave and other three are positive waves. 'A', 'B' and 'C' waves occur when light stimulus falls on retina. 'D' wave occurs when light stimulus is stopped. 'A' and 'B' waves arise from rods and cones. 'C' wave arises from pigment epithelial layer and 'D' wave arises from inner nuclear layer.

■ ACUITY OF VISION

■ DEFINITION

Acuity of vision is the ability of eye to determine the precise shape and details of the object. It is also called **visual acuity.** Acuity of vision is also defined as the ability

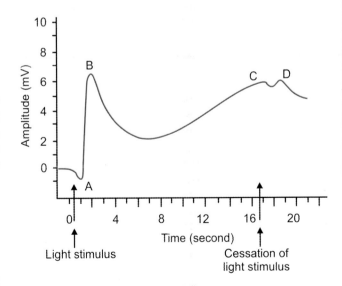

FIGURE 166.6: Electroretinogram

to recognize the separateness of two objects placed together. Cones of retina are responsible for acuity of vision. Visual acuity is highly exhibited in fovea centralis, which contains only cones. It is greatly reduced during the refractory errors.

■ TEST FOR VISUAL ACUITY

Acuity of vision is tested for distant vision as well as near vision. If there is any difficulty in seeing the distant object or the near object, the defect is known as **error of refraction.** Refractive errors are described separately in Chapter 171.

Distant Vision

Snellen chart is used to test the acuity of vision for distant vision in the diagnosis of refractive errors of the eye.

Near Vision

Jaeger chart is used to test the visual acuity for near vision.

Field of Vision

- ■ **DEFINITION**
- ■ **BINOCULAR AND MONOCULAR VISION**
  - ■ **BINOCULAR VISION**
  - ■ **MONOCULAR VISION**
- ■ **DIVISIONS OF VISUAL FIELD**
  - ■ **TEMPORAL AND NASAL FIELDS**
  - ■ **UPPER AND LOWER FIELDS**
- ■ **CORRESPONDING RETINAL POINTS**
  - ■ **DIPLOPIA**
- ■ **BLIND SPOT**
- ■ **VISUAL FIELD AND RETINA**
- ■ **MAPPING OF VISUAL FIELD**

■ DEFINITION

Part of the external world seen by one eye, when it is fixed in one direction is called field of vision or visual field of that eye. According to **Traquair**, the visual field is described as **'island of vision,** surrounded by a sea of blindness'.

■ BINOCULAR AND MONOCULAR VISION

■ BINOCULAR VISION

Binocular vision is the vision in which both the eyes are used together, so that a portion of external world is seen by the eyes together. In human and some animals, eyeballs are placed in front of the head. So, the visual fields of both the eyes overlap. Because of this, a portion of the external world is seen by both the eyes.

■ MONOCULAR VISION

Monocular vision is the vision in which each eye is used separately. In some animals like dog, rabbit and horse, the eyeballs are present at the sides of head. So, the visual fields of both eyes overlap to a very small extent. Because of this, different portion of the external world is seen by each eye.

■ DIVISIONS OF VISUAL FIELD

Visual field of the human eye has an angle of 160° in horizontal meridian and 135° in vertical meridian. Visual filed is divided into four parts:
1. Temporal field
2. Nasal field
3. Upper field
4. Lower field.

■ TEMPORAL AND NASAL FIELDS

Visual field of each eye is divided into two unequal parts, namely outer or temporal field and the inner or nasal field, by a vertical line passing through the fixation point (Fig. 167.1). The fixation point is the meeting point of visual axis with the object.

Temporal part of visual field extends up to about 100° but the nasal part extends only up to 60°, because it is restricted by nose.

■ UPPER AND LOWER FIELDS

Visual field of each eye is also divided into an upper field and a lower field by a horizontal line passing through the fixation point. Extent of the upper field is about 60°, as it is restricted by upper eyelid and orbital margin. Extent of lower field is about 75°. It is

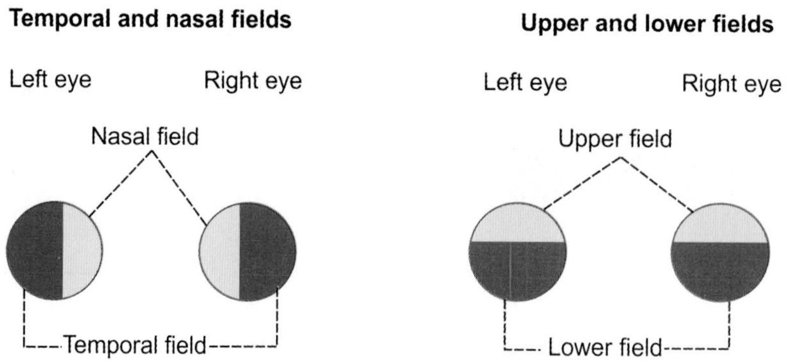

Temporal and nasal fields

Left eye   Right eye

Nasal field

Temporal field

Upper and lower fields

Left eye   Right eye

Upper field

Lower field

FIGURE 167.1: Divisions of visual field

restricted by cheek. Thus, the visual field is restricted in all the sides, except in the temporal part.

CORRESPONDING RETINAL POINTS

Corresponding retinal points are the area in retina of both eyes, on which the light rays from the object falls. It occurs in the binocular vision. The two images developed on retina of both eyes are fused into a single sensation. So, we see the objects with single image.

The single sensation is because of the ocular muscles, which direct the axes of the eyes in such a way that the light rays from the object fall upon the corresponding points of both retinas. If the light rays do not fall on the corresponding retinal points, diplopia occurs.

DIPLOPIA

Diplopia means **double vision.** While looking at an object, if the eyeballs are directed in such a way that the light rays from the object do not fall upon the corresponding point on the retina of both eyes, a double vision occurs, i.e. one single object is seen as two.

Causes of Diplopia

1. Permanent diplopia occurs during paralysis or weakness of ocular muscles. It occurs in myasthenia gravis also.
2. In alcoholic intoxication, the imbalanced actions of ocular muscles produce temporary diplopia
3. Lesions in III, IV and VI cranial nerves, oculomotor nucleus, red nucleus and cerebral peduncles also results in diplopia.

Experimental Diplopia

Diplopia can be produced experimentally, by the following methods:
1. Applying pressure from outer side of one eye and thus displacing the eye from its normal position

2. By holding an object like pen or pencil vertically in front of face, at about 5 cm from the root of nose. It is not possible for the convergence of the eyeballs sufficiently. The light rays from the object do not fall on the corresponding retinal points and diplopia occurs.

BLIND SPOT

Blind spot is the small area of retina where visual receptors are absent. The optic disk in the retina does not have any visual receptors and if the image of any object falls on the optic disk, the object cannot be seen. So this part of the retina is blind hence the name blind spot.

Normally, the darkness in the visual field due to the blind spot does not cause any inconvenience because, the fixation of each eye is at different angles. Even when one eye is closed or blind, the person is not aware of blind spot. However, one can recognize blind spot by some experimental procedures.

VISUAL FIELD AND RETINA

Light rays from different halves of each visual field do not fall on the same halves of the retina. Light rays from temporal part of visual field of an eye fall on the nasal half of retina of that eye. Similarly, the light rays from nasal part of visual field fall on the temporal half of retina of the same side.

MAPPING OF VISUAL FIELD

The shape and extent of visual field is mapped out by means of an instrument called **Goldmann perimeter** and this technique is called **perimetry.** Visual field is also determined by **Bjerrum (Tangent)** screen or by **confrontation test. Humphrey field analyzer** is also used to map visual field and it is more useful to test the central portion of visual fields.

Visual Pathway

■ INTRODUCTION

Visual pathway or **optic pathway** is the nervous pathway that transmits impulses from retina visual center in cerebral cortex.

In binocular vision, the light rays from temporal (outer) half of visual field fall upon the nasal part of corresponding retina. The rays from nasal (inner) half of visual field fall upon the temporal part of retina.

■ VISUAL RECEPTORS

Rods and cones which are present in the retina of eye form the visual receptors. Fibers from the visual receptors synapse with dendrites of bipolar cells of inner nuclear layer of the retina.

■ FIRST ORDER NEURONS

First order neurons (primary neurons) are **bipolar cells** in the retina. Axons from the bipolar cells synapse with dendrites of ganglionic cells.

■ SECOND ORDER NEURONS

Second order neurons (secondary neurons) are the **ganglionic cells** in ganglionic cell layer of retina. Axons of the ganglionic cells form optic nerve. Optic nerve leaves the eye and terminates in lateral geniculate body.

■ THIRD ORDER NEURONS

Third order neurons are in the **lateral geniculate body.** Fibers arising from here, reach the visual cortex.

■ CONNECTIONS OF VISUAL RECEPTORS TO OPTIC NERVE

Two pathways exist between the visual receptors and optic nerve:

1. Private pathway
2. Diffuse pathway.

■ PRIVATE PATHWAY

The individual cones in fovea centralis are connected to separate bipolar cells. Each bipolar cell is connected to separate ganglionic cell, namely **midget ganglionic cell.** Thus, individual cone is connected to an individual optic nerve fiber. This type of private pathway is responsible for **visual acuity** and **intensity discrimination.**

■ DIFFUSE PATHWAY

A number of cones and rods are connected with a polysynaptic bipolar cell. The bipolar cells are connected to **diffused ganglionic cells.** So, there is great overlapping. This type of pathway is present outside the fovea.

■ COURSE OF VISUAL PATHWAY

Visual pathway consists of six components:

1. Optic nerve
2. Optic chiasma
3. Optic tract
4. Lateral geniculate body
5. Optic radiation
6. Visual cortex.

■ OPTIC NERVE

Optic nerve is formed by the axons of ganglionic cells (Fig. 168.1). Optic nerve leaves the eye through optic disk. The fibers from temporal part of retina are in lateral part of the nerve and carry the impulses from nasal half of visual field of same eye. The fibers from nasal part of retina are in medial part of the nerve and carry the impulses from temporal half of visual field of same eye.

■ OPTIC CHIASMA

Medial fibers of each optic nerve cross the midline and join the uncrossed lateral fibers of opposite side, to form

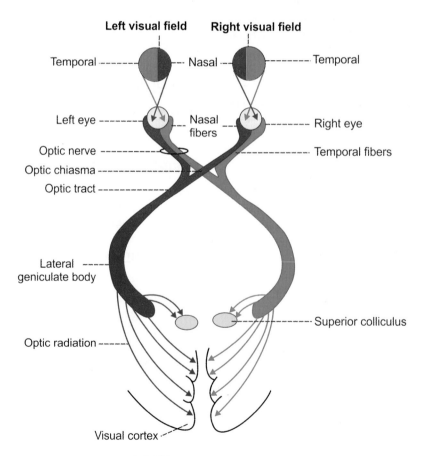

FIGURE 168.1: Visual pathway

the optic tract (Fig. 168.1). This area of crossing of the optic nerve fibers is called optic chiasma.

■ OPTIC TRACT

Optic tract is formed by uncrossed fibers of optic nerve on the same side and crossed fibers of optic nerve from the opposite side. All the fibers of optic tract run backward, outward and towards the **cerebral peduncle.** While reaching the peduncle, the fibers pass between **tuber cinereum** and **anterior perforated substance.** Then, the fibers turn around the peduncle to reach the **lateral geniculate body** in thalamus. Here, many fibers synapse while few fibers just pass through this and run towards superior colliculus in midbrain. Fibers from fovea do not enter **superior colliculus.**

Some fibers from fovea of each side pass through the optic tract of same side and others through the optic tract of opposite side. Due to crossing of medial fibers in optic chiasma, the left optic tract carries impulses from temporal part of left retina and nasal part of right retina, i.e. it is responsible for vision in nasal half of left visual field and temporal half of right visual field. The right optic tract contains fibers from nasal half of left retina and temporal half of right retina. It is responsible for vision in temporal half of left visual field and nasal half of right visual field.

■ LATERAL GENICULATE BODY

Majority of the fibers of optic tract terminate in lateral geniculate body, which forms the **subcortical center** for visual sensation. From here, the **geniculocalcarine tract** or **optic radiation** arises. This tract is the last relay of visual pathway.

Some of the fibers from optic tract do not synapse in lateral geniculate body, but pass through it and terminate in one of the following centers:
  i. *Superior colliculus:* It is concerned with reflex movements of eyeballs and head, in response to optic stimulus
  ii. *Pretectal nucleus:* It is concerned with light reflexes
  iii. *Supraoptic nucleus of hypothalamus:* It is concerned with the retinal control of pituitary in animals. But in human, it does not play any important role.

■ OPTIC RADIATION

Fibers from lateral geniculate body pass through **internal capsule** and form optic radiation. The fibers between lateral geniculate body and visual cortex are also called **geniculocalcarine fibers.** Optic radiation ends in visual cortex (Fig. 168.2).

■ VISUAL CORTEX

Primary **cortical center** for vision is called visual cortex, which is located on the medial surface of occipital lobe. It forms the walls and lips of calcarine fissure in medial surface of occipital lobe.

There is a definite localization of retinal projections upon visual cortex. In fact, the point to point projection of retina upon visual cortex is well established. The peripheral retinal representation occupies the anterior part of visual cortex. **Macular representation** occupies the posterior part of visual cortex near occipital pole.

Areas of Visual Cortex and their Function

Three areas are present in visual cortex:
  i. Primary visual area (area 17), which is concerned with the perception of visual impulses
  ii. Secondary visual area or visual association area (area 18), which is concerned with the interpretation of visual impulses
  iii. Occipital eye field (area 19), which is concerned with the movement of eyes (Chapter 152).

■ APPLIED PHYSIOLOGY – EFFECTS OF LESION AT DIFFERENT LEVELS OF VISUAL PATHWAY

Injury to any part of optic pathway causes visual defect and the nature of defect depends upon the location and extent of injury. Loss of vision in one visual field is known as **anopia.** Loss of vision in one half of visual field is called **hemianopia** (Figs. 168.3 to 168.5).

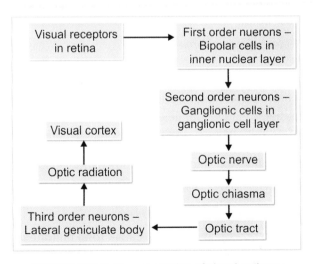

FIGURE 168.2: Representation of visual pathway

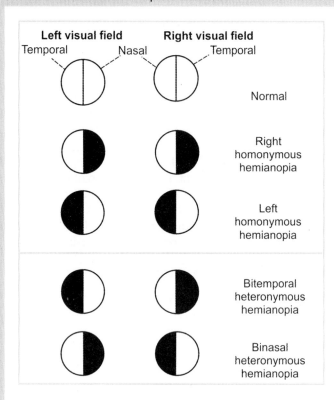

Left visual field   Right visual field
Temporal   Nasal   Temporal

Normal

Right homonymous hemianopia

Left homonymous hemianopia

Bitemporal heteronymous hemianopia

Binasal heteronymous hemianopia

FIGURE 168.3: Types of hemianopia

Hemianopia is classified into two types:
1. Homonymous hemianopia
2. Heteronymous hemianopia.

1. Homonymous hemianopia

Homonymous hemianopia means loss of vision in the same halves of both the visual fields. Loss of vision in right half of visual field of both eyes is known as right homonymous hemianopia. Similarly, left homonymous hemianopia means loss of vision in left half of visual field of both eyes.

2. Heteronymous hemianopia

Heteronymous hemianopia means loss of vision in opposite halves of visual field. For example, binasal heteronymous hemianopia means loss of vision in right half of left visual field and left half of right visual field (nasal half of both visual fields). Bitemporal heteronymous hemianopia is the loss of sight in left side of left visual field and right side of right visual field (temporal half of both visual fields).

Effects of Lesion of Optic Nerve

Lesion in one optic nerve will cause **total blindness** or anopia in the corresponding visual field. Lesion occurs due to increased **intracranial pressure.**

Effects of Lesion of Optic Chiasma

Nature of defect depends upon the fibers involved:
  i. Pressure on uncrossed lateral fibers by aneurysmal dilatation of carotid artery causes blindness in the temporal part of retina of same side, i.e. the retina cannot receive light stimulus from the objects in nasal half of same visual field. So, the hemianopia developed is called **left or right nasal hemianopia.**
  ii. If lateral fibers of both sides are affected, the vision is lost in nasal half of both visual fields, causing **binasal hemianopia.** It occurs due to dilated third ventricle, which forces the angle of chiasma against carotid arteries. It also occurs due to dilatation of carotid artery on both sides.
  iii. Compression of nasal fibers, i.e. crossed fibers by pituitary tumor causes **bitemporal hemianopia.**

Effects of Lesion of Optic Tract, Lateral Geniculate Body and Optic Radiation

Lesion of optic tract or lateral geniculate body or optic radiation causes **homonymous hemianopia.** In the right-sided lesion, there is loss of vision in right side of both retina, i.e. in left side of both visual fields – left homonymous hemianopia. In the left-sided lesion, there is loss of vision in left half of retina of both eyes and loss of sight on right half of both visual fields – right homonymous hemianopia.

Effects of Lesion of Visual Cortex

Lesion of upper or lower part of visual cortex leads to inferior or superior homonymous hemianopia.

Macular sparing

In all the conditions mentioned above, total blindness does not occur because, the macular vision is not lost. This phenomenon in which the macular vision is retained (unaffected) in conditions of hemianopia is called macular sparing.

Macular sparing occurs because of the following reasons:
  i. Fibers from macula project into the visual cortex of both sides
  ii. Fibers from macular region are projected into both anterior and posterior parts of each visual cortex.

Only the bilateral lesion of visual cortex causes total blindness.

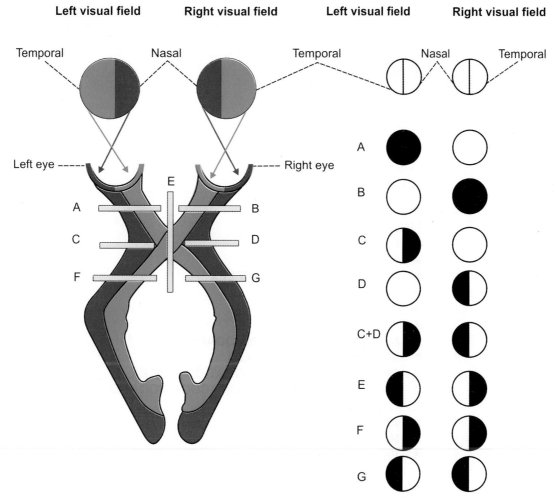

FIGURE 168.4: Effects of lesions of optic pathway. Dark shade in circles indicates blindness.
A. Lesion of left optic nerve: Total blindness of left eye
B. Lesion of right optic nerve: Total blindness of right eye
C. Lesion of lateral fibers in left side of optic chiasma: Left nasal hemianopia
D. Lesion of lateral fibers in right side of optic chiasma: Right nasal hemianopia
   C + D. Lesion of lateral fibers in both sides of optic chiasma: Binasal hemianopia
E. Lesion of medial fibers in optic chiasma: Bitemporal hemianopia
F. Lesion of left optic radiation: Right homonymous hemianopia
G. Lesion of right optic radiation: Left homonymous hemianopia.

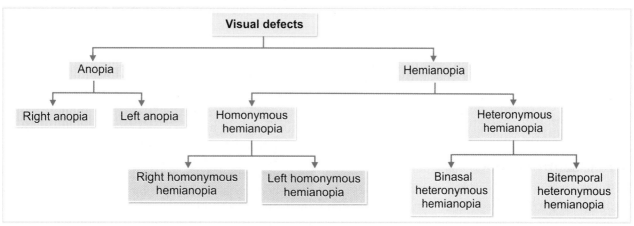

FIGURE 168.5: Visual defects

Pupillary Reflexes

■ INTRODUCTION

Pupillary reflexes are the **visceral reflexes,** which alter the size of pupil. Pupillary reflexes are classified into three types:

1. Light reflex
2. Ciliospinal reflex
3. Accommodation reflex.

■ LIGHT REFLEX

Light reflex is the reflex in which pupil constricts when light is flashed into the eyes. It is also called **pupillary light reflex.** Light reflex is of two types:

1. Direct light reflex
2. Indirect light reflex.

■ DIRECT LIGHT REFLEX

Direct light reflex is the reflex in which there is constriction of pupil in an eye when light is thrown into that eye. It is also called the **direct pupillary light reflex** or the direct reaction to light.

■ INDIRECT LIGHT REFLEX

Indirect light reflex is the reflex that involves constriction of pupil in both eyes when light is thrown into one eye. If light is flashed into one eye, the constriction of pupil occurs in the opposite eye, even though no light rays falls on that eye. It is otherwise called **consensual light reflex.**

■ PATHWAY FOR LIGHT REFLEX

Pathway for light reflex is slightly deviated from visual pathway. Fibers of light reflex pathway and the fibers of visual pathway are the same up to optic tract. Beyond that, these two sets of fibers are separated.

When light falls on the eye, the **visual receptors** are stimulated. Afferent (sensory) impulses from the receptors pass through the **optic nerve, optic chiasma** and **optic tract.** At the midbrain level, few fibers get separated from optic tract and synapse on the neurons of **pretectal nucleus,** which lies close to the superior colliculus. Pretectal nucleus of midbrain forms the **center for light reflexes.** Efferent (motor) impulses from this nucleus are carried by short fibers to **Edinger-Westphal nucleus** (parasympathetic nucleus) of **oculomotor nerve** (third cranial nerve). From Edinger-Westphal nucleus, preganglionic fibers pass through oculomotor nerve and reach the **ciliary ganglion.** Postganglionic fibers arising from ciliary ganglion pass through short ciliary nerves and reach the eyeball. These fibers cause contraction of constrictor pupillae muscle of iris (Fig. 169.1).

Reason for consensual light reflex is that, some of the fibers from pretectal nucleus of one side cross to the opposite side and end on opposite Edinger-Westphal nucleus.

■ CILIOSPINAL REFLEX

Ciliospinal reflex is the dilatation of pupil in eyes caused by painful stimulation of skin over the neck. It is due to the

contraction of dilator pupillae muscle. Sensory impulses pass through cutaneous afferent nerve. The center is in first thoracic spinal segment. Efferent impulses pass through sympathetic fibers and reach dilator pupillae.

■ ACCOMMODATION

■ DEFINITION

Accommodation is the adjustment of eye to see either near or distant objects clearly. It is the process by which light rays from near objects or distant objects are brought to a focus on sensitive part of retina. It is achieved by various adjustments made in the eyeball.

■ MECHANISM OF ACCOMMODATION

Light rays from distant objects are approximately **parallel** and are less refracted while getting focused on retina. But, the light rays from near objects are divergent. So, to be focused on retina, these light rays should be **refracted (converged)** to a greater extent. There are three possible ways by which, accommodation occurs:

1. Retina must be moved towards or away from the lens. It is done by shortening or elongation of eyeball. So, the divergent, parallel or convergent rays are focused accurately. This mechanism is present only in some molluscs and not in human beings.
2. Lens must be moved towards or away from the retina. It is done in photography. This mechanism exists in some fishes.
3. Convexity of lens must be altered, so that the refractory power of lens is altered according to the need. This mechanism is present in human eye and it was first suggested by **Young** and later supported by **Helmholtz** (Fig. 169.2).

Young-Helmholtz Theory

Young-Helmholtz theory describes how the curvature of lens increases and thereby, the refractive power of lens is enhanced. When the eyes are fixed on a distant object (distant vision) lens is flat due to the traction of suspensory ligaments, which extend from the capsule of lens and are attached to ciliary processes. Ciliary processes are attached to choroid through the ciliary muscle (Refer Fig. 169.1).

When vision is shifted from the distant object to a near object (near vision), ciliary muscle contracts and draws the choroid forward. Ciliary processes are brought closer to lens, i.e. these processes form a small circle. Suspensory ligaments are slackened. Now, the tension on lens is released. Lens, due to its elastic property, bulges forward. **Anterior curvature** (convexity) of lens

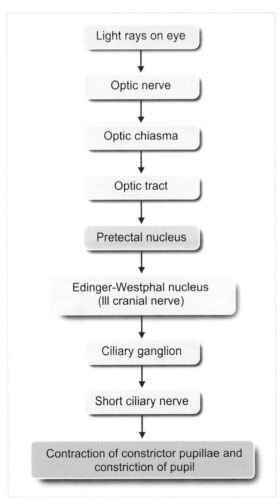

FIGURE 169.1: Pathway for light reflex

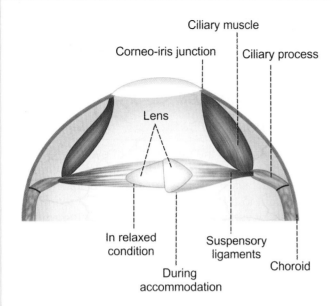

Ciliary muscle

Corneo-iris junction | Ciliary process

Lens

In relaxed condition

Suspensory ligaments

During accommodation

Choroid

FIGURE 169.2: Accommodation

increases greatly. A very little change occurs in posterior curvature. This can be demonstrated by using Purkinje-Sanson images.

In resting eye, the intraocular pressure sets up tension in choroids and pulls the ciliary processes backward and outward. Suspensory ligaments are tensed up and the lens becomes flat.

Purkinje-Sanson Images

Purkinje-Sanson images are used to demonstrate the change in convexity of lens during accommodation for near vision. A subject is made to sit in a darkroom. A lighted candle is held in front. One eye is opened and the other eye is closed. Three images of the flame are seen in the opened eye (Fig. 169.3).

First image is upright and bright. It shines from the surface of cornea, which acts as a mirror. Second image is upright, but dim. It is reflected from the anterior convex surface of the lens. Third image is inverted and small. It is formed by posterior surface of the lens, which acts as a concave mirror.

When the person looks at a distant object, the second image reflected from anterior surface of lens is near the third image from posterior surface. During accommodation for near vision, no change occurs either in first image or the third image. But, the second image becomes smaller and moves towards the first image.

Thus, the increased convexity of the anterior surface of lens during accommodation for near vision

is evident by the change in the size and the position of second image.

Other Adjustments in Eyeball during Accommodation

In addition to increase in anterior curvature of the lens, two more adjustments are made in the eyeball during accommodation for near vision.

1. Convergence of both eyeballs: It is necessary to bring the retinal images on to the corresponding points
2. Constriction of pupil: It is necessary to:
   i. Increase the visual acuity by reducing lateral chromatic and spherical aberrations
   ii. Reduce the quantity of light entering eye
   iii. Increase the depth of focus through more central part of lens as its convexity is increased.

During distant vision

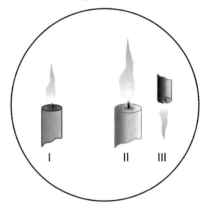

I II III

During near vision

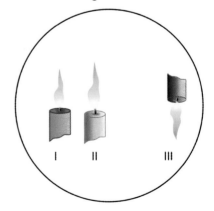

I II III

FIGURE 169.3: Purkinje-Sanson images

■ ACCOMMODATION REFLEX

Accommodation is a reflex action. When a person looks at a near object after seeing a far object, three adjustments are made in the eyeballs:

1. Convergence of the eyeballs due to contraction of the medial recti
2. Constriction of the pupil due to the contraction of constrictor pupillae of iris
3. Increase in the anterior curvature of the lens due to contraction of the ciliary muscle.

Thus, the accommodation reflex involves both skeletal muscle (medial recti) and smooth muscle (ciliary muscle and sphincter pupillae).

During accommodation, all the adjustments are carried out simultaneously. Although accommodation is a reflex action, it can be controlled by willpower to a certain extent.

■ PATHWAY FOR ACCOMMODATION REFLEX

Afferent Pathway

Visual impulses from retina pass through the optic nerve, optic chiasma, optic tract, lateral geniculate body and optic radiation to visual cortex (area 17) of occipital lobe. From here, the association fibers carry the impulses to frontal lobe (Fig. 169.4).

Center

The center for accommodation lies in frontal eye field (area 8) that is situated in the frontal lobe of cerebral cortex.

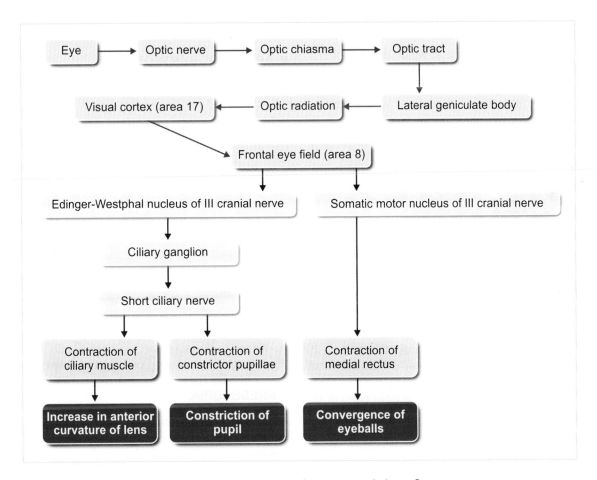

FIGURE 169.4: Pathway for accommodation reflex

Efferent Pathway

1. *Efferent fibers to ciliary muscle and sphincter pupillae*

From area 8, the corticonuclear fibers pass via internal capsule to the Edinger-Westphal nucleus of third cranial nerve. From here, the preganglionic fibers pass through the third cranial nerve to ciliary ganglion. Postganglionic fibers from ciliary ganglion pass via the short ciliary nerves and supply the ciliary muscle and the constrictor pupillae.

2. *Efferent fibers to medial rectus*

Some of the fibers from frontal eye field terminate in the somatic motor nucleus of oculomotor nerve. The fibers from motor nucleus supply medial rectus.

■ RANGE AND AMPLITUDE OF ACCOMMODATION

The farthest point from the eye at which the object can be seen is called **far point** or **punctum remotum.** In the normal eye, it is infinite, i.e. at a distance beyond 6 meters or 20 feet. It is limited only by the size of object, clearness of the atmosphere and the curvature of earth.

The nearest point from eye at which the object is seen clearly is called **near point** or **punctum proximum.** It is about 7 to 40 cm, depending upon the age. Distance between far point and near point is called **range of accommodation.**

Since, the focal length of eye is different in near vision and far vision, the refractive power of eye is also altered. The refractive power during far vision is called **static refraction** (R) and that during near vision is called **dynamic refraction** (P). The difference between these two refractive powers (P – R) is called **amplitude of accommodation,** which is expressed in diopter.

The **refractive power** is reciprocal of focal length and the unit for focal length is 1 meter or 100 cm. The refractory power is expressed as diopter (D).

For example, in a normal eye, if the near point is 10 cm, the dynamic refraction is:

$$P = \frac{1 \text{ meter}}{10 \text{ cm}} = \frac{100 \text{ cm}}{10 \text{ cm}} = 10 \text{ D}$$

In **emmetropic** (normal) **eye,** since the far point is at infinite distance, the static refraction is taken as zero. Now,

Amplitude of accommodation = P – R
= 10 – 0
= 10 D

Amplitude of Accommodation at Different Ages

Amplitude of accommodation varies with age. Amplitude of accommodation at different age groups is:

10 years	=	11.0 D
20 years	=	9.5 D
30 years	=	7.5 D
40 years	=	5.5 D
50 years	=	2.0 D
60 years	=	1.2 D
70 years	=	1.0 D

■ APPLIED PHYSIOLOGY

■ ARGYLL ROBERTSON PUPIL

Argyll Robertson pupil is a clinical condition in which the light reflex is lost but the accommodation reflex is present. It is common in tertiary syphilis. It also occurs because of lesion in Edinger-Westphal nucleus, diabetes and alcoholic neuropathy.

■ HORNER SYNDROME

Horner syndrome is an eye disorder caused by damage to cervical sympathetic nerve. It is also called **Bernard-Horner syndrome,** Claude Bernard-Horner syndrome or **oculosympathetic palsy.**

Symptoms of Horner syndrome appear on the affected side. The symptoms are:
1. **Ptosis** (drooping of upper eyelid)
2. Swelling of lower eyelid
3. **Miosis** (abnormal constriction of pupil)
4. **Enophthalmos** (sinking of eyeball into its cavity)
5. Absence of sweating on affected side of the face.

■ PRESBYOPIA

In old age, the amplitude of accommodation is decreased and the near point is away from the eye. This condition is called presbyopia. Details are given in Chapter 171.

Color Vision

■ INTRODUCTION

Human eye can recognize about 150 different colors in the visible spectrum. Discrimination and appreciation of colors depend upon the ability of receptors in retina.

■ VISIBLE SPECTRUM

■ SPECTRAL COLORS

When sunlight or white light is passed through a glass **prism,** it is separated into different colors. Series of colored light produced by the prism is called the visible spectrum. Colors that form the spectrum are called spectral colors. Spectral colors are red, orange, yellow, green, blue, indigo and violet (**ROYGBIV** or **VIBGYOR**). In the spectrum, colors occupy the position according to their wavelengths. **Wavelength** is the distance between two identical points in the wave of light energy. Accordingly, red has got the maximum wavelength of about 8,000 Å and the violet has got the minimum wavelength of about 3,000 Å.

Light rays longer than red are called **infrared rays.** Rays shorter than violet are called **ultraviolet rays.** But, these two extraordinary types of rays do not evoke the sensation of vision. Refraction of spectral colors by the prism also depends on wavelengths. Red is refracted less and violet is refracted more. So, longer the light rays, lesser is the refraction by the prism.

Purkinje Phenomenon

Purkinje phenomenon is the shift of brightest part of spectrum, when the intensity of illumination is changed.

When white light is passed through a prism, it splits into spectral colors from red to violet and if the colors are viewed at high illumination, the brightest part of the spectrum is the yellow, i.e. the brightest part of the spectrum is shifted to left. But when the light intensity is reduced to that of twilight, the color of the spectrum fades. Now the brightest part of spectrum is green, i.e. the brightest part of spectrum is shifted to right. It is called **Purkinje shift** or effect.

According to Purkinje, this effect is due to the maximal stimulation of cones by yellow and the maximal stimulation of rods by green.

■ EXTRASPECTRAL COLORS

Extraspectral colors are the colors other than those present in visible spectrum. These colors are formed by the combination of two or more spectral colors. For example, purple is the combination of violet and red. Pink is the combination of red and white.

■ PRIMARY COLORS

Primary colors are those, which when combined together produce the white. Primary colors are red, green and blue. These three colors in equal proportion give white.

■ COMPLEMENTARY COLORS

Complementary colors are the pair of two colors, which produce white when mixed or combined in proper proportion. Examples of complementary colors are red and greenish blue; orange and cyan blue; yellow and indigo blue; violet and greenish yellow; purple and green.

■ THEORIES OF COLOR VISION

Many theories are available to explain the mechanism of perception of color by eyes. However, most of the theories are not accepted universally. Following are the five theories, which are recognized:

■ 1. THOMAS YOUNG TRICHROMATIC THEORY

According to Thomas Young, retina has three types of cones. Each one possesses its own photosensitive substance. Each cone gives response to one of the primary colors – red, green and blue. Different color sensations are produced by the stimulation of various combinations of these three types of cones. For sensation of white light, all the three types of cones are stimulated equally.

■ 2. HELMHOLTZ TRICHROMATIC THEORY

Helmholtz substituted the **sensitive filaments** of optic nerve for cones. The sensitive filaments of nerves give response selectively to one or other of the three primary colors. It is also called Young-Helmholtz theory.

■ 3. GRANIT DOMINATOR-MODULATOR THEORY

Granit observed that the ganglionic cells of retina are stimulated by the whole of the visual spectrum. He studied the action potentials in ganglionic cells, which are stimulated by light and obtained some sensitivity curves. Sensitivity curves were recorded by using different wavelengths of light both in light-adapted and dark-adapted eyes. On the basis of these sensitivity curves, Granit classified the ganglionic cells into two groups namely, dominators and modulators.

Dominators

Dominators are responsible for brightness of light. Dominators are further divided into two types:
  i. Dominators for cones, which respond in light-adapted eye and a broad sensitivity curve is produced with the maximum response around the wavelengths 55 Å
  ii. Dominators for rods, which respond in dark-adapted eye and in the sensitivity curve the maximum response is given at the wavelengths of 500 Å.

Modulators

Modulators are responsible for different color sensations. Modulators are of three types:
  i. Modulators of blue, which are stimulated by light with wavelengths of 450 to 470 Å
  ii. Modulators of green, which are stimulated by light with wavelengths of 520 to 540 Å
  iii. Modulators of red-yellow, stimulated by light with wavelengths of 580 to 600 Å.

If green light falls on retina, modulators of green are stimulated and other two are less affected. Thus, according to Granit, the dominators are responsible for brightness or intensity of light, both in dark-adapted (rods) and light-adapted (cones) eyes. The modulators are responsible for color vision in light-adapted eyes.

■ 4. HARTRIDGE POLYCHROMATIC THEORY

According to this theory, human retina has seven types of receptors. All the seven receptors are divided into three units:

First Unit

First unit is a tricolor unit consisting of receptors for orange, green and blue.

Second Unit

Second unit is a dicolor unit with receptors for yellow and blue colors. Receptors for yellow and blue are complementary to each other.

Third Unit

Third unit is another dicolor unit with red and blue-green receptors.

■ 5. HERING'S THEORY OF OPPOSITE COLORS

According to Hering, retina has three photochemical substances. Each substance produces the sensation of a particular color by its breakdown or resynthesis.

First Substance

First substance is white-black substance. Its breakdown causes sensation of white and resynthesis causes sensation of black.

Second Substance

Second substance is yellow-blue substance. Its breakdown causes sensation of yellow and resynthesis causes sensation of blue.

Third Substance

Third substance is red-green substance. Its breakdown causes sensation of red and resynthesis causes sensation of green.

This theory explains the successive contrast and afterimages, but not the simultaneous sensation of antagonistic colors.

■ COLOR SENSITIVE AREAS IN RETINA

Peripheral part of retina is devoid of cones and is insensitive to color and gives sensation of white, black and grey only. Central portion of retina, fovea centralis

has more cones so, it is more sensitive to color. In extrafoveal regions, cones are mingled with rods.

Retinal area sensitive to blue is largest and to green is smallest. Red comes next to blue and then comes yellow. All the color areas of retina are mapped out by using perimeter.

■ CONTRAST EFFECTS

■ SIMULTANEOUS CONTRAST

Simultaneous contrast is the effect that intensifies the contrast (difference) between two colors, which are placed against each other. When black is placed against white or white against black, these two colors set one another off, i.e. the black looks blacker and the white looks whiter. Similarly, the green is enhanced by red and red by green.

Maximum effect of simultaneous contrast is obtained when the complementary colors are paired. Reason for simultaneous contrast is that, the stimulation of an area of retina by one color modifies the response in the surrounding or neighboring areas. It increases the sensitivity to other colors in the surrounding receptors. This action is probably due to horizontal cells.

■ SUCCESSIVE CONTRAST

Successive contrast is the effect of previously viewed color field on the appearance of currently viewed color field. When a person looks at a green object after looking at a bright red, the green object appears to be more greenish. There is an increase in the sensitivity to the complementary color.

Reason for successive contrast is that, the stimulation of an area of retina modifies its sensitivity to the successive stimuli. Thus, there is an increase in the sensitivity to the second color.

■ AFTERIMAGE

Afterimage is the phenomenon in which retention of image occurs even after cessation of light stimulus. After looking at a bright object, if the eyes are closed, the image remains more distinct for some time and then fades away gradually. Afterimage is of two types:

■ 1. POSITIVE AFTERIMAGE

Positive afterimage is an afterimage persisting after closure of eyes or turning towards a dark background. After looking at a bright object, if the eyes are closed or fixed on a black surface, the afterimage appears to be bright and with same color of the object.

■ 2. NEGATIVE AFTERIMAGE

Negative afterimage is an afterimage that persists while turning towards a bright background. After looking at bright object, if the eyes are fixed on white surface (instead of closing or fixing on a black surface), the afterimage appears in complementary color. Reason for negative afterimage is the persistence of activity in retina, even after the particular stimulus ceases to act.

■ APPLIED PHYSIOLOGY – COLOR BLINDNESS

Color blindness is the failure to appreciate one or more colors. It is common in 8% of males and only in 0.4% of females, as mostly the color blindness is an inherited sex-linked recessive character. In addition to hereditary conditions, color blindness occurs due to acquired conditions also such as ocular diseases or injury or disease of retina.

The term 'color blind' does not mean that objects are seen only in black and white. Total color blindness is very rare. There are many types and degrees of color blindness. The most appropriate term for color blindness is deficiency of color vision.

■ CAUSES FOR ACQUIRED COLOR BLINDNESS

1. Trauma

Injury to eye due to accidents or strokes results in color blindness.

2. Chronic Diseases

Color blindness is caused by chronic diseases such as:
  i. Glaucoma
  ii. Degeneration of macula of eye
  iii. Retinitis
  iv. Sickle cell anemia
  v. Leukemia
  vi. Diabetes
  vii. Liver diseases
  viii. Parkinson disease
  ix. Alzheimer disease
  x. Multiple sclerosis.

3. Drugs

Frequent use of some drugs leads to color blindness:
  i. Antibiotics
  ii. Antihypertensive drugs
  iii. Antituberculosis drugs
  iv. Barbiturates
  v. Drugs used to treat psychological problems and neural disorders.

4. Toxins

Industrial toxins or strong chemicals cause color blindness. Common substances causing color blindness are:
  i. Fertilizers
  ii. Carbon monoxide
  iii. Carbon disulfide
  iv. Chemicals with high lead content.

5. Alcoholism

Chronic alcoholism results in color blindness.

6. Aging

Color blindness can occur after 60 years of age due to various changes in eye.

■ CLASSIFICATION OF COLOR BLINDNESS

Based on Young-Helmholtz trichromatic theory, color blindness is classified into three types (Fig. 170.1):

1. Monochromatism

Monochromatism is the condition characterized by total inability to perceive color. It is also called **total color blindness** or **achromatopsia**. Monochromatism is very rare. Persons with monochromatism are called **monochromats.** Retina of monochromats is totally insensitive to color and they see the whole spectrum in only black, white and different shades of grey. So, their vision is similar to black and white photography. Monochromatism is divided into two types:

i. Rod monochromatism

Rod monochromatism is the condition in which cones are functionless and the vision depends purely on rods. So, **rod monochramats** are totally color blind. They are dazzled by light but definitely are not blind during daylight. Their visual acuity is lowered and foveal vision is absent which results in **central scotoma.** Central scotoma is the formation of big blind spot in fovea centralis due to the non-functioning of cones. Rods are also absent in fovea.

ii. Cone monochromatism

Cone monochromatism is the condition in which vision depends upon one single type of cone. Central scotoma does not occur in this condition.

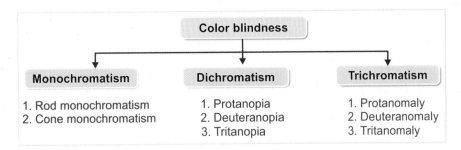

FIGURE 170.1: Color blindness

2. *Dichromatism*

Dichromatism is the color blindness in which the subject can appreciate only two colors. Persons with this defect are called **dichromats.** They can match entire spectrum of colors by only two primary colors because the receptors for third color are defective. The defects are classified into three groups:

i. *Protanopia*

Protanopia is the type of dichromatism caused by the defect in receptor of first primary color, i.e. red. So, the red color cannot be appreciated. Persons having protanopia are called **protanopes.** They use blue and green to match the colors. Thus, they confuse red with green.

ii. *Deuteranopia*

Deuteranopia is the dichromatism caused by the defect in receptor of second primary color, i.e. green. **Deuteranopes** use blue and red colors and they cannot appreciate green color.

iii. *Tritanopia*

Tritanopia is the dichromatism caused by the defect in receptor of third primary color, i.e. blue. **Tritanopes** use red and green colors and they cannot appreciate blue color.

3. *Trichromatism*

Trichromatism is the color blindness in which intensity of one of the primary colors cannot be appreciated correctly though the affected persons are able to perceive all the three colors. Persons with this defect are called **trichromats.** Even the dark shades of one particular color look dull for them. Trichromatism is classified into three types:

i. *Protanomaly*

Protanomaly is the type of trichromatism in which the perception for red is weak. So to appreciate red color, the person requires more intensity of red than a normal person.

ii. *Deuteranomaly*

Deuteranomaly is the trichromatism in which the perception for green is weak.

iii. *Tritanomaly*

Tritanomaly is the trichromatism with weak perception for blue.

■ TESTS FOR COLOR BLINDNESS

Three methods are available to determine the color blindness:
1. By using **Ishihara color charts**
2. By using **Holmgren colored wool**
3. By using **Edridge-Green lantern.**

Errors of Refraction

- ■ AMETROPIA
  - ■ MYOPIA OR SHORT SIGHTEDNESS
  - ■ HYPERMETROPIA OR LONG SIGHTEDNESS
- ■ ANISOMETROPIA
- ■ ASTIGMATISM
  - ■ CAUSE
  - ■ TYPES
  - ■ CORRECTION
- ■ PRESBYOPIA
  - ■ CAUSES
  - ■ CORRECTION

■ AMETROPIA

The eye with normal refractive power is called **emmetropic eye** and the condition is called **emmetropia**. Any deviation in the refractive power from normal condition, resulting in inadequate focusing on retina is called **ametropia** and the eye is called **ametropic eye**. The defect is due to the change in shape of the eyeball.

Ametropia is of two types:
1. Myopia
2. Hypermetropia.

■ MYOPIA OR SHORT SIGHTEDNESS

Myopia is the eye defect characterized by the inability to see the distant object. It is otherwise called short sightedness because the person can see near objects clearly but not the distant objects. In emmetropia, the far point is infinite. In myopia, the near vision is normal but the far point is not infinite, i.e. it is at a definite distance (Fig. 171.1 and Table 171.1). In extreme conditions, it may be only a few centimeter away from the eye (myo = half closed; ops = eye).

Cause

In myopia, the refractive power of lens is usually normal. But, the **anteroposterior diameter** of the eyeball is abnormally long. Therefore, the image is brought to focus a little in front of retina. Light rays, after coming to a focus, disperse again so, a blurred image is formed upon retina.

Correction

In myopic eye, in order to form a clear image on the retina, the light rays entering the eye must be divergent and not parallel. Thus, the myopic eye is corrected by using a **biconcave lens.** Light rays are diverged by the concave lens before entering the eye (Fig. 171.1).

■ HYPERMETROPIA OR LONG SIGHTEDNESS

Hypermetropia is the eye defect characterized by the inability to see near object. It is otherwise known as long sightedness because the person can see the distant objects clearly but not the near objects. It is also called **hyperopia.** In this defect, distant vision is normal but, near vision is affected (metras = measure).

Cause

Hypermetropia is due to **decreased anteroposterior diameter** of the eyeball. So, even though the refractive power of lens is normal, the light rays are not converged enough to form a clear image on retina, i.e. the light rays are brought to a focus behind retina. It causes a blurred image of near objects. Hypermetropia occurs in childhood, if the eyeballs fail to develop the correct size. It is common in old age also.

Correction

Hypermetropia is corrected by using **biconvex lens.** Light rays are converged by convex lens before entering the eye (Fig. 171.1).

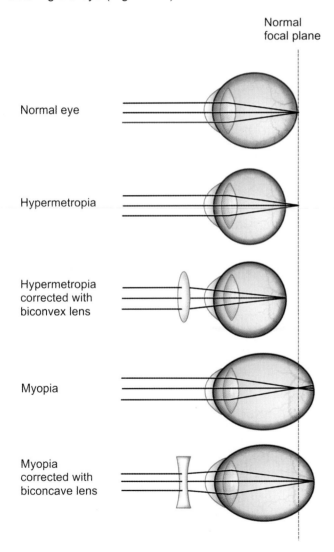

Normal focal plane

Normal eye

Hypermetropia

Hypermetropia corrected with biconvex lens

Myopia

Myopia corrected with biconcave lens

FIGURE 171.1: Errors of refraction

■ ANISOMETROPIA

Anisometropia is the condition in which the two eyes have **unequal refractive power.** It is corrected by using different appropriate lens for each eye (Table 171.1).

■ ASTIGMATISM

Astigmatism is the condition in which light rays are not brought to a sharp point upon retina. It is the common optical defect. This defect is present in all eyes. When it is moderate, it is known as **physiological astigmatism.** When it is well marked, it is considered abnormal. For example, the stars appear as small dots of light to a person with normal eye. But in astigmatism, the stars appear as radiating short lines of light (A = not; stigma = point).

■ CAUSE OF ASTIGMATISM

Light rays pass through all meridians of a lens. In a normal eye, lens has approximately same curvature in all meridians. So, the light rays are refracted almost equally in all meridians and brought to a focus.

If the curvature is different in different meridians, vertical, horizontal and oblique, the refractive power is also different in different meridians. The meridian with greater curvature refracts the light rays more strongly than the other meridians. So, these light rays are brought to a focus in front of the light rays, which pass through other meridians. Such irregularity of curvature of lens causes astigmatism.

■ TYPES OF ASTIGMATISM

Astigmatism is of two types:
1. Regular astigmatism
2. Irregular astigmatism.

1. Regular Astigmatism

In regular type of astigmatism, the refractive power is unequal in different meridians because of alteration of curvature in one meridian. But, it is uniform in all points throughout the affected meridian.

2. Irregular Astigmatism

In irregular type of astigmatism, the refractive power is unequal not only in different meridians, but it is also unequal in different points of same meridian.

TABLE 171.1: Errors of refraction

Type of error	Cause	Correction
Myopia	Increase in anteroposterior diameter of the eyeball	Biconcave lens
Hypermetropia	Decrease in anteroposterior diameter of the eyeball	Biconvex lens
Anisometropia	Difference in refractive power of both eyes	Separate lens (biconcave or biconvex) for each eye as required
Astigmatism	Refractory power of lens is different in different meridians	Cylindrical lens
Regular astigmatism	Refractory power of lens is unequal in different meridians but uniform in one single meridian	
Irregular astigmatism	Refractory power of lens is unequal in different meridians as well as in different points in same meridian	
Presbyopia	Loss of elasticity in lens and weakness of ocular muscles due to old age	Biconvex lens

■ CORRECTION OF ASTIGMATISM

Astigmatism is corrected by using **cylindrical glass** lens having the convexity in the meridians, corresponding to that of lens of eye having a lesser curvature, i.e. if the horizontal curvature of lens is less, the person should use cylindrical glass lens with the convexity in horizontal meridian.

■ PRESBYOPIA

Presbyopia is the condition characterized by progressive diminished ability of eyes to focus on near objects with age. It is due to the gradual reduction in the amplitude of accommodation. It progresses as the age advances (presbyos = old; ops = eye). Presbyopia starts developing after middle age. In presbyopia, the distant vision is unaffected. Only the near vision is affected. The near point is away from eye. In presbyopia, the anterior curvature of lens does not increase during near vision. So, the light rays from near objects are not brought to focus on retina.

■ CAUSES OF PRESBYOPIA

1. Decreased elasticity of lens is because of the physical changes in lens and its capsule during old age. So, the anterior curvature is not increased during near vision.
2. Decreased convergence of eyeballs due to the concomitant weakness of ocular muscles in old age.

■ CORRECTION OF PRESBYOPIA

Presbyopia is corrected by using **biconvex lens.**

Structure of Ear

■ **EXTERNAL EAR**
    ■ **AURICLE OR PINNA**
    ■ **EXTERNAL AUDITORY MEATUS**
■ **MIDDLE EAR**
    ■ **AUDITORY OSSICLES**
    ■ **AUDITORY MUSCLES**
    ■ **EUSTACHIAN TUBE**
■ **INTERNAL EAR**
    ■ **COCHLEA**
    ■ **COMPARTMENTS OF COCHLEA**
    ■ **ORGAN OF CORTI**

■ EXTERNAL EAR

Ear consists of three parts, namely external ear, middle ear and internal ear (Fig. 172.1).

External ear is formed by two parts:

1. Auricle or pinna
2. External auditory meatus.

■ AURICLE OR PINNA

Auricle or pinna of the external ear consists of **fibrocartilaginous plate** covered by connective tissue and skin. This plate is characteristically folded and ridged. Skin covering this plate is thin and contains many fine hairs and sebaceous glands. On the posterior surface of auricles, many sweat glands are present.

In many animals, auricle can be moved and turned to locate the source of sound or the auricle can be folded to avoid unwanted sound. But in man, extrinsic and intrinsic muscles of auricles are rudimentary and the movement is not possible. The depression of auricle, which forms the orifice of external auditory meatus, is called **concha.**

■ EXTERNAL AUDITORY MEATUS

External auditory meatus starts from the concha and extends inside as a slightly curved canal, with a length of about 55 mm.

Meatus consists of two parts:

i. Outer cartilaginous part
ii. Inner bony part.

i. *Outer Cartilaginous Part*

Cartilaginous part is the initial part of external auditory meatus and is made up of cartilage. It is covered by thick skin, which contains stiff hairs. These hairs prevent the entry of foreign particles.

Large **sebaceous glands** and **ceruminous glands** are also present in the skin covering this portion. These glands are coiled and tubular in nature and open on the surface of the skin. Columnar epithelial cells of the glands contain brown pigment granules and fat droplets. Secretions of ceruminous glands, sebaceous glands and desquamated epithelial cells form the earwax.

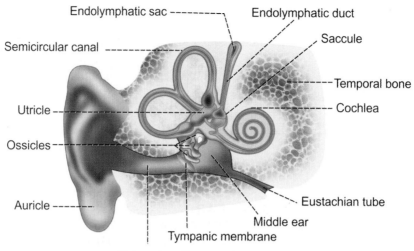

FIGURE 172.1: Diagram showing the structure of ear

ii. *Inner Bony Part*

Inner part of the external auditory meatus is also covered by skin, which adheres closely to periosteum. Only sebaceous glands are present here. Small fine hairs are present on the superior wall of the canal. Skin covering this portion is continuous with cuticular layer of tympanic membrane.

■ MIDDLE EAR

Middle ear or tympanic cavity is a small, narrow, irregular, laterally compressed chamber, situated within the temporal bone. It is also known as **tympanum.** It is separated from external auditory meatus by **tympanic membrane.**

Middle ear consists of the following structures:
1. Auditory ossicles
2. Auditory muscles
3. Eustachian tube.

Tympanic Membrane

Tympanic membrane is a thin, semitransparent membrane, which separates the middle ear from external auditory meatus. Periphery of the membrane is fixed to tympanic sulcus in the surrounding bony ring, by means of fibrocartilage (Fig. 172.2).

Structure of Tympanic Membrane

Tympanic membrane is formed by three layers:
1. Lateral cutaneous layer, which is the continuation of the skin of auditory meatus

2. Intermediate fibrous layer, which contains collagenous fibers
3. Medial mucus layer or tympanic mucosa, which is composed of single layer of cuboidal epithelial cells.

■ AUDITORY OSSICLES

Auditory ossicles are the three miniature bones, which are arranged in the form of a chain, extending across the middle ear from the tympanic membrane to oval window (Fig. 172.2).

Auditory ossicles are:
i. Malleus
ii. Incus
iii. Stapes.

i. *Malleus*

Malleus is otherwise called **hammer.** It has a handle, head and neck. **Hand** is called **manubrium** and it is attached to tympanic membrane. Neck extends from handle to the head. **Head** or **capitulum** articulates with the body of incus.

ii. *Incus*

Incus is also known as **anvil.** It looks like a premolar tooth. Incus has a body, one long process and one short process. Anterior surface of the body articulates with the head of malleus. The **short process** is attached to a ligament. The **long process** runs parallel to handle of malleus. Tip of the long process is like a knob called **lenticular process** and it articulates with the next bone, stapes.

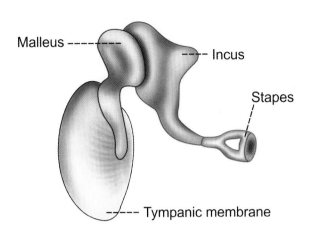

Malleus

Incus

Stapes

Tympanic membrane

FIGURE 172.2: Tympanic membrane and auditory ossicles

iii. *Stapes*

Stapes is also called **stirrup.** It is the smallest bone in the body. It has a head, neck, anterior crus, posterior crus and a footplate. **Head** articulates with incus. **Footplate** fits into oval window.

■ AUDITORY MUSCLES

Two skeletal muscles are attached to ossicles:
  i. Tensor tympani
  ii. Stapedius.

i. *Tensor Tympani*

Tensor tympani is larger of the two muscles of tympanic cavity.

Origin, insertion and nerve supply

Tensor tympani arises from cartilaginous portion of eustachian tube (see below), adjacent to great wing of sphenoid bone and osseous canal. Its tendon is inserted on manubrium of malleus, which is in turn attached to tympanic membrane. Thus, the tensor tympani is attached to tympanic membrane through malleus. It is supplied by mandibular division trigeminal nerve.

Function

Tensor tympani muscle pulls and keeps the tympanic membrane stretched or tensed constantly. This constant stretching of tympanic membrane is essential for the transmission of sound waves, which may reach any part of the tympanic membrane. Paralysis of tensor tympani causes hearing impairment.

ii. *Stapedius*

Stapedius is the **smallest skeletal muscle** in human body with a length of just over 1 mm. It lies in a conical bony cavity, on the posterior wall of the tympanic cavity.

Origin, insertion and nerve supply

Stapedius arises from interior pyramid of tympanic cavity. Its tendon is inserted into the posterior surface of neck of stapes. It is supplied by branch of facial nerve.

Function

Stapedius prevents excess movements of stapes. When it contracts, it pulls the neck of stapes backwards and reduces the movement of footplate against the fluid in cochlea. Paralysis of stapedius allows wider range of oscillation of stapes, leading to **hyper-reaction** of auditory ossicles to sound vibrations This condition is called **hyperacusis.** Paralysis of stapedius occurs in the lesion of facial nerve.

Tympanic Reflex

Tympanic reflex is an **attenuation reflex** characterized by involuntary contraction of tensor tympani and stapedius muscles, in response to a loud noise. It has a latent period of 40 to 80 millisecond.

When both the muscles contract, manubrium of malleus moves inward and stapes is pulled outward. These two actions result in stiffness of auditory ossicles, so that the transmission of sound is decreased.

Significance of tympanic reflex

  i. Tympanic reflex protects the tympanic membrane from being ruptured by loud sound
  ii. It also prevents fixation of footplate of stapes, against oval window, during exposure to loud sound
  iii. It helps to protect the cochlea from damaging effects of loud sounds. Contraction of tensor tympani and stapedius during exposure to loud sound develops stiffness of the auditory ossicles so that, the transmission of sound into cochlea is decreased.

■ EUSTACHIAN TUBE

Eustachian tube or the **auditory tube** is the flattened canal extending from the anterior wall of middle ear to nasopharynx. Its upper part is surrounded by the bony wall and the lower part is surrounded by fibrocartilaginous plate.

Eustachian tube connects middle ear with posterior part of nose and forms the passage of air between middle ear and atmosphere. So, the pressure on both sides of tympanic membrane is equalized.

■ INTERNAL EAR

Internal ear or labyrinth is a membranous structure, enclosed by a bony labyrinth in petrous part of temporal bone. It consists the sense organs of hearing and equilibrium. Sense organ for hearing is the cochlea and the sense organ for equilibrium is the vestibular apparatus. Vestibular apparatus is already explained in Chapter 158.

■ COCHLEA

Cochlea is a coiled structure like a snail's shell (cochlea = snail's shell). It consists of two structures:
1. Central conical axis formed by spongy bone called **modiolus**
2. Bony canal or tube, which winds around the modiolus.

In man, the **bony canal** makes two and a half turns, starting from the base of the cochlea and ends at the top (apex) of cochlea. End of the canal is called **cupula.** Base of modiolus forms the bottom of internal auditory meatus, through which cochlear nerve fibers pass and enter the modiolus. Thus, a section through the axis of cochlea reveals the central **bony pillar,** modiolus and **periotic or osseous canal,** which coils around the modiolus.

From modiolus, a bony ridge called **osseous spiral lamina** projects into the canal, winding around modiolus like the thread of a screw. Spiral lamina follows the spiral turns of cochlea and ends at the cupula in a hook-shaped process called **hamulus.**

■ COMPARTMENTS OF COCHLEA

Two membranous partitions extend between the osseous spiral lamina and outer wall of the **spiral canal.** Both the membranes divide the spiral canal of cochlea into three compartments.

Membranes of cochlea:
1. Basilar membrane
2. Vestibular membrane.

1. *Basilar Membrane*

Basilar membrane is a connective tissue membrane. It stretches from the tip of the osseous spiral lamina to tough dense fibrous band called **spiral ligament,** which lines the outer wall of the canal. Basilar mem-

brane is also called **membranous spiral lamina.** Along the basilar membrane are twenty thousand to thirty thousand tiny fibers that are called **basilar fibers.** Each fiber has different size and shape. Fibers near the oval window are short and stiff. While approaching towards **helicotrema** (see below) the basilar fibers gradually become longer and soft.

2. *Vestibular Membrane*

Vestibular membrane is also known as **Reissner membrane** and it is a thin membrane. It is placed obliquely between the upper surface of osseous spiral lamina and upper part of spiral ligament.

Basilar membrane and vestibular membrane divide the spiral canal of cochlea into three compartments called scalae (Fig. 172.3).

Compartments of spiral canal of cochlea:
   i. Scala vestibuli
   ii. Scala tympani
   iii. Scala media.

All the three compartments are filled with fluid. Scala vestibuli and scala tympani contain **perilymph.** Scala media is filled with **endolymph.**

i. *Scala vestibuli*

Scala vestibuli lies above scala media. It arises from **oval window (fenestra vestibuli),** which is closed by the

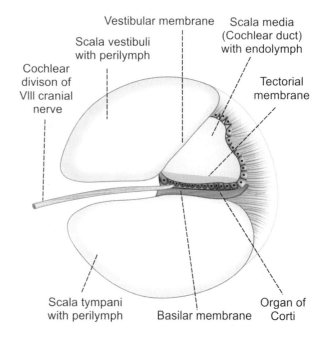

Vestibular membrane Scala media (Cochlear duct) with endolymph
Scala vestibuli with perilymph
Cochlear divison of VIII cranial nerve
Tectorial membrane
Scala tympani with perilymph   Basilar membrane   Organ of Corti

FIGURE 172.3: Cross-section of spiral canal of cochlea

footplate of stapes. It follows the bony canal up to its apex. At the apex, it communicates with the scala tympani through a small canal called **helicotrema.**

ii. Scala tympani

Scala tympani lies below scala media. It is parallel to scala vestibuli and ends at the round window. **Round window** is closed by a strong thin membrane known as **secondary tympanic membrane.**

iii. Scala media

Scala media is otherwise called **cochlear duct, membranous cochlea** or **otic cochlea.** It is a triangular compartment enclosed by basilar and vestibular membranes. It ends blindly at the apex and at the base of cochlea. A slender **ductus reuniens** arises from the basal end and connects scala media with the saccule of otolith organ.

Scala media is formed by upper, outer and lower walls. Upper wall or vestibular wall is formed by **vestibular membrane.** Outer wall is formed by spiral ligament, which is the thickening of periosteum. Lower wall is called **tympanic wall.** It is formed by **basilar membrane** (membranous spiral lamina) and a part of osseous spiral lamina. Scala media stretches between the tip of osseous spiral lamina and spiral ligament.

Basilar membrane consists of straight unbranched connective tissue fibers, which are called basilar fibers or the auditory fibers. On the upper surface of the basilar membrane, epithelial cells are arranged in the form a special structure called the organ of Corti. It is the sensory part of cochlea.

■ ORGAN OF CORTI

Organ of Corti is the **receptor organ** for hearing. It is the neuroepithelial structure in cochlea (Fig. 172.4).

Situation and Extent

Organ of corti rests upon the lip of osseous spiral lamina and basilar membrane. It extends throughout the cochlear duct, except for a short distance on either end. Roof of the organ of Corti is formed by **gelatinous tectorial membrane.**

Structure

Organ of Corti is made up of sensory elements called **hair cells** and various supporting cells. All the cells of organ of Corti are arranged in order from center towards the periphery of the cochlea.

Cells of organ of Corti:

1. Border cells
2. Inner hair cells
3. Inner phalangeal cells
4. Inner pillar cells
5. Outer pillar cells
6. Outer phalangeal cells
7. Outer hair cells
8. Cells of Hensen
9. Cells of Claudius
10. Tectorial membrane and lamina reticularis.

1. Border Cells

Border cells are the slender columnar cells, arranged in a single layer on the tympanic lip along the inner side of inner hair cells. Surfaces of the border cells have **cuticle.**

2. Inner Hair Cells

Inner hair cells are flask-shaped cells and are broader than the outer hair cells. Inner hair cells are arranged in a single row and occupy only the upper part of epithelial layer. Rounded base of each cell rests on the adjacent supporting cells called the inner phalangeal cell. Surface of the inner hair cell bears a **cuticular plate** and a number of short stiff hairs, which are called **stereocilia.** Each hair cell has about 100 sterocilia. One of the sterocilia is larger and it is called **kinocilium.** Stereocilia are in contact with the **tectorial membrane.** Inner hair cells and outer hair cells together form the receptor cells. Sensory nerve fibers are distributed around the hair cells. Both inner hair cells and outer hair cells have afferent and efferent nerve fibers (Chapter 173).

3. Inner Phalangeal Cells

Inner phalangeal cells are the supporting cells of inner hair cells and are arranged in a row along the inner surface of inner pillar cells. Their bases rest on the basilar membrane. Cuticular plate of cells (formed by the lower portion of cells) look like the finger bones, phalanges.

4 and 5. Inner and Outer Pillar Cells – Rods of Corti

Inner and outer pillar cells are called rods of Corti. Each pillar cell has a broader base, an elongated body

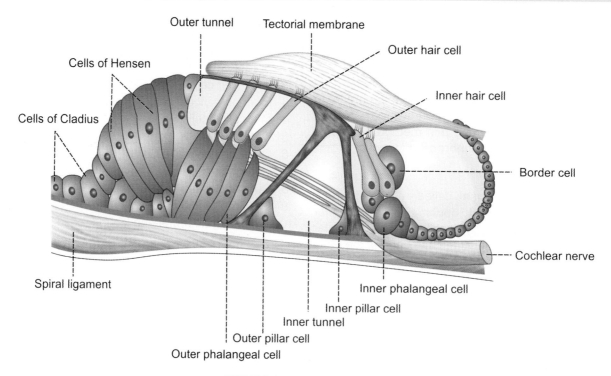

FIGURE 172.4: Organ of Corti

or pillar and a head at the tip of pillar. Bases of inner pillar cells are close to the lip of osseous spiral lamina (tympanic lip), whereas the bases of outer pillar cells are close to basilar membrane. Pillars of inner and outer pillar cells slope towards each other and their heads articulate. Thus, the pillars of cells form series of arches, which enclose a triangular tunnel called **inner tunnel** or **tunnel of Corti.**

6. *Outer Phalangeal Cells*

Outer phalangeal cells or the cells of Deiters are the supporting cells of outer hair cells. Outer phalangeal cell is the tall columnar cell. It sends stiff phalangeal processes upward between the hair cells, to form the part of **lamina reticularis.**

Rows of outer phalangeal cells vary in different regions of cochlear duct like the outer hair cells, i.e. from three to five rows. Between the inner most outer phalangeal cells and outer pillar cells, is a fluid space known as the **space of Nuel.**

7. *Outer Hair Cells*

Outer hair cells are the columnar cells occupying the superficial part of epithelium of organ of Corti. Their bases are supported by outer phalangeal cells. Structure of outer hair cells is similar to that of inner hair cells (see above).

8. *Cells of Hensen*

Cells of Hensen are tall columnar cells forming the outer border cells of organ of Corti. These cells are arranged in several rows on basilar membrane, lateral to outer phalangeal cells. The space between outer phalangeal cells and cells of Hensen is called outer tunnel.

9. *Cells of Claudius*

Cells of Claudius are cuboidal in nature and line the lower surface of external spiral sulcus. In certain areas, some groups of cells are present between the cells of Claudius and basilar membrane. These cells are called Boettcher cells.

10. *Tectorial Membrane and Lamina Reticularis*

Tectorial membrane extends from vestibular lip to the level of cells of Hensen. It forms the roof of organ of Corti. It is in contact with the processes of hair cells. It is assumed that the processes of hair cells are stimulated by the movements of tectorial membrane, in relation to vibrations in endolymph.

Cuticular plates of all the supporting cells collectively form a reticular membrane, which is known as lamina reticularis. It covers the organ of Corti. It looks like a mosaic and has rows of holes, through which the heads of hair cells are inserted.

Auditory Pathway

```
■ INTRODUCTION
■ RECEPTORS
■ FIRST ORDER NEURONS
■ SECOND ORDER NEURONS
■ THIRD ORDER NEURONS
■ CORTICAL AUDITORY CENTERS
■ APPLIED PHYSIOLOGY – EFFECT OF LESION
```

■ INTRODUCTION

Fibers of auditory pathway pass through **cochlear division** of **vestibulocochlear nerve** (VIII cranial nerve). It is also known as **auditory nerve.** Major part of the auditory pathway lies in medulla oblongata, midbrain and thalamic region.

Higher center for hearing is in temporal lobe of cerebral cortex, where the fibers of auditory pathway finally terminate. Fibers are both crossed and uncrossed, so that each cochlea is represented in the cortex on both sides.

■ RECEPTORS

Hair cells in organ of Corti are the receptors of the auditory sensation. Hair cells are of two types, outer hair cell and inner hair cell. All the hair cells are innervated by afferent and efferent nerve fibers. Afferent nerve fibers from the hair cells form auditory nerve (see below).

■ FIRST ORDER NEURONS

First order neurons of auditory pathway are the **bipolar cells of spiral ganglion,** situated in modiolus of cochlea (Fig. 173.1).

Peripheral short processes (dendrites) of the bipolar cells are distributed around hair cells of organ of Corti as afferent nerve fibers. Their long processes

(axons) leave the ear as cochlear nerve fibers and enter medulla oblongata. In medulla oblongata, these fibers divide into two groups, which end on ventral cochlear nucleus and dorsal cochlear nucleus of the same side in medulla oblongata.

Efferent Nerve Fibers to Hair Cells

Efferent nerve fibers of hair cells arise from **superior olivary nucleus.** Fibers from this nucleus reach the hair cells by passing through the ventral and dorsal cochlear nuclei and cochlear nerve of the same side.

Efferent nerve fiber to outer hair cell terminates directly on the cell body and controls the motility of this cell (Chapter 174). Efferent nerve fiber to inner hair cell terminates on the auditory (afferent) nerve fiber, where it leaves the inner hair cell. It controls the impulse output from this hair cell.

■ SECOND ORDER NEURONS

Neurons of **dorsal** and **ventral cochlear nuclei** in the medulla oblongata form the second order neurons of auditory pathway. Axons of the second order neurons run in four different groups:
1. First group of fibers cross the midline and run to the opposite side, to form **trapezoid body.** Fibers from trapezoid body go to the **superior olivary nucleus.**

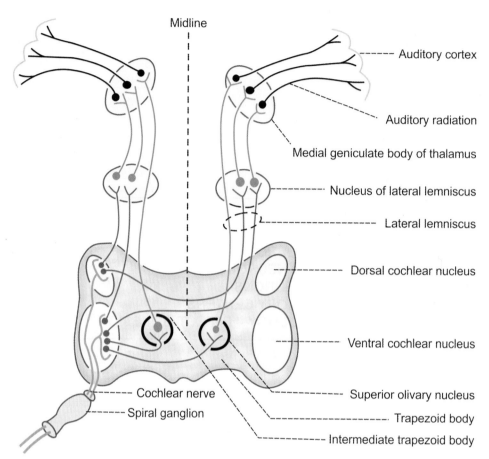

Midline

- - - - Auditory cortex

- - - - Auditory radiation

Medial geniculate body of thalamus

- - - - Nucleus of lateral lemniscus

- - - - Lateral lemniscus

- - - - Dorsal cochlear nucleus

- - - - Ventral cochlear nucleus

- - - - Superior olivary nucleus

- - - - Trapezoid body

- - - - Intermediate trapezoid body

- - - - Cochlear nerve
- - - - Spiral ganglion

FIGURE 173.1: Auditory pathway. Blue = First order neuron, Red = Second order neuron, Green = Third order neuron, Black = Auditory radiation.

2. Second group of fibers terminate at superior olivary nucleus of same side via trapezoid body of the same side
3. Third group of fibers run in lateral lemniscus of the same side and terminate in **nucleus of lateral lemniscus** of same side
4. Fourth group of fibers run into reticular formation, cross the midline as **intermediate trapezoid fibers** and finally join the nucleus of lateral lemniscus of opposite side.

■ THIRD ORDER NEURONS

Third order neurons are in the **superior olivary nuclei** and **nucleus of lateral lemniscus.** Fibers of the third order neurons end in medial **geniculate body,** which forms the **subcortical auditory center.**

Fibers from medial geniculate body go to the temporal cortex, via internal capsule as **auditory**

radiation. Some fibers from medial geniculate body go to **inferior colliculus** of tectum in midbrain. The fibers of auditory radiation are involved in reflex movement of head, in response to auditory stimuli.

■ CORTICAL AUDITORY CENTERS

Cortical auditory centers are in the temporal lobe of cerebral cortex (Chapter 152).
Auditory areas are:
1. Primary auditory area, which includes area 41, area 42 and Wernicke area
2. Secondary auditory area or auditopsychic area, which includes area 22.
Areas 41 and 42 are the primary auditory areas situated in the anterior transverse gyrus and lateral surface of superior temporal gyrus. Wernicke area is in upper part of superior temporal gyrus, posterior to areas 41 and 42. Area 22 occupies the superior temporal gyrus.

■ FUNCTIONS OF CORTICAL AUDITORY CENTERS

Cortical auditory centers are concerned with the perception of auditory impulses, analysis of pitch and intensity of sound and determination of source of sound.

Areas 41 and 42 are concerned with the perception of auditory impulses only. However, analysis and interpretation of sound are carried out by Wernicke area, with the help of area 22.

■ APPLIED PHYSIOLOGY – EFFECT OF LESION

1. Lesion of cochlear nerve causes **deafness** of the ear
2. Unilateral lesion of auditory pathway, above the level of cochlear nuclei causes **diminished hearing**
3. Degeneration of hair cells in the organ of Corti leads to **presbycusis.** Presbycusis is the gradual loss of hearing. It is common in old age.
4. Lesion in superior olivary nucleus results in **poor localization of sound.**

Mechanism of Hearing

Chapter 174

■ INTRODUCTION

Sound waves travel through external auditory meatus and produce vibrations in the tympanic membrane. Vibrations from tympanic membrane travel through malleus and incus and reach the stapes resulting in the movement of stapes. Movements of stapes produce vibrations in the fluids of cochlea. These vibrations stimulate the hair cells in organ of Corti. This, in turn, causes generation of action potential (auditory impulses) in the auditory nerve fibers. When auditory impulses reach the cerebral cortex, the perception of hearing occurs.

Thus, during the process of hearing, ear converts energy of sound waves into action potentials in auditory nerve fibers. This process is called **sound transduction.**

■ ROLE OF EXTERNAL EAR

External ear directs the sound waves towards tympanic membrane. Sound waves produce pressure changes over the surface of tympanic membrane. Accumulation of wax prevents conduction of sound. In many animals, the auricle (pinna) can be turned to locate the source of sound. Auricle can be folded to avoid unwanted sound. But in man, the extrinsic and intrinsic muscles of auricle are rudimentary and the movement is not possible.

■ ROLE OF MIDDLE EAR

■ ROLE OF TYMPANIC MEMBRANE

Due to the pressure changes produced by sound waves, tympanic membrane vibrates, i.e. it moves in and out of middle ear. Thus, tympanic membrane acts as a **resonator** that reproduces the vibration of sound.

■ ROLE OF AUDITORY OSSICLES

Vibrations set up in tympanic membrane are transmitted through the malleus and incus and reach the stapes, causing to and fro movement of stapes against oval window and against perilymph present in scala vestibuli of cochlea.

Impedance Matching

Impedance matching is the process by which tympanic membrane and auditory ossicles convert the sound energy into mechanical vibrations in cochlear fluid with minimum loss of energy by matching the impedance offered by fluid.

Impedance means obstruction or opposition to the passage of sound waves. When sound waves reach inner ear, the fluid (perilymph) in cochlea offers impedance, i.e. the fluid resists the transmission of sound due to its own inertia. Tympanic membrane and auditory ossicles effectively reduce the sound impedance.

Sound waves are conducted from external ear to inner ear, with an impedance of only 40%. Remaining 60% of sound energy developed in tympanic membrane is transmitted to cochlear fluid by the ossicles. Thus, along with the help of tympanic membrane, ossicles match the impedance offered by fluid to a great extent. It is because, the ossicles act like a **lever system** so that stapes exerts a greater force (pressure) against the cochlear fluid. This results in generation of vibrations in the cochlear fluid. The increased force is very essential to set up the vibrations in cochlear fluid because of higher inertia of the fluid.

Force exerted by footplate of stapes on cochlear fluid is 17 to 22 times greater than the force exerted by sound waves at the tympanic membrane. It is because of two structural features of ossicles:

1. Head of malleus is longer than long process of incus so that a higher force is generated in small structure
2. Surface area of tympanic membrane (55 sq mm) is larger compared to that of footplate of stapes (3.2 sq mm). So the pressure increases when force is applied to small area.

Thus, the tympanic membrane and the auditory ossicles are capable of converting the sound energy into mechanical vibrations in cochlear fluid with minimum loss of energy.

Significance of impedance matching

Impedance matching is the most important function of middle ear. Because of impedance matching the sound waves (stimuli) are transmitted to cochlea with minimum loss of intensity. Without impedance matching conductive deafness occurs.

Types of Conduction

Conduction of sound from external ear to internal ear through middle ear occurs by three routes:
1. Ossicular conduction
2. Air conduction
3. Bone conduction.

1. Ossicular conduction

Ossicular conduction is the conduction of sound waves through middle ear by auditory ossicles. In normal conditions, the sound waves are conducted through auditory ossicles.

2. Air conduction

Air conduction is the conduction of sound waves through air in middle ear. If the ossicular chain is broken, conduction occurs in an alternate route of air conduction. Air conduction is common in otosclerosis. **Otosclerosis** is the disease associated with fixation of stapes to oval window.

3. Bone conduction

Bone conduction is the conduction of sound waves through middle ear by bones. It occurs when middle ear is affected. In this type of conduction, sound waves are transmitted to cochlear fluid by the vibrations set up in skull bones. Bone conduction is tested by placing vibrating tuning forks or other vibrating bodies directly on the skull. This route plays a role in transmission of extremely loud sounds.

■ ROLE OF EUSTACHIAN TUBE

Eustachian tube is not concerned with hearing directly. However, it is responsible for **equalizing the pressure** on either side of tympanic membrane.

■ ROLE OF INNER EAR

■ TRAVELING WAVE

Movement of footplate of stapes against oval window causes movement of perilymph in scala vestibuli. This fluid does not move all the way from oval window to round window through helicotrema. It immediately hits the vestibular membrane near oval window. This causes movement of fluid in scala media, since the vestibular membrane is flexible.

Movement of fluid in scala media causes bulging of basal portion of basilar membrane towards scala tympani (Fig. 174.1).

Bulging of basilar membrane increases the elastic tension in basilar fibers in that portion of basilar membrane. Elastic tension in basilar fibers initiates a wave, which travels along basilar membrane towards the helicotrema like that of arterial pulse wave. It is called **traveling wave.**

Resonance Point

Resonance point is the part of basilar membrane, which is activated by traveling wave. In the beginning, each traveling wave is weak (Fig. 174.2). While traveling through basilar membrane from base towards apex (helicotrema), the wave becomes stronger and stronger and at one point (resonance point) of basilar membrane, it becomes very strong and activates the basilar membrane. This resonance point of basilar membrane immediately vibrates back and forth. The traveling wave stops here and does not travel further.

Distance between stapes and resonance point is inversely proportional to frequency of sound waves reaching the ear. Traveling wave generated by high-pitched sound disappears near the base of the cochlea. Wave generated by medium-pitched sound reaches half of the way and the wave generated by low-pitched sound travels the entire distance of basilar membrane.

■ EXCITATION OF HAIR CELLS

Stereocilia of hair cells in organ of Corti are embedded in tectorial membrane. Hair cells are tightly fixed by cuticular lamina reticularis and the pillar cells or rods of Corti.

When traveling wave causes vibration of basilar membrane at the resonance point, the basilar fiber, rods of Corti, hair cells and lamina reticularis move as a single unit. It causes movements of stereocilia leading to excitement of hair cells and generation of receptor potential.

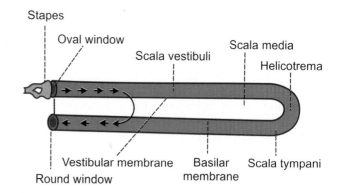

FIGURE 174.1: Diagrammatic representation of cochlea. Arrows show displacement of fluid

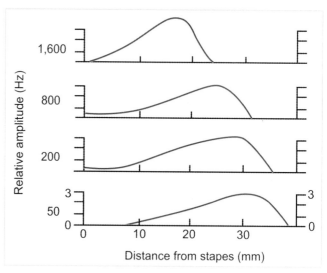

FIGURE 174.2: Traveling waves for different frequencies of sound

■ ELECTRICAL EVENTS DURING PROCESS OF HEARING

■ SOUND TRANSDUCTION

Sound transduction is a type of sensory transduction (Chapter 139) in the hair cell (receptor cells) in organ of Corti by which the sound energy is converted into action potentials in the auditory nerve fiber.

Electrical Events of Sound Transduction

Three types of electrical events that occur during sound transduction are:

1. Receptor potential or the cochlear microphonic potential
2. Endocochlear potential or endolymphatic potential
3. Action potential in auditory nerve fiber.

■ RECEPTOR POTENTIAL OR COCHLEAR MICROPHONIC POTENTIAL

Receptor potential or cochlear microphonic potential is the **mild depolarization** that is developed in the hair cells of cochlea when sound waves are transmitted to internal ear. Resting membrane potential in hair cells is –60 mV. Sensory transduction mechanism in cochlear receptor cells is different from the mechanism in other sensory receptors.

When sound waves reach internal ear traveling wave is produced. It causes vibration of basilar membrane, which moves stereocilia of hair cells away from modiolus (towards kinocilium). It causes opening of mechanically gated potassium channels (Chapter 3) and influx of potassium ions from endolymph, which contains large amount of potassium ions. Influx of potassium ions causes development of **mild depolarization** (receptor potential) in hair cells up to –50 mV.

Cochlear microphonic potential is non-propagative. But, it causes generation of action potential in auditory nerve fiber. Due to depolarization hair cells release a neurotransmitter, which generates action potential in the auditory nerve fibers. Probable neurotransmitter may be **gulatamate.**

Movement of stereocilia away from modiolus (towards kinocilium) causes **depolarization** in hair cells. Movement of stereocilia in the opposite direction (away from kinocilium) causes **hyperpolarization.** Ionic basis of hyperpolarization is not clearly known. It is suggested that **calcium** plays an important role in this process. Hyperpolarization in hair cells stops generation of action potential in auditory nerve fiber.

■ ROLE OF HAIR CELLS

Inner hair cells and outer hair cells have different roles during sound transduction.

Role of Inner Hair Cells

Inner hair cells are responsible for sound transduction, i.e. these receptor cells are the primary sensory cells, which cause the generation of action potential in auditory nerve fibers.

Role of Outer Hair Cells

Outer hair cells have a different action. These hair cells are shortened during depolarization and elongated during hyperpolarization. This process is called electromotility or mechanoelectrical transduction. This action of outer hair cells facilitates the movement of basilar membrane and increases the amplitude and sharpness of sound. Hence, the outer hair cells are collectively called **cochlear amplifier.** The electromotility of hair cell is due to the presence of a contractile protein, **prestin** (named after a musical notation **presto**).

Role of Efferent Nerve Fibers of Hair Cells

Efferent nerve fibers (Chapter 173) of hair cells also play important role during sound transduction by releasing acetylcholine.

Efferent nerve fiber to inner hair cell terminates on the auditory (afferent) nerve fiber where it leaves the inner hair cell. It controls the generation of action potential in auditory nerve fiber by inhibiting the release of glutamate from inner hair cells.

Efferent nerve fiber to outer hair cell terminates directly on the cell body. It inhibits the electromotility of this cell.

■ ENDOCOCHLEAR POTENTIAL OR ENDOLYMPHATIC POTENTIAL

Endocochlear or endolymphatic potential is the electrical potential developed in fluids outside the hair cells.

Cochlear Fluids

Cochlear fluids are the extracellular fluids in the inner ear. These fluids are perilymph and endolymph, which have different composition.

Perilymph

Scala vestibuli and scala tympani are filled with perilymph, which is similar to ECF in composition with high concentration of sodium ions.

Endolymph

Scala media is filled with endolymph, which contains high concentration of potassium and low concentration of sodium. It is due to continuous secretion of potassium ions by stria vascularis into scala media.

Electrical Potential

Difference in potassium concentration is responsible for the development of an electrical potential difference between endolymph and perilymph. Potential in endolymph is positive up to +80 mV.

Significance of Endocochlear Potential

Lower portion of the hair cells is bathed by perilymph. Head portion of hair cells penetrates the lamina reticularis and it is bathed by endolymph (Fig. 172.3). Endolymph has a positive potential (+80 mV).

So inside the hair cells, the electrical potential is –60 mV in comparison to that of perilymph and –140 mV in comparison to that of endolymph. High potential difference sensitizes the hair cells so that, the excitability of hair cells increases. It also increases the response of cells even to slight movement of stereocilia.

■ ACTION POTENTIAL IN AUDITORY NERVE FIBER

Action potential in auditory nerve fiber is generated by cochlear microphonic potential. It obeys **all-or-none law** and has a definite threshold and refractory period.

Action potential to a click sound with moderate intensity level consists of three successive spike potentials called N_1 N_2 N_3 representing synchronous repetitive firing in many fibers.

At high frequency, the synchronization of action potential disappears and single spike occurs. Action potential appears 0.5 to 1 millisecond after the development of cochlear microphonic potential.

■ PROPERTIES OF SOUND

Sound has two basic properties:
1. **Pitch,** which depends upon the frequency of sound waves. Frequency of sound is expressed in **hertz.** Frequency of sound audible to human ear lies between 20 and 20,000 Hz or cycles/second. The range of greatest sensitivity lies between 2,000 and 3,000 Hz (cycles/second).
2. **Loudness** or **intensity,** which depends upon the amplitude of sound waves. It is expressed in **decibel** (dB). The threshold intensity of sound wave is not constant. It varies in accordance to the frequency of sound.

■ APPRECIATION OF PITCH OF THE SOUND – THEORIES OF HEARING

Many theories are postulated to explain the mechanism by which the pitch of the sound is appreciated or the frequency is analyzed. These theories are generally classified into two groups. According to the first group, the analysis of sound frequency is the function of cerebral cortex and the cochlea merely transmits the sound.

According to the second group of theories, the frequency analysis is done by cochlea, which later sends the information to cerebral cortex.

■ THEORIES OF FIRST GROUP

1. *Telephone Theory of Rutherford*

Telephone theory was postulated by **Rutherford** in 1880. It is also called **frequency theory.** According to this

theory, the cochlea plays a simple role of a **telephone transmitter.**

In telephone, sound vibrations are converted into electrical impulses, which are transmitted by cables to the receiving end. There the receiver instrument converts the electrical impulses back into sound waves. Similarly, cochlea just converts the sound waves into electrical impulses of same frequency. Impulses are transmitted by auditory nerve fibers to cerebral cortex, where perception and analysis of sound occur.

It is believed that, the nerve fibers can transmit maximum of 1,000 impulses per second. Thus, the telephone theory fails to explain the transmission of sound waves with frequency above 1,000 cycles per second. So, a second theory was postulated.

2. *Volley Theory*

In 1949, **Wever** postulated this theory. **Volley** means groups. According to this theory, the impulses of sound waves with frequency above 1,000 cycles per second are transmitted by different groups of nerve fibers. However, this theory has no evidence to prove it. Thus, these two theories were not accepted by many physiologists.

■ THEORIES OF SECOND GROUP

1. *Resonance Theory of Helmholtz*

Resonance theory was the first theory of hearing to emerge in 1863. According to **Helmholtz,** analysis of sound frequency is the function of cochlea. Basilar membrane contains many basilar fibers. Helmholtz named these basilar fibers resonators and compared them with the resonators of piano.

When a string in piano is struck, sound with a particular note is produced. Similarly, when the sound with a particular frequency is applied, the basilar fibers in a particular portion of basilar membrane are stimulated.

Resonance theory was not accepted because the individual resonators could not be identified in cochlea. Gradually, this theory was modified into another theory called the place theory, which is more widely accepted.

2. *Place Theory*

According to this theory, nerve fibers from different portions (places) of organ of Corti on basilar membrane give response to sounds of different frequency. Accordingly, corresponding nerve fiber from organ of Corti gives information to the brain regarding the portion of organ of Corti that is stimulated. Many experimental evidences are available to support place theory.

Experimental evidences supporting place theory

   i. If a person is exposed to a loud noise of a particular frequency for a long period, he becomes deaf for that frequency. It is found that the specific portion of organ of Corti is destroyed as in the case of **boilermaker's disease.**

   ii. In experimental animals, destruction of a portion of organ of Corti occurs by exposing the animal to loud noise of a particular frequency

   iii. In human **high-tone deafness,** there is degeneration of organ of Corti near the base of cochlea or degeneration of nerve supplying the cochlea near the base

   iv. During exposure to high-frequency sound, cochlear microphonic potentials show greater voltage in hair cells near base of the cochlea. Also, during the exposure to low-frequency sound, cochlear microphonic potentials show greater voltage in hair cells near apex of the cochlea.

   v. There is point-to-point representation of basilar membrane in auditory cortex.

3. *Traveling Wave Theory*

From place theory, emerged yet another theory called the traveling wave theory. This theory explains how the traveling wave is generated in the basilar membrane. Development, generation, movement and disappearance of traveling wave are already described earlier in this chapter.

■ APPRECIATION OF LOUDNESS OF SOUND

Appreciation of loudness of sound depends upon the activities of auditory nerve fibers. Intensity or loudness of sound correlates with two factors:

1. Rate of discharge from the individual fibers of auditory nerve
2. Total number of nerve fibers discharging.

When loudness of sound increases, it produces large vibrations, which spread over longer area of basilar membrane. This activates large number of hair cells and recruits more number of auditory nerve fibers. So, the frequency of action potential is also increased.

■ LOCALIZATION OF SOUND

Sound localization is the ability to detect the source from where sound is produced or the direction through which sound wave is traveling. It is important for survival and it helps to protect us from moving objects such as vehicles.

Cerebral cortex and medial geniculate body are responsible for localization of sound.

Auditory Defects

```
■ TYPES AND CAUSES OF AUDITORY DEFECTS
    ■ CONDUCTION DEAFNESS
    ■ NERVE DEAFNESS
■ TESTS FOR HEARING
    ■ RINNE TEST
    ■ WEBER TEST
    ■ AUDIOMETRY
```

■ TYPES AND CAUSES OF AUDITORY DEFECTS

Auditory defects may be either partial or complete. Auditory defects are of two types:
1. Conduction deafness
2. Nerve deafness.

■ CONDUCTION DEAFNESS

Conduction deafness is the type of deafness that occurs due to impairment in transmission of sound waves in the external ear or middle ear.

Causes for Conduction Deafness

i. Obstruction of external auditory meatus with dry wax or foreign bodies
ii. Thickening of tympanic membrane due to repeated middle ear infection
iii. Perforation of tympanic membrane due to inequality of pressure on either side
iv. **Otitis media** (inflammation of middle ear)
v. **Otosclerosis** (fixation of footplate of stapes against oval window) due to ankylosis. **Ankylosis** means the abnormal immobility and consolidation of a joint.

■ NERVE DEAFNESS

Nerve deafness is the deafness caused by damage of any structure in cochlea, such as hair cell, organ of Corti, basilar membrane or cochlear duct or the lesion in the auditory pathway.

Causes for Nerve Deafness

i. Degeneration of hair cells due to some antibiotics like streptomycin and gentamicin
ii. Damage of cochlea by prolonged exposure to loud noise
iii. Tumor affecting VIII cranial nerve.

■ TESTS FOR HEARING

There are various tests to assess the sensation of hearing. However, some simple tests called bedside tests are usually carried before doing conventional types of hearing tests. Such simple tests are useful to know whether the hearing is normal or less.

Bedside tests:
1. Whispering test
2. Tickling of watch test.

Whispering Test

The examiner stands about 60 cm away from the subject at his side and whispers some words. If the subject is not able to hear the whisper, then hearing deficit is suspected.

Tickling of Watch Test

Wrist watch with tickling sound is kept near the ear of the subject. The subject suffering from hearing defects cannot hear the tickling sound of watch.

Routine Tests for Hearing

Routine tests for hearing are of three types:
1. Rinne test
2. Weber test
3. Audiometry.

First two tests are done by using a tuning fork with high frequency. Mostly, a tuning fork with 512 cycles per second is used. By turning fork tests, only the nature of auditory defect is determined. By audiometry, both nature and severity of auditory defects can be determined.

■ RINNE TEST

Base of a vibrating tuning fork is placed on mastoid process, until the subject cannot feel the vibration and cannot hear the sound. When the subject does not hear the sound any more, the tuning fork is held in air in front of the ear of same side. Normal person hears vibration in air even after the bone conduction ceases because, in normal conditions, air conduction via ossicles is better than bone conduction. But in conduction deafness, the vibrations in air are not heard after cessation of bone conduction. Thus in conduction deafness, the bone conduction is better than air conduction.

In nerve deafness, both air conduction and bone conduction are diminished or lost.

■ WEBER TEST

Base of a vibrating tuning fork is placed on the vertex of skull or the middle of forehead. Normal person hears the sound equally on both sides. In unilateral conduction deafness (deafness in one ear), the sound is heard louder in diseased ear. In unaffected ear, there is a masking effect of environmental noise. So, the sound through bone conduction is not heard as clearly as on the affected side. In affected side, the sound is louder due to the absence of masking effect of environmental noise.

During unilateral nerve deafness, sound is heard louder in the normal ear.

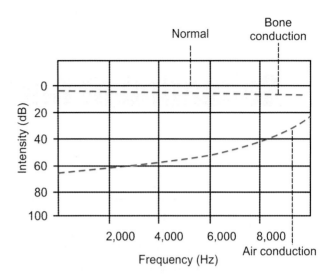

FIGURE 175.1: Audiogram in a patient with conductive deafness

■ AUDIOMETRY

Audiometry is the technique used to determine the nature and the severity of auditory defect. An instrument called **audiometer** is used. This instrument is an electronic **function generator** or **oscillator,** connected to an ear phone. This instrument is capable of generating sound waves of different frequencies from lowest to highest.

Intensity (loudness or volume) of sound at each frequency is adjusted on the basis of previous studies in normal persons.

Thus, before calibrating the instrument, minimum (threshold) volume or intensity or loudness, for each frequency of sound heard by normal persons is determined. Minimum intensity is set in the instrument as zero. Now, while testing the patient, the loudness is increased above zero level (Fig. 175.1). Intensity of sound is expressed in decibel (dB).

At a particular frequency, if the patient hears the sound with loudness of 30 dB above zero level, the person is said to have hearing loss of 30 dB for that particular frequency. During the tests by audiometer, the subject's ability to hear the sounds with 8 to 10 different frequencies is observed and the hearing loss is determined for each frequency. By using these values, the audiogram is plotted.

Audiometer has an **electronic vibrator** also. It is used to test the bone conduction from mastoid process into the cochlea.

Sensation of Taste

- ■ TASTE BUDS
- ■ PATHWAY FOR TASTE
- ■ PRIMARY TASTE SENSATIONS
- ■ DISCRIMINATION OF DIFFERENT TASTE SENSATIONS
- ■ TASTE SENSATIONS AND CHEMICAL CONSTITUTIONS
- ■ TASTE TRANSDUCTION
- ■ APPLIED PHYSIOLOGY – ABNORMALITIES OF TASTE SENSATION

■ TASTE BUDS

Sense organs for taste or **gustatory sensation** are the taste buds. Taste buds are ovoid bodies with a diameter of 50 μ to 70 μ. In adults, about 10,000 taste buds are present and the number is more in children. In old age, many taste buds degenerate and the taste sensitivity decreases.

■ SITUATION OF TASTE BUDS

Most of the taste buds are present on the papillae of tongue. Taste buds are also situated in the mucosa of epiglottis, palate, pharynx and the proximal part of esophagus.

Types of papillae located on tongue:
1. Filiform papillae
2. Fungiform papillae
3. Circumvallate papillae.

1. *Filiform Papillae*

Filiform papillae are small and conical-shaped papillae, situated over the dorsum of tongue. These papillae contain less number of taste buds (only a few).

2. *Fungiform Papillae*

Fungiform papillae are round in shape and are situated over the anterior surface of tongue near the tip. Numerous fungiform papillae are present. Each papilla contains moderate number of taste buds (up to 10).

3. *Circumvallate Papillae*

Circumvallate papillae are large structures present on the posterior part of tongue and are many in number. These papillae are arranged in the shape of 'V'. Each papilla contains many taste buds (up to 100).

■ STRUCTURE OF TASTE BUD

Taste bud is a bundle of taste receptor cells, with supporting cells embedded in the epithelial covering of the papillae (Fig. 176.1). Each taste bud contains about 40 cells, which are the modified epithelial cells. Cells of taste bud are divided into four groups:

Type of Cells in Taste Bud

1. Type I cells or sustentacular cells
2. Type II cells
3. Type III cells
4. Type IV cells or basal cells.

Type I cells and type IV cells are supporting cells. Type III cells are the **taste receptor cells.** Function of type II cell is unknown. Type I, II and III cells have microvilli, which project into an opening in epithelium covering the tongue. This opening is called **taste pore.** Neck of each cell is attached to the neck of other. All the cells of taste bud are surrounded by epithelial cells. There are tight junctions between epithelial cells and the neck portion of the type I, II and III cells, so that only the tip of these cells are exposed to fluid in oral cavity.

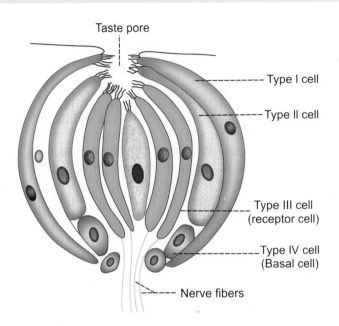

FIGURE 176.1: Taste bud

Cells of taste buds undergo constant cycle of growth, apoptosis and regeneration.

■ PATHWAY FOR TASTE

■ RECEPTORS

Receptors for taste sensation are the type III cells of taste buds. Each taste bud is innervated by about 50 sensory nerve fibers and each nerve fiber supplies at least five taste buds through its terminals.

■ FIRST ORDER NEURON

First order neurons of taste pathway are in the nuclei of three different cranial nerves, situated in medulla oblongata. Dendrites of the neurons are distributed to the taste buds. After arising from taste buds, the fibers reach the cranial nerve nuclei by running along the following nerves (Fig. 176.2):

1. **Chorda tympani fibers** of facial nerve, which run from anterior two third of tongue
2. **Glossopharyngeal nerve fibers,** which run from posterior one third of the tongue
3. **Vagal fibers,** which run from taste buds in other regions.

Axons from first order neurons in the nuclei of these nerves run together in medulla oblongata and terminate in the nucleus of **tractus solitarius.**

■ SECOND ORDER NEURON

Second order neurons are in the nucleus of tractus solitarius. Axons of second order neurons run through **medial lemniscus** and terminate in **posteroventral nucleus** of thalamus.

■ THIRD ORDER NEURON

Third order neurons are in the posteroventral nucleus of thalamus. Axons from third order neurons project into **parietal lobe** of the cerebral cortex.

■ TASTE CENTER

Center for taste sensation is in opercular insular cortex, i.e. in the lower part of postcentral gyrus, which receives cutaneous sensations from face. Thus, the taste fibers do not have an independent cortical projection.

■ PRIMARY TASTE SENSATIONS

Primary or fundamental taste sensations are divided into five types:
1. Sweet
2. Salt

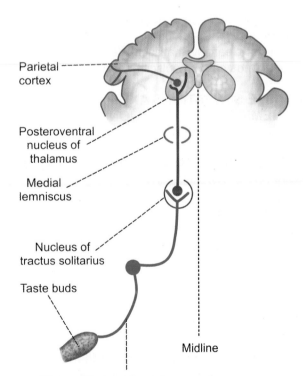

FIGURE 176.2: Pathway for taste sensation

3. Sour
4. Bitter
5. Umami.

Man can perceive more than 100 different tastes. Other taste sensations are just the combination of two or more primary taste sensations.

Combination of Taste Sensation with Other Sensations

Sometimes, taste sensation combines with other sensations to give rise to a different sensation. For example, combination of taste, smell and touch senses, gives rise to **sensation of flavor**. Combination of taste with pain gives rise to **sensation of ginger**.

■ DISCRIMINATION OF DIFFERENT TASTE SENSATIONS

Earlier, it was believed that different areas of tongue were specialized for different taste sensation. Now it is clear that all areas of tongue give response to all types of taste sensations. Usually, in low concentration of taste substance, each taste bud gives response to one primary taste stimulus. However, in high concentration, the taste buds give response to more than one type of taste stimuli.

It is also clear now that each afferent nerve fiber from the taste buds carry impulses of one taste sensation.

■ TASTE SENSATIONS AND CHEMICAL CONSTITUTIONS

Substances causing sour or salt tastes are mostly electrolytes. Bitter and sweet tastes are caused by electrolytes or non-electrolytes.

■ SWEET TASTE

Sweet taste is produced mainly by organic substances like monosaccharides, polysaccharides, glycerol, alcohol, aldehydes, ketones and chloroform. Inorganic substances, which produce sweet taste are lead and beryllium.

■ SALT TASTE

Salt taste is produced by chlorides of sodium, potassium and ammonium, nitrates of sodium and potassium. Some sulfates, bromides and iodides also produce salt taste.

■ SOUR TASTE

Sour taste is produced because of hydrogen ions in acids and acid salts.

■ BITTER TASTE

Bitter taste is produced by organic substances like quinine, strychnine, morphine, glucosides, picric acid and bile salts and inorganic substances like salts of calcium, magnesium and ammonium. Bitterness of the salts is mainly due to cations.

■ UMAMI

Umami is the recently recognized taste sensation. Umami is a Japanese word, meaning 'delicious'. Receptors of this taste sensation respond to glutamate, particularly **monosodium glutamate (MSG)**, which is a common ingredient in Asian food. However, excess MSG consumption is proved to produce Chinese restaurant syndrome in some people taking Chinese food regularly. Common symptoms are headache, flushing, sweating, perioral numbness, chest pain. In severe conditions, airway swelling and obstruction and cardiac arrhythmia occur.

Threshold for Taste Sensations

Sweet taste Sugar   : 1 in 200 dilution
Salt taste   Sodium chloride : 1 in 400 dilution
Sour taste   Hydrochloric acid : 1 in 15,000 dilution
Bitter taste Quinine   : 1 in 2,000,000 dilution.

Bitter taste has very low threshold and sweet taste has a high threshold. Threshold for umani is not known.

■ TASTE TRANSDUCTION

Taste transduction is the process by which taste receptor converts chemical energy into action potentials in the taste nerve fiber. Receptors of taste sensation are chemoreceptors, which are stimulated by substances dissolved in mouth by saliva. The dissolved substances act on microvilli of taste receptors exposed in the taste pore. It causes the development of receptor potential in the receptor cells. This in turn, is responsible for the generation of action potential in the sensory neurons.

Taste Receptor

Generally, taste receptor is a **G-protein coupled receptor** (GPCR). It is also called **G protein gustducin**.

However, several other receptors are also involved in taste sensation. Transduction mechanism is different in each taste receptor cells.

■ SWEET RECEPTOR

Receptor for sweet taste is **GPCR**. The sweet substances bind to receptor and cause depolarization via cyclic AMP.

■ SALT RECEPTOR

Receptor for salt taste is called **epithelial sodium channel (ENaC).** It acts like ENaC receptors in other parts of the body. When sodium enters, this receptor releases glutamate, which causes depolarization.

■ SOUR RECEPTOR

Sour sensation also has the same ENaC receptor. The proton (hydrogen) enters the receptor and causes depolarization. It is believed that besides ENaC, other receptors such as **hyperpolarization-activated cyclic nucleotide-gated cation channel (HCN)** also are involved in sour sensation.

■ BITTER RECEPTOR

Bitter receptor is a GPCR. In bitter receptor, the sour substances activate phospholipase C through G proteins. It causes production of inositol triphosphate (IP_3), which initiates depolarization by releasing calcium ions.

■ UMAMI RECEPTOR

Umami receptor is called **metabotropic glutamate receptor (mGluR4).** Glutamate causes depolarization of this receptor. Exact mechanism of depolarization is not clearly understood. Activation of umami taste receptor is intensified by the presence of guanosine monophosphate (GMP) and inosine monophosphate (IMP).

■ APPLIED PHYSIOLOGY – ABNORMALITIES OF TASTE SENSATION

■ AGEUSIA

Loss of taste sensation is called ageusia. Taste buds in anterior two thirds of the tongue are innervated by the chorda tympani branch of facial nerve. Chorda tympani nerve receives taste fibers from tongue via lingual branch of mandibular division of trigeminal nerve. So, the lesion in facial nerve, chorda tympani or mandibular division of trigeminal nerve causes loss of taste sensation in the anterior two third of the tongue. Lesion in glossopharyngeal nerve leads to loss of taste in the posterior one third of the tongue.

Temporary loss of taste sensation occurs due to the drugs like captopril and penicillamine, which contain sulfhydryl group of substances.

■ HYPOGEUSIA

Hypoguesia is the decrease in taste sensation. It is due to increase in threshold for different taste sensations. However, the taste sensation is not completely lost.

■ TASTE BLINDNESS

Taste blindness is a rare genetic disorder in which the ability to recognize substances by taste is lost.

■ DYSGEUSIA

Disturbance in the taste sensation is called dysgeusia. It is found in temporal lobe syndrome, particularly when the anterior region of temporal lobe is affected. In this condition, the paroxysmal hallucinations of taste and smell occur, which are usually unpleasant.

Sensation of Smell

Chapter 177

- OLFACTORY RECEPTORS
- VOMERONASAL ORGAN
  - VOMERONASAL ORGAN IN HUMAN BEINGS
- OLFACTORY PATHWAY
- OLFACTORY TRANSDUCTION
- CLASSIFICATION OF ODOR
- THRESHOLD FOR OLFACTORY SENSATION
- ADAPTATION
- APPLIED PHYSIOLOGY – ABNORMALITIES OF OLFACTORY SENSATION
  - ANOSMIA
  - HYPOSMIA
  - HYPEROSMIA

■ OLFACTORY RECEPTORS

Olfactory receptors are situated in **olfactory mucus membrane,** which is the modified mucus membrane that lines upper part of nostril. Olfactory mucus membrane consists of 10 to 20 millions of olfactory receptor cells supported by the sustentacular cells. Mucosa also contains mucus-secreting **Bowman glands** (Fig. 177.1).

Olfactory receptor cell is a bipolar neuron. Dendrite of this neuron is short and it has an expanded end called olfactory rod. From olfactory rod, about 10 to 12 cilia arise. Cilia are non-myelinated, with a length of 2 µ and a diameter of 0.1 µ. These cilia project to the surface of olfactory mucus membrane.

Mucus secreted by Bowman glands continuously lines the olfactory mucosa. Mucus contains some proteins, which increase the actions of odoriferous substances on receptor cells.

■ VOMERONASAL ORGAN

Vomeronasal organ is an **accessory olfactory organ** found in many animals including mammals. This organ was discovered in 1813, by a Danish physician

Ludwig Jacobson, hence it is also called **Jacobson organ.** It is enclosed in a cartilaginous capsule, which opens into the base of nasal cavity. Olfactory receptors of this organ are sensitive to non-volatile substances such as scents and pheromones. Vomeronasal organ helps the animals to detect even the trace quantities of chemicals. Impulses from this organ are sent to amygdala and hypothalamus via accessory olfactory bulb.

■ VOMERONASAL ORGAN IN HUMAN BEINGS

In human beings, the vomeronasal organ was considered as vestigial or non-functional. Recently, it is found that this organ is present in the form of vomeronasal pits on the anterior part of nasal septum. Receptors of vomeronasal pit detect odorless human **pheromones** or **vomeropherins,** at a very low concentration in air. Refer Chapter 62 for details of pheromones. The subconscious detection of odorless chemical messengers in air is considered as the **sixth sense** in human beings.

■ OLFACTORY PATHWAY

Axons of **bipolar olfactory receptors** pierce the **cribriform plate** of ethmoid bone and reach the

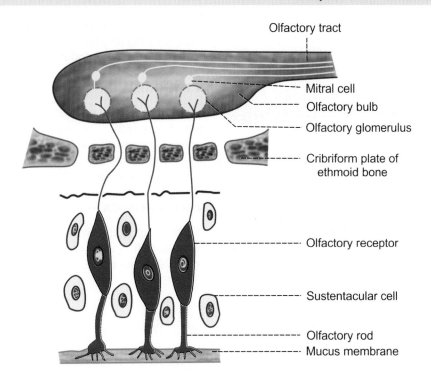

FIGURE 177.1: Olfactory mucus membrane and pathway for olfactory sensation

olfactory bulb. Here, the axons synapse with dendrites of **mitral cells.** Different groups of these synapses form globular structures called **olfactory glomeruli.**

Axons of mitral cells leave the olfactory bulb and form **olfactory tract.** Olfactory tract runs backward and ends in **olfactory cortex,** through the intermediate and lateral **olfactory stria.**

Olfactory cortex includes the structures, which form a part of limbic system. These structures are anterior olfactory nucleus, prepyriform cortex, olfactory tubercle and amygdala.

■ OLFACTORY TRANSDUCTION

Olfactory transduction is the process by which olfactory receptor converts chemical energy into action potentials in olfactory nerve fiber. The odoriferous substance stimulates the olfactory receptors, only if it dissolves in mucus, covering the olfactory mucus membrane. Molecules of dissolved substance, bind with receptor proteins in the cilia and form substance-receptor complex. Substance-receptor complex activates adenyl cyclase that causes the formation of cyclic AMP. Cyclic AMP in turn, causes opening of sodium channels, leading to influx of sodium and generation of receptor potential.

Receptor potential causes generation of action potential in the axon of bipolar neuron.

■ CLASSIFICATION OF ODOR

Odor is classified into various types. Substances producing different types of odor are:
1. Aromatic or resinous odor: Camphor, lavender, clove and bitter almonds
2. Ambrosial odor: Musk
3. Burning odor: Burning feathers, tobacco, roasted coffee and meat
4. Ethereal odor: Fruits, ethers and beeswax
5. Fragrant or balsamic odor: Flowers and perfumes
6. Garlic odor: Garlic, onion and sulfur
7. Goat odor: Caproic acid and sweet cheese
8. Nauseating odor: Decayed vegetables and feces
9. Repulsive odor: Bed bug.

■ THRESHOLD FOR OLFACTORY SENSATION

Ethyl ether	: 5.8 mg/L of air
Chloroform	: 3.3 mg/L of air
Peppermint oil	: 0.02 mg/L of air
Butyric acid	: 0.009 mg/L of air
Artificial musk	: 0.00004 mg/L of air
Methyl mercaptan	: 0.0000004 mg/L of air.

Thus, **methyl mercaptan** produces olfactory sensation even at a low concentration of 0.0000004 mg/L of air.

■ ADAPTATION

Olfactory receptors are phasic receptors and adapt very rapidly. Within one second, the adaptation occurs up to 50%.

■ APPLIED PHYSIOLOGY – ABNORMALITIES OF OLFACTORY SENSATION

■ ANOSMIA

Anosmia refers to total loss of sensation of smell, i.e. inability to recognize or detect any odor. It may be temporary or permanent. **Temporary anosmia** is due to obstruction of nose, which occurs during common cold, nasal sinus and allergic conditions.

Permanent anosmia occurs during lesion in olfactory tract, meningitis and degenerative conditions such as Parkinson disease and Alzheimer disease.

■ HYPOSMIA

Hyposmia is the reduced ability to recognize and to detect any odor. The odors can be detected only at higher concentrations. It is the most common disorder of smell. Hyposmia also may be temporary or permanent. It occurs due to same causes of anosmia.

■ HYPEROSMIA

Hyperosmia is the increased or exaggerated olfactory sensation. It is also called **olfactory hyperesthesia.** It occurs in brain injury, epilepsy and neurotic conditions.

QUESTIONS IN SPECIAL SENSES

■ LONG QUESTIONS

1. Draw a diagram of visual pathway and explain it. Indicate the effects of lesions at different levels of optic pathway.
2. Give an account of accommodation. Add a note on presbyopia.
3. Explain the auditory pathway with suitable diagram. Add a note on auditory defects.
4. Explain the mechanism of hearing.
5. What is sound transduction? Explain the electrical events, which occur during sound transduction
6. Describe how the pitch of the sound is analyzed in human ear (theories of hearing).

■ SHORT QUESTIONS

1. Retina.
2. Ocular muscles.
3. Ocular movements.
4. Visual receptors.
5. Aqueous humor.
6. Intraocular pressure.
7. Glaucoma.
8. Fundus oculi.
9. Lens of eye.
10. Cataract.
11. Lacrimal glands.
12. Rhodopsin.
13. Phototransduction.
14. Dark adaptation.
15. Light adaptation.
16. Nyctalopia.
17. ERG.
18. Diplopia.
19. Hemianopia.
20. Effects of lesion in optic pathway.
21. Accommodation reflex.
22. Presbyopia.
23. Theories of color vision.
24. Color blindness.
25. Errors of refraction.
26. Auditory ossicles.
27. Tympanic reflex.
28. Cochlea.
29. Organ of Corti.
30. Role of middle ear in hearing (Functions of middle ear).
31. Role of inner ear in hearing (Functions of internal ear).
32. Impedance matching.
33. Traveling wave.
34. Electrical potentials in cochlea.
35. Theories of hearing.
36. Auditory defects.
37. Tests for hearing.
38. Audiometry.
39. Taste buds.
40. Taste transduction.
41. Taste pathway.
42. Olfactory transduction.
43. Olfactory pathway.

Index

Page numbers followed by *f* for figure and *t* for table, respectively.

Gonorrheal vaginitis 478
Good cholesterol 295
Goormaghtigh cells 309
Gorilla face 384
Gower tract 810
G-protein coupled
    oxytocin receptor 384
    receptor 1026
Graafian follicle 380, 484, 484f, 492
Graded potential 193, 193t, 767
Graded potentials, different 193
Gram-negative bacteria 661
Grand mal 935
Grand mal, causes of 936
Granit dominator-modulator theory 1000
Granular
    cells 310
    layer 866
    pneumocytes 675
Granule cells 866
Granules 969
Granulocytes 97
Granulocytopenia 99
Granulocytosis 99
Granulosa cells 483, 485
Granulosa cells, changes in 483
Granulose cells 476
Granzymes 10
Graphical registration 551
Graves' disease 120, 395
Graveyard of rbcs 67
Gravindex test 509
Gravitational force 740
Gravity 575, 618, 680
Gray matter of
    cerebellum 865
    spinal cord 804
Graying of vision 740
Grayout 740
Greater
    circulation 524
    curvature 230
Growth
    factors 16
    hormone 377, 408, 460, 461f
        actions of 377
        inhibiting hormone 285, 377, 420
        receptor 379
        releasing hormone 377, 793
        releasing polypeptide 377
        secretagogue 379
    of ductile system 510
    of glandular tissue 510
    plate 409
Guanosine
    diphosphate 313f, 373
    triphosphate 313f

Guillain-Barré syndrome 65
Gustatory sensation 1024
Gutter 201

■ H

H substance 647
Hagen-poiseuille equation 598
Hair
    cells 921, 922, 1013
        of vestibular apparatus 922f
    distribution 478
    follicle 356
Hairpin bend 307
Haldane effect 715
Haldane effect, causes for 715
Haldane-priestely tube 704
Half-life of hormones 370
Hallucination 935
Hamburger phenomenon 714
Hammer 1008
Hamulus 1010
Haploid 459, 484, 498
    cells 13
    number of chromosomes 459
    or half number of chromosomes 459
Harmful stimuli 796
Harrison sulcus 414
Harsh blowing sound 550
Hartridge polychromatic theory 1001
Hashimoto's thyroiditis 119, 396
Haustra 266
Haversian
    canal 410
    lamellae 410
    systems 410
Hazards of blood transfusion 146
HCG
    actions of 506
    antiserum 509
HCS, actions of 506
Head 471
    or capitulum 1008
    portion 5
        of myosin molecule 172
Headache 741
Health benefits of dietary fiber 289
Hearing 1022
Heart 441, 446, 519, 601
    actions of 522
    attack 297
    block 565, 590
    disease 295
    failure 654, 662, 663
        acute 662
        causes of 662
        compensated 663

rate 392, 557, 575, 587, 594f, 666, 821, 931
    decreases 799
    regulation of 588, 858
    variability 557
    re-excitation of 568
    sounds 544, 545t
        description of 544
        different 544
        importance of 544
Heartbeat 600
Heartburn 240
Heart-lung preparation 582, 583f
Heat
    balance 360
    cramps 747
    exhaustion 747
    gain
        center 361, 858
        or heat production in body 360
    loss
        center 361, 858
        from body 361
        prevention of 361, 362, 746
    of activation 199
    of activity 360
    of metabolism 360
    of relaxation 199
    of shortening 199
    production 255, 746
        prevention of 361
        promotion of 362
    rigor 183
Heatstroke 747, 748
Heidenhain pouch 235
Helicobacter pylori 239
Helicotrema 1010, 1011
Helium dilution technique 694
Helmholtz trichromatic theory 1000
Hematemesis 240
Hematinic principle 76
Hematocrit value 59, 149
Hematoma 412
Hematospermia 472
Hematuria 334, 335, 337
Heme 78, 80
Heme iron 82
Hemianesthesia 854
Hemianopia 854, 991
Hemiballismus 883
Hemidesmosome 25
Hemihyperesthesia 854
Hemiplegia 837t
Hemisection of spinal cord 823
Hemodromography 599
Hemodynamics 595
Hemofilter 346